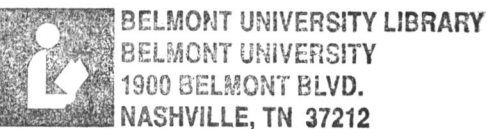

D1221904

The Practice of Medicinal Chemistry

The Practice of Medicinal Chemistry

Edited by

CAMILLE G. WERMUTH
Laboratoire de Pharmacochimie Moléculaire, Faculté de Pharmacie,
Université Louis Pasteur, Illkirch, France

ACADEMIC PRESS
Harcourt Brace and Company, Publishers
London   San Diego   New York
Boston   Sydney   Tokyo   Toronto

ACADEMIC PRESS
24–28 Oval Road
LONDON NW1 7DX

U.S. Edition Published by
ACADEMIC PRESS INC.
San Diego, CA 92101

This book is printed on acid free paper

A catalogue record for this book is available from the British Library

ISBN 0-12-744640-0

Typeset by Mackreth Media Services, Hemel Hempstead
Printed in Great Britain by The University Printing House, Cambridge

Contents

Contents

A colour plate section can be found between pages 446 and 447.

Contributors

Bradley D. Anderson   Department of Pharmaceutics and Pharmaceutical Chemistry, University of Utah-University Research Park, 421 Wakara Way, Room 321, Salt Lake City, UT 84108, USA

Peter R. Andrews   Centre for Drug Design and Development, The University of Queensland, Brisbane, Qld 4072, Australia

Kurt H. Bauer   Pharmazeutisches Institut, Albert-Ludwig-Universität, Hermann Herder Strasse, 9, D-79104 Freiburg, Germany

Frans M. Belpaire   Heymans Institute of Pharmacology, University of Gent Medical School, De Pintelaan 185, B-9000 Gent, Belgium

Marc G. Bogaert   Heymans Institute of Pharmacology, University of Gent Medical School, De Pintelaan 185, B-9000 Gent, Belgium

Jean-Jacques Bourguignon   Laboratoire de Pharmacochimie Moléculaire, Centre de Neurochimie du CNRS, 5, Rue Blaise Pascal, Strasbourg, France

Jacques A. Dangoumau   Département de Pharmacologie-Université de Bordeaux II, UFR Victor PACHON, 33076 Bordeaux Cedex, France

Karl P. Flora   Division of Research and Testing, Center for Drug Evaluation and Research, Food and Drug Administration, MOD 1, Room 2008, 8301 Mulkirk Road, Laurel, MD 20708, USA

Jean-Cyr Gaignault   Roussel-UCLAF, 111, Route de Noisy, 93230 Romainville, France

Jean-Pierre Gies   Laboratoire de Neuroimmuno-Pharmacologie, Université Louis Pasteur, Faculté de Pharmacie, 74, Route du Rhin, 67401 Illkirch Cedex, France

Phillip A. Hart   School of Pharmacy, University of Wisconsin–Madison, 425 North Charter Street, Madison, WI 53706-1515, USA

Marcel F. Hibert   Marion Merrell Dow Research Institute, 16, Rue d'Ankara, 67000 Strasbourg, France

Fumitoshi Hirayama   Faculty of Pharmaceutical Sciences, Kumamoto University, 5-1 Oe Honmachi, Kumamoto 862, Japan

Sheila Hobbs de Witt   Parke-Davis Pharmaceutical Research, 2800 Plymouth Road, Ann Arbor, MI 48105, USA

Adrian N. Hobden   GLAXO Research and Development, Greenford Road, Greenford, UB6 0HE, Middlesex, UK

Hans-Dieter Höltje   Fachbereich Pharmazie, WE 1, Freie Universität Berlin, Königin-Luise-Strasse, 2+4, D-14195 Berlin, Germany

Victor J. Hruby   Department of Chemistry, University of Arizona, Tucson, AZ 85721, USA

Michael Kahn   Department of Pathobiology, University of Washington, Seattle, Washington 98195, and The Molecumetics Institute, 2023 120th Avenue North East–Suite 400, Bellvue, Washington 98005, USA

Jean-Paul Kan   Sanofi Recherche, Centre de Montpellier, 371, Rue du Professeur J. Blayac, 34184 Montpellier Cedex 04, France

David G. I. Kingston   Department of Chemistry, Virginia Polytechnic Institute and State University, Blacksburg, Virginia 24061-0212, USA

Sabine E. Kopp-Kubel   DMP-RGS, World Health Organization, 20, Avenue Appia, 1211 Genève-27, Switzerland

C. Thomas Lin   D-431, Abbott Laboratories, AP-9A, Abbott Park, IL 60064-3500, USA

Anne-Christine Macherey   UPS 831-Prévention du Risque Chimique, ICSN-CNRS, Avenue de la Terasse, 91198 Gif-sur-Yvette Cedex, France

Gábor Maksay   Central Research Institute for Chemistry, Hungarian Academy of Sciences, Budapest, Pf 17, H-1525, Hungary

Christian Marchandeau   Roussel-UCLAF, 111, Route de Noisy, 93230 Romainville, France

Yvonne Connolly Martin   Abbott Laboratories, D-47E, AP-10A, Abbott Park, IL 60064-3500, USA

Philippe Meyer   Medical Epistemology, Faculté de Médecine Necker-Enfants Malades, 156, rue de Vaugirard, 75015 Paris, France

Hiroshi Nakanishi   Department of Pathology, University of Washington, Seattle, Washington 98195, and The Molecumetics Institute, 2023, 120th Avenue N.E., Suite 400, Bellevue, Washington 98005, USA

André Picot   UPS 831-Prévention du Risque Chimique, ICSN-CNRS, Avenue de la Terasse, 91198 Gif-sur-Yvette Cedex, France

Bryan G. Reuben   South Bank University, School of Applied Science, 103, Borough Road, London SE1 0AA, UK

Daniel H. Rich   School of Pharmacy and Department of Chemistry, University of Wisconsin-Madison, 425 North Charter Street, Madison, WI 53706-1515, USA

Jean-Michel Rondeau   Marion Merrell Dow Research Institute, 16, Rue d'Ankara, 67080 Strasbourg, France

Etienne H. Schacht   Biomaterial and Polymer Research Group, University of Gent, Krijgslaan, 281 S4bis, B-9000 Gent, Belgium

Herman Schreuder   Marion Merrell Dow Research Institute, 16, Rue d'Ankara, 67080 Strasbourg, France

Len Seymour   University of Birmingham Clinical Oncology, Queen Elizabeth Hospital, Edgbaston, Birmingham B15 2TH, UK

Miklós Simonyi   Central Research Institute for Chemistry, Hungarian Academy of Sciences, Budapest, Pf 17, H-1525, Hungary

Maria Souleau   Sanofi Recherche, Division de la Propriété Industrielle, Direction Juridique Corporate, 32–34, Rue Marbeuf, 75008 Paris Cedex 08, France

Bernard Testa Université de Lausanne, École de Pharmacie, B.E.P., CH-1015 Lausanne-Dorigny, Switzerland

David J. Triggle State University of New York, School of Pharmacy, Amherst Campus, Buffalo, NY 14260, USA

Kaneto Uekama Faculty of Pharmaceutical Sciences, Kumamoto University, 5-1 Oe Honmachi, Kumamoto 862, Japan

Stefan Vansteenkiste Biomaterial and Polymer Research Group, University of Gent, Krijgslaan, 281 S4bis, B-9000 Gent, Belgium

Han van de Waterbeemd F. Hoffmann-La Roche Ltd, Pharma Research New Technologies, CH-4002 Basel, Switzerland

Hans-Peter Weber Sandoz Pharma AG, Gebäude 503–560, CH-4002 Basel, Switzerland

Camille G. Wermuth Laboratoire de Pharmacochimie Moléculaire, Faculté de Pharmacie, Université Louis Pasteur, 74, Route du Rhin, 67401 Illkirch Cedex, France

Foreword

One more book on medicinal chemistry, you will say to yourselves! It is true, but this one purports to be different from the others and it is, unquestionably, from many points of view. The principal author and also the chief organizer of this work, Professor Camille G. Wermuth, is a craftsman of medicinal chemistry. He has been responsible for the development of two commercial CNS drugs and is the author of major studies in the domain of gabaergic receptors and their ligands. Molecular modelling, of which he has made reasonable use during his career, holds no secrets for him.

Thus, this work brings together over forty chapters truly covering every area of modern medicinal chemistry. The co-authors are all well-known specialists in their field and the overall effect is harmonious.

Medicinal chemistry has, like all disciplines, evolved rapidly over the last two decades. Originally based on the exploitation of natural resources such as plants and, more rarely, animals and minerals, medicinal chemistry has followed an evolutionary course parallel to that of 'chemistry triumphant' during the 19th century and a large part of the 20th century.

The recent advent of molecular biology, also presently 'triumphant', has somewhat masked the importance of so-called classical medicinal chemistry. However, the functional control of complex biological systems is, quite naturally, the result of the intervention of molecules often quite simple structurally, compared to the substrates to which they bind. We can thus confidently predict a bright future for 'classical' medicinal chemistry, still aided as ever by the often fortuitous (though increasingly guided) discovery of new drugs, most notably from natural sources. The use of predictive methods that are increasingly satisfying to the spirit and to logic but also with regard to the results obtained, will also enjoy exponential development over the next decade.

This work, elaborated under the direction of Camille Wermuth, thus represents, in many respects, a major contribution to the field. If this were all, it would already be very good. However, as the reader will discover with interest, there is in fact much more.

Finally, this book is particularly addressed to chemists who, due to their training, have not received much exposure to medicinal chemistry and in whom basic notions of biology are often lacking. It will prove to be a precious tool for them, different from most known works in this field. This book will doubtlessly and deservedly have much success.

P. Potier
Member of the French Academy of
Sciences and of the Academia Europae

Preface

The role of chemistry in the manufacture of new drugs, and also of cosmetics and agrochemicals, is essential. It is doubtful, however, whether chemists have been properly trained to design and synthesize new drugs or other bioactive compounds. The majority of medicinal chemists working in the pharmaceutical industry are organic synthetic chemists with little or no background in medicinal chemistry who have to acquire the specific aspects of medicinal chemistry during their early years in the pharmaceutical industry. This book is precisely aimed to be their 'bedside book' at the beginning of their career.

After a concise introduction covering background subject matter, such as the definition and history of medicinal chemistry, the measurement of biological activities and the three main phases of drug activity, the second part of the book discusses the most appropriate approach to *finding a new lead compound or an original working hypothesis*. This most uncertain stage in the development of a new drug is nowadays characterized by high-throughput screening methods, synthesis of combinatorial libraries, data base mining and a return to natural product screening. The core of the book (Parts III to V) considers the *optimization of the lead in terms of potency, selectivity, and safety*. In 'Primary Exploration of Structure-Activity Relationships', the most common operational stratagems are discussed, allowing identification of the portions of the molecule that are important for potency. 'Substituents and functions' deals with the rapid and systematic optimization of the lead compound. 'Spatial Organization, Receptor Mapping and Molecular Modelling' considers the three-dimensional aspects of drug–receptor interactions, giving particular emphasis to the design of peptidomimetic drugs and to the control of the agonist–antagonist transition. Parts VI and VII concentrate on the definition of satisfactory drug-delivery conditions, i.e. means to ensure that the molecule reaches its target organ. Pharmacokinetic properties are improved through adequate chemical modifications, notably prodrug design, obtaining suitable water solubility (of utmost importance in medical practice) and improving organoleptic properties (and thus rendering the drug administration acceptable to the patient). Part VIII, 'Development of New Drugs: Legal and Economic Aspects', constitutes an important area in which chemists are almost wholly self taught following their entry into industry.

This book fills a gap in the available bibliography of medicinal chemistry texts. There is not, to the author-editor's knowledge, any other current work in print which deals with the practical aspects of medicinal chemistry, from conception of molecules to their marketing. In this single volume, all the disparate bits of information which medicinal chemists gather over a career, and generally share by word-of-mouth with their colleagues, but which have never been organized and presented in coherent form in print, are brought together. Traditional approaches are not neglected and are illustrated by modern examples and, conversely, the most recent discovery and development technologies are presented and discussed by specialists. Therefore, *The Practice of Medicinal Chemistry* is exactly the type of book to be recommended as a text or as first reading to a synthetic chemist beginning a career in medicinal chemistry. And, even if primarily aimed at organic chemists entering into pharmaceutical research, all medicinal chemists will derive a great deal from reading the book.

The involvement of a large number of authors presents the risk of a certain lack of cohesiveness and of some overlaps, especially as each chapter is written as an autonomic piece of information. Such a situation was anticipated and accepted, especially for a first edition. It can be defended because each contributor is an expert in his/her field and many of them are 'heavyweights' in medicinal chemistry. In editing the book I have tried to ensure a balanced content and a more-or-less consistent style. However, the temptation to influence the personal views of the authors has been resisted. On the contrary, my objective was to combine a plurality of opinions, and to present and discuss a given topic from different angles. Such as it is, this first edition can still be improved and I am grateful in advance to all colleagues for comments and suggestions for future editions.

Special care has been taken to give complete references and, in general, each compound described has been identified by at least one reference. *For compounds for which no specific literature indication is given, the reader is referred to the Merck Index.*

The cover picture of the book is a reproduction of a copperplate engraving designed for me by the late Charles Gutknecht, who was my secondary school chemistry teacher in Mulhouse. It represents an extract of Brueghel's engraving *The alchemist ruining his family in pursuing his chimera*, surmounted by the aquarius symbol. Represented on the left-hand side is my lucky charm castor oil plant *(Ricinus communis L., Euphorbiaceae)*, which was the starting point of the pyridazine chemistry in my laboratory. The historical cascade of events was as follows: cracking of castor oil produces n-heptanal and aldolization of n-heptanal — and, more generally, of any enolisable aldehyde or ketone — with pyruvic acid leads to α-hydroxy-γ-ketonic acids. Finally, the condensation of these keto acids with hydrazine yields pyridazones. Thus, all our present research on pyridazine derivatives originates from my schoolboy chemistry, when I prepared in my home in Mulhouse n-heptanal and undecylenic acid by cracking castor oil!

Preparing this book was a collective adventure and I am most grateful to all authors for their cooperation and for the time and the effort they spent to write their respective contributions. I appreciate also their patience, especially as the editing process took much more time than initially expected.

I am very grateful to Brad Anderson (University of Utah, Salt Lake City), Jean-Jacques André (Marion Merrell Dow, Strasbourg), Richard Baker (Eli Lilly, Erl Wood, UK), Thomas C. Jones (Sandoz, Basle), Isabelle Morin (Servier, Paris), Bryan Reuben (South Bank University, London) and John Topliss (University of Michigan, Ann Arbor) for their invaluable assistance, comments and contributions.

My thanks go also to the editorial staff of Academic Press in London, particularly to Susan Lord, Nicola Linton and Fran Kingston, to the two copy editors Len Cegielka and Peter Cross, and finally, to the two secretaries of our laboratory, Françoise Herth and Marlyse Wernert.

Last but not least, I want to thank my wife Renée for all her encouragement and for sacrificing evenings and Saturday family life over the past year and a half, to allow me to sit before my computer for about 2500 hours!

Camille G. Wermuth

PART I

General Aspects of Medicinal Chemistry

Medicinal Chemistry: Definition and Objectives. Drug and Disease Classifications

CAMILLE G. WERMUTH

Medicinal chemistry remains a challenging science, which provides profound satisfaction to its practitioners. It intrigues those of us who like to solve problems posed by nature. It verges increasingly on biochemistry and on all the physical, genetic and chemical riddles in animal physiology which bear on medicine. Medicinal chemists have a chance to participate in the fundamentals of prevention, therapy and understanding of diseases and thereby to contribute to a healthier and happier life.

A. Burger[1]

I. DEFINITION AND OBJECTIVES

A. Medicinal chemistry

Taken in the *prospective* sense medicinal chemistry relates to the design and production of compounds that can be used in medicine for the prevention, treatment or cure of human and animal diseases. Thus, from a purely etymological standpoint medicinal chemistry may be said to be a part of pharmacology ('pharmakon' + 'logos' = study of drugs; Fig. 1). Taken in the *retrospective* sense, medicinal chemistry includes the study of already existing drugs, of their biological properties and of their structure–activity relationships.

THE PRACTICE OF MEDICINAL CHEMISTRY
ISBN 0-12-744640-0

Pharmacology	Medicinal chemistry
	Molecular and cellular pharmacology
	Systemic pharmacology
	Clinical pharmacology

Fig. 1.1 The domains of pharmacology.

An early definition of medicinal chemistry was given by a IUPAC specialized commission:[2] 'Medicinal chemistry concerns the discovery, the development, the identification and the interpretation of the mode of action of biologically active compounds at the molecular level. Emphasis is put on drugs, but the interests of the medicinal chemistry are not restricted to drugs but include bioactive compounds in general. Medicinal chemistry is also concerned with the study, identification, and synthesis of the metabolic products of these drugs and related compounds.'

The main activities of medicinal chemists may be observed from a study of their most important scientific journals (*Journal of Medicinal Chemistry, European Journal of Medicinal Chemistry, Il Farmaco, Arzneimittelforschung, Chemical and Pharmaceutical Bulletin*, etc.). Thus, medicinal chemistry covers three critical steps:[3]

- A **discovery step**, consisting of the *identification and production* of new active substances, usually called lead compounds. The lead compounds can originate from synthetic organic chemistry, from natural sources, or from biotechnological processes.
- An **optimization step** that deals mainly with the synthetic modification of the lead structure in order to improve potency, selectivity and lessen toxicity. Its characteristics are the establishment and analysis of *structure–activity relationships*.
- A **development step** consisting of the optimization of the synthetic route for bulk production and the modification of the pharmacokinetic and the pharmaceutical properties of the active substance to render it suitable for clinical use. This process can involve the preparation of chemical formulations that are better absorbed, or are more water-soluble, or have sustained release properties. Additionally, it may result in the elimination of properties which may compromise patient compliance, such as an unpleasant taste, irritation, or pain at the site of injection.

B. Molecular and cellular pharmacology

This is the study of the pharmacological action of drug at the molecular or at the cellular level. The first objective is to identify the cellular levels of action. Three levels important for drug activity can be distinguished: (i) the cell membrane, which is very rich in potential targets, notably in receptors; (ii) the cytosol with its enzymatic systems and the organelle membranes with their particular ion transporters; (iii) the nucleus, which responds to the steroid hormones, to anticancer drugs and to gene therapy. The second objective is to elucidate the precise biochemical and biophysical sequence of events that results from the drug–target interaction. All these studies are performed *in vitro* and therefore yield generally rather reliable quantitative data.

They are also free from factors such as pharmacokinetics and metabolism between the site of administration of the drug and the site of action. Finally, they save the use of animals and are thus more acceptable to the animal protection organizations.

C. Systemic pharmacology

Systemic pharmacology considers the effects of biologically active substances in integrated systems (cardiovascular, skeletal, central nervous, gastrointestinal, pulmonary, etc.). Experiments are performed in intact animals or in isolated organs (isolated heart, isolated arteries, perfused kidney, etc.). The main difficulty resides in the design of animal experimental models that are predictive of an activity in a human disease. As many pharmacological experiments are performed on healthy animals or on disease-simulating paradigms, their extrapolation to clinical situations is questionable. Moreover, intra- and interspecific physiological variations are responsible for rather imprecise results, the margins being often as high as ± 50%.

D. Clinical pharmacology

Clinical pharmacology deals with the examination in humans of the effects of a new drug candidate. The tests are performed under the responsibility of the clinical pharmacologist, who is usually a medical doctor and who has to report to an ethical committee. Phase I tests take place in healthy volunteers. They aim to assess the level of dosing and the tolerance ('dose ranging') and to initiate metabolic studies in humans. Once the safety margin has been determined, phase II, III and IV studies examine successively the beneficial effects in patients, the possible side-effects, the comparison of the drug with reference drugs and the emergence of new therapeutic indications.

II. CONTENT AND COVERAGE

Originally, medicinal chemistry dealt mainly with *ad hoc* chemical modifications of small molecules. The present trend is much more guided by interaction studies between active substances and their molecular targets. Access to increasingly sophisticated molecules is facilitated due to the progress of organic synthesis on the preparative level (e.g. stereoselective reactions, new carbon–carbon coupling reactions, easy chromatographic separations, automated syntheses, etc.) as well as on the level of structural identification (e.g. high-field NMR, X-ray analyses, etc.). Knowledge of the molecular targets (enzymes, receptors, nucleic acids) has, in turn, benefited from the progress in molecular biology and in genetic engineering. For an increasing number of targets the three-dimensional structure and the precise location of the active site are known. The design of new active substances is therefore increasingly based on results obtained from ligand–receptor modelling studies. One can indeed consider the discipline of molecular pharmaco*chemistry*, making a pair with molecular pharmaco*logy*.

Comments Medicinal chemistry is an interdisciplinary science situated at the interface of organic chemistry with life sciences such as biochemistry, pharmacology, molecular biology, immunology, pharmacokinetics and toxicology on one side, and chemistry-based disciplines such as physical chemistry, crystallography, spectroscopy and computer-based information technologies on the other.

Since the objective is the discovery of new drug candidates, medicinal chemistry is also concerned with the fate of drugs in living organisms ('ADME' studies: absorption, distribution, metabolism, excretion). A number of terms more or less synonymous with medicinal chemistry are used: pharmacochemistry, molecular pharmacochemistry, drug design, selective toxicity. The French equivalent to medicinal chemistry is 'chimie thérapeutique' and the German is 'Arzneimittelforschung'.

III. DRUG CLASSIFICATIONS

All attempts to establish clear-cut drug classifications lead to failure owing to the complex nature of the medicaments, which do not fit into simplified systems. The best way to illustrate how drugs are related to one another is to use several classification systems, based on different criteria.

A. Classification systems

The commonest classifications take the following into account.[4-7]

(1) **The origin of the drug**.   Drugs of natural origin can come from three sources. They can originate from minerals: various simple inorganic substances are still in use in medicine, such as sulfur, iodine, phosphates and arsenicals, calcium, sodium, magnesium, iron and bismuth salts, etc. From the animal kingdom some hormones (e.g. insulin) and fish liver oils (vitamins A and E) are still extracted. Biliary salts yield precursors for steroid hemisynthesis (corticoids, sexual hormones). However, the majority of natural compounds are of vegetable origin (alkaloids, cardiac glycosides, antibiotics, anticancer drugs).

Drugs of synthetic origin replace the natural compounds in providing improved and or simplified synthetic analogues, the production of which is not dependent on unpredictable botanical supplies.

In an intermediate position between natural and synthetic compounds are the various fermentation products (vitamins, antibiotics, amino acids) and the products of genetic engineering (e.g. recombinant insulin).

(2) **The mode of action.**   One can distinguish between medicaments that treat the cause of a disease, medicaments that compensate for deficiency of a given substance, and medicaments that aim only to alleviate the symptoms of disease.

Drugs acting directly on the causal agent of a disease are called *aetiological* drugs and represent 'true' medicaments. Presently most of them belong to the class of chemotherapeutic drugs, that is to compounds used to treat infectious diseases (antibacterials, antifungals and antivirals) and parasitic diseases. The principle of their activity resides in their *selective toxicity*: destroying the invader without destroying the host. To this group can logically be added substances used by healthy persons in a preventive way as protection against future illness (vaccinotherapy, aspirin and anticoagulants to prevent cardiac infarcts, vitamins and antioxidants against neurodegenerative disorders). Other drugs can temporarily modify a physiological process (steroidal contraceptives).

Substitutive drugs take the place of a *missing substance*: the deficiency can be due to dietary reasons (vitamin deficiency) or to a physiological disturbance (insulin in diabetes, estrogens in menopause). Substitutive treatment can cover a very short period (intravenous rehydration in case of haemorrhages and diarrhoea) or can last a whole life time (hormonal treatment in Addison's disease).

Symptomatic treatments are given to attenuate or to neutralize disorders that result from a pathological state. They abolish 'general' symptoms such as fever, pain or insomnia. However, their activity can be much more specific and targeted to a particular system: thus symptomatic drugs are available for cardiovascular, neuropsychiatric, respiratory or digestive diseases and so on.

As a rule, a symptomatic treatment is not supposed to cure the patient but rather to render daily life more comfortable and to prolong life. In fact, the distinction between substitutive, preventive and symptomatic treatment is not always easy. Antihypertensive drugs, for example, abolish, or at least diminish, the symptoms associated with arterial hypertension but they also play a preventive role against the cardiovascular complications of hypertension (notably myocardial infarct).

(3) **The nature of the illness**. The so-called *physiological classification* was adopted by the World Health Organization (WHO) in 1968. It classifies drugs by the body system on which they act (drugs affecting the central nervous system, the genitourinary tract or the musculoskeletal system, for example). WHO requests member countries that report to it to classify diseases according to the scheme laid down in the *Manual of the International Statistical Classification of Diseases*, 9th revision (1975), WHO, Geneva, 1977. There are 17 main categories of drugs and each individual disease is represented by a three-digit number. For example, cholera is denoted 001 and mental disorders such as schizophrenic psychoses are found under entries 295 to 299 (see Table 1.1).

Table 1.1   International classification of diseases.

1.	Infectious and parasitic diseases
2.	Neoplasms (cancers)
3.	Endocrine, nutritional and metabolic diseases, and immunity disorders
4.	Diseases of blood and blood-forming organs
5.	Mental disorders
6.	Diseases of the nervous system and sense organs
7.	Diseases of the circulatory system
8.	Diseases of the respiratory system
9.	Diseases of the digestive system
10.	Diseases of the genitourinary system
11.	Complications of pregnancy, childbirth and puerperium
12.	Diseases of the skin and subcutaneous tissue
13.	Diseases of the musculoskeletal system and connective tissue
14.	Congenital anomalies
15.	Conditions originating in the prenatal period
16.	Symptoms, signs and ill-defined conditions
17.	Injury and poisoning

(4) **The chemical structure** Classification by chemical structure is important to those doing pharmaceutical research. An expert in peptide or prostaglandin chemistry will be primarily concerned with the various chemical manipulations that can be performed on these molecules and will rely on someone else to screen them for effects against the various illnesses amenable to peptide or prostaglandin therapy. On the other hand, the chemical classification allows an excellent overview of all the congeners and analogues derived from an initial lead and thus facilitates structure–activity considerations.

B. Practical classifications

In practice the most powerful and useful system developed so far is a compromise between these methods, known as the anatomical–therapeutic–chemical (ATC) system. The system divides products into 14 general groups (Table 1.2) according to the body system on which they act: A, alimentary system; B, blood and blood-forming organs, and so on. This is usually followed by the name of the disease they cure and finally by a description of the chemical classes involved.

Table 1.2 Drug classification by general anatomical groups.[5]

Code letter	Code heading	Examples
A	Alimentary tract and metabolism	Antipeptic ulcerants, anticholinergics antidiarrhoeals, antiemetics, vitamins, anorectics, hypoglycaemics
B	Blood and blood-forming organs	Anticoagulants, thrombolytics, hypolipaemics
C	Cardiovascular system	Cardiovascular drugs
D	Dermatologicals	Antifungals, antibiotics, corticosteroids, antiacne
G	Genitourinary system and sex hormones	Antibacterials, corticosteroids, sex hormones
H	Other systemic hormonal preparations	Glucocorticoids, thyroid therapy
J	General systemic anti-infectives	Antibacterials and antibiotics, antivirals, antifungals
L	Antineoplastic and immunosuppressive drugs	Antineoplastics
M	Musculoskeletal system	Corticosteroids, antigout agents, non-steroidal anti-inflammatory agents, muscle relaxants
N	Central nervous system	Psychotropic drugs, neurological drugs (e.g. anti-Parkinson drugs), analgesics
P	Antiparasitic products	Drugs for tropical diseases
R	Respiratory system	Antihistamines, antiasthmatics, cough and cold preparations
S	Sensory organs	
V	Various	

An even simpler classification is usual among the medicinal chemical community; it distinguishes between four major classes of drugs as follows.

(1) **Agents acting on the central nervous system: psychotropic and neurological drugs.** In man the central nervous system (CNS) comprises the brain and the spinal cord and it

controls the thoughts, the emotions, the sensations and the motor functions. The CNS-active drugs comprise (i) *psychotropic drugs* consisting of the antidepressants, the antipsychotics, the anxiolytics and the psychomimetics, which all affect mood or mental functioning; (ii) *neurological drugs* such as anticonvulsants intended for the treatment of epilepsy, sedatives and hypnotics used for sleep disorders; analgesics as painkillers; and anti-Parkinson drugs.

(2) **Pharmacodynamic agents**.   Pharmacodynamic agents are drugs affecting the normal dynamic processes of the body, such as the cardiovascular domain. This group is composed of the antiarrhythmics, the antianginals, the vasodilators, the antihypertensives, the diuretics and the antithrombotics, which all, directly or indirectly, concern the heart or the blood circulation.

   Traditionally the antiallergic drugs and drugs acting on the gastrointestinal tract and on the respiratory and urogenital systems are also included in the class of pharmacodynamic agents.

(3) **Chemotherapic agents**.   Initially the term chemotherapy referred to treatment by means of drugs selectively preventing the development of various kinds of infesting hosts: protozoa (amoebae, leishmania, hematozoa, treponema, trypanosoma), microbes, fungi, viruses, and as a rule all parasites that propagate infectious diseases. In the context of selective toxicity, anticancer treatments also belong to the class of chemotherapeutic agents.

(4) **Agents acting on metabolic diseases and on endocrine functions**.   This category of drugs comprises a collection of agents that do not fit easily into the previous classes. It consists of the anti-inflammatory drugs, the antiarthritics, the antidiabetics, the hypolipaemic agents, the anorectics and most of the peptide and steroidal hormones.

IV.   CONCLUSION

About 6000 chemical entities can be used, in various pharmaceutical formulations, to treat human or animal diseases; all attempts towards their classification represent arbitrary procedures. The primary reason is that no single drug has ever been encountered that exhibits only one biological activity: for example, antimalarial drug chloroquine is also active on some inflammatory processes, the anxiolytic benzodiazepines possess antiepileptic properties, and so on. On the other hand, the communities have different needs: a chemical classification which may be very useful to a medicinal chemist could be of no relevance to a community care worker, for example. Similarly, pharmacologists, pharmacists and physicians will probably prefer a physiological classification, which would be of less relevance to a medicinal chemist.

REFERENCES

1.   Burger, A. (1990) Preface. In Hansch, C., Sammes, P. G. and Taylor, J. B (eds) *Comprehensive Medicinal Chemistry*, vol. I, p. 1. Pergamon Press, Oxford.
2.   Anonymous. (1974) *Technical Report No. 13*. IUPAC Information Bulletin.
3.   Wermuth, C. G. (1993) Preface. In *Trends in QSAR and Molecular Modeling '92*. ESCOM, Leiden.
4.   Burger, A. (1990) Classification of drugs. In Hansch, C., Sammes, P. G. and Taylor, J. B. (eds)

Comprehensive Medicinal Chemistry, vol. I, pp. 249–260. Pergamon Press, Oxford.
5.   Reuben, B. G. and Wittkoff, H. A. (1989) *Pharmaceutical Chemicals in Perspective.* Wiley, New York.
6.   Taylor, J. B. and Kenewell, P. D. (1993) *Modern Medicinal Chemistry.* Ellis Horwood, London.
7.   Pradal, H. (1975) *Les Grands Médicaments.* Editions du Seuil, Paris.

2

Discovering New Drugs: The Legacy of the Past, Present Approaches, and Hopes for the Future

PHILIPPE MEYER

Ceux qui vivront dans cent ans, dans deux cent ans après nous...
est-ce qu'ils auront seulement un mot gentil pour nous?
Those who will live in one hundred years, in two hundred years after us...
will they even have one nice word for us?
Chekov, *Uncle Vanya*

I. INTRODUCTION

For many centuries the search for therapeutic substances centred on the investigation of herbs grown in the gardens of religious establishments where the sick found shelter. In the nineteenth century, the advent of analytical and synthetic chemistry signalled an important change in direction in that alkaloids were purified, and simple molecules such as acetylsalicylic acid were synthesized. However, the true era of medicinal chemistry really began in the 1930s with the preparation and use of the anti-bacterial sulfonamide drugs. The history of medicine was, from that time on, to be dominated by medicinal therapeutics. Today, a large number of diseases are

THE PRACTICE OF MEDICINAL CHEMISTRY
ISBN 0-12-744640-0

cured, or at least controlled by drug therapy. Thus, the fight against bacterial and fungal infections, has been largely won, and significant progress has been made in treating mental, pulmonary, gastrointestinal, inflammatory, and cardiovascular conditions. In addition, some cancers and certain forms of leukaemia are cured by chemotherapy.

At the outset of this century, a physician needed to know the characteristics of perhaps a dozen or so drugs. Nowadays, human memory is no longer sufficient, and the clinician routinely resorts to consulting pharmacopoeias since the field of drugs is constantly on the move. Although the search for new entities is being increasingly governed by rational and high-throughput techniques, serendipitous discoveries do still occur, as in the old days of medicinal herbs. Criteria by which the quality of a drug is judged have changed, since not only do efficiency and safety matter, but the patient's quality of life must also be taken into account. This stiffening in the drug policy by the Regulatory Authorities has had obvious consequences for the pharmaceutical industry.

For a historical survey of medicinal observations and discoveries from 1785 to 1975 (more than 1300 references) the reader is referred to the exhaustive compilation made by Alfred Burger.[1] Another recommended book is Robert A. Maxwell's and Shohreh B. Eckhardt's excellent 'Drug Discovery, A Casebook and Analysis'.[2] It presents, for about thirty major therapeutic breakthroughs, a description of the innovative therapeutic agent, its early clinical research history, the scientific breakthrough that led to it and the background contributions that preceded it. In addition, the authors comment on the events having led to the compound and on the developments subsequent to its introduction in therapeutics. Other useful sources are Jasjit Bindra's and Dan Lednicer's two volumes 'Chronicles of Drug Discovery',[3,4] Bryan Reuben's and Harold Wittcoff's book 'Pharmaceutical Chemicals in Perspective',[5] Walter Sneader's book on the evolution of modern medicines[6] and the second edition of 'Medicinal Chemistry' by Ganellin and Roberts.[7]

II.   THE LEGACY OF THE PAST

From the early ages of antiquity medicine aimed at healing, and besides the summons to the gods of health its main concern was to find new drugs. On the world's oldest prescription, a clay tablet dating back to 2100 BC and found in Sumeria, two columns of recommendations were written in cuneiform. The left column prescribes carpenter grains and gum resin from thyme ground to powder and dissolved in beer; in the right column 'lunar plant' and 'white pear-tree' roots are prescribed. In Homeric Greece, doctors would prescribe hellebore and lentil broth. Great Hippocrates' favourite recipes were oils, herb potions, opium and *jusquiamus*. Likewise, Galen had his own recipes for his medicinal potions. The therapeutic (and toxic) properties of herbs were gradually discovered through an empirical approach. Plutarch reported how starving soldiers from Marcus Aurelius' army died after eating turnip-shaped roots. These must have been monkshood, *Aconitum napellus*, containing aconitin which has curative properties when taken in small quantities but is toxic when taken in larger amounts. Step by step, accurate therapeutic methods based on medicinal herbs were implemented and largely used until the nineteenth century: in 1882, the French Pharmacopoeia gave a list of 52 herbs used to make medicaments.

During the Middle Ages, healing herbs were chosen according to Graeco-Latin traditions completed through Eastern and mainly Arabic methods. Moreover, these herbs were grown on religious premises sheltering the sick population. In the fourteenth century, young physicians from Montpellier learned the *Corpus Simplicium Medicamentarum* by Ibn al Beiter, which is no more than the *Materia Medica* by Dioscorides, or the *Precious Book* by Donnoba to which a hundred more new plants have been added.

In the Renaissance, gardens of *simples* flourished all over Europe outside Arabic and Mediterranean spheres of influence, and became secular. In Paris, in 1580, Master Nicolas Houël founded a garden to teach botany and the use of medicinal herbs. This was the beginnings of the Pharmaceutical Faculty. The discovery of maritime routes to India and America contributed still further to enriching the pharmacopoeia, and the Aztec and the Mayan civilisations were especially active in this field. Thanks to Le Gras, Europe discovered the *ipecacuanha*, a golden root that treats dysentery; and thanks to Juan de Vega, cinchona bark which contains quinine and is effective against malaria.

Urged by his doctors, Louis XIII established the Royal Garden for Medicinal Herbs in Paris in 1635, so that theoretical courses could be completed through practical studies. The study of botany was enriched thanks to the work of the Garden's directors, from Daquin to Bernardin de Saint-Pierre and Buffon. They set the stage for taxonomists such as Joseph Pitton de Tournefort in Paris in the seventeenth century, Hermann Boerhave and Carl von Linné in Leyden and in Uppsala in the seventeenth century.

The first apothecaries were established in Venice in the thirteenth century. During the following century, many shops where pre-cut herbs were kept and herb teas, syrups and balms were prepared opened throughout Europe. The often difficult relationships between the medical and the pharmaceutical world were ruled by royal decrees, such as the Codex of Augsburg (1538), or by traditions such as those in the kingdom of Sicily where drugs had to be prepared in front of the doctors who had prescribed them in order to avoid any possible fraudulent activities. The invention of printing naturally contributed to the boom of herbal pharmacopoeia: starting with the *Receptario fiorentino* which was the first printed list of useful drugs, published in Florence on 10 January 1499, to the *Dictionary of Simple Drugs* by Nicolas Lemery, published in 1761, there were at least a dozen publications in Europe.

Syphilis, brought to Europe by Columbus' seamen and soldiers was first treated by a plant called the *gaiac*, according to the traditions set up by Ferdinand and Isabelle of Spain. To increase its efficiency, which was virtually zero, other plants were investigated but all in vain; among them were China roots, convolvulus, sassafras from Florida and dill tea. During the next two centuries the idea of chemical therapy was advanced, and this proved to be slightly more efficacious albeit somewhat toxic. Initiated by alchemists, it used mercury, arsenic, antimony, copper, zinc and tartar emetic. Given in inappropriate dosage the cure often proved to be more deadly than the disease.

The nineteenth century saw a great expansion in the use of chemistry which, in about one hundred years' time, was to so greatly extend the herbal pharmacopoeia that had been established for many centuries. Building on the work of Lavoisier, chemists throughout Europe refined and extended the techniques of chemical analysis. In addition, the synthesis of acetic acid by Kolbe in 1845, and that of methane by Berthelot some eleven years later, established the principle of organic chemistry as a preparative tool. Also in the nineteenth century, pharmacognosy was replaced by physiological chemistry; the main concern was no longer to find new medicaments from the huge world of plants, but rather to find the active ingredients that accounted for the particular properties of a given plant.

One breakthrough came after another. In 1803, Friedrich Sertürner, a German pharmacist, isolated morphine from opium — this was the first ever isolation of a pure alkaloid. In 1816, the French pharmacist Pierre Pelletier extracted emetine, the emetic principle of ipecacuanha. With the collaboration of his colleague, Joseph Caventou, Pelletier's research led, in 1819, to the purification of strychnine, caffeine and quinine, and of colchicine in 1820. Thus, within the space of less than twenty years several of the major herbal alkaloids had been identified. In 1828 nicotine was isolated, followed by codeine and atropine in 1832. In 1875 William Withering, an English physician and botanist, had used foxglove, *Digitalis purpurea*, to treat dropsy, and in 1799 Ferriar had ascribed the therapeutic action of foxglove to its cardiac effects. Subsequently, Homolle and Quevenne (1840), Nativelle (1869) and Arnaud (1888) separated increasingly pure glycosidal preparations from digitaline. In 1860 Niemann isolated cocaine and noticed that it numbed his tongue; Von Arep (1879) discovered that subcutaneous injection produced anaesthesia and Hall (1884) used it in dentistry; Halstead (1885) used it to study nerve block. The Calabar bean, seed of *Physostigma venenosum*, had been used by primitive African societies for trial by ordeal — if vomited up, so that symptoms were aborted, the verdict was not guilty — and in 1864 the active ingredient, physostigmine, was first isolated. In 1875 a crystalline mixture, ergotinine, was isolated from ergot fungus, *Claviceps purpura*, that grows on rye. In 1877 yohimbine was isolated, followed by sparteine in 1885, and ouabain in 1888. In 'La révolution des médicaments', the reader will find a detailed history of the discovery of many of these alkaloids.[8] By the middle of the century the first synthetic halogenated drugs had begun to appear, and the use of chloroform as a general anaesthetic was pioneered in 1847 by the Scottish obstetrician James Simpson. This was followed in 1869 by the German physician, Liebrich, using chloral and bromural to produce sedation and hypnosis.

As a result of these discoveries, and allied to the progress made in organic chemistry, the drugs industry came into being at the end of the nineteenth century. Throughout the Western world bulk production of pharmaceuticals sprang up from modernized dispensaries, or from the diversification of already existing industries, such as those of textiles and dyestuffs in the Rhine valley. Thus, by the dawn of the twentieth century several purely synthetic drugs were available for use. Among them, salicylic acid, acetylsalicylic acid, acetanilide and aminopyrine which were used as analgesics, chloroform and ether as anaesthetics, chloral hydrate as hypnotic and amyl nitrite as a vasodilator. In 1888, the pharmaceutical division of the firm Bayer launched a very efficacious analgesic called *phenacetine*, and also one of the first sleeping pills, *sulfonal*. In addition, the popular anti-inflammatory/analgesic drug *aspirin* was first marketed amid exceptional publicity in 1899.

Later, various substances derived from morphine were prescribed as cough mixtures and medicines against malaria. In 1907 Paul Ehrlich synthesized *salvarsan*, one of the great drugs of all time in that it introduced the concept of chemotherapy. *Salvarsan* was the first effective treatment against syphilis, and it resulted in Ehrlich being awarded the Nobel Prize for Medicine in 1908. Experimental biologists and medicinal research began also at the end of the 19th century with Claude Bernard, Louis Pasteur, Robert Koch, Joseph Lister and Paul Ehrlich. Ehrlich's studies on the receptor theory and on structural modifications of active compounds opened the way for modern medicinal chemistry.

In spite of the vagaries caused by two World Wars, some of the most advanced drug industries are still to be found in the Ruhr region. Basel's drug industry introduced its first products at the Universal Exhibition in Paris in 1889: antiseptics, drugs against rheumatism, digitalis and alkaloids derived from rye ergot. For the first time in the history of medicine, industrial research added its results to those of university-based laboratories and other research institutions run by the state. It soon turned out to be extremely powerful, becoming more efficienct throughout the twentieth century and achieving amazing results against more and more serious diseases. The period from 1900 to 1935 saw the introduction of drugs against parasitic diseases, of barbiturates as hypnotics, of organomercurials as diuretics and of highly iodinated substrates as X-ray contrast agents. At approximately the same period the isolation and structural identification of endogenous compounds such as neurotransmitters, vitamins, steroidal and peptidic hormones was achieved and the first partial or total syntheses of some of them was effected. A new phase in medicinal chemistry research began in 1933 with the discovery of the antibacterial sulfonamides by Mietzsch, Klarer and Domagk. Thanks to these compounds a spectacular effect of the decline in mortality from infectious diseases was observed.

Starting in the 1940s the antibiotics took over from the sulfonamides with major discoveries such as penicillin, tetracycline and streptomycin. The discovery of penicillin (which will be dealt with again in the coming pages), of other antibiotics and of drugs against tuberculosis during the Second World War and the following years was the starting point of an era of success for the world's pharmacopoeia. New antibiotics challenge bacterial resistance; fungal infections are cured; cardiac and arterial diseases can be foreseen and in some cases controlled by some twenty therapeutic classes; mental disorders are transformed, some cancers can be stemmed, and the secondary effects of anticancer chemotherapy considerably reduced. Remarkable progress has also been made in the treatment of inflammatory, pulmonary and gastrointestinal diseases.

If the 1940s was the decade of antibiotics, the 1950s was the decade of psychotropic medicines. The first major tranquillizer, chlorpromazine, was discovered in 1950, followed in 1954 by the minor tranquillizer meprobamate, and in 1960 by another minor tranquilizer, chlordiazepoxide, which was the first representative of the benzodiazepine class of compounds. By 1960 there were also available two groups of antidepressants, the monoamine oxidase inhibitors and the tricyclics (imipramine). For the first time there were medicines available for the treatment of schizophrenia, anxiety, and acute depression. Another area where the advances have been slower but also impressive is heart disease. Reserpine was discovered in 1952 and methyldopa in 1960. The golden age for heart drugs, however, was the late 1960s and the early 1970s (β-blockers, calcium antagonists, hypotensive agents). However, despite decades of effort, cancer remains a major killer disease, with chemotherapy only really successful in a few instances.

Figures from the various pharmacopoeias clearly show the boom that is adding to the noticeable progress in surgery, endoscopy and the rise of medical technology. The controversy initiated in 1975 by Ivan Illich on the effectiveness of medicine (and drugs) as compared to hygiene on mankind's well-being[9] seems totally irrelevant today. In particular, the pretence that medical progress stems only from the adoption of new rules of life, and not from medicine, is no longer accepted. Nobody can question that the unprecedented increase in human life expectancy, which has almost doubled in a hundred years, is mainly due to drugs and to those who discovered them.

The modern era is characterized by the fact that new drugs are being developed within a much stricter regulatory framework, with greater emphasis being placed on the quality of life.

'Most significant of all, new drugs are being designed . . . on the basis of an understanding of the biochemistry of the systems they are intended to influence. Although drug design still relies on the intuitive feel of the scientist, development of receptor theory (the modern equivalent of Ehrlich's 'magic bullet' hypothesis) provided a way to escape from molecular roulette. This new approach gathered momentum in the 1970s and the results are seen in some of the pharmaceutical innovations of the 1970s and in most innovations of the 1980s. This seminal period truly represents a second chemotherapeutic revolution.'[5]

Table 2.1 collects the present status of some diseases; it shows clearly that many very important diseases are not completely cured today.

All these achievements in the twentieth century's medicinal therapeutics have significantly influenced medical practice and the training of doctors. At a time when it was deprived of effective drugs, medicine's main concern was sympathy with the sick, diagnosis and interpretation of morbid disorders. During the last 30 to 40 years, drugs have become the centre of medical activity. The clinician now has to choose from a wide range of drugs, and has to be acquainted with pharmacopoeias detailing new mechanisms of action, side effects, and

Table 2.1   Status of some diseases

1. **Diseases largely cured or avoided**
   Cholera
   Diphtheria
   Lobar pneumonia
   Erysipelas
   Measles
   Meningococcal meningitis
   Pertussis (whooping cough)
   Plague
   Poliomyelitis
   Rheumatic fever
   Scarlet fever
   Smallpox
   Staphylococcal septicaemia
   Subacute bacterial endocarditis
   Tuberculosis
   Typhoid fever
   Vitamin deficiency

2. **Diseases alleviated**
   Asthma
   Diabetes
   Heart disease
   Schizophrenia
   Syphilis and other veneral diseases

3. **Diseases that still present challenges**
   AIDS
   Alzheimer's disease
   Arthritis
   Cancer
   Cirrhosis
   Common cold
   Genetically transmitted diseases
   Genital herpes
   Huntingdon's chorea
   Influenza
   Multiple sclerosis
   Parkinson's disease
   Pulmonary fibrosis
   Senility, geriatric problems

interactions with other medicines. In addition, the costs of treatment have to be taken into account as governments try to rein in the burgeoning price of healthcare.

A.   The signature theory

The first drugs were discovered as a result of a sustained and desperate search for natural products capable of treating disease. Numerous examples have been given above. In this search, men believed in symbols, in imprints ('signatures'), one might say in nature's winks. Ivy, since it embraces the trees and makes them slimmer, could perhaps contain some active principle against obesity; the bitter taste of artichokes could possibly be useful against liver diseases, and blueberries useful to the sight. Some phallus-shaped roots (European asparagus, African sausage tree, Chinese ginseng) might have aphrodisiac properties.

The history of aspirin is the best example of how a natural substance was discovered as a result of an impression from the environment. Willows always live near water; their branches lean towards its surface and their roots choose humid soil. Willows are hospitable trees; their leaves are perfect shelters; most of all, it seems that people who have lived in their surroundings have always been protected against fevers that held sway in marsh lands and other flooded lands. By analogy, willows, which 'grow with their feet in water without suffering' seemed useful against 'diseases caused by wet feet'. The 'imprint', the sign left by the willows, led to the discovery of the drug which is still today the most commonly used. On 2 June 1763, a British cleric, Edward Stone confirmed the legend in front of the Royal Society in London: he considered willow bark tea as a suitable treatment against fevers. Because it was highly bitter, his claims sounded even more believable. Had not cinchona bark tea, which had just been brought back from Peru and which was so effective against fevers, the same taste? Decoctions made of willow bark and quinquina bark did not treat the same fevers, cinchona being more specific to malaria, but, in those days malaria and fevers of all kinds were confounded, and Stone's message was not forgotten. The 'imprint' of the willow had left another indication: its bark could be used against rheumatisms since it 'came from flexible and malleable branches'. In 1829, H. Leroux, a pharmacist from Vitry-le-François, isolated the active principle of willow bark, which he called salicin. It is actually a molecule derived from a sugar (a salicylic). Salicin may also be extracted from a flower, the meadowsweet, which is plentiful in many parts of the world. Pagenstecher from Switzerland, Cahours in France, and Procter in the United States transformed salicin into an aldehyde and then into salicylic acid. In 1853, Charles Gerhardt in Strasburg transformed the compound into acetylsalicylic acid. A salicylic acid salt, sodium salicylate, was given for the first time in 1853 to a child who suffered from articular rheumatism. The child's fever and articular aches clearly diminished.

In 1893, Felix Hoffman, working for the drug company Bayer, achieved the first commercial synthesis of acetylsalicylic acid and bulk production began. The substance was given the name aspirin, 'a' standing for acetyl and 'spir' for Spirae, the Latin name for the family of herbs to which the meadowsweet belongs. After the First World War, Bayer's rights were seized and the word 'aspirin' became public property. In 1983, 30 000 tonnes, that is 75 billion aspirin pills, were manufactured throughout the world. Recently, its properties have been extended to the possible prevention of a myocardial infaction by virtue of its effect on thromboxane A_2 production.

Even if it is sustained by allegories, the discovery of natural substances used for therapeutical purposes is often the result of serendipity. Important drugs, many of which are still in widespread use today, have come about by this route. Thus, a chance observation or an unexpected side-effect have played a significant part in the drug discovery process.

B. The drugs of chance

Sweet clover is a large and beautiful plant with fragrant flowers, that smell like honey when it is fresh, but which quickly wither once cut. If cattle are fed on the faded plant it can cause lethal stomach bleeding. This is because the fermentation of sweet clover produces a hemorrhagic substance, *dicumarol*, that results from the dimerization of two molecules of coumarin with one molecule of formaldehyde. Subsequently, it was shown that *dicumarol* acts as an antagonist of vitamin K that is essential for blood coagulation. Analogues of *dicumarol* have since become first-choice anti-coagulants for use in postoperative thrombophlebitis, pulmonary embolism and coronary thrombosis.

Sulfur mustard gas was used as an offensive weapon in Europe during World War I,[10] and the related nitrogen mustards were manufactured by both sides for the same purpose in World War II. During the war against Japan an American ship carrying such gas exploded in the Pacific Ocean. It was found that those survivors who had breathed the ensuing cloud of toxic gas had lost their natural defences against microbes and were threatened by bacterial infections. On further investigation it was discovered that the toxic gases had destroyed the blood's white cells. Regrettable though this incident was, it did lead to the discovery of drugs which are now used in leukaemia therapy.

Another story connected to the use of explosive materials resulted in a drug that is widely used to relieve the symptoms of angina pectoris. It was noted that workers in the explosives industry who were handling trinitroglycerine experienced severe vascular headaches. This proved to be due to the ability of trinitroglycerine to produce a marked dilation of the blood vessels. During an anginal attack the coronary vasculature is unable to supply the heart muscle with adequate oxygen and nutrient for it to function properly. Immediate relief from pain is achieved by dilatation of the coronary blood vessels. Trinitroglycerine is readily absorbed through the skin or the sublingual mucosa and consequently affords rapid symptomatic relief.

Finally, a story related to the rubber industry resulted in a drug, *antabuse*, which is used in the treatment of chronic alcoholism. Workers in the industry were at one time very surprised indeed to discover that they had apparently spontaneously developed a strong disgust for alcohol. Careful investigation revealed that this was not a spontaneous phenomenon but was in fact due to an antoxidant, di(diethylcarbamoyl) disulfide which had contaminated both food and atmosphere. This agent prevented the on-going oxidation of alcohol in the liver, thereby producing a build-up of acetaldehyde in the body. The acetaldehyde caused flushing, a pounding sensation in the heart and head, dyspnoea and nausea, which not surprisingly discouraged further drinking.

C. Unforeseen drugs

Penicillin is the best example of those unforeseen drugs that were discovered during medically oriented research that was not aimed specifically at obtaining them. In 1878, Pasteur put forward the concept of 'antagonism' between two strains of microorganisms, so that the development of one strain prevented that of the other; some nonpathogenic aerobic bacteria can, for example, stop the development of the golden staphylococcus that causes skin infections.

Nearly twenty years later, his student, Roux, revived the idea and entrusted a young physician, Ernest Duchesne from the Military Health School, with the research. Duchesne was undertaking an elective in Roux' laboratory and was looking for a job to be able to finance his PhD thesis. The thesis was presented on 17 December 1897; at that time Duchesne was 23 years old. His thesis was entitled 'Contribution to the study of vital competition among microorganisms. Antagonism between moulds and microbes'. It was shown that under certain experimental conditions some moulds can prevent the growth of certain bacteria and that 'certain moulds, such as that of *Penicillium glaucum*, when inoculated in an animal at the same time as highly virulent cultures of some pathogenic microbes (bacillus coli and bacillus typhosus of Eberth) can alleviate to quite a significant extent the virulence of bacterial cultures'.[11]

A new and brilliant idea by Pasteur, or by Roux as Duchesne used to say ('It was Professor Sir Roux who first came up with the idea'), had been demonstrated. The experiments had been carried out with full care and they indicated the existence and the activity of antibiotic substances. Yet the realization of the discovery of the antibiotic failed on this occasion. Ernest Duchesne, who had to face various pressures due to his career as a military doctor and also had health problems, gave up his research immediately after the presentation of his thesis. Roux focused his own attention on other fields of research.

Some thirty years later in London, in September 1928, Alexander Fleming was working as a bacteriologist at St Mary's Hospital. There, the growth of microbial colonies was being studied in flat glass boxes containing a layer a few millimetres deep of nutrient gelatin. At this time it was known that an orderly and clean environment was essential to efficient bacteriological research: thus, culture boxes containing the microbes to be studied were placed in incubators at 37°C where the sustaining nutrient medium and the heat contributed to the development of germs; once the proliferation of microbes is analysed, the boxes were washed and sterilized. Fleming, though, had a most unusual habit: he would leave the boxes on the laboratory's draining board and wash them some time later. Some say he was somewhat careless and untidy; others that he was only being cautious, checking the boxes before they were washed. Whatever the case, this is how he made his discovery. Fleming observed that in old culture boxes where moulds had had time to develop, colonies of microbes were inhibited and destroyed, to the point that they had disappeared. The destruction can be replicated through the use of the mould broth filtrate, which Fleming called penicillin, after *penicillium*, the name of one of the more common moulds. Penicillin appeared to be active, when used *in vitro*, against golden staphylococci in culture boxes, and *in vivo*, with no toxic secondary effects on mice and rabbits.

Fleming reported all these results clearly in a note published in 1929.[12] It should have been realized there and then that penicillin had all the properties of a new anti-infective drug, being much more effective than the then existing sulfonamides and further studies should have been undertaken as soon as the note was published. But Fleming's publication did not arouse the interest that might logically have been expected.

According to André Maurois,[13] Fleming's shyness prevented him from convincing the chemists of the necessity to launch a programme of work for the purification of a substance that he knew was extremely interesting to medicine. Ernst Chain, who later discovered the chemical nature of penicillin and produced the first clinically usable antibiotic from it, gave a less amicable explanation. Fleming, according to Chain, had not carried out all the experiments that would have undeniably proved the antibiotic action of penicillin *in vivo*: if these had been done, and detailed reports produced, the chemists would have undoubtedly been attracted by the substance. More, his lack of perseverance would have been due to the prejudices of Professor Almroth Wright, Fleming's chief of department, on the future therapeutic role of antibacterial chemical substances: 'His Head of Department, Professor Sir Almroth Wright . . . has a rigid outlook and for whom the concept of chemotherapy was taboo and treated as such throughout his whole scientific career.'[14]

The truth of the whole story will probably never be known. One thing is sure: a jinx was to remain on penicillin and when it was discovered by chance a second time, it once again fell into oblivion for several more years. Even more amazing is that its third, and this time successful, discovery was the result of a random approach. In the middle of 1935, a young biochemist of German background, Ernst Chain, who was just back from two happy years of studies at Cambridge University, decided that he would carry on his research in England. He therefore joined a team run by Professor H. W. Florey, who had just obtained the chair of pathology at Cambridge. In the course of his chemical studies, working on the principles of the venom of certain snakes, Chain had acquired a fair knowledge of enzymes. More specifically, he had demonstrated that the snakes' venom can become toxic to the nervous system as a result of the activity of a nucleotide enzyme, nucleotidase. In Cambridge his studies focused on a recently isolated substance, lysozyme, which can be found in certain microbes and in the digestive liquid of the duodenum, and which seemed to react as an enzyme. It was known that lysozyme could kill certain microbes, but it was mainly thought that it might be held responsible for duodenal ulcers. Thirty years before, Fleming also had done much work on bacterial lysozymes. He had even discovered a lysozyme inside a quite common saprophyte, *Bacillus lysodeicticus.*

This was how Chain ended up studying Fleming's work. He discovered his publication on penicillin, which, by that time, was totally forgotten, and he wondered whether it had common characteristics with lysozyme. Florey and Chain began purifying penicillin. In August 1940, their publication appeared in the well-known British journal of Medicine, *The Lancet,*[15] and it listed the main chemical properties of penicillin, showing its amazing antibiotic effects on animals, and its good tolerance. This was the end of the chaotic history of penicillin. The work which was done from then on, led to the final form of the first antibiotic.

Penicillin soon turned out to be just as effective in humans as in animals. Within a few days infections that were hitherto considered incurable were abating and then disappearing. This was nothing less than a major landmark in the field of medicine, and it was to transform the lives of millions of people throughout the entire world. Understandably, a large number of pharmaceutical laboratories were attracted by the promise of this new drug. A systematic search was soon launched for other antibiotics of microbial origin, and this led to the discovery of the cephalosporins; tetracyclines, erythromycin, streptomycin, poypeptides and macrolides. Knowing the chemical structure of these agents, it became possible to carry out synthetic modifications and thereby to produce a wide range of novel semi-synthetic analogues. So far these have enabled mankind to keep just ahead of the growing problem of bacterial resistance.

D. Some other unexpected drugs

Many pharmaceutical products have revealed properties that were unforseeable at the time of their discovery and consequently their use has changed. These unexpected effects have been observed for the most part during clinical trials that preceded marketing, but some were discovered post-launch.

Beta-blockers were initially produced to alleviate the pain of angina by reducing the burden of work on the heart. However, thanks to the careful work of the English cardiologist, Pritchard,[16] these drugs were subsequently found to have excellent antihypertensive properties, and this is now their main clinical use.

Clonidine, is another example of an antihypertensive drug that was discovered by chance. At Boehringer, the German pharmaceutical company where clonidine was discovered, the drug was designed as an alpha agonist to be used either as a nasal vasoconstrictor and/or as an additive to shaving soaps.[17,18] However, the first clinical trials with clonidine resulted in hypotensive collapse due to a marked fall in blood pressure. The mechanism by which this came about was discovered several years later: a neuronal adrenergic system in the brain is involved in the regulation of blood pressure, and the stimulation of its alpha-receptors by clonidine had the effect of causing a lowering of the blood pressure. Clonidine in fact has both a central and a peripheral effect. Early in treatment blood pressure reduction is associated with a central reduction of sympathetic outflow, but long-term treatment reduces the responsiveness of peripheral blood vessels to vasoconstrictor and vasodilator substances. Thus, from originally being a drug designed for nasal drops and shaving soaps, clonidine progressed to being an important antihypertensive agent. In addition, it became an exceedingly useful pharmacological tool for the study of the central regulation of blood pressure.

The origins of the first *antidepressant drugs* are yet another fortuitous story. The hydrazide of isonicotinic acid was synthesized in 1912, but another forty years were to elapse before its remarkable clinical properties were discovered. In 1945 it was shown that an amide, nicotinamide, had useful tuberculostatic activity, and this prompted a systematic search for even better agents from among those compounds related to this lead. It was not long before isoninzid was evaluated and its excellent tuberculostatic properties confirmed. Very quickly isoninzid became the first choice treatment in tuberculosis, administered in combination with aminosalicylic acid and/or streptomycin in order to delay the appearance of resistant bacteria. Interestingly, it was noticed that patients treated with isoninzid were excessively cheerful, and this observation led to isoninzid being evaluated for psychiatric depression.[19] Following the successful outcome of this work, superior analogues for the treatment of depression were discovered, and these included isocarboxazid, nialamide and the phenethylamines, tranylcypromine and phenelzine. These drugs are known as MAO's (monoamine oxidase inhibitors) and their mode of action is to delay the metabolism of primary amines such as noradrenalines and serotonin. Elevation of mood is assumed to result from the accumulation of these amines in the central nervous system.

In 1933 Fourneau and Bovet reported that some simple benzodioxans with basic side chains had antihistaminic activity. Following this observation several groups of chemists attempted to improve on the potency of the original benzodioxans, and this led to the discovery of the well-known series of H_1-antihistamines such as diphenhydramine, pyrilamine and pheniramine. One of the structural classes that was investigated in the course of this work was a series of compounds based on the tricyclic phenothiazine ring. The best compound of the series was eventually marketed under the name of promethazine. Promethazine though had a problem in that it produced quite significant sedative effects at the higher doses. However, this unforeseen side-effect did not deter research workers at Rhône-Poulenc, who decided that they would continue synthesizing and studying phenothinizine analogues in the hope of finding superior antihistimines and antiparkinsonian agents. One of the compounds that they produced was different from the others in that it was virtually devoid of antihistamic effects, but it reduced motor activity, induced quietness, and caused mild drowsiness. The compound was named chlorpromazine and it was the first of the neuroleptic drugs, i.e. it was a major tranquillizer, very effective in psychotic conditions such as schizophrenia.[20-22] Psychiatry was revolutionized by this discovery. Hitherto the only 'treatment' for the bizarre behaviour sometimes manifested by schizophrenics had been restraint by straitjacket or in the padded cell. The advent of chlorpromazine brought new hope to the treatment of mental disease. Further research work, most particularly by Janssen in Belgium, led to the discovery of other neuroleptics such as the butyrophenomes and the benzamides. Another very major spin-off resulting from the discovery of chlorpromazine was the subsequent discovery of the tricyclic antidepressants (see Chapter 6).

The *hypoglycaemic drugs* experienced similar good fortune with regard to their discovery. In 1942 a clinician in Montpellier was treating typhoid patients with sulfonamide antibacterial drugs. In the course of the treatment he noticed that his patients were experiencing quite marked hypoglycaemic effects. A pharmacologist, Loubatières, who was alerted to these findings carried out some research and confirmed that certain of the sulfonamides did indeed produce hypoglycaemia. Thus once again a serendipitous finding was the key to an important advance in medicine. The sulfonylurea drug carbutamide, introduced by Loubatières, was the forerunner of the presentday antidiabetic compounds such as chlorpropamide and tolbutamide. These drugs lower blood sugar by activating the release of insulin by the pancreatic B-cells.

'Chance favours the prepared mind' said Pasteur, and the history of drug discovery this century fully testifies to the truth of that dictum. Yet further examples of drugs discovered in this way are to be found in the identification of the anti-leukamia alkaloids vinblastine and vincristine from the periwinkle plant;[23-25] aminoglutethimide, originally prepared as a potential antiepileptic agent but now used as an anticancer agent due to its ability to inhibit production of corticosteroids by the adrenal glands; mifepristone, synthesized as an antagonist of cortisol receptors but used as a medical alternative to surgical termination of pregnancy by virtue of its effect on progresterone receptors.[26]

A particularly noteworthy achievement in the field of empirical research was the discovery of cyclosporine A by the Swiss firm Sandoz. Like most other pharmaceutical companies, Sandoz were looking for new antibiotics by growing cultures from the microorganisms found in different soil samples. In order to widen the range of soil samples being examined, Sandoz' research workers were encouraged to bring back a few grams of soil whenever they went abroad on holiday. In 1969 some soil from a region in Norway called Hardanger Vida was examined and it proved interesting because the microorganism in the soil secreted a novel polypeptide. This was evaluated in the usual manner but it quickly became apparent that there was no significant antibiotic activity. Neither had the substance any properties that might cause it to be considered as an anticancer agent. Unexpectedly though the polypeptide turned out to have potent immunosuppressive properties. Its mode of action was to specifically and reversibly inhibit the production of lymphokines that stimulate T-cell growth.[27,28] Since T-cell lymphocytes are part of the immune system, being concerned with attacking foreign, invading cells, the Sandoz research team had discovered a drug with a previously unknown and unforeseen mechanism. The polypeptide was found to consist of eleven amino acids arranged in cyclic fashion, and was named cyclosporine A. Its discovery represented a landmark in immunopharmacology, and launched the era of organ and bone marrow transplant surgery.[29]

III.   PRESENT APPROACHES AND HOPES FOR THE FUTURE

Contemporary medicinal research operates both upstream and downstream of endogenous organic molecules. Downstream, it involves processes which modify the behaviour of cellular constituents. By neutralizing, inhibiting, activating or facilitating the intervention of a messenger, an enzyme, or a receptor, pharmacology aims to correct the cellular perturbation that initiates the pathology of an organ. Upstream, research is concerned with the synthesis of endogenous cellular compound through the intervention of genes. Several strategies are now used at this level.

Genetic engineering, by modification of the genome of unicellular organisms so as to enable them to produce foreign substances helpful to ill people; for example the production of insulin or human growth hormone by *Escherichia coli*. Fears of the proliferation of mutated bacteria as expressed in Asilomar, are no longer justified. The production by this method of pure products free of toxic viral contamination stimulates the development of this technique.

Somatic gene therapy, by the utilization of a carrier virus, adenovirus or retrovirus, introduces a healthy gene in place of a defective gene responsible for a given pathology. Successes have been obtained against melanomas and strong hopes are already expressed regarding the most serious diseases such as cancers, AIDS or synthesis defects of genetic origin (hereditary diseases of the blood). This new therapeutic method, which poses no ethical problems, despite difficulties of insertion of the beneficial gene to the right place, is doubtless destined for a considerable expansion. Somatic gene therapy must be clearly distinguished from the *germinal gene therapy*, which is the replacement of a gene in the gamete. Ethical and technical questions impose considerable limits on this process. Does it not accelerate mutations simply for reasons of convenience? Does it not introduce the risk of genomic destabilization of the gamete with the danger, among others, of carcinogenic mutations?

The molecular evolution of medicine, besides therapeutic progress, will improve the understanding of morbid processes. It is far simpler, indeed, to follow a morbid process from the gene to the organic damage, than to start with the anatomochemical inventory of the problems caused by a lesion, an operation that is always complicated by unpredictable molecular interactions. The simultaneous growth of fundamental knowledge and therapeutic processes will have as a consequence a stunning acceleration of medicine.

REFERENCES

1. Burger, A. (1980) Introduction: History and economics of medicinal chemistry. In Wolff, M. E. (ed.) *The Basis of Medicinal Chemistry — Burger's Medicinal Chemistry*, pp. 1–54. Wiley, New York.
2. Maxwell, R. A. and Eckhardt, S. B. (eds) (1990) *Drug Discovery — A Casebook and Analysis*. Humana Press, Clifton.
3. Bindra, J. S. and Lednicer, D. (1982) *Chronicles of Drug Design I*, vol. 1. Wiley, New York.
4. Bindra, J. S. and Lednicer, D. (1983) *Chronicles of Drug Design II*, vol. 2. Wiley, New York.
5. Reuben, B. G. and Wittcoff, H. A. (1989) *Pharmaceutical Chemicals in Perspective*. Wiley, New York.
6. Sneader, W. (1985) *Drug Discovery: The Evolution of Modern Medicines*. Wiley, Chichester.
7. Ganellin, C. R. and Roberts, S. M. (1993) *Medicinal Chemistry, The Role of Organic Chemistry in Drug Research*, 2nd edn. Academic Press, London.
8. Meyer, P. (1984) *La Révolution des Médicaments*, pp. 54–72. Fayard, Paris.
9. Illich, Y. (1975) *Némésis Médicale*. Seuil, Paris.
10. Bernard, J. (1978) *L'espérance*, p. 97. Buchet-Chastel, Paris.
11. Duchesne, E. (1897) *Contribution à l'étude de la concurrence vitale chez les microorganismes. Antagonisme entre les moisissures et les microbes* (Thesis). Alexandre Rey, Lyon.
12. Fleming, A. (1929) On antibacterial action of cultures of *Penicillium*, with special reference to their use in isolation of *B. influenzae*. *Br. J. Exp. Pathol.* **10**: 226–236.
13. Maurois, A. (1959) *La vie de Sir Alexander Fleming*. Hachette, Paris.

14. Chain, E. (1979) The early years of the penicillin discovery. *Tr. Pharmacol. Sci.* **1**: 6–11.
15. Chain, E., Florey, H. W., Gardner, A. D., Heatley, N. G., Jennings, M. A., Orr-Ewing, J. and Sanders, A. G. (1940) Penicillin as chemotherapeutic agent. *The Lancet.* **2**: 226–228.
16. Pritchard, B. N. C. (1964) Hypotensive action of pronethalol. *Br. Med. J.* **1**: 1227–1228.
17. Stähle, H. (1982) Clonidine. In Bindra, J. S. and Lednicer, D. (eds) *Chronicles of Drug Discovery*, pp. 87–111. Wiley, New York.
18. Zeile, K., Stähle, H. and Hauptmann, K.-H. (1961–73) Disubstituierte 2-Phenylamino-1,3-diazacyclopentene-(2). Ger. Pat. 1,303,141, to C. H. Boehringer Sohn, Ingelheim/Rhein.
19. Mauvernay, R. Y. and Moleyre, J. (1975) *La seconde révolution thérapeutique.* Editions du Rocher, Paris.
20. Laborit, H., Huguenard, P. and Alluaume, R. (1952) Un nouveau stabilisateur végétatif (le 4560 R.P.). *Presse Méd.* **60**: 206–208.
21. Delay, J., Deniker, P. and Harl, J. M. (1952) Utilisation en thérapeutique psychiatrique d'une phénothiazine d'action centrale élective (4560 R.P.). *Ann. Méd.-Psychol. (Paris)* **110**: 112–117.
22. Delay, J., Deniker, P. and Harl, J. M. (1952) Traitement de états d'excitation et d'agitation par une méthode medicamenteuse dérivée de l'hibernothérapie. *Ann. Méd.-Psychol.* **110**: 267–273.
23. Noble, R. L., Beer, C. T. and Cutts, J. H. (1958) Role of chance observations in chemotherapy: *Vinca rosea. Ann. N.Y. Acad. Sci.* **76**: 882–894.
24. Johnson, I. S., Wright, H. F., Svoboda, G. H. and Vlantis, J. (1960) Antitumour Principles Derived from *Vinca rosea* (Linn.) I. Vinca leucoblastine and leurosine. *Cancer Res.* **20**: 1016–1022.
25. Johnson, I. S., Armstrong, J. G., Gorman, M. and Burnett, J. P. J. (1963) The Vinca alkaloids: a new class of oncolytics. *Cancer Res.* **23**: 1390–1427.
26. Couzinet, B., Le Strat, N., Ulmann, A., Baulieu, E. E. and Schaison, G. (1986) Termination of early pregnancy by the progesterone antagonist RU 486 (Mifepristone). *N. Engl. J. Med.* **315**: 1565–1570.
27. Borel, J. F. (1982) The History of Cyclosporin A and its Significance. In White, D. J. G. (ed) *Cyclosporin A.*, pp. 5–17. Elsevier, Amsterdam.
28. Maxwell, R. A. and Eckhardt, S. B. (1990) Cyclosporine. In Maxwell, R. A. and Eckhardt, S. B. (eds) *Drug Discovery — A Casebook and Analysis.*, pp. 95–108. Humana Press, Clifton.
29. Borel, J. F. (1983) Cyclosporin: historical perspectives. *Transplant Proc.* **15**(supp 1): 2219–2229.

3

Measurement and Expression of Drug Effects

JEAN-PAUL KAN

To most of the modern pharmacologists the receptor is like a beautiful but remote lady. He has written her many a letter and quite often she has answered the letters. From these answers the pharmacologist has built himself an image of this fair lady. He cannot, however, truly claim ever to have seen her, although one day he may do so

D.K. de Jongh, 1964[1]

THE PRACTICE OF MEDICINAL CHEMISTRY
ISBN 0-12-744640-0

I. INTRODUCTION

The knowledge of the full sequence of the biochemical and pharmacological effects of a given drug, and the understanding of its mechanism of action, are of basic utility for the chemist, the pharmacologist and the clinician. Identification, description and quantification of each step leading from the primary action of a drug to the resulting effects provides the basis for a rational therapeutic use and the design of improved or original chemical agents. In addition, the study of the effects of drugs and the analysis of their modes of action also provide essential clues for the discovery and elucidation of biochemical and physiological mechanisms. The aim of this chapter is to describe the main strategies used to assess drug effects at various levels of complexity of organization: cell, tissue, organ and living animal. Kinetic analysis of drug–receptor interactions and drug–receptor effects will be presented briefly. The main classical terms and expressions commonly used in describing drug effects will also be defined. For further information, a dictionary of pharmacology can be consulted.[2]

II. MECHANISMS OF DRUG EFFECTS

Since the situation picturesquely described by de Jongh,[1] not only has the concept of *receptor* first proposed by Langley[3] and Ehrlich[4] at the turn of the nineteenth century been universally accepted, but the powerful techniques used in modern pharmacology have allowed us to truly see 'the fair lady'.[5]

Thus, the effects of drugs basically result from their interaction with functional macromolecules — generally cellular proteins termed receptive substances or, more simply, receptors[3,4] — which normally serve as natural targets for endogenous regulatory *ligands*. The latter are mostly cell-to-cell information-transferring molecules (e.g. hormones, neurotransmitters) acting on specific *membrane* receptors. Receptor activation induces a cascade of biochemical responses that depends both on the type of the receptor and on the type of the *effector* cell. These unitary responses are then integrated by the cell to yield a specific *cellular response* (e.g. release of Ca^{2+} from the sarcoplasmic reticulum of the myocyte and contraction of the myofibrils). Finally, the individual cellular responses are summed up by the functional tissue or organ to generate the *physiological response* (e.g. contraction of the muscle) (Fig. 3.1). In theory a drug can interfere with any step of this process. In this respect, it does not create effects but merely modulates ongoing cellular functions.

It must be noted that the term ligand concerns any molecule — endogenous or exogenous — able to bind to a receptor. Any drug usually refers to exogenous chemicals, however. In addition, a ligand can bind to *acceptor sites* that are not coupled to effector systems. They are often circulating proteins (e.g. plasma albumin) that trap the ligand thus preventing its effects.

For a given effector cell, the drug–receptor interaction initiates a series of biochemical and physiological changes that are characteristic of the *effect* of, or *response* to, the drug. If most of these changes are identical to those induced by the endogenous ligand, the drug is termed an *agonist*. A compound that is itself devoid of intrinsic activity but causes effects by inhibition of the action of the endogenous ligand or a specific agonist, is designated as an *antagonist*. Generally, during interaction with the receptor the chemical structures of both the regulatory ligand and the drug remain unchanged.

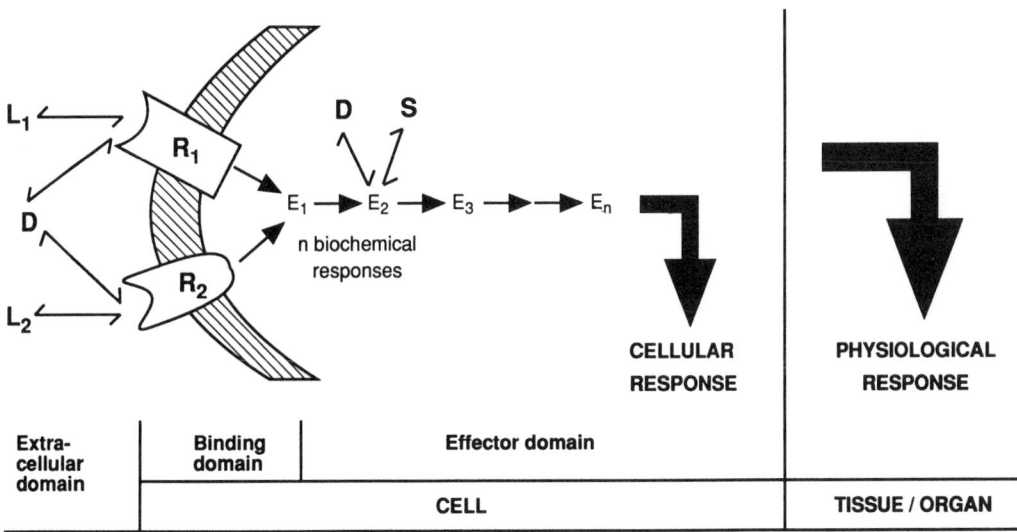

Fig. 3.1   Schematic representation of the series of biochemical steps leading from ligand–receptor interaction to the cellular and physiological responses. L_1, L_2 and D stand for ligands and drug, respectively. R_1 and R_2 represent specific membrane receptors that recognize L_1 and L_2. $E_1 \rightarrow E_n$ are effector proteins (generally enzymes) modulated by receptor activation or by drugs acting as inhibitors. S is a specific substrate.

Agonist-induced effects can also be defined with reference to those typically caused by the endogenous ligand itself. For example, noradrenergic (from the Greek *ergon,* work) drugs are compounds that initiate the typical effects induced by the endogenous neurotransmitter noradrenaline (norepinephrine). They are also termed sympathomimetics since noradrenaline triggers part of its effects on peripheral organs (e.g. heart, vascular, visceral and bronchial smooth muscles, secretory glands) by stimulating the sympathetic peripheral nerves (autonomic nervous system). Corresponding antagonists may be termed adrenolytics or sympatholytics. Pharmacological effects can also be classified according to the specific activation of receptor subtypes. For example, the effects of acetylcholine that are mimicked by the alkaloid muscarine and selectively antagonized by atropine are termed muscarinic effects. Other effects of acetylcholine that are mimicked by nicotine and selectively blocked by *d*-tubocurarine are described as nicotinic effects. These effects are actually mediated by activation of muscarinic and nicotinic cholinergic receptors, which are two distinct molecular entities buried in the surface of the effector cell (see below).

The suffix -*ergic* is also used to characterize nerve endings that work by releasing a particular neurotransmitter (e.g. neurons that release noradrenaline are termed noradrenergic, serotonin/serotoninergic, acetylcholine/cholinergic, dopamine/dopaminergic, and so on).

Finally, the expression *synergistic action* is used when two or more drugs work together to produce an effect greater than the sum of their individual effects.

Enzymes of critical metabolic or regulatory pathways of the cell (e.g. acetylcholinesterase, monoamine oxidase) are also receptors for many drugs. These compounds interact with the endogenous substrate of the enzyme to inhibit the catalytic activity of the protein. Conversely to the ligand, the substrate combines with the active site of the enzyme during the course of the reaction (enzyme–substrate complex) to produce a new, chemically distinct compound.

Of equal interest are proteins of the cytoskeleton that serve structural roles (e.g. tubulin) or those involved in transport processes. For example, many drugs act indirectly by releasing — or preventing the release of — pharmacologically active molecules (e.g. neurotransmitters) concentrated in cytoplasmic vesicles. Such compounds can also interact with autoreceptors, which respond to the neurotransmitter by modulating the release of the neurotransmitter (e.g. noradrenergic nerve endings possess α_2-adrenergic receptors mediating suppression of noradrenaline release).

Nucleic acids are important drug receptors, for example, for chemicals controlling malignancy. Finally, general anaesthetics interact with and alter the structure and function of the lipids of the cellular membrane.

The binding of drugs to receptors involves all known types of interaction: ionic, hydrogen bonding, hydrophobic, Van der Waals and covalent. In the last case, the duration of action of the drug will be prolonged. Covalent interactions of a highly specific and tightly bound drug will be essentially irreversible.

A.   Sites of drug effects

Drug effects can be measured at various levels of complexity: from the cell to the living animal a wide spectrum of biological preparations are accessible to the pharmacologist. As already pointed out, most drugs interfere at the membrane receptors with physiological regulatory molecules, to modulate the response of the cell and, ultimately, that of a particular tissue (Fig. 3.1). Complex pathways involving integrated control systems, i.e. homeostasis, are often essential in order to lead from receptor activation to the observable effect (e.g. drug–receptor interaction → n integrated steps → alteration of cardiac contractility and blood pressure). Thus, the more complex the biological preparation is (e.g. isolated organ → *in situ* organ), the more complicated is the stimulus–effect relationship (see below). It is therefore necessary to have access, at the molecular level, to the actual primary effects of a drug by measuring its interaction with the receptor and the direct consequences on cellular regulatory effectors.

1.   The receptor–effector complex of the cell

The eukaryotic plasma membrane is the cellular switchboard responsible for receiving all sorts of extracellular messengers, mainly hormones and neurotransmitters but also growth factors, pheromones, odours and light. These messengers must be detected, decoded, amplified, integrated with each other and with cellular metabolism, and conveyed to the cytoplasm as intracellular chemical messengers. Thus, for a given cell, a particular *receptor–effector complex* (Figs. 3.1 and 3.2) regulates information received from other neighbouring and distant cells. Despite the diversity of extracellular signals, cell surface receptor proteins utilize only a few biochemical mechanisms for these processes. In fact, two main transducing mechanisms of the signal can be considered: (1) the same molecular entity recognizes the extracellular messenger and transduces the signal (e.g. transmitter-gated ion channels and receptor tyrosine kinases); (2) distinct molecular entities coupled by regulatory G-proteins recognize the extracellular messenger and transduce the signal.

Transmitter-gated ion channels form a class of multisubunit membrane-spanning receptors concerned with rapid signal transduction. The transmitter molecule (e.g. acetylcholine (nicotinic receptors), glutamate, γ-aminobutyric acid), itself operates the opening or closing of the ion channel enclosed inside the receptor. The subsequent exchange of ions (Na^+, K^+, Ca^{2+}, Cl^-, HCO_3^-) between the extracellular and intracellular compartments affects the cell membrane potential. Receptor tyrosine kinases mediate the response of cells to insulin and growth factors. In response to ligand binding, the intracellular domain phosphorylates itself on specific tyrosines. These individual phosphotyrosyl residues serve as highly selective binding sites for cytoplasmic regulatory proteins.

All receptors transducing the signal via coupling to guanine (G) nucleotide-dependent regulatory proteins (G-proteins) consist of a single polypeptidic chain forming seven transmembrane domains joined by intracellular and extracellular loops. They include receptors for biogenic amines (e.g. noradrenaline, dopamine, serotonin and histamine), prostaglandins, many peptide hormones, neuropeptides (e.g. substance P, neurotensin, cholecystokinin), muscarinic receptors for acetylcholine and metabotropic glutamate receptors. This family also includes visual rhodopsin and receptors for odorants and pheromones. *G-proteins*, which link cell-surface receptors to effector proteins of the plasma membrane, are membrane proteins composed of three subunits ($\alpha\beta\gamma$). At least twenty distinct α-subunits have been discovered, generating four G-protein families (Gs, Gi, Gq and G_{12}). α-Subunits strongly bind G-nucleotides (GTP and GDP). Upon activation by the ligand, the receptor interacts with the G-protein and triggers a complex regulatory cycle where among other steps, one leads to the release of the GTP-bound α-subunit. This complex activates effector proteins of the membrane (e.g. enzymes or ion channels) that mobilize chemical *second messengers*. Two classes of enzymes play a major role in the synthesis of these second messengers: adenylylcyclases and phospholipases.

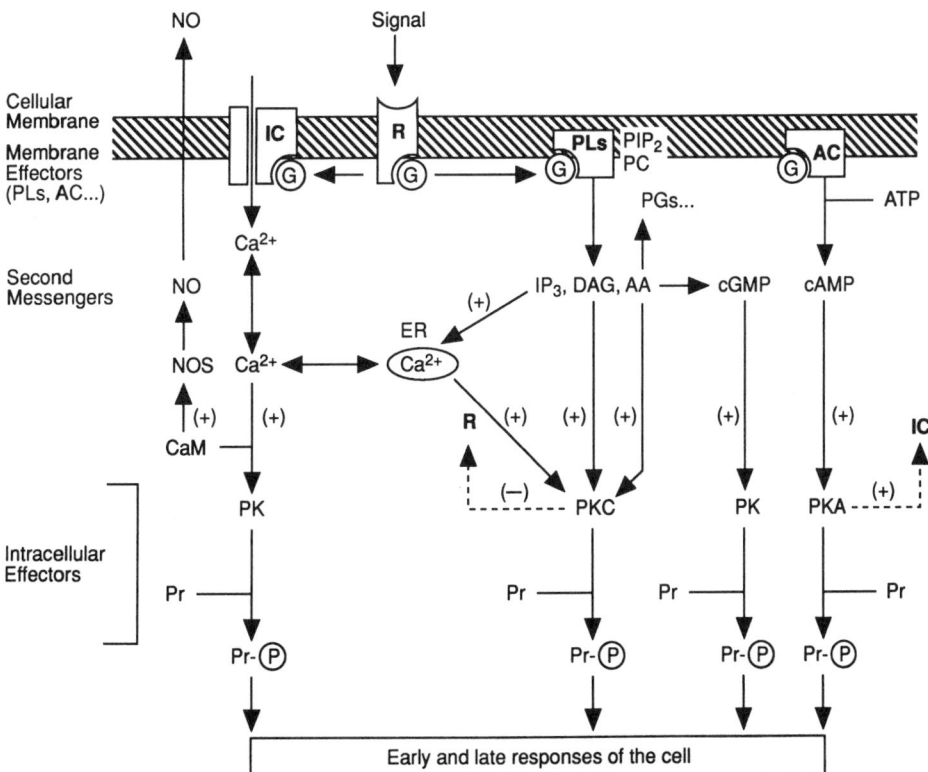

Fig. 3.2 The main transduction signal pathways in eukaryotic cells initiated by activation of G-protein-coupled membrane receptors. ER, endoplasmic reticulum; (+) activation; (−), inhibition; Pr, effector protein phosphorylated (P) by protein kinases (see text for other abbreviations).

Adenylylcyclases catalyse the synthesis of cyclic AMP (cAMP) from ATP stores. Inhibition or activation of cAMP formation depends on the G-protein type involved in the coupling: Gi and Gs lead to inhibition and stimulation of adenylylcyclase, respectively. Phospholipases (PLs) are enzymes that degrade membrane phospholipids. For example, PLC hydrolyses phosphatidylinositol 4,5-bisphosphate (PIP_2) into diacylglycerol (DAG) and inositol trisphosphate (IP_3). Diacylglycerol can also be formed from phosphatidylcholine (PC) by PLD. Another phospholipase, PLA_2, cleaves PC to give arachidonic acid (AA).

Second messengers initiate characteristic actions within the cell. Cyclic AMP stimulates a particular class of *protein kinase,* termed protein kinase A (PKA), which catalyses the phosphorylation of numerous enzymes and other proteins including ionic channels (IC). For example, voltage-dependent Ca^{2+} channels of cardiac cells are phosphorylated by PKA, thus increasing their opening probability and Ca^{2+} entry. These channels may also be directly activated by Gs. IP_3 binds to specific receptors that cause the release of Ca^{2+} from intracellular stores (endoplasmic or sarcoplasmic reticulum). Diacylglycerol and AA, in the presence of Ca^{2+}, activate a distinct protein kinase, termed protein kinase C (PKC). PKC will phosphorylate other intracellular effectors and, in turn, the G-protein-coupled receptor itself to inactivate it (Fig. 3.2). The released arachidonic acid may be metabolized by oxygenases to form further intracellular messengers such as prostaglandins (PGs), eicosanoids, leukotrienes and epoxides (Fig. 3.2). Arachidonate and its metabolites stimulate and amplify other second messenger systems as cyclic GMP (cGMP) synthesized from GTP by guanylylcyclase. This cyclic nucleotide activates cGMP-dependent protein kinases (Fig. 3.2). Bound to calmodulin (CaM), Ca^{2+} forms a complex able to activate another distinct group of protein kinases. Furthermore, CaM may activate nitric oxide (NO) synthase (NOS), an enzyme that catalyses the synthesis of NO from arginine. These gaseous molecules diffuse out to neighbouring cells to stimulate a particular class of guanylylcyclases (Fig. 3.2).

Various transducing pathways regulate the expression of *immediate early genes* (e.g. the proto-oncogene c-*fos*) which, through their corresponding oncoproteins, will modulate the transcription of other appropriate genes. The latter can also be regulated by various steroid-receptor complexes that cross the nuclear membrane and bind to the nuclear chromatin.

The use of discriminant ligands and, more recently, molecular cloning, have led to the discovery of many subtypes for G-protein-coupled receptors. For example, noradrenaline binds to two types of adrenergic receptors (or adrenoceptors) designated α and β. Type α adrenoceptors are divided into two subtypes α_1 and α_2, each corresponding to several different molecular entities (α_{1A} to α_{1D} receptors and α_{2A} to α_{2C} receptors). Regarding the coupled cellular effectors, α_1 receptors are linked to the IP_3/DAG pathway and α_2 receptors to the cAMP pathway and/or ion channels. Type β adrenoceptors are divided into three subtypes, β_1, β_2 and β_3, all controlling cAMP formation.

The ability of membrane receptors to be regulated in response to their level of activation is well documented. For example, sustained stimulation of cells with agonists generally results in a state of desensitization such that the effect that follows subsequent exposure to the same concentration of drug is diminished, that is it appears to result from an apparent loss of intrinsic efficacy or efficiency coupling (see below). This can be very important in therapeutic situations (e.g. treatment of asthma by the β-adrenergic agonist isoproterenol). Various mechanisms may give rise to receptor desensitization. For example, receptors may become less efficiently coupled with a particular enzyme that they normally activate (e.g. adenylylcyclase). Under prolonged stimulation, there may be *down-regulation* of receptor numbers by internalization of the receptor protein into the cell. Finally, receptor desensitization may lead to *tachyphylaxis,* a rapid diminution in response to each of a succession of repeated doses of a drug. Conversely, *supersensitivity* to receptor agonist, or *up-regulation,* is also frequently observed following a reduction in the chronic level of receptor stimulation. Such a situation is observed after long-term treatment with certain antagonists (e.g. propranolol) or after chronic denervation. In both cases, the cell compensates by inserting new receptors into its membrane.

This brief description of the receptor–effector complex is not exhaustive, but shows that cellular homeostasis is continually regulated by numerous membrane receptors linked to a network of multiply interacting pathways (cross-talk) which control both extra- and intracellular information. A complete overview of the dynamic regulation of signalling at the plasma membrane has been published.[6]

Specific markers (e.g. selected radiolabelled ligands or substrates, specific antibodies, hybridization probes) associated with powerful analytical techniques (separation by chromatography or electrophoresis, blotting, highly sensitive immunoassays, etc.) are utilized to determine the cellular sites of action of endogenous ligands and drugs at the molecular level. These methods are applied on various biological preparations including subcellular structures, cell membrane suspensions and tissue homogenates. Cell and tissue culture preparations are also widely used to assess biological processes and drug actions. They have a number of general advantages: cells are more accessible for study, diffusion delays and barriers to applied substances are minimized, the humoral and cellular components of the culture environment can be controlled, and progressive changes in intracellular and intercellular events can be monitored directly. Primary cell cultures from various embryonic tissues (e.g. brain structures) can be achieved. A number of transformed cell lines derived from tumoral tissues are also available. Cells (e.g. Chinese hamster ovarian cells, or CHO cells) transfected with the cloned gene of a particular receptor, including human clones, generally express a large amount of this receptor on their cell surface. These cells, all identical, are useful preparations for assessing the transducing pathways linked to the receptor and for screening specific drugs.

2.   *From the cell to the living animal*

Although many drugs are known to act at well-defined cellular receptor–effector systems, more complex biological preparations are needed to reveal their subsequent physiological effects. Isolated tissues or organs, generally smooth muscles, are routinely used *in vitro* to classify drugs as agonists or antagonists. For example, cholinergic agonists (e.g. arecaidine) acting at peripheral muscarinic receptors, induce a concentration-dependent contraction of the uterine horn of the guinea-pig. This response is antagonized by muscarinic antagonists.[7] Once isolated, such organs are free from the nervous and regulatory influences that complicate their functions *in vivo*. Using standardized test conditions, typical reactions can be reproduced reliably.

Isolated organs have also permitted the discovery of the two main classes of adrenoceptors. Indeed, Ahlquist,[8] comparing the relative potencies on different tissues of a number of sympathomimetics, found that the order of potency on smooth muscles that responded with contraction was adrenaline > noradrenaline > isoprenaline, whereas on smooth muscles responding with relaxation the order of potency was isoprenaline > adrenaline > noradrenaline. To explain these findings, he postulated the existence of two classes of receptors, which he designated α- and β-adrenoceptors (see above). Later, the observation that noradrenaline, an effective stimulant of cardiac β-receptors, had little or no ability to stimulate β-receptors mediating vasodilation in the smooth muscles of blood vessels, suggested the existence of β_1 (heart) and β_2 (bronchial, vascular and uterine) β-adrenoceptor subtypes.

In addition, there are still many examples of drug action where the knowledge is less precise (e.g. unknown receptor–effector complexes), and the action is recognized as a response involving a tissue, an organ or even a living animal. The action of the drug may be on many cells rather than on a particular type of cell. For example, a drug that acts as a diuretic can only act in that way on an organized tissue, namely the kidney, although the mechanism of action may be known at the molecular or cellular level. Although apparently simple, isolated preparations have a relative degree of local regulatory control systems that play a role in the understanding of drug action.

Living animals are also needed to assess secondary effects of drugs resulting from homeostatic mechanisms. For example, a drug that relaxes smooth muscle in the walls of blood vessels and so causes vasodilation may thereby elicit a reflex acceleration of the heart rate. Thus, the direct action of acetylcholine or of a muscarinic agonist on the heart is to decrease the rate of beating (bradycardia), yet the intravenous injection of small amounts produces the opposite effect, providing that cardiovascular reflexes are operating.

Finally, chemicals aimed at relieving symptoms observed in psychiatric illnesses (e.g. anxiety, depression, schizophrenia) are studied in various animal models, which reveal typical behaviours claimed to mimic those exhibited by human patients. Animal tests are also needed to discover and develop drugs to treat cognitive decline. Recent studies of the effects of certain brain lesions on learning in rats or monkeys as animal models of Alzheimer's disease may go some way towards developing an experimental model for this disorder.

III.   MEASUREMENT OF DRUG EFFECTS

A.   Kinetic analysis of ligand–receptor interactions

1.   Theoretical background

The simplest assumption about the reversible formation of a ligand–receptor complex is that it may be expressed, according to the mass-action law, as the following chemical reaction:

$$\text{Ligand} + \text{Receptor} \rightleftharpoons \text{Ligand–receptor complex}$$

or

$$[L] + [R] \underset{k_{-1}}{\overset{k_1}{\rightleftharpoons}} [LR] \tag{1}$$

Where k_1 and k_{-1} are the rate constants for association and dissociation of the LR complex. Square brackets signify the concentration of the entity they enclose.

At equilibrium or steady state, the rates of association and dissociation of the complex are equal:

$$k_1 [L] [R] = k_{-1} [LR] \tag{2}$$

The equilibrium binding constant may then be defined as a *dissociation binding constant* (K_d)

such as

$$k_{d} = \frac{k_{-1}}{k_1} = \frac{[L]\,[R]}{[LR]} \tag{3}$$

The total number of receptors (R_T) is the maximum number of receptors on which the drug is able to specifically bind. This finite number, termed B_{max}, is the sum of the receptors engaged in forming the complex (LR), plus the free receptors (R);

$$[R_T] = [LR] + [R] = B_{max} \tag{4}$$

From equations (3) and (4) after rearrangement:

$$[LR] = \frac{B_{max}\,[L]}{[L] + K_d} \tag{5}$$

In these equations, L may represent any specific ligand that binds to the receptor, i.e. a biologically active agonist or an appropriate antagonist, as well as the endogenous ligand itself (hormone or neurotransmitter).

If we now define [LR] as bound ligand = B, and [L] as free ligand = F, then from equation (5),

$$B = \frac{B_{max}\,F}{F + K_d} \tag{6*}$$

and

$$\frac{B}{F} = \frac{B_{max} - B}{K_d} \tag{7}$$

Equation (7) is the Scatchard equation.

2.   The binding experiment

Receptor labelling studies involve binding of a radioactive form of the ligand to membrane preparations of target tissues. Radiolabelled ligands must be pure and stable and have a high radiochemical specific activity. The most commonly used isotopes are tritium [³H] and radioactive iodine [¹²⁵I]. Radioactive ligand and membrane suspension are incubated in appropriate conditions: tissue concentration, temperature, pH and ionic strength. At the end of the incubation period, while the binding reaction is at equilibrium, bound and free ligands are promptly separated using filtration or centrifugation.

Experimental determination of K_d and B_{max} for a given radioligand and tissue receptor requires incubation of various concentrations of the radioligand with a fixed concentration of tissue: this is the so-called *saturation* experiment. Such experiments can be performed in the absence (control) or presence of various concentrations of nonradioactive ('cold') ligand or drug — also termed the *displacer* — able to compete with the radioligand for the same receptor. Finally, interaction of displacers with a given receptor can also be studied by incubating various

---

* Equation (6) is actually identical to the Michaelis–Menten equation used in enzyme kinetics, i.e. $v = V_{max}\,[S]/[S] + K_m$, where v = initial velocity; V_{max} = limiting maximal velocity; [S] = substrate concentration; K_m = dissociation constant of the enzyme–substrate complex.

concentrations of the displacer with fixed concentrations of radioligand and tissue: this is the so-called *displacement* experiment. In all cases, the *nonspecific binding* is measured by the bound radioactivity remaining in the presence of a large excess of cold ligand.

3. Analysis of binding data

In most cases, data generated from a saturation experiment are analysed according to equation (7). When the radioactive ligand interacts with a single population of noninteracting receptors, the Scatchard plot,[8] (i.e. B/F versus F) leads to a linear curve. K_d is estimated as the negative reciprocal of the slope of the line of best fit, and B_{max} by the abscissa intercept of the line (Fig. 3.3A). The reciprocal of K_d measures the *affinity constant* (K_a) of the radioligand for the receptor. Thus, for a given ligand–receptor pair, the smaller the K_d (generally 0.1–10 nmol l^{-1} or nM) the higher is its *affinity*. B_{max} is expressed as pmol or fmol per mg tissue or protein. A downwards concave Scatchard plot may indicate that there is more than one type of binding site, and that the different types differ in their dissociation constants for binding with the radiolabelled ligand under investigation. Alternatively, the binding of ligand to its receptors may inhibit further binding and hasten dissociation from the receptor (e.g. insulin receptor). This latter phenomenon is called *negative cooperativity. Positive cooperativity* also occurs; that is the binding of ligand facilitates the fixation of subsequent molecules to the receptors (e.g. nicotinic receptor). In this case, the Scatchard plot is upwards concave. Cooperativity generally involves the ligand behaving as an allosteric modifier that induces a conformational change in the structure of the receptor protein.

When the saturation experiment is performed in the presence of a displacer, the line of best fit of the Scatchard plot can be modified in a manner that depends on the type of receptor interaction exhibited by the displacer. Two main cases exist: (1) decreased slope and unchanged B_{max}, the displacement is of the *competitive* type; (2) unchanged slope and decreased B_{max}, the displacement is of the *noncompetitive* type (Fig. 3.3A). Intermediate cases where both the slope and B_{max} are modified, also exist.

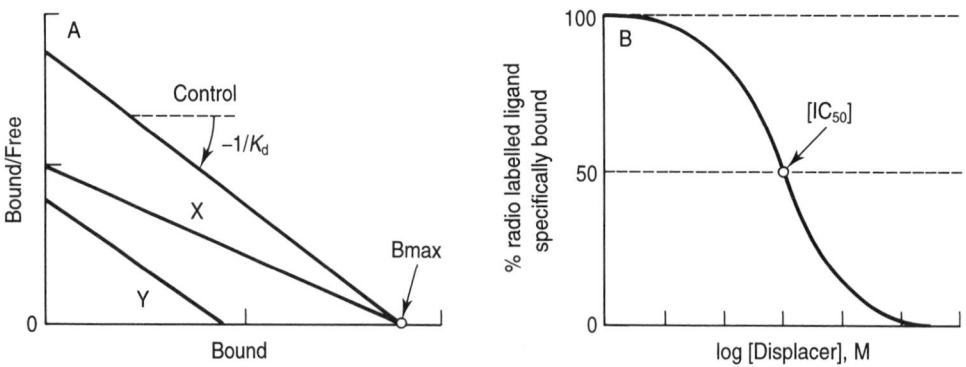

Fig. 3.3 Analysis of ligand–receptor interactions. (A) Scatchard plot in absence (control) or presence of two different displacers. X and Y are competitive and noncompetitive displacers, respectively. (B) Displacement curve.

Data generated from a displacement experiment are generally fitted by a sigmoidal curve termed the *displacement* or *inhibition curve,* that is the percentage radioalabelled ligand specifically bound versus log[Displacer] (in M) (Fig. 3B). The abscissa of the inflexion point of the curve gives the IC_{50} value, the concentration of displacer that displaces or inhibits 50% of the radioactive ligand specifically bound. IC_{50} is a measure of the *inhibitory* or *affinity constant* (K_i) of the displacer for the receptor. IC_{50} and K_i are linked as follows: if the displacement is of the competitive type, then

$$K_i = \frac{IC_{50}}{1 + [L]/K_d}$$

This is the Cheng–Prusoff[10] equation, where [L] is the concentration of radioactive ligand used in the experiment and K_d its dissociation constant determined from the Scatchard plot. Finally, if the displacement is of the noncompetitive type, then $K_i = IC_{50}$.

B.   Kinetic analysis of drug–receptor effects

1.   Theoretical background

The chemical reaction expressing any ligand–receptor interaction (cf. equation 1) can be completed as follows, assuming that L is an agonist molecule:

$$\text{Agonist} + \text{Receptor} \rightleftharpoons \text{Agonist–receptor complex} \rightarrow \text{Effect}$$

or

$$[A] + [R] \underset{k_{-1}}{\overset{k_1}{\rightleftharpoons}} [AR] \rightarrow E \qquad (8)$$

whatever the number of steps leading from the agonist–receptor complex to the effect observed (E).

Substituting A for L in equation (4) gives

$$[R] = [R_T] - [AR] \qquad (9)$$

Finally, substituting for [R] in equation (3) and rearranging,

$$\frac{[AR]}{[R_T]} = r = \frac{[A]}{[A] + K_d} \qquad (10)$$

where r is the proportion of receptors occupied by the agonist, i.e. $0 \leqslant r \leqslant 1$, and K_d its dissociation constant.

Assuming that the effect observed (E) is linearly proportional to receptor occupancy and that the maximum response is reached when the total number of receptors is occupied,

$$r = \frac{[AR]}{[R_T]} = \frac{[A]}{[A] + K_d} = \frac{E}{E_{max}} \qquad (11)$$

where E_{max} is the maximum effect and E/E_{max} is the fraction of maximum response, i.e. $0 \leqslant E/E_{max} \leqslant 1$.

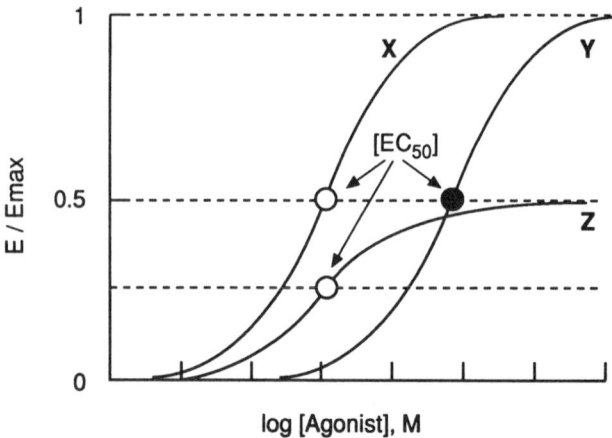

Fig. 3.4 Analysis of drug–receptor effects. Concentration–effect relationships in various situations. In all cases agonists act on the same receptor. Curves X and Y may concern full agonists acting on two different tissues X and Y, the efficiency of receptor coupling being higher for X than for Y ; alternatively, X and Y may concern two full agonists acting on the same tissue, but where the affinity of X is higher than that of Y. Curves X and Z may concern two agonists acting on the same tissue, where X is a full agonist and Y a partial agonist having the same potency. X and Y may also concern the same agonist: it behaves as a full agonist on tissue X and as a partial agonist on tissue Z, the efficiency of receptor coupling being higher for X than for Z.

This rationale, developed by Clark in the 1930s,[11] implies the following criteria: (1) An all-or-nothing stimulus is elicited by the combination of each receptor site with an agonist molecule. (2) There is summation of these individual stimuli. (3) The effect is linearly proportional to the number of stimuli. (4) The maximum stimulus occurs when every receptor site is occupied by an agonist molecule. (5) The drug–receptor complex is formed by readily and rapidly reversing chemical bonds. (6) The occupation of one receptor does not affect the tendency of other receptors to be occupied.

Equation (11) indicates that the fractional response (E/E_{max}) will vary as a rectangular hyperbolic function of the agonist concentration. When [A] is such that half the maximum effect is obtained, [A] is equal to K_d. In addition, the plot of E/E_{max} versus log[A] produces a symetrical sigmoid curve from which the abscissa of the inflexion point gives K_d. In fact, K_d values obtained from concentration–effect curves can be different from the apparent affinity determined from binding studies using radiolabelled ligands (see below). For this reason, the abscissa of the inflexion point of the sigmoid is usually termed EC_{50}, i.e. the concentration which causes 50% of the maximum possible effect induced by a given agonist on a particular target tissue (Fig. 3.4). EC_{50} reflects the potency, which depends on the intrinsic efficacy of the agonist and the efficiency of receptor coupling (see below). In practice, however, the pD_2 value is usually considered:

$$pD_2 = -\log EC_{50}$$

2.   Full agonists, partial agonists, antagonists

As already suggested, a complex sequence of reactions is often involved in the production of the ultimate effect induced by an agonist, especially when traditional bioassay systems are used (e.g. isolated organs). Numerous factors are therefore involved in the production of a response by an agonist. They can be divided into two general categories termed drug-related and tissue-related factors. The drug-related factors are *intrinsic efficacy* (ε) and the equilibrium dissociation constant of the agonist–receptor complex (K_d). Those related to tissue are the number of viable specific receptors in a particular tissue [R_T] and the *efficiency* of the mechanisms which convert stimulus (S) into effector response. Thus, there exists for a given target tissue, a complex function $f(S)$ that determines the magnitude of the response:[12,13]

$$\text{Response} = f(S) = f\left(\frac{[A]\ \varepsilon\ [R_T]}{[A] + K_d}\right) \tag{12}$$

More simply, equation (12) signifies that the response is a function of both the stimulus produced by agonist interaction with the receptor and the efficiency of the transduction of that stimulus by the tissue. Stimulus is proportional to the intrinsic efficacy of the agonist and the number of receptors. Consequently, variations in receptor density in different tissues can affect the stimulus for response. Furthermore, some tissues have very efficiently coupled receptors and others relatively inefficient coupling. This has been termed 'receptor reserve' (or spare receptor) since, in the first case, a maximum effect can be achieved when a relatively small fraction of receptor is apparently occupied and further receptor occupancy can produce no additional effect. The magnitude of the response will thus depend on the intrinsic efficacy value so that, by classical definition, *full agonists* ($\varepsilon = 1$) produce the maximum response for a given tissue, *partial agonists* produce a maximum response that is below that induced by the full agonist ($0 \leqslant \varepsilon \leqslant 1$), and *antagonists* produce no visible response and block the effect of agonists ($\varepsilon = 0$) (Fig. 3.4). These activities can be completely dependent upon the tissue, i.e., upon the *efficiency coupling*. For example, the low-efficacy β_1-adrenoceptor agonist prenalterol[14] can be nearly a full agonist in thyroxine-treated guinea-pig atria, a partial agonist in rat atria, and an antagonist in canine coronary artery, indicating that efficiency coupling increases from dog coronaries to rat atria and guinea-pig atria. In comparison, isoproterenol behaves as a full agonist in the three tissues, with increasing potency from dog coronaries to rat atria and guinea-pig atria (see also Fig. 3.4).

The comparison between binding (K_d) and potency (EC_{50}) also reveals the efficiency of receptor coupling. For example, in intact S49 lymphoma cells, the stimulation of adenylylcyclase activity by the full agonist adrenaline, through activation of β-adrenoceptors, exhibits a wide gap between the K_d (2 µM) and the EC_{50} (10 nM). The existence of this apparent 'receptor reserve' actually reveals an amplification step between adrenaline binding and the observed response. In this case, the amplification effect seems to be mainly due to the mobility of the β-receptor and of the G-protein, which makes it possible for one receptor to activate numerous α-GTP/adenylylcyclase complexes.[15] A recent exhaustive review discusses the theoretical concepts and methods used for *in vitro* measurement of agonist affinity and relative efficacy, when G-protein-coupled receptors are involved.[16]

3.   Interaction between agonist and antagonist: the Schild analysis

A competitive antagonist may be regarded as a drug that interacts reversibly with a set of receptors to form a complex that does not elicit any response. The antagonist–receptor interaction is characterized by a dissociation constant, but the intrinsic efficacy is zero. *Schild analysis*[17] allows the determination of the dissociation constant (K_d) of a competitive antagonist. Practically, several concentration–response curves are generated for a given agonist–tissue pair in the absence or presence of increasing concentrations of the antagonist (Fig. 3.5A).

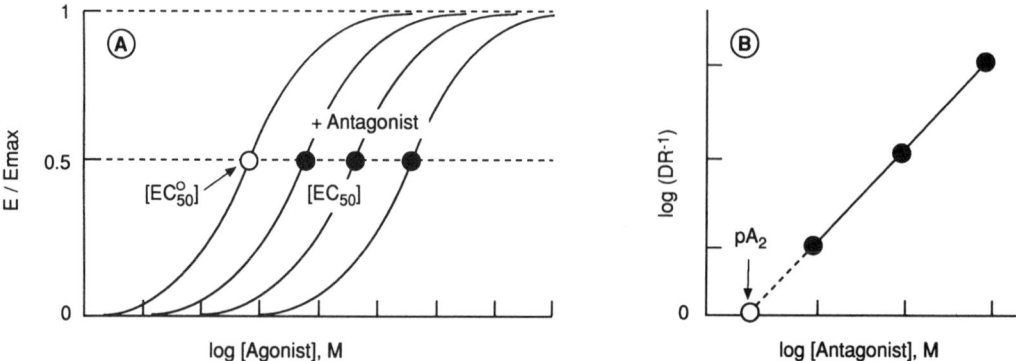

Fig. 3.5 Schild analysis of agonist–antagonist competition. (A) Concentration–effect relationship for an agonist in the absence (○) and the presence (●) of three increasing concentrations of antagonist. (B) Schild plot generated from curve (A) (see text for explanation).

A Schild plot (Fig. 3.5B) is constructed by plotting log(dose ratio − 1), or log(DR − 1), versus log[Antagonist], where 'dose ratio' is the ratio of equiactive agonist concentrations in the absence and presence of antagonist concentrations.[18] In other words, if an agonist causes a 50% effect at a concentration of $[EC_{50}^0]$ in the absence of antagonist, and at a concentration of $[EC_{50}]$ in the presence of a fixed concentration of antagonist, then the dose ratio is $[EC_{50}]/[EC_{50}^0]$ (Fig. 3.5A). The Schild plot is analysed by linear regression. This line meets the abscissa at a point that provides an estimate of pA_2 (Fig. 3.5B). Assuming that $pA_2 = -\log K_d$, Schild analysis is therefore a useful method for calculating the dissociation constant of a given antagonist in fixed conditions (agonist, tissue).

C.   Relationship between dose and effect

When drugs are administered *in vivo* to living animals or humans, there is no single characteristic relationship between intensity of drug effect and drug dosage. A dose–effect curve may be linear, concave upwards or downwards, or sigmoid. In addition, differences appear in the magnitude of response among individuals in the same population for the same dose of a given drug; that is, drug effects are never identical in all animals or all patients. In other words, a range of doses is required to produce a specified intensity of effect in all individuals; alternatively, a range of effects will be produced if a given dose is administered to a group of individuals. It is possible to determine the dose of a drug required to produce a specified effect in an individual, i.e. the individual effective dose for which the specified intensity of effect is present (e.g. animals injected with a hypnotic sleep or do not sleep). The percentage of individuals who exhibit the specified effect plotted as a function of log dose (mg kg^{-1}), gives the so-called sigmoidal *dose–effect curve* (Fig. 3.6).

The dose required to produced a specified intensity of effect in 50% of individuals is known as the *median effective dose,* or ED_{50} (Fig. 3.6). If death is the specified effect, the median effective dose is termed the *median lethal dose,* or LD_{50}. The ratio LD_{50}/ED_{50} leads to the *therapeutic index* (or therapeutic ratio). This index has limited usefulness since it cannot be calculated for man and data relating to one species cannot reliably be transferred to another.

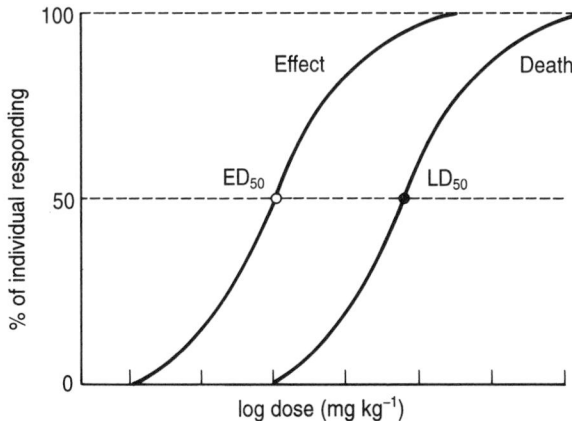

Fig. 3.6   Examples of dose–effect curves.

REFERENCES

1. de Jongh, D. K. (1964) Introductory remarks. In Ariëns E.J. (ed) *Molecular Pharmacology.* Academic Press, New York.
2. Bowman, W. C., Bowman, A. and Bowman A, (1986) *Dictionary of Pharmacology.* Blackwell Scientific Publications, Oxford.
3. Langley, J. N. (1878) On the physiology of the salivary secretion. *J. Physiol. (London)* **1:** 339–369.
4. Ehrlich, P. (1913) Chemotherapeutics: scientific principles, methods and results. *Lancet* **2:** 445–451.
5. Giraudat, J. and Changeux, J. P. (1981) The acetylcholine receptor. In Lamble JW (ed) *Towards Understanding Receptors; Current Reviews in Biomedicine 1,* pp. 34–41. Elsevier, North-Holland Biomedical Press, Amsterdam.
6. Signal transduction: crosstalk. *Trends Biochem. Sci.* (1992) **17:** 367–443.
7. Dörje, F., Friebe, T., Tacke, R., Mutschler, E. and Lambrecht, G. (1990) Novel pharmacological profile of muscarinic receptors mediating contraction of the guinea-pig uterus. *Naunyn-Schmiedeberg's Arch. Pharmacol.* **342:** 284–289.
8. Ahlquist, R. P. (1966) The adrenergic receptor. *J. Pharm. Sci.* **155:** 359–367.
9. Scatchard, G. (1949) The attraction of proteins for small molecules and ions. *Ann. N. Y. Acad. Sci.* **51:** 660–672.
10. Cheng, Y. C. and Prusoff, W. H. (1973) Relationship between the inhibition constant (K_i) and the concentration of inhibitor which causes 50 percent inhibition (I_{50}) of an enzymatic reaction. *Biochem. Pharmacol.* **22:** 3099–3108.
11. Clark, A. J. (1937) General pharmacology. *Heffner's Handbuch des Experimentellen Pharmakologie,* Ergiband 4. Springer, Berlin.
12. Stephenson, R. P. (1956) A modification of receptor theory. *Br. J. Pharmacol.* **11:** 379–393.
13. Furchgott, R. F. (1966) The use of β-haloalkylamines in the differentiation of receptors and in the determination of dissociation constants of receptor agonist complexes. *Adv. Drug Res.* **3:** 21–55.
14. Kenakin, T. (1984) The classification of drugs and drug receptors in isolated tissues. *Pharmacol. Rev.* **36:** 165–222.
15. Stickle, D. and Barber, R. (1989) Evidence for the role of epinephrine binding frequency in activation of adenylate cyclase. *J. Pharmacol. Exp. Ther.* **36:** 437–445.

16. Kenakin, T. (1990) Drugs and receptors, an overview of the current state of knowledge. *Drugs* **40:** 666–687.
17. Schild, H.O. (1957) Drug antagonism and pA$_2$. *Pharmacol. Rev.* **9:** 242–246.
18. Lazareno, S. and Birdsall, N.J.M. (1993) Estimation of competitive antagonist affinity from functional inhibition curves using the Gaddum, Schild and Cheng–Prusoff equations. *Br. J. Pharmacol.* **109:** 1110–1119.

4

The Three Main Phases of Drug Activity: The Pharmaceutical, the Pharmacokinetic and the Pharmacodynamic Phases

CAMILLE G. WERMUTH

'Aller guten Dinge sind Drei'
All good things go by threes
German proverb

THE PRACTICE OF MEDICINAL CHEMISTRY
ISBN 0-12-744640-0

The activity of a given drug depends on a sequence of physicochemical events that begin when the active molecule penetrates into the living organism and which culminates when the active molecule reaches its target and elicits the appropriate biological response. Classical wisdom is that three characteristic phases govern the biological activity of a drug in a living organism:[1] the pharmaceutical phase, the pharmacokinetic phase, and the pharmacodynamic phase (Table 4.1).

Table 4.1   The three phases that govern the activity of a drug.

Phase	Events involved	Objectives
Pharmaceutical phase	Selection of the administration route Preparation of the most appropriate pharmaceutical formulation	Optimize distribution Facilitate absorption Eliminate unwanted organoleptic properties
Pharmacokinetic phase	Fate of the drug in the organism: absorption, distribution metabolism, excretion ('ADME')	Control the *bioavailability*, i.e. the ratio of the administered dose to the concentration at the site of action, as a function of time
Pharmacodynamic phase	Quality of the drug–receptor interaction Nature and intensity of the biological response	Maximal activity Maximal selectivity Minimal toxicity

I.   THE PHARMACEUTICAL PHASE

The *pharmaceutical phase*, sometimes also called *biopharmaceutical phase*, deals with the choice of the appropriate *route of administration* and with the choice of the *pharmaceutical formulation* most suited to the desired medical effects.

A.   Routes of administration

Possible routes of administration are divided into two major classes: *enteral*, whereby drugs are absorbed from the alimentary canal, and *parenteral*, in which drugs enter the bloodstream directly (intravenous injection) or by some other nonenteral absorptive route (intramuscular or subcutaneous injection, transdermal delivery systems, nasal sprays, etc.). Below we describe briefly the intravenous and the oral route; other routes of administration are considered in Chapter 28.

1.   Intravenous injection

Intravenous injection is the route of administration which produces the fastest effects. The drug preparation is directly injected into the bloodstream and from there the active principle is carried along to its site of action. The intravenous route bypasses the natural barriers of the body

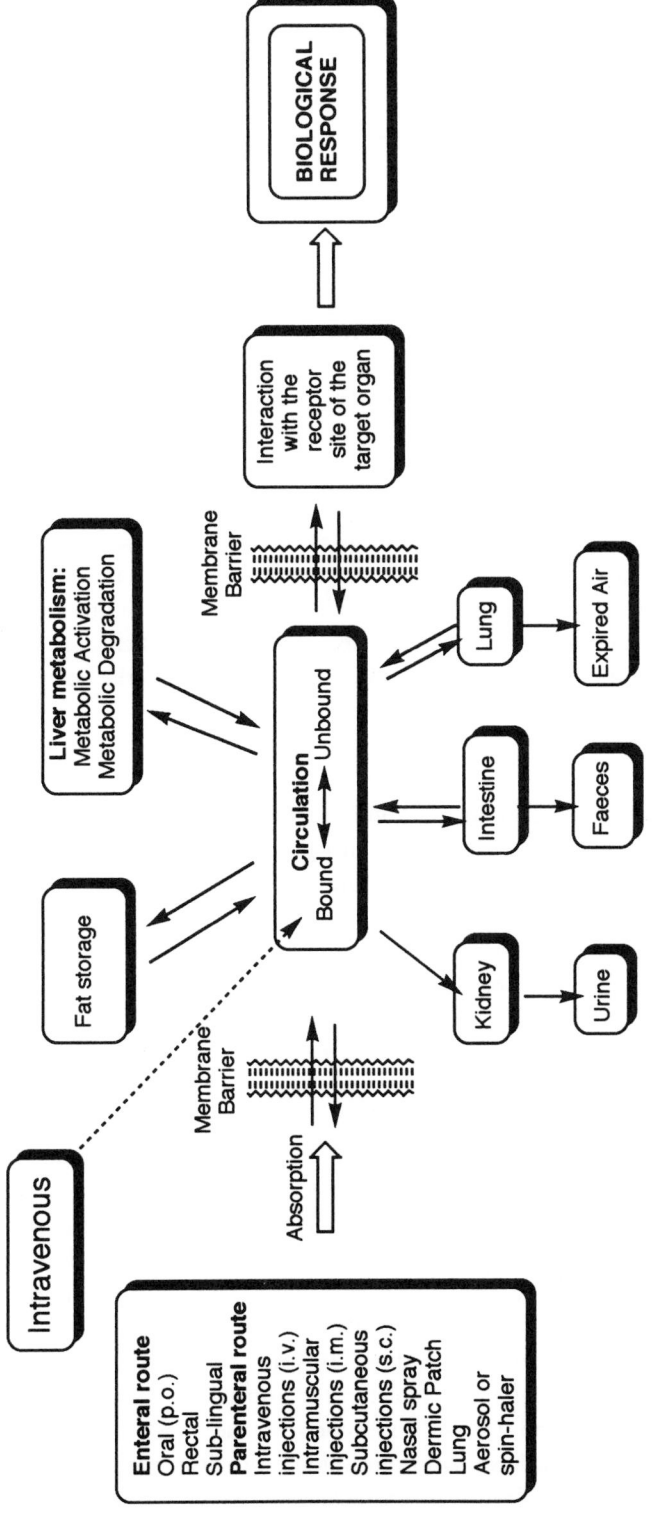

Fig. 4.1 Schematic diagram of *in vivo* events and compartments. (After Kier[5] and Ariëns.[6])

to absorption, and therapeutic blood levels are reached almost instantaneously. The drug solution must be completely clear with no particulate matter present. Injection solutions should be sterile to avoid any infection, and also isotonic and at a pH close to that of the plasma (pH 7.4) to avoid local pain and tissue necrosis.[2–4] Once arrived at the target, the drug can trigger its receptor mechanism and induce the desired biological response. Actually the situation is not usually as simple as this, and many additional and unwanted events can occur (Fig. 4.1):

1. In the bloodstream the drug can bind to the plasma proteins, to the blood cells, or to the platelets and may never reach the target organs in sufficient concentration.
2. Owing to its ionized character or to inadequate partition coefficient, the drug may be unable to cross the lipid biomembranes.
3. Instead of being carried to the biophase, the drug may be concentrated in the fat storage compartment.
4. The drug may also be rapidly altered by metabolic processes. Drug metabolism usually yields more water-soluble, less active and much less toxic derivatives of the parent drug. However, it is not unknown for metabolic processes to generate more active or possibly more toxic molecules.
5. Owing to exchanges with the intestine, the kidneys and the lungs, the parent drug or its metabolites may be tremoved from the organism much too rapidly.
6. On the practical side, only water-soluble drugs can be administered by the intravenous route, and the injections have to be done slowly to avoid excessively high concentrations (as much as 400 times the final blood level) of the drug in the heart tissue.

2.   Oral route

The most common route of administration is the oral route. In this case, the passage of the drug from the gastrointestinal track to the bloodstream, and hence to the site of action, involves several additional steps. The drug preparation is swallowed and the active principle is absorbed through the mucous membrane of the small intestine or, to a limited extent, from the stomach. As absorption is maximal for un-ionized drugs, acidic drugs are rather well absorbed through the stomach epithelium (pH of the gastric juice is 2–3) and weakly basic drugs through the small intestine epithelium (pH varying progressively from 5 to 7). Once absorbed, drugs are carried to the portal vein and from there into the liver, where they may be subjected to chemical attack (oxidation, reduction, hydrolysis, coupling with solubilizing moieties) before being released into the bloodstream. This metabolic attack, taking place before the drug reaches the general circulation, is called 'the first pass effect'; it is avoided when using intravenous injections and thus represents the major difference between the intravenous and the oral route. A drug that is completely broken down by this 'first pass effect' is clearly unsuitable for oral use.

For oral administration the active compound is usually incorporated into tablets, soft or hard gelatine capsules, or coated tablets. As a rule, a tablet is a compressed preparation that contains approximately 5–10% of the active principle, 80% of various excipients (fillers, disintegrants, lubricants, glidants and binders) and about 10% of compounds ensuring easy disintegration, disaggregation and dissolution of the tablet in the stomach or the intestine. Tablets are relatively simple to manufacture and to use and represent the most used formulation. Thanks to appropriate pharmaceutical formulation techniques the disintegration time can be modified so that a rapid effect or a sustained release is achieved. Special coatings can also render the tablet gastro-resistant, the disintegration taking place only in the duodenum, under the combined action of the intestinal enzymes and of the change in pH. The range also includes pills which are coated with sugar and a fine layer of varnish or wax in order to disguise the taste. Recently, films have replaced the sugar and the dyestuffs. Capsules are constituted of a gelatinous envelope that encloses the active substance in the form of powder or granules. The most used forms are capsules in hard or soft gelatine, chewable capsules and capsules for rectal use.

3.   Other pharmaceutical preparations (see also Chapter 28)

Suppositories are composed of an excipient that melts at the body temperature. This can be a natural fat (cocoa butter) or a poly(ethylene glycol) (Carbowax). They are exclusively destined to be introduced in the anus and allow a rapid action because the rectum is richly irrigated. Moreover, they avoid loading of the digestive system.

Pessaries are for introduction into the vagina so as to exert a local action there. They are usually constituted of a dissolution of the active principle in a soft gelatine.

Ointments are coatings to be spread on the skin or on mucous membranes. They are generally used for the treatment of cutaneous or subcutaneous lesions.

Aerosols are sprays for local application. Their therapeutic advantages are the ability to treat large surface areas, good resorption and simple and easy utilization. Aerosols are also of particular importance for inhalation therapies for the respiratory system.

Liquid medicines, sterile for the most part, are composed of active substances in solution. Besides those for intravenous injection, other liquid medicines are perfusions for parenteral nutrition after surgical intervention or traumatic coma, or solutions for stomach washings after intoxication. Finally, drinkable ampoules also belong to the group of liquid medicines.

4.   The bioequivalence problem

A given formulation procedure for an active principle ensures the corresponding bioavailability in patients (bioavailability is the fraction of a drug that reaches the general circulation in a given time). A slight modification in procedure (change of one excipient, changes in the granulation process before tableting, changes in the drying process, modification of the ageing or storage conditions) can sometimes dramatically influence the drug release from the final product. The same is true for changes in the final purification process of the active principle. Thus, recrystallization from a different solvent system or under other temperature and/or concentration conditions can produce mesomorphic crystalline forms, exhibiting different solubilities and as a consequence different bioavailability (see Chapter 38). As stated by Kellaway:[7] 'When a patient is successfully treated or stabilized on a branded product, it is therefore undesirable to change to a chemically equivalent product from an alternative manufacturer unless bioequivalence has been proven. Economic pressures advocating change of product should be resisted — at least until bioequivalence data are presented.'

When the pharmaceutical formulation of an active compound is ineffective, slight chemical modifications or the formation of bioreversible derivatives (esters, amides, peptides) can improve its physicochemical properties (lipophilicity, pK, polarity) and optimize the dissolution rates in the biological fluids and the passage through the first biological membranes (cutaneous, intestinal, etc.). The end result is better penetration into the organism. Compared to the pharmaceutical formulation discussed above, this process can be considered as chemical formulation; it will be treated in Chapters 31, 32 and 38.

II.   THE PHARMACOKINETIC PHASE

The pharmacokinetic phase controls the different parameters that govern the random walk of the drug between its application point and its final site of action and which ensure its destruction and/or elimination once the effect is produced. The site of action is often separated in space and time from the site of administration or penetration. In chronological order the events of the pharmacokinetic phase are as follows.

A.   Absorption

The processes of absorption through the different biological membranes and compartments, are highly dependent on the physical properties of the drug (ionized or un-ionized state, partition coefficient, molecular size) and can proceed simply through passive diffusion or by more sophisticated physiological transport mechanisms (Chapter 28).

B.   Distribution

The distribution of the drug into the various compartments is ensured by the blood and, to a lesser extent, by the lymphatic, circulation. Blood plasma contains suspended blood cells and platelets and is essentially a solution of $70 \, gl^{-1}$ of proteins (albumin and globulins), $9 \, gl^{-1}$ of mineral salts (essentially sodium chloride) and $\sim 1 \, gl^{-1}$ of glucose (for the exact composition see Table 4.2 due to Rettig[8]).

The proteins, especially albumin, are able to bind various drugs and thus to temporarily extract them from their pharmacological destination. Albumin has a molecular weight of 69 000 kDa and is mainly negatively charged at the physiological pH of the blood (7.4). At pH 5, its isoelectric point, the molecule has 100 negative and 100 positive charges; this explains its important role as a physiological buffer molecule.

Table 4.2   Constitution of blood.[8]

Constituent	gl^{-1}	Percentage of the total
Blood cells (haematocrit)		45
Erythrocytes	446	
Leukocytes	1.5	
Thrombocytes	2.5	
Plasma		55
Fibrinogen	3	
Serum		54.7
Proteins	35	
Electrolytes	~4.5	
Carbohydrates	~0.5	
Hormones	traces	
Enzymes	traces	
Vitamins	traces	
Antibodies	traces	
Gases, dyestuffs	traces	
Water	~507	

C. Metabolism

The usual end-point of metabolism is the chemical transformation of drugs or other substances that are foreign to the organism (xenobiotics) into water-soluble derivatives to facilitate their urinary elimination. This change normally produces a diminution, or even suppression, of the pharmacological activity and of the eventual toxicity. However, it can happen that the metabolism activates the parent molecule (see Chapters 31 and 32) or even generates highly reactive intermediates (mostly electrophiles) that induce toxicity mechanisms (see Chapter 30). If metabolic activation is involved, drugs that are inactive *in vitro* may be found to be active *in vivo*. Sulfamidochrysoidine ('Prontosil rubrum'), converted *in vivo* to the anti-infectious agent sulfanilamide, is the historical example. In its turn the active metabolite is inactivated through acetylation (Fig. 4.2).

Metabolic reactions take place largely in the liver, but other organs such as the kidneys, the lungs or the brain can also effect drug transformations.

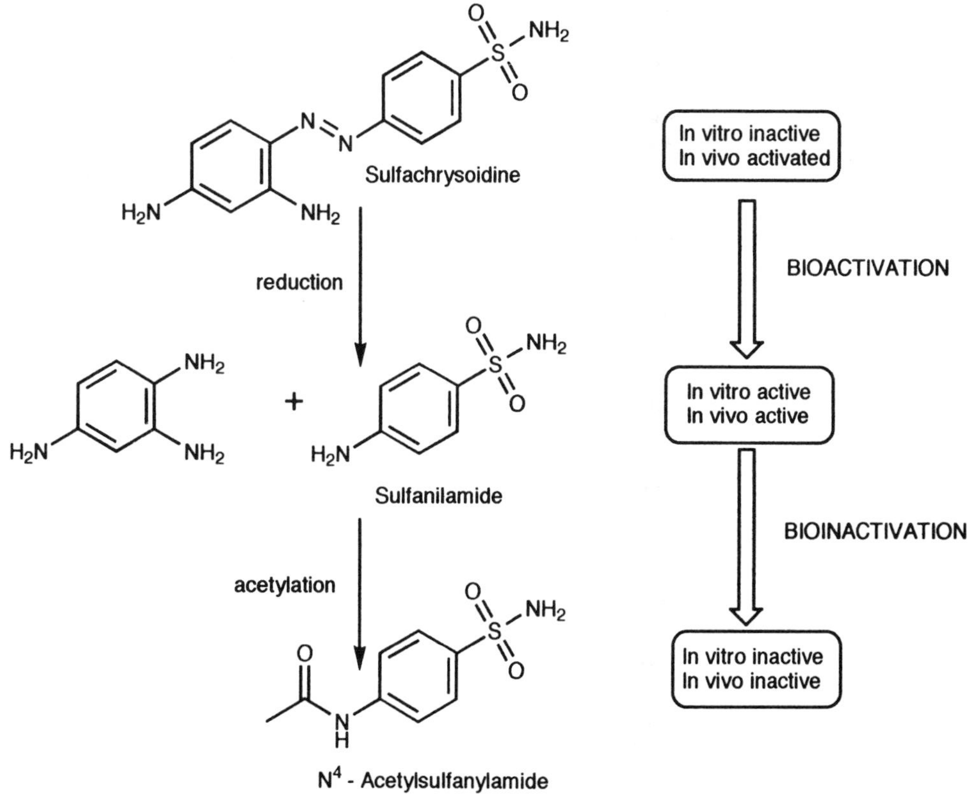

Fig. 4.2 Metabolic activation and inactivation.

D. Elimination

Once the desired pharmacological effect is produced, drugs and their metabolites have to be eliminated from the organism at a suitable rate. Too slow an elimination process produces a progressive accumulation of the drug and the appearance of toxic effects. Conversely, too rapid elimination necessitates repeated daily administration and low patient acceptance. The main elimination routes are renal (urine) and rectal (faeces). They can occasionally include pulmonary (expired air), oral (salivary) and cutaneous (sweat) routes. The elimination kinetics is very seldom of order zero (Figure 4.3a). One of the best known example is the linear elimination of ethanol (that allows the calculation of the ethanol blood level at the moment of a car accident even when the blood sample was taken some time after the accident).

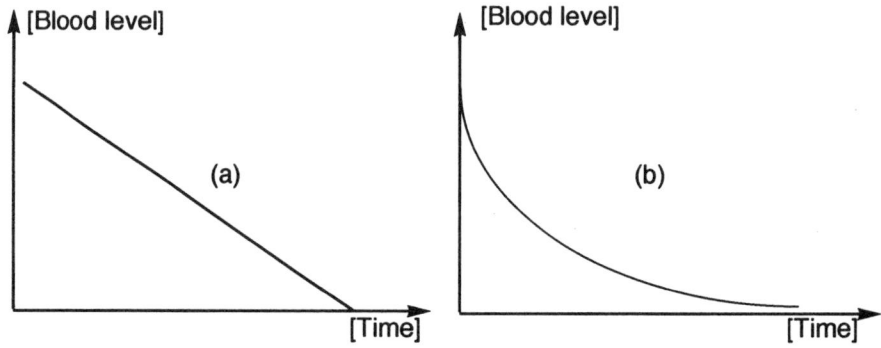

Fig. 4.3   Elimination kinetics (a) of order zero and (b) of order 1.

The usual elimination kinetics of a drug from the circulating blood is of first order (Fig. 4.3b). In this case the time at which the drug is completely cleared from the blood is relatively difficult to determine, since the curve does not intersect the x axis but only approaches it asymptotically. Much easier is the determination of the biological half-life ($t_{1/2}$), i.e. the time after which the blood level has reached half of the original level. Table 4.3 gives some examples of elimination half-lives.

Table 4.3   Examples of drugs possessing very different elimination half-times (taken from references 9–11).

Compound	t½ (h)
Pyridostigmine	0.1
Fentanyl	0.2
Morphine	2–3
Clonidine	8
Adamantine	10
Griseofulvin	20
Phenobarbital	35–96
Chloroquine	48
Reserpine	150
Sulfamethoxine	200
Bromide ion	280–340

These four pharmacokinetic processes (ADME: absorption, distribution, metabolism, excretion) account for the bioavailability of a given drug. Since the bioavailability expresses the percentage of drug that reaches the general circulation in a given time, intravenous administration represents, by definition, 100% bioavailability. After an oral dosage, 100% bioavailability would signify a complete absorption and no first pass destruction.

III. THE PHARMACODYNAMIC PHASE

The pharmacodynamic phase is the phase of greatest interest to the medicinal chemist as it deals directly with the nature and the quality of the interaction of the drug with its biological target. Starting often with a relatively weak and nonselective compound, the challenge is to maximize the potency and to minimize the deleterious or undesired effects of the molecule. The biological response obtained is maximal when the active principle shows precise stereoelectronic complementarity with the target site. Ideally the medicinal chemist, from the knowledge of the characteristics of the target (enzyme, receptor, transport protein, nucleic acid), tries to design drugs with the optimal size, shape, hydrophilic–lipophilic ratio, and disposition of functional groups. The closer the fit obtained between the receptor site and the molecule, the more selective will be the drug in eliciting only the expected biological response.

A. Dose–effect relationships

During the search for relationships between the concentration of an active compound and its effects it is essential to resort to quantitative data describing the potency of the compound and allowing comparisons with other substances. In classical pharmacological studies the activity of the compound is often examined towards isolated organs maintained at appropriate temperature in nutritive and oxygenated solutions. In cardiovascular pharmacology, for example, the changes in the diameter of an isolated blood vessel (portal or mesenteric vein, coronary artery) represent a means of measuring vasodilating or vasoconstrictive properties. Experimental research conducted on isolated organs presents many advantages such as the precise knowledge of the concentration of the active substance in the nutritive solution, easy observation conditions, elimination of the compensation reactions found in whole animals through feedback reactions, and the possibility of studying a given compound to its maximum effect. The inconveniences are unavoidable lesions caused to the tissue during preparation, loss of the physiological control of the function of the isolated organ, and the artificial character of the environment.

B. Dose–response curves

When the drug concentration is increased in a stepwise manner, the increase of the effect is initially constant, but it tends progressively towards zero on approaching maximal active concentration. Consequently, the concentration that triggers the maximal effect is difficult to measure precisely, whereas the concentration producing half of the maximal effect can be determined exactly. This value (EC_{50}; EC = effective concentration) corresponds to the inflexion point of the sigmoid curve obtained in plotting the effect–concentration data in semilogarithmic coordinates (see Chapter 3). To fully characterize a dose–response curve, the E_{max} (maximal possible effect) and the slope of the curve (concentration range used to establish the curve) also have to be considered.

C.   Binding curves

In molecular pharmacology, when biochemical tests are performed on tissue homogenates or partially purified preparations, and also on isolated enzymes or on cloned receptors, the binding curves are based on the mass-action law. This describes the hyperbolic function (B) that links the binding to the ligand concentration (c). This curve is characterized by the affinity $1/K_d$ and the maximal binding B_{max} (which corresponds to the total number of binding sites contained per unit weight of the preparation):

$$B = B_{max} - \frac{c}{c + K_d}$$

In this equation K_d is the equilibrium dissociation constant and corresponds to the ligand concentration for which 50% of the binding sites are occupied by the ligand. As discussed in Chapter 3, the biological response can be an activation mechanism (postsynaptic agonists, presynaptic antagonists) or an inhibition (postsynaptic antagonists, enzyme inhibitors). Therefore, compounds having the same affinity for a receptor site do not necessarily produce the same response, one possessing an agonist and the other one an antagonist profile. Moreover, two agonists with similar affinities can induce quantitatively different biological responses depending on their intrinsic activity (also called efficacy).[12,13]

D.   Criteria for the expression of pharmacological results

Quantitative dose–effect relationships alone do not provide enough information; ideally a well-conceived pharmacological study should comply with the following criteria.[14]

1. There should be a relationship between the dose and the observed effect. Increase in the concentration of the compound must be accompanied by an increase in activity.
2. The results should always be presented with confidence limits (for example, ED_{50} = 5.8 ± 1.7 mg kg^{-1}). This avoids considering as different two values that in fact have overlapping intervals.
3. The results should always be published in comparison with one or more reference substances serving as internal standards.
4. For tests performed in whole animals, an activity kinetic study is highly recommended. This will allow determination of the time of the peak action and comparison of the different molecules at the optimal time.

E.   Medicinal chemistry approaches as a function of the therapeutic class

The approaches employed by medicinal chemists do not follow strict rules, and in daily practice they vary with the therapeutic class.

1.   *Agents acting on the central nervous system: psychotropic and neurological drugs*

Regulation at the level of the central nervous systems is effected by neurotransmitters. Such substances can be simple molecules (acetylcholine, γ-aminobutyric acid, noradrenaline, etc.) or neuropeptides (substance P, vasopressin, corticotrophin releasing factor, neurotensin, etc.). Pharmacological interventions aim to correct dysregulations, either in reducing excessive neuronal activity or in stimulating a weak working system. The easiest ways for medicinal chemists to intervene are at the enzymatic level (inhibition of biosynthesis or biodegradative enzymes), at the receptor level (activation or blockade by a synthetic analogue of the endogenous neurotransmitter) and at the level of transport systems (blockade of the neurotransmitter reuptake by a structural analogue). As these systems are well characterized, most of the initial testing can be performed *in vitro* on a practically unlimited number of compounds, thus making the search for and the discovery of new CNS agents fairly simple. The real difficulties in the development of CNS drugs reside in the pharmacokinetics. A CNS drug must be able to enter the central nervous system, in other words to cross the blood–brain barrier (BBB). On the other hand, the molecule has to resist premature metabolic degradation and it should not be distributed mainly towards peripheral sites of action.

2.   *Pharmacodynamic agents*

Despite the increasing possibility of biochemical approaches, the design of pharmacodynamic agents in the cardiovascular, antiasthmatic and antiallergic domains is still heavily dependent on animal models or animal-derived models such as isolated organs, perfused hearts or kidneys. Mass screening can therefore be somewhat limited. Conversely, access to the target organs is facilitated by their peripheral location. In some rare instances pharmacodynamic agents can be used in a preventive way (e.g. aspirin to diminish the risks of heart infarct).

3.   *Chemotherapy*

Chemotherapeutic treatments rely predominantly on selective toxicity approaches aiming to kill the invader without killing the host. Albert distinguishes three selectivity principles:[15] favourable differences in drug distribution, favourable differences in biochemistry and favourable differences in cell structure. Certainly the most seductive of these is the difference in biochemistry. A practical application is the inhibition of bacterial cell wall construction by β-lactam antibiotics; the activity is absolutely restricted to the bacteria because similar cell walls do not exist in mammals.

4.   *Agents acting on metabolic or immunological diseases and on endocrine functions*

In this group we find deficiency diseases (vitamin deficiencies, diabetes, Addison's disease, etc.). The logical treatment is to compensate these deficiencies by an exogenous supply of the missing molecule (vitamin or hormone). In hormonology modified versions of the original endogenous hormone have often been developed. Examples are modified vitamins (menadione, benfotiamine), steroids (fluocinolone acetonide, flumethasone) and modified peptides (modified TRH, angiotensin, somatostatin, etc.).

Immunological diseases have benefited recently from the advances in knowledge of protein structure and protein chemistry. Immunostimulant and immunosupressant drugs are now available and immunological approaches to rheumatoid arthritis and to some autoimmune diseases are underway. Vaccines and serums represent other aspects of immunological therapies, vaccination acting in a preventive manner.

REFERENCES

1. Ariëns, E. J. (1974) *Drug Design and Cancer*. In *27th Annual Symposium on Fundamental Cancer Research*, pp. 127–152. The University of Texas M. D. Anderson Hospital and Tumor Institute: The Williams and Wilkins Company.
2. Taylor, J.B. and Kennewell P.D. (1993) The pharmaceutical phase. In Taylor, J. B. and Kennewell P. D. (eds) *Modern Medicinal Chemistry*, pp. 49–71. Ellis Horwood, New York.
3. Trissel, L. A. (1986) *Handbook on Injectable Drugs*, 4th edn. American Society of Hospital Pharmacists, Bethesda, MD, USA.
4. Sinkula, A. A.. and Yalkowsky, S. H. (1975) Rationale for design of biologically reversible drug derivatives: prodrugs. *J. Pharm. Sci.* **64:** 181–210.
5. Kier, L. B. (1971) Molecular orbital theory in drug research. In: DeStevens, G. (ed.) *Medicinal Chemistry*, vol. 10. Academic Press, New York.
6. Ariëns, E. J. (1966) Some of the principal processes that take place in drug action. In Jucker, E. (ed.) *Progress in Drug Research*, pp. 429. Karger Verlag, Basel.
7. Kellaway, I. W. (1983) The indluence of formulation on drug availability. In Smith, H. J. and Williams, H. (eds) *Introduction to the Principles of Drug Design*, pp. 39–51. Wright PSG, Bristol.
8. Rettig, H. (1981) Physiologische Transportvorgänge. In Meier, J. Rettig, H. and Hess, H. (eds) *Biopharmazie-Theorie und Praxis der Pharmakokinetik*, pp. 93–124. Georg Thieme Verlag, Stuttgart and New York.
9. Forth, W. Henschler, D. and Rummel, W. (1987) *Pharmakologie und Toxicologie* 5th edn. B.I. Wissenschaftsverlag, Mannheim.
10. Bennet, W. M., Singer, I. and Coggins, C. H. (1970) A practical guide to drug usage in adult patients with impaired renal function. *J. Am. Med. Assoc.* **214:** 1468–1475.
11. Bennet, W. M., Singer, I. and Coggins, C. H. (1973) Guide to drug usage in adult patients with impaired renal function. *J. Am. Med. Assoc.* **223:** 991–997.
12. Ariëns, E. J. and Simonis, A. M. (1964) A molecular basis for drug action. *J. Pharm. Pharmacol.* **16:** 137.
13. Ariëns, E. J. and Simonis, A. M. (1964) A molecular basis for drug action. The interaction of one or more drugs with different receptors. *J. Pharm. Pharmacol.* **16:** 289–312.
14. Bizière, K. (1984) The Biological Activity. Lecture given at the Louis Pasteur University, 8 March.
15. Albert, A. (1975) The selectivity of drugs. In Ashworth J. M. (ed.) *Outline Studies in Biology*. Chapman and Hall, London.

PART II

Drug Targets and Lead Compound Discovery Strategies

5

Drug Targets — Molecular Mechanisms of Drug Action

JEAN-PIERRE GIES

*Only such substances can be anchored at any particular part of the organism, as fit into
the molecules of the recipient complex like a piece of mosaic finds its place in a pattern*
Paul Ehrlich, 1956[1]

THE PRACTICE OF MEDICINAL CHEMISTRY
ISBN 0-12-744640-0

I.   INTRODUCTION

To understand drug actions it is necessary to consider the effects produced by the drug on the biological system at various levels of complexity of organization. The main levels, from the most complex to the simplest, can be designated as follows: intact organism, organized cells (tissues and organs), cells, subcellular structures and biological molecules. The effects produced by a drug can be recognized only as an alteration in a function or process that maintains the existence of the living organism, since all drugs act by producing changes in some known physiological function or process. Drugs may increase or decrease the normal function of tissues or organs, but they do not endow them with new functions. Thus the particular effect of a drug is always expressed in relative terms — relative to the physiological conditions at the time of administration of the drug.

The action of the drug may be specific, i.e. aimed directly at the agent responsible for the disease, or nonspecific, i.e. ameliorating a symptom of the disease (fever, for example) without getting to the cause of the disorder. Clearly, the distinction between what is produced by an agent — its effect — and where and how the effect is produced — its action — becomes of consequence in determining the purpose for which the drug may be used.[2] To even begin to

How can the properties of drugs be discriminated at a molecular level? To even begin to answer this question, manipulations of the structure of the ligand (drug, hormone, neurotransmitter) have often been performed by chemists. Moreover, a comprehensive understanding of pharmacological selectivity and responses cannot be dissociated from a knowledge of the fundamentals of the molecular structure of the drug binding sites. The recent cloning of the genes for numerous drug receptors as well as the development of recombinant DNA technology, i.e. site-specific mutagenesis and chimeric receptor constructs, are throwing light on how to describe the precise mechanism of the specificity of drug action.

The functional macromolecular structures that are targets for drug action can be arbitrarily divided into receptors, enzymes, proteins involved in the transport, and nucleic acids. A number of other molecular interactions between drugs and the components of the biological system may occur, such as the binding of drugs to plasma albumin or other constituents of the tissues. Serum albumin can transport drugs in the circulation to various organs, and it can hold drugs up, preventing them from binding to their site of action. These interactions have secondary rather than primary consequences for pharmacodynamic actions, since the duration of the drug action or its rate of action is affected. Albumin might then be considered as an acceptor site for the drug rather than a receptor. In this chapter we do not deal with these acceptor or binding sites but we focus interest on the molecular level of drug action on cell membrane receptors.

A.   Induction of drug responses

The common event in the induction of pharmacological responses is the formation of a complex between the ligand, or the drug, molecule and its site of action. The component of the organism with which the drug interacts is termed the *receptor*. Such interaction alters the function of the pertinent component and thereby initiates biochemical and physiological changes that are characteristic of the response to the drug. The statement that the receptor for a drug can be any functional macromolecular component of the organism has several fundamental corollaries. One is that a drug is potentially capable of altering the rate at which any bodily function proceeds.

Another is that drugs do not create effects but merely modulate ongoing functions; a drug does not impart a new function to a cell. Although gene therapy may soon challenge this principle, it remains valid for the immediate future.

The vast majority of drugs produce their effects by interacting with cells, either with components of the interior of the cell or with those on the surface of the cell comprising the cellular membrane. Some others act extracellularly on noncellular constituents of the body without involving a drug–receptor interaction.[3] The simplest example is that of the neutralization of gastric acid by antacid drugs. In this reaction the excess of gastric acid is neutralized by the base sodium bicarbonate. The base reacts chemically with the hydrochloric acid and removes the acid by inducing the formation of a salt, water and carbon dioxide. This reaction is not considered as a drug–receptor interaction, since no macromolecular cell component is involved. Other types of extracellular mechanisms, where the action of the drug is the result of a chemical reaction, can be illustrated, for example, by the action of heparin, which prevents blood coagulation, or by antidotes used to treat poisoning. There are still other mechanisms of drug action that are not mediated by receptors. These actions may occur at cellular sites and may involve macromolecular components, but the biological effects produced are nonspecific consequences of the chemical properties of the drugs. Detergents, alcohol, oxidizing agents and phenol derivatives act by destroying the integrity of the cell by disrupting the cellular constituents, such as proteins or nucleic acids. These actions are not treated in the present chapter, which gives emphasis to the drug actions on cell membrane receptors.

B. Chemistry of drug binding to receptors

The receptor concept was formulated by Langley and the term 'receptor' was proposed by Ehrlich.[4] The concept of receptor binding, *Corpora non agunt nisi fixata* (compounds do not act unless bound), has been subject to refinement but is still valid.

According to the receptor theory of drug action, the common event in the initiation of pharmacological responses is the formation of a complex between the drug molecule and its site of action. Since most pharmacological responses are mediated through receptors, recognition of the more mobile drug molecules by the cellular receptor is the critical element determining the specificity of the response. There must be some forces that not only attract the drug to its receptor but also hold it in combination with the receptor long enough to initiate the chain of events leading to the effect. Thus the combination of various chemical bonds is of great interest in drug potency.

- Hydrophobic binding plays an important role in stabilizing the conformation of proteins and in the association of hydrophobic structure between the drug and the receptor.
- Hydrogen bonding, which is strongly directional, has considerable importance in stabilizing structures by intramolecular bond formation. The formation of such bonds between a drug and a receptor can result in a relatively stable and reversible interaction. Such bonds are also involved in the maintenance of the tertiary structure of receptor macromolecules and are thought to be involved in the specificity and selectivity of drug–receptor interaction.
- Drug–receptor interaction often involves charge–transfer complexes formed between electron-rich donor molecules and electron-deficient acceptors.
- Ionic bonds, which are very ubiquitous, are of importance in the actions of ionizable drugs since they act over long distances. The formation of an ionic bond results from the

electrostatic attraction that occurs between oppositely charged ions. Most receptors have a number of ionizable groups (COO^-, OH^-, NH_3^+) at physiological pH that are available for the binding with charged drugs.

- Covalent bonds are less important in drug–receptor interaction. Since bonds of this type are so stable at physiological temperatures, the binding of a drug to a receptor through covalent bond formation results in the formation of a long-lasting complex. Although most drug–receptor interactions are readily reversible, some drugs, such as anticancer nitrogen mustards and alkylating compounds, form reactive cationic intermediates (i.e. aziridinium ion) that can react with electron-donor groups on the receptor. Covalent bonds are also seen, for example, in the case of penicillin, which acylates a transpeptidase enzyme that is essential to bacterial cell-wall synthesis. In this case a long-lasting inhibition of bacterial replication is needed. Most drugs, however induce brief formation of a reversible drug–receptor complex.

C.   Drug receptors and physiological mediators

The drug–receptor complex formed in the first stage triggers, in the second stage, the formation of intracellular messengers or induces the opening of ion channels. In a third stage, other members of the chain reaction such as protein kinases can be activated. This cascade of events finally results in the physiological change attributed to the drug. Since most drugs have a considerable degree of selectivity or specificity in their action, it follows that the receptors with which they interact must be equally specific. It is generally accepted that endogenous or exogenous agents interact specially with a specific receptor site. Thus receptors will interact with only a limited number of structurally related or complementary compounds. This cascade of events also occurs with endogenous agents such as hormones and neurotransmitters.

It is generally assumed that all receptors with which drugs combine exist to function as receptors for neurotransmitters, hormones, or other physiological substances.[5] Many drugs act on such physiological receptors. Those that mimic the effects of endogenous regulatory compounds are termed *agonists*. Other compounds may bind to the receptor but have no intrinsic regulatory activity. These drugs usually prevent the neurotransmitter from reaching the receptor, by competition at the agonist binding site, and are termed *antagonists*.

The differential capacity to induce responses is attributed either to conformational changes in the receptor or to different states of association of the receptor with active complexes of coupling proteins (Fig. 5.1).

II.   RECEPTORS AS PRIMARY TARGETS FOR DRUG ACTION

Receptors are commonly classified according to the mediator to which they respond and hence according to their chemical specificity. The name given to a receptor is often derived from this classification (e.g. cholinergic receptors, glutamic receptors). In some cases, when the endogenous mediator is unknown, the receptor is named according to a exogenous compound to which the receptor respond (this was the case for the opioid receptors).

At present a large number of cell surface receptors for transmitters have been identified and purified, and corresponding amino acid sequences of short stretches have been determined. These sequences have been used to design synthetic oligonucleotides in order to screen cDNA

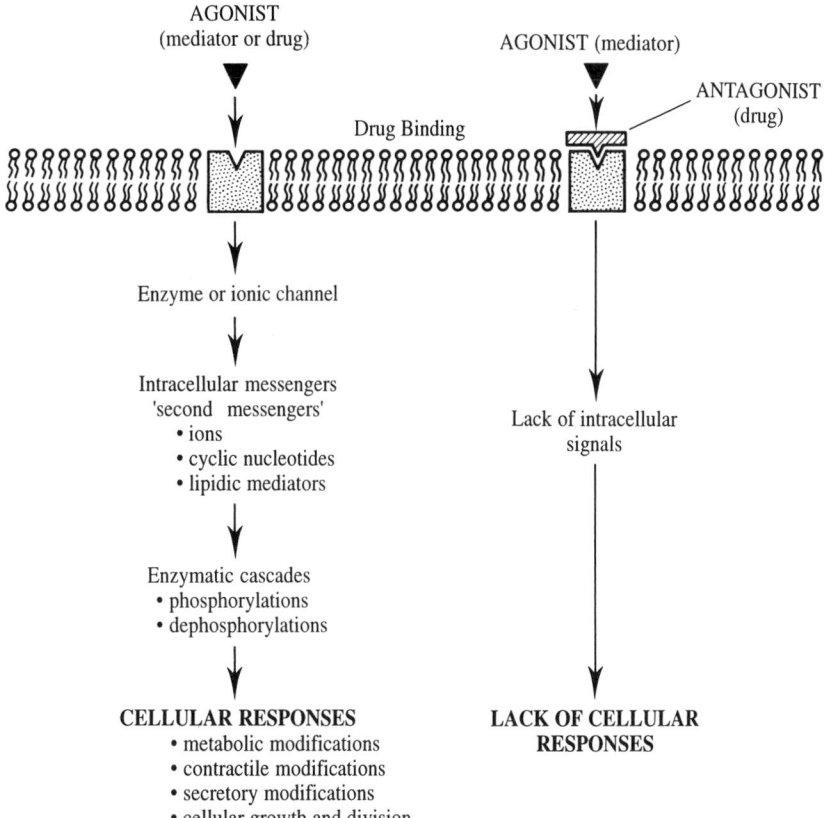

Fig. 5.1   Mode of action of agonists and antagonists. (Adapted, with permission from Gies, J. P. (1993) *Bases de pharmacologie moléculaire*. Published by Ellipses–Édition Marketing, Paris.)

libraries by conventional gene cloning methods. Sequencing of long stretches of cDNA has been the route to obtaining complete amino acid sequences for the receptor polypeptides. These molecular biology techniques have demonstrated that receptors for different mediators are similar in sequence; they may be derived from common ancestors and have allowed a possibility for the development of informative models above the three-dimensional structure of the receptors. Molecular pharmacology has allowed detailed analysis of structure–function relationships of signalling proteins through site-directed mutagenesis. The classification inherent in the primary amino acid sequence of the receptor shows a small number of receptor subfamilies that share homologous structures and common mechanisms of action (Fig. 5.2). These different subfamilies correspond to (1) the receptors that gate ion channels; (2) the receptors that contain enzymatic activity; (3) the G-protein-coupled receptors; and (4) the nuclear receptors that regulate the transcription of different genes. These receptor subfamilies are coupled to different effectors, yielding different cellular effects. The effects produced by the ionic receptors are very fast (milliseconds); those produced by steroids and thyroids hormones are very slow; and those induced by the G-coupling receptors occupy an intermediate timescale.

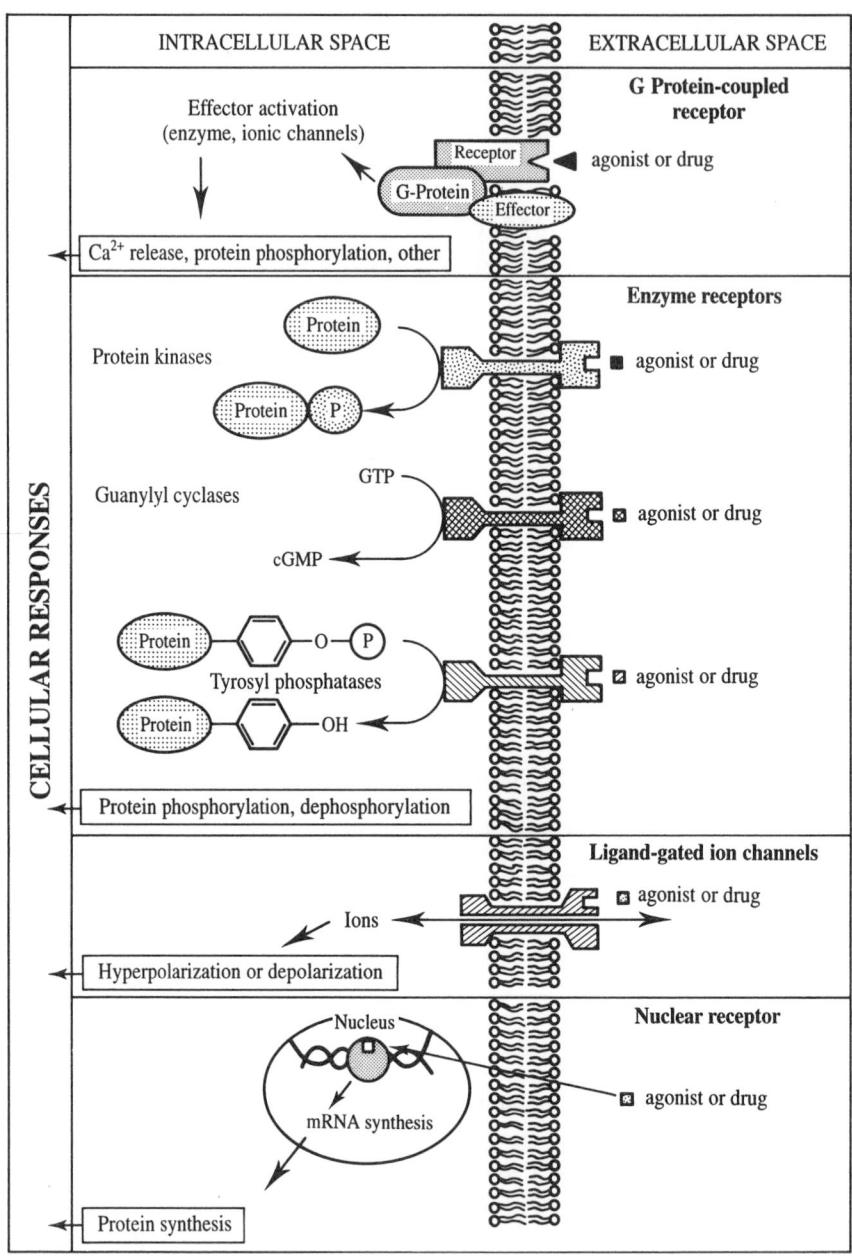

Fig. 5.2 Physiological receptor–effector linkage. (Adapted, with permission from Gies, J. P. (1993) *Bases de pharmacologie moléculaire.* Published by Ellipses–Édition Marketing, Paris.)

A. Ligand-gated ion channels

Receptors for several neurotransmitters form ion-selective channels in the plasma membrane and diffuse their signals by altering the cell's membrane potential or the cytoplasmic ionic composition. This subfamily of receptors includes the well-characterized nicotinic acetylcholine receptor from the electric organ of *Torpedo marmorata,* muscle and brain,[7] the receptors for the excitatory amino acids (aspartate and glutamate), the inhibitory amino acids (γ-aminobutyrate, glycine),[8] and the serotoninergic 5HT3 receptors.[9] Structural and functional evidence supports the view that these membrane-bound allosteric proteins are heteropentameric oligomers. The nicotinic receptor contains five families of peptides designated α, β, γ, δ, ε. In the muscle, the α-subunit is α_1 and two distinct types (α_1A and α_1B) have been cloned; additional α-subunits (α_2 to α_8) and β-subunits (β_2 to β_4) have been cloned from chick and rat autonomic and central nervous systems. These are not all pharmacologically identical. There are also two variant species in the rat (α_{4-1}) and (α_{4-2}), which are derived from the α_4 gene. The nicotinic receptor from the electric organ of *Torpedo marmorata*, or embryonic muscle appears to consist of a pentamer $(\alpha_1)_2$-β_1-γ-δ, while the neuronal type is a pentamer $(\alpha)_2$-$(\beta)_3$. The distinct pharmacological and electrophysiological properties are associated with defined combinations of subunits. Chemical labelling and site-directed mutagenesis show that the various members of the superfamily are composed of subunits sharing the same conformational pattern and showing a great sequence homology with the nicotinic acetylcholine receptor. The receptors for these rapid-acting neurotransmitters, both excitatory (glutamate, aspartate) and inhibitory (glycine, γ-aminobutyric acid (GABA)), appear as a superfamily that has probably arisen by duplication and divergence of an ancestral neurotransmitter receptor. The significance of this is that knowledge obtained about the function of any one of these receptors can also be applied to all the receptors belonging to the same family.

The neuromuscular nicotinic acetylcholine receptor is a pentamer in which five structurally related subunits are assembled to form an integral ion channel. Each subunit is believed to contain four transmembrane domains inserted in the plasma membrane (Fig. 5.3). The second transmembrane domain of each subunit forms the ion channel lining. This is also true for the glycine and glutamate receptors.[10,11] Thus, unlike the G-protein-coupled receptors, the

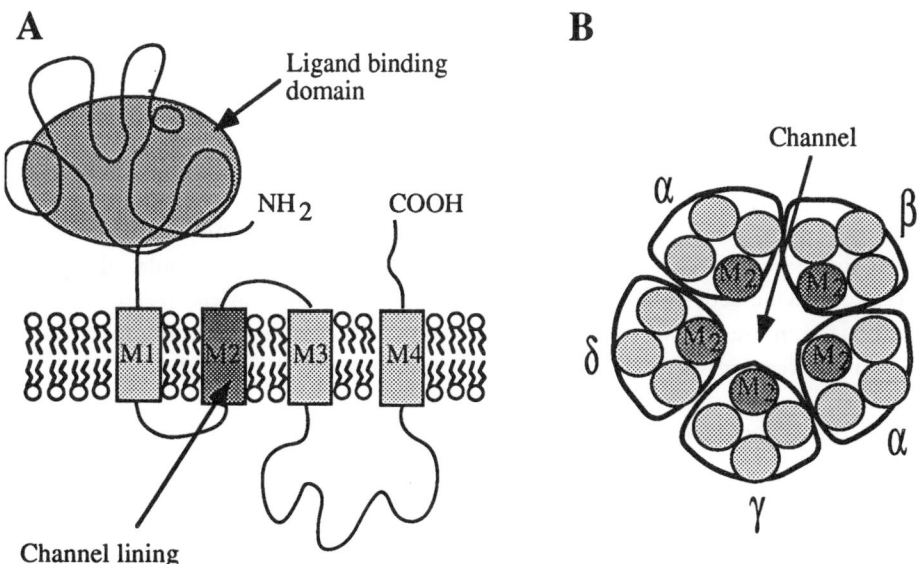

Fig. 5.3 Proposed topography of the nicotinic acetylcholine receptor. (A) The different subunits are composed of four membrane-spanning helices. Only the α-subunit contains the ligand binding site. (B) Cross section in the plane of the membrane. The receptor complex contains 20 membrane-spanning segments surrounding the central ion channel. Only the M2 membrane-spanning helices form the inner wall of the central channel. (Adapted, with permission from Gies, J.-P. (1993) *Bases de pharmacologie moléculaire.* Published by Ellipses–Édition Marketing, Paris.)

ligand-gated ion channel receptors do not appear to form the ligand binding site. The nicotinic acetylcholine receptor possess two primary acetycholine binding sites that mediate both the channel gating and desensitization responses to agonists. Covalent labelling of these sites and α-toxin binding studies with subunits expressed from the corresponding cDNA in frog oocytes show that the acetylcholine binding sites are located at the long extracellular N-terminal tails of the two α-subunits. The two sites differ in the binding of cholinergic ligands. Photolabelling studies performed on torpedo nicotinic receptors support the notion that the site for the noncompetitive blockers chlorpromazine and triphenylmethylphosphonium are located in the second transmembrane segment. Recent mutagenesis data reveal that the picrotoxine (a noncompetitive blocker of the glycine receptor channel) binding site also extended over a large portion of the second transmembrane domain.[12] The nicotinic, glutamate and $5HT_3$ receptors contain channels that discriminate poorly between permeant cations.[13] The channel selectivity among monovalent cations may be confined to a layer located at the cytoplasmic end of the channel domain as well as to the geometry of the quaternary structure.

The receptors of this family control the fastest synaptic events in the nervous system by increasing transient permeability to particular ions. Excitatory neurotransmitters such as acetylcholine at the neuromuscular junction or glutamate in the central nervous system induce an opening of cation channels. These channels are relatively unselective for cations, but, because of the electrochemical gradient across the plasma membrane, the major effect of channel opening is a increase in Na^+ and K^+ permeability. This results in a net Na^+ inward current, which depolarizes the cell and results in the generation of an action potential. The action of the transmitter occurs in a fraction of a millisecond and decays within a few milliseconds. In this way the receptor converts a chemical signal (neurotransmitter) into an electrical signal (depolarization). The firing of the action potential is inhibited by other receptor-gated channels such as $GABA_A$ or glycine. Stimulation of these receptors induces the opening of anionic channels (Cl^-), which results in a inward influx of Cl^-. The opening of these channels causes slight hyperpolarization and will resist depolarization induced by excitatory ligands.

B.   Receptors with intrinsic enzymatic activity

The receptors of this family possess an intrinsic enzymatic activity and are quite different in structure and function from either the G-protein coupled receptors or the channel-linked receptors discussed above. The binding of an agonist on the extracellular domain directly activates an enzyme activity located on the intracellular domain of the receptor. The present subfamily is composed of the tyrosine kinase-linked receptors that phosphorylate tyrosine residues in the receptors themselves and the receptors linked to the guanylyl cyclase.

1.   Tyrosine kinase-linked receptors

These receptors mediate the actions of several hormonal agonists such as insulin, insulin-like growth factor, epidermal growth factor and platelet-derived growth factor. These receptors contain a very large extracellular domain rich in cysteine residues, and a cytoplasmic domain containing the tyrosine kinase activity as well as the sites of autophosphorylation. There are about 400–700 aminoacyl residues in each domain. These receptors span the plasma membrane only once. While certain of these receptors possess a single polypeptide chain (epidermal growth factor receptors, platelet-derived growth factor receptors), others like the insulin receptor possess two chains (α-β) linked as a dimer by disulphide bounds. In this case the α chain possess the ligand-binding site and the β chain the tyrosyl kinase activity. The tyrosine kinase domain seems to be similar among these receptors while the ligand-binding domain shows very little sequence homology between the members of this family. At present we do not know the mechanism by which the extracellular binding site communicates with the intracellular enzymatic site. The autophosphorylation of tyrosine residues, which promote the phosphorylation of other proteins, appears to be a unique mode of cellular regulation, much less common compared to the phosphorylation of the serine and threonine residues in cellular proteins. These receptors are able to produce both rapid and slower effects on target cells. The cellular actions are complex. The activation of these receptors can lead to stimulation of the transcription of DNA sections (oncogenes) that produce oncogene products which are themselves related to the growth factor receptors, possessing a tyrosine kinase activity stimulated without a ligand presence (v-*erb*, v-*ros*).

2. Guanylyl cyclase-linked receptors

Some receptors appear to be linked to the stimulation of guanylyl cyclase. These membrane receptors mediate the action of the atrial natriuretic peptide (ANP), the heat-stable enterotoxin of *E. coli* and the receptors involved in fertilization in some species. These membrane receptors are glycoproteins of about 130–160 kDa spanning the membrane only once.[14] The binding of the peptides occur at the extracellular domain, while the intracellular regions contain both cyclase catalytic domains, converting GTP to cGMP, and a protein kinase-like domain.

A second family of G-cyclases is found in the cytosol. These enzymes contain a tightly bound haem group as a 'co-factor' and are activated by organic and inorganic nitrate (nitric oxide, nitroprusside).

As with adenylyl cyclases it is now clear that many families of guanylyl cyclase catalyse cGMP formation.[15] The membrane-associated G-cyclases contains at least three different isoenzymes that appear to be coded for by different genes. They are currently termed GC-A, GC-B and GC-C forms.

C. Receptors linked to JAKs and STATs

We saw in Section II.B that a number of growth factors bind to receptors and mediate their biological responses by activating the receptor intrinsic protein kinase activity. By contrast, a large number of cytokines bind to receptors of the cytokine receptor superfamily.[16] Cytokines and growth factors serve as signal carriers in a dynamic cellular communication network. These pleiotropic mediators act synergistically or antagonistically to orchestrate the proliferation and death of cells by acting directly and/or by regulating the expression of other cytokines. The cytokines bind to the extracellular domain of the transmembrane receptors and induce intracellular responses. Unlike the receptor protein tyrosine kinases, receptors of the cytokine receptor superfamily do not possess kinases domains. Despite the absence of such cytoplasmic domains, cytokines induce a rapid tyrosine phosphorylation of the cellular substrate proteins and of the receptors. This leads to the hypothesis that a protein tyrosine kinase associates with the receptor and is activated after ligand binding. It is well known that cytokine receptors associate with and activate members of the Janus kinase (JAK) family of protein tyrosine kinases. These JAKs possess two domains; the first is associated with a protein tyrosine kinase catalytic activity and the second is a kinase-like domain without kinase activity. These kinase domains bear no homology to the Src homology 2 (SH2) or Src homology 3 (SH3) domains of cytoplasmic protein tyrosine kinases.[17,18] In the case of receptors containing a single chain (prolactin, granulocyte colony-stimulating factor (G-CSF), growth factor), the binding of a ligand induces receptor dimerization and oligomerization. This molecular rearrangement increases the affinity of the cytoplasmic domain of the receptor for the JAKs and results in a ligand-dependent increase of receptor-coupled JAKs.

The receptors with two chains (α and β chains) (interleukin 3 (IL-3), interleukin 5 (IL-5), interleukin 6 (IL-6)) associate with JAK with the β chain while the α chain binds the ligand.

The activated JAKs phosphorylate the receptors as well as the cytoplasmic proteins belonging to a family of transcription factors called the signal transducers and activators of transcription (STATs), providing a new signalling pathway that is shared by all the members of the cytokine receptor superfamily. JAKs must be present to obtain tyrosine phosphorylation of the STAT proteins, which suggests that STAT proteins are direct substrates of the JAKs. The STATs are directly involved in the regulation of gene transcription.[19]

D. G-Protein-coupled receptors

A large range of neurotransmitters, polypeptides and inflammatory mediators transduce their signal into the interior of the cell by a specific interaction with receptors coupled to G-proteins. The most familiar are the muscarinic acetylcholine receptors, the adrenergic receptors, the dopaminergic receptors and the opioid receptors, as well as many peptide receptors. However, the rapid acquisition of structural information on the members of this subfamily indicates a much greater diversity than previously suspected. The diversity of these receptors is reflected by the cloned sequences reported to date (see Table 5.1). The characterization of novel molecular receptor subtypes and their corresponding pharmacological properties has extended the existing definitions of receptor diversity based on pharmacological criteria. This is the case with the cloning of the D_4[20] and D_5[21] subtypes of the dopamine receptors, the third subtype of the human β_3-adrenoceptor,[22] or the cloning of the rat α_{1A}[23] and α_{1D}[24] adrenoceptor which increases the number to four α_1 adrenoceptor subtypes (α_{1A} to α_{1D}).

Table 5.1 Illustration of the diversity of the G-protein-coupled receptor family. Numbers in parentheses refer to the number of receptor subtypes identified to date.

Neurotransmitter receptors	Peptides/peptide hormones
Adenosine (4)	Angiotensin (2)
α_1-Adrenergic (4)	Bombesin (3)
α_2-Adrenergic (3)	Bradykinin (2)
β-Adrenergic (3)	Chemokine-α (2)
Dopamine (5)	Chemokine-β (2)
Glutamate metabotropic (7)	Cholecystokinin (2)
Histamine (3)	Endothelin (2)
Serotonin (13)	Neuropeptide Y (2)
Muscarinic acetylcholine (5)	Opioid (3)
	Somatostatin (5)
	Tachykinin (3)

The receptors of this subfamily are characterized by a common topology and by varying degrees of primary sequence similarities. Most of the receptors are formed by a single polypeptide chain of 400–500 residues (Fig. 5.4). Hydropathy plots reveal seven hydrophobic regions. They are likely to correspond to transmembrane α-helices which are membrane-spanning domains. This topology is highly conserved between the members of the family. The amino-terminal extracellular domain contains potential N-linked glycosylation sites in most receptors. The carboxyl-terminal cytoplasmic end is involved in the coupling to G-proteins and contain a palmitoylation site (Cys) and phosphorylation sites (Thr, Ser), both involved in receptor desensitization. The transmembrane domains possess the residues involved in the binding of ligands. The three cytoplasmic loops are implicated in coupling with G-proteins and the third confers the specificity of the coupling to different G-proteins.

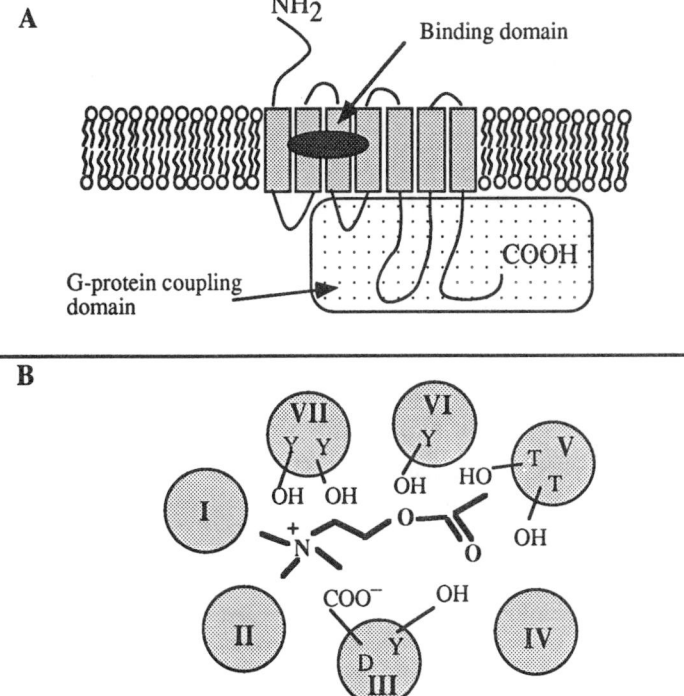

Fig. 5.4   Structure of the G-protein-coupled receptor. (A) α-Helical segments of the protein (about 20 amino acids), represented by rectangles, form the membrane-spanning domains of the receptor. (B) Residues that are important for high-affinity acetylcholine binding to the muscarinic m3 receptor are indicated: Y; Tyr; T, Thr; D; aspartate residues. (Adapted, with permission from Gies, J.-P. (1993) *Bases de pharmacologie moléculaire.* Published by Ellipses–Édition Marketing, Paris.)

1.   Ligand-binding domains

The receptors for the glycoprotein hormones follicle-stimulating hormone (FSH), luteinizing hormone/chorionic gonadotropin (LH/CG) and thyroid-stimulating hormone (TSH) show a very large extracellular extremity NH$_2$ terminal (>300 amino acids). The construction of chimeric receptors of this subfamily has established that this extremity represented the ligand-binding site.[25,26]

The ligand-binding sites for the neurotransmitter receptors lack the significant amino acid extracellular domain. Chimeric α_2-β_2 adrenoceptor constructs indicate, by switching the transmembrane domains, that these domains are important in determining ligand-binding specificity. Consistent with findings obtained with the adrenergic receptors,[27] ligand binding to muscarinic receptors as well as the other biogenic amine receptors occurs in a pocket formed by a ring-like arrangement of seven transmembrane α-helices. Site-directed mutagenesis studies and construction of chimeric adrenoceptors have pointed to the importance of negatively charged aspartic acid residues in transmembrane segments III[28,29] in the ligand binding (Fig. 5.4). The role of these negatively charged residues appears to be in binding positively charged ligands (e.g. muscarinic, adrenergic) into the centre of the receptor. Interestingly, these residues seem to be conserved among all other biogenic amine receptors. However, additional molecular interactions can be required to determine the specificity of the binding of a given amine for a particular receptor.[30,31]

2.   Coupling of the receptors to G-proteins

Several lines of evidence suggest that multiple intracellular receptor domains (particularly the cytoplasmic loop between transmembrane segments III–IV and V–VI) are involved in G-protein coupling. In order to delineate receptor domains responsible for the G-protein coupling selectivity displayed by the individual muscarinic receptor subtypes, chimeric m1/m2 and m2/m3 muscarinic receptors have been constructed and functionally characterized in different expression systems. Biochemical and electrophysiological studies have shown that the exchange of the third intracellular loop between two functionally different muscarinic receptor subtypes results in mutant receptors that display qualitatively the same coupling properties as the wild type receptor from which the third intracellular loop is derived. These data indicate that the third intracellular loop represents the primary structural determinant dictating G-protein coupling selectivity.[32,33] Similar findings obtained with the chimeric human β_2-α_{2A} adrenoceptor, where segments of the β_2 adrenoceptor, which normally couples to Gs (stimulation of adenylyl cyclase), have been replaced with the corresponding segments of the α_{2A} adrenoceptor, coupled to Gi (inhibition of adenylyl cyclase), indicate that the carboxy-terminal segment of the third cytoplasmic loop is involved in the coupling with Gs.[34] Interestingly, synthetic peptides as short as 15 amino acids in length that mimic those sequences can activate purified G-proteins in vitro.[35] Thus one function of the intact receptor structure must be to prevent these small activating domains from interacting with G-proteins until an agonist binds to the receptor.[35] How this happens is not known.

3.   Mechanism of multifunctional signalling by G-proteins

Addition of a drug to a cell frequently results in the regulation of multiple cellular signalling cascades. In a number of cases these effects are the reflection of an initial stimulation that produces multiple signals by regulating the transmembrane signalling apparatus at a proximal level. G-proteins represent the level of middle management in the organizational hierarchy, able to communicate between the receptors and the effectors (enzymes or ion channels).

Around ten different genes have been found to code for G-proteins, and the family is expected to grow. Five principal classes of G-proteins, designated Gi, Gs, Go, Gt, and Gp have been described, based on both functional and structural criteria of the α-subunit. All display a common, heterotrimeric structure; the three subunits are designated α, β, and γ, in order of

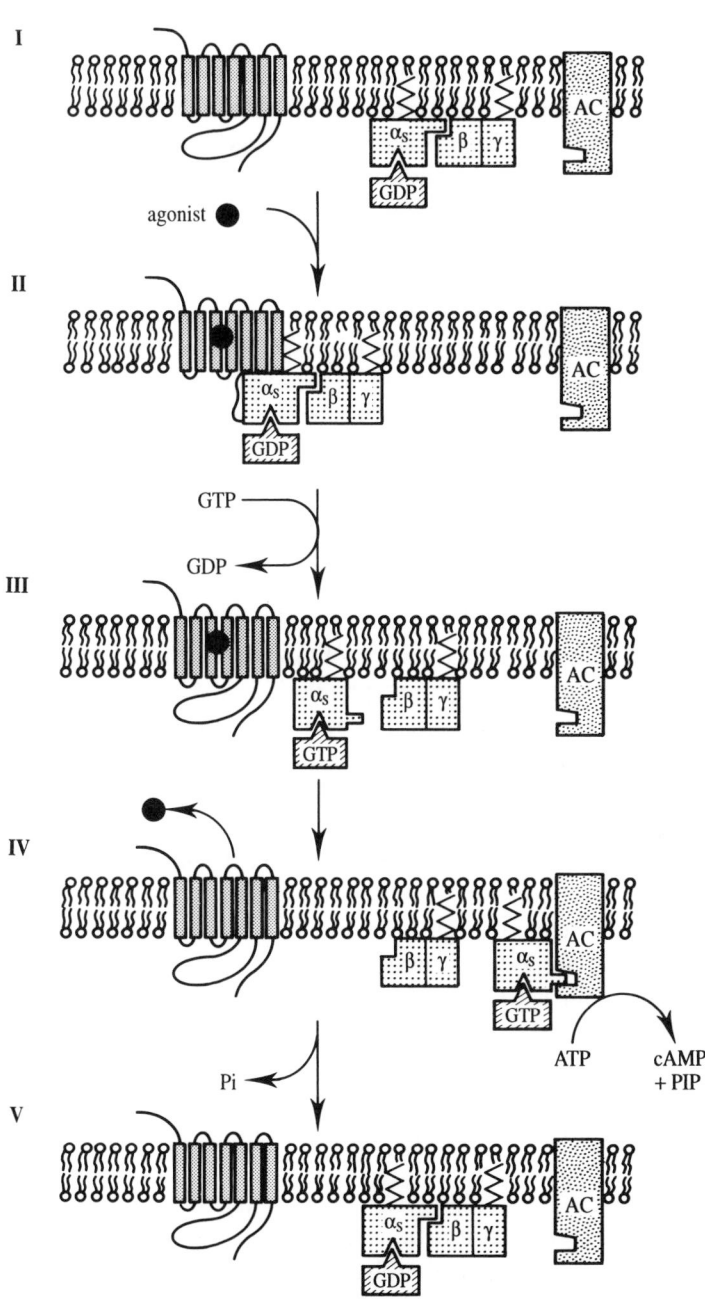

Fig. 5.5 Activation of G-proteins. G-proteins are compounds of three subunits (α, β and γ). Interaction of the α-subunit with an agonist-stimulated receptor (I) causes exchange of the bound GDP with GTP (II–III). The α-GTP complex dissociates and interacts with an effector (for instance adenylyl cyclase) (IV). The α-subunit catalyses hydrolysis of the bound GTP to GDP (V) and reassociates with the β-δ dimer (I). (Adapted, with permission from Gies, J.-P. (1993) *Bases de pharmacologie moléculaire*. Published by Ellipses–Édition Marketing, Paris.)

decreasing mass. The trimer is necessary for interaction with the receptor, but dissociation of the subunits is required for activation.

Interaction of the G-protein with an appropriate agonist–receptor complex promotes the dissociation of GDP and permits binding of the more prevalent cellular guanine nucleotide, GTP. This interaction between GTP and the G-protein's α-subunit is believed to promote dissociation of α-GTP from a complex of the β and γ subunits. In this dissociated state the G-protein modulates the activity of an effector. Slow hydrolysis of bound GTP by the GTPase intrinsic to the α-subunit leads to reassociation of the oligomer and cessation of the signal (Fig. 5.5). At present, there is an ongoing debate about which subunit is the active mediator of hormonal signal to effector. There are arguments for the variant α-subunit and also for the invariant β-γ dimer.

The key aspect in the function of G-proteins is that they are freely diffusible in the plane and can interact with several different receptors and effectors in a promiscuous fashion. A number of G-protein-linked receptors have recently been shown to regulate multiple effector pathways both when expressed endogenously and, more frequently, following transfection into heterologous systems. Direct evidence for the interaction of a single receptor with multiple classes of G-proteins has been obtained. The thyrotrophin-releasing hormone (THR) G-protein-linked receptor has, for example, recently been shown to be able to activate both adenylyl cyclase and phosphoinositidase C, probably by interacting with two different G-proteins.[36] In another case, a single receptor can modulate two distinct effectors by interacting with a single G-protein. In particular the α_2-adrenoceptor, when expressed at high level in fibroblasts, has been shown to inhibit adenylyl cyclase and to stimulate phosphoinositidase C. This may be a reflection of Gi-α-mediated inhibition of adenylyl cyclase and a Gi-β-γ-mediated activation of phosphoinositidase C.[37] Many other receptors have recently been shown to have multifunctional signalling that varies with the cell type.[38]

Thus, the receptor–G-protein–effector systems are complex networks of convergent and divergent interactions that permit extraordinarily versatile regulation of cell function.

4.   Effectors modulated by the G-protein-coupled receptors

This family of membrane receptors regulates distinct effector proteins through the activation of GTP-binding proteins known as G-proteins. The targets of G-proteins include enzymes such as adenylyl cyclase, phospholipases C and A_2, and channels that are specific for Ca^{2+} or K^+. An individual cell may express one or more G-proteins, each of these responding to several different receptors and regulating several different effectors with selectivity patterns. It is not unusual that a cell has either several receptors that activate a common G-protein or several G-proteins regulated by a same receptor. We will now consider in more detail several effector systems (see also Chapter 3).

(a) Adenylyl cyclase/cAMP system.   Sutherland's studies revealed that the intracellular messenger cyclic 3',5'-adenosine monophosphate (cAMP) is a nucleotide synthesized within the cell from ATP by the action of adenylyl cyclase. Receptors linked to Gs activate adenylyl cyclase and those linked to Gi inhibit the enzyme and reduce the cAMP formation.

Cloning and the modelled topography revealed that this enzyme contained a pair of six membrane-spanning segments separated by a large cytoplasmic loop and one major extracellular loop containing one of the four possible glycosylation sites in the sequence. Two similar cytoplasmic domains of around 250 amino acids should be the nucleotide binding sites. These domains appeared to be similar to a cytoplasmic domain present in the four guanyl cyclases that have also been cloned. The adenylyl cyclase bears a striking resemblance to proteins of markedly different function such as transporters, channels (dihydropyridine-sensitive Ca^{2+} channel) and the drug efflux pump (P-glycoprotein) whose synthesis is enhanced in multidrug-resistant cells.[39]

The cAMP is broken down by phosphodiesterases that hydrolyse the 3'-phosphate ester to give the common inactive metabolite, 5'-AMP. There are also several pharmacological agents that elevate cAMP itself inside the cell, such as caffeine, the mild stimulant drug found in coffee, cocoa and tea. Isobutylmethylxanthine is another phosphodiesterase inhibitor which increases the cAMP content of the cells. The plant terpenoid forskolin stimulates cAMP formation by acting directly on the adenylyl cyclase.

A large number of drugs and neurotransmitters exert their effects by increasing or decreasing the catalytic activity of adenylyl cyclase and thus raising or lowering the cAMP content in the cell. There are numerous and varied regulatory effects of cAMP on cellular function, including, for example, enzymes involved in energy metabolism, ion transport, ion channel function leading to changes in neuronal excitability, cell differentiation, or contractile proteins. The biological effects can be as diverse as gluconeogenesis (glucagon in liver), lipolysis (adrenaline on β_1-receptors in adipocytes), Na^+/water reabsorption (vasopressin on V2 receptors in kidney), contraction (adrenaline on α_2 vascular smooth muscle receptors), and relaxation (acetylcholine on muscarinic M_2 receptors in the heart). These various effects are, however, all brought about by a common mechanism, namely the activation of protein kinases by the intracellular mediator, cAMP.

(b) Phosphoinositidase-C/diacylglycerol-inositol phosphate system.

The phospho-inositide system is an important intracellular messenger system. It is well established that receptor-dependent activation of phosphoinositidase C (PLC) results in the hydrolysis of phosphatidylinositol 4,5-bisphosphate (PIP_2) and the formation of two intracellular mediators: inositol 1,4,5-triphosphate (IP_3) and diacylglycerol (DAG). IP_3 binds to endoplasmic membrane receptors and liberates the calcium from the sequestered stores (intracellular vesicles), inducing an increase of cytoplasmic calcium. An increase in cytoplasmic calcium occurs in many cells in response to a wide variety of agonists or drugs. It is the most important pathway by which cellular effects are produced. An elevation of free calcium in the cell can induce, for example, a smooth muscle contraction, secretion from exocrine glands, and release of transmitters. The range of pharmacological effects induced by calcium elevation is too broad to be discussed on the present chapter.

DAG is the principal endogenous regulator of membrane-bound protein kinase C. So far, ten different PKC isoenzymes have been identified in different species, tissues and cell lines and more are being identified by reverse transcription of RNA.[40] It is now known to consist of a family of isoenzymes that differ in their structures, cofactor requirements and substrate specificities. These enzymes control phosphorylation of serine and threonine residues of a variety of intracellular proteins, also inducing a wide range of pharmacological effects: tumour propagation, inflammatory responses, contraction or relaxation of smooth muscle, increase or decrease of neurotransmitter release, increase or decrease of neuronal excitability (by phosphorylating ion channels), and receptor desensitization. There are other types of kinases involved in these pharmacological effects, such as those regulated by cAMP or cGMP and those controlled directly by the family of receptor-protein kinases (discussed later). This multitude of pharmacological effects underlines the importance of protein phosphorylation regulation. Potent and selective inhibitors of PKC have been shown to block activation of human T cells both *in vitro* and *in vivo*. Therefore, inhibition of PKC might represent a target mechanism for a new class of therapeutic agents aimed at T-cell-driven chronic inflammatory or autoimmune diseases, such as rheumatoid arthritis, and could be used to prevent graft rejection.[41]

(c) Regulation of ion channels.   G-protein-coupled receptors can control ion channel function by interacting directly with the channel. Intracellular messengers (cAMP or any others) are not involved in this pathway of activation. For example, muscarinic agonists relax the heart directly by causing opening of K^+ channels located in the pacemaker region of the atrium, and thus hyperpolarization. This mechanism of direct activation may be quite general. The G-proteins involved seems to be isoforms of the Gi family (Gi_1-α, Gi_2-α, Gi_3-α).

E.   Intracellular receptors

The question of how agonists and antagonists differ at the molecular level was approached most directly by the studies of steroid hormone receptors. Unlike membrane-bound peptide receptors, steroid receptors (glucocorticoids, mineralocorticoids, sex steroids, vitamin D), thyroid hormone and inducers of drug metabolism (tetrachlorodibenzodioxan, dioxin) are found in intracellular locations.

Following steroid binding, the complex is activated and binds to specific sequences in the chromatin (HRE; hormone responsive element) and initiates transcription and protein synthesis. These receptors are organized into three major domains:[42] a variable amino-terminal domain responsible for antigenic properties of the receptors; a relatively well-conserved carboxy-terminal domain which represents the hormone-binding domain; and a well-conserved, cysteine-rich central domain containing two Zn^{2+}-stabilized fingers, which mediates binding to specific sites on nuclear DNA to activate or inhibit transcription of the nearby gene.

It is therefore not surprising that the steroids are identified in many quarters of modern biology as agents that regulate gene expression. Another area of steroid action is related to their lipophilic character and their effect on cell surface events. For example, the efficacy of both synthetic and natural relatives of progestational steroids as local anaesthetics has been known for many years. However, the relatively high concentrations of steroids needed to produce such effects put such apparent membrane actions on the back burner. There is now some evidence that steroids affect the surface of cells and alter ion permeability as well as releasing of neurohormones and neurotransmitters.

Certain steroids positively modulate GABA-induced Cl^- flux in a manner that resembles that of the barbiturates, although the steroid modulatory site is believed to differ from that of the barbiturates.[43] Steroids are also able to activate different genes and thus activate varying patterns of protein synthesis. For instance, glucocorticoids enhance the production of anti-inflammatory compounds like annexins (lipocortin); mineralocorticoids stimulate the production of transport proteins (sodium channels) involved in renal tubular function.

There is also an impressive array of genomic and nongenomic effects of steroids on neural activity.[44]

III.   DRUGS ACTING THROUGH VOLTAGE-SENSITIVE ION CHANNELS

Ion channels are essential for a great range of functions such as muscle contraction, sensory transduction, and endocrine and exocrine secretions. The ion channels mediate Na^+, Ca^{2+}, K^+

VOLTAGE-GATED Na⁺ CHANNEL (α-subunit)

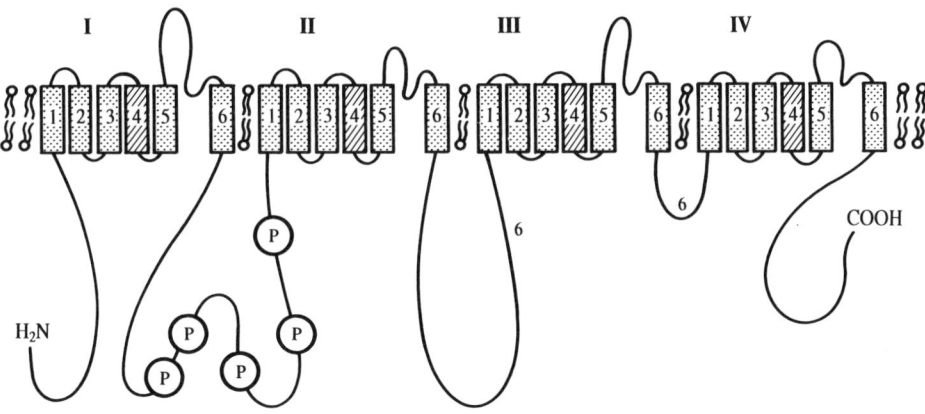

VOLTAGE-GATED Ca²⁺ CHANNEL (α-subunit)

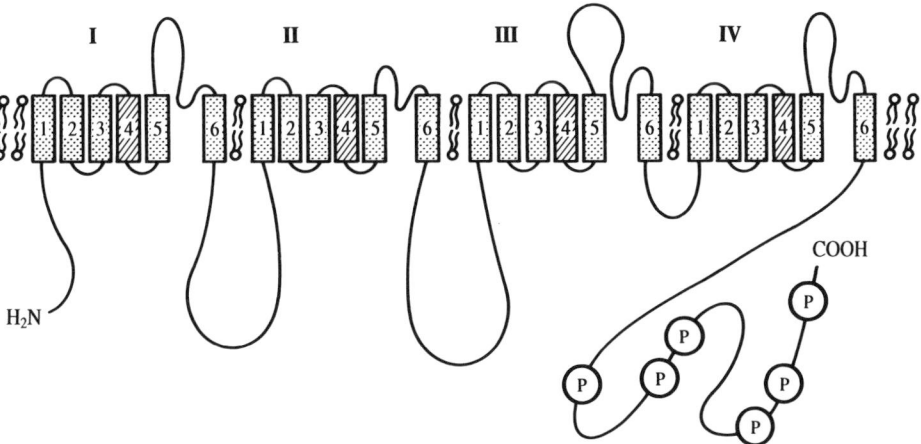

VOLTAGE-GATED K⁺ CHANNEL (α-subunit)

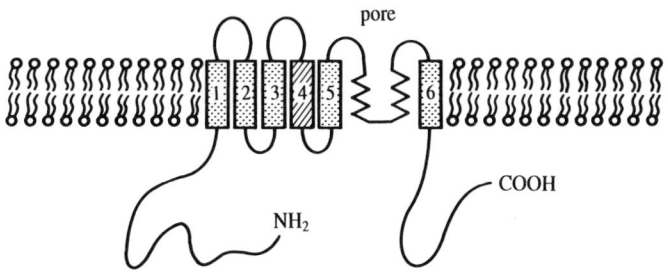

Fig. 5.6 Putative topology of the Na⁺ voltage-gated channel, the Ca²⁺ voltage-gated channel and the K⁺ voltage-gated channel. (Adapted, with permission from Gies, J.-P. (1993) *Bases de pharmacologie moléculaire.* Published by Ellipses–Édition Marketing, Paris.)

and Cl^- conductance induced by membrane potential changes. These channels propagate action potentials in excitable cells and are also involved in the regulation of membrane potential and intracellular Ca^{2+} transients in most eukaryotic cells. The molecular structures of the ion channels differ from those of the ligand-gated ion channels (or neurotransmitter channels) in which the ligand receptor and the ion channel form a single functional entity. Moreover, the voltage-gated channels reveal some common structural and functional features with the ligand-gated channels (Fig. 5.6). In this chapter we consider the main types of ion channels.[45]

A.   The Na⁺ channels

These play a critical role in initiating the action potential. The activation of the channels allows for the inward movement of Na^+ from the extracellular space of the cell. The Na^+ channels from brain and skeletal muscle are hetero-oligomeric and composed of α- and β-subunits. The α-subunit determines the major functional characteristics of Na^+ channels. It consists of an 1800–2000 residue polypeptide composed of four repeats, each containing six putative transmembrane helices.

The α-subunit shares significant homology with other voltage-gated ion channels, particularly the α_1-subunit of the Ca^{2+} channel.

Site-directed mutagenesis studies sugggest that: (1) the fourth membrane segment may act as the voltage sensor; (2) the cytoplasmic loop linking repeats III and IV is essential for inactivation and the region between segment V and VI forms the permeation pathway.

B.   The Ca²⁺ channels

The L-type Ca^{2+} channels are the best characterized of the voltage-gated Ca^{2+} channels. They are hetero-oligomeric and composed of α_1-, α_2-, β-, δ- and γ-subunits. The α_1-subunit provides the binding site for the L-channel blockers. Different types of the α_1-subunit, present in skeletal and cardiac muscle and brain, are encoded by distinct genes; alternative splicings may also occur. Each α_1-subunit includes four homologous repeats containing six transmembrane segments, and shares significant homology with other voltage-gated ion channels, particularly the Na^+ channel.

The Ca^{2+} channels of intracellular membranes, which regulate Ca^{2+} release from internal stores, comprise the ryanodin and inositol trisphosphate receptor families.[46] The sarcoplasmic reticulum Ca^{2+}-release channel of the skeletal muscle is the best ryanodin receptor that has been studied so far. It occupies a central position in excitation–contraction coupling in skeletal muscle by linking T-tubule depolarization to sarcoplasmic reticulum Ca^{2+} release.

C.   The K⁺ channels

The K^+ channel gene encodes only a single repeat and four polypeptides come together to form the channel. Four types can be distinguished:

- Voltage-dependent K^+ channels
- Ca^{2+}-activated K^+ channels
- Receptor-coupled K^+ channels
- Other K^+ channels (ATP-sensitive K^+ channels, Na^+-activated K^+ channels, etc.)

D. The Cl⁻ channels

Chloride channels have also been identified, for instance, one in epithelial cells and another in skeletal muscle. Malfunction of these channels is respectively responsible for cystic fibrosis and myotonia congenita.

The epithelial Cl⁻ channel is activated by cAMP. It is composed of 12 putative transmembrane helices, two hydrophilic nucleotide-binding domains and a large cytosolic regulatory domain containing phosphorylation sites. The most common mutation, found in over 70% of patients, is a single amino acid deletion in the first nucleotide-binding domain (Phe 508), which induces a decrease of the epithelial chloride conductance and is responsible for causing cystic fibrosis.[47]

The mammalian skeletal Cl⁻ channel belongs to a voltage-gated Cl⁻ channel and is formed by 12–13 putative transmembrane domains belonging to an 800–1000 amino acid sequence.[48] The deficit in the Cl⁻ conductance induces hyperexcitability of the skeletal muscle.

IV. DRUGS ACTING THROUGH TRANSPORTERS

For many years there was little information about these integral membrane proteins, but cloning and sequencing have considerably increased knowledge in this field. Transporter genes encode proteins, generally constituted of 12 transmembrane-spanning regions. These mediate Na⁺- or H⁺-dependent accumulation of small molecules such as neurotransmitters and antibiotics, and also ions, into the cells or organelles. The transport is achieved by different mechanisms: uniport, substrate–ion symport, substrate–ion antiport, substrate–substrate antiport or ATP-dependent translocation. The transporters can be classified into families and subfamilies based on ion dependence. The family that is of key importance for neurotransmitter uptake is that of the Na⁺/Cl⁻ dependent neurotransmitter transporters (see ref. 49). This contains monoamine-recognizing (dopamine, noradrenaline, 5HT) and amino acid-like (GABA, glycine, betaine, taurine, proline) subfamilies. Other families have been described such as the Na⁺/K⁺/glutamate transporter, the Na⁺-dependent glucose transporter, and the H⁺-dependent vesicular monoamine transporters.[50] These transporters, which are transmembrane proteins, represent sites of action of several drugs such as antidepressants or psychostimulants like cocaine. Portions of the Na⁺-dependent neurotransmitter transporter family that are important for activities in recognizing substrates and inhibitors are being defined by mutagenesis. Mutations on the single aspartic acid residue in the first transmembrane-spanning domain of the dopamine transporter reduce both dopamine and cocaine affinities, while mutation on serine residues of the seventh transmembrane domain reduces the transporter's affinity for dopamine without affecting that for cocaine.[51] This ability to dissociate cocaine-binding sites from dopamine ones is a key to the development of anticocaine drugs (molecules that will prevent cocaine binding without interfering with transport function). Some neurotoxins appear to bind onto transporters to enter the cell cytoplasm, where they exert their nerve-killing action. The possibility that neurodegenerative diseases such as Parkinson's disease may be triggered by such a process remains an attractive hypothesis. For instance, sensitivity to MPTP-induced toxicity can be conferred on normal cells by tranfection with the dopamine transporter, and this toxicity can be blocked by mazindol. Since nontoxic transport inhibitors block the toxicity of transported toxins, there is the possibility of preventing, by stopping or slowing, the progression of the neurotoxin-induced neurodegenerative diseases. These growing transporter families might represent templates for drug screening in the discovery of new therapeutic agents.

V.   DRUG ACTION MEDIATED THROUGH ENZYMES

Several families of drugs do not act on receptors, and their therapeutical properties are attributed to inhibition or activation of enzyme activities. A number of drugs in clinical use exert their effect by inhibiting a specific enzyme present either in tissues of individual under treatment or in those of an invading organism. The basis of using enzyme inhibitors as drugs is that inhibition of a suitable selected target enzyme leads to a build-up in concentration of substrate and a corresponding decrease in concentration of the metabolite, which leads to a useful clinical response. The type of inhibitor selected for a particular target enzyme may be important in producing a useful clinical effect. Enzyme-inhibiting processes may be divided into two main classes, reversible and irreversible, depending upon the manner in which the inhibitor is attached to the enzyme.

Reversible inhibition occurs when the inhibitor is bound to the enzyme through a suitable combination of Van der Vaals', electrostatic, hydrogen bonding and hydrophobic attractive forces. Reversible inhibitors may be competitive, noncompetitive, uncompetitive, or of mixed type.

During irreversible inhibition, after initial binding of the inhibitor to the enzyme, covalent bonds are formed between a functional group on the enzyme and the inhibitor. This is the case, for exemple, for the active-site-directed inhibitors (affinity labelling).

The inhibitors used in therapy must possess a high specificity towards the target enzyme, since inhibition of closely related enzymes with different biological functions could lead to a range of side-effects.

The importance of enzymes as drug targets is enormous and has long been an area of interest for structure-based drug design. For instance, reversible phosphorylation of proteins on serine, threonine and tyrosine residues by protein kinases and phosphatases is widely accepted as a principal mechanism by which eukaryotic cells respond to extracellular signals.[52] Many protein kinases and phosphatases have multiple substrates *in vivo*, enabling a diversity of responses to these extracellular stimuli. In view of the pleiotropic actions of the protein phosphatases involved in cellular regulation, compounds that regulate their activity may affect the phosphorylation state and thus the activity of many proteins. Two important enzymes are the serine/threonine protein phosphatases of type 1 (PP-1) and type 2A (PP-2A), for which an important range of potent inhibitor molecules has been described.[53]

There is a very large area of enzyme targets, as selectively illustrated in Table 5.2. For example dihydrofolate reductase (DHFR) catalyses the NADPH-linked reduction of dihydrofolate to tetrahydrofolate. The tetrahydrofolates are cofactors for the biosynthesis of nucleic acids and amino acids. Reduction of their level induces a limitation of cell growth.[54]

Thymidylate synthase methylates deoxyuridylate into thymidylate using 5,10-methylenetetrahydrofolate as a cofactor. This reaction is the rate-limiting step in the *de novo* synthetic pathway to thymidine nucleotide. Antitumoral effects are obtained with antifolate compounds.[55]

A functional HIV protease is required for the production of infective virions; this key role of the protease in the viral life cycle makes the inhibition of this enzyme a potential way for

Table 5.2 Selective illustration of enzymes inhibitors.

Enzyme	Inhibitor	Disease
Dihydrofolate reductase	Methotrexate	Cancer
Thymidylate synthase	Fluorouracyl	Cancer
HIV reverse transcriptase	Zidovudine (AZT)	AIDS
HIV protease	U75875	AIDS
Angiotensin-converting enzyme	Captopril, enalapril	Hypertension
Cyclooxygenase	Aspirin	Inflammation, pain
Catechol-O-methyltransferase	Ro41-0960	Parkinson's disease
Acetylcholinesterase	Organophosphorus	Myasthenia gravis, glaucoma, Alzheimer's disease
H^+/K^+ ATPase 'proton pump'	Omeprazol	Gastric secretion, ulcers

therapeutic intervention in the treatment of AIDS.[56] The HIV-RT inhibitor zidovudine is an approved drug for use in combating AIDS. However, the toxicity and the rapid development of resistance is rate limiting for the use of such compounds.

Angiotensin-converting enzyme (ACE) inhibitors have been used for the treatment of high blood pressure,[57] and were designated using the carboxypeptidase structure as a model for Zn^{2+} protease action.[58] Captopril is a small, potent, orally available, dipeptidyl inhibitor of ACE. Acetylcholinesterase (AchE) hydrolyses the neurotransmitter acetylcholine and yields acetic acid and choline. AchE is a serine hydrolase inhibited by organophosphorus poisons as well as by carbamates and sulfonyl halides which form a covalent bond to a serine residue in the active site.[59] AchE inhibitors are used in the treatment of various disorders.[60]

VI. DRUGS INFLUENCING SYNAPTIC TRANSMISSION

Synaptic transmission is rapid and brief. As soon as the neurotransmitter interacts with its receptor, it is whisked away. Some kinds of neurotransmitters are destroyed by enzymes located in the vicinity of the synapse. More frequently, however, cells that release neurotransmitters have sites that recognize the particular type of neurotransmitter and activate an energy-requiring enzymatic system that pumps the transmitter into the interior of the cell. In some situations glial cells remove transmitter molecules from the synaptic space using a similar pump system. After the neurotransmitter is recognized by a receptor site on the postsynaptic cell, a number of biochemical events take place that translate the original message (recognition of the transmitter) into metabolic alteration into the cell. Drugs can influence the process of synaptic transmission in a number of ways (Fig. 5.7).

Because all neurotransmitters must be synthesized from precursor molecules in the presence of specific enzymes, a drug that inhibited one of those enzymes would impede the formation of neurotransmitters. For instance, certain drugs that treat high blood pressure stop the formation of noradrenaline, a neurotransmitter that increases blood pressure.

Some drugs interfere with the storage of neurotransmitters by causing them to leak out of synaptic vesicles. Once out of the vesicles, the transmitters are degraded by enzymes, leaving the nerve ending devoid of messenger molecules. Reserpine, a tranquillizer that also lowers blood

PRESYNAPTIC NEURON   POSTSYNAPTIC CELL
                                               (Cell or neuron)

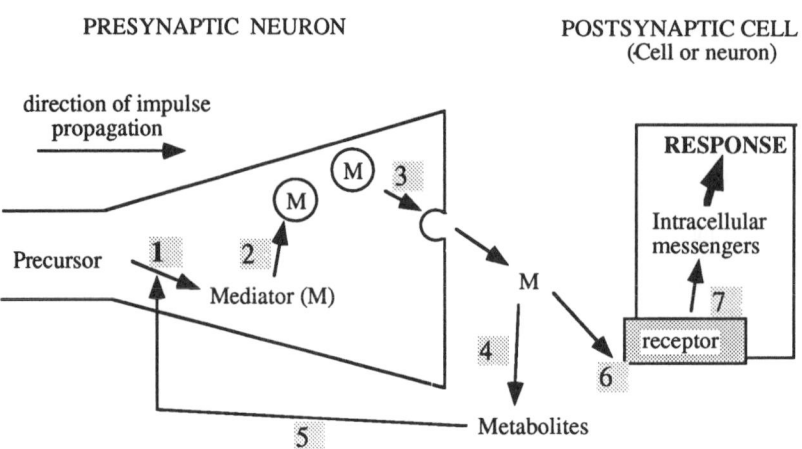

Fig. 5.7 Drugs influencing synaptic transmission by: (1) inhibiting enzymes that synthesize neurotransmitters; (2) preventing neurotransmitter storage in synaptic vesicles; (3) blocking the release of neurotransmitter into the synapse; (4) blocking enzymes that degrade neurotransmitters; (5) blocking neurotransmitter reuptake; (6) binding to the receptor and either mimicking or blocking neurotransmitters; (7) interfering with second-messenger activity. (Adapted, with permission from Gies, J.-P. (1993) *Bases de pharmacologie moléculaire*. Published by Ellipses–Édition Marketing, Paris.)

pressure, acts by interfering with the storage of noradrenaline.

Other drugs affect the release of neurotransmitters from nerve endings. Some of these compounds resemble the neurotransmitter in chemical structure and are thus able to slip into the vesicles in place of the transmitter molecules, virtually pushing the transmitters out into the synaptic cleft. Amphetamines act in this way to release noradrenaline or dopamine, for instance. In contrast, drugs like bretylium, a hypertensive agent, block the release process itself.

Some therapeutic compounds act by inhibiting enzymes that degrade neurotransmitters, thus augmenting levels of the transmitters and facilitating synaptic transmission. Certain antidepressants inhibit the enzyme monoamine oxidase, which degrades transmitters responsible for mood regulation. Other drugs facilitate synaptic transmission by blocking the reuptake inactivation process. Examples include the most widely used antidepressants, known as tricyclic antidepressants.

Some drugs bear a chemical resemblance to the neurotransmitter and mimic its effects at receptors, while others may occupy the receptor without causing any second-messenger response. These drugs generally block the access of the neurotransmitter to the receptor.

VII.   FUTURE DEVELOPMENT OF DRUG TARGETS

Oligonucleotides offer attractive potential alternatives to conventional drugs. The most significant is the relative ease of synthesis and the possibility of elaborating an oligonucleotide than can bind specifically and with high affinity to its target nucleic acid sequence either by Watson–Crick base pairing or by Hoogsteen base pairing. Both models have the potential to regulate gene expression and are under investigation in modulating human diseases.[61,62] The basic idea of these approaches is to interfere with the information flow from gene to protein, and to do so in a very specific manner. Agents that bind to single- or double-stranded nucleic acids are potential candidates for therapeutics targeted at specific genes, either at the mRNA (antisense) or the double-stranded DNA (antigene) level. Antisense oligonucleotides have potential as antiviral or anticancer agents.[63] For instance, antisense oligonucleotides have been designated for use against viruses, and especially retroviruses that are responsible for human infections. The human immunodeficiency virus (HIV) is associated with AIDS, the human T-cell lymphotropic virus (HTLV) is implicated in some human T-cell leukaemias. The specificity of the antisense oligonucleotides is derived from both its sequence and its length. The combination of specificity and affinity lowers the toxicity, owing to interference with other essential cellular metabolic functions, of the other antiviral agents such as nucleoside analogues or AZT (3'-azido-3'-deoxythymidine).

The antiviral properties of antisense oligonucleotides, their low toxicity and favourable pharmacokinetics provide an opportunity to design true isotypically selective pharmacological tools, and should allow the testing of many types of hypotheses in biomedicine.

REFERENCES

1. Ehrlich, P. (1956) The relation existing between chemical constitution, distribution and pharmacological action. In *The Collected Papers of Paul Ehrlich*, vol. 1. Pergamon Press, London.
2. Levine, R. R. (1990) *Pharmacology: Drug Actions and Reactions*, 4th edn. Little, Brown and Company, Boston.
3. Ross, E. M. and Gilman, A. G. (1990) Pharmacodynamics: mechanisms of drug action and the relationship between drug concentration and effect. In Gilman, A. G., Nies, A. S., Rall, T. W. and Taylor, P. (eds) *The Pharmacological Basis of Therapeutics*, pp. 35–48. Macmillan, New York.
4. Ehrlich, P. (1913) Chemotherapeutics: scientific principles, methods and results. *Lancet* **2**: 445–451.
5. Taylor, P. and Insel, P. A. (1990) Molecular basis of drug action. In Pratt, W. B. and Taylor, P. (eds) *The Principles of Drug Action: The Basis of Pharmacology*, 3rd edn, pp. 103–200. Churchill, New York.
6. Gies, J. P. (1993) *Bases de pharmacologie moléculaire*. Ellipses–Édition Marketing, Paris.
7. Sargent, P. B. (1993) The density of neuronal nicotinic acetylcholine receptors. *Annu. Rev. Neurosci.* **16**: 403–443.
8. Wisden, W. and Seeburg, P. H. (1992) GABA-A receptor channels: from subunits to functional entities. *Curr. Biol.* **2**: 263–269.
9. Peters, J. A., Malone, H. M. and Lambert, J. L. (1992) Recent advances in the electrophysiological characterization of 5-HT3 receptors. *Trends Pharmacol. Sci.* **13**: 392–397.
10. Mori, H., Masaki, H., Yamakura, T. and Mishina, M. (1992) Identification by mutagenesis of Mg^{++}-block site of the NMDA receptor channel. *Nature* **358**: 673–675.
11. Giraudat, J., Dennis, M., Heidmann, T., Chang, J. Y. and Changeux, J. P. (1986) Structure of the high affinity site for noncompetitive blockers of the acetylcholine receptor: serine-262 of the delta subunit is labeled by ³H-chlorpromazine. *Proc. Natl. Acad. Sci. USA* **83**: 2719–2723.
12. Pribilla, I., Takagi, T., Langosch, D., Bormann, J. and Betz, B. (1992) The atypical M2 segment of the beta subunit confers picrotoxin resistance to inhibitory glycine receptor channels. *EMBO J.* **11**: 4305–4311.
13. Yang, J., Mathie, A. and Hille, B. (1992) 5-HT3 receptor channels in dissociated rat superior cervical ganglion neurons. *J. Physiol.* **448**: 237–256.
14. Garbers, D. L. (1989) Guanylate cyclase, a cell-surface receptor. *J. Biol. Chem.* **264**: 9103.
15. Koesling, D., Boehme, E. and Schultz, G. (1991) Guanyl cyclases, a growing family of signal-transducin enzymes. *FASEB J.* **5**: 2785–2791.
16. Bazan, J. F., (1990) Structural design and molecular evolution of a cytokine receptor superfamily, *Proc. Natl. Acad. Sci. USA* **87**: 6934–6938.

17. Pawson, T. and Schlessinger, J. (1993) SH2 and SH3 domains. *Curr. Biol.* **3**: 434–442.
18. Marengere, L. E. M., Songyang, Z., Gish, G. D., Schaller, M. D., Parsons, J. T., Stern, M. J., Cantley, L. C. and Pawson, T. (1994) SH2 domain specificity and activity modified by a single residue, *Nature* **369**: 502–505.
19. Ihle, J. N., Witthuhn, B. A., Quelle, F. W., Yamoto, K., Thierfelder, W. E., Kreider, B. and Silvennoinen, O. (1994) Signaling by cytokine receptor superfamily: JAKs and STATs. *Trends Biochem. Sci.* **19**: 222–227.
20. Van Toi, H. H. M., Bunzow, J. R., Guan, H. C., Sunahara, R. K., Seeman, P., Niznik, H. B. and Civelli, O. (1991) Cloning of the gene for human dopamine D4 receptor with high affinity for the antipsychotic clozapine. *Nature* **350**: 610–614.
21. Sunahara, R. K., Guan, H. C., O'Dowd, B. F., Seeman, P., Laurier, L. G., Ng, G., George, S. R., Torchia, J., Van Toi, H. H. M. and Niznik, H. B. (1991) Cloning of the gene for the human dopamine D5 receptor with higher affinity for dopamine than D1, *Nature* **350**: 614–619.
22. Emorine, L. J., Marullo, S., Briend-Sutren, M. M., Patey, G., Tate, K., Delavier-Klutchko, C. and Strosberg, A. D. (1989) *Science.* **245**: 1118–1121.
23. Lomansey, J. W., Cotecchia, S., Lorenz, W., Leung, W. Y., Schwinn, D. A., Yang-Feng, T. L., Brownstein, M., Lefkowitz, R. J. and Caron, M. G. (1991) Molecular cloning and expression of the cDNA for the alpha-1A-adrenergic receptor: the gene for which is located on human chromosome 5. *J. Biol. Chem.* **266**: 6365–6369.
24. Perez, D. M., Piascik, M. T. and Graham, R. M. (1991) Solution-phase library screening for the identification of rare clones: isolation of an alpha-1D-adrenergic receptor cDNA. *Molec. Pharmacol.* **40**: 876–883.
25. Nagayama, Y., Wadsworth, H. L., Chazenbalk, G. D., Russo, D., Seto, P. and Rapoport, B. (1991) Thyrotropin-luteinizing hormone/chorionic gonadotropin receptor extracellular domain chimeras as probes for thyrotropin receptor function. *Proc. Natl. Acad. Sci. USA* **88**: 902–905.
26. Braun, T., Schofield, P. R. and Sprengel, R. (1991) Amino-terminal leucine-rich repeats in gonadotropin receptors determine hormone selectivity. *EMBO J.* **10**: 1885–1890.
27. Dohlman, H. G., Thorner, J., Caron, M. G. and Lefkowitz, R. J. (1991) Model systems for the study of seven-transmembrane-segment receptors. *Annu. Rev. Biochem.* **60**: 653–688.
28. Strader, C. D., Sigal, I. S., Register, R. B., Candelore, M. R., Rands, E. and Dixon, R. A. F. (1987) Identification of residues required for ligand binding to the beta-adrenergic receptor. *Proc. Natl. Acad. Sci. USA* **84**: 4384–4388.
29. Kobilka, B. K., Kobilka, T. S., Daniel, K., Regan, J. W., Caron, M. G. and Lefkowitz, R. J. (1988) Chimeric alpha-2, beta-2 adrenergic receptors: delineation of domains involved in effector coupling and ligand binding specificity. *Science* **240**: 1310–1316.
30. Wess, J. (1993) Mutational analysis of muscarinic acetylcholine receptors: structural basis of ligand/receptor/G protein interactions. *Life Sci.* **53**: 1447–1463.
31. Haddad E. B., Landry, Y. and Gies, J. P. (1990) Sialic acid residues as catalysts for M2-muscarinic agonist receptor interactions. *Mol. Pharmacol.* **37**: 682–688.
32. Lechleiter, J., Hellmiss, R., Duerson, K., Ennulat, D., David, N., Clapham, D. and Peralta, E. (1990) Distinct sequence elements control the specificity of G-protein activation by muscarinic acetylcholine receptor subtypes. *EMBO J.* **9**: 4381–4390.
33. Wess, J., Bonner, T. I., Dörje, F. and Brann, M. R. (1990) Delineation of muscarinic receptor domains conferring selectivity of coupling to guanine nucleotide-binding proteins and second messengers. *Mol. Pharmacol.* **38**: 517–523.
34. Ligget, S. B., Caron, M. G., Lefkowitz, R. J. and Hnatowich, M. (1991) Coupling of a mutated form of the human beta-2 adrenergic receptor to Gi and Gs; requirement for multiple cytoplasmic domains in the coupling process. *J. Biol. Chem.* **266**: 4816–4821.
35. Okamoto, T., Murayama, Y., Hayashi, Y., Inagaki, M., Ogata, E. and Nishimoto, I. (1991) Identification of a Gs activator region of the beta 2-adrenergic receptor that is autoregulated via protein kinase A-dependent phosphorylation. *Cell* **67**: 723–730.
36. Paulssen, R.H., Paulssen, E.J., Gautvik, K.M. and Gordeladze, J.O. (1992) The thyroliberin receptor interacts directly with a stimulatory guanine-nucleotide-binding protein in the activation of adenylyl cyclase in GH3 rat pituitary tumor cells. Evidence obtained by the use of antisense RNA inhibition and immunoblocking of the stimulatory guanine-nucleotide-binding protein. *Eur. J. Biochem.* **204**: 413–418.

37. Cotecchia, S., Kobilka, B. K., Daniel, K. W., Nolan, R. D., Lapetina, E. Y., Caron, M. G., Lefkowitz, R. J. and Regan, J. W. (1990) Multiple second messenger pathways of alpha-adrenergic receptor subtypes expressed in eukaryotic cells. *J. Biol. Chem.* **265**: 63–69.

38. Milligan, G. (1993) Mechanisms of multifunctional signalling by G protein-linked receptors. *Trends Pharmacol. Sci.* **14**: 239–244.

39. Gottesman, M. M. and Pastan, I. (1988) Resistance to multiple chemotherapeutic agents in human cancer cells. *Trends Pharmacol. Sci.* **9**: 54–58.

40. Chang, J. D., Xu, Y., Raychowdhury, M. K. and Ware, J. A. (1993) Molecular cloning and expression of a cDNA encoding a novel isoenzyme of protein kinase C (nPKC). *J. Biol. Chem.* **268**: 14208–14214.

41. Birchall, A. M., Bishop, J., Bradshaw, D. *et al.* (1994) Ro 32-0432, a selective and orally active inhibitor of protein kinase C prevents T-cell activation. *J. Pharm. Exp. Ther.* **268**: 922–929.

42. Beato, M. (1989) Gene regulation by steroid hormones. *Cell.* **56**: 335–344.

43. Turner, D. M., Richard, W. R., Yang, J. S. J. and Olsen and R. W. (1989) Steroid anesthetics and naturally occuring analogs modulates the gamma-aminobutyric acid receptor complex at a site distinct from barbiturates. *J. Pharmacol. Exp. Ther.* **248**, 960–966.

44. McEwen, B. S. (1991) Non-genomic and genomic effects of steroids on neural activity. *TIPS* **12**: 141–147.

45. Watson, S. and Girdlestone, D. (1994) Receptor and ion channel nomenclature. *Trends Pharmacol. Sci.* suppl 43–48.

46. Ehrlich, B. E., Kaftan, E., Bezprozvannaya, S. and Bezprozvanny, L. (1994) The pharmacology of intracellular Ca^{++} release channels. *Trends. Pharmacol. Sci.* **15**: 145–149.

47. Denning, G. M., Anderson, M. P., Amara, J. F., Marshall, J., Smith, A. E. and Welsh, M. J. (1992) Processing of mutant cystic fibrosis transmembrane conductance regulator is temperature sensitive. *Nature* **358**: 761–764.

48. Steinmeyer, K., Ortland, C. and Jentsch, T. J. (1991) Primary structure and functional expression of a developmentally regulated skeletal muscle chloride channel. *Nature* **354**: 301–304.

49. Landry, Y. and Gies, J. P. (1993) *Pharmacologie moléculaire: mécanisme d'action des médiateurs et des médicaments*, 2nd edition. Arnette Edition, Paris.

50. Henderson, P. J. F. (1993) The transmembrane helix transporters. *Curr. Opinion Cell Biol.* **5**: 708–721.

51. Kitayama, S., Shimada, S. and Uhl, G. R. (1992) Parkinsonism-inducing neurotoxin MPP+: uptake and toxicity in nonneuronal COS cells expressing dopamine transporter cDNA. *Ann. Neurol.* **32**: 109–111.

52. Fisher, E. H., Charbonneau, H. and Tonks, N. K. (1991) The control of cellular signalling mechanisms by tyrosyl phosphoprotein phosphatases. *Science* **253**: 401–406.

53. Quinn, R. J., Taylor, C., Suganuma, M. and Fujiki, H. (1993) The conserved acid binding domain model of inhibitors of protein phosphatase-1 and phosphatase-2-A. Molecular modelling aspects. *Bioorg. Med. Chem. Lett.* **3**: 1029–1034.

54. Roth, B. (1986) Design of dihydrofolate reductase inhibitors from X-ray crystal structures. *Fed. Proc.* **45**: 2765–2772.

55. Appelt, K., Bacquet, R. J., Bartlett, C. A. *et al.* (1991) Design of enzyme inhibitors using iterative protein crystallographic analysis. *J. Med. Chem.* **34**: 1925–1934.

56. Thompson, W. J., Fitzgerald, P. M. D., Hollowag, M. K. *et al.* (1992) Synthesis and antiviral activity of a series of HIV-1 protease inhibitors with functionality tethered to the P1 or P1' phenyl substituents: X-ray crystal structure assisted design. *J. Med. Chem.* **35**: 1685–1701.

57. Greenlee, N. J. and Siegl, P. K. S. (1991) Angiotensin/renin modulators. *Annu. Rep. Med. Chem.* **26**: 63–72.

58. Hooper, N. M. (1991) Angiotensin converting enzyme: implications from molecular biology for its physiological functions. *Int. J. Biochem.* **23**: 641–647.

59. Quinn, D. M. (1987) Acetylcholinesterase: enzyme, structure, reaction dynamics and virtual transition states. *Chem. Rev.* **87**: 955–975.

60. Taylor, P. (1990) Anticholinesterase agents. In Gilman, A. G., Nies, A. S., Rall, T. W. and Taylor, P. (eds) *The Pharmacological Basis of Therapeutics*, pp. 131–150. Macmillan, New York.

61. Erickson, E. P. and Izant, J. G. (1992) *Gene Regulation: Biology of Antisense RNA and DNA*. Raven Press, New York, 1992.

62. Agrawal, S. (1991) In Wickstrom, E. (ed) *Prospect for Antisense Nucleic Acid Therapy of Cancer and AIDS*, pp. 143–158. Wiley-Liss, New York.
63. Crooke, S. T. (1992) Therapeutic applications of oligonucleotides. *Annu. Rev. Pharmacol. Toxicol.* **32**: 329–376.

6

Strategies in the Search for New Lead Compounds or Original Working Hypotheses

CAMILLE G. WERMUTH

So ist denn in der Strategie alles sehr einfach, aber darum nicht auch alles sehr leicht.
Thus, in the strategy everything is very simple, but not necessarily very easy.
Carl von Clausewitz[1]

THE PRACTICE OF MEDICINAL CHEMISTRY
ISBN 0-12-744640-0

I. INTRODUCTION

Medicinal chemists have efficient methods for optimizing the potency and the profile of a given active substance. These methods may consist of more or less intuitive approaches such as the synthesis of analogues, isomers and isosteres, or the modification of ring systems. They may also rest on computer-assisted design, such as identifying pharmacophores by molecular modelling or optimizing activity by means of quantitative structure–activity relationships. In each case, at the start of the process, whether one is to identify a new chemical structure or a new mechanism of action, the medicinal chemist is responsible for developing as rapidly as possible more active molecules that are also both more selective and less toxic.

The real challenge is the absolute requirement to discover or identify an original research track. Indeed, no codified recipe exists for this major step, and the creativity of a laboratory cannot be planned. As a result, the discovery of a new lead substance represents the most uncertain stage in a drug development programme. Up to the 1970s the discovery of lead compounds depended essentially upon random occurrences such as accidental observations, fortuitous findings, hearsay or laborious screening of a large number of molecules. Since then, more rational approaches have become available, based on the knowledge of structures of the endogenous metabolites, the enzymes and the receptors, or on the nature of the biochemical disorder implied in the disease.

An analysis of the ways discoveries are made allows one to distinguish four strategies leading to new chemical entities usable as lead compounds. The first is based on the modification and improvement of already existing active molecules. The second strategy consists of the systematic screening of sets of arbitrarily chosen compounds in selected biological assays. The third approach involves the retroactive exploitation of various pieces of biological information that sometimes result from new discoveries made in biology and medicine, and sometimes are simply the fruits of more or less fortuitous observation. Finally, the fourth route to new active compounds is a rational design based on the knowledge of the molecular cause of the pathological dysfunction.

II. FIRST STRATEGY: IMPROVEMENT OF EXISTING DRUGS

The objective of this strategy is, starting from already known active principles, to prepare by various chemical transformations new molecules for which can be claimed an increase in potency, a better specific activity profile, an improved safety profile, or a formulation that is more easily handled by physicians and nurses or more acceptable to the patient.

In the pharmaceutical industry, motivations for this approach are often driven by competitive and economic factors. Indeed, if the sales of a given medicine are high and the firm is in a monopolistic situation, protected by patents and trademarks, other companies will want to produce similar medicines, if possible with some therapeutic improvements. They will therefore use the already commercialized drug as a lead compound and search for ways to modify its structure and some of its physical and chemical properties while retaining or improving its therapeutic properties. This approach lacks originality and has often been a source of criticism of the pharmaceutical industry. Each laboratory wants to have its own antiulcer drug, its own antihypertensive, and so on. These drug copies are referred to as 'me-too' products. Generally the firm that owns the original drug also continues to prepare new analogues, both to ensure a maximum perimeter of protection of its patents and to remain the leader in a given area. For these reasons, the chemical transformation of known active molecules constitutes the most widespread practice in pharmaceutical research (Fig. 6.1).

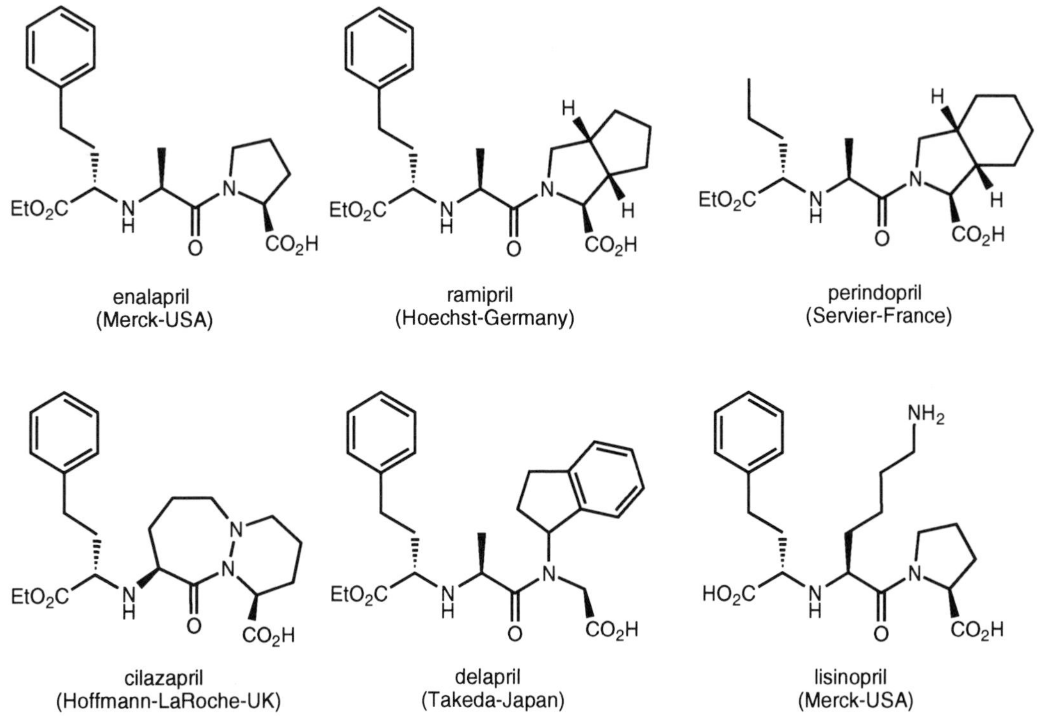

enalapril
(Merck-USA)

ramipril
(Hoechst-Germany)

perindopril
(Servier-France)

cilazapril
(Hoffmann-LaRoche-UK)

delapril
(Takeda-Japan)

lisinopril
(Merck-USA)

Fig. 6.1   Me-too copies derived from the angiotensin-converting enzyme inhibitor captopril.

A.   Pros and cons of therapeutic copies

A reassuring aspect of making a therapeutic copy is the certainty of ending with an active drug in the desired therapeutic area. It is indeed extremely rare, and practically very improbable, that a given biological activity is unique to a single molecule. Molecular modifications allow the preparation of additional products for which one can expect, if the investigation has been sufficiently prolonged, a comparable activity to that of the copied model and perhaps even a better one. This is comforting for the copiers as well as for the financiers that subsidize them. It is necessary, however, to keep in mind that the original inventor of a new medicine possesses a technological and scientific advantage over the copier and that he, too, had been able to design a certain number of copies of his own compound before selecting the molecule that provides the best compromises between activity, secondary effects, toxicity and monetary investment.

A second element that favours the copy derives from the information already gained, which then facilitates subsequent pharmacological and clinical studies. As soon as the pharmacological models that serve to identify the activity profile of a new prototype are known, it suffices to apply them to the therapeutic copies. In practical terms, the pharmacologist will know in advance what kind of activity is desired and which tests will have to be applied to select the desired activity profile. In addition, during clinical studies the original research undertaken with the lead compound will serve as a reference and can be adopted unchanged to the evaluation of the copy. Criticism of this approach is a result of the obvious fact that, in selecting a new active molecule using the same pharmacological models as were used for the original compound, one will inevitably end with a compound presenting an identical activity profile, and thus the innovative character of a such research is practically nil.

Finally, financial arguments may favour the therapeutic copy. Thus it may be important, and even vital, for a pharmaceutical company or for a national industry, to have its own drugs rather than to subcontract a licence. Indeed, in paying licence dues, an industry impovishes its own research. Moreover, the financial profitability of research based on me-too drugs can appear to be higher because no investment in fundamental research is required. The counterpart is that the placement of the copy on the market will naturally occur later than that of the original drug, and thus it will make it more difficult to achieve a high sales ranking, all the more so because the me-too drug will be in competition with other copies targeting a similar market.

In reality the situation is more subtle because very often the synthesis of me-too drugs is justified by a desire to improve the existing drug. Thus for penicillins, the chemical structure that surrounds the β-lactamate cycle is still being modified. Current antibiotics that have been derived from this research are more selective, more active against resistant strains, and can be administered by the oral route. They are as different from the parent molecule as a recent car compared to a forty-year-old model. Innovation can result from the sum of a number of stepwise improvements as well as from a major breakthrough.

It can also happen that during the pharmacological or clinical studies of a me-too compound a totally new property, not present in the original molecule, appears unexpectedly. Thanks to the emergence of such a new activity, the therapeutic copy becomes in turn a new lead structure. This was the case for imipramine, initially synthesized as an analogue of chlorpromazine and presented to investigators for study of its antipsychotic profile.[2] During its clinical evaluation this substance demonstrated much more activity against depressive states than against psychoses. Imipramine has truly opened, since 1954, a therapeutic avenue for the pharmacological treatment of depression.

III. SECOND STRATEGY: SYSTEMATIC SCREENING

This method consists in screening new molecules, whether synthetic or of natural origin, on animals or in any biological test without regard to hypotheses on its pharmacological or therapeutic potential. It rests on the systematic use of selective batteries of experimental models destined to mimic closely the pathological events. The trend is to undertake *in vitro* rather than *in vivo* tests: binding assays, enzyme inhibition measurements, activity on isolated organs or cell cultures, and so on. In practice, systematic screening can be achieved in two different ways. The first is to apply to a small number of chemically sophisticated and original molecules a very exhaustive pharmacological investigation: this is 'extensive screening.' The second method, in contrast, strives to find among a great number of molecules (several hundreds or thousands) one that could be active in a given indication: this is 'random screening'.

A. Extensive screening

Extensive screening is generally applied to totally new chemical entities coming from an original effort of chemical research or from a laborious extraction from a natural source. For such molecules, the high investment in synthetic or extractive chemistry justifies extensive pharmacological study (central nervous, cardiovascular, pulmonary and digestive systems, antiviral, antibacterial or chemotherapeutic properties, etc.) to detect whether there is interesting potential in these new structures. In summary, a limited number of molecules is studied in a thorough manner (vertical screening). It was by such an approach that the antihistaminic, and later the neuroleptic properties of the amines derived from phenothiazine, were identified. Initially these compounds had been submitted to a limited screening study directed towards possible chemotherapeutic, antimalarial, trypanocidal and anthelmintic activities, with negative results.

Original chemical research is also at the origin of the discovery of the benzodiazepines by Sternbach.[3] This author specifies that the class of compounds he was seeking had to fulfil the following criteria: (i) the chemical series had to be relatively unexplored; (ii) it had to be easily accessible; (iii) it had to allow a great number of variations and transformations; (iv) it had to offer some challenging chemical problems; (v) it had to 'look' as if it could lead to biologically active products.

The extensive screening approach has often led to original molecules; it is, however, highly dependent on the skill and the intuition of the medicinal chemist, and even more on the talents of the pharmacologist who has to be able to adapt and reorient the tests as soon as findings evolve to reveal the real therapeutic potential of the molecule under study.

B. Random screening

In this case the therapeutic objective is fixed in advance and, in contrast to the preceding case, a great number (several thousands) of molecules are tried, but on a limited number of experimental models. With this method one practises so-called random screening. This method has been used for the discovery of new antibiotics. It was by submitting samples of earth collected in countries from all over the world to selective antibacterial and antifungal screening, that the rich arsenal of anti-infectious drugs was developed that is presently at the disposal of the clinicians.

During the Second World War, an avian model in chickens infected with *Plasmodium gallinaceum* was used for the mass screening of thousands of potential antimalarials. The objective was to solve the problem of the shortage of quinine by finding a synthetic antimalarial. Unfortunately, no satisfactory drug was found. Presently massive screening is implemented in Europe and the United States to discover new anticancer and antiepileptic drugs. Here again the problem is to select some predictive but cheap animal model. It is a common criticism of these methods that, in the absence of a rational lead, they constitute a sort of fishing. Besides, the results are very variable: nil for the discovery of new antimalarials, rather weak for the anticancer drugs, but excellent, in their time, for the discovery of antibiotics.

More recent examples are seen in the discovery through systematic screening programmes of the cyclopyrrolones (e.g. zopiclone, Fig. 6.2) as ligands for the central benzodiazepine receptor,[4,5] or of taxol as an original and potent anticancer drug (for a review, see Suffness[6]). Other examples are the discovery by systematic screening of the antiherpetic properties of quinoline-3-carboxamides related to the antibacterial quinolones,[7] and by the discovery of the nonpeptidic neurotensin antagonist SR 48692.[8]

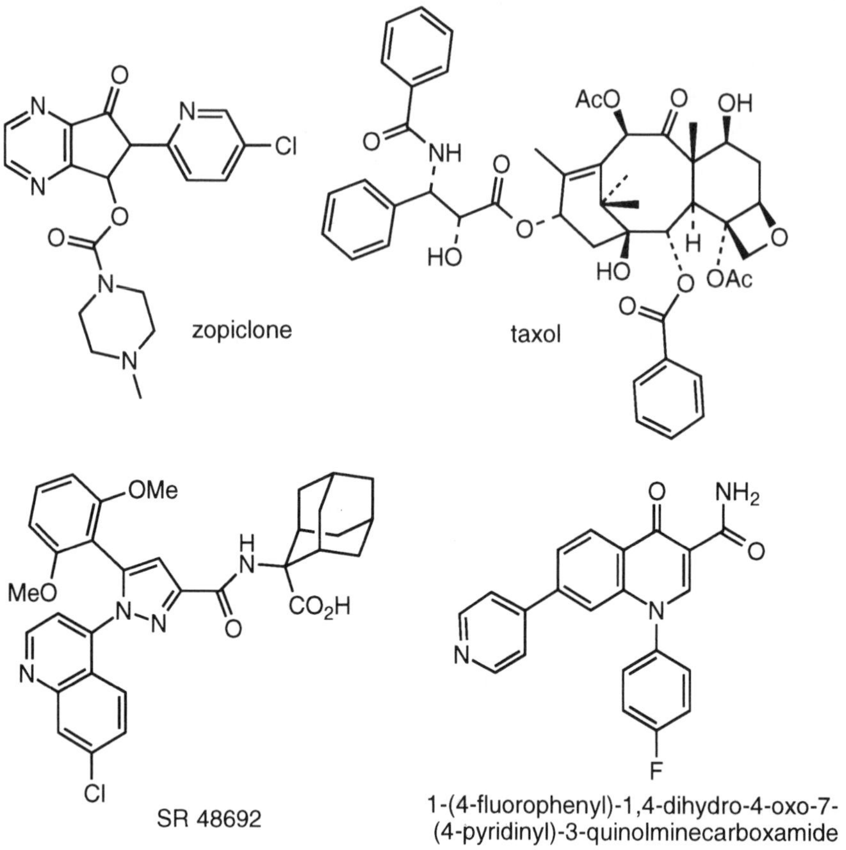

Fig. 6.2 Drugs discovered by random screening.

C. High-throughput screening

With the arrival of robotics and with the miniaturization of *in vitro* testing methods, it became possible in the 1980s to combine the two preceding approaches; in other words, to screen thousands of compounds on a large number of biological targets. This high-throughput screening is usually applied to the displacement of radioligands and to the inhibition of enzymes. As it now is possible for a pharmaceutical company to screen several thousand molecules simultaneously in 30 to 50 different biochemical tests, the problem becomes one of feeding the robots with interesting molecules. Primary sources are chemicals coming from company compound libraries or from commercial collections, but the samples can also be crudely purified vegetal extracts or fermentation fluids. In this latter case one proceeds to the isolation and identification of the responsible active principle[9,10] only when an interesting activity is observed.

Among the recent successes of this approach one can mention the discovery of lovastatin, also called mevinolin (Fig. 6.3),[11,12] which was the basis of a new generation of hypocholesterolaemic agents, acting by inhibition of hydroxymethylglutaryl-CoA reductase (HMG-CoA reductase), or that of asperlicin,[13] which is a nonpeptidic competitive antagonist of cholecystokinin (CCK)

lovastatin (mevinolin)   asperlicin

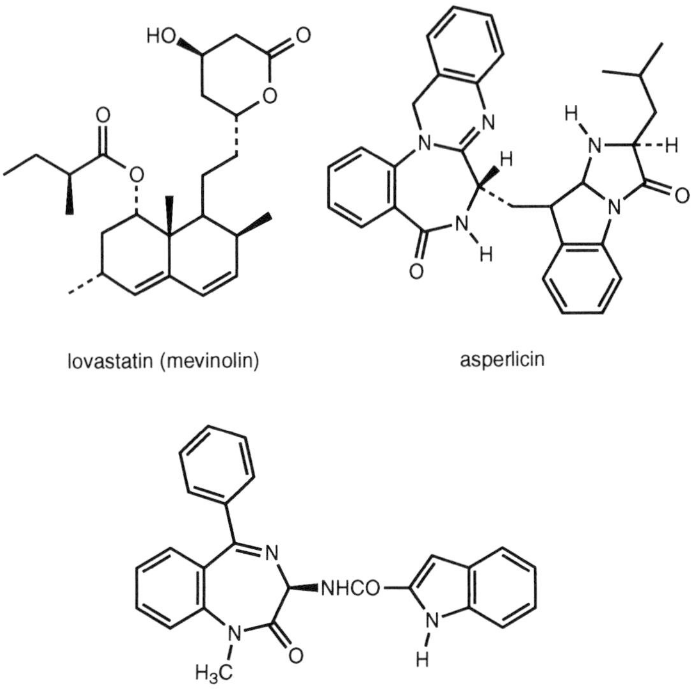

indolylcarboxamide

Fig. 6.3   Structures of lovastatin, asperlicin and a synthetic asperlicin analogue. Note a benzodiazepinic structure of natural origin in asperlicin. This structure was conserved in the synthetic indolylcarboxamide analogue.

and which has served as a model in the development of simplified, but extremely powerful, synthetic analogues such as the indolylcarboxamides.[14]

Very recently an extraordinary acceleration of synthesis technologies has occurred, rendering possible the simultaneous synthesis of hundreds or thousands of diverse molecules that are necessary to supply enough samples to the biochemical screening robots. As stated by Moos et al.,[15] 'The power of multiple compound synthesis methodologies suggests that more compounds have been synthesized and screened in the 1990s than in the combined histories of the pharmaceutical and biotechnology industries pre-1990.' Generation and screening of molecular diversity has become a major tool in the search for novel lead structures. Besides chemical laboratory synthesis, molecular diversity may derive from biological systems. The exploitation of biological systems is outside the scope of this book, but references can be found in the review of Bull et al.[16] On the other hand, biodiversity resulting from natural sources is treated in Chapter 7 and in refs 9 and 10. More chemistry-oriented approaches such as synthesis of peptide and of nonpeptide combinatorial libraries[15,17] for lead structure screening are detailed in Chapters 8 and 9. Finally, so-called electronic screening, which means finding the lead by database mining, is described in Chapter 11.

D.   A particular case: the screening of synthesis intermediates

As synthesis intermediates are chemically connected to final products, and as they often present some common groupings with them, it is not inconceivable that they also share some pharmacological properties. For this reason it is always prudent also to submit these compounds to pharmacological evaluation. Among drugs discovered in this way are the tuberculostatic semicarbazones: they were initially used in the synthesis of antibacterial sulfathiazoles. Subsequent testing of isonicotinic acid hydrazide, destined for the synthesis of a particular thiosemicarbazone, revealed the powerful tuberculostatic activity of the precursor, which has since become a major antitubercular drug (isoniazid).

IV. THIRD STRATEGY: EXPLOITATION OF BIOLOGICAL INFORMATION

A major contribution to the discovery of new active principles comes from the exploitation of biological information. By this is meant information that relates to a given biological effect (fortuitous or intentional) provoked by some substances in man, in animals, or even in plants or bacteria. When such information becomes accessible to the medicinal chemist, it can serve to initiate a specific line of therapeutic research. Originally, the observed biological effect might simply be noted without any rational knowledge of how it works.

A. Observations made in man

The activity of exogenous chemical substances on the human organism can be observed in various contexts: ethnopharmacology, popular medicines, clinical observation of secondary effects or adverse events, fortuitous observation of activities of industrial chemical products, and so on. Since in all cases the information harvested is observed directly in man, this approach represents a notable advantage.

1. Study of indigenous medicines (ethnopharmacology)

Natural substances were for a long time the unique source of medicines. At present, they constitute 30% of the active principles used and probably more (approximately 50%) if one considers the number of prescriptions that utilize them, particularly since use of antibiotics plays a major role.[18] Behind most of these substances one finds indigenous medicines. As a consequence ethnopharmacology represents a useful source of lead compounds. Historically, we are indebted to this approach for the identification of the cardiotonic digitalis glycosides, the opiates and the cinchona alkaloids. Curare was obtained from a South American plant long used by natives to make arrow poisons. The cardiotonic glycosides of *Strophantus* seeds and eserine from Calabar beans are other examples of useful drugs originally used by natives as poisons. *Rauwolfia serpentina* was used for centuries in India before Western medicine became interested in its tranquillizing properties and extracted reserpine from it. Atropine, pilocarpine, nicotine, ephedrine, cocaine, theophylline and innumerable other medicines have similarly been extracted from plants to which the popular medicine attributed therapeutic virtues.

Despite its extremely useful contributions to the modern pharmacopoeia, folk medicine is a rather unreliable guide in the search for new medicines. This is illustrated by the example of antifertility agents: according to the natives of some islands of the Pacific, approximately 200 plants would be efficient in reducing male or female fertility. Extracts have been prepared from 80 of these plants and have been administered at high doses to rats for periods of 4 weeks and more, without observing the slightest effect upon pregnancies or litter sizes.[19] When ethnopharmacology and the chemistry of natural substances result in the discovery of a new active substance, it is first reproduced by total synthesis. It is then the object of systematic modifications and simplifications aiming to recognize by trial and error the minimal requirements that are responsible for the biological activity.

2. Clinical observation of side-effects of medicines

The clinical observation of entirely unexpected side-effects constitutes a quasi-inexhaustible source of tracks in the search for lead compounds. Indeed, in addition to the desired therapeutic action, most drugs possess side-effects. These are either accepted from the beginning as a necessary evil, or recognized only after some years of use. When side-effects present a medical interest in themselves, one strategy may be to dissociate the primary from the side-effect activities: enhance the activity originally considered as secondary and diminish or nullify the activity that was initially dominant. For example, promethazine, an antihistaminic derivative of phenothiazine, has significant sedative effects. Like Laborit,[20] a clinician might promote the utilization of this side-effect and direct research towards better-profiled analogues. This impulse was the origin of chlorpromazine, the prototype of a new therapeutic series, the neuroleptics, whose existence was previously unsuspected and which has revolutionized the practice of psychiatry.[2,21] Innumerable other examples can be found in the literature, such as the hypoglycaemic effect of some antibacterial sulfonamides, the uricosuric effect of the coronary-dilating drug benziodarone, the antidepressant effect of isoniazid, an antitubercular drug, and the hypotensive effect of β-blocking agents.

This last example is beautifully illustrated by the discovery of the potassium channel activator cromakalim.[22] Cromakalim is the first antihypertensive agent shown to act exclusively through potassium channel activation.[23] This novel mechanism of action involves an increase in the outward movement of potassium ions through channels in the membranes of vascular smooth muscle cells, leading to relaxation of the smooth muscle. The discovery of this compound can be summarized as follows. β-Adrenergic receptor blocking drugs were not thought to have antihypertensive effects when they were first investigated. However, pronethalol, a drug that was never marketed, was found to reduce arterial blood pressure in hypertensive patients with angina pectoris. This antihypertensive effect was subsequently demonstrated for propranolol and all other β-adrenergic antagonists.[24] Later there were some doubts that blockade of the β-adrenergic receptors was responsible for the hypotensive activity and attempts were made, in the classical β-blocking molecules, to dissociate the β-blockade from the antihypertensive activity. Among the various conceivable molecular variations that are possible for the flexible β-blockers, it was found that conformational restriction obtained in cyclizing the carbon atom bearing the terminal amino group onto the aromatic ring yielded derivatives devoid of β-blocking activity, but retaining the antihypertensive activity (Fig. 6.4).

One of the first compounds prepared (compound 1, Fig. 6.4) was indeed found to lower blood pressure in hypotensive rats by a direct peripheral vasodilator mechanism; no β-blocking activity was observed. Optimization of the activity led to the 6-cyano-4-pyrrolidinylbenzopyran (compound 2), which was more than a hundredfold more potent than the nitro derivative. The replacement of the pyrrolidine by a pyrrolidinone (which is the active metabolite) produced a threefold increase in activity and the optical resolution led to the (−)-3S,4R enantiomer of cromakalim (BRL 38227), which concentrates almost exclusively the hypotensive activity.[22,25,26]

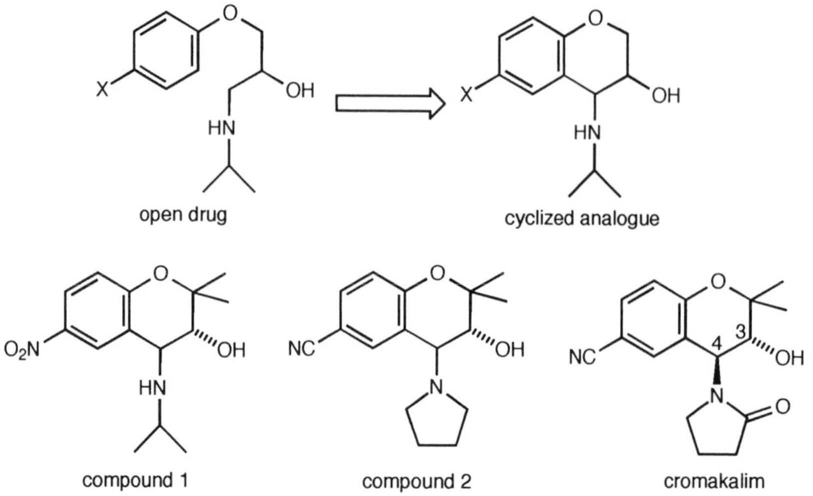

Fig. 6.4 Clinical observation of the hypotensive activity of the 'open' (and therefore flexible) β-blocking agents was the initial lead to cyclized analogues devoid of β-blocking activity, but retaining the antihypertensive activity.[22]

In many therapeutic families each generation of compounds induces the birth of the following one. This happened in the past for the sulfonamides, penicillins, steroids, prostaglandins, and tricyclic psychotropics families, and one can draw real genealogical trees representing the progeny of the discoveries. More recent examples are found in the domain of ACE inhibitors (Fig. 6.1) and in the family of histaminergic H_2 antagonists (see Figs. 6.9 and 13.7). Research programmes based on the exploitation of side-effects are of great interest in the discovery of new tracks in so far as they depend on information about activities *observed directly in man* and not in animals. On the other hand they allow detection of new therapeutic activities *even when no pharmacological models in animals exist.*

3.   Fortuitous discovery of activities of industrial chemical products

During the industrial manufacture of nitroglycerine, toxic manifestations due to this compound, i.e., particularly strong vasodilating properties, were observed in workers. From this observation came the clinical utilization of this substance, and later of other nitric esters of aliphatic alcohols, in angina pectoris and as cerebral vasodilators. In an analogous manner it observed during the manufacture of the sulfa drug sulfathiazole that 2-amino-4-thiazole, one of the starting materials, was endowed with antithyroidal properties. This observation fostered the use of this compound, and of aminothiazoles in general, for the treatment of thyroid gland hyperactivity. Tetraethylthiurame disulphide was originally used as antioxidant in the rubber industry. After having handled this product, workers felt an intolerance to alcohol and it was proposed for alcohol withdrawal cures (disulfiram). On the molecular level, the mode of action of disulfiram rests on the inhibition of the enzyme aldehyde dehydrogenase that normally ensures the oxidation of acetaldehyde to acetic acid. The intake of alcohol under disulfiram medication provokes an accumulation of acetaldehyde that produces flushing, pounding of the heart, dyspnoea and nausea.

B. Observations made in animals

We find here all the research done by physiologists that has been the basis of the discovery of vitamins, hormones and neurotransmitters. We also find here the outcomes of various pharmacological studies performed *in vivo*. Other observations made on animals, often in a more or less fortuitous manner, have led to useful discoveries. An example is provided by the dicumarol-derived anticoagulants described in Chapter 2.

The discovery of the anticancer properties of the alkaloids of *Vinca rosea*, periwinkle, constitutes a particularly beautiful example of pharmacological feedback. Preparations from this plant had the reputation in some popular medicines of possessing antidiabetic virtues. During a controlled pharmacological test these extracts were proved to be devoid of hypoglycaemic activity. On the other hand, it was frequently observed that the treated rats died from acute septicaemia. A study of this phenomenon showed that it was due to massive leukopenia. Taking the leukocyte count as the activity end-point criterion, it became possible to isolate the main alkaloid, vinblastine.[27] At the same time, in another laboratory, routine anticancer screening had revealed the activity of the crude extract on murine leukaemia.[28] Subsequently the antileukaemic activity became a screening tool. Out of 30 alkaloids isolated from various periwinkles, four (vinblastine, vinleurosine, vincristine and vinrosidine) were found active in human leukaemias.[29]

Remember too that it was research on insecticides that led to the discovery of the organophosphorus acetylcholinesterase inhibitors by Schrader at the Bayer laboratory.[30] Study of their mechanism of action has shown that they act by acylation of a serine hydroxyl in the catalytic site of the enzyme. This was one of the first examples describing a molecular mechanism for an enzymatic inhibition.

C. Observations made in the plant kingdom and in microbiology

Among the numerous discoveries that we owe to the botanists and the pharmacognosts are the developments of tryptophan metabolites, and especially of indolylacetic acid.[31] This compound acts as a growth hormone in plants. *Para*-chlorinated phenoxyacetic acids (MCPA or methoxone, 2,4-D or chloroxone) are mimics of indolylacetic acid (bioisostery) and show similar phytohormonal properties. However, at high doses they serve as weedkillers. Ring-chlorinated phenoxyacetic acids were later introduced in molecules as varied as meclofenoxate (cerebral metabolism), clofibrate (lipid metabolism), and ethacrynic acid (diuretic).

The 5-hydroxylated analogue of indolylacetic acid is the principal urinary metabolite of serotonin. On the basis of two biochemical observations — the possible role serotonin in inflammatory processes and the increase of urinary metabolites of tryptophan in rheumatic patients — Shen, from the Merck Laboratories, designed anti-inflammatory compounds derived from indolylacetic acid. Among them in 1963 he found indomethacin, one of the most powerful non-steroidal anti-inflammatory drugs currently known.[32]

A particularly rich contribution of this approach in the therapeutic area has been the discovery and the development of penicillin (see Chapter 2). It initiated the discovery of many other major antibiotics such as chloramphenicol, streptomycin, tetracyclines, cephalosporins and rifampicin.

In conclusion, whatever its origin, the use of biological information constitutes a preferential source for original molecular research. It offers creative approaches that do not rest on the exploitation of routine pharmacological models. Once the lead molecule is identified, it will immediately be the object of thorough studies to elucidate its mechanism of action. Simultaneously, one will proceed to the synthesis of structural analogues, as well as to the establishment of structure–activity relationships and to the optimization of all the important parameters for its development: potency, selectivity, metabolism, bioavailability, toxicity, cost price, etc. Thus, even if the initial discovery was purely fortuitous, subsequent research must be thoroughly rational.

V.   FOURTH STRATEGY: PLANNED RESEARCH AND RATIONAL APPROACHES

The approaches that we have described so far leave too great a place to chance (screening, fortuitous discoveries) or they lack originality (therapeutic copies). The progress of pharmacology resulting from the development of very sensitive biochemical methods based on use of radiolabelled elements, from the contributions of molecular biology allowing better characterization of receptors, or from the possibilities offered by computer methods, has allowed us to envisage the design of drugs on a more scientific basis.

In spite of the technological advances, the key information that permits rational approaches to drug design is knowledge of the aetiology of a given disease, or at least of the biochemical processes that are disturbed. Thus, from the moment it was observed in patients suffering from parkinsonism that the dopamine levels in the basal ganglions were much lower than those found in the brains of healthy persons,[33] a symptomatic but rational therapy became possible. This therapy consists of administering L-3,4-dihydroxyphenylalanine (L-dopa); this amino acid is able to cross the blood–brain barrier, then to be decarboxylated to dopamine by brain dopa-decarboxylase. Initial clinical studies were undertaken by Cotzias, Van Woert and Schiffer.[34] Several hundred thousand patients have benefited from this treatment. However, 95% of the dopa administered by the oral route is decarboxylated in the periphery before crossing the blood–brain barrier. To preserve the peripheral dopa from this unwanted premature degradation, a peripheral inhibitor of dopa-decarboxylase is usually added to the treatment.

Other examples of the rational approach in pharmacology are the discovery of the inhibitors of the angiotensin-converting enzyme or of antagonists of histaminergic H_2-receptors.

A.   Example of the inhibitors of the angiotensin-converting enzyme

The angiotensin-converting enzyme catalyses two reactions that are supposed to play an important role in the regulation of arterial pressure: (i) conversion of angiotensin I, which is an inactive decapeptide, into angiotensin II, an octapeptide with a very potent vasoconstrictor activity; (ii) inactivation of the nonapeptide, bradykinin, which is a potent vasodilator (Fig. 6.5).

An inhibitor of the converting enzyme would therefore constitute a good candidate for the treatment of patients suffering from hypertension. The first substance developed in this sense was teprotide, a nonapeptide presenting an identical sequence to that of some peptides isolated in 1965 by Ferreira from the venom of *Bothrops jararaca*, a Brazilian viper (Fig. 6.6). Teprotide inhibits in a competitive manner the degradation of angiotensin by the converting enzyme. The presence of four prolines and a pyroglutamate renders this peptide relatively resistant to

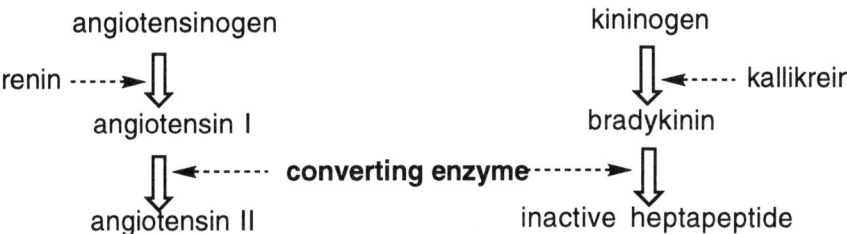

Fig. 6.5 Scheme of the renin–angiotensin and of the kallikrein–kinin systems. The converting enzyme (a carboxydipeptidyl hydrolase) is common to the two systems.

---

pyro-Glu-Trp-Pro-Arg-Pro-Glu-Ile-Pro-Pro-OH

Fig. 6.6   The structure of the nonapeptide teprotide.

hydrolysis, but not sufficiently to render it administrable by the oral route. In the search for a molecule offering better bioavailability, the reasoning of the Squibb scientists rested on the analogy of the angiotensin-converting enzyme to the bovine carboxypeptidase A.[35] Both enzymes are carboxypeptidases; carboxypeptidase A detaches only one C-terminal amino acid, while the converting enzyme detaches two. Furthermore, it was known that the active site of carboxypeptidase A comprises three important elements for the interaction with the substrate (Fig. 6.7): an electrophilic centre, establishing an ionic bond with a carboxylic function, a site capable of establishing a hydrogen bond with a peptidic C-terminal function, and an atom of zinc, solidly fixed on the enzyme and serving to form a coordinating bond with the carbonyl group of the penultimate (the scissile) peptidic function.

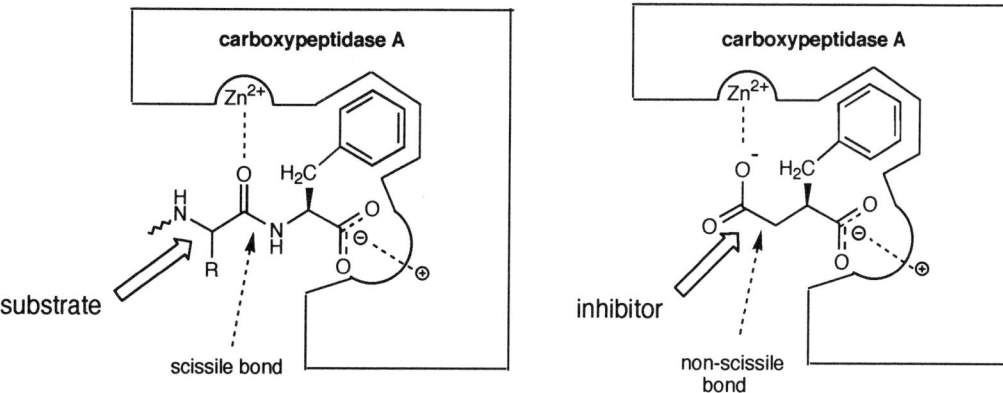

Fig. 6.7   Interactions between carboxypeptidase A and a substrate (left) or an inhibitor (right). (Adapted from Cushman ref. 35.)

By identifying that the conversion enzyme had a similar function, but altered by one amino acid unit (cleavage of the second peptidic bond instead of the first, departing from the terminal carboxyl group), scientists of the Squibb company elaborated the model shown in Fig. 6.8. According to this model, N-succinyl amino acids such as the succinyl prolines shown in Fig. 6.8 (left) should be able to interact with each of the above-mentioned sites based on first their proline carboxyl (ionic bond), their amide function (hydrogen bond) and then on the carboxyl of the succinyl moiety (coordination with the zinc atom). These compounds should then be able to act as competitive and specific inhibitors of the converting enzyme. A series of N-succinyl amino acids was then prepared and the N-succinyl-L-proline derivative (**1**) (Fig. 6.9) showed some activity (IC$_{50}$ = 330 μM). Amino acids other than L-proline lead to less active

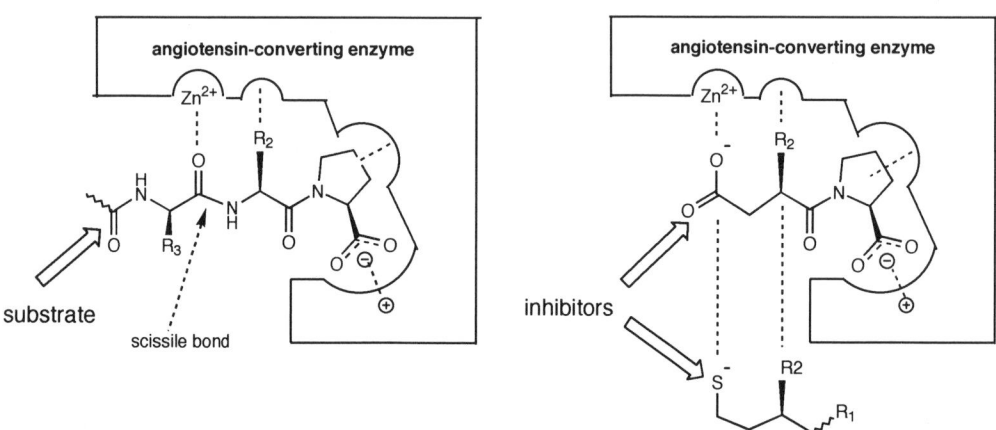

Fig. 6.8   Interactions between angiotensin-converting enzyme (a dipeptidyl carboxypeptidase) and a substrate (left) or inhibitors (right). (Adapted from ref. 35.)

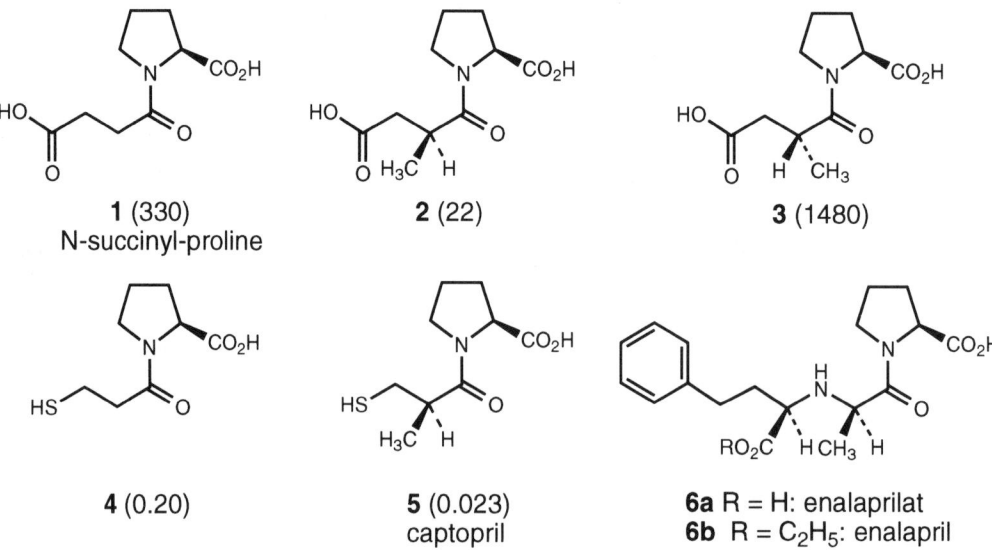

Fig. 6.9   Structures of some key compounds in the development of captopril and enalapril.[35]

succinyl derivatives; this result is in agreement with the fact that several peptidic inhibitors (notably teprotide) also possess a proline in the C-terminal position. In the present example N-succinyl-L-proline was selected as lead compound. The next task was then to optimize its activity. This was done by identifying the best interaction with the active site of the enzyme. Two steps were decisive in this quest: 'fishing for hydrophobic pockets' and the search for a better coordinant for the zinc atom (Fig. 6.9). The exploration of hydrophobic pockets was achieved by substituting the succinyl moiety with methyl groupings (four possibilities, taking account the regio- and the stereoisomers). The structure (**2**), methylated at position α to the amide, appeared clearly more active than (**1**) ($IC_{50} = 22$ instead of $330\,\mu M$). In this process, one observes an important stereoselectivity, since the IC_{50} value of epimer (**3**) of compound (**2**) falls to $1480\,\mu M$. The best coordination with the zinc was achieved by replacing the carboxyl function by a mercapto group. The gain resulting from this modification has been extremely important as shown by the comparison of compounds (**1**) and (**4**) or also (**2**) and (**5**). Compound (**5**) (SQ 14225) with an IC_{50} of $0.023\,\mu M$, and a K_i of $0.0017\,\mu M$ is active by the oral route and has been introduced into therapeutic use under the designation of captopril.

It is interesting to observe that the loss in affinity caused by the replacement of the mercapto function by a carboxyl rest was compensated with the help of an additional hydrophobic interaction. Thus, scientists from Merck developed enalaprilat (**6a**), a compound of comparable power to captopril in which the additional hydrophobic interaction is brought by a phenethyl substituent. Enalaprilat is poorly absorbed orally, and therefore the commercial compound is enalapril (**6b**), the corresponding ethyl ester.

B. Example of the H₂-receptor antagonists

Research to develop specific antagonists of the H_2 histamine receptor with a view to the treatment of gastric ulcers also proceeded through a rational process.[36,37] Starting from the observation that the antihistaminic compounds known at that time (antagonists of H_1-receptors) were not capable of antagonizing the gastric secretion provoked by histamine, Black and his collaborators envisaged the existence of an unknown subclass of the histamine receptor (the future H_2-receptor). From 1964 on, they initiated a programme of systematic search for specific antagonists for this receptor.

The starting point was guanylhistamine (**7**) (Fig. 6.10), which possesses weak antagonistic properties against the gastric secretion induced by histamine. The lengthening of the side-chain of this compound clearly increased the H_2-antagonistic activity, but a residual agonist effect remained. In replacing the strongly basic guanidino function by a neutral thiourea, burimamide (**8**) was obtained. Although very active, this compound was rejected for its low oral bio-availability. The addition of a methyl grouping in position 4 of the imidazolic ring, followed by the introduction of an electron-withdrawing sulfur atom in the side-chain, led finally to a compound that was both very active and less ionized, properties which improved its absorption by the oral route. The derivative thus obtained, metiamide (**9**) was excellent and, moreover, ten times more potent than burimamide. However metiamide, because of its thiourea grouping, was tainted with side-effects (agranulocytosis, nephrotoxicity), that would limit its clinical use. The replacement of the thiourea by an isosteric grouping having the same pK_a (N-cyanoguanidine) led finally to cimetidine (**10**) which became a medicine of choice in the treatment of gastric ulcers. Later it appeared that the imidazolic ring, present in histamine and in all H_2-antagonists

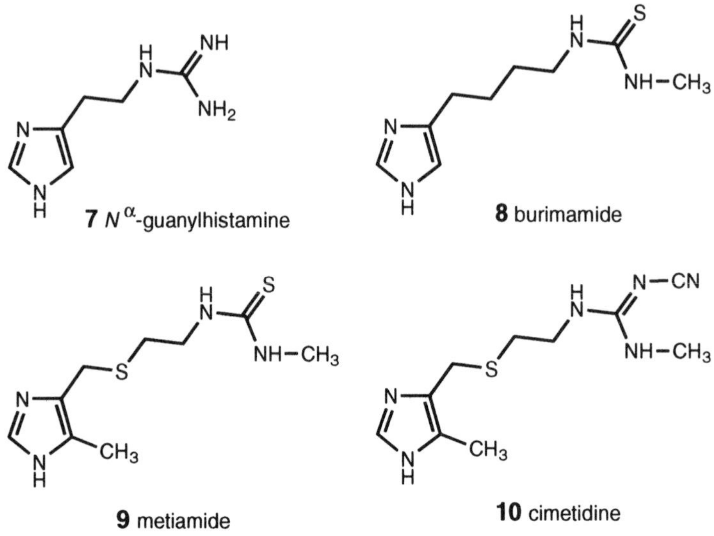

Fig. 6.10 Structures of some key compounds in the development of H_2-receptor antagonists.

discussed hitherto, was not indispensable to the H_2-antagonistic activity. Thus, the competitor products ranitidine, famotidine and roxatidine possess furan, thiazole and aryl rings, respectively (see Fig. 13.7, Chapter 13).

C.   Computer-assisted drug design

Computer-assisted drug design represents today one of the new developments in medicinal chemistry. It can be applied to any active molecule for which an interaction with a precise molecular target (receptor, enzyme, ion channel, transport protein, etc.) is postulated. In practice molecular modelling uses two approaches: the *direct* and the *indirect design* of active substances.[38] Direct design can be envisaged when the three-dimensional structure of the target macromolecule (enzyme, receptor) is known (see Chapters 24 and 25). The computer scientist is able, based on the structure determined by X-ray crystallography, to build the macromolecule with the help of the computer. He can then optimize the fit of the host molecule with its receptor and establish the best geometric and electronic complementarity between the ligand and its receptor. The structure of the ligand, its substituents and its conformation can be modified, and the most favourable conditions for interaction ('docking') can be simulated on the screen. However, this direct approach is limited by the small number of known three-dimensional structures of receptors. On the other hand, interesting examples of application to enzymes have been described (see Chapter 24).

When the three-dimensional structure of the target macromolecule is unknown (which is presently the case for most pharmacological receptors), indirect design constitutes the only possible approach. The strategy that is then employed has been described by Marshall *et al.*[39] as 'the active analogue approach'. One proceeds here to the comparison of a set of ligands selective for a given receptor, in order to reveal the molecular information that the compounds have in common despite apparently different chemical formulae (see Chapter 22). The objective is to determine the greatest common denominator (the 'pharmacophore') for the set under study.

The contribution of computer-assisted drug design to the discovery of new lead compounds is of somewhat limited value. This is due to the fact that molecular modelling studies only identify new ligands of already known biological systems. Similarly, quantitative structure–activity relationship (QSAR) methods only optimize already discovered series. Computer-assisted drug design nevertheless presents various advantages and even possesses some heuristic (inventive) power:[40]

(1) It can account for the lack of activity of certain analogues of the active structures. The knowledge of structural or electronic parameters leading to poorly active or inactive compounds is a cost-lowering factor that allows reduction of the number of compounds to be synthesized.

(2) It can discriminate stereoisomers. Stereospecificity is one of the principal attributes of pharmacological receptors and a perfect stereochemical complementarity between the ligand and the binding-site protein is an essential criterion for high affinity and selectivity.

(3) It can distinguish between agonists and antagonists. This is relatively easy for the specific category of antagonists which, according to Ariëns's theory,[41] derive from the agonists simply through the addition of some supplementary aromatic rings that play the role of additional binding sites (e.g. the passage from muscarinic agonists to muscarinic antagonists[42] or from GABA agonists to GABA antagonists).[43] The discrimination between the two categories becomes less evident when the passage from agonist to antagonist relies on relatively subtle changes such as as one observes for glutamate, oxotremorine and benzodiazepine antagonists.

(4) Molecular modelling can explain apparently paradoxical observations, e.g. the unexpected affinity reversal found in R and S enantiomers of the sulpiride series when changing N-ethyl to N-benzyl derivatives.[44]

(5) Molecular modelling can show some predictive power and lead to the design of new, more potent compounds or, better, of totally novel chemical structures, not evidently deriving from the translation of structural elements from one active series into another.

VI. CONCLUSION

The means leading to the discovery of new lead compounds, and possibly to new drugs, can be schematically classified into four approaches. These consist of the improvement of already existing drugs, of systematic screening, of retroactive exploitation of biological information, and of attempts towards rational design. According to which of these four strategies they apply, medicinal chemists can be seen as copiers, industrious, intuitive and deductive. It would be imprudent to compare hastily the merits of each of these characteristics. Indeed, 'poor' research can end with a universally recognized medicine and, conversely, a brilliant rational demonstration can remain sterile. It is therefore of the highest importance, given the random character of discovery and the virtual impossibility of planned invention of new active principles, that decision makers in the pharmaceutical industry appeal to all the four strategies that have been described and that they realize that they are not mutually exclusive. On the other hand, it would be inappropriate if, once a lead compound was discovered and characterized, its molecular mechanism of action were not studied: every effort possible should be made in this direction. In conclusion, all strategies resulting in identification of lead compounds are *a priori* equally good, provided that the research they subsequently induce is done in a rational manner.

REFERENCES

1. von Clausewitz, C. (1832) *Vom Kriege, Drittes Buch, 1. Kapitel Strategie.* 18th edn. Ferdinand Dümmlers Verlag, Bonn, 1973.
2. Thuilier, J. (1981) *Les dix ans qui ont changé la folie,* pp. 253–257. Robert Laffont, Paris.
3. Sternbach, L. H. (1979) The benzodiazepine story. *J. Med. Chem.* **22**: 1–7.
4. Jeanmart, C. and Cotrel, C. (1978) Synthèse de (chloro-5 pyridyl-2)-6-méthyl-4-pipérazinyl-1) carbonyloxy-5-oxo-7-dihydro-6,7-5*H*-pyrrolo[3,4-*b*]pyrazine. *Compt. Rend. Acad. Sci. Paris Ser. C.* **287**: 377–378.
5. Blanchard, J. C., Boireau, A., Garret, C. and Julan, L. (1979) *In vitro* and *in vivo* inhibition by zopiclone of benzodiazepine binding to rodent brain receptors. *Life Sci.* **24**: 2417–2420.
6. Suffness, M. (1993) Taxol: from discovery to therapeutic use. In Bristol, J. A. (ed.) *Annual Reports in Medicinal Chemistry,* pp. 305–314. Academic Press, San Diego,
7. Wentland, M. P., Perni, R. B., Dorff, P. H. *et al.* (1993) 3-Quinolinecarboxamides. A series of novel orally-active antiherpetic agents. *J. Med. Chem.* **36**: 1580–1596.
8. Gully, D., Canton, M., Boigegrain, R. *et al.* (1993) Biochemical and pharmacological profile of a potent and selective nonpeptide antagonist of the neurotensin receptor. *Proc. Natl. Acad. Sci. USA* **90**: 65–69.
9. Nisbet, L. J. and Westley, J. W. (1986) Developments in microbial products screening. In Bristol, J. A. (ed.) *Annual Reports in Medicinal Chemistry,* pp. 149–157. Academic Press, San Diego.
10. Hylands, P. J. and Nisbet, L. J. (1991) The search for molecular diversity (I). In Bristol, J. A. (ed.) *Annual Reports in Medicinal Chemistry,* pp. 259–269. Academic Press, San Diego.
11. Endo, A. (1985) Compactin (ML-236B) and related compounds as potential cholesterol-lowering agents that inhibit HMG-CoA reductase. *J. Med. Chem.* **28**: 401–405.
12. Lee, T. J. (1987) Synthesis, SARs and therapeutic potential of HMG-CoA reductase inhibitors. *Trends Pharmacol. Sci.* **8**: 206–208.
13. Chang, R. S. L. and Lotti, V. Y. (1986) Biochemical and pharmacological characterization of an extremely potent and selective nonpeptide CCK antagonist. *Proc. Natl. Acad. Sci. USA* **83**: 4923–4926.
14. Evans, B. E., Rittle, K. E., Bock, M. G. *et al.* (1988) Methods for drug discovery: Development of potent, selective, orally effective cholecystin antagonists. *J. Med. Chem.* **31**: 2235–2246.
15. Moos, W. H., Green, G. D. and Pavia, M. R. (1993) Recent advances in the generation of molecular diversity. In Bristol, J. A. (ed.) *Annual Reports in Medicinal Chemistry,* pp. 315–324. Academic Press, San Diego.
16. Bull, A. T., Goodfellow, M. and Slater, J. H. (1992) Biodiversity as a source of innovation in biotechnology. *Ann. Rev. Microbiol.* **46**: 219–252.
17. Dower, W. J. and Fodor, A. P. (1991) The search for molecular diversity (II): recombinant and synthetic randomized peptide libraries. In Bristol, J. A. (ed.) *Annual Reports in Medicinal Chemistry,* pp. 271–280. Academic Press, San Diego.
18. Kleemann, A. and Engel, J. (1982) *Pharmazeutische Wirkstoffe-Synthese, Patente, Anwendungen* (Preface). Georg Thieme Verlag, Stuttgart.
19. Price, J. R. (1965) Antifertility agents of plant origin. In Austin, C. R. and Perry, J. S. (eds) *A Symposium on Agents Affecting Fertility,* pp. 3–17. Little, Brown and Co, Boston.
20. Laborit, H., Huguenard, P. and Alluaume, R. (1952) Un nouveau stabilisateur végétatif, le 4560 R.P. *Presse Méd.* **60**: 206–208.
21. Maxwell, R. A. and Eckhardt, S. B. (1990) *Drug Discovery — A Casebook and Analysis.* Humana Press, Clifton.

22. Stemp, G., and Evans, J. M. (1993) Discovery and development of cromakalim and related potassium channel activators. In Ganellin, C. R. and Roberts, S. M. (eds) *Medicinal Chemistry, the Role of Organic Chemistry in Drug Research,* 2nd edn, pp. 141–162. Academic Press, London.

23. Hamilton, T. C., Weir, S. W. and Weston, A. H. (1986) Comparison of the effects of BRL 34915 and verapamil on electrical and mechanical activity in rat portal vein. *Br. J. Pharmacol.* **88**: 103–111.

24. Gerber, J. G. and Nies, A. S. (1990) Antihypertensive agents and the drug therapy of hypertension. In Gilman, A., Rall, T. W., Nies, A. S. and Taylor, P. (eds) *Goodman and Gilman's The Pharmacological Basis of Therapeutics,* 8th edn, pp. 784–813. Pergamon Press, New York.

25. Evans, J. M., Fake, C. S., Hamilton, T. C., Poyser, R. H. and Watts, E. A. (1983) Synthesis and antihypertensive activity of substituted *trans*-4-amino-3,4-dihydro-2,2-dimethyl-2*H*-1-benzopyran-3-ols. *J. Med. Chem.* **26**: 1582–1589.

26. Evans, J. M., Fake, C. S., Hamilton, T. C., Poyser, R. H. and Showell, G. A. (1984) Synthesis and antihypertensive activity of 6,7-disubstituted *trans*-4-amino-3,4-dihydro-2,2-dimethyl-2*H*-1-benzopyran-3-ols. *J. Med. Chem.* **27**: 1127–1131.

27. Noble, R. L., Beer, C. T. and Cutts, J. H. (1958) Role of chance-observations in chemotherapy: *Vinca rosea. Ann. N.Y. Acad. Sci.* **76**: 882–894.

28. Johnson, I. S., Wright, H. F., Svoboda, G. H. and Vlantis, J. (1960) Antitumor principles derived from *Vinca rosea* Linn. I. vincaleukoblastine and leurosine. *Cancer Res.* **20**: 1016–1022.

29. Johnson, I. S., Armstrong, J. G., Gorman, M. and Burnett Jr., J. P. (1963) The Vinca alkaloids: a new class of oncolytic agents. *Cancer Res.* **23**: 1390–1427.

30. Schrader, G. (1952) *Die Entwicklung neuer Insektizide auf Grundlage von Organischen Fluor und Phosphorverbindungen.* Monographie n.62. Verlag Chemie, Weinheim.

31. Albert, A. (1979) *Selective Toxicity.* 6th edn, p. 221. Chapman and Hall, London.

32. Shen, T. Y. (1972) Perspectives in non-steroidal antiinflammatory agents. *Angew. Chem. Int. Ed.* **11**: 460–472.

33. Ehringer, H. and Hornykiewicz, O. (1960) Verteilung von Noradrenalin und Dopamin (3-Hydroxytyramin) im Gehirn des Menschen und ihr Verhalten bei Erkrankungen des extrapyramidalen Systems. *Klin. Wochenschr.* **38**: 1236–1239.

34. Cotzias, G. E., Van Woert, M. H. and Schiffer, L. M. (1967) Aromatic amino acids and modification of parkinsonism. *N. Engl. J. Med.* **276**: 374–379.

35. Cushman, D. W., Cheung, H. S., Sabo, E. F. and Ondetti, M. A. (1977) Design of potent competitive inhibitors of angiotensin-converting enzyme. Carboxyalkanoyl and mercaptoalkanoyl amino acids. *Biochemistry* **16**: 5485–5491.

36. Black, J. W., Duncan, W. A. M., Durant, J. C., Ganellin, C. R. and Parsons, M. E. (1972) Definition and antagonism of histamine H_2-receptors. *Nature* **236**: 385–390.

37. Ganellin, C. R. (1982) Cimetidine. In Bindra, J. S. and Lednicer, D. (eds) *Chronicles of Drug Discovery*, pp. 1–38. John Wiley and Sons, New York.

38. Cohen, N. C. (1985) Rational drug design and molecular modeling. *Drugs Fut.* **10**: 311–328.

39. Marshall, G. R., Barry, C. D., Bosshard, H. E., Dammkoehler, R. A. and Dunn, D. A. (1979) The conformational parameter in drug design: The active analog approach. In Olson, E. C. and Christoffersen, R. E. (eds) *Computer-Assisted Drug Design*, pp. 205–226. American Chemical Society, Washington, DC.

40. Wermuth, C. G. and Langer, T., (1993) *Pharmacophore identification*. In Kubinyi, H. (ed.) *3D QSAR in Drug Design. Theory Methods and Applications*, pp. 117–136. ESCOM, Leiden.

41. Ariëns, E. J., Rodrigues de Miranda, J. F. and Simonis, A. M. (1979) The pharmacon-receptor-effector concept: A basis for understanding the transmission of information in biological systems. In O'Brien, R. D. (ed) *The Receptors*, pp. 33–91. Plenum Press, New York.

42. Wermuth, C. G. (1993) Aminopyridazines — An alternative route to potent muscarinic agonists with no cholinergic syndrome. *Il Farmaco* **48**: 253–274.

43. Rognan, D., Boulanger, T., Hoffmann, R., Vercauteren, D. P., André, J. M., Durant, F. and Wermuth, C. G. (1993) Structure and molecular modeling of $GABA_A$ antagonists. *J. Med. Chem.* **35**: 1969–1977.

44. Rognan, D., Sokoloff, P., Mann, A., Martres, M. P., Schwartz, J. C., Costentin, J. and Wermuth, C. G. (1990) Optically active benzamides as predictive tools for mapping the dopamine D_2 receptor. *Eur. J. Pharmacol. — Mol. Pharmacol. Sect.* **3**: 59–70.

7

Natural Products as Pharmaceuticals and Sources for Lead Structures

DAVID G. I. KINGSTON

The leaves of the tree were for the healing of the nations
Revelation 22:2, RSV
Accuse not Nature, she hath done her part; do thou but thine
Milton, *Paradise Lost*

THE PRACTICE OF MEDICINAL CHEMISTRY
ISBN 0-12-744640-0

I. INTRODUCTION

Despite major advances in the treatment of human sickness and disease with drugs over the past sixty years, many diseases remain which are presently untreatable. The ravages of cancer, although ameliorated to a large extent in some cases by surgery, radiation or chemotherapy, continue unchecked in other cases. The scourge of AIDS continues unabated by any curative treatment. Even bacterial diseases such as tuberculosis, once thought to have been conquered, at least in Western countries, have reared their pestilential heads again. It is small wonder, then, that both the medical profession and the pharmaceutical industries of the western world are vigorously continuing their quest for new and more effective pharmaceuticals to combat both old and new diseases. In the quest for new pharmaceuticals, the realm of natural products has frequently been overlooked. Natural products have, however, a unique contribution to make to new pharmaceuticals, either as the actual drug or as lead compounds for drug development. This chapter will thus address the contributions of natural products to drug discovery and development.

II. THE IMPORTANCE OF NATURAL PRODUCTS IN DRUG DISCOVERY AND DEVELOPMENT

The existence of bioactive compounds in plants and other natural sources has been known for millennia, and history records the use of poisons such as the hemlock that Socrates drank and the yew that a Gallic chieftain took to avoid captivity at the hands of Julius Caesar. The medicinal use of natural products is also very ancient, dating back at least to the first millennium BC, where the use of plants to treat cancer is recorded in the Ebers papyrus. The opium poppy has been used for thousands of years, and Sumerian tablets of 2500 BC noted that small balls of opium induced sleep and relieved pain. The quina tree of the Peruvian Andes, later renamed *Cinchona officinalis* by Linnaeus, was found to produce a substance that could cure malaria, and Charles II of England, among others, was treated with the so-called 'Jesuit powder', or cinchona bark. The active principle of this bark is the alkaloid quinine, useful for treatment of some forms of malaria.

  Given this history of the efficacy of plant-derived pharmaceuticals (and until this century essentially all pharmaceuticals were natural products), three questions cry out to be asked. In the first place, why do plants and other organisms produce compounds that are effective in human medicine? Secondly, why did the search for naturally occurring pharmaceuticals fall into disfavour in recent decades? Thirdly, what has brought about the present resurgence of interest in natural products as lead compounds in the pharmaceutical industry? Each of these questions will be discussed in turn.

A.   The origin of natural products

The question of the origin of natural products, often referred to as secondary metabolites, has long intrigued chemists and biochemists. Six major hypotheses have been proposed, and these have been well summarized by Haslam.[1] (1) Secondary metabolites are simply waste products, with no particular physiological role. (2) Secondary metabolites are compounds which at one point had a functional metabolic role, but which no longer do. (3) Secondary metabolites are products of random mutations, and have no real function in the organism. (4) Secondary metabolites are an example of 'evolution in progress', and provide a pool of compounds out of which new biochemical processes can emerge. (5) Secondary metabolism provides a way of enabling the enzymes of primary metabolism to function when they are not needed for their primary purpose. 'It is the *processes* of secondary metabolism, rather than the *products* (secondary metabolites) which are important.' (6) Secondary metabolites play a key role in the organism's survival, providing defensive substances or other physiologically important compounds.

Although each of these hypotheses has (or has had) its supporters, Williams[2] and Harborne[3] argue convincingly that the weight of evidence favours the sixth hypothesis. This hypothesis is consistent with the fact that most secondary metabolites are produced by plants and other organisms that cannot move, and must thus rely on chemical means of defence and attraction. In addition, annual plants like grasses, which can regenerate themselves readily each year, tend to have fewer secondary metabolites than more permanent plants such as shrubs and trees. A further consideration is that plants lack the immune system of vertebrates, and must thus rely on chemical means to defend against viruses. In addition, this hypothesis is consistent with the fact that the biosynthesis of secondary metabolites requires much metabolic energy and the storage of much genetic information, and it makes intuitive sense that all this energy and information should be used for some specific purpose. Put another way, there are simpler pathways that could have been used to get rid of waste products or to keep the enzymes of primary metabolism functioning, and the very complexity of many secondary metabolites thus argues for some specific function.

Finally, however, and most importantly in the present context, many secondary metabolites do indeed 'trigger very specific physiological responses . . . in many cases by binding to receptors with a remarkable complementarity'.[2] This incontrovertible fact provides a powerful incentive to search for bioactive compounds in the microbial, plant, and animal kingdoms, since it is assured that such compounds do exist and that some of them will be effective in treating human disease.

B.   The decline of natural products research

Given the history of the use of natural products as pharmaceuticals, coupled with the arguments for finding new bioactive constituents indicated above, it is surprising to learn that many of the major pharmaceutical companies, particularly in the United States, discontinued their research efforts in the plant-derived natural products field during the period 1960–1985. The reasons for this probably varied in detail from case to case, but underlying them all probably lay the perception that the natural products approach to drug discovery was slow, expensive and inefficient. In addition, the problems of scale-up of the isolation process and of the acquisition of adequate amounts of biomass undoubtedly served as additional deterrents to work in this area. Many pharmaceutical companies thus dropped research programmes on natural products, except for fermentation programmes where the logistics were already well worked out, in favour of chemical synthesis programmes where compounds could be produced much more readily than by the natural products approach. Even the US National Cancer Institute, long a bulwark of natural products research in the anticancer area, discontinued its plant collection and fractionation contracts in 1979. The prospects for natural products research in the pharmaceutical area thus appeared to be particularly gloomy in the 1980s.

C.   The rise of natural products research

Natural products research, especially in the pharmaceutical industry, has enjoyed a resurgence of interest over the last ten years. The reasons for this are varied, but the following stand out as particularly significant.

1.   The success of the natural products approach

The data of Table 7.1, dating from 1991, indicate that over half of the world's 25 best-selling pharmaceuticals are either themselves natural products or are derived from natural products.[4] Thus captopril was derived from the lead nonapeptide inhibitor SQ20,881, isolated from the

Table 7.1   The World's 25 best selling pharmaceuticals.

Position 1991	Product	Therapeutic class	Sales $m
1	Ranitidine	H_2 antagonist	3,032
2	[a]Enalapril	ACE inhibitor	1,745
3	[a]Captopril	ACE inhibitor	1,580
4	[a]Diclofenac	NSAID	1,185
5	Atenolol	β-antagonist	1,180
6	Nifedipine	Ca^{2+} antagonist	1,120
7	Cimetidine	H_2 antagonist	1,097
8	[a]Mevinolin	HMGCoA-R inhibitor	1,090
9	[a]Naproxen	NSAID	954
10	[a]Cefaclor	β-lactam antibiotic	935
11	Diltiazem	Ca^{2+} antagonist	912
12	Fluoxetine	5HT reuptake inhibitor	910
13	Ciprofloxacin	Quinolone	904
14	Amlodipine	Ca^{2+} antagonist	896
15	[a]Amoxycillin/clavulanic acid	β-lactam antibiotic	892
16	Acyclovir	Anti-herpetic	887
17	[a]Ceeftriaxone	β-lactam antibiotic	870
18	Omeprazole	H^+ pump inhibitor	775
19	Terfenadine	Anti-histamine	768
20	[a]Salbutamol	$β_2$-agonist	757
21	[a]Cyclosporin	Immunosuppressive	695
22	[a]Piroxicam	NSAID	680
23	Famotidine	H_2 antagonist	595
24	Alprazolam	Benzodiazepine	595
25	[a]Oestrogens	HRT	569

[a]Natural product-derived.
Reproduced with permission from ref. 4. Copyright 1993.

venom of the Brazilian snake *Bothrops jararaca*.[5] Lovastatin, an HMGCoA reductase inhibitor, was isolated from the fungi *Monascus ruber* and *Aspergillus terreus*.[6] The cyclic oligopeptide cyclosporin A, an immunosuppressant used to prevent organ transplant rejection, was isolated from the fungus *Trichoderma polysporum*.[7]

Not included in Table 7.1, but making a major contribution to cancer chemotherapy, are such natural products as vinblastine, vincristine, and paclitaxel (Taxol®) as well as the natural product derivatives etoposide, teniposide, and topotecan.[8] It is thus clear that the use of natural products as pharmaceuticals or as lead compounds for the development of pharmaceuticals has been a worthwhile endeavour, and there is every reason to believe that it will continue to be so.

2.   The uniqueness of the natural products approach

Natural products are often highly complex chemical structures, whether cyclic oligopeptides like cyclosporin A, or complex diterpenoids like paclitaxel. A perusal of the structures discussed in Section 4 is enough to convince any skeptic that few of them would have been discovered without application of natural products chemistry.

Not only are natural products structurally diverse, but they often provide highly specific biological activities based on novel mechanisms of action. This is illustrated by the HMG-CoA reductase inhibition of lovastatin, or the tubulin-assembly promotion activity of paclitaxel, for example; these activities would not have been discovered without the natural product lead. This bioactivity of natural products stems from the previously discussed hypothesis that essentially *all* natural products have some receptor-binding capacity. It thus remains simply to determine which receptor a given natural product is binding to.

Viewed another way, a given plant or other organism provides the scientist with a complex 'library' of unique bioactive constituents, analogous to the 'library' of synthetic products produced by combinatorial chemistry. The natural products approach can thus be seen as complementary to the synthetic approach, each providing access to very different types of lead compounds. The task of the natural products researcher is thus to select out those compounds of pharmacological interest from this 'natural combinatorial library'. Fortunately, the means to do this are now at hand.

3.   The impact of new screening methods

In the early days of natural products research, new compounds were simply isolated at random, or at best by the use of simple broad-based bioactivity screens such as antimicrobial screens or cytotoxicity screens. Although these screens did result in the isolation of bioactive compounds, including many of those described earlier, they have increasingly been seen as too nonspecific for the next generation of drugs. Fortunately, a number of robust and specific biochemical screens have been developed which can be used to detect bioactive compounds in complex matrices with great precision. The targets of the screens may be a particular cell type, a key regulatory enzyme, a receptor–ligand interaction, or a compound involved in gene transcription.

One interesting feature of these screens has increased the attractiveness of natural products to the pharmaceutical industry. The screens themselves are almost all highly automated and high-throughput screens. Because of this, the screening capacity at many companies is actually significantly larger than the potential input from in-house chemical libraries. For this reason, the major pharmaceutical companies are very interested in screening crude extracts as a low-cost means of discovering novel lead compounds; screening capacity is no longer a barrier to drug discovery.

4. The impact of new analytical techniques

The science of natural product isolation has undergone significant advances over the last 20 or so years. Chief among these advances has been the advent of routine high-performance liquid chromatography (HPLC), but other techniques such as thin-layer chromatography (TLC) and various liquid–liquid distribution methods have also shown significant advances. Although the isolation of a new bioactive natural product can still be a challenging task, this task can now be performed with greater speed and ease than ever before.

Similarly, advances in chemical instrumentation, particularly nuclear magnetic resonance (NMR) and mass spectrometry, have made the structure elucidation of even small amounts of complex molecules feasible. The isolation of a bioactive but highly complex natural product, in other words, is no longer a matter of despair, but instead a matter of excitement and hope, as the structure can be elucidated relatively rapidly and efficiently, and its very complexity may indicate a highly specific biochemical action.

III.   THE DESIGN OF AN EFFECTIVE NATURAL PRODUCTS-BASED APPROACH TO DRUG DISCOVERY

There are four major elements in the design of a successful natural products-based drug discovery programme: acquisition of biomass, effective screening, bioactivity-directed fractionation, and effective structure elucidation. Although some of these items have been touched on in the preceding section, it is instructive to bring them together here.

A.   Acquisition and extraction of biomass

The acquisition of biomass has undergone a significant transformation from the days when drug companies and others routinely collected microorganisms, plants, or marine specimens without any thought of reimbursement to the country of origin. Today, thanks to the Rio Treaty on Biodiversity and to an increased consciousness of the need to preserve and protect the world's biodiversity, all ethical biomass acquisition now includes provisions for the country of origin to be recompensed in some way for the use of its biomass. Such recompense is best provided through formal agreements with governments and collectors in the host country, such agreements providing not only for reimbursement of collecting expenses, but also for further benefits (often in the form of a percentage of product sales) in the event that a drug is developed from a collected species. Such financial benefit should be shared with the host country, and also with any indigenous peoples in cases where the biomass can be attributed to an area occupied by a particular indigenous group. A sample legal agreement which includes these and other provisions has been published.[9]

It goes without saying that the samples collected, be they microbial, plant, animal or marine, must be fully identified as to genus and species. Voucher specimens should be provided to an appropriate herbarium or other depository in the host country, as well as to an appropriate repository in the home country of the purchaser.

In the case of microbial and marine samples, extraction is normally carried out on the whole organism. In the case of plants, however, which may be large and have clearly differentiated parts, it is common to make separate extracts of different parts, such as root, stems, leaves and, in some cases, bark and fruit.

The procedure for extraction varies with the nature of the organism and, in some cases, with the type of bioassay being run. Some screens, for example, are sensitive to common and rather useless plant components such as tannins, and an extraction process which removes tannins may be necessary as a precursor to such a screen. In the simplest cases, however, extraction can be carried out with a solvent such as ethanol or methanol, which will extract most natural products of interest. Some workers prefer to carry out a sequential extraction, using a nonpolar solvent such as hexane followed by a moderately polar solvent such as ethyl acetate, and finishing with methanol or ethanol.

The selection of plant samples raises the question of the ethnobotanical approach versus a random approach. The ethnobotanical approach, which involves the selection of (usually) plants which have a documented use by native healers, is attractive in that it taps into the empirical knowledge developed over centuries of use by large numbers of people. The benefits of this approach have been extolled in several recent articles,[10-12] and one author provides personal verification of the effectiveness of some jungle medicines.[13] The weakness of the ethnobotanical approach has always been that it is a slow approach, requiring careful interviewing of native healers by skilled ethnobotanists. In addition, the presumed folkloric activity in the collected plant(s) may not be detectable, given the particular screens in use by the screening laboratory.

For these reasons many workers prefer to rely on a random approach, in which a skilled botanist collects plants on a random or semirandom basis. This approach yields the highest number of plant samples in the shortest time, but of course gives no assurance that any of them will be active.

One interesting experiment to test the relative effectiveness of the ethnobotanical and the random approaches to plant collection is currently underway in Suriname. In this study funded jointly by the NIH and NSF, two collection teams will be collecting plants in Suriname based either on an ethnobotanical approach or on a random approach. Extracts from both sets of collections will be tested by Bristol-Myers Squibb in the same group of screens, so it should be possible to draw some conclusions about the relative effectiveness of these two approaches.

B. Screening methods

As mentioned earlier, the advent of new robust and high-throughput screens has had a major impact on natural products research in the pharmaceutical industry. Most of the screens employed today are highly proprietary, and published information is thus rare, although general summaries of this approach have been published.[14-18] One screen that has been described in detail is the National Cancer Institute's 60 cell-line cytotoxicity screen for anticancer agents;[19] although this is not a receptor-based screen it is automated and high-throughput. A simple yeast screen to detect antitumour agents has also been described.[20] Workers in academia who may not have or need access to high-volume screens can develop their own individual assays, depending on the activity being sought. In the anticancer area, for example, simple brine shrimp and potato disk assays have been described,[21] while simple antimicrobial assays can still be used for the discovery of antibiotic compounds.[22]

C.   Isolation of active compounds

The isolation of the bioactive constituent(s) from a given biomass can be a challenging task, particularly if the active constituent is a minor component of the extract. The actual procedure used will depend to a large extent on the nature of the extract: a marine sample,[23] for example, may require a somewhat different extraction and purification process from a plant sample.[24] Nevertheless, the key feature in all fractionation processes is the use of an appropriate bioassay to guide the purification and ensure the isolation of the active compound. In many cases, HPLC will be needed to obtain the pure active compound, but other techniques such as countercurrent chromatography and planar chromatography also play important roles.

D.   Structure elucidation

Structure elucidation of the bioactive constituent depends almost exclusively on the application of modern instrumental methods, particularly NMR and MS. These powerful techniques, coupled in some cases with selective chemical manipulations, are usually adequate to solve the structures of most secondary metabolites of molecular weight up to about 2000. X-ray crystallography is also a valuable tool, but its application is often hindered by the difficulty of obtaining suitable crystals. However, it has made and will continue to make major contributions in situations where it can be applied.

E.   Biological assessment

Once the bioactive constituent has been obtained in pure form, it must be tested thoroughly in a range of biological assays to determine its efficacy, its toxicity, and its pharmacology. These tests will determine the new compound's spectrum of biological activity, and may also give some insight into its mechanism of action.

F.   Procurement of large-scale supplies

If the active compound successfully completes evaluation in the secondary and tertiary assays described above, then large amounts of material will be needed for preclinical toxicology and formulation trials and for eventual clinical use. The large supplies could be made available by cultivation of the plant or marine starting material, or by large-scale fermentation in the case of a microbial product. Chemical synthesis or partial synthesis may also be possible if the structure of the active compound is not too complex. The example of paclitaxel is instructive here: after initial large-scale production by direct extraction from *Taxus brevifolia* bark, it is now also produced by a semisynthetic procedure starting from the more readily available precursor baccatin III.[25]

Another method of obtaining adequate supplies of a natural plant product is by plant tissue culture methods. Although there are a few examples of the commercial production of secondary metabolites by plant cell culture (shikonin is perhaps the best-known one[26]), the application of this technique to commercial production of pharmaceuticals has yet to find general acceptance, primarily for economic reasons.[27] It is quite probable, however, that this approach will find wider acceptance in the future, as yields are improved and costs reduced.

G. Determination of structure–activity relationships

The lead compound isolated from the biomass, whether microbial, plant, marine or animal, is not necessarily the best compound for pharmaceutical use. Once the lead compound has been obtained, however, analogues can be prepared either by total synthesis or by chemical modification of the natural product, and various structure–activity relationships can be worked out. In many cases these studies have led to semisynthetic or synthetic products which surpass the natural product in efficacy or in lack of side-effects or in other ways, and some examples will be discussed in Section IV below.

IV. EXAMPLES OF NATURAL PRODUCTS OR ANALOGUES AS PHARMACEUTICALS

A. Cromolyn sodium

This synthetic product (**1**), which has achieved wide usage as an antiasthmatic drug, was developed after observations on the vasodilator effects of khellin (**2**), a chromone isolated from the umbelliferous plant *Ammi visnaga*.[28]

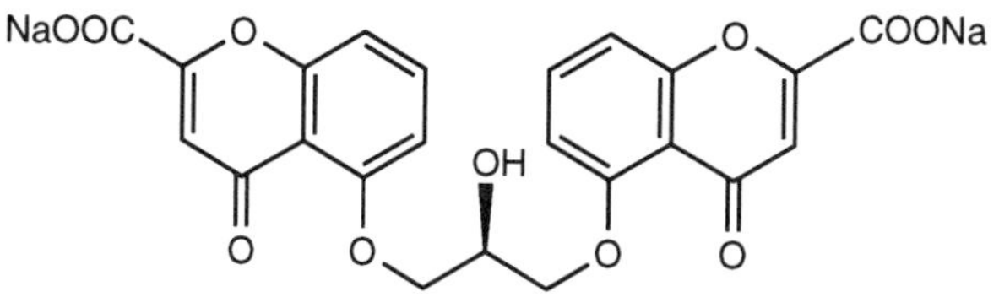

1

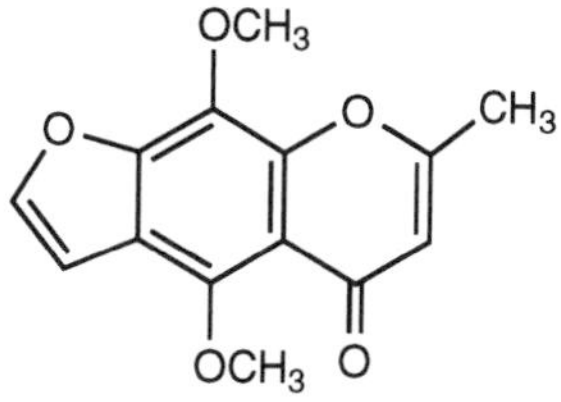

2

B. Captopril

This synthetic product (**3**) was derived from a nonapeptide inhibitor SQ 20,881 (**4**), which was isolated from the venom of the Brazilian snake *Bothrops jararaca*.[5] Careful and extensive studies of structure–activity relationships led to the synthesis of Captopril and its development as a blood pressure lowering agent by virtue of its angiotensin converting enzyme (ACE) inhibition activity (Chapter 6).

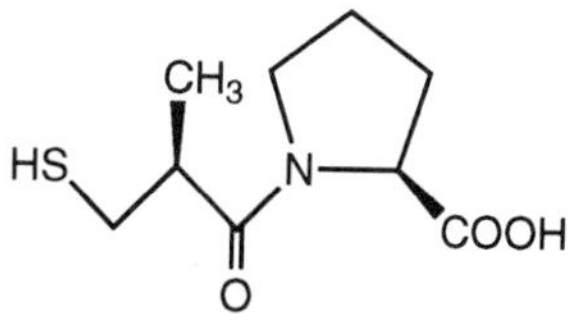

3

pyroGlu-Trp-Pro-Arg-Pro-Gln-Ile-Pro-Pro

4

C. Lovastatin

Elevated serum cholesterol levels are an important risk factor in cardiac disease, and drugs which lower these levels are thus important in prophylaxis against heart attacks and other manifestations of cardiac problems. Although a significant amount of cholesterol is ingested in the normal diet, cholesterol is also biosynthesized in the liver, and the control of this biosynthesis is thus important in lowering serum cholesterol levels. The rate-limiting step of cholesterol biosynthesis involves the reduction of β-hydroxy-β-methylglutaryl-Coenzyme A (HMG-CoA) to mevalonic acid (**5**, shown as its lactone), mediated by the enzyme HMG-CoA reductase. A search for inhibitors of this enzyme led to the isolation of lovastatin (mevinolin) (**6**) from the fungi *Monascus ruber* and *Aspergillus terreus*,[6] and this compound has become a major drug for the reduction of serum cholesterol levels.

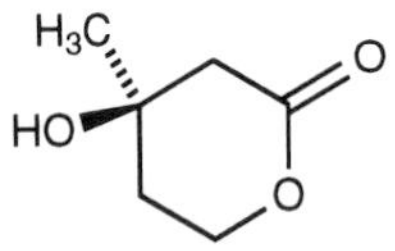

5

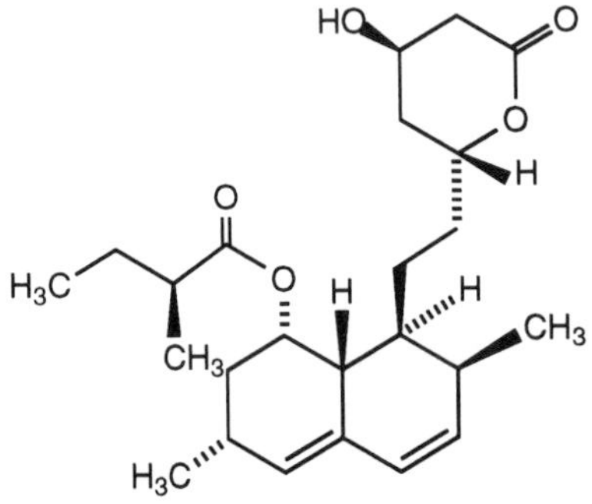

6

D. Cyclosporin A

The cyclic oligopeptide cyclosporin A (**7**) was isolated from the fungus *Trichoderma polysporum*.[7] It has found wide use as an immunosuppressant to prevent organ transplant rejection.

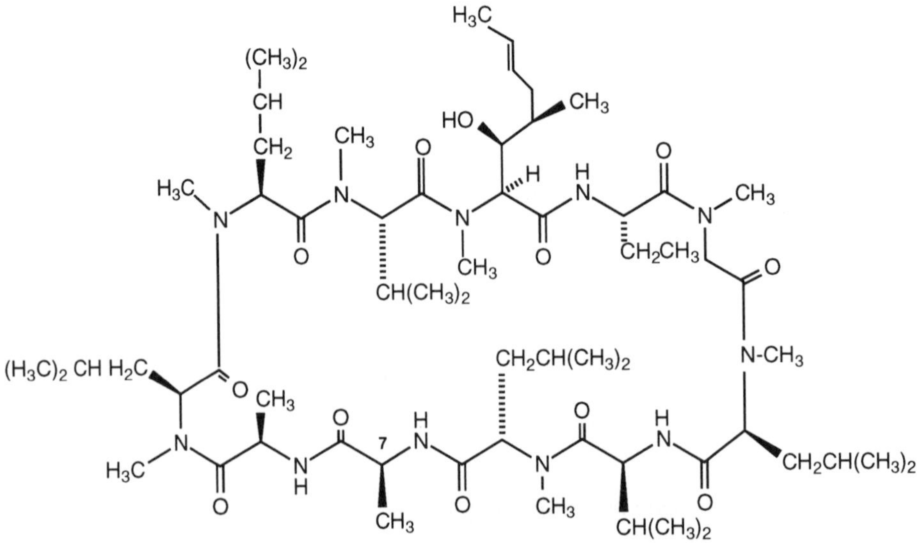

7

E. Avermectin

The avermectins are a group of broad-spectrum antiparasitic antibiotics of which avermectin A_{1a} (**8**) is an example. They were isolated from the actinomycete *Streptomyces avermitilis*,[29] and have both antiparasitic and pesticidal properties.[30]

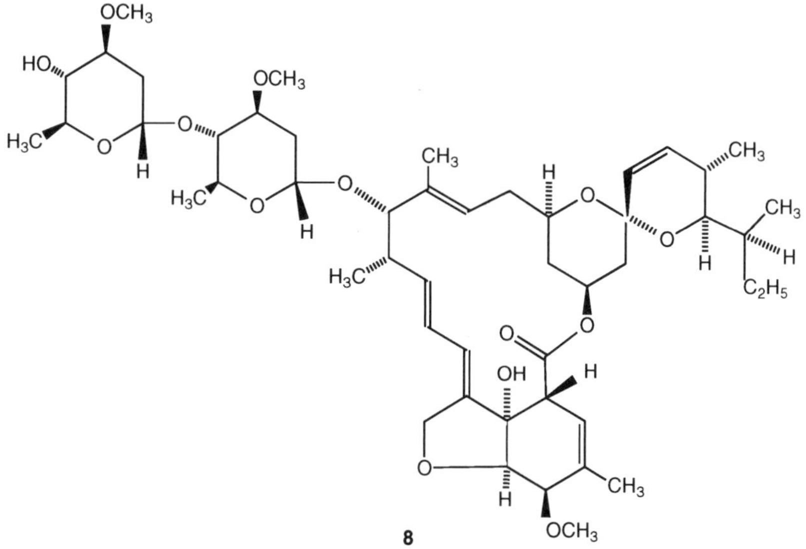

8

F. Paclitaxel (Taxol®)

The most exciting new drug in the anticancer area in recent years is the plant-derived compound paclitaxel (Taxol®) (**9**). First isolated from the Pacific Yew, *Taxus brevifolia*, in the late 1960s as a cytotoxic agent, it was later found to be a tubulin-assembly promoter. Its development as an anticancer drug was delayed by problems with its availability and its solubility, but these were overcome and it has been shown to be an effective treatment for both ovarian and breast cancer.[31,32] A large number of analogues have been prepared, and it is very probable that an improved second-generation analogue will be developed. [33–35]

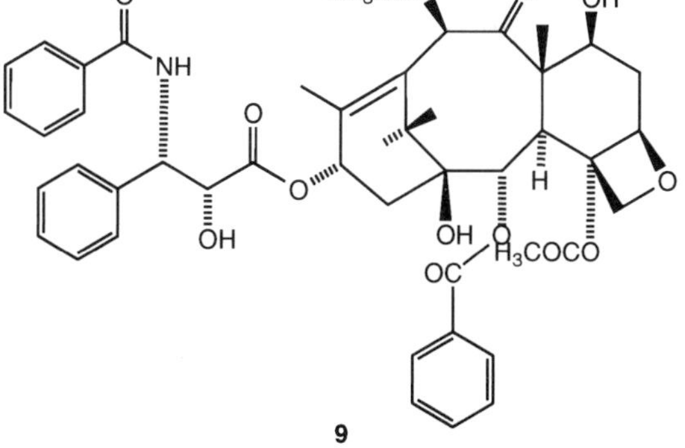

9

G.   Etoposide and teniposide

The cytotoxic agent podophyllotoxin (**10**) has been known for many years as the major cytotoxic isolate of the may apple, *Podophyllum peltatum*.[36] Detailed structure–activity relationship studies led to the development of the podophyllotoxin analogues etoposide (**11**) and teniposide (**12**) as effective anticancer agents.[37] Interestingly, although podophyllotoxin itself is an antimitotic agent and tubulin-polymerization inhibitor, etoposide and teniposide function as DNA topoisomerase II inhibitors.[38]

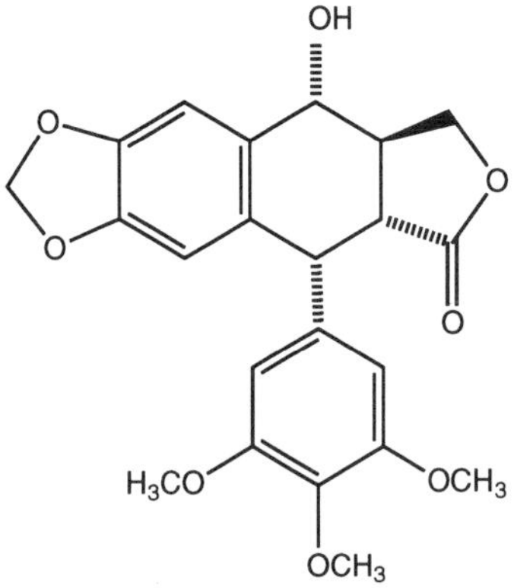

10

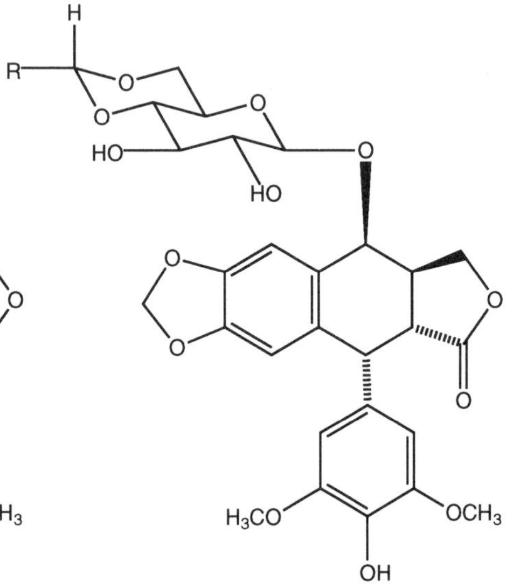

11   R = CH₃   **12**   R =

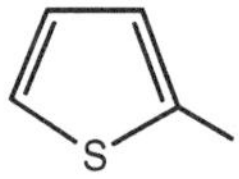

H.   Vinblastine and vincristine

The anticancer activity of the vinca alkaloids vinblastine (**13**) and vincristine (**14**) was discovered serendipitously as a result of a search for compounds with hypoglycaemic activity[39] and also independently as part of a directed search for plant-derived anticancer agents.[40] Both alkaloids are effective anticancer agents, and vincristine in particular is used as part of the effective MOPP therapy (Nitrogen Mustard, Oncovin (vincristine), Procarbazine, Prednisone) for Hodgkin's disease.[41] Their mechanisms of action are probably directly related to their functions as tubulin polymerization inhibitors, and hence they act as antimitotic agents.

I.   Camptothecin and analogues

The alkaloid camptothecin (**15**) was first isolated from the Chinese tree *Camptotheca acuminata*, and showed very encouraging initial results in animal models. Because of its water insolubility, clinical trials were carried out on the lactone ring-opened sodium salt, and these had to be halted because of severe toxicity. Later studies then focused on the development of agents with

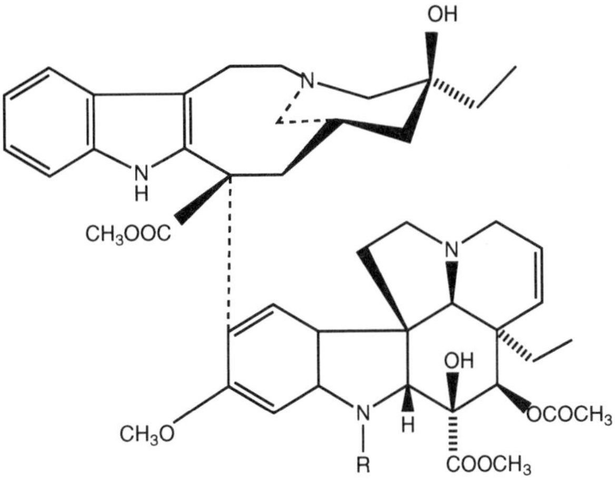

13 R = CH$_3$ **14** R = CHO

improved water-solubility and/or activity, and three such analogues are now in clinical trial. CPT-11 (**16**) developed in Japan, has shown promising results in leukaemia and lymphoma,[42] and also in lung, colorectal, ovarian and cervical cancers.[43] Topotecan (**17**),[44] has shown activity against lung, ovarian and colorectal cancer.[43] 9-Aminocamptothecin (**18**) is still in the early stages of clinical trial,[43] and no data on its effectiveness are available.

One interesting and important finding on camptothecin and its analogues is that they act as inhibitors of DNA topoisomerase I. In this respect they differ from etoposide, teniposide and other known DNA topoisomerase II inhibitors, and provide a new approach to cancer chemotherapy.

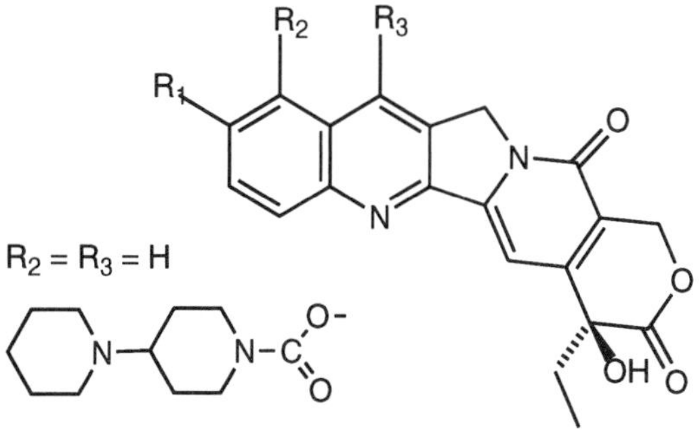

15   R$_1$ = R$_2$ = R$_3$ = H

16   R$_1$ = [structure]

R$_2$ = H; R$_3$ = CH$_3$CH$_2$

17   R$_1$ = OH; R$_2$ = CH$_2$N(CH$_3$)$_2$; R$_3$ = H

18   R$_1$ = R$_3$ = H; R$_2$ = NH$_2$

J. Magainins

The magainins illustrate the truth that bioactive compounds can be obtained from animals as well as plants and microorganisms. The magainins are a family of peptides isolated from the skin of the African clawed frog *Xenopus laevis*, and they have excellent antibiotic activity. They were discovered after a researcher noted that the frogs seldom developed infections after surgery, despite the use of nonsterile surgical procedures and holding tanks. Magainin 1 and magainin 2 each have 23 amino acids, and differ only in the amino acids of positions 10 and 22.[45] They are good candidates for development as topical or locally administered anti-infective drugs.[46]

K. Other natural products

The previous examples are only a selection of natural products and natural product analogues which have entered clinical use or are in preclinical investigation. In the cancer area alone several additional natural products continue to provide effective drugs, including the actinomycins, anthracyclines such as adriamycin and daunorubicin, bleomycin A_2 and bleomycin B_2, and the mitomycins,[47] and the use of natural products as lead compounds has been described.[48] Other promising natural antitumour agents have been reviewed.[8] In other pharmaceutical areas, promising new lead compounds have been described in various recent reviews and books.[49–51] The contribution of older natural products as drugs should not be forgotten either; medicine would be immeasurably poorer without the alkaloids morphine and quinine, without the cardiotonic steroids found in digitalis, and without antibiotics such as the penicillins and the cephalosporins, to name just a few examples.

V. SUMMARY

The preceding pages have given just a small glimpse into the importance of natural products as pharmaceutical agents. With the use of modern screening and isolation tools, the potential for the discovery of new natural product drugs or lead compounds has been significantly enhanced, and the future of natural products in the pharmaceutical industry is a bright one.

REFERENCES

1. Haslam, E. (1986) Secondary metabolism — fact and fiction. *Nat. Prod. Rep.* **3**: 217–249.
2. Williams, D. H., Stone, M. J., Hauck, P.R. and Rahman, S. K. (1989) Why are secondary metabolites (natural products) biosynthesized? *J. Nat. Prod.* **52**: 1189–1208.
3. Harborne, J. B. (1990) Role of secondary metabolites in chemical defence mechanisms in plants. In Chadwick, D. J., and Marsh, J. (eds) *Bioactive Compounds from Plants*, pp. 126–139. Wiley, Chichester.
4. O'Neill, M. J. and Lewis, J. A. (1993) The renaissance of plant research in the pharmaceutical industry. In Kinghorn, A. and Balandrin, D. (eds.) *Human Medicinal Agents from Plants*, pp. 48–55. American Chemical Society, Washington.
5. Ondetti, M. A., Rubin, B. and Cushman, D. W. (1977) Design of specific inhibitors of angiotensin-converting enzyme: a new class of orally active antihypertensive agents. *Science.* **196**: 441–444.
6. Endo, A. (1985) Compactin (ML-236B) and related compounds as potential cholesterol-lowering agents that inhibit HMG-CoA reductase. *J. Med. Chem.* **28**: 401–405.
7. Borel, J. F. (ed.) (1986) *Progress in Allergy*, vol. 38. *Cyclosporin*, pp. 1–465. Karger, Basel.
8. Kingston, D. G. I. (1992) Taxol and other anticancer agents from plants. In Coombes, J. D. (ed.) *New Drugs from Natural Sources*, pp. 101–119. IBC Technical Services Ltd., London.

9. Downes, D., Laird, S. A., Klein, C. and Carney, B. K. (1993) Biodiversity prospecting contract. In Reid, W. V., Laird, S. A., Meyer, C. A., Gámez, R., Sitterfeld, A., Janzen, D. H., Gollin, M. A. and Juma, C. (eds) *Biodiversity Prospecting: Using Genetic Resources for Sustainable Development*, pp. 255–287. World Resources Institute, Washington.

10. Farnsworth, N. R. (1990) The role of ethnopharmacology in drug development. In Chadwick, D. J. and Marsh, J. (eds) *Bioactive Compounds from Plants*, pp. 2–21. Wiley, Chichester.

11. Balick, M. J. (1990) Ethnobotany and the identification of therapeutic agents from the rainforest. In Chadwick, D. J. and Marsh, J. (eds) *Bioactive Compounds from Plants*, pp. 22–39. Wiley, Chichester.

12. Cox, P. A. (1990) Ethnopharmacology and the search for new drugs. In Chadwick, D. J. and Marsh, J. (eds) *Bioactive Compounds from Plants*, pp. 40–55. Wiley, Chichester.

13. Plotkin, M. J. (1988) Conservation, ethnobotany, and the search for new jungle medicines: pharmacognosy comes of age . . . Again. *Pharmacotherapy* **8**: 257–262.

14. Harris, T. J. R., Hayes, M. V. and Hobden, A. N. (1992) Molecular genetics in natural product screen design. In Coombes, J. D. (ed.) *New Drugs From Natural Sources*, pp. 3–12. IBC Technical Services Ltd., London.

15. Stein, R. B. (1992) Intracellular receptors as targets for drug discovery. In Coombes, J. D. (ed.) *New Drugs From Natural Sources*, pp. 13–19. IBC Technical Services Ltd., London.

16. Schindler, P. W. (1992) The design and operation of enzyme inhibitor screens. In Coombes, J. D. (ed.) *New Drugs From Natural Sources*, pp. 20–35. IBC Technical Services Ltd., London.

17. Wolff, M. E. and Maggio, E. T. (1992) Antibody directed drug design and screening. In Coombes, J. D. (ed.) *New Drugs From Natural Sources*, pp. 36–45. IBC Technical Services Ltd., London.

18. Hertzberg, R. P., Johnson, R. K., Caranfa, M. J., Myers *et al.* (1992) Mechanism-based strategies for the discovery of natural product inhibitors of HIV. In Coombes, J. D. (ed.) *New Drugs From Natural Sources*, pp. 46–58. IBC Technical Services Ltd., London.

19. Boyd, M. R. (1989) Status of the NCI preclinical antitumor drug discovery screen. *Princ. Pract. Oncol. Updates* **3**: 1–12.

20. Johnson, R. K., Bartus, H. F., Hofmann, G. A., Bartus, J. O., Mong, S.-M., Faucette, L. F., McCabe, F. L., Chan, J. A. and Mirabelli, C. K. (1986) Discovery of new DNA-reactive drugs. In Hanka, L. J., Kondo, T. and White, R. J. (eds) *In Vitro and In Vivo Models for Detection of New Antitumor Drugs*, pp. 15–26. Organizing Committee of the 14th International Congress of Chemotherapy.

21. McLaughlin, J. L., Chang, C.-J. and Smith, D. L. (1990) Simple bench-top bioassays (brine shrimp and potato discs) for the discovery of plant antitumor compounds: review of recent progress. In Chadwick, D. J. and Marsh, J. (eds) *Bioactive Compounds from Plants*, pp. 112–137. Wiley, Chichester.

22. Mitscher, L. A., Leu, R.-P., Bathala, M. S., Wu, W.-N. and Beal, J. L. (1972) Antimicrobial agents from higher plants. I. Introduction, rationale, and methodology. *Lloydia* **35**: 157–166.

23. Shimizu, Y. (1985) Bioactive marine natural products, with emphasis on handling of water-soluble compounds. *J. Nat. Prod.* **48**: 223–235.

24. Marston, A. and Hostettmann, K. (1991) Modern separation methods. *Nat. Prod. Rep.* **8**: 391–413.

25. Cragg, G. M., Schepartz, S. A., Suffness, M. and Grever, M. R. (1993) The Taxol supply crisis. New NCI policies for handling the large-scale production of novel natural anticancer and anti-HIV agents. *J. Nat. Prod.* **56**: 1657–1668.

26. Fujita, Y. (1988) Industrial production of shikonin and berberine. In Bock, G. and Marsh, J. (eds) *Applications of Plant Cell and Tissue Culture*, pp. 228–238. Wiley, Chichester.

27. Fowler, M. W., Cresswell, R. C. and Stafford, A. M. (1990) An economic and technical assessment of the use of plant cell cultures for natural product synthesis on an industrial scale. In Chadwick, D. J. and Marsh, J. (eds) *Bioactive Compounds from Plants*, pp. 157–174. Wiley, Chichester.

28. Cox, J. S. G. (1977) Cromolyn sodium. In Goldberg, M. E. (ed.) *Pharmacological and Biochemical Properties of Drug Substances*, vol. 1, pp. 277–310. American Pharmaceutical Association, Washington.

29. Albers-Schönberg, G., Arison, B. H., Chabala, J. C., Douglas, A. W., Eskola, P., Fisher, M. H., Lusi, A., Mrozik, H., Smith, J. L. and Tolman, R. L. (1981) *J. Am. Chem. Soc.* **103**: 4216–4221.

30. Babu. J. R. (1988) Avermectins: biological and pesticidal activities. In Cutler, H. G. (ed.) *Biologically Active Natural Products*, pp. 91–108. American Chemical Society, Washington.

31. Slichenmyer, W. J. and von Hoff, D. D. (1991) Taxol: a new and effective anti-cancer drug. *Anti-Cancer Drugs* **2**: 519–530.

32. Rowinsky, E. K., Onetto, N., Canetta, R. M. and Arbuck, S. G. (1992) Taxol: the first of the taxanes, an important new class of antitumor agents. *Semin. Oncol.* **19**: 646–662.
33. Kingston, D. G. I. (1991) The chemistry of Taxol. *Pharmac. Ther.* **52**: 1–34.
34. Kingston, D. G. I., Molinero, A. A. and Rimoldi, J. M. (1993) The taxane diterpenoids. In Herz, W., Kirby, G. W., Moore, R. E., Steglich, W. and Tamm, Ch. (eds) *Progress in the Chemistry of Organic Natural Products*, vol. 61, pp. 1–206. Springer-Verlag, Vienna.
35. Nicolaou, K. C., Dai, W.-M. and Guy, R. K. (1994) Chemistry and biology of Taxol. *Angew. Chem. Int. Ed.* **33**: 5–44.
36. Hartwell, J. L. and Schrecker, A. W. (1958) Chemistry of podophyllum. In Zechmeister, L. (ed.) *Fortschritte Chemie der Organische Naturstoffe*, vol 15, pp. 83–166. Springer-Verlag, Vienna
37. Jardine, I. (1980) Podophyllotoxins. In Cassady, J. M. and Douros, J. D. (eds) *Anticancer Agents Based on Natural Product Models*, pp. 319–351. Academic Press, New York
38. Chen, G. L., Yang, L., Rowe, T. C., Halligan, B. D., Tewey, K. and Liu, L. (1984) Nonintercalative antitumor drugs interfere with the breakage-reunion reaction of mammalian DNA topoisomerase II. *J. Biol. Chem.* **259**: 13560–13566.
39. Noble, R. L., Beer, C. T. and Cutts, J. H. (1958) Role of chance observations in chemotherapy: *Vinca Rosea. Ann N.Y. Acad. Sci.* **76**: 882–894.
40. Johnson, I. S., Wright, H. F., Suoboda, G. H. and Lantis, J. (1960) Antitumor principles derived from *Vinca rosea* Linn. I. Vincaleukoblastine and leurosine. *Cancer Res.* **40**: 1016–1022.
41. Neuss, N. and Neuss, M. N. (1990) Therapeutic use of bisindole alkaloids from *Catharanthus*. In Brossi, A. and Suffness, M. (eds) *The Alkaloids*, vol. 37, pp. 229–239. Academic Press, New York.
42. Ohno, R., Okada, K., Masaoka, T. *et al.* (1990) An early phase II study of CPT-11, a new derivative of camptothecin, for the treatment of leukemia and lymphoma. *J. Clin. Oncol.* **8**: 1907–1912.
43. Wall, M. E. and Wani, M. C. (1993) Camptothecin and analogues: synthesis, biological in vitro and in vivo activities, and clinical possibilities. In Kinghorn, A. D. and Balandrin, M. F. (eds) *Human Medicinal Agents from Plants*, pp. 149–169. American Chemical Society, Washington.
44. Kingsbury, W. D., Boehm, J. C., Jakas, D. R. *et al.* (1990) Synthesis of water-soluble (aminoalkyl) camptothecin analogues: inhibition of topoisomerase I and antitumor activity. *J. Med. Chem.* **34**: 98–107.
45. Zasloff, M. (1987) Magainins, a class of antimicrobial peptides from *Xenopus* skin: isolation characterization of two active forms, and partial cDNA sequence of a precursor. *Proc. Natl Acad. Sci. USA* **84**: 5449–5453.
46. Berkowitz, B. A. (1992) Magainins: novel and effective peptide anti-infective and immunomimetics. In Coombes, J. D. (ed.) *New Drugs From Natural Sources*, pp. 176–182. IBC Technical Services, Ltd., London.
47. Remers, W. A. (1979) *The Chemistry of Antitumor Antibiotics*, vol. 1, pp. 1–276. Wiley-Interscience, New York.
48. Cassady, J. M. and Douros, J. D. (eds) (1980) *Anticancer Agents Based on Natural Product Models*, pp. 1–487. Academic Press, New York.
49. Coombes, J. D. (ed.) (1992) *New Drugs From Natural Sources*, pp. 1–190. IBC Technical Services, Ltd., London.
50. Kinghorn, A. D. and Balandrin, M. F. (eds) (1993) *Human Medicinal Agents from Plants*, pp. 1–340. American Chemical Society, Washington.
51. Hylands, P. J. and Nisbet, L. J. (1991) The search for molecular diversity (I): natural products. In Bristol, J. A. (ed.) *Annual Reports in Medicinal Chemistry*, vol. 26, pp. 259–269. Academic Press, San Diego.

8

Combinatorial Libraries and High-Throughput Synthesis

SHEILA HOBBS DE WITT

An important scientific innovation rarely makes its way by gradually winning over and converting its opponents: it rarely happens that Saul becomes Paul. What does happen is that its opponents gradually die out and that the growing generation is familiarized with the idea from the beginning.
Max Planck (1936) *The Philosophy of Physics*

THE PRACTICE OF MEDICINAL CHEMISTRY
ISBN 0-12-744640-0

I. INTRODUCTION

A. The drug discovery process

The pharmaceutical industry has a continued commitment to discovering, developing and marketing new medicines. Over the years, innovation in new drug therapy has become significantly more complex, time-consuming and costly. For example, the discovery and development of a new drug requires, on average, the preparation and evaluation of approximately 10 000 compounds over a period of 12 years at a cost of $359 million.[1] These figures, combined with increasing global competition and government regulations have demanded more efficient and accelerated approaches to drug discovery.

B. Chemical diversity: the need

Historically, compound collections or 'chemical libraries' for testing in biological assays were obtained from proprietary databases of compounds accumulated over many years, natural products, fermentation broths, or rational drug design. Recently, advances in molecular biology and automation have resulted in the development of rapid, high-throughput biological assays which have significantly affected the drug discovery process (Fig. 8.1). Consequently, the synthesis of compounds for both lead generation and lead optimization has become a rate-limiting step in the drug discovery effort. This need for large chemical libraries has initiated combinatorial and high-throughput synthesis methods.[2-6] A combinatorial library is generated by a systematic and comprehensive construction of molecular 'building blocks'. The building blocks represent a variety of reactive components or reagents which are incorporated into the final molecules. For example, benzodiazepines can be chemically synthesized to result in five or more sites for diversity (Fig. 8.2). As the number of building blocks introduced at each location increases, the potential number of target molecules increases dramatically.

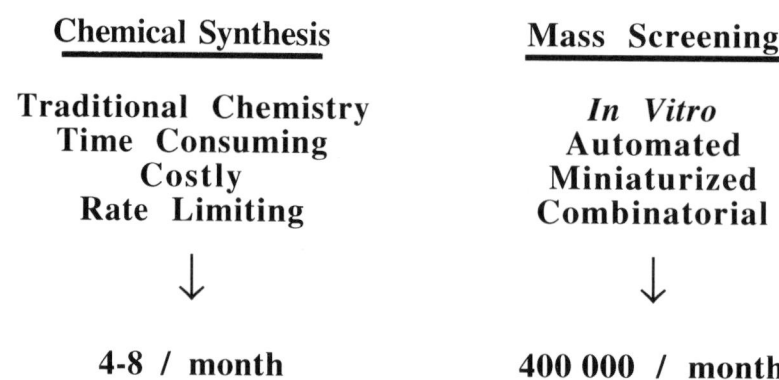

Fig. 8.1   Chemical diversity: The need.

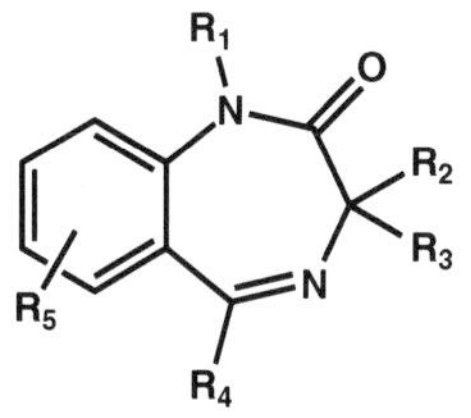

Building Blocks/Step	Potential Compounds
2	$2^5 = 32$
10	$10^5 = 100\,000$
20	$20^5 = 3.2$ million

Fig. 8.2 The potential for small-molecule diversity: Benzodiazepines.

C. Lead generation versus lead optimization

Compound collections have utility both for the generation of lead candidates and for the optimization of structure–activity relationships (SAR). Lead generation resulting from mass screening of a proprietary database of compounds often generates a variety of interesting 'hits'. However, these collections of compounds within a single company are still biased. The typical pharmaceutical databases of 50 000 to 500 000 compounds still represent only a small fraction of potential diversity. Therefore, a more *de novo* synthesis approach using combinatorial and high-throughput synthesis methods can begin to provide a large and more uniform source of chemical diversity for lead generation. On the other hand, lead optimization requires a more focused synthesis and testing approach. Often, a variety of structural and electronic modifications are designed into one unique core or template structure to generate tens or hundreds of compounds. This facilitates the efficient optimization of a SAR in a single chemical series.

II. SYNTHESIS AND TESTING METHODS

The synthesis of compounds requires chemical methods. However, the traditional methods of solution-phase or homogeneous reactions are yielding to more rapid and efficient methods for the generation of large libraries of compounds. The exploitation of solid-phase synthesis, parallel processing, automation and deconvolution strategies for compound mixtures have enabled and enhanced the synthesis and evaluation of large compound collections (i.e. >100 000). Chemical diversity may be presented in a variety of ways. The products may be soluble or still attached to a solid support (resin-bound) as single products or as a mixture. The utility of each approach is dependent upon the biological assay and the objectives for lead generation versus lead optimization.

A.   Solid-phase synthesis

The synthetic construction of compounds on a solid support was pioneered by Bruce Merrifield in 1963.[7] In contrast to traditional solution-phase synthesis, solid-phase synthesis obviates the need for the isolation and purification of reaction intermediates. Purification is achieved by extensive washing of the solid support to remove residual reagents, by-products and solvents. This also enables the use at intermediate steps of reagents, catalysts, or solvents that are difficult to remove. Additionally, intermediate reactions may be driven to completion with excess equivalents of reagents or catalysts.

A wide variety of solid supports has been utilized since the original work of Merrifield[7] with cross-linked polystyrene–divinylbenzene. Other solid supports include cellulose, in the form of functionalized paper,[8] cellulose disks,[9–11] or cotton,[9,12] controlled pore glass (CPG),[13] silica gel,[14] and polystyrene-grafted polyethylene films (PS-PE).[15] A representative reaction scheme and methods of cleavage for solid-phase synthesis are illustrated in Fig. 8.3. Building blocks (or reagents) react with resin-bound functionality to assemble the desired compound covalently on the solid support. Cleavage can be achieved by several methods. Displacement by intramolecular cyclization has the advantage of cleaner products since unreacted resin-bound intermediates are not amenable to cyclization (Fig. 8.3, cleavage 1). Cleavage of the penultimate resin-bound intermediate can also proceed through nucleophilic displacement (Fig. 8.3, cleavage 2) or hydrolysis (Fig. 8.3, cleavage 3) at the resin-bound linkage.

Solid-phase synthesis methods have dramatically impacted both peptide and oligonucleotide synthesis over the past 30 years. Although some non-peptide and non-nucleotide chemistry has been demonstrated on a solid support,[16–19] the wide range of chemistries common to the field of organic chemistry has not been fully exploited. The investment of time and resources to adapt chemistry to a solid support have to be weighed against the more well-known and better-developed methods for chemical synthesis in solution. However, as parallel synthesis strategies become more attractive and amenable to the laboratory, the investment will be warranted. Furthermore, as the repertoire of chemistries amenable to solid-phase synthesis increases, the development time necessary for implementation will become more competitive with traditional solution-phase synthesis methods.

B.   Combinatorial mixtures

Mixtures of compounds are easy to generate. Synthetic organic chemists have been synthesizing 'crude' product mixtures for years. However, knowledge of the content and distribution of the mixture is often elusive. The intentional generation of 'controlled' product mixtures becomes a paradigm for innovative synthesis and testing strategies. Most current methods for generating compound mixtures utilize solid-phase chemistry for the reasons summarized above. Three methods exist for the generation of compound mixtures on a solid support (Fig. 8.4): introduction of a mixture of soluble building blocks to a single resin-bound intermediate,[20,21] introduction of a single soluble building block to a mixture of resin-bound intermediates,[22–24] or introduction of a mixture of soluble building blocks to a mixture of resin-bound intermediates.

1.   Mixed building block strategy

The reaction between one resin-bound intermediate and a mixture of reactive building blocks provides a mixture of either resin-bound or soluble products with a product distribution

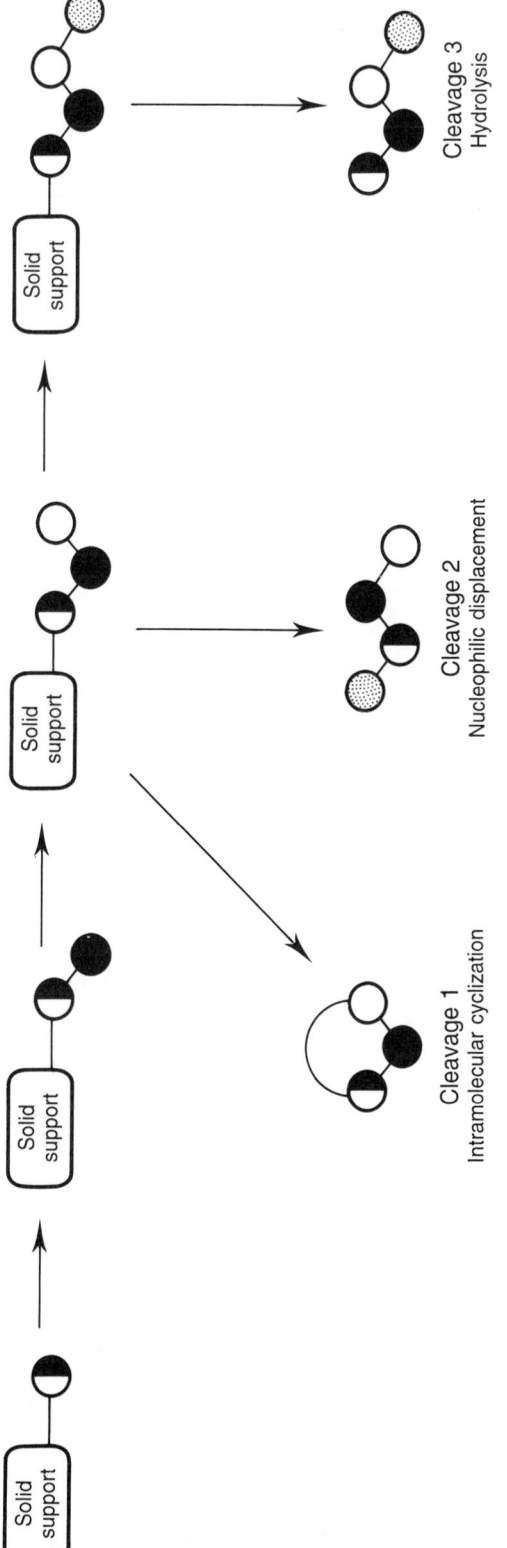

Fig. 8.3 Solid-phase synthesis: A representative approach.

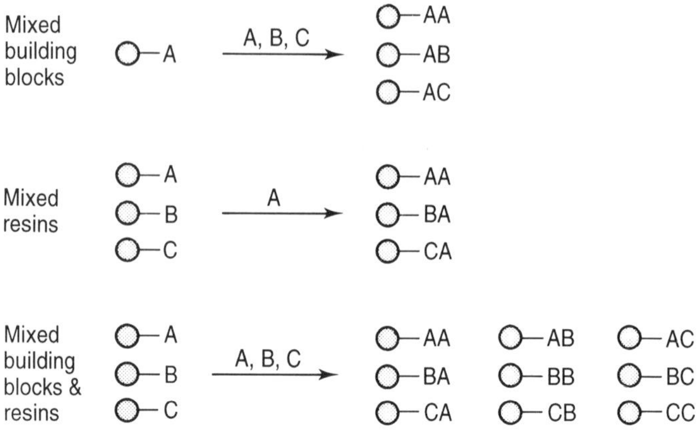

Fig. 8.4   Methods for generating combinatorial mixtures on a solid support.

dependent upon the competing reaction kinetics of the incoming building blocks. The equimolar distribution of products is important to make even semiquantitiative determinations of the biological activity with compound mixtures. A more uniform distribution is achieved through the use of sub-equimolar amounts of each building block, which drives each individual reaction to completion. For example, if a mixture of three building blocks is reacted with one resin-bound intermediate, the use of 0.33 equivalents of each building block should result in a mixture containing three resin-bound products each representing 33% of the final product mixture (Fig. 8.4).

2.   Mixed resin strategy

An equimolar distribution of final products can be difficult to achieve by the mixed building block approach, even through the use of controlled reaction kinetics and subequimolar building block mixtures. The 'mixed resin' approach overcomes the differing reactivities of building blocks by physically mixing and separating the solid support to achieve mixtures of resin-bound intermediates which are reacted with only one soluble building block (Figs. 8.4 and 8.5). This 'portion-mixing' approach was first demonstrated by Furka et al.[24,25] and is also referred to as the 'split synthesis'[23] or 'divide couple, and recombine' (DCR)[22] process.

3.   Testing and deconvolution strategies

As discussed above, methods for the high-throughput testing of millions of compounds have changed the face of drug discovery. In addition to *in vitro* analyses, automation and miniaturization, the testing of compound mixtures containing from ten to thousands of compounds while still attached to a solid support has emerged. The limiting feature of these approaches is the ability to assess the active constituents in large mixtures. This is analogous to searching for a 'needle in a haystack'. A variety of strategies aimed at identifying and isolating active components in a resin-bound product mixture have emerged.[23,26–32] However, the 'deconvolution' strategies of resin-bound products are limited to soluble receptors such as

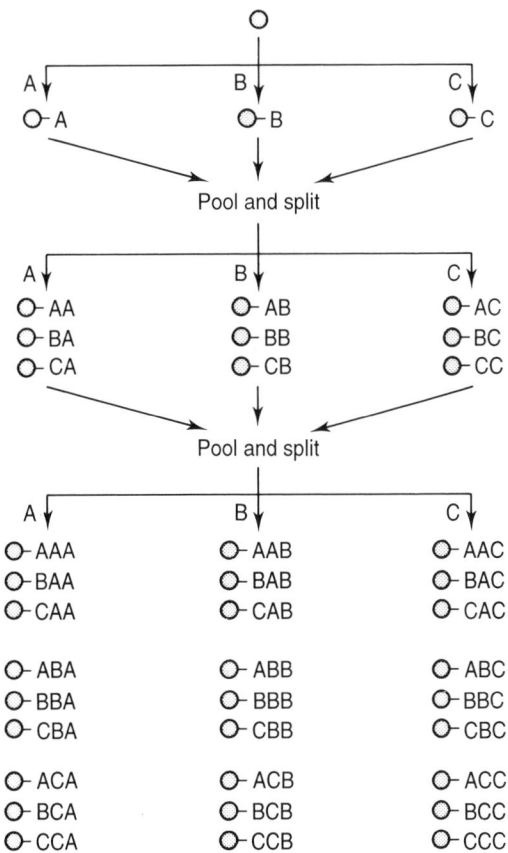

Fig. 8.5 The split synthesis method for combinatorial mixtures.

antibodies or enzymes. Continued development of these methods or alternative strategies for soluble libraries is necessary to identify active ligands to insoluble receptors (such as G-protein-linked receptors).

(a) Reporter groups. Combinatorial mixtures generated with non-cleavable linkages to the solid support are comprised of particles each of which ideally bears a single resin-bound product. Exposure of these libraries to soluble receptor assays requires methods for determining the identity of the resin-bound product which demonstrates biological activity. Reporter groups on the receptor in combination with a method for sequencing and determining the product on the solid support have been utilized for peptide libraries. Typical reporter groups are enzymes which elicit a detectable response (e.g. fluorescence) when a receptor binds to an active ligand, enabling visualization and manual separation of the active particles from the compound mixture (e.g. ELISA). Identification of the resin-bound product of peptide or oligonucleotide libraries can be achieved by Edman degradation or Sanger dideoxy sequencing, respectively. Additionally, soluble libraries of mixtures can be generated by using chemically labile linkages to the resin and cleaving a small portion of the resin-bound product from single particles. After testing the soluble library, the corresponding resin-bound product can be sequenced for identification of the active ligand.

(b) Encoded synthesis. The use of reporter groups in combination with sequencing methods has been limited to peptide (Edman degradation) or oligonucleotide (Sanger dideoxy sequencing) libraries. The nature of unnatural oligomeric or small molecule libraries prohibits direct sequencing methods. Furthermore, as the number of components in a combinatorial mixture increases, the likelihood that each component of the mixture is present and represented on a single particle in the mixture is suspect. The alternative, iterative testing and resynthesis of the libraries and sublibraries to identify the active components, is a tedious and labour-intensive process.

The process of explicitly identifying products generated on individual particles is made possible by coincident attachment of an identifier tag or code during the synthesis of the libraries (Fig. 8.6).[27] These encoded libraries can be fully deconvoluted by chemically reading the sequence of codes corresponding to each building block or reaction step to identify the resin-bound or cleaved product. The variety of codes incorporated to date include nucleotides for encoding peptides,[27,29,30] amino acids for encoding unnatural amino acids,[28,31] and photolabile aromatics for encoding peptides[26,32] (Table 8.1).

The encoding method of Ohlemeyer *et al.*,[32] which utilizes photolabile aromatics as 'molecular tags' differs from the former approaches through the use of a binary coding strategy which uses defined mixtures of tagging molecules to represent each building block uniquely at each reaction step. Following testing of the resin-bound products, the tags are cleaved by photolysis and analysed by electron-capture gas chromatography (ECGC). The chemically inert

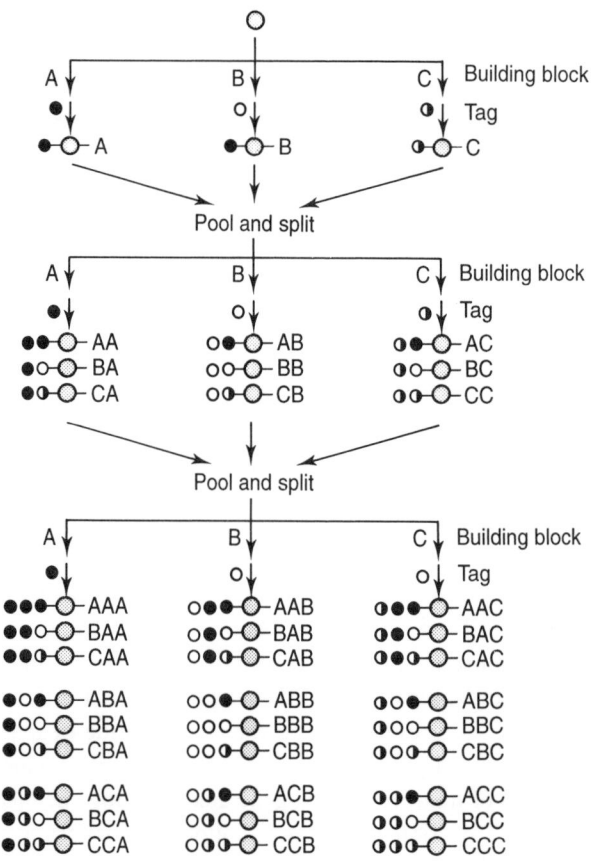

Fig. 8.6 Encoded libraries: A representative approach.

Table 8.1 Approaches to encoded libraries.

Reference	Unnatural amino acids	Molecular tag	Ligand:tag	Solid support	Products	Biological assay
Nielsen et al.[30]	No	Nucleotide	1:1 and 2:1	Controlled pore glass	Pentamers (resin–bound)	mAb endorphin[a]
Nikolaiev et al.[31]	Yes	Amino acid	1:1 and 2:1	Tentagel	820 000 heptamers (resin–bound)	mAb endorphin and streptavidin
Kerr et al.[28]	Yes	Amino acid	1.0:1.0	Polystyrene	200 decamers (cleaved)	mAb gp120
Needels et al.[29]	No	Nucleotide	1.0:1.0	Polystyrene	823 000 heptamers (resin–bound)	mAb dynorphin B
Ohlmeyer et al.[32]	No	Photolabile aromatics	1:0.05	Polystyrene	117 000 pentamers (resin–bound)	mAb cMYC

[a]mAb = monoclonal antibody.

nature of the tags is an attractive feature of this approach and should facilitate the screening of organic molecules prepared in resin-bound or cleaved combinatorial mixtures.

C.   Automation and integration

The objectives of automated synthesis within a laboratory are to increase productivity, to improve quality, to increase precision, to liberate scientists from tedious and labour-intensive tasks, and to provide the means to execute comprehensive and exhaustive experimental studies. The repetitive nature of oligomeric synthesis has enabled the implementation of automated methods.[33–42] Using these systems, multiple reaction vessels numbering 36,[38–42] 48,[34] or 96[37] can be manipulated. Additionally, the system of Zuckermann *et al.* has resin mixing and splitting capabilities for generating combinatorial mixtures by the mixed resin approach.[40] Although these systems are effective for oligonucleotide or oligopeptide syntheses, the more diverse chemistries and sample manipulations of general organic synthesis have hindered the design and use of automated systems. Recently, more flexible systems for automation of both solution-phase and solid-phase organic synthesis have emerged.[43–50]

As more efficient and productive automated synthesis systems are designed, automated data handling and integration between instruments and operating systems are desirable. For example, a four-step synthesis of 96 compounds simultaneously, including four-point reaction monitoring at each step and analysis of the final products by two methods, can involve more 1700 discrete pieces of data. Therefore, systems designed to control, communicate and handle various types of data input and output are necessary. The full exploitation of automation in a synthetic chemistry laboratory has not been realized. Future enhancements should lead to new, innovative systems and commercial products for high-throughput synthesis.

III.   COMPOUND LIBRARIES

Oligomeric forms of chemical diversity are derived from repetitive bond-forming reactions (Fig. 8.7). These compounds include oligonucleotides, oligopeptides, and oligosaccharides. Additionally, a variety of novel oligomeric compound libraries have been generated. On the other hand, nonoligomeric or small-molecule compounds generated from a diverse repertoire of chemical reactions and building blocks explore an even wider range of potential diversity (Figs 8.3 and 8.8).

A.   Oligonucleotides

The utility of oligonucleotide libraries to discover new ligands for biologically relevant targets is enhanced by their conformational complexity. These DNA and RNA oligonucleotide libraries may be generated by both biological and synthetic methods. The advantage of oligonucleotide libraries as sources of chemical diversity is the ability to isolate and identify the active components by amplification (by the polymerase chain reaction). Several workers have demonstrated the utility of DNA oligonucleotide libraries in biological assays.[51] Two methods of systematically evaluating a library of single-stranded RNA sequences generated from randomized DNA oligonucleotides have recently been reported by Tuerk and Gold[52] and Ellington and Szostak.[53]

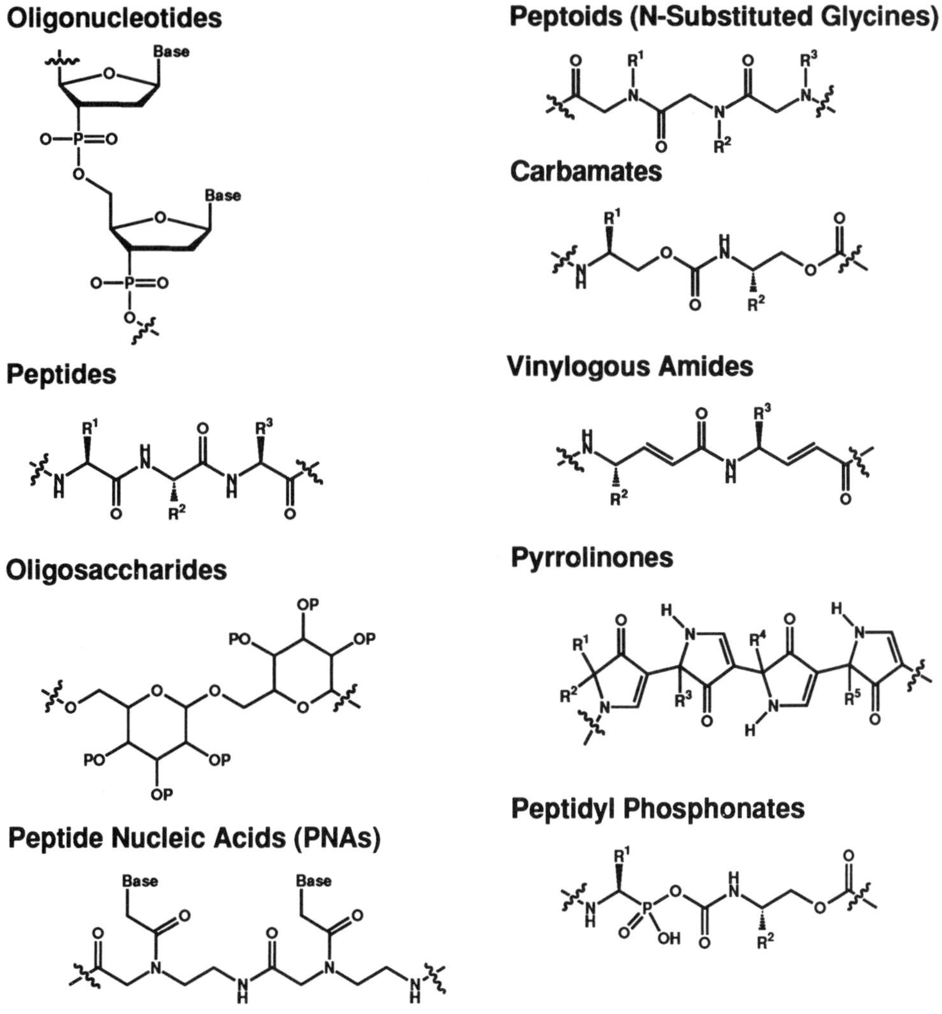

Oligonucleotides

Peptoids (N-Substituted Glycines)

Carbamates

Peptides

Vinylogous Amides

Oligosaccharides

Pyrrolinones

Peptide Nucleic Acids (PNAs)

Peptidyl Phosphonates

Fig. 8.7   Oligomeric libraries.

B.   Peptides

Combinatorial chemistry and high-throughput synthetic methods have historically been applied in the development of peptide libraries. A number of reviews[2,38,41,54,55] on this subject, in addition to the following chapter, preclude a discussion here.

C. Oligosaccharides

The synthesis of oligosaccharides has lagged behind oligonucleotide and oligopeptide synthesis owing to stereospecificity requirements in glycosidation, and differential protection of competing hydroxyl functionality. Traditional solution-phase synthesis methods for generating oligosaccharides results in (1) glycosidic linkage yields of 50–80%, (2) low-reactivity and

Table 8.2 Solid-phase synthesis of oligosaccharides and glycopeptides.

Reference	Polymer	Linkage	Results	Yields
Danishefsky et al.[56]	Polystyrene copolymer	To hydroxyl groups as silyl ether. Attachment at secondary hydroxyl tolerated. Cleavage with TBAF[a]	Stereospecific glycosidation. Interior deletions avoided. Average yield/coupling cycle = 70%. Amenable to D-glucal units	32% (overall of tetrasaccharide)
Douglas, et al.[57]	Poly(ethylene glycol) monomethyl ether (PEG). Soluble polymer during glycosylation. Insoluble polymer during workup	To anomeric carbon as aglycon or hydroxyl groups as ester. Cleavage with acetic acid	Anomeric control of solution chemistry. Ease and speed of solid phase workup. Reaction monitoring by proton NMR	85–95% (unoptimized of isolated di- and trisaccharides)
Schuseter et al.[58]	Aninopropyl silica with hexaglycine spacer. Compatible with aqueous and organic solvents	To amino groups of amino acids. Cleavage with chymotrypsin	Rapid, iterative formation of peptide bonds chemically. Rapid, iterative formation of glycosidic bonds enzymatically. No protection of sugar hydroxyl groups required	95% (crude product containing 20% of desired glycopeptide)

[a]TBAF = tetra-n-butylammonium fluoride.

unstable reactants, and (3) complex reaction mixtures. Historically, solid-phase synthesis approaches have been hampered by (1) the lack of effective differential protection and deprotection strategies, (2) incomplete coupling reactions, and (3) the lack of stereospecific reactions. Recently, innovative approaches in solid-phase synthesis techniques[56–58] have dramatically enhanced the synthesis of oligosaccharides and glycopeptides (Table 8.2) and provided the tools for the high-throughput synthesis of these molecules.

D. Novel oligomeric compounds

The generation of chemical diversity can be significantly enhanced by the repetitive coupling of unique building blocks to create novel oligomeric compounds. The resistance to proteolysis introduced by these novel backbone structures is a desirable characteristic for therapeutic potential and the design of peptidomimetic targets. A variety of methods using oligomeric backbones comprised of carbamates,[59] *N*-substituted glycines (peptoids),[60,61] peptidyl phosphonates,[62,63] vinylogous amides,[64] and pyrrolinones[65] (Fig. 8.7) have been reported.

E. Small molecules

While large numbers of oligomeric compounds can be synthesized rapidly using solid-phase techniques and automation, the repetitive coupling reactions and limited building blocks from which they are formed inherently limit their potential diversity. In fact, true chemical diversity is only realized by exploiting unlimited reaction types and building blocks. Furthermore, the vast majority of drugs on the market today are small molecules (MW < 700), as opposed to oligomeric compounds, which are generally unsuitable as stable, orally active drugs.

Construction of small organic molecules, however, requires a wider range of chemical reactions, more diverse building blocks, and more flexible equipment and automation design. Currently, this results in extended development and implementation time.

Some initial approaches for the high-throughput synthesis of nonoligomeric, small molecules are illustrated by the syntheses of benzodiazepines,[45,47,66,67] hydantoins,[45,47] and β-mercapto ketones[68] (Figs 8.8–8.11). Each of these libraries was synthesized on a polystyrene support to generate soluble compounds. Individual compounds were multiply and simultaneously synthesized in 40- or 96-unit arrays by DeWitt *et al.*[45] and Bunin *et al.*,[67] respectively. Mixtures containing nine compounds each were generated by Chen *et al.*[68] using the mixed resin approach described above. These small-molecule libraries have been referred to as DIVERSOMERS™ by DeWitt *et al.*[45] and 'analogous' organic synthesis by Chen *et al.*[68]

Although the chemistries can be achieved in ordinary laboratory glassware, the use of equipment capable of multiple, simultaneous organic synthesis on a milligram scale is desirable. To address the physical handling of 40 compounds, the DIVERSOMER™ approach utilizes custom-designed equipment interfaced with a liquid-sample handling robot for a semi-automated system.[45,47] In contrast, Bunin *et al.* utilize Geysen's pin apparatus[69] to synthesize 96 compounds simultaneously.[67] Furthermore, the compounds generated by both the DIVERSOMER™ approach[45] and Bunin *et al.*[67] demonstrated the utility of the libraries for the efficient and comprehensive evaluation of SAR.

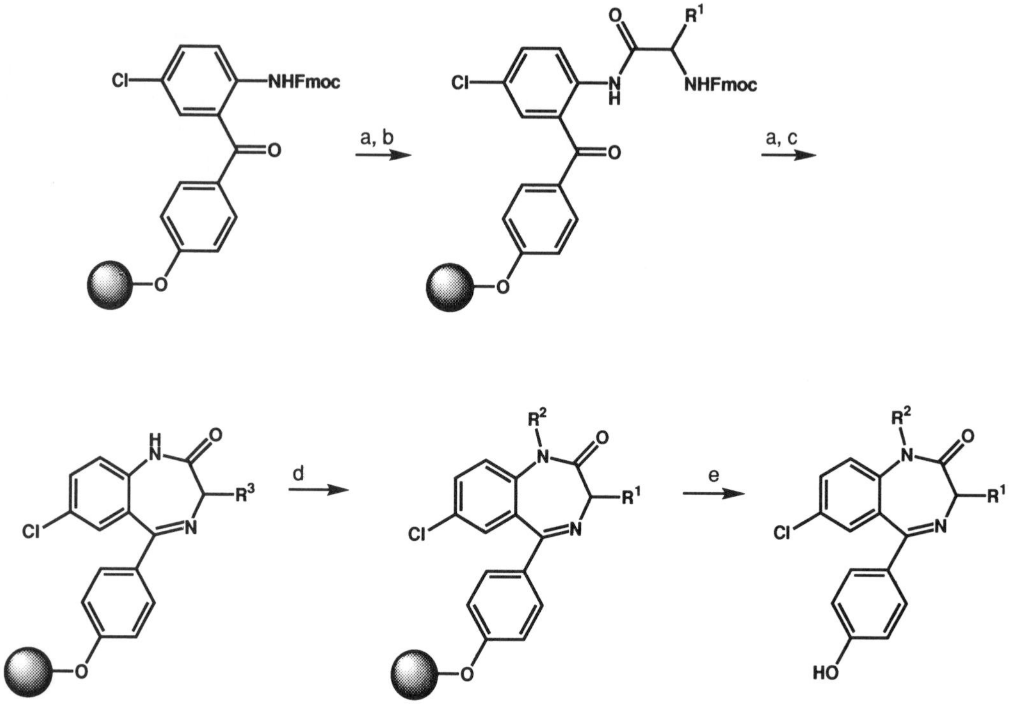

Fig. 8.8 Solid-phase synthesis of benzodiazepines by Bunin *et al.*[66,67] Conditions: (a) 20% piperidine in dimethyl formamide (DMF), 1 min then 20 s; (b) *N*-Fmoc-amino acid fluoride in CH_2Cl_2, 3 days, room temperature; (c) 5% acetic acid in DMF, 60–80°C, 12 h; (d) two alkylation treatments with lithiated 5-phenylmethyl-2-oxazolidinone in DMF/tetrahydrofuran (1 : 10 v/v) for 30 min at 0°C, followed by alkylating agent in DMF for 1 h at 0°C then warmed slowly to room temperature; (e) trifluoroacetic acid/H_2O/dimethyl sulfide (95:5:10 v/v), 24 h, room temperature.

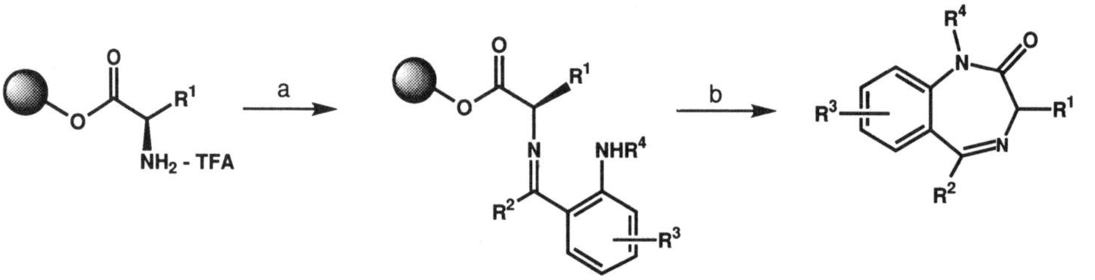

Fig. 8.9 Solid-phase synthesis of benzodiazepines by DeWitt *et al.*[45] Conditions: (a) substituted 2-aminobenzophenone imine in dichloroethane, 60°C, 24 h, (b) trifluoroacetic acid, 60°C, 20 h.

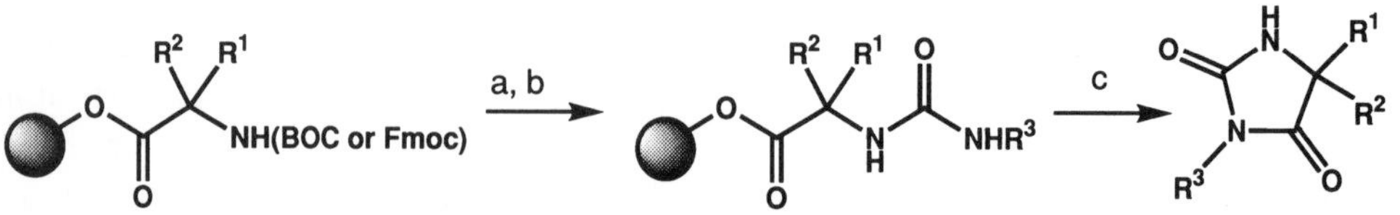

Fig. 8.10 Solid-phase synthesis of hydantoins.[45] Conditions: (a) 25% piperidine in DMF with anthracene as an internal standard or 50% trifluoroacetic acid, 6 h, room temperature; (b) substituted isocyanate in DMF with anthracene as an internal standard, 6 h, room temperature; (c) 6 M HCl, 85–100°C, 2 h.

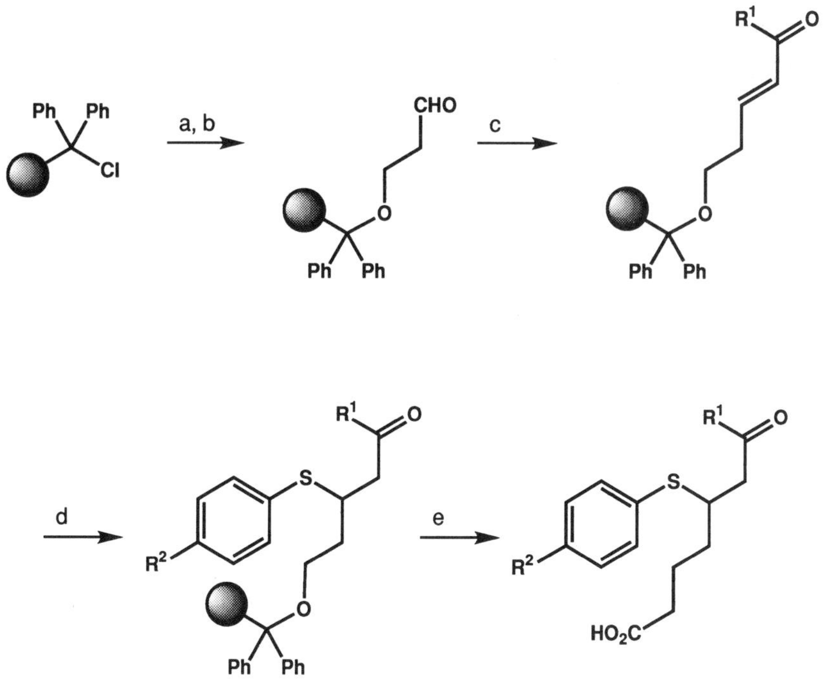

Fig. 8.11   Solid-phase synthesis of β-mercapto ketones.[68] Conditions: (a) butanediol, pyridine, 2 days, room temperature; (b) sulfur trioxide–pyridine, dimethyl sulfoxide, triethylamine, 2 h, room temperature; (c) ylide reagent, tetrahydrofuran (THF), 60°C, 2 days; (d) aromatic thiol, sodium methoxide (cat.), THF, 2 days, room temperature; (e) formaldehyde, THF, 2 h, room temperature.

IV.   SUMMARY AND CONCLUSIONS

As the future of medicinal chemistry and drug discovery unfolds, the advent of new technologies such as combinatorial libraries and high-throughput synthesis is guaranteed to alter traditional approaches to chemical synthesis (one step at a time, one compound at a time). Solid-phase synthesis, encoding strategies, and automation are new tools for medicinal chemistry. These and additional innovative methods for synthesizing and evaluating large collections of compounds will continue to be developed and implemented for many years to come.

The final impact of combinatorial libraries and high-throughput synthesis on the pharmaceutical industry has yet to be realized. However, preliminary indications suggest that these technologies will dramatically enhance and accelerate the drug discovery process. A time reduction of only six months in lead generation and lead optimization within a therapeutic project could significantly influence the competitive and costly process for moving a compound through the drug development pipeline.

REFERENCES

1. Pharmaceutical Manufacturers Association (1993) 'Facts at a Glance', Washington DC.
2. Gallop, M. A., Barrett, R. W., Dower, W. J., Fodor, S. P. W. and Gordon, E. M. (1994)

Applications of combinatorial technologies to drug discovery. 1. Background and peptide combinatorial libraries. *J. Med. Chem.* **37**: 1233–1251.

3. Gordon, E. M., Barrett, R. W., Dower, W. J., Fodor, S. P. W. and Gallop, M. A. (1994) Applications of combinatorial technologies to drug discovery. 2. Combinatorial organic synthesis, library screening strategies, and future directions. *J. Med. Chem.* **37**: 1385–1401.

4. Liskamp, R. M. J. (1994) Opportunities for new chemical libraries: Unnatural biopolymers and Diversomers. *Angew. Chem. Int. Ed. Engl.* **33**: 633–636.

5. Moos, W. H., Green, G. D. and Pavia, M. R. (1993) Recent advances in the generation of molecular diversity. *Annu. Rep. Med. Chem.* **28**: 315–324.

6. Pavia, M. R., Sawyer, T. K. and Moos, W. H. (1993) The generation of molecular diversity. *Bioorg. Med. Chem. Lett.* **3**: 387–396.

7. Merrifield, R. B. (1963) Solid phase peptide synthesis. I. The synthesis of a tetrapeptide. *J. Am. Chem. Soc.* **85**: 2149–2154.

8. van 't Hof, W., van den Berg, M. and Aalberse, R. C. (1993) The use of T bag synthesis with paper disks as the solid phase in epitope mapping studies. *J. Immunol. Methods* **161**: 177–186.

9. Eichler, J., Bienert, M., Stierandova A. and Lebl, M. (1991) Evaluation of cotton as a carrier for solid-phase peptide synthesis. *Pept. Res.* **4**: 296–307.

10. Frank, R. (1992) Spot-synthesis: An easy technique for the positionally addressable, parallel chemical synthesis on a membrane support. *Tetrahedron* **48**: 9217–9232.

11. Frank, R. (1993) Strategies and techniques in simultaneous solid phase synthesis based on the segmentation of membrane type supports. *Bioorg. Med. Chem. Lett.* **3**: 425–430.

12. Rinnova, M., Jezek, J., Malon P. and Lebl, M. (1993) Comparative multiple synthesis of fifty linear peptides: evaluation of cotton carrier vs. T bag-benzhydrylamine resin. *Peptide Res.* **6**: 88–94.

13. Adams, S. P., Kavka, K. S., Wykes, E. J., Holder, S. B. and Galluppi, G. R. (1983) Hindered dialkylamino nucleoside phosphite reagents in the synthesis of two DNA 51-mers. *J. Am. Chem. Soc.* **105**: 661–663.

14. Koster, H. (1972) Polymer support oligonucleotide synthesis VI: Use of inorganic carriers. *Tetrahedron Lett.* **16**: 1527–1530.

15. Berg, R. H., Almdal, K., Pedersen, W. B., Holm, A., Tam, J. P. and Merrifield, R. B. (1989) Long-chain polystyrene-grafted polyethylene film matrix: A new support for solid-phase peptide synthesis. *J. Am. Chem. Soc.* **111**: 8024–8026.

16. Camps, F., Cartells, J. and Pi, J. (1974) Organic synthesis with functionalized polymers. *Anales De Quimica* **70**: 848–849.

17. Crowley, J. I. and Rapoport, H. (1976) Solid-phase organic synthesis: Novelty or fundamental concept? *Acc. Chem. Res.* **9**: 135–144.

18. Leznoff, C. C. (1974) The use of insoluble polymer supports in organic chemical synthesis. *Chem. Soc. Rev.* **3**: 65–85.

19. Leznoff, C. C. (1978) The use of insoluble polymer supports in general organic synthesis. *Acc. Chem. Res.* **11**: 327–333.

20. Geysen, H. M., Rodda, S. J. and Mason, T. J. (1986) A priori delineation of a peptide which mimics a discontinuous antigenic determinant. *Mol. Immunol.* **23**: 709–715.

21. Pinilla, C., Appel, J. R., Blanc, P. and Houghten, R. A. (1992) Rapid identification of high affinity peptide ligands using positional scanning synthetic peptide combinatorial libraries. *Biotechniques* **13**: 901–905.

22. Houghten, R. A., Pinilla, C., Blondelle, S. E., Appel, J. R., Dooley, C. T. and Cuervo, J. H. (1991) Generation and use of synthetic peptide combinatorial libraries for basic research and drug discovery. *Nature* **354**: 84–86.

23. Lam, K. S., Salmon, S. E., Hersh, E. M., Hruby, V. J., Kazmierski, W. M. and Knapp, R. J. (1991) A new type of synthetic peptide library for identifying ligand-binding activity. *Nature* **354**: 82–84. [published erratum appears in *Nature*. (1992) **358** (6385): 434].

24. Sebestyen, F., Dibo, G., Kovacs, A. and Furka, A. (1993) Chemical synthesis of peptide libraries. *Bioorg. Med. Chem. Lett.* **3**: 413–418.

25. Furka, A., Sebestyen, F., Asgedom, M. and Dibo, G. (1991) General method for rapid synthesis of multicomponent peptide mixtures. *Int. J. Peptide Protein Res.* **37**: 487–493.

26. Borchardt, A., and Still, W. C. (1994) Synthetic receptor binding elucidated with an encoded combinatorial library. *J. Am. Chem. Soc.* **116**: 373–374.

27. Brenner, S. and Lerner, R. A. (1992) Encoded combinatorial chemistry. *Proc. Natl. Acad. Sci. USA* **89**: 5381–5383.

28. Kerr, J. M., Banville, S. C. and Zuckermann, R. N. (1993) Encoded combinatorial peptide libraries containing non-natural amino acids. *J. Am. Chem. Soc.* **115**: 2529–2531.

29. Needels, M., Jones, D., Tate, E., Heinkel, G., Kocherspergerer, L., Dower, W., Barrett, R. and Gallop, M. (1993) Generation and screening of an oligonucleotide-encoded synthetic peptide library. *Proc. Natl. Acad. Sci. USA* **90**: 10700–10704.

30. Nielsen, J., Brenner, S. and Janda, K. D. (1993) Synthetic methods for the implementation of encoded combinatorial chemistry. *J. Am. Chem. Soc.* **15**: 9812–9813.

31. Nikolaiev, V., Stierandova, A., Krchnak, V., Seligmann, B., Lam, K. S., Salmon, S. E. and Lebl, M. (1993) Peptide-encoding for structure determination of nonsequenceable polymers within libraries synthesized and tested on solid-phase supports. **6**: 161–170.

32. Ohlmeyer, M. H. J., Swanson, R. N., Dillard, L. W., Reader, J. C., Asouline, G., Kobayashi, R., Wigler, M. and Still, W. C. (1993) Complex synthetic chemical libraries indexed with molecular tags. *Proc. Natl. Sci. USA.* **90**: 10922–10926.

33. Andrus, A., Huynh, V., Ramstad, P. and Pallas, M. (1991) Large scale automated synthesis of oligodeoxyribonucleotides. *Nucleic Acids Symp. Ser.* **24**: 41–42.

34. Gausepohl, H., Boulin, C., Kraft, M. and Frank, R. W. (1992) Automated multiple peptide synthesis. *Peptide. Res.* **5**: 315–320.

35. Kaplan, B. E. and Itakura, K. (1987) DNA synthesis on solid supports and automation. In Narang, S. A. (ed.) *Synthesis and Applications of DNA and RNA*, pp 9–45. Academic Press, Orlando.

36. Neimark, J. and Briand, J. P. (1993) Development of a fully automated multichannel peptide synthesizer with integrated TFA cleavage capability. *Peptide Res.* **6**: 219–228.

37. Schnorrenberg, G. and Gerhardt, H. (1989) Fully automatic simultaneous multiple peptide synthesis in micromolar scale—rapid synthesis of series of peptides for screening in biological assays. *Tetrahedron* **45**: 7759–7764.

38. Zuckermann, R. N. (1993) The chemical synthesis of peptidomimetic libraries. *Curr. Opin. Struct. Biol.* **3**: 580–584.

39. Zuckermann, R. N. and Banville, S. C. (1992) Automated peptide-resin deprotection/cleavage by a robotic workstation. *Peptide Res.* **5**: 169–174.

40. Zuckermann, R. N., Kerr, J. M., Siani, M. A. and Banville, S. C. (1992) Design, construction and application of a fully automated equimolar peptide mixture synthesizer. *Int. J. Peptide Protein Res.* **40**: 497–506.

41. Zuckermann, R. N., Kerr, J. M., Siani, M. A., Banville, S. C. and Santi, D. V. (1992) Identification of highest-affinity ligands by affinity selection from equimolar peptide mixtures generated by robotic synthesis. *Proc. Natl. Acad. Sci. USA* **89**: 4505–4509.

42. Zuckermann, R. N., Siani, M. A. and Banville, S. C. (1992) Control of the Zymate robot with an external computer. Construction of a multiple peptide synthesizer. *Lab. Rob. Autom.* **4**: 183–192.

43. Corkan, L. A. and Lindsey, J. S. (1992) Experiment manager software for an automated chemistry workstation, including a scheduler for parallel experimentation. *Chemom. Intell. Lab. Syst.* **17**: 47–74.

44. Corkan, L. A., Plouvier, J. C. and Lindsey, J. S. (1992) Application of an automated chemistry workstation to problems in synthetic chemistry. *Chemom. Intell. Lab. Syst.* **17**: 95–105.

45. DeWitt, S. H., Kiely, J. K., Stankovic, C. J., Schroeder, M. C., Cody, D. M. R. and Pavia, M. R. (1993) 'Diversomers': an approach to nonpeptide, nonoligomeric chemical diversity. *Proc. Natl. Acad. Sci. USA.* **90**: 6909–6913.

46. DeWitt, S. H., Schroeder, M. C., Stankovic, C. J., Strode, J. E. and Czarnik, A. W. (1994) DIVERSOMER™ technology: solid phase synthesis, automation, and integration for the generation of chemical diversity. *Drug Dev. Res.* **33**: 116–124.

47. DeWitt, S. H., Stankovic, C. J. and Schroeder, M. C. (1993) The DIVERSOMER approach: Integration and automation of multiple, simultaneous solid phase synthesis. In Stimatitis, J. R. and Hawk, G. L. (eds) *Advances in Laboratory Automation—Robotics*, pp. 248–263. Zymark Corporation, Hopkinton, MA.

48. Lantrip, D. A., Fuchs, P. L. and Kramer, G. W. (1989) Controlling the Purdue automated synthesis system. *Adv. Lab. Autom. Rob.* **5**: 115–137.

49. Lindsey, J. S. (1992) A retrospective on the automation of laboratorysynthetic chemistry. *Chemom. Intell. Lab. Syst.* **17**: 15–45.

50. Metivier, P., Josses, P., Bulliot, H., Corbet, J. P. and Joux, B. (1992) Automation of organic synthesis in industrial research laboratories. *Chemom. Intell. Lab. Syst.* **17**: 137–143.
51. Sherman, M. I., Bertelsen, A. H. and Cook, A. F. (1993) Protein epitope targeting: Oligonucleotide diversity and drug discovery. *Bioorg. Med. Chem. Lett.* **3**: 469–475.
52. Tuerk, C. and Gold, L. (1990) Systematic evolution of ligands by exponential enrichment: RNA ligands to bacteriophage T4 DNA polymerase. *Science* **249**: 505–510.
53. Ellington, A. D. and Szostak, J. W. (1990) *In vitro* selection of RNA molecules that bind specific ligands. *Nature* **346**: 818–822.
54. Houghten, R. A. (1993) Peptide libraries: Criteria and trends. *Trends Genet.* **9**: 235–239.
55. Jung, G. and Beck-Sickinger, A. G. (1992) Multiple peptide synthesis methods and their applications. *Angew. Chem. Int. Ed. Engl.* **31**: 367–383.
56. Danishefsky, S. J., McCure, K. F., Randolph, J. T. and Ruggeri, R. B. (1993) A strategy for the solid-phase synthesis of oligosaccharides. *Science* **260**: 1307–1309.
57. Douglas, S. P., Whitfield, D. M. and Krepinsky, J. J. (1991) Polymer-supported solution synthesis of oligosaccharides. *J. Am. Chem. Soc.* **113**: 5095–5097.
58. Schuster, M., Wang, P., Paulson, J. C. and Wong, C.-H. (1994) Solid-phase chemical-enzymatic synthesis of glycopeptides and oligosaccharides. *J. Am. Chem. Soc.* **116**: 1135–1136.
59. Cho, C. Y., Moran, E. J., Cherry, S. R., Stephans, J. C., Fodor, S. P. A., Adams, C. L., Sundaram, A., Jacobs, J. W. and Schultz, P. G. (1993) An unnatural biopolymer. *Science* **261**: 1303–1305.
60. Simon, R. J., Kania, R. S., Zuckermann, R. N. *et al.* (1992) Peptoids: A modular approach to drug discovery. *Proc. Natl Acad. Sci. USA* **89**: 9367–9371.
61. Zuckermann, R. N., Kerr, J. M., Kent, S. B. H. and Moos, W. H. (1992) Efficient method for the preparation of peptoids (oligo(N-substituted glycines)) by submonomer solid-phase synthesis. *J. Am. Chem. Soc.* **114**: 10646–10647.
62. Campbell, D. A. (1992) The synthesis of phosphonate esters, and extension of the Mitsunobu reaction. *J. Org. Chem.* **57**: 6331–6335.
63. Campbell, D. A. and Bermak, J. C. (1994) Phosphonate ester synthesis using a modified Mitsunobu condensation. *J. Org. Chem.* **59**: 658–660.
64. Hagihara, M., Anthony, N. J., Stout, T. J., Clardy, J. and Schreiber, S. L. (1992) Vinylogous polypeptides: An alternative peptide backbone. *J. Am. Chem. Soc.* **114**, 6568–6570.
65. A.B. Smith, I., Keenan, T. P., Holcomb, R. C., Sprengler, P. A., Guzman, M. C., Wood, J. L., Carroll, P. J. and Hirschmann, R. (1992) Design, synthesis and crystal structure of a pyrrolinone-based peptidomimetic possessing the conformation of a β-strand: Potential applications to the design of novel inhibitors of proteolytic enzymes. *J. Am. Chem. Soc.* **114**: 10672–10674.
66. Bunin, B. A. and Ellman, J. A. (1992) A general and expedient method for the solid-phase synthesis of 1,4-benzodiazepine derivatives. *J. Am. Chem. Soc.* **114**: 10997–10998.
67. Bunin, B. A., Plunkett, M. J. and Ellman, J. A. (1994) The combinatorial synthesis and chemical and biological evaluation of a 1,4-benzodiazepine library. *Proc. Natl. Acad. Sci. USA* **91**: 4708–4712.
68. Chen, C., Randall, L. A. A., Miller, R. B., Jones, A. D. and Kurth, M. J. (1994) 'Analogous' organic synthesis of small-compound libraries: Validation of combinatorial chemistry in small-molecule synthesis. *J. Am. Chem. Soc.* **116**: 2661–2662.
69. Geysen, H. M., Rodda, S. J., Mason, T. J., Tribbick, G. and Schoofs, P. G. (1987) Strategies for epitope analysis using peptide synthesis. *J. Immunol. Methods* **102**, 259–274.

9

Synthesis of Peptide Libraries for Lead Structure Screening

VICTOR J. HRUBY

I. INTRODUCTION

The idea of using various combinatorial mathematical methods to help prepare very large chemical 'libraries', and then to use these libraries to screen for binding, enzyme antagonist properties, hormone agonist or antagonist activity, cell growth promoting or inhibiting activities, anti-viral activities, cell adhesion properties, etc., has become a 'hot' area of organic, bio-organic and medicinal chemistry. In a sense this is a somewhat unexpected development. Organic chemists, who only a few years ago would have loudly criticized the creation of complex mixtures or populations of organic molecules without particular and specific knowledge of the precise chemical nature of each chemical entity, now appear to be highly enthusiastic regarding any synthetic effort that in principle, though *often* not in practice, can

THE PRACTICE OF MEDICINAL CHEMISTRY
ISBN 0-12-744640-0

produce a structurally diverse mixture of organic compounds. The realization, primarily with peptides, that it is possible to create very large (>1 000 000) diverse peptide libraries by *chemical methods*[1,2] and that these libraries could be used to screen for binding and other biologically relevant interactions with biological macromolecules, such as receptors, antibodies, enzymes, etc., has led to an explosion of activity both to develop synthetic approaches to a variety of other organic molecular classes and to develop rapid screening methods that would allow evaluation of millions of individual organic structures for their interactions with a wide variety of biological targets.

Though few examples can be cited where dramatic new discoveries of ligands with immediate potential as new drugs have been made, and outside of the peptide area the chemical purity of the libraries usually has not been rigorously demonstrated, enough new and provocative discoveries have been made to elicit a virtual stampede into this technologically enticing area.

Clearly this area of chemical research has enormous potential and is especially enticing because it provides synthetic chemists for the first time with an approach that, in principle, can effectively complete with biologists in producing and evaluating large and diverse chemical populations. Biologists simultaneously have been developing very large combinatorial 'libraries' using microbiological and molecular biological approaches (e.g. see refs 3–7). These latter methods will not be discussed here except for comparison with chemical methods. Both biological and chemical approaches have advantages and disadvantages, some intrinsic to the limitations of living systems and chemical reactivity, respectively, and the current limitations of technologies currently available by these approaches. At present, perhaps the most critical limitations of biological systems are related to the inherent limitations of the genetic machinery that uses limited numbers of nucleic acids and amino acids as its building blocks (with the ability to also incorporate certain carbohydrates and lipids into polypeptide structures). The major limitations of the organic synthetic approach is that relatively few classes of compounds can be synthesized with high (>95%) chemical and stereochemical fidelity. These limitations will be revisited on occasion during our discussions, but the major focus of the rest of this chapter will be on the design, synthesis and use of peptide libraries, which thus far have been the most widely used and developed synthetic organic combinatorial chemistry approach. A good overview of the possibilities and potential of other biological approaches has recently appeared.[8]

A major question that might be asked is 'Why peptides?' Peptides constitute a class of organic molecules that nature has used to recognize essentially all the rest of the known chemical world; peptides can control, catalyse and modulate most biological processes; and peptides are highly compatible with and generally nontoxic to living systems. Furthermore, synthetic peptide chemistry is perhaps the most highly developed, high-yield, stereospecific synthetic methodology available to synthetic chemistry. Thus large (>10^6) peptide libraries can be prepared with a high degree of confidence that the peptides present will be those designed to be present, with few other compounds as a result of side reactions. Under optimized conditions, a 99.9% yield for the peptide bond formation reaction without racemization is common. Thus, in a 'typical' library synthesis, only a small amount of truncated or deletion peptides will be obtained. This is important for the screening process used to evaluate most libraries, since it generally will be difficult or impossible to detect and determine the structure of a 1% or even a 10% impurity that happens to be superpotent or have antagonist activities. In these cases, binding or other activity may be observed, but on determining the structure of the major component it may be found as resynthesis that this component is inactive or only weakly active. Finally, peptides are diverse structures both in terms of chemical functionality and in terms of conformational space that can be explored both with the peptide backbone (*phi–psi space*,

Ramachandran space) and the peptide side-chain groups (*chi space*), both of which are quite conformationally flexible. Hence, a simple hexapeptide not only has its unique chemical structure but also has hundreds or even tens of thousands of available conformations at physiological temperature. In fact it is now well established that a biological system can use several of these conformations during its biological life, depending on the environment (solvent, pH, etc.), and the acceptor molecule (enzyme, receptor, antibody, etc.) with which it is interacting. Thus, in addition to the enormous chemical diversity possible for a relatively small peptide, the conformational diversity that can be examined by these peptides is enormous. Moreover, synthetic chemists are not limited to the 20 α-amino acids that biological systems can utilize via the genetic machinery of the cell, but can utilize hundreds or even thousands of additional amino acids or amino acid mimetics to greatly expand the diversity.

In addition to the mathematical and chemical considerations that must go into the construction of combinatorial peptide libraries, the availability of methods to examine the biological properties of these compounds is critical. Most biological acceptor molecules, receptors, enzymes, antibodies, nucleic acids, etc. are large complex structures, and therefore there is the possibility (certainty) that interactions of the peptide with the acceptor will occur at sites completely independent from sites important for biological activity. Thus, so-called false positive results are likely to be common in a screening process involving millions of potential binders. Obviously this can seriously interfere with the discovery process. Screening strategies must be developed that will minimize the 'nonspecific' binding of a compound or compounds to the acceptor. When a good deal is known about the properties of the acceptor molecule *before* a screening process is initiated, then the controls and conditions that were utilized previously can be used to avoid such interactions. However, usually the case is that very little is known about the acceptor molecule except for some specific chemical, biochemical, pharmacological or physiological process it displays or modulates. In these cases, the acceptor molecule often is not a pure chemical entity but rather is part of a membrane or a component of a cell, or is part of some even more complex tissue system. In this case, a good many of nonspecific interactions are to be expected, and efforts to minimize them by choice of experimental conditions as well as by well-designed controls are needed.

II. THE CHEMICAL CONSTRUCTION OF COMBINATORIAL PEPTIDE LIBRARIES

As already discussed, the central importance of peptides and proteins in almost all important biological processes, though well known for over forty years, has not been recognized and used by many organic and medicinal chemists. To a considerable extent the reason can be traced back to the lack of training in synthetic amino acid, peptide and peptidomimetic chemistry, and to a lack of appreciation of the stereostructural and conformational properties of peptides. However, this has changed considerably in recent years. Interestingly, though much of the technology necessary to construct and use large synthetic peptide libraries has been available for some time, their introduction and use in biology is of much more recent origin. The idea of making peptide mixtures has been discussed for many years, but this use was frowned upon by most synthetic chemists and medicinal chemists owing to a lack of quality control and the difficulty of interpreting the results. However, a couple of developments in the mid 1980s apparently served as stimuli for the creation and use of large peptide libraries. A major stimulus was the need to produce ever increasing numbers of peptides as a result of the discovery of many new peptide hormones, neurotransmitters, enzymes, cytokines, growth factors, adhesion proteins, glycoproteins, receptors, antigenic sites, antibodies, structural proteins, oncogenes, ion channels, and so on. This explosion of peptides and proteins was of critical interest to a diverse scientific community ranging from biophysicists and chemists to molecular biologists and medical doctors, and created a tremendous demand for the synthesis of peptides. In part, this was met by tremendous advances in synthesis of peptides using primarily the solid-phase method of peptide chemistry developed by Merrifield.[9–11] A major reason for its utilization for these purposes was the ability to automate peptide synthesis and the rapid availability of synthesizers. The development of these methods and the more recent developments in rapid multiple peptide synthesis has been reviewed.[12] Despite these developments, the ability to synthesize large numbers of individual peptides became increasingly an issue owing to advances in immunology, in the genome project, and in the molecular cloning of numerous bioactive receptors, enzymes, hormones, oncogenes, etc., which led to the need to discover agonist or antagonist ligands for these acceptors. This need became especially acute in the area of immunology, where rapid developments in molecular biology, in biochemical investigations of the immune system and its mechanism(s) of action, in the development of monoclonal antibodies as diagnostic, scientific and medicinal tools, and so forth, led to the need for unprecedented numbers of peptides to evaluate and investigate these issues. The development of multiple peptide synthesis by Geysen and co-workers, and the 'tea bag method' by Houghton and co-workers (see below) to help deal with these issues serves as a convenient starting point for discussing methods used for the synthesis of relatively large, chemically specific peptide libraries using optimized methods of peptide synthesis.

A.   The multipin method

As with all processes that have been developed for multiple peptide synthesis in formats that are useful for evaluation of biologically or biochemically relevant interactions of the synthesized peptides with acceptor and receptor molecules or cells, the simultaneous application of several diverse technologies has been critical to their successful development and utilization for a wide variety of problems. The development of the multipin method by Geysen and co-workers is an excellent example of bringing together several technologies to create a whole greater than its parts.

The Geysen method[13–15] starts with the synthesis of 96 *different* peptide sequences by parallel synthesis on the pinhead surface of polyacrylic acid-grafted polyethylene pins arrayed in a 96 microtitre plate format. As originally developed, the peptide material (about 50 nanomoles) was synthesized on a solid support covalently linked to the spherical head of each pin. By exposing each pinhead to only one activated amino acid at each coupling step of the synthetic process, it was possible to synthesize 96 different peptides (one for each pinhead) simultaneously, and to know the structure of the individual peptide on each pinhead. A common synthetic strategy is used for the construction of each of the 96 peptides, with common reagents and solvents for the removal of the N^α temporary protecting groups and subsequent neutralization (if necessary) and washing steps. Using several plates, several hundred to several thousand individual peptides with a specific spatial location on a particular pinhead can be synthesized in a relatively short time. Though only small amounts of peptide ($\leq$ 50 nmol) were initially prepared, much larger quantities ($\sim$2 μmol)[16] can now be 'loaded' on the pinheads. Having now a unique peptide (assuming the synthesis has been done in very high yields) on each pinhead, the interactions of each peptide with an acceptor molecule can be examined by a direct binding assay. In practice, this usually means some kind of ELISA assay that produces a colour reaction that can be readily visualized. In principle, other types of detection such as radioactivity measurements or fluorescence measurements might be used, but these present safety problems or technological difficulties. In any case, the coupling of sophisticated polymer technology, optimized solid-phase peptide chemistry methodology, and highly sensitive state-of-the-art analytical biochemistry and molecular pharmacology methodology has made possible the development of this approach into a highly useful method.

As with the introduction of the solid-phase method of peptide synthesis, the introduction of this methodology was met with considerable criticism by the synthetic community. Criticisms regarding the purity of the peptides and the general applicability of the methods led Geysen and co-workers to develop several techniques to assess the synthetic methodology, improve it, and evaluate the chemical structure and purity of the peptides attached to the pinheads. Of particular importance was the utilization of linker moieties that allowed cleavage of the peptides from the pinheads into solution so that the purity and structural integrity of the peptide on the pinhead could be carefully evaluated. An additional bonus was that the peptides could now be examined in solution in competitive binding experiments and/or functional bioassays with isolated acceptor molecules or whole cells.[17–19] This powerful methodology has been applied since its inception to an ever-widening array of molecular recognition processes in biological systems. Among the most important applications to date one can include epitope analysis for antibody–antigen (protein) interaction,[20,21] binding sites to viral proteins,[13,22–24] endothelin structure–activity relationships,[25,26] and substance P structure–activity studies.[27,28]

B.   The tea-bag method

In order to more rapidly synthesize large numbers of peptides simultaneously, Houghton[29] devised an ingenious method using the solid-phase synthesis methodology but physically separating the resin into a number (a few to a few hundred) of individual porous polypropylene bags (since these bags resemble tea bags, the methodology has been subsequently dubbed the 'tea-bag' method). The idea, similar to that of Geysen's methods (and analogous to the subsequently developed proportioning-mixing or split synthesis method (see below)), was to segregate a growing peptide chain for coupling to different individual amino acids at each individual step of the synthesis, while performing all other steps such as α-amino group deprotection, washing, neutralizations steps if needed, etc., to a single reaction method. In this way, specific individual peptides would be synthesized in each tea bag, and by appropriate 'bookkeeping' throughout the synthesis the structure of the peptide in each tea bag would be known. The method had several major advantages. Most importantly there was no need for inventing any new solid supports, synthetic methodologies, and so on; optimized Merrifield solid-phase synthesis methods could be used throughout. Second, the amount of peptide to be made could be varied easily by the size of the tea bag and the amount and substitution level of the resin placed in the tea bag. Third, classical linkers could be used for the synthesis, so the peptide could be released from the resin by well-known and well-evaluated methods to provide a single peptide moiety whose purity, structure, biological activity, etc., could be completely evaluated. Finally the synthesis could be automated.[30] The method is widely applicable to a wide variety of problems, and essentially can use any synthetic methodology for producing peptides of interest. Finally the tea-bag synthetic method can be used in conjunction with combinatorial methods for synthesis of diverse chemical libraries containing hundreds of thousands to millions of peptides, generally put into solution.[1] This method will be discussed further later in this chapter.

Before proceeding to a discussion of the synthesis and use of large combinational libraries for obtaining lead structures in biological systems, a few additional comments regarding the limitations of peptide synthesis should be stated. These fall into essentially three categories: (a) considerations regarding the activated amino acid component; (b) considerations regarding the nucleophilicity of the peptide component; and (c) problems of racemization. Point (c) can be handled by a simple statement that, except for histidine and occasionally other amino acids (e.g. Ser and Cys), if N^α-urethane protected amino acids are used in conjunction with highly developed peptide bond-forming methods, little or no racemization will occur in solid-phase peptide synthesis. In general, highly activated α-amino acids will condense readily with simple amino acid or small peptides (2 or 4 residues) on resins. In simple dipeptide cases, relative rates generally vary over a few orders of magnitude and often much less when large excesses of the activated amino acids are used. It has been suggested that equimolar mixtures of peptides can be made by adjusting the ratios of the amino acid coupling to the peptide mixture. Although this can be made to work with relatively small peptides (dipeptides or tripeptides), as a general strategy it will not work, for well-known reasons. First and foremost is point (b) above, namely that peptides have enormous differences in nucleophilicity depending on their sequence, secondary structure, solvation, flexibility and other factors. The formation of even the same bond (say Phe–Val) in one peptide can be significantly different from that in the next. Thus, the attempt to prepare an equimolar mixture of peptides by such an approach will generally be unsuccessful for large ($>10^6$) peptide mixtures, and is likely to give complex mixtures of peptides of different concentrations if mixtures of activated amino acids are used for coupling.

The desire to prepare many peptides simultaneously so as to meet the needs of chemists and biologists at a reasonable cost has led to the development of automated multiple peptide synthesizers. As mentioned previously, the solid-phase method of peptide synthesis lends itself to automation, and it was only a matter of time before the synthesis of more than one peptide at a time was introduced. At first this meant two or three peptides at a time, but recently a number of groups have applied various robotic techniques[31-36] to the synthesis of a larger number (over 30–100) of peptides simultaneously. These instruments are generally capable of making 10–100 micromolar quantities or more of desired peptides, that is milligram quantities, which can be used to satisfy many analytical and assay requirements. In addition, in some cases it is possible to manipulate the resins so as to use various combinatorial strategies (see above) to produce large peptide libraries as well.

III. SYNTHESIS OF COMBINATORIAL PEPTIDE LIBRARIES AND THEIR USE FOR LARGE-SCALE SCREENING FOR BIOLOGICAL ACTIVITY

The ability to synthesize peptides on solid supports in a stepwise manner with nearly quantitive yields for each step in the synthesis has made it possible to synthesize relatively large peptides (10 or more amino acid residues) with high fidelity (>95% overall yield) when optimized conditions are used. In addition, numerous methods have been developed to tether the peptide to the resin so that the peptide can be released either in protected or unprotected form.[11] Thus, a peptide containing no protecting groups (except for the point of attachment) can be left on the solid support and used in an assay, and can then be released from the resin and examined in solution. From the standpoint of structure determination for the active component of a large mixture, leaving the peptide on the resin has the advantage that the resin particle or surface can be isolated and the structure determined directly. If the peptide is part of a large mixture of released peptides, then in general additional interactive synthesis and biological screening will be necessary to determine the structure of the active component. Strategies have been developed so that this can be done quickly.

When these methods are combined with various statistical (combinatorial) mathematical approaches that were developed several centuries ago, it is possible to synthesize millions of peptides in a small volume, either attached to a solid support and spatially resolvable or released into solution at concentrations that are suitable for screening. We will discuss here some of the approaches that have been used for rapid synthesis of large (>10^6) peptide libraries that are used in conjunction with rapid screening methods and state-of-the-art analytical procedures to detect bioactive peptides of interest in these large libraries and determine the structure of the bioactive peptides. There are two keys to success using a methodology in which millions of peptides are generated and then evaluated by some screening process. First, the synthesis needs to be done in a statistical manner such that many compounds can be produced simultaneously. Obviously, if several million peptides are to be produced, this can only be done in a reasonable length of time if exponential statistics are applied to the synthetic process. Equally important is the development of methods that can simultaneously screen thousands to millions of compounds. Again, if only one compound can be assayed at a time, it will take too long and be too costly to screen large libraries of millions of individual compounds.

One such method that has been developed for the synthesis and biological evaluation of very large peptide libraries (>10^6) is the Selectide process.[2,37] In this methodology, also referred to as the 'one-bead one-peptide' process, millions of peptides are produced on a solid support (bead). Then the protecting groups are removed and the peptides on the surface are evaluated for their ability to interact with biologically important acceptor molecules. Alternatively, or after the binding assay, the peptides can be partially released from the beads and utilized in a soluble form for an assay. Sufficient peptide material is on the bead initially, and after partial release, that the structure of the peptide can be determined by modern microsequencing methods. The overall process is illustrated in Fig. 9.1.

The first step in the process is the synthesis of a large peptide library. The keys to success in the construction of the library are: (1) that at any given time all beads in the library are only reacting with a single coupling reagent (removal of temporary protecting groups can be done in the combined pool); (2) that the number and the size of the beads in each pool are essentially identical (this is done so that a Poisson distribution is obtained; of course other statistical distributions can be used); (3) that optimized solid-phase synthesis methods be used to provide 'clean' libraries. The choice of a suitable bead is important both for synthesis and later for biological screening. Of particular importance, if one is to provide the peptides at more or less equal molar concentrations, is that the beads be of uniform size and surface characteristics, since, in most cases where macromolecular acceptor molecules are the targets, these targets will not enter the polymer matrix but will interact with those peptides on the surface of the beads. These requirements can be met by some of the currently available solid supports such as Tentagel.

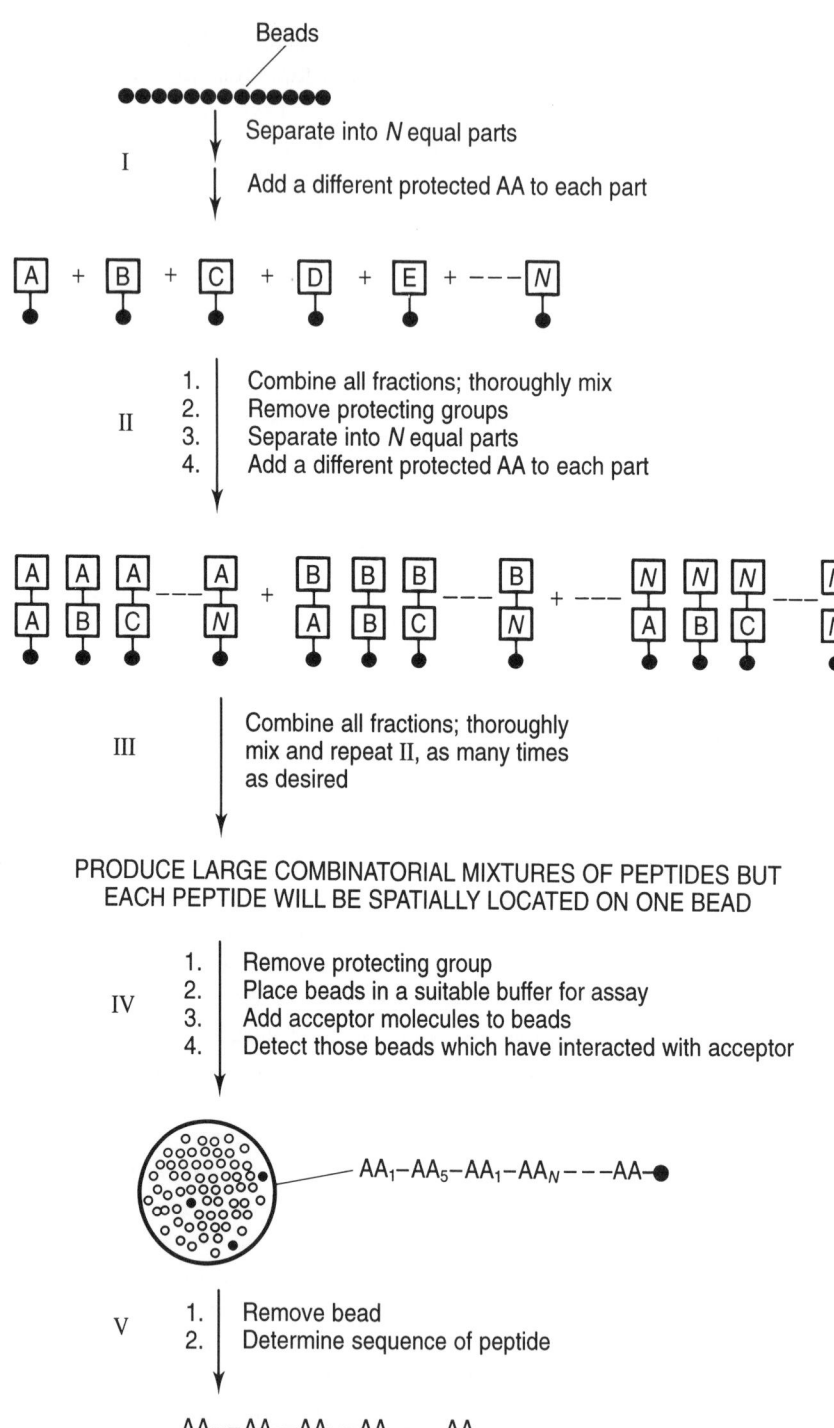

Fig. 9.1 An outline of the procedures necessary to synthesize a large (>10⁶) peptide library on beads, utilize it for detecting interactions with a receptor/acceptor, and determine the structure of the interacting peptides.

The first criterion is met by splitting of the resin into N equal portions and reacting each portion with an individual single amino acid or peptide. The earliest description of this method of synthesis was reported by Furka and co-workers.[38] It was referred to as 'proportioning mixing'[38–41] and used to produce solution mixtures of peptides following synthesis. A similar approach was suggested by Houghton et al.[1] and was referred to as a 'divide, couple and recombine' process, and was used to produce solution mixtures which were used for screening for binding or biological activity. In these approaches the size of the library in terms of numbers of individual chemical structures that are possible depends on the value of N and the chemical diversity of structures A to N. If each α-amino acid is a different chemical species, then a very large chemical library can be produced very quickly as shown in Table 9.1. If 20 different amino acids are chosen, at the pentapeptide stage over three million different species are possible, and at the heptapeptide level over a billion different peptides are possible.

Table 9.1 Size of a peptide library from number of amino acids used at each step.

Number of iterations	Number of distinct amino acids	Theoretical size of library
1	20	20
2	20	400
3	20	8 000
4	20	160 000
5	20	3 200 000
6	20	64 000 000
7	20	1 380 000 000
1	60	60
2	60	3 600
3	60	216 000
4	60	12 960 000
1	20	20
2	40	800
3	10	8 000
4	100	800 000
5	40	3 200 000

The extent to which the entire population of peptides is present depends on how many beads are present during the synthesis. Which peptides individually are present among all those possible also depends on how many beads are present throughout the synthetic assembly. Since the synthetic scheme is such that each bead in the mixture will contain only one peptide, obviously one cannot have more peptides than beads. However, there will actually have fewer because of the statistical nature of the synthetic procedure. Whereas in the tea-bag method every peptide (tea bag) can be singly and independently made to follow a unique synthetic route, in the statistical procedure some beads out of the several million of a typical synthesis will follow exactly the same route and thus have the same structure. In order not to have too much redundancy, large libraries often are synthesized using approximately the same number of beads (or fewer) as the theoretical number that could be formed according to the iterative synthetic process used (Table 9.1), counting on the highly redundant nature of the synthetic process to provide most sequences. However, it must be kept in mind that unless one uses five or six times the number of beads as the number of theoretical chemical compounds, a significant percentage of the possible compounds that could be synthesized will not be present (the exact percentage can be calculated from the Poisson distribution or from whatever statistical distribution method is used for the synthesis).

The number of beads per unit volume will depend on several factors, including the size of the beads (for solid phase peptide synthesis (SPPS) the most common beads are 50–120 μm in diameter) and the extent to which they swell in the solvent used (beads generally swell from a few fold to 10-fold or more). Typically 1 million beads of 80 μm take up about 1–2 ml, so when in solvent they will occupy 2–20 ml. From a practical point of view (reagent costs, solvents costs, instrumental limitations, etc.), a library of 500 000 to 5 000 000 is the most practical. The choice of resin and the linker group depends very much on the application. If the peptides are to be released into solution then almost any polymer matrix that is compatible with the synthetic methodology can be used. However, in this case it must be kept in mind that, unless a large excess of beads is used in relation to the number of possible chemical entities, some peptides may be present at 2–3 or more times the concentration of others when the library is released into solution because there can be two or more beads of one entity and only one of another. The linker in this case should be simple, compatible with the synthetic methodology, and generally cleavable under the same conditions as the side-chain protecting groups for the amino acids. Typically this involves some acid or base procedure,[11] but in general any well-developed method of solid-phase peptide synthesis can be used.[11,42,43] These peptide mixtures then can be used in a wide variety of assays.

On the other hand, if the peptide is to be retained on the resin (perhaps to be released later), then other criteria must be considered. From the standpoint of synthesis the resin must be compatible with and inert to the synthetic methodology. In addition, the resin, or at least the resin surface, must be compatible with the biological macromolecule or more complex biological system to be assayed. In terms of the linker arm it must be stable to (orthogonal to) the conditions used for removal of N^α-protecting groups, and to the subsequent conditions that will be used to remove the side-chain protecting groups. For this reason the N^α-Fmoc strategy[43] is generally used for library construction. Several considerations apply to the linker. The linker can have an important effect on how the peptide is 'presented' to the acceptor molecule while still attached to the resin. Since most acceptor molecules of interest are high-molecular-weight polymers (proteins, nucleic acids, etc.), and the binding pockets can be several angstroms deep, it is important that the linker be extended away from the solid support matrix and be 'biocompatible'. In addition, if the peptide is to be released into solution, the linker must either come off the resin with the peptide and not interfere seriously with the peptides binding or biological activity, or it must remain on the resin independently of the peptide. Linkers for doing this have been developed,[44–47] and one also can utilize release mechanisms already developed as part of the developments for segment solid-phase peptide synthesis.[11,42,43]

If the peptides are retained on the solid support in the one-bead one-peptide format, a variety of methods can be used for assaying the library. In general, these involve a binding interaction. Thus, the ability to detect specific binding and distinguish it from nonspecific binding is critical. A comprehensive discussion of binding assay methods is beyond the scope of this chapter; however, a few important points should be emphasized. First, having a pure acceptor molecular or multimolecular entity can greatly facilitate the assay since its nonspecific interactions with the library and the solid support can be examined directly and largely controlled. Second, the availability of the native ligand or an analogue or compound that is known to bind specifically and potently at the desired site of interaction is critical for establishing controls, and evaluating whether the binding interaction observed in the library is specific or non-specific. Third, proper choice of the experimental conditions such as salt concentrations, temperature, solvents, etc., is critical.

A wide variety of possibilities exist for detection. Since most of the acceptor molecules (receptors, enzymes, antibodies, etc.) are large macromolecules, they can often be linked to a variety of enzymes in a manner that will not interfere with the binding pocket for the acceptor. The enzyme system is chosen so as to provide a coupled chemical reaction that provides a coloured product that can be readily seen. Alternatively, the acceptor can be labelled with fluorescent or radioactive labels for detection. In any case, those beads that possess a peptide that can interact with the acceptor molecule can readily be distinguished from those that do not, and separated by manual procedures using a micromanipulator or by other techniques. Once the individual beads are obtained, each bead can be washed with 8 M guanidine hydrochloride or treated in some other manner to remove the binding moiety from the surface of the peptide. Then the peptide sequence can be determined using, for example a microsequencer. Since for the most part acceptor molecules are large macromolecules that do not penetrate into the bead but only interact with the peptide on the surface of the bead, most of the peptide in the bead is available for structural analysis even if the acceptor molecule is not removed. In addition to microsequencing methods, other methods for structure determination are being examined, including mass spectroscopy, various encoding methods and other methods.[48-55] These methods will become essential as one increasingly prepares and utilizes nonpeptide libraries, but they can be useful even for peptide libraries, especially when the library is made on small beads and when the lower level of detection in micropeptide sequencing (1–5 picomoles) is reached. Generally the structures are determined one bead at a time so as to examine the diversity of structures that can bind to the acceptor molecule. However, owing to the redundancy of the libraries, one often obtains a 'consensus sequence', especially when the binding moiety is located on a continuous sequence (though in principle the method also should work for a discontinuous sequence). In this approach a number of beads can be sequenced simultaneously and the consensus sequence determined in a much faster fashion.[47] Using these methods, the binding peptides (or nonpeptides) for a variety of acceptor molecules can be discovered, and in some cases several different kinds of ligands for the same binding site are obtained, including both linear and cyclic peptides for the same acceptor molecule.[2,47,56-59]

Another method for preparing and utilizing large combinatorial libraries for discovering peptide ligands that bind and interact with receptors, antibodies and other acceptor molecules of biological importance has been developed by Houghton and co-workers.[1] In part it is based on the Houghton tea bag method,[29] but uses a further combinatorial approach[1] in which peptide solutions, generally each containing hundreds of thousands of peptides, are constructed. The libraries are construcuted in such a way that all of the possible structures of a peptide of a particular size are made in a series of sublibraries that are used for assay. For example, all hexapeptides made up of the 20 common amino acids (64 million) are included in 400 libraries, each containing 160 000 peptides. Each solution containing 160 000 peptides is than screened for binding or some other biochemical or bioassay end point, and the active fractions are resynthesized in a modified combinatorial form such that, by a process of iteration, the most favoured amino acid at each residue position in the peptide sequence is obtained. This generally results in an increasingly potent hexapeptide during the process. As it is generally practised to date, only the most potent mixture is chosen for iteration at each step, so that to some extent the final ligand obtained may depend on where one begins the search. On the other hand, this method has certain inherent advantages including the substantial flexibility in synthesis that it allows, the possibility of more readily integrating different combinatorial approaches in the discovery process, and the ability to work in solution for all assays so that even whole cells are readily studied. In addition, the use of positional scanning combinatorial synthetic approaches allows for some optimization in an early stage of the discovery process. This approach has been used to obtain active compounds for a wide variety of receptors/acceptors including antibodies, receptors and whole cells.[60-64]

IV. COMBINATORIAL LIBRARIES ON SURFACES PREPARED BY LIGHT-DIRECTED SPATIALLY ADDRESSABLE PARALLEL CHEMICAL SYNTHESIS AND OTHER METHODS

The complexity of combinatorial chemistry and its application to biological systems and medical problems has stimulated the application of high technology to the problem. The application of multipeptide synthesizers, robotics and novel polymer technology to the synthesis problem and ELISA technology, FACS methodology and related methods to the detection problem are all examples of the use of state-of-the-art technologies.

One of the most sophisticated applications along these lines is the suggested utilization of solid-state peptide synthetic methodology in conjunction with photolithography as suggested by Fodor *et al.*[65] Synthesis of the peptide is accomplished on a flat surface using a material suitable for solid-phase peptide synthesis and compatible photolithographic methods. The key for success in this methodology from a synthetic point of view is the ability to photochemically remove the N^α-amino protecting group at a specifically defined portion of the surface. Thus only that portion of the surface previously exposed to light will react with the protected amino acid when it is provided to the full surface. Using technology already available, it is possible to expose only a very small part of the surface, say 0.5 mm $\times$ 0.5 mm, and create a synthetic grid on which numerous peptides can be prepared (400 on a 10 mm $\times$ 10 mm surface with the spatial resolution of 0.5 mm $\times$ 0.5 mm). In principle, much higher resolution is possible, further increasing the number of peptides that can be prepared on a fairly small surface in spatially discrete locations (much as the peptides on beads are each in a spatially discrete location — a particular bead). Following the first reaction and suitable washings, a different area of the surface can be exposed to light and a different amino acid added, and so on until the entire surface is substituted with a variety of amino acids. The entire process can be repeated N times in a predetermined synthetic scheme until the entire array of desired peptides is produced. Using combinatorial approaches of synthesis, all possible examples of a particular combination can in principle be prepared. Once the peptides have been assembled on the surface, the protecting groups are removed and the peptides are exposed to the molecule to be assayed, which generally must possess a fluorescent reporter group for detection. As with the bead methodology, an advantage of this method is that each peptide can be assembled and evaluated in a small spatial location of 50–100 μm (about the size of the SPPS beads discussed previously) and evaluated for interaction with the acceptor molecule of interest. The key to success, assuming the peptide synthesis has gone well, is whether the peptides on the surface of the plates are accessible for interaction with the acceptor molecules, and the ability of the acceptor molecule to bind to the peptides in this format. The nonquantitative nature of the removal of the photochemical protecting groups currently in use provides a challenge to chemists to find better ones so that the full power of this technology can be utilized. Thus far, its major uses appear to be binding of peptides to monoclonal antibodies.[65,66]

In the meantime, other solid supports are being developed for use in a library format that are suitable for assay while the peptide is attached to the solid support. These include arrays attached to a modified polyethylene surface,[67] and controlled porous glass modified surfaces.[68] Undoubtedly many others are currently under investigation.

V.   FURTHER INVESTIGATION ON SCREENING

With the ability to synthesize very large complex libraries on a variety of surfaces and in solution, and in a variety of formats, the technology of screening becomes central. Many aspects of screening such as binding (specific and nonspecific), second messenger determination, enzyme cleavage or inhibition, and antigen–antibody interactions are chemical in nature, and aspects of kinetics, thermodynamics, molecular recognition, and so forth, are critical for success. Thus, it is surprising that chemists have not paid more attention to the need for new developments in this area as well. The ability to manipulate assay methods and systems in ways compatible with various library formats is of great importance. This is especially critical when the peptide libraries are attached to solid supports, but even in solution critical developments in preventing nonspecific binding, in eliminating background, whether from fluorescence or visible colour, are needed. In any case, a large number of approaches have been suggested for creating diversity and evaluating the structure in addition to those already discussed (see for example refs 69–72). However, the basic science necessary to rapidly optimize screening so that the best peptide ligands that interact with the acceptor system can be detected and quantitatively evaluated has not been as well developed. It requires major input from chemists.

VI.   CONCLUDING COMMENTS

The concept of using large peptide and nonpeptide arrays of compounds in a library format that can be used to screen for specific biological activities has great potential. Though the technology and the basic science are still in their infancy, it is clear that very powerful methods for examining and evaluating biological systems using chemical principles will be developed. Chemists are devising the tools that will allow them to compete with nature in exploring the physical and chemical basis for biological activity and control and explore new aspects of structure in relation to the possibilities for affecting biological properties. Both structural complexity and chemical diversity will be able to be examined in new and unique ways currently not available. This creates enormous challenges, opportunities and excitement for scientists and technologists.

ACKNOWLEDGEMENTS

The partial support of the US Public Health Service and National Institute of Drug Abuse is gratefully acknowledged. The help of Charlene Morgan in preparing this manuscript is gratefully acknowledged. I also thank Drs Kit Lam, Fahad Al-Obeidi and Sydney Salmon, colleagues at Selectide Corporation, and many others for their stimulating dicussions regarding this area.

REFERENCES

1. Houghton, R. A., Pinella, C., Blondelle, S. E., Appel, J. R., Dooley, C. T. and Cuervo, J. H. (1990) Generation and use of synthetic peptide combinatorial libraries for basic research and drug discovery. *Nature* **354**: 84–86.

2. Lam, K. S., Salmon, S. E., Hersh, E. M., Hruby, V. J., Kazmierski, W. M. and Knapp, R. J. (1991) A new type of synthetic peptide library for identifying ligand-binding activity. *Nature* **354**: 82–84.

3. Scott, J. K. and Smith, G. P. (1990) Searching for peptide ligands with an epitope library. *Science* **249**: 386–390.

4. Parmley, S. F. and Smith, G. P. (1988) Antibody-selected filamentous fd phage vectors: affinity purification of target genes. *Gene* **73**: 305–318.

5. Cwirla, S., Peters, E. A. Barrett, R. W. and Dower, W. J. (1990) Peptides on phage: a vast library of peptides for identifying ligands. *Proc. Natl Acad. Sci. USA* **87**: 6378–6382.

6. Devlin, J. J., Panganiban, L. C. and Devlin, P. E. (1990) Random peptide libraries: a source of specific binding molecules. *Science* **249**: 404–406.

7. Greenwood, J., Willis, A. E. and Perham, R. N. (1991) Multiple display of foreign peptides on a filamentous bacteriophage. *J. Mol. Biol,* **220**: 821–827.

8. Gordon, E. M., Barrett, R. W., Dower, W. J., Fodor, S. P. A. and Gallop, M. A. (1994) Applications of combinatorial technologies to drug discovery. 2. Combinatorial organic synthesis, library screening strategies, and future directions. *J. Med. Chem.* **37**: 1385–1401.

9. Merrifield, R. B. (1963) Solid phase peptide synthesis. I. The synthesis of a tetrapeptide. *J. Am. Chem. Soc.* **85**: 2149–2154.

10. Merrifield, R. B. (1986) Solid phase synthesis. *Science* **232**: 341–347.

11. For a recent review of peptide synthesis, see Hruby, V. J. and Meyer, J.-P. (1995) Chemical synthesis of peptides. In Hecht, S. (ed.) *Peptides and Proteins*, Academic Press (and references therein). In press.

12. Jung, G. and Beck-Sickinger, A. G. (1992) Multiple peptide synthesis methods and their applications. *Angew. Chem. Int. Ed. Engl.* **31**: 367–383.

13. Geysen, M. H., Meloen, R. H. and Barteling, S. J. (1984) Use of peptide synthesis to probe viral antigens for epitopes to a resolution of a single amino acid. *Proc. Natl Acad. Sci. U.S.A* **81**: 3998–4002.

14. Geysen, H. M., Rodda, S. J., Mason, T. J., Tribbick, G. and Schoofs, P. G. (1987) Strategies for epitope analysis using peptide synthesis. *J. Immunol. Methods* **102**: 259–274.

15. Geysen, H. M., Rodda, S. J. and Mason, T. J. (1986) A priori delination of a peptide which mimics a discontinuous antigenic determinant. *Mol. Immunol* **23**: 709–715.

16. Valerio, R. M., Bray, A. M., Campbell, R. A., Dipasquale, A., Margellis, C., Rodda, S. J., Geysen, H. M. and Maeji, N. J. (1993) Multipin peptide synthesis at the micromole scale using 2-hydroxyethyl methacrylate grafted polyethylene supports. *Int. J. Peptide Protein Res,* **42**: 1–9.

17. Bray, A. M., Maeji, N. J. and Geysen, H. M. (1990) The simultaneous multiple production of solution phase peptides: assessment of the Geysen method of simultaneous peptide synthesis. *Tetrahedron Lett.* **31**: 5811–5814.

18. Bray, A. M., Maeji, N. J., Jhingran, A. G. and Valerio, R. M. (1991) Gas phase cleavage of peptides from a solid support with ammonia vapor. Application in simultaneous multiple peptide synthesis. *Tetrahedron Lett.* **32**: 6163–6166.

19. Valerio, R. M., Benstead, M., Bray, A. M., Campbell, R. A. and Maeji, N. J. (1991) Synthesis of peptide analogs using the multipin peptide synthesis method. *Anal. Biochem.* **197**: 168–177.

20. Geysen, H. M. (1993) Generation of diverse chemically synthesized peptide libraries. In Yanaihara, N. (ed.) *Peptide Chemistry 1992*, pp. 3–10. Escom, Leiden.

21. Geysen, H. M. and Mason, T. J. (1993) Screening chemically synthesized peptide libraries for biologically relevant molecules. *Bioorg. Med. Chem. Lett.* **3**: 397–404.

22. Geysen, H. M., Barteling, S.-J. and Meloen, R. H. (1985) Small peptides induce antibodies with a sequence and structural requirement for binding antigen comparable to antibodies raised against native protein. *Proc. Natl Acad. Sci. U.S.A.* **82**: 178–182.

23. Gombert, F., Blecha, W. and Tahtinen, M. *et al.* (1990) Antigenic epitopes of NEF proteins from different HIV-1 strains as recognized by sera from patients with manifest and latent HIV infection. *Virology,* **176**: 458–466.

24. Gammon, G., Geysen, H. M., Apple, R. J., Pickett, E., Palmer, M., Ametani, A. and Sercarz, E. E. (1991) T cell determinant structure: cores and determinant envelopes in three mouse major histocompatibility complex halotypes. *J. Exp. Med.* **173**: 609–617.

25. Spellmeyer, D. C., Brown, S., Stauber, G. B., Geysen, H. M. and Valerio, R. (1993) Endothelin receptor ligands. Replacement net approach to SAR determination of potent hexapeptides. *Bioorg. Med. Chem. Lett.* **3**: 519–524.

26. Spellmeyer, D. C., Brown, S., Stauber, G. B., Geysen, H. M. and Valerio, R. (1993) Endothelin receptor ligands. Multiple D-amino acid replacement net approach. *Bioorg. Med. Chem. Lett.* **3**: 1253–1256.

27. Wang, J.-X., Bray, A. M., DiPasquale, A. J., Maeji, N. J. and Geysen, H. M. (1993) Application of the multipin peptide synthesis technique for peptide receptor binding studies: substance P as a model system. *Bioorg. Med. Chem. Lett.* **3**: 447–450.

28. Wang, J.-X., Pasquale, A. J., Bray, A. M., Maeji, N. J. and Geysen, H. M. (1993) Study of stereorequirements of stubstance P binding to NK1 receptors using analogs with systematic D-amino acid replacements. *Bioorg. Med. Chem. Lett.* **3**: 451–456.

29. Houghton, R. A. (1985) General method for the rapid solid-phase synthesis of large numbers of peptides: specificity of antigen–antibody interaction at the level of individual amino acids. *Proc. Natl. Acad. Sci. U.S.A.* **82**: 5131–5135.

30. Beck-Sickmeyer, A. G., Durr, H. and Jung, C. (1991) Semi-automated T-bag peptide synthesis using 9-fluorenylmethoxycarbonyl strategy and benzotriazole-1-yl-tetramethyluronium tetrafluoroborate activation. *Peptide Res.* **4**: 88–94.

31. Schnorrenberg, G. and Gerhardt, H. (1989) Fully automatic simultaneous multiple peptide synthesis in micromolar-scale rapid synthesis of series of peptides for screening in biological assays. *Tetrahedron* **45**: 7759–7765.

32. Zuckermann, R. N., Kerr, J. M., Siani, M. A. and Banville, S. C. (1992) Design, construction and application of a fully automated equimolar peptide mixture synthesizer. *Int. J. Peptide Protein Res.* **40**: 497–506.

33. Gausepohl, H., Boulin, C., Kraft, M. and Frank, R. W. (1992) Automated multiple peptide synthesis. *Peptide Res.* **5**: 315–320.

34. Krchnak, V., Vagner, J. and Mach, O. (1989) Multiple continuous-flow solid-phase peptide synthesis. Synthesis of an HIV antigenic peptide and its omission analogues. *Int. J. Peptide Protein Res.* **33**: 209–213.

35. Meldal, M., Holm, C. B., Bojesen, G., Havsteen-Jakobsen, M. and Holm, A. (1993) Multiple column peptide synthesis. Part 2. *Int. J. Peptide Protein Res.* **41**: 250–260.

36. Neimark, J. and Briand, J.-P. (1993) Development of a fully automated nulti-channel peptide synthesizer with integrated TFA cleavage capability. *Peptide Res.* **6**: 219–228.

37. Lam, K. S., Salmon, S., Hersh, E. M., Hruby, V. J., Al-Obeidi, F., Kazmierski, W. M. and Knapp, R. J. (1992) The selectide process: rapid generation of large synthetic peptide binding ligands. In Smith, J. A. and Rivier, J. E. (eds) *Peptides: Chemistry and Biology*, pp. 442–495. Escom, Leiden.

38. Furka, A., Sebestyen, F., Asgedom, M. and Dibo, G. (1988) *Abstracts 14th Int. Congr. Biochem.*, Prague, Czecholsalvakia, 1988, vol. 5, p. 47. Furka, A., Sebestyen, F., Asgedom, M. and Dibo, G. (1988) *Abstracts 10th Int. Symp. Med. Chem.* p. 288. Budapest, Hungary.

39. Furka, A., Sebestyen, F., Asgedom, M. and Dibo, G. (1991) General method for rapid synthesis of multicomponent peptide mixtures. *Int. J. Peptide Protein Res.* **37**: 487–493.

40. Sebestyen, F., Dibo, G. and Furka, A. (1993) Proportioning mixing: A multi–purpose technique in peptide synthesis. In Yanaihara, N. (ed.) *Peptide Chemistry 1992*, pp. 84–86. Escom, Leiden.

41. Furka, A., Sebestyen, F. and Campian, E. (1994) The use of sub-library kits in a new screening strategy. Hodges, R. S. and Smith, J. A. (eds) *Peptides: Chemistry Structure Biology*, pp. 986–988. Escom, Leiden.

42. Barany, G. and Merrifield, R. B. (1979) In Gross, E. and Meienhofer, J. (eds) *The Peptides: Analysis, Synthesis, Biology*, vol. 2, pp. 1–284. Academic Press, New York.

43. Fields, G. B. and Noble, R. L. (1990) Solid phase peptide synthesis using 9-fluorenylmethoxycarbonyl amino acids. *Int. J. Peptide Protein Res.* **35**: 161–214,

44. Lebl, M., Patek, M., Kocis, P., Krchnak, V., Hruby, V. J., Salmon, S. E. and Lam, K. S. (1993) Multiple release of equimolar amounts of peptides from a polymeric carrier using orthogonal linkage cleavage chemistry. *Int. J. Peptide Protein Res.* **41**: 201–203.

45. Kočiš, P., Krchňák, V. and Lebl, M. (1993) Symmetrical structure allowing the selective release of a defined quantity of peptide from a single bead of polymeric support. *Tetrahedron Lett.* **45**: 7251–7252.

46. Salmon, S. E., Lam, K. S. and Lebl, M. *et al.* (1994) An orthogonal partial cleavage approach for solution-phase identification of biologically active peptides from larger chemically synthesized peptide libraries. In Hodges, R. S. and Smith, J. A. (eds) *Peptides: Chemistry, Structure and Biology*, pp. 1001–1002. Escom, Leiden.

47. Lebl, M., Lam, K. S., Kočiš, P., Krchňák, V., Patek, M., Salmon, S. E. and Hruby, V. J. (1993) Methods for building libraries of peptide structures and determination of consensus sequences. In Schneider, C.H. and Eberle, A.W. (eds) *Peptides 1992*, pp. 67–69. Escom, Leiden.

48. Brenner, S. and Lerner, R. A. (1993) Encoded combinatorial chemistry. *Proc. Natl Acad. Sci. U.S.A.* **90**: 10700–10704.

49. Nielsen, J., Bremer, S. and Janda, K. D. (1993) Synthetic methods for the implementation of encoded combinatorial chemistry. *J. Am. Chem. Soc.* **115**: 9812–9813.

50. Needels, M. N., Jones, D. G., Tate, E. H., Heinbel, G. L., Kochersperger, L. M., Dower, W. J., Barrett, D. W. and Gallop, M. A. (1993) Generation and screening of an oligonucleotide-encoded synthetic peptide library. *Proc. Natl Acad. Sci. U.S.A.* **90**: 10700–10704.

51. Sebestyen, F., Dibo, F. and Furka, A. (1993) Efficiency and limitations of the portioning-mixing peptide synthesis. In Schneider, C. H. and Eberle, A. N. (eds) *Peptides 1992*, pp. 63–64. Escom, Leiden.

52. Nikolaev, V., Stierandova, A., Krchňák, V., Seligmann, B., Lam, K. S., Salmon, S. E. and Lebl, M. (1993) Peptide-encoded for structure determination of non-sequenceable polymers within libraries synthesized and tested on solid phase supports. *Peptide Res.*, **6**: 161–170.

53. Kerr, J. M., Banville, S. G. and Zuckermann, R. E. (1993) Encoded combinatorial peptide libraries containing non-natural amino acids. *J. Am. Chem. Soc.* **115**: 2529–2531.

54. Ohlmeyer, M. H. J., Swanson, R. N., Dillard, L. W., Reader, J. C., Asouline, G., Kobayashi, R., Wigler, M. and Still, W. C. (1993) Complex synthetic chemical libraries indexed with molecular tags. *Proc. Natl Acad. Sci. U.S.A.* **90**: 10922–10929.

55. Kassarpan, A., Schellenberger, V. and Turck, C. W. (1993) Screening of synthetic peptide libraries with radiolabeled acceptor molecules. *Peptide Res.* **6**: 129–133.

56. Lam, K. S., Hruby, V. J., Lebl, M., Knapp, R. J., Kazmierski, W. M., Hersh, E. M. and Salmon, S. E. (1993) The chemical synthesis of large random peptide libraries and their use for the discovery of ligands for macromolecular acceptors. *Bioorg. Med. Chem. Lett.* **3**: 419–424.

57. Lam, K. S., Lebl, M., Krchňák, V., Lake, D. F., Smith, J., Wade, S., Ferguson, R., Ackermann-Perrier, M. and Wertman, K. (1994) Application of selectide technology in identifying (i) aminotope for a discontinuous epitope, and (ii) D-amino acid ligands. In Hodges, R. S. and Smith, J. A. (eds) *Peptides: Chemistry, Structure and Biology*, pp. 1003–1004. Escom, Leiden.

58. Lebl, M., Krchňák, V. and Stierandová, A. *et al.* (1994) Nonsequenceable and/or nonpeptide libraries. In Hodges, R. S. and Smith, J. A. (eds) *Peptides: Chemistry, Structure and Biology*, pp. 1007–1008. Escom, Leiden.

59. Lam, K. S., Lebl, M., Wade, S., Stierandová, A., Khattri, P. S., Collins, N. and Hruby, V. J. (1993) Streptavidin-peptide interaction as a model system for molecular recognition. In Hodges, R. S. Smith, J. A. (eds) *Reptides: Chemistry, Structure and Biology*, pp. 1005–1006. Escom, Leiden.

60. Houghton, R. A., Appel, J. P., Blondelle, S. E., Cuerva, J. H., Dooley, C. T. and Purella, C. (1992) The use of synthetic combinatorial libraries for the identification of bioactive peptides. *Biotechniques* **13**: 412–421.

61. Pinilla, C., Appel, J. R., Blanc, P. and Houghton, R. A. (1992) Rapid indentification of high affinity peptide ligands using positional scanning synthetic combinatorial libraries. *Biotechniques* **13**: 901–905.

62. Dooley, C. T., Chung, N. N., Schiller, P. W. and Houghton, R. A. (1993) Acetalins, opioid receptor antagonists determined through the use of synthetic peptide combinatorial libraries. *Proc. Natl Acad. Sci. U.S.A.* **90**: 10811–10815.

63. Dooley, C. T. and Houghton, R. A. (1993) The use of positional scanning synthetic peptide combinatorial libraries for the rapid determination of opioid receptor ligands. *Life Sciences* **52**: 1509–1517.

64. Houghton, R. A. and Dooley, C. T. (1993) The use of synthetic peptide cominatorial libraries for the

determination of peptide ligands in radio-receptor assays, opioid peptides. *Bioorg. Med. Chem. Lett.* **3**: 405–412.

65. Fodor, S. P. A., Read, J. L., Pirrung, M. C., Stryer, L., Lu, A. T. and Solar, D. (1991) Light-directed, spatially addresssable parallel chemical synthesis. *Science* **251:** 767–773.

66. Adam, C. L., Kochersperger, L. M., Martinsen, R. B., Aldwin, L. A. and Holmes, C. P. (1994) New methodologies in the preparation of peptide libraries. In Crabb, J. W. (ed.) *Techniques in Protein Chemistry V*, pp. 525–532. Academic Press, San Diego.

67. Cass, C., Dreyer, M. L., Giebel, L. B., Hudson, D., Johnson, C. R., Ross, M. J., Schaeck, J. and Shoemaker, K. R. (1994) Pilot, a new peptide lead optimization technique and its application as a general library method. In Hodges, R. S. and Smith, J. A., (eds) *Peptides: Chemistry Structure and Biology*, pp. 975–977. Escom, Leiden.

68. Ator, M. A., Beigel, S., Dankanovich, T. C. *et al.* (1994) Immolulized peptide assays: a new technology for the characterization of protease function. In Hodges, R. S. and Smith, J. A. (eds) *Peptides: Chemistry Structure and Biology*, pp. 1012–1015. Escom, Leiden.

69. Pinilla, C., Appel, J. R. and Houghton, R. A. (1994) Positional scanning synthetic peptide combinatorial libraries. In Schneider, C. H. and Eberle, A. N. (eds) *Peptides 1992*, pp. 65–66. Escom, Leiden.

70. Houghton, R. A. and Dooley, C. T. (1993) Novel *N*-acetylated opioid peptides determined through the use of synthetic peptide combinatorial libraries. In Yanaihara, N. (ed.) *Peptide Chemistry 1992*, pp. 11–13. Escom, Leiden.

71. Salmon, S. E., Lam, K. S., Lebl, M. *et al.* (1993) Discovery of biologically active peptides in random libraries: solution phase testing after staged orthogonal release from resin beads. *Proc. Natl Acad. Sci. U.S.A.* **90**: 11708–11712.

72. Saneii, H. H., Shannon, J. P., Miceli, R. M., Fischer, H. D. and Smith, C. W. (1994) The peptide librarian: fully automated selection and synthesis of peptide libraries. In Hodges, R. S. and Smith, J. A. (eds) *Peptides: Chemistry, Structure and Biology*, pp. 1018–1020. Escom, Leiden.

10

The Contribution of Molecular Biology to Drug Discovery

ADRIAN N. HOBDEN

If one considers the purpose of a drug to be to restore the normal function of some particular
process in the body, then DNA would be considered to be the ultimate drug
Aposhian (1970)

I. INTRODUCTION

Over the past fifty years the pharmaceutical industry has been extremely successful in its search for new and improved medicines. However, a survey of the world's best-selling drugs rapidly reveals that the majority are small molecules that were discovered using natural product screening, medicinal chemistry and animal testing but without the aid of molecular biology. If that technology existed and was so successful, why do we need molecular biology? Of course, we should not forget that genetic engineering is a relatively new science dating only from 1975[1] and the process of drug discovery, refinement and testing can take a long time. It is,

THE PRACTICE OF MEDICINAL CHEMISTRY
ISBN 0-12-744640-0

therefore, not surprising that the current drugs do not reflect the revolution that has occurred in the pharmaceutical industry. It is most unlikely that any of tomorrow's drugs will not have benefited from molecular biology at some stage in their discovery. Indeed, for most, molecular biology will have been used, directly or indirectly, at all stages in the medicine discovery process.

In its infancy, genetic engineering was considered to be useful only for the production of therapeutic proteins. Many companies, e.g. Genentech and Biogen, were founded solely with that objective in mind. However, proteins do not make ideal drugs, being difficult to administer, rapidly cleared and potentially immunogenic. Thus far, only a handful of such 'recombinant' proteins have been commercially successful drugs. Nonetheless, the pharmaceutical industry has begun to recognize a much bigger role for molecular biology than simply expressing therapeutic proteins. There cannot now be a major pharmaceutical company that does not employ considerable numbers of staff with expertise in these techniques.

It is not my intention in this chapter to describe in great detail the techniques of genetic engineering. There are numerous specialized textbooks available to those who wish to learn them. Nor do I want to describe the process of drug discovery. That is covered elsewhere within this book. Rather, I will illustrate the various uses of molecular biology in the industry (Table 10.1). Some of these applications are well-established, almost mature for such a young science, others are now being applied, and still more applications will be thought of in the future. The essence of pharmaceutical research is innovative thought and competition. The winners will be those who have the best ideas and can most rapidly exploit them by bringing a drug to market. Molecular biology is critical to that process.

Table 10.1   Uses of molecular biology in drug discovery.

Dissection of disease aetiology
Target identification and validation
Therapeutic proteins
Protein structure determination
Provision of reagents for screening
Screening organisms
Transgenic animals
Drug metabolism
Toxicology

II. DISSECTION OF DISEASE AETIOLOGY

It is self-evident that all drug discovery programmes require a disease and a therapeutic target. In the past, that target did not need to be defined too closely. Antibacterial therapy required the discovery of a compound, often a natural product, that killed the organism. The exact molecular target did not need to be known. However, the limitations of this approach have become apparent as pathogenic strains of bacteria remained immune to the best cephalosporin or as previously sensitive strains became resistant. It has become obvious that an understanding of antibiotic resistance is required in order to overcome it and that new antibacterial targets are required. Equally, many of today's drugs effectively combat the symptoms of disease, e.g. captopril for hypertension, but do nothing to modify the causes leading to the development of the disease. In other diseases, our understanding of their aetiology is so poor that we do not even have good drugs to treat the symptoms, e.g. rheumatoid arthritis.

Genetic engineering has enormously expanded our ability to explore disease processes, to dissect the aetiology of these disease and, ultimately, to identify new molecular targets for drug discovery.

There are some 5000 known inherited disorders in man[2] leading to a wide range of diseases. In general, these diseases are so rare that a drug discovery programme cannot be commercially viable. However, in addition to these rare disorders, it is well known that many common diseases show familial predispositions. These are the so-called polygenic diseases where one cannot point to a simple Mendelian inheritance of the disease. Rather, inheritance of a specific mutation in a particular gene leads to a predisposition to the disease. A simple example is loss of the retinoblastoma gene which, as the name implies, predisposes to cancer — often first presenting in the eye.[3,4] Since cancer is believed to be a multistep process resulting from a series of somatic mutations, and leading to uncontrolled cell division, any individual who is born without one gene required to regulate the process of cell division presumably needs to accumulate a fewer number of mutations. Hence, the disease can appear earlier than it might in a normal individual. Equally, we know that many genes are involved in the control of blood pressure and that particular mutations in some of these genes predispose the individual to hypertension. A greater knowledge of all the genes involved in a disease and how they interact should allow us to define the critical new drug targets of the future.

The rapid advancement in the mapping and sequencing of all the human genes, the vast majority of which will have been completed in 5–10 years' time[5] will greatly facilitate this process. Naturally this knowledge will need to be placed alongside information on the frequency of genetic mutations in these genes, their impact upon the incidence of disease, and an understanding of the function of the gene. This latter process is poorly developed at present and will, undoubtedly, demand the attention of large numbers of molecular biologists in the future.

III.   PRODUCTION OF PROTEIN

As mentioned in the introduction, the ability to move DNA from man to bacteria or, indeed, from bacteria to man made it possible, suddenly, to do what had previously been impossible. Human proteins could be produced in sufficient quantities for it to be possible to use them as drugs. The first commercial example was human insulin, which has now taken over from porcine insulin as the drug of choice for type 1 diabetics.

The techniques of genetic engineering started to reveal a whole range of proteins that could be used as drugs. But their structure did not always allow successful production in bacteria. As a general rule, *Escherichia coli* do not readily secrete proteins nor will they glycosylate them. As a consequence, if the protein required a large number of specific disulphide bonds or glycosylation for activity, *E. coli* were unsuitable hosts for their production. Although it was possible to produce the protein, it was unfolded and usually precipitated within the cell. No amount of protein re-folding *in vitro* could produce reasonable quantities of active product. It became necessary to use other protein expression systems. Nowadays we have a vast array of systems from which to choose, each with its own advantages and disadvantages. For example, the yeast *Saccharomyces cerevisiae* is easy to grow and to manipulate genetically and will secrete proteins. However, quantities of secreted protein tend to be low and the glycosylation profile of proteins secreted from yeast is distinct from that of mammalian cells. Most of the therapeutic proteins currently on the market, e.g. erythropoietin, G-CSF and tPA, are produced in mammalian cell expression systems. Obviously these cells will secrete and glycosylate the protein in a manner similar to the natural protein. However, the cells are harder to manipulate and much more expensive to grow than their microbial counterparts. Furthermore, the expression levels have until recently been relatively low. Recently, expression systems based upon viruses have started to make expression in complex eukaryotic cells much more straightforward owing to the ease of getting foreign DNA into the cells and the high level of expression of recombinant protein following infection of the cells. Particular systems of great merit are baculovirus,[6] which will infect certain insect cells, and the more recent semliki forest virus system,[7] which has a very broad host range allowing a large number of different cell lines to be used.

Whilst therapeutic proteins were an obvious use for the technology, it is evident that any protein can be produced provided the right system is chosen. Drug discovery requires that, if small molecules are the objective, they should work against the correct target, i.e. the human protein or specific viral enzyme. Genetic engineering often provides the only mechanism to acquire sufficient protein for screening or X-ray crystallography. The technology is in routine

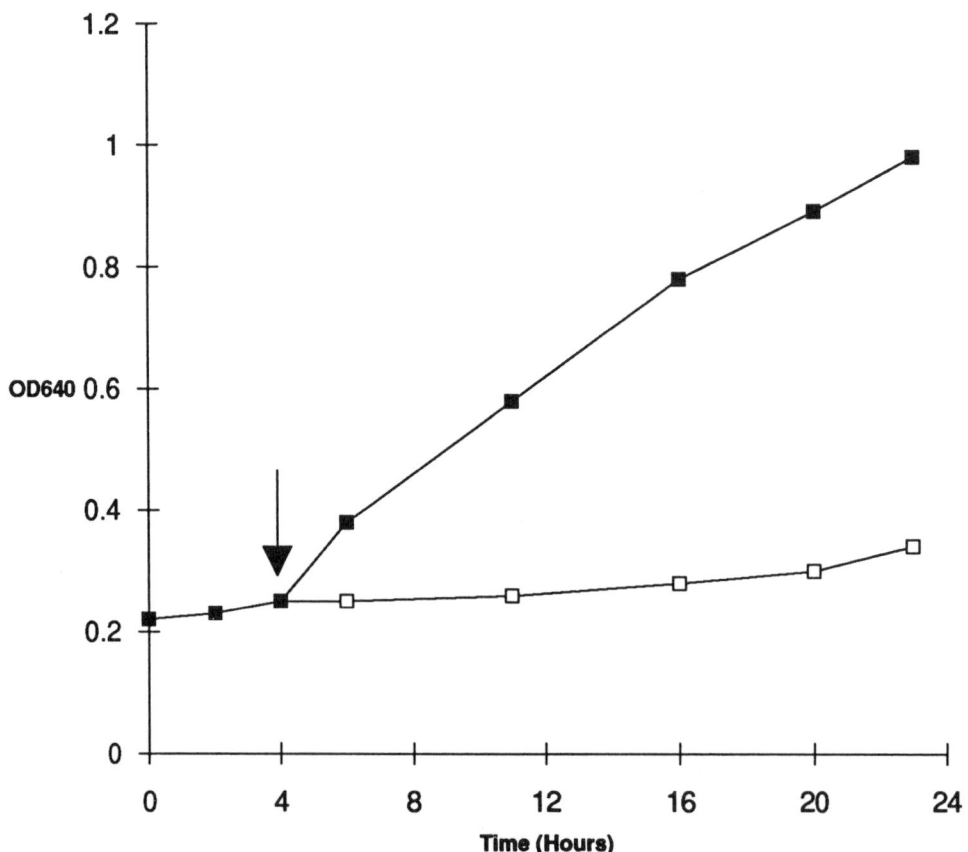

Fig. 10.1 Growth response of *E. coli* to the expression of HIV protease. *E. coli* containing the HIV protease gene were either induced (□) or uninduced (■) to express HIV protease at 4 hours (arrow) and their subsequent growth was measured.

use to supply proteins for these purposes. However, expression of recombinant proteins is not always a neutral event for the host cell. Some years ago, we attempted to express HIV protease in *E. coli* in order to acquire sufficient material for high-throughput screening. It proved impossible, however, to express large quantities since the moment the cell was induced to make the protein it stopped growing (Fig. 10.1). If the active site aspartic acid was mutated to asparagine (making the protein inactive), large quantities of protein were produced by actively growing cells. It became apparent that production of active protein prevented cell growth, presumably because of the protease activity of the recombinant product, and it occurred to us and others[8] that it was unnecessary to purify large quantities of HIV protease for use in some biochemical screen for inhibitors of the enzyme. The recombinant *E. coli* could act as the screen. The bacteria would grow while expressing HIV protease provided an inhibitor of the enzyme was present.

The use of molecular biology to alter the phenotype of a host cell and thus permit the use of that cell in high-throughput screening is the subject of the next section.

IV.   WHOLE CELL SCREENS

In the process of drug discovery, we can envisage two types of compound screening. The first phase is the screening of vast numbers of randomly selected compounds, whether as single molecular entities, e.g. from companies' compound libraries, or as mixtures of compounds such as may be present in multisynthesis chemical libraries or in microbial broths. In either case, the primary objective is to run through as many compounds, broths, etc., in as short a period as possible to identify a few molecules that may act as leads for further chemical synthesis. It does not matter, at this stage, whether the compounds are particularly potent or selective. Medicinal chemistry will address these issues. However, if possible, the screen should avoid identifying too many false positives. They can be time-consuming to identify and eliminate.

In the second phase, the lead compound has been identified and the medicinal chemist is seeking, in collaboration with pharmacologists, to identify a potent, selective compound to take forward into development. At this stage, it is important that the assay is predictive of what will be seen when the compound ultimately is tested in man.

Molecular biology has been used extensively for both these activities. Its utility appears limited only by the imagination and inventiveness of the molecular biologists. Below are a few examples of its use. They are but the tip of a large iceberg of work, most of which goes unreported by the pharmaceutical industry.

V.   INTRACELLULAR RECEPTORS

We have come to recognize that the intracellular receptor gene family is both large and diverse. Its best-characterized members are the sex hormone receptors, estrogen, progesterone and testosterone, but also included are receptors for corticosteroids, vitamin D_3, thyroxine and retinoids. In addition, molecular biology has revealed a number of 'orphan' receptors, i.e. proteins known to be produced that carry a sequence motif suggestive of the ability to bind a small molecule but for which the ligand is currently unknown.

This family of receptors expressed, as their name suggests, within the cell are already the targets for many drug discovery programmes. For example, tamoxifen is widely used for the treatment of breast cancer and is an antagonist of the estrogen receptor. Many synthetic analogues of corticosteroids are used in asthma treatment. The estrogen receptor is present in the cytoplasm in association with HSP90 (heat shock) protein. Upon binding estrogen, the complex dissociates and the receptor enters the nucleus where it binds to specific DNA sequences and activates transcription of certain genes. This chain of events has been reconstructed in the yeast, *S. cerevisiae*.[9] The estrogen responsive DNA sequence was inserted into a yeast promoter upstream of a reporter gene. The reporter, in this case β-galactosidase, is usually an enzyme whose presence can be detected simply by a colorimetric indicator. The effect of inserting the DNA sequence into the yeast promoter is to render it inactive until bound by an estrogen receptor/estradiol complex. Obviously, therefore, the yeast must also express the receptor. With this combination of receptor, responsive element and indicator (Fig. 10.2), the yeast is ready to be used as a screen for estrogen agonists or antagonists. Similar systems have been reported for corticosteroids[10] and androgens.[11]

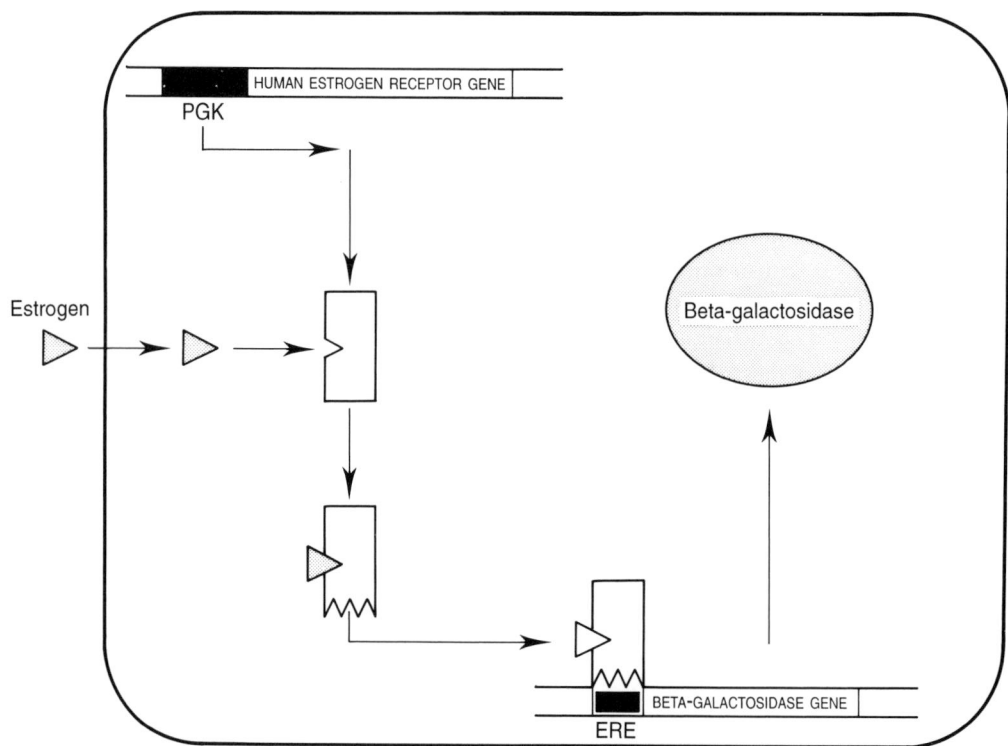

Fig. 10.2 Yeast intracellular receptor screen. Yeast screening organism containing the human estrogen receptor. The hormone (estradiol) binds to the estrogen receptor which is expressed from a gene driven by the PGK promoter. The hormone receptor complex binds to an estrogen-responsive element that controls the expression of β-galactosidase. The assay measures the activity of the enzyme using a substrate that forms a coloured product on conversion.

Of course, the above description is rather simplistic in its description of the screen. In reality, the screener is seeking to achieve stability and sensitivity in the screen. The recombinant yeast must, therefore, be 'fine-tuned' to ensure that the 'foreign' DNA is not lost upon frequent growth of the cells and the concentration of estrogen receptor is sufficient, but not too high, so as to detect small quantities of active material. Once a therapeutic opportunity has been defined for the orphan receptors, it is likely that agonists and antagonists will be sought using this technology.

VI. INTRACELLULAR ENZYMES

I have already mentioned that the expression of HIV protease within *E. coli* gives rise to a phenotype. In a similar fashion, it has been observed that phosphodiesterases when expressed in yeast affect the cells. These enzymes function to modulate intracellular concentrations of the cyclic mononucleotides cAMP or cGMP. Yeast has two genes encoding phosphodiesterases (PDEs) which, when deleted, lead to elevated levels of cAMP within the cell. The consequence, to the yeast, of elevated cAMP is increased sensitivity to heat shock and inability to utilize acetate as sole carbon source. Yeast mutants may be complemented by the human PDE gene and the phenotype reversed (Fig. 10.3). The use of such yeast in the search for inhibitors of PDEs with utility in, for example, asthma has been proposed[12] and certainly works with the known type IV phosphodiesterase inhibitor rolipram.

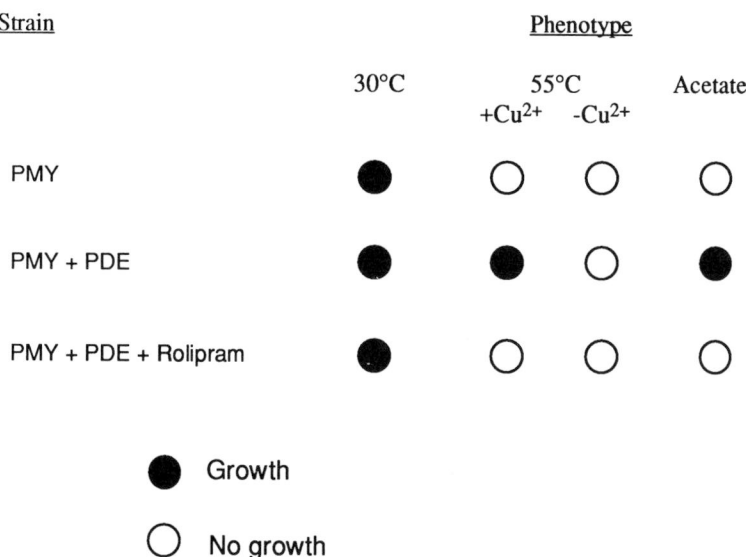

Fig. 10.3 Yeast phosphodiesterase screen. A phosphodiesterase-(PDE-) deficient yeast (PMY) will not utilize acetate as a sole carbon source and is sensitive to heat shock (55°C). Complementation with a human type IV PDE (PMY + PDE) expressed from a copper-dependent (CUP1) promoter reverses the mutant phenotype. Addition of type IV PDE inhibitor (rolipram) to the complemented yeast restores the mutant phenotype (PMY + PDE + rolipram).

In a similar fashion, it is evident that the estrogen screen described above could be modified to include enzymes required for the synthesis or degradation of estradiol. An alternative therapeutic objective for estradiol inhibition might be to prevent its synthesis. Thus, a yeast already built to be sensitive to estradiol could be supplied instead with the precursor to estradiol, 19-nortestosterone, and the enzyme, aromatase, required for its conversion to estradiol. An inhibitor of the enzyme would obviously lead to the inability to synthesise estradiol and the loss of production of β-galactosidase.

A major potential objection to the above approaches is that the compound is required to cross the yeast cell wall and membrane. Failure of a compound to do so would lead it to not being identified it in this type of screen. Obviously, an *in vitro* biochemical screen does not suffer from this constraint. There is no simple argument to counter this objection but a series of observations should allow the reader to make some judgement on the relative merits of the two approaches. Firstly, biochemical assays can be expensive and complicated, preventing their use in high-throughput screening. Secondly, screening of random compounds rarely results in a complete failure to identify leads. Rather, it is often difficult to decide which, of a series of structurally diverse but relatively inactive leads, should be progressed into medicinal chemistry. The mechanism by which compounds enter cells is poorly defined but there is considerable overlap in their ability to cross microbial and mammalian cell membranes. Starting with a compound already able to cross the membrane may well be advantageous to the medicinal chemist.

There are, of course, a number of targets for drug discovery which are not located within the cell. Rather, they are located within the cytoplasmic membrane, where they serve to tell the cell about its environment. They are the cell surface receptors and have been, over the years, the targets of many of the world's best-selling drugs.

VII.   G-PROTEIN-COUPLED RECEPTORS

The G-protein-coupled receptors are a superfamily of structurally related proteins, located in the cell membrane and consisting of seven transmembrane segments. Their primary amino acid sequence, however, can be quite diverse. Agonists or antagonists acting at these receptors constitute a large number of today's best-selling pharmaceuticals. Examples include the H_2 antagonists for ulcer therapy, β-blockers for hypertension, β-agonists for asthma and serotonin agonists for migraine.

In addition to the extensive families of these receptors that have small molecules as their agonists, e.g. histamine, prostaglandins, acetylcholine, many have peptides or even proteins as their ligand, e.g. angiotensin II, gastrin, luteinizing hormone. There is, in addition, an extensive collection of 'orphan' 7-transmembrane receptors, identified by molecular biology techniques but for which a ligand has not yet been identified. Table 10.2 gives an impression of the diversity of this family.

There is enormous activity worldwide seeking to identify nonpeptide agonists or antagonists for both the peptide receptors and the orphans, since it is expected that this will be a fruitful area for drug discovery. Indeed, we will shortly see nonpeptide angiotensin II antagonists licensed for the treatment of hypertension.

The standard approach to finding such molecules has been to express the cloned human receptor in mammalian cells and look for molecules able to inhibit ligand binding. This method can be successful — witness the angiotensin II antagonists. However, it is most useful for identifying antagonists and requires both the ligand to be known and for a radiolabelled derivative to be available. Recently two novel approaches have been reported that potentially should facilitate the whole process.

The first system makes use of yeast. It has been known for some time that *S. cerevisiae* can

Table 10.2   Diversity of ligands for cloned G-protein coupled receptors.

Ligand	Example
Amines	Adrenalin Histamine Dopamine
Protein hormones	Luteinizing hormone Follicle-stimulating hormone
Peptide hormones	Angiotensin Bradykinin Substance P Endothelin Gastrin
Sensory stimuli	Light Odorants Calcium ions
Others	Thrombin Low-density lipoprotein cAMP

exist as two sexual types, a and α cells, which communicate with each other via sex pheromones, a-factor and α-factor. The receptors for these two pheromones are members of the 7-transmembrane family although their amino acid sequences are quite distinct from their mammalian counterparts. The consequence of the binding of the pheromone to its receptor is to set in train a wide range of biochemical events that lead ultimately to mating of the two opposite cell types. However, there are two principal events that can readily be detected. The cells undergo rapid, but transient, cell cycle arrest and express on their cell surface a variety of proteins that aid fusion of the mating types. Unlike their mammalian counterparts, the intracellular signal is transmitted via the β- and γ-subunits of the trimeric G-protein complex and not by the α-subunit. A detailed description of this pathway can be found elsewhere.[13] More importantly, from the point of view of this chapter, the system has been adapted so that the yeast expresses the β_2-adrenergic receptor and its cognate Gα subunit instead of the yeast homologues.[14] The yeast responds to the presence of a β_2-agonist by inducing the FUS1 promoter which, in turn, has been connected to β-galactosidase. The yeast, therefore, turns blue, in the presence of the indicator 5-bromo-4-chloro-3-indolyl-β-D-galactopyranoside (X-gal) (Fig. 10.4).

It is evident that the yeast could be used to look for agonists or antagonists of this receptor and, because of the ease with which the yeast can be grown, has the potential to be used for very high-throughput screens.

Many companies are seeking to exploit this technology for their favourite 7-transmembrane receptors and, indeed, a biotechnology company, Cadus Pharmaceutical Corporation, has recently been founded with this technology as its central theme. As a cautionary note, however, it is worth pointing out that these are very complex yeasts to construct and not all receptors will be as amenable to this approach as the β_2-adrenergic receptor.

As an alternative approach, the second system uses frog melanophores. This is an immortalized cell line derived from frog melanophores which responds to melanocyte-stimulating hormone

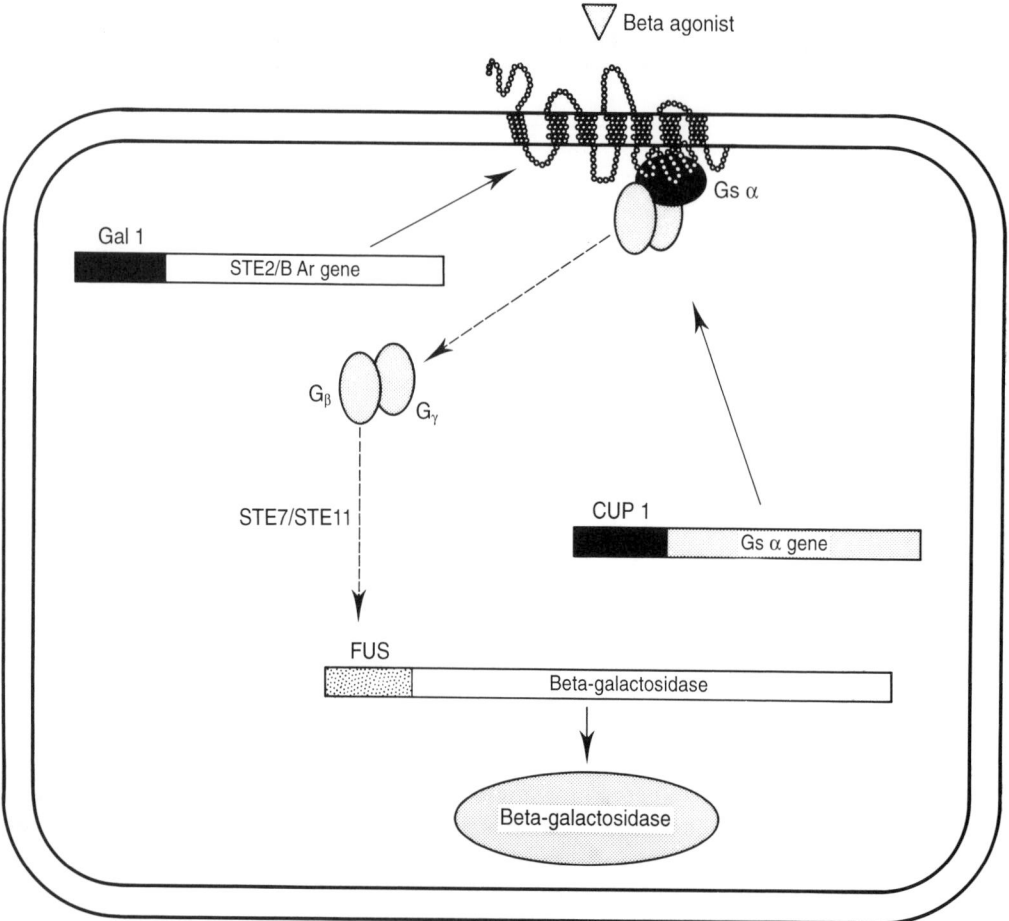

Fig. 10.4 Receptor super-expression in yeast. The β_2-adrenoceptor expressed from a GAL1 promoter links to the mating type response via Gsα expressed off the CUP1 promoter, by complementation of GPA-1. The detection of signalling is by induction of the FUS promoter linked to a reporter gene.

or melatonin by, respectively, a dispersal or aggregation of pigment.[15] The consequence of addition of these ligands, which act at 7-transmembrane receptors, is that the cells change colour within 30 minutes. Indeed, a dose–response curve for agonists or antagonists can be constructed using the cells in a 96-well plate in combination with an ELISA plate reader. Human 7-transmembrane receptors, such as the β_2-adrenergic receptor, have been expressed in these cells.

The system is especially powerful when one wishes to determine structure–activity relationships for compounds derived in a medicinal chemistry programme. Dose–response curves can be constucted versus the human receptor in less than 1 hour. However, the system is not without its problems. First, the cells need special conditions to grow. They are amphibian and, therefore, need lower temperatures and a frog-derived growth factor supplement. Second, they have an endogenous background of frog 7-transmembrane receptors which may complicate analysis. Third, they are as difficult as mammalian cells to transfect with exogenous DNA. Nonetheless, the system has great promise and may even have application for high-throughput screening of random compounds.

In the process of drug discovery, one can imagine running the initial, lead discovery, part of the programme in yeast, then switching to frog melanophores for the lead refinement stage. There is still, of course, a requirement that the compound must work *in vivo*. This is a combination of drug absorption, secretion and metabolism activity of the compound at its target *in vivo* and lack of other activities, i.e. toxicity. Molecular biology is starting to address all of these issues.

VIII.   TRANSGENIC ANIMALS

It has become possible to manipulate the genetic material of mice so that extra genes can be expressed or mice genes deleted. Obviously, this allows also for mouse genes to be replaced by their human homologues. It is only a matter of time before it will be possible to do this for other animal species. Such manipulations make it possible to screen *in vivo* against the human target or predispose the animal to a particular disease. For example, a mouse has been constructed that develops breast cancer at a high frequency.[16] Because the change that has induced the phenotype is known, it allows drugs directed against the tumour-promoting gene to be tested. Equally, it is no longer necessary to treat animals with carcinogens in order to induce tumours.

Mice and other animal models of disease are often poor mimics of the human condition. However, the expression of human genes in these animals can initiate development of the disease. In mice, the distribution of cholesterol between low-density lipoproteins (LDL) and high-density lipoproteins (HDL) is quite distinct from that in humans. However, if the human enzyme, cholesterol ester transfer protein (CETP), is expressed in mice, the LDL:HDL ratio becomes more human in profile.[17] Inhibition of CETP is a target for antiatherosclerotic drugs and there now exists an animal model in which to test them.

Rodents are used extensively in toxicity evaluation of drugs and transgenic mice are now being considered for this use. This area is addressed later.

IX.   DRUG METABOLISM

A major problem in all drug discovery programmes is to discover compounds with good pharmacokinetics. Although it is possible to examine the metabolism of the drug in animals, it has often been difficult to predict what would happen in man. The obvious implications of drug metabolism are an effect on half-life *in vivo* and the production of toxic metabolic products.

In seeking to establish an effective dose for a new drug, the clinician needs to know what ranges of abilities humans will have to metabolize the drug and what effect the drug will have on the metabolizing enzymes. Failure to metabolize the drug may lead to overdose, whereas rapid metabolism could lead to lack of clinical benefit. Equally, inhibition of the metabolism of another drug could cause problems in a patient receiving several medications.

A large proportion of the metabolizing enzymes are members of the P450 superfamily[18] and a large number of these genes have now been cloned and their metabolic potential determined. Increasingly, the enzymes are being expressed in microbial systems, e.g. yeast, where their ability to metabolize the drug can be evaluated. It would not be surprising if in a few years all new drugs were 'typed' for their P450 metabolism profile. Equally, their metabolic products can be determined and their biological activity and toxicity determined.

An additional application is likely to be the P450 genotyping of patients. As 'poor metabolizers' become recognized in the population, the problem is often found to be mutations in one or more of their P450 genes. Once identified, such mutations are easily screened for and it is entirely likely that some degree of P450 'profiling' will take place for patients in the future. Armed with knowledge on the metabolic fate of new drugs, the physician will, in the future, be able to prescribe the best drug for an individual depending on their P450 profile.

X. TOXICOLOGY

Toxicity testing for new drugs is an essential part of drug discovery and, of course, reflects our ignorance of biological processes. Toxicity constitutes the unwanted effects of the molecule. While it is hard to imagine that long-term testing of compounds in animals will not always need to be performed, molecular biology is starting to impact on genetic toxicology, i.e. the ability of compounds to induce mutations in DNA and, thus, carcinogens. Systems have been constructed that permit identification of genetic mutation *in vitro* and *in vivo* extremely rapidly. Potentially, therefore, a compound's potential as a carcinogen can be identified rapidly, with concomitant savings in numbers of animals, human effort and the supply of compound needed for the larger-scale animal studies.

Most systems reported so far depend upon the detection of mutations either in an indicator gene, e.g. β-galactosidase, or a gene controlling the expression of β-galactosidase.[19,20] The bacteriophage λ which normally infects and lyses the bacterium *E. coli* has been altered genetically such that the β-galactosidase gene is contained within its DNA. This gene will only be expressed when the phage infects *E. coli*. The phage λ DNA is then incorporated into the mouse genome so that it is inherited in subsequent generations of mice. Since, the phage λ DNA is not capable of expressing any proteins in the mouse, it is effectively neutral in the mouse's growth and development. However, the λ DNA may be rescued from mouse by extracting total DNA and adding a 'λ packaging extract' *in vitro*. This complex, which is commercially available, finds and extracts the λ DNA and packages it into infectious phage particles. The phages are then used to infect *E. coli*, where they replicate and lyse the bacteria. The lysed 'plaques' can be stained for β-galactosidase. Mutations within the λ DNA are scored by proportion of plaques scoring negative for β-galactosidase.

In practice, the transgenic mice are given the new drug over a period of a few days before sacrifice. DNA is then extracted from a variety of organs and the mutation frequency is scored by counting λ plaques. It therefore becomes possible to demonstrate the ability of the drug to induce mutations and determine whether it shows any tissue selectivity. Furthermore, since the λ packaging can be repeated several times for each DNA sample, far fewer animals are required to obtain a statistically significant result.

It can be expected that several refinements to this system will be developed with time, allowing, for example, the scoring of mutation frequency to be automated.

XI. CONCLUSIONS

Molecular biology is already having an enormous impact on the process drug discovery and its influence can only become greater. Its enormous power will facilitate the discovery and development of novel pharmaceuticals and shorten the period from idea to market. The pharmaceutical industry is very competitive and companies will prosper through a combination of hard work, innovation and serendipity. Companies that fully adopt molecular biology as part of their drug discovery strategy and use it in imaginative and inventive ways will find ultimately that serendipity has a less important role to play.

REFERENCES

1. Cohen, S. N. and Boyer, H. W. (1980) Process for producing biologically functional molecular chimeras. US Patent 4 237 224 (Stanford University).
2. McKusick, V. A. (1990) *Mendelian Inheritance in Man. Catalogs of Autosomal Dominant, Antosomal Recessive and x-linked Phenotypes,* 9th edn. The Johns Hopkins Press, Baltimore.
3. Lee, W. H., Bookstein, R., Hong, F., Young, L. J., Shaw, J. Y. and Lee, E. Y. (1987) Human retinoblastoma susceptibility gene: cloning, identification and sequence. *Science* **235**: 1394–1399.
4. Ewen, M. E. (1994) The cell cycle and the retinoblastoma protein family. *Cancer Metastasis Rev.* **13**: 45–66.
5. Collins, F. and Galas, D. (1993) A new five year plan for the US human genome project. *Science* **262**: 43–46.
6. Miller, L. K. (1989) Insect baculoviruses: powerful gene expression to vectors. *Bioessays* **11**: 91–95.
7. Liljestrom, P. and Gargoof, H. (1991) A new generation of animal cell expression vectors based on the semliki forest virus replicon. *Bio/Technology* **9**: 1356–1361.
8. Baum, E. Z., Bebernitz, G. A. and Gluzman, Y. (1990) Isolation of mutants of human immunodeficiency virus protease based on the toxicity of the enzyme in *Esherichia coli. Proc. Natl Acad. Sci. USA* **87**: 5573–5577.
9. Metzger, D., White, J. H. and Chambon, P. (1988) The human oestrogen receptor functions in yeast. *Nature* **334**. 31–36.
10. Schena, M. and Yamamoto, K. R. (1988) Mammalian glucorticoid receptor derivatives enhance transcription in yeast. *Science* **241**: 965–967.
11. Purvis, I. J. Chotai, D., Dykes, C. W., Lubatin, D. B., French, F. S., Wilson, E. M. and Hobden, A. N. (1991) An androgen inducible expression system for *Saccharomyces cerevisiae. Gene.* **106**: 35–42.
12. McHale, M. M., Cieslinski, L. B., Eng, W. K., Johnson, R. K., Trophy, J. J. and Livi, G.P. (1991) Expression of human recombinant cAMP phosphodiesterase isozyme reverses growth arrest phenotypes in phosphodiesterase-deficient yeast. *Mol. Pharmacol.* **39**: 109–113.
13. Konopka, J. B. and Fields, S. (1992) The pheromone signal pathway in *Saccharomyces cerevisiae. Antonie Van Leeuwenhoek.* **62**: 95–108.
14. King, K., Dohlman, H. G., Thorner, J., Caron, M. G. and Lefkowitz, R.J. (1990) Control of yeast mating signal transduction by a mammalian β2-adrenergic receptor and Gsα subunit. *Science* **250**: 121–123.
15. Putenza, M. N. and Lerner, M. R. (1992) A rapid quantitative bioassay for evaluating the effects of ligands upon receptors that modulate cAMP levels in a melanophore cell line. *Pigment Cell Res.* **5**: 372–378.
16. Muller, W. J., Sinn, E., Pattengale, P. K., Wallace, R. and Leder, P. (1988) Single step induction of mammary adenocarcinoma in transgenic mice bearing the activated c-*neu* oncogene. *Cell.* **54**: 105–115.
17. Hayek, T., Azrolan, N., Verdeny, R. B., Walsh, A., Shajek-Shaul, J., Agellon, L. B., Jall, A. R. and Breslow, J. L. (1993) Hypertension and cholesteryl ester transfer protein interact to dramatically alter high density lipoprotein levels, particle sizes and metabolism. Studies in transgenic mice. *J. Clin. Invest.* **92**: 1143–1152.
18. Nebert, D. W. (1991) Proposed role of drug-metabolising enzymes: Regulation of steady state levels of the ligands that affect growth, homeostasis, differentiation and neuroendocrine functions. *Mol. Endocrinol.* **5**: 1203–1214.

19. Myhr, B. C. (1991) Validation studies with Muta mouse: a transgenic mouse model for detecting mutations *in vivo. Environ. Mol. Mutatagens.* **18**: 308–315.
20. Shepherd, S. E., Sengstag, C., Lutz, W. K. and Schlatter, C. (1993) Mutations in liver DNA of *lac* I transgenic mice (Big Blue) following subchronic exposure to z-acetylaminofluorene. *Mutat. Res.* **302**: 91–96.

11

Electronic Screening:
Lead Finding from Database Mining

HANS-PETER WEBER

I. INTRODUCTION

Most drugs in current use have been developed through optimization of *lead compounds*. The source of lead compounds used to be primarily natural products from plants, microorganisms, and higher species, including hormones, transmitters, etc., which were discovered by screening techniques. This approach to drug development was highly successful and is still being successfully applied in most pharmaceutical companies. However, the rapid development of biotechnology has offered other promising routes towards the same goal; the present chapter discusses one of these new routes.

THE PRACTICE OF MEDICINAL CHEMISTRY
ISBN 0-12-744640-0

Biotechnology can provide, in principle, material for any protein target, and modern X-ray crystallography can, again in principle, determine the crystalline structure at near-atomic resolution for any protein of therapeutic interest. This allows a direct approach to the design of, or search for, biologically active compounds, i.e. *structure-based drug design*.

With the knowledge of the target protein in atomic detail, there are two basically different strategies that can be applied in structure-based drug design:

1. Design of a novel ligand for a receptor binding site by applying (graphical) *molecular modelling* methods. This approach, which involves mainly interactive use of modelling systems, may be helped by special programs to place small to medium fragments into strategic positions in the binding site, e.g. making favourable H-bonds, and extending the fragment with the same strategy to a 'receptor-site-filling' molecule. Among the many specialized computing tools for this purpose a few are particularly helpful, e.g. programs like LUDI,[1] CLIX,[2] or CAVEAT.[3] The special character of this approach is the direct control and navigation of all steps in the design of one or a few active molecules by the medicinal chemist. There is some automation involved in the process, but it is mostly based on individual know-how and expertise in graphical structure-based drug design.

2. The second route to structure-based drug discovery is *electronic screening of 3D databases*. In this approach, a large 3D database containing organic compounds is screened by a computer program that tests each compound in the database in an *automated* fashion for how well it would fit into a defined receptor binding site and calculates a score according to the fit. The top-scoring compounds will be potential candidates for biological testing.

The pioneering work in this field was done by I.D. Kuntz and co-workers[4] with the development of a computer program called DOCK. He was well ahead of his time, but a few years later derivatives of his work quickly followed, for example, ALADDIN[5] and FLOG.[6] The approach has gained great interest among pharmaceutical companies because two of the prerequisites for electronic database screening are now available: (1) large chemical databases, in electronic format, containing all (or a large part of) the compounds that have been synthesized in the company since its foundation, and (2) the biotechnology and the crystallographic techniques to establish 3D models of any protein targets of interest, either in-house or in collaboration with an external company.

In this context, focus will be on lead finding by electronic screening of 3D databases, although the other approach, molecular modelling, would be equally important and interesting. In fact, the two methods are complementary and have a lot in common.

One of the prerequisites for this approach is the knowledge of the 3D structure of the receptor of interest in atomic detail. Although the biotechnological production of a protein and its structure elucidation by X-ray analysis or NMR are major research projects, this aspect will not be discussed here. Just one comment will be made concerning an obvious but sometimes overlooked detail: the timing. When a new, therapeutically interesting target protein has been identified, a period of about two years has to be anticipated for biotechnology to produce the protein and for crystallography (or NMR) to determine the structure. Only then can structure-based design start. This period may be shortened if, for example, the protein is already physically available, or if a reliable model can be built by homology from a related, known protein structure. Otherwise, a two-year horizon is realistic for planning a novel structure-based project.

II.   3D DATABASES

There are a number of 'experimental' 3D databases publicly available, which need not be generated. The most prominent among these are the *Cambridge Crystal Database* (CSD), containing the collected results of some 120000 published X-ray crystal structure analyses, and the *Brookhaven Protein Data Base* (PDB) containing about 2500 entries of protein crystal structures (and some NMR solution structures). Both 3D databases are most valuable sources for reliable structural data on both organic and biopolymer molecular conformations as they exist in the solid state.

For the purpose of electronic screening the CSD can be a useful 3D database for lead finding; it contains a broad spectrum of diverse molecular structures in reliable low-energy conformations. However, its use as a source for lead compounds for pharmaceutical purposes is somewhat limited for three reasons: (1) many of the CSD compounds may have an 'unbiological chemistry', e.g. undesirable physical or chemical properties such as containing metals, (2) many other compounds of *a priori* interesting molecules are chemically 'corrupted' — i.e. derivatives made for purely crystallographic purposes, and (3) most of the compounds will either be unavailable or difficult to obtain.

The PDB database is, of course, the primary source for receptor structures. However, a derivative of the PDB database might also be a useful source of potential lead candidates: peptides in the conformation in which they exist in proteins, particularly in surface loops, may be interesting peptide leads, since they are in a conformation that biologically may be more relevant than the conformation of the same peptides as found, for example, in a crystal structure or modelled *in vacuo*. The preparation of a 3D database containing such peptides could be a very valuable ligand source in structure-based drug design.

Next to these 'experimental' 3D databases there are a few 'theoretical', or 'modelled' ones. Four such 3D databases, commercially (publicly) available, do exist and are useful for lead finding. Molecular Design Ltd. has prepared and maintains three such modelled databases: the *MACCS Drug Data Report file* (MDDR, containing some 47000 compounds), the *Available Chemicals Database* (ACD, containing about 130000 commercially available compounds), and *Compounds of Medicinal Chemistry* (CMC, with approximately 6500 compounds). Also, *Chemical Abstracts* has created a huge 3D database of about 6 million compounds in its prime database. The methods and problems involved in creating such 'modelled' 3D databases will be discussed briefly.

A.   Generation of 3D databases from 2D databases

Most pharamceutical companies, and some university institutes, have large proprietary 2D chemical databases. These databases, originally in a hard copy registry form and now converted into electronic form containing a full description of each compound by chemical topology (CT), bond type (BT) and chirality information, may well contain over 100000 compounds, and they represent one of the company's (or institute's) most valuable resources: the compiled and electronically accessible results of the work of many hundreds of medicinal chemists, biologists and pharmacologists, accumulated in many years of research. Obviously, re-evaluation of this data as new assays and drug design projects emerge is of highest importance to pharmaceutical research, because (1) these compounds are (usually) available in-house, and

(2) most of them are compounds of biological potential.

For the purpose of electronic screening, these 2D databases have to be converted into 3D databases by automated procedures. The basic requirements for such procedures are, (1) robustness (i.e. they should not crash with an unexpected type of molecule), (2) the ability to produce stereochemically acceptable and thermodynamically favourable conformations, and (3) to be fast, i.e. using less than, say, 1 CPU-second per 2D→3D conversion. Two types of such programs have been developed.

- Programs applying basic stereochemical principles to build a rough 3D molecular model of the compound atom by atom using the stored CT, BT and chirality information followed by an abbreviated form of geometry optimization to straighten out the somewhat rough conformation. Popular programs of this type are e.g. CONCORD[7,8] and CORINA,[9] which both meet the criteria mentioned above. Problems only arise with larger cyclic compounds (higher than 7-membered rings), and with occasional overlap of topologically distant atoms.
- Programs using a database of fragments (e.g. ring systems, (semi)rigid groups, etc.) that are able to be assembled into a full molecule fragment by fragment, by applying empirical rules for fragment connection. Typical programs of this type are WIZARD/COBRA,[10] AIMB,[11] and CHEM-X BUILDER.[12] Many of the fragment-joining rules have been derived from crystal structures, and some learning mechanisms are implemented into a knowledge base to produce crystal-like low-energy conformations. This approach is potentially superior to the atom-by-atom approach. However, such programs are relatively slow, using typically about 10 times the CPU-time of the atom-by-atom programs, and are not yet as highly developed as to deal with all (or most) classes of organochemical compounds.

Both types of 2D→3D converting programs have the same limitation: they are able to produce one, and only one conformation for a particular molecule. This particular conformation may be a stereochemically reasonable one, it may even be a low-energy conformation; but the ultimate requirement for the purpose of electronic screening is to have the conformation of the molecule when bound to the receptor of interest in the database! And for a potentially flexible molecule the 'modelled' conformation in the database may well be different from the required one. This basic problem of electronic screening leads to the next point: how to address *conformational flexibility* in electronic database screening.

B.   Conformational flexibility in 3D databases

All presently used docking procedures in electronic screening of 3D databases use the *rigid ligand–rigid receptor docking* approach. An obvious, and at first glance attractive solution to conformational flexibility in this case is to use a 2D→3D conversion program that will produce multiple conformations of a compound. Clearly, the size of the 3D database would then increase by a factor of, say, 20 if on average 20 conformers of a compound were generated. With today's computer resources, such a multiconformer 3D database, containing some 1 000 000 original compounds, would require about 6 GB of disk space, which is large but realizable. The time to search such a multiconformer 3D database would, of course, also increase by the same factor. However, as attractive and elegant as this way would appear, the problem of conformational flexibility is only partly solved with such a multiconformer 3D database: clearly the probability of having the 'right' receptor-bound conformation of the molecule among the conformers is now increased, but there is still no guarantee that the 'right' one is among them!

To my knowledge, there is only one public program to date, CATALYST,[13] which will produce up to a user-defined number of conformers per compound whose internal energy will lie within a defined energy range. In our laboratory we have converted a 2D database of some 150 000 compounds with CATALYST (Version 2.0) into a multiconformation 3D database. The quality of the conformers generated is difficult to assess ojectively, but from looking at random at some of the structures in our 3D database one gets the impression that in general the generated conformations are reasonable and conformational space is well explored, but some badly distorted ring structures that were found have cast some doubt on the quality of the algorithms, and we suspect that there are still some systematic faults in either recognition or building of molecular conformers. However, since the authors of CATALYST do not provide detailed documentation on their methods, neither on how they generate the starting conformation nor on how they explore conformational space for diverse conformers, it is not possible to say much more at this point.

Another solution to conformational flexibility would be to generate diverse conformers 'on the fly' during the docking procedure. There is an interesting approach already in use for flexible ligand searching by TRIPOS:[14] starting with a random (but reasonable) conformation of a molecule (as it is in the 3D database), the algorithm tries to change the conformation in a directed way through bond rotations (excluding ring bonds!) so as to achieve a conformation satisfying some predefined constraints without producing excessive internal strain. Clearly the ideal application of this method is the search for compounds containing a particular pharmacophoric pattern, defined with interatomic distances and angles. However, in the case of 3D database screening for compounds fitting into a receptor binding site, it is usually difficult to define distance or angle constraints in advance, and the method may find application only in special cases of electronic screening.

In summary, the approaches as discussed above do not provide a satisfactory solution to the problem of conformational flexibility. At present, the (rigid) multiple conformer 3D database seems to be the best available and most practical way. New original approaches have still to developed.

III. DEFINING THE RECEPTOR BINDING SITE

Let us assume that a 3D database and a binding site in a protein (in atomic detail) are at hand. The next problem then is to characterize the binding cavity in such a way that computational docking of a compound (from the database) into the binding site can be done. The basic idea is to place a number of discrete, strategically distributed points into the receptor cavity, forming the so-called 'cluster of centres', and then try to fit the atoms of a ligand on to these points.

In the pioneering work of Kuntz and co-workers,[4] a general method for producing such a 'cluster of centres' was proposed, based on the use of Connolly's[15] solvent-accessible surface. It proved to be a very useful method and Kuntz and his collaborators were able to show that with their method some crystallographically determined protein–ligand complexes could be reproduced quite accurately.[16]

Many refinements and variations of his original method have been proposed subsequently. One of these variants developed in our laboratory[17] places the 'centres' in closest contact with the receptor surface, postulating that fitting ligand atoms to such points will also produce a most effective fit of a ligand. Such 'closest' points are situated at approximatly the double van der Waals distance from receptor surface atoms, i.e. they are close to or on the Lee–Richards surface[18] of the receptor binding site. In fact we used a modified Lee–Richards surface that is obtained with a probe atom whose radius varies with the receptor atom in contact (assuming that the best contacts between ligand and receptor atoms occur when both are of similar type).

Other schemes for defining a 'cluster of centres' for the receptor site use points of an evenly spaced 'potential energy grid' placed over the site; at every grid point the interaction energies of various probe atoms with the receptor are calculated. The grid points with the highest interaction energy may then be retained as 'centres' defining the receptor site.[6]

Clearly, a good definition of the receptor binding site is an important aspect of such docking procedures and great care should be taken in this step; the choice of method will also depend to some extent on particular features of the receptor binding site of interest, e.g. whether it is a deep hydrophobic pocket, or a rather shallow cavity with polar residues. Some of the considerations are discussed in the next section.

IV.   DOCKING PROCEDURES

The fundamental problem of docking a ligand molecule into a receptor cavity is to fit n ligand atoms (out of N_l atoms in the ligand) onto n centres in the receptor binding site (out of N_r receptor centres). This is a formidable combinatorial problem. The number of possible pairing sets Z is

$$Z = {}^nC(N_r) \times {}^nP(N_l) \sim (N_r)^n \times (N_l)^n$$

C and P represent combinations and permutations, respectively.[19] The approximation is valid for $n \ll N_r, N_l$, which in practice is normally the case, since the number of ligand atom–receptor center pairs, n, to be matched, usually 4 (minimum) to 8, is much smaller than the number of atoms in the ligand (typically 30) or centres in the binding site (typically 100–200). In any case, the number Z is so enormous that a systematic and exhaustive docking procedure is beyond any practical relevance.

Therefore, some heuristic approaches to this combinatorial problem have to be applied: for detailed descriptions see, for example, Shoichet et al.[19] or Miller et al.[6] Here we summarize a general scheme of the heuristics as implemented in most docking procedures (Fig. 11.1).

Variations in this procedure can be introduced at all stages. An interesting modification, for example, can be introduced at stage (1) as follows.[17] Selected receptor centres can be given 'properties', e.g. H-bond donor/acceptor property, or lipophilic/hydrophilic property. If receptor centres of a particular property match with ligand atoms of the same property, it will be positively scored, but scored negatively if they do not match. In another interesting variation, a few receptor centres (or small clusters of centres) may be assigned to be always occupied with a ligand atom of a particular type, e.g. a H-bond acceptor atom of the ligand so that a H-bond to the receptor is possible. Such modifications will speed up the procedure tremendously by rejecting in an early check many of the docking attempts. Such restrictions will produce much fewer successful dockings, but all of the few successful dockings will each show the particular required feature.

In phase (3) also many variations are possible; for example, the selection of the next intraligand distance need not be the next longest but could be chosen so as to be at maximum

(0) $k = 0$ (k, l are receptor centre numbers)
(1) $k => k + 1$ (loop on centres)
             select (and flag as used) receptor centre k

             if $k > N_r$ then continue procedure with the next ligand (0)

             $i = 0$ (i, j are ligand atom numbers)
(2) $n = 0$ (number of matching intraligand/intracentre vector pairs found)
             $i => i + 1$ (loop on atoms)
             select (and flag as used) ligand atom i,
(3)   select the longest intraligand distance d_{ij} (j not flagged)
             search the best-matching intracentre distance d_{kl} (l not flagged)

             if $| d_{kl} - d_{ij} | < e_d$ then $n => n + 1$
             else continue with (2)

             check on the $(n-1)$ 'cross vector differences'
             if all $(n-1)$ cross-vector-diff $< e_c$
                 then flag ligand atom j and receptor centre l, $j => i$, continue (4)
             else continue with (1)

(4)   if $n = n_{max,}$ then (5)
             else *continue* (3)

(5)   found one match:
             do docking,
             do scoring, store and restart with (2)

Fig. 11.1   Heuristics for rigid ligand–rigid receptor docking procedures.

distance from all previous points. Or variation in the tolerance for distance checks (e_d and e_c in Fig. 11.1) could be introduced, depending on the type of ligand atom and property of the receptor center.[17]

A comment on phase (5): After a matching set of intraligand and intracenter distances has successfully been found, a superposition — usually a least squares fit — of the selected ligand atoms onto the matching receptor centres is done. Since up to this point only intraligand and intracenter *distances* have been mtached, it is possible that the fit is much worse than one would expect from the tolerances (e_d, e_c), which would indicate that the enantiomer of the original ligand should be fitted.

V.   SCORING OF DOCKED LIGANDS

After a successful docking has been achieved, the calculation of a score must be done to assess quantitatively the 'goodness of fit'. A good scoring function should take into account (1) the shape fitting of ligand and receptor, which basically is a measure of the contact surface, and (2) the 'chemical fit', i.e. checking on the presence of matching or nonmatching ligand atom/receptor atom properties, respectively, such as whether contacting H-bond partners are of donor–acceptor type, or whether polar interactions are of opposite charge, or lipophilic ligand atoms are in contact with lipophilic receptor atoms, and so on. All these features would be positively scored if true, but negatively scored if false.

Obviously, the calculation of the van der Waals and Coulombic interaction energy between ligand and receptor would be a good score to assess both shape and chemical fit quantitatively. A prerequisite for such a scoring calculation is the choice of an appropriate force field and the complete assignment of atom types and of partial atomic charges for ligand and receptor atoms.

An 'all-H included' force field, or even an 'only polar-H included' force field for scoring would be an adequate choice. However, there is a serious problem with such force fields in the current 'rigid ligand–rigid receptor' docking procedures: the position of the freely-rotatable OH-hydrogens. Assumptions on these positions have to be made in advance of docking. This, however, may lead to bad scoring since a OH-hydrogen may be pointing towards a HB-donor and hence cause a negative scoring, although only a small flick on the HB-hydrogen would be needed to restore a good score. This may be so bad that an otherwise good docking position may be lost. The elegant way to eliminate such a situation is of course to make a search for the best positioning for every freely-rotatable OH-hydrogen, or even better to do a full energy minimzation of the receptor–ligand complex. These extra calculations, however, which would have to be done for every ligand and every fit in turn, are computationally so expensive that such a procedure becomes impractical.

A remedy to this situation could be the choice of a 'no-H included' force field. Such a force field is certainly a poorer choice than either of the other two, but it effectively eliminates the problems mentioned above. An additional advantage of a 'no-H included' force field is that no assignment of partial atomic charges to atoms is needed, since the calculation of a Coulombic energy for H-bonds without a hydrogen would be meaningless. We have been working with such a 'no-H force field' and found good experience with the following scoring function.

(1)   A (negative) van der Waals potential is calculated between all (non-H) atoms of the ligand and of the receptor binding site (with a receptor atom cutoff-distance of, e.g., 6 Å).
(2)   A hydrophobicity and hydrogen-bond scoring function of the form

$$C \exp\left[-A(d - d_{opt})^2\right]$$

where C, A, and d_{opt} are parameters depending on the atom types, and d is the distance between a pair of ligand and receptor atoms.

A very interesting scoring function has recently been published by Bohm,[1] where the author proposes a function to estimate the ligand–receptor affinity. A relatively simple 'ansatz' for $\Delta G_{binding}$ was proposed consisting of only five terms:

(1)   a basic ground value, ΔG_0, independent of any interactions;
(2)   a term ΔG_{HB}, describing the contribution of H-bonds (depending on the geometry of the H-bond: $d = d(D \cdots A)$, $\alpha = (D–H \cdots A)$);
(3)   a term for lipophilic interactions, ΔG_{lipo}, depending on the lipophilic contact surface;
(4)   a term for ionic interactions, ΔG_{ionic}, depending on the geometry of the interaction; and
(5)   a term accounting for freezing internal degrees of freedom in the ligand, ΔG_{rot}, linearly dependent on the number of rotational bonds.

The few parameters in the equation

$$\Delta G_{binding} = \Delta G_0 + \Delta G_{HB}\, f(d,\alpha) + \Delta G_{lipo}\, A + \Delta G_{ionic}\, f(d,\alpha) + \Delta G_{rot}\, N_{rot}$$

were calibrated using some 40 ligand–protein complexes from the Brookhaven database with published K_D values. The cross-validated r^2 for the resulting function was 0.696, i.e. the predictive power for $\Delta G_{binding}$ was about 2.3 kcal mol^{-1}, corresponding to about 1.6 in K_D. The simplicity of the estimate, and the speed with which it can be calculated at the end of a ligand docking, make this scoring function look very promising. Further refinement of the method has been announced.

Another interesting development that has been published recently[6] concerns optimization of the fitted ligand after successful initial docking: as pointed out above, a straight energy minimization of the ligand–receptor complex is impractical in screening large databases owing to exessive computing time. However Miller *et al.*[6] propose a simplex optimization of the rigid ligand in the (rigid) receptor, which significantly improves the scoring with only modest additional CPU-time.

Most newer DOCK programs are using a 'potential energy grid' for the calculation of the ligand–receptor interaction energy. The basic idea is to pre-calculate the interaction energy of the receptor with various atom types placed in turn on the grid points of a grid covering the binding site, i.e. a 3D table containg an interaction energy vector on each grid point. The score for a fitted ligand is then a simple sum of the appropriate values from the interaction energy vectors at the grid points closest to the ligand atoms. A tridimensional interpolation between the ligand atom and the eight nearest grid points can be used for higher precision, which will of course also be achieved by reducing the grid spacing. The size of the grid and memory size available will ultimately define the choice of the grid spacing (typically 0.2 to 0.5 Å).

VI.   POST-PROCESSING OF ELECTRONIC SCREENING RESULTS

The primary post-processing of the docking results is of course sorting according to the scores. If the scoring function were absolutely reliable, and if the docking procedures were perfect too, the top-scoring compounds could go straight for biological testing without further inspection. But in practice the, say, 300 top-scoring compounds have to be inspected graphically/visually by a medicinal chemist for various aspects such as (1) What is the conformation of the ligand? (2) How is the ligand docked into the binding site? (3) What kind of interactions between ligand and receptor exist? (4) What kind of chemical class is the ligand? etc. This is both a tedious and a subjective process. Clearly, automated post-processing would be useful.

Automated post-processing could, for example, collect families of chemically similar ligands, so that one could visualize family by family via their best representatives, and select the most promising candidates for testing from each family. This would also improve the chances of finding chemically diverse new leads, rather than wasting time assaying dozens of compounds all basically alike.

Another approach, which might rather be called pre-processing, would be to re-sort the original large 3D database according to chemical diversity and work with a subset of, say, the 10% most diverse compounds. This would have the additional advantage of reducing the computing time (which might be used for improved scoring and optimizing ligand fitting).

However, there may always remain a final visual (graphical) inspection of the top-scoring candidates, since some of the criteria for selection will remain to be assessed by the medicinal chemist himself, e.g. solubility of a compound, chemical stability, synthetic possibilities of derivation, chemical intuition — in short, criteria that are difficult to program.

VII.   SOME COMPUTING ASPECTS

The most demanding computing part of electronic screening of large 3D databases with one of the methods described is the docking procedure. Improvement in efficiency without sacrificing too much accuracy is the goal. Two main parameters govern this part: (1) The number of centres defining the receptor binding site; clearly the higher the density of these centres, the better the chances of finding matching distances, but also the higher the CPU-time consumed per ligand. (2) The heuristics of matching intraligand distances to intracentre distances; in particular, specifying receptor centres that have to be occupied by ligand atoms at the start of the docking procedure can greatly reduce the computing time.

The second demanding aspect of computing is the scoring. In this phase, the 'potential energy grid' concept is much more efficient than a repetitive van der Waals or Coulombic interaction energy calculation. Implemeting a short (rigid) ligand position optimization before scoring, or even a partial energy relaxation of ligand and receptor, will add some computing time but improve on scoring.[6,20]

Although optimizing a DOCK program according to the points above will improve performance, the most effective, and fortunately the easiest, way of speeding-up is achieved by parallelization of the whole process. The nature of the procedure is such, that this can be done in either of two ways: (1) operating on one single database, and forking into child processes, each handling one ligand at the time with a master process watching over the number of active child processes and opening a new one as soon as one dies, or (2) splitting the original database into N subsets and having N processors running simultaneously, each working on a different subset. Both methods have advantages and which one to choose depends on the type of computing facility available.

VIII.   FUTURE ASPECTS AND POTENTIAL IN PHARMACEUTICAL RESEARCH

The most severe deficiency of the present DOCK methods is its restriction to 'rigid ligand to rigid receptor' fitting. While a mulitconformer database relaxes this limitation at least partially on one side, no practical method has yet emerged to deal with a fully flexible system.

A single, exploratory experiment was done in our laboratory with a 'flexible ligand to (semi)flexible receptor' fit, using the modified X-PLOR scripts *random* and *sa*.[21] The first script randomizes the coordinates of the ligand, and the second script reconstitutes a molecular conformation by simulated annealing procedures. To ensure that the molecule is generated within the binding cavity interacting with the receptor, the centre of mass can be tethered to some point in the middle of the cavity, and the side-chains lining the binding site were flexible. Such a procedure was successful in regenerating correctly the X-ray structure of an HIV-P/inhibitor complex by restarting the script 30 times, which took 30 hours of CPU-time on an Alliant FX2800 using eight processors in parallel. It was clearly a success, but at an enormous expense of computer time, and hardly a direction to follow in the future for screening 3D databases.

Since no real breakthrough of practical relevance for flexible ligand–flexible receptor docking is in sight, the impact of electronic screening in pharmaceutical research may for the time being be somewhat reduced. However, what is available and practical should be used and applied; only experience will tell how useful the methods are, regardless of their scientifically unsatisfactory state. It is up to the experts to keep expectations at a realistic level, and to motivate further development.

With today's docking methods, the best results may be expected by use of a multiconformer 3D database, applying state-of-the-art rigid ligand to rigid receptor docking, followed by a fit-optimzation, and using a scoring function based on a force field–energy grid (or an affinity scoring as proposed by Bohm).[1] These procedures will work best if the receptor binding site is a deep and and almost closed cavity, as is the case for many enzymes (e.g. for HIV-protease, thrombin, sialidase, etc.). In most of these cases the side-chains in the cavities are tightly packed, and the 'rigid receptor' restriction is an adequate assumption. The worst case for the present methods is the search for ligands for a rather flat binding site (e.g. above a β-sheet), lined with long and polar side-chains that are floppy and can move independently. An example of this situation is the putative binding surface of the co-receptors CD2/CD58. There are, however, also intermediate cases with a shallow, but still distinct, binding cavity lined with more or less tightly packed side-chains, e.g. cyclophillin, or FKBP12.

A last comment: Electronic screening of 3D databases has to compete with biological screening. Both electronic and biological screening have the same purpose: to discover new leads. Electronic screening relies on 3D databases, powerful computing resources, and a target structure known in atomic detail. Application is relatively cheap and fast, but it produces 'theoretical' results of limited reliabilty, which first have to be tested experimentally before being useful. Biological screening, on the other hand, relies on the availability of a 'physical' compound store (i.e. a vast collection of diverse compounds to test), and of highly automated assays. Its application is relatively expensive and slow, but it produces experimental results which are of immediate use. Rather than being competitors, I suggest that these two approaches to drug discovery are complementary; while electronic screening provides potentially active candidates for special targets to be tested in special assays, biological screening is searching with a battery of general assays of high capacity and automation for leads of a more general interest.

REFERENCES

1. Bohm, H. J. (1992) The computer program LUDI: a new method for the *de novo* design of enzyme inhibitors. *J. Computer-Aided Mol Design.* **6**: 593–601.
2. Lawrence, M. C. and Davis, P. C. (1992) CLIX: a search algorithm for finding novel ligands capable of binding proteins of known three-dimensional structure. *Proteins Struct. Funct. Genet.* **12**: 31–42.
3. Lauri, G. and Bartlett, P. A. (1994) CAVEAT: a program to facilitate the design of organic molecules. *J. Computer-Aided Mol. Design* **8**: 51–66.
4. Kuntz, I. D., Baney, J. M., Oatley, S. J., Langridge, R and Ferrin, T. E. (1982) A geometric approach to macromolecule–ligand interactions. *J. Mol. Biol.* **161**: 269–288.
5. Van Drie, J. H., Weininger, H. and Martin, Y. C. (1989) ALADDIN: an integrated tool for computer-assisted molecular design and pharmacophore recognition from geometric, steric, and substructure searching of three-dimensional molecular structures. *J. Computer-Aided Mol. Design* **3**: 225–237.
6. Miller, M. D., Kearsley, D. J., Underwood, D. J. and Sheridan, R. P. (1994) FLOG: A system to select 'quasi-flexible' ligands complementary to a receptor of known three-diemnsional structure. *J. Computer-Aided Mol. Design* **8**: 153–174.
7. Pearlman, R. S. (1987) CONCORD: from connectivity to 3D-coordinates of organic compounds. *Chem. Design. Auto. News* **2**: 1–14.

8. Pearlman, R. S. (1993) Three-dimensional structures: How do we generate them and what can we do with them? *Chem. Design. Auto. News* **8**: 3–15.

9. Gasteiger, J., Rudolph, C. and Sadowski, I. J. (1990) Automatic generation of 3D-atomic coordinates for organic molecules. *Tetrahedron Comput. Method.* **3**: 537.

10. Dolata, D. P. and Carter, R. E. (1987) WIZARD: applications of expert system techniques to conformational analysis. 1. The basic algorithms exemplified on simple hydrocarbons. *J. Chem. Info. Comp. Sci.* **27**: 36–45.

11. Wipke, W. T. and Hahn, M. A. (1988) Artificial intelligence model builder. *Tetrahedron Comput. Method.* **1**: 141–153.

12. Davies, K. and Upton, R. (1990) Experiences building and searching the Chapman & Hall dictionary of drugs. *Tetrahedron Comput. Method.* **3**: 665–681.

13. BioCAD Corporation, (1994), Sunnyvale, CA: CATALYST Documentation Version 2.1.

14. TRIPOS Assoc., St Louis, MO (1994), *UNITY 2D/3D*. A 3D database management system.

15. Connolly, M. L. (1983) Analytical molecular surface calculation. *J. Appl. Crystallogr.* **16**: 548–558.

16. DesJarlais, R. L., Sheridan, R. P., Seibel, G. L., Dixon, J. S. and Kuntz, I. D. (1988) DOCK: a program to search molecule databases. *J. Med. Chem.* **31**: 722–734.

17. Burkhard, P. unpublished work.

18. Lee, B. and Richards, F. M. (1971) The interpretation of protein structures: estimation of static accessibility. *J. Mol. Biol.* **55**: 379–400.

19. Shoichet, B. K., Bodian, D. L. and Kuntz, I. D. (1991) New methods for matching ligands to the receptor sites. *J. Comput. Chem.* **13**: 380–397.

20. Meng, C. M., Gschwend, A., Blaney, J. M. and Kuntz, I. D. (1993) Orientational sampling and rigid-body minimization in molecular docking. *Proteins.* **17**: 266–278.

21. Brunger, A. T. (1992) X-PLOR Version 3.1, Yale Univesity Press.

PART III

Primary Exploration of Structure–Activity Relationships

12

Molecular Variations in Homologous Series: Vinylogues and Benzologues

CAMILLE G. WERMUTH

Methyl, Ethyl, Propyl, Butyl, ... Futile
Old adage

THE PRACTICE OF MEDICINAL CHEMISTRY
ISBN 0-12-744640-0

I.   HOMOLOGOUS SERIES

The concept of a homologous series was introduced into organic chemistry by Gerhardt.[1] In medicinal chemistry the term has the same meaning, namely molecules differing one from another by only a methylene group.

II.   CLASSIFICATION OF HOMOLOGOUS SERIES

The most frequently encountered homologous series in medicinal chemistry are monoalkylated derivatives, cyclopolymethylenic compounds, straight-chain difunctional, polymethylenic compounds and substituted cationic head groups.

A.   Monoalkylated derivatives

$$R—X \rightarrow R—CH_2X \rightarrow R—CH_2—CH_2—X, \text{ etc...}$$

An example is provided by the 1-methyl-1,2,3,4-tetrahydropyridylpyrazines described by Ward et al.,[2] which are M_1-muscarinic agonists. For the sequence from O-methyl to O-butyl, the affinity for the M_1 receptor varies from 850 nM to 17 nM (Fig. 12.1).

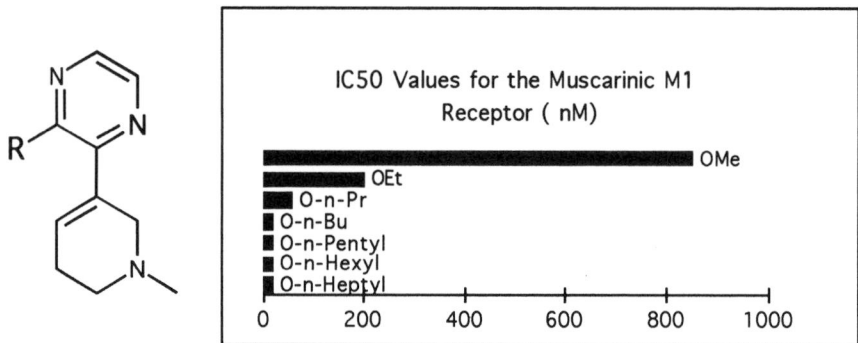

Fig. 12.1   Monoalkylated homologous series.

A similar behaviour was observed for a series of 2-pyrone-derived elastase inhibitors.[3]

B.   Cyclopolymethylenic compounds

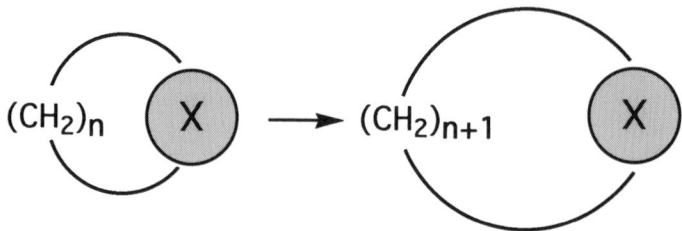

Examples of such structures with regularly increasing ring sizes are found for guanethidine (see Chapter 14), or for enalaprilat analogues (Fig. 12.2).[4] In the latter example, a 4000-fold increase in inhibition of angiotensin converting enzyme is obtained when changing from the five-membered ring ($n = 2$) to the eight-membered ring ($n = 5$).

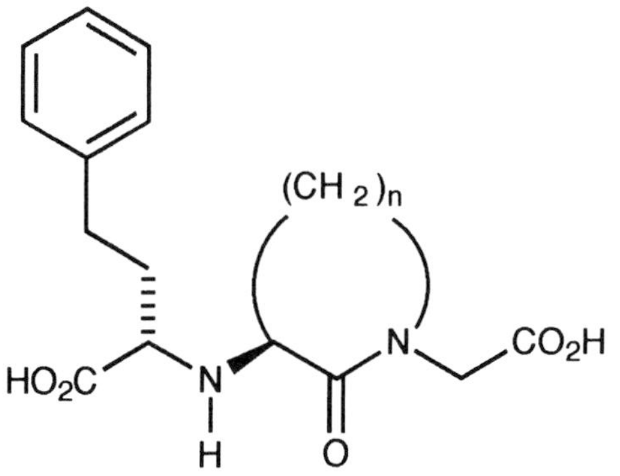

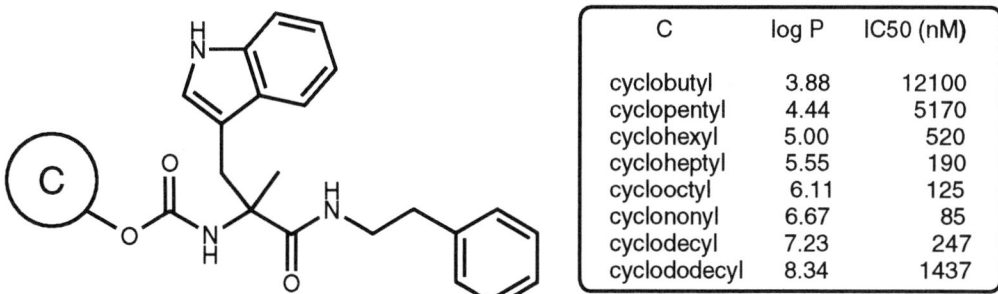

Size	IC$_{50}$ (nM)
n = 2	19,000
n = 3	1,700
n = 4	19
n = 5	4.8
n = 6	8.1

Fig. 12.2 Angiotensin-convertase inhibiting potency of enalaprilat analogues.[4]

Another example, published by scientists from Parke-Davis, relates to a series of 'dipeptoid' analogues of cholecystokinin.[5] These compounds are α-methyltryptophan derivatives, *N*-substituted by carbamic esters of cyclanols with ring sizes increasing from cyclobutyl to cyclododecyl (Fig. 12.3). Here again an optimal size was found (cyclononyl).

C	log P	IC50 (nM)
cyclobutyl	3.88	12100
cyclopentyl	4.44	5170
cyclohexyl	5.00	520
cycloheptyl	5.55	190
cyclooctyl	6.11	125
cyclononyl	6.67	85
cyclodecyl	7.23	247
cyclododecyl	8.34	1437

Fig. 12.3 Optimal ring size for a series of cyclanol carbamates.[5]

C. Open, difunctional, polymethylenic series

$$X\text{---}(CH_2)_n\text{---}Y \rightarrow X\text{---}(CH_2)_{n+1}\text{---}Y$$

In the above general formula, X and Y can represent very diverse functional elements. The compounds can be symmetrical (X = Y; 'dimers') or nonsymmetrical (X π Y); see Chapter 15. Usually X and Y represent *polar functions* or *functionalized cyclic systems*.

When X and Y are polar functions, they are essentially functional groups such as alcohols, amines, acids, amides, amidines or guanidines (Fig. 12.4). A classical representative of a difunctionalized, symmetrical compound is decamethonium.

When X and Y are functionalized cyclic systems, they can be alicyclic or aromatic as well as homocyclic or heterocyclic (Fig. 12.5). In any case, they bear some polar function or polar element. An example of this type of compound is pentamidine.

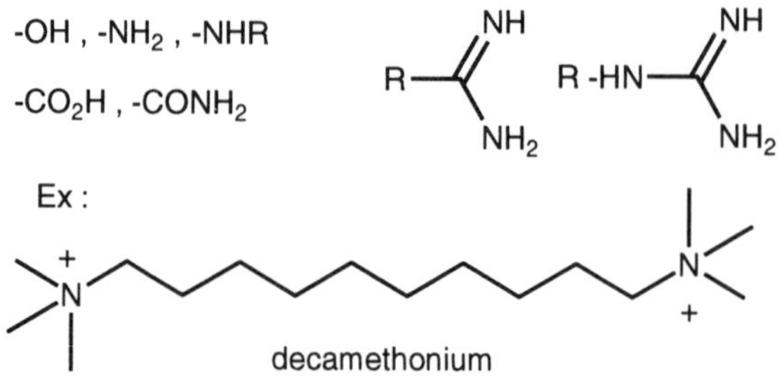

Fig. 12.4 Examples of functional groups encountered in open, difunctional, polymethylenic compounds and structure of decamethonium.

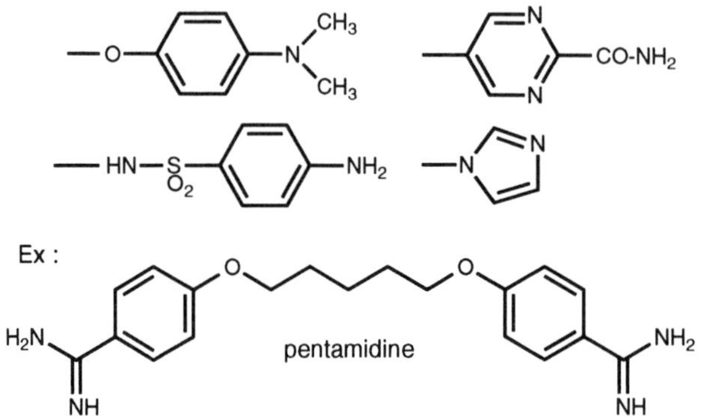

Fig. 12.5 Examples of functionalized rings found in straight-chain, difunctional, polymethylenic compounds. Structure of pentamidine.

Other examples are symmetrical bradykinin antagonists[6] and symmetrical lexitropsines (netropsine, distamycine), active against HIV-I viruses.[7] Nonsymmetrical polymethylenic thromboxane synthetase inhibitors have been described by Press *et al.*[8] The compounds contain a thiophen-2-carboxamide moiety, separated from an imidazole ring by 3 to 8 methylene units. Surprisingly, whereas most of the compounds show similar thromboxane-synthetase-inhibiting activities, only the two medium-sized ones ($n = 3$ and $n = 4$) showed hypotensive effects in spontaneously hypertensive rats (Fig. 12.6).

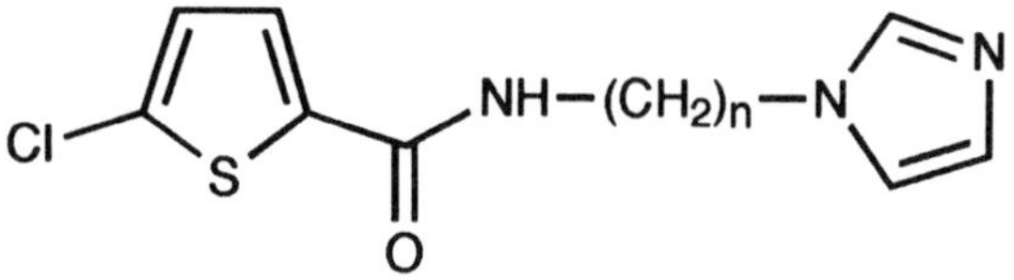

Size	IC$_{50}$ (nM)
$n = 3$	600
$n = 4$	200
$n = 5$	200
$n = 6$	200
$n = 8$	70

Fig. 12.6 Thromboxane synthetase inhibiting activity of a series of *N*-(imidazolylalkyl)thiophene-5-carboxamides.[8]

In a series of benzimidazole-derived thromboxane A$_2$-receptor antagonists described by Nicolai *et al.*,[9] the crucial element is the distance between the carboxylic group and the benzimidazole ring. A 200-fold increase in affinity was observed when changing from a propionic to a butyric side-chain (Fig. 12.7).

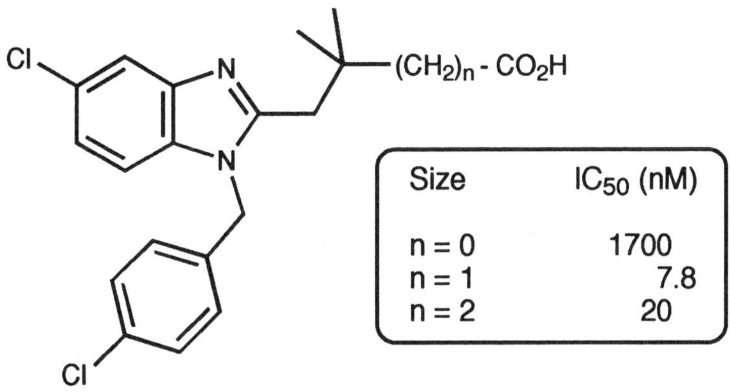

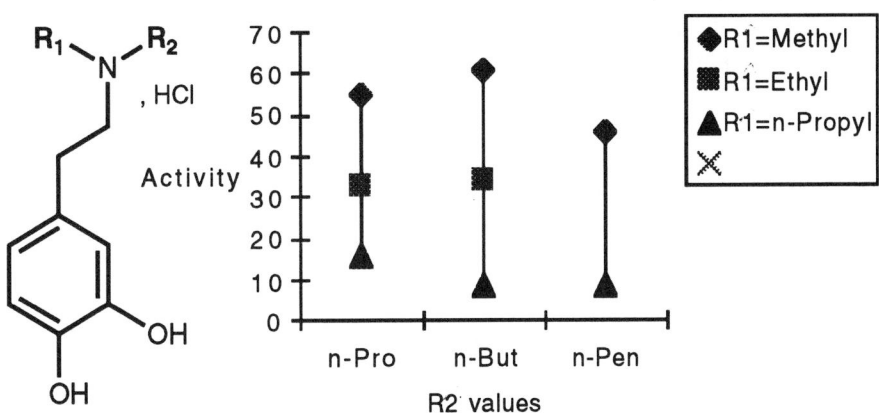

Size	IC$_{50}$ (nM)
n = 0	1700
n = 1	7.8
n = 2	20

Fig. 12.7   Affinity for the thromboxane A$_2$ receptor.[9]

D.   Substituted cationic heads

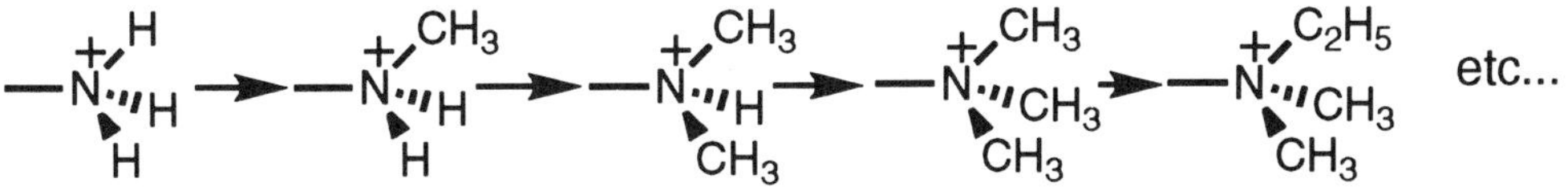

With cationic head groups, homology achieves a simultaneous progressive increase in bulkiness and lipophilicity. Figure 12.8 illustrates the influence of increasing bulkiness around the dopamine nitrogen in the antagonism of reserpine-induced catalepsy in mice.[10]

Fig. 12.8   Anticataleptic activity of substituted dopamines.[10]

III. SHAPES OF BIOLOGICAL RESPONSE CURVES

The most common curves are bell-shaped, the peak activity corresponding to a given value of the number n of carbon atoms (curve A, Fig. 12.9). However many other relationships have been found among homologous series:

1.   The activity can increase, without any particular rule, with the number of carbon atoms (curve B).

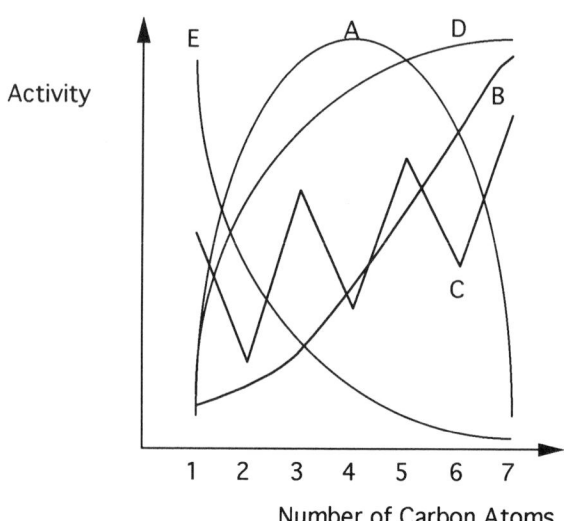

Fig. 12.9 Shapes of the biological response curves in homologous series.

2. The biological activity can alternate with the number of carbon atoms, resulting in a zigzag pattern (curve C).

3. In other series the activity first increases with the number of carbon atoms and then reaches a plateau (curve D).

4. The activity can also decrease regularly, starting with the first member of the series (curve E). This was found for the toxicity of aliphatic nitriles and for the antiseptic properties of aliphatic aldehydes.

5. A final possibility is inversion of the pharmacological activity accompanying increase in the number of carbon atoms (not shown on Fig. 12.9; this will be discussed below).

IV. RESULTS AND INTERPRETATION

A. Curves with a maximum activity peak (bell-shaped curves) and curves with a continuous increase of activity

In such series the continuous growth of an alkyl chain or of methylene units increases the hydrophobic part of the molecule. Various physicochemical parameters, such as solubility in water, partition coefficients, chromatographic R_f values, and critical micellar concentration, are precisely governed by the same fundamental property: the hydrophobic character.

1. Bell-shaped curves

Curves with an activity maximum are the most common; it is presumed that they reflect the existence of an optimal partition coefficient associated with the easiest crossing of biological membranes. The relationship between the biological response and the partition coefficient is then illustrated by a parabolic or bilinear curve. An example is found in structural analogues of PAF-acether.[11] In varying the length of the alkoxy chain from n-butyl to n-eicosanyl, the authors observed peak activity for the n-hexadecyl chain, with a 1200-fold interval between the most active and the least active compounds (Fig. 12.10). The drop in activity observed for the descending branch is usually attributed to insufficient solubility in water (corresponding inability to cross the aqueous biophases), but can also be due to the formation of micelles. In this case, the concentration of the free drug, which represents the directly available form, lies under the critical threshold level.

Bell-shaped curves are also seen when using isolated cells, for which it can be demonstrated that the receptor is outside the membrane. In this case the dominant factor is probably not the crossing of biological membranes. Changes in critical micellar concentration with increasing chain length could explain the effect in some cases; however the curve is often too steep for this to be an acceptable explanation. Another possibility is that there is a lipophilic pocket of finite size. In many cases this pocket is not actually in the receptor protein. An argument in favour of this explanation is that the top of the bell is at C_{16} or C_{18}, which fits with the length of the alkyl chains making up part of the bilayer, examples being PAF-acether analogues[11] and leukotriene D_4- agonists/antagonists. Another bit of evidence that supports this idea is the observation that the position of the peak of the curve can vary depending on which cell type is expressing the same receptor protein.

The study of the activities of *some* homologous compounds, can, through interpolation, identify which term is associated with the highest potency. The optimization method proposed by Bustard,[12] makes use of the Fibonacci numbers, and allows the identification of the most active compound (presumed to exist in a given interval) with the smallest possible number of syntheses (see also refs. 13,14).

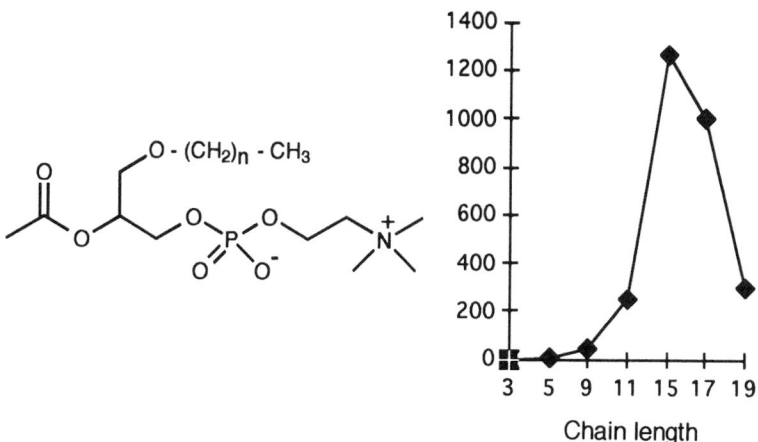

Fig. 12.10 Antiaggregant activity of structural analogues of PAF-acether.[11]

2. Apparently continuous increase

Actually, an apparently continuous increase of activity may correspond simply to the ascending branch of the parabola (see the two curves in Fig. 12.11). The observed 'pseudolinear' curve usually occurs in an insufficiently explored series. A true linear correlation would imply the existence of compounds of infinite potency!

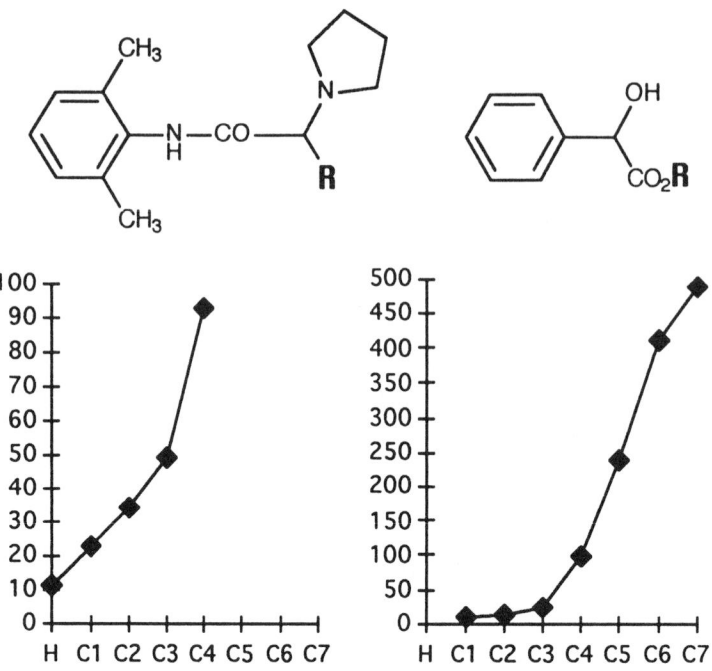

Fig. 12.11 Local anesthetic activity[15] and spasmolytic activity[16] in homologous series.

R	Duration of anaesthesia in rabbit cornea (min)
Hydrogen	11
Methyl	23
Ethyl	34
Propyl	49
Butyl	93

R	Spasmolytic activity on guinea-pig isolated gut
Methyl	8
Ethyl	12
Propyl	24
Butyl	98
Pentyl	240
Hexyl	410
Heptyl	490

B. Nonsymmetrical curves with a maximum activity peak

In some instances curves with maximum activity peaks are not symmetrical and one side shows very sharp activity variations whereas the other corresponds to a progressive variation. The shape of such a curve is represented in Fig. 12.12.

For the GABA$_A$ antagonists represented in Fig. 12.13, the peak activity corresponds to the attachment of a *butyric* side-chain on the aminopyridazine system. The affinity diminishes drastically for shorter chains, but very gradually for longer chains.[17]

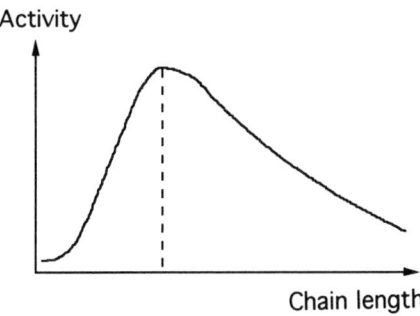

Fig. 12.12   Nonsymmetrical curve with a maximum activity peak.

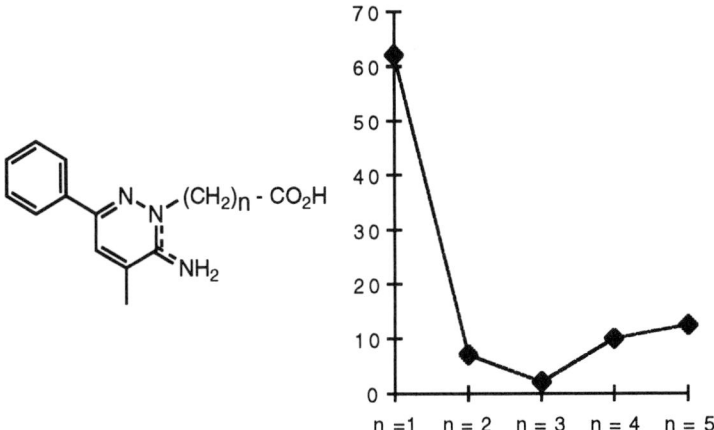

Fig. 12.13   Affinity of GABA$_A$ antagonists for the GABA$_A$ receptor site.[17]

1.   *The particular case of polymethylenic bisammonium compounds*

Compounds having the general formula $(CH_3)_3N^+$—$(CH_2)_n$—$N^+(CH_3)_3$ usually have high affinity for cholinergic receptors. When the values of n are intermediate ($n = 5$ or 6: penta- or hexamethonium), such compounds behave like cholinergic *agonists* (towards the sympathetic ganglions). For higher values ($n = 10$: decamethonium) the compounds become *antagonists* of acetylcholine (at the muscular end plate). In both cases, increasing acetylcholine levels displaces them from their binding sites. When considering neuromuscular blockade, one observes again a curve with an asymmetric profile: sudden changes between $n = 6$ and $n = 8$, and then progressive diminution between $n = 9$ and $n = 12$.

To explain this, if we suppose that compounds of general structure X—$(CH_2)_n$—Y interact by means of their polar groups X and Y with complementary groups at the receptor, four interaction schemes can be envisaged, depending on the value of n (Fig. 12.14a: (1–5)):

1.   *n is small*: The molecule is too short and only one of its polar ends can establish an interaction with the complementary sites of the receptor (Fig. 12.14: (1)). The molecule will be inactive or poorly active. This is the case for the pyridazinyl-glycine of Fig. 12.13.
2.   *n is large enough*: A good interaction can be established with complementary sites of the

receptor, which triggers the biological response (Fig. 12.14: (2)). This represents the optimal case.

3. *n is too large*: Two situations are possible. If the molecule is rigid or if there is steric hindrance, interaction is not possible for Y (Fig. 12.14: (3)). If the molecule is flexible and if the steric tolerance is sufficient, the fit can be entirely satisfactory (Fig. 12.14: (4)).

4. *n is very large*: In this case (Fig. 12.14: (5)), the fit with the receptor is again very good, but with a more distant subsite Y" instead of Y'. The substance can then behave as an *antagonist* (this was the case discussed above of decamethonium).

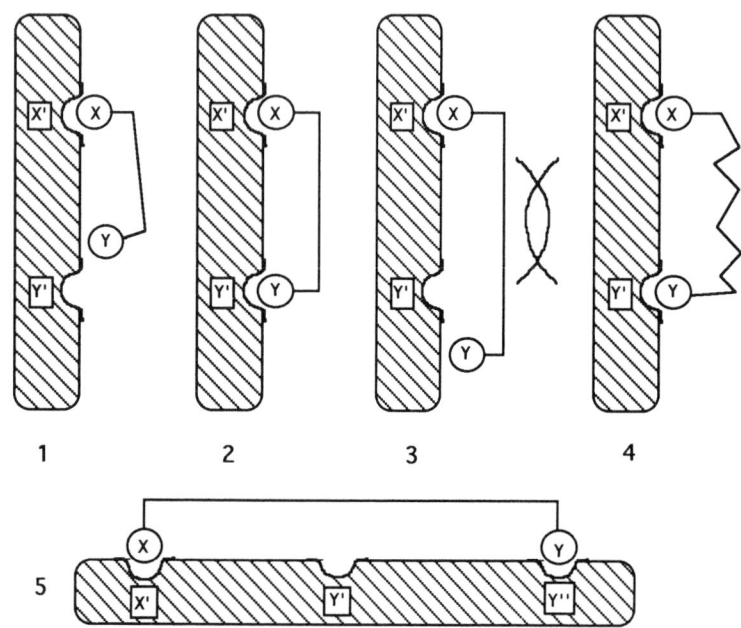

Fig. 12.14 Different modes of interaction of bifunctional molecules according to their length.

C. Serrated variations

One sometimes observes alternating (serrated) variations of activity (zig-zag curves) according to whether the number of carbon atoms is even or odd. Such examples are found for antimalarials derived from methoxy-6-amino-8-quinoline (Fig. 12.15). For these derivatives the antimalarial activity is greater if n is odd (for studied values that vary from $n = 4$ to $n = 10$).[18] Similar observations were made in a series of 4,4'-dimethylaminodiphenoxyalkanes tested as potential schistosomicides.[19] For diamines with $n = 4$ up to $n = 10$, the activity on the schistosomes varies in alternating manner (Fig. 12.16). Alkyl-linked bis(amidinobenzimidazoles) with an even number of methylenes connecting the benzimidazole rings have a higher affinity for the minor groove of DNA than those with an odd number of methylenes.[20]

Zig-zag variations are well known in homologous series for physical properties such as melting points and solubilities. In the previous examples the alkyl chain represents a spacer group between two binding groups. In some cases it can be shown that the energy required to fold the molecule to obtain the required separation should change in a zig zag manner with increasing chain length. An example is found in the leukotriene B_4 antagonists derived from

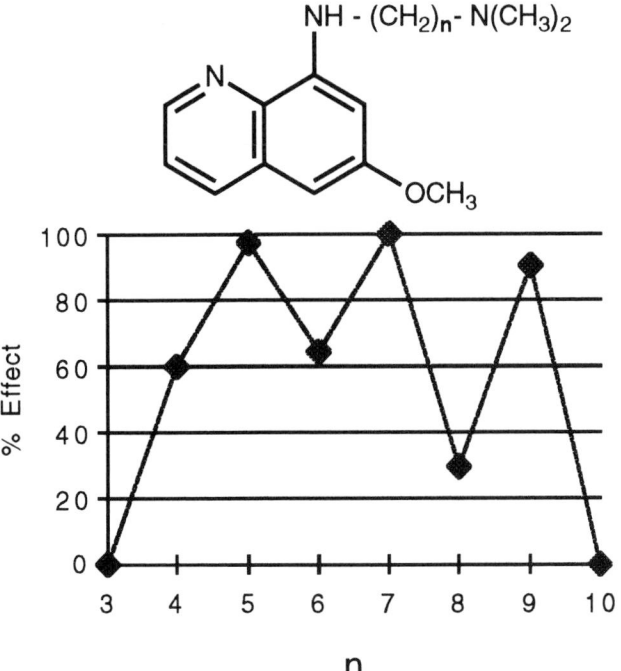

Fig. 12.15 Antimalarial activity in a homologous series of bifunctional methoxy-6-amino-8-quinolines. (After Magidson and Strukov.[18])

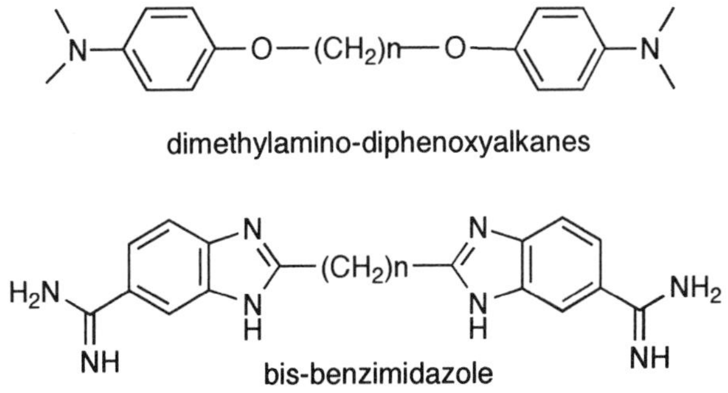

dimethylamino-diphenoxyalkanes

bis-benzimidazole

Fig. 12.16 Schistosomicidal 4,4'-dimethylaminodiphenoxyalkanes.[19]

hydroxyacetophenones[21] (Table 12.1). This is just a reflection of the rotational energy curves for adjacent CH_2 groups.

In the biological domain, variations of activity are not necessarily linked to the induction of effects at the level of a given receptor, but could have come from a pharmacokinetic factor (urinary or biliary excretion, plasma protein binding, differential metabolism). A case of differential metabolism is illustrated by comparison of the toxicities of odd and even ω-fluoro acids.[22] The β-oxidation of odd-chain-length compounds leads to the extremely toxic fluoroacetic acid, while acids with even numbers of carbon atoms generates β-fluoropropionic acid which is clearly less toxic (Table 12.2).

Table 12.1 Zig-zag variations of the affinity of hydroxyacetophenone derivatives for the human peripheral neutrophils. Inhibition of [^{3}H]LTB$_4$ binding at 0.1 mM.[21]

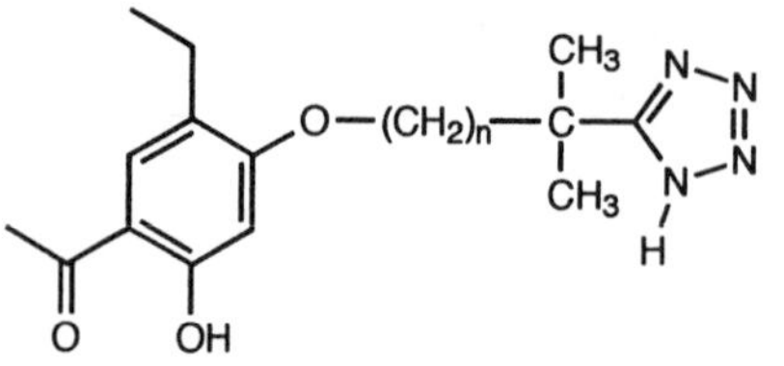

Length of methylene chain, n	Percentage inhibition of [^{3}H]LTB$_4$ binding at 0.1 µM
3	28
4	17
5	56
6	13
7	49

Table 12.2 Zig-zag variations of the toxicity of aliphatic ω-fluoro derivatives (LD$_{50}$ for mice in mg/kg intraperitoneally).[22]

	F(CH$_2$)$_n$COOH		F(CH$_2$)$_n$CO		F(CH$_2$)$_n$COH		F(CH$_2$)$_n$CH$_3$	
n	Odd	Even	Odd	Even	Odd	Even	Odd	Even
1	6.6		6		10			
2		60				46.5		
3	0.65		2		0.9			
4		>100		81		>100		
5	1.35		0.58		1.2		1.7	
6		40		>100		80		35
7	0.64		2		0.6		2.7	
8		>100		53		32		21.7
9	1.5		1.9		1		1.7	
10		57		>40		>100		15.5
11	1.25				1.5		2.5	

D. Inversion of the activity

It can happen that the lower members of a series possess one activity profile and that the higher members possess a different profile, contrasting with that of the lower members. This phenomenon is particularly observed when the bulkiness of cationic heads is progressively increased. In N-alkylated derivatives of norepinephrine,[23] progressive alkylation reduces the hypertensive activity according to the sequence: —NH$_2$, —NHMe, —NHEt, —NHPr^n. Finally, the molecules become hypotensive for —NHPr^i, —NHBu^n and —NHBu^i (Table 12.3).

This anomaly is explained by the fact that norepinephrine can interact with two subclasses of receptors (α- and β-adrenergic receptors). The less hindered derivatives are able to bind to both

Table 12.3 Gradual inversion of the activity in a homologous series.[22]

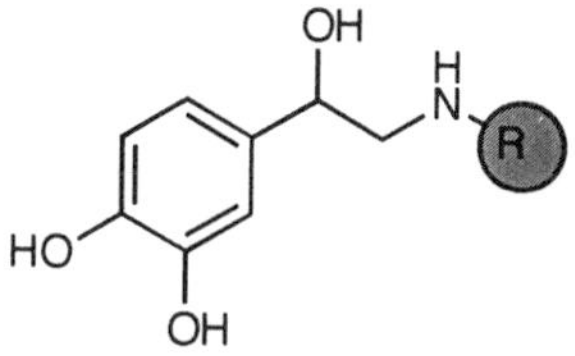

	Blood pressure in the cat	
R	Hypertensive	Hypotensive
Hydrogen	++	–
Methyl	++	–
Ethyl	+	+
Propyl	–	+
Isopropyl	–	++
Butyl	–	++
Isobutyl	–	++

α- and β-receptors, hindered ones solely to β-receptors. A similar inversion of properties is observed when the cholinergic agonist carbachol is modified by dibutylation at the carbamate function and exchange of one of its methyl groups for an ethyl group (Fig. 12.17). The analogue, dibutoline, is a powerful cholinolytic.

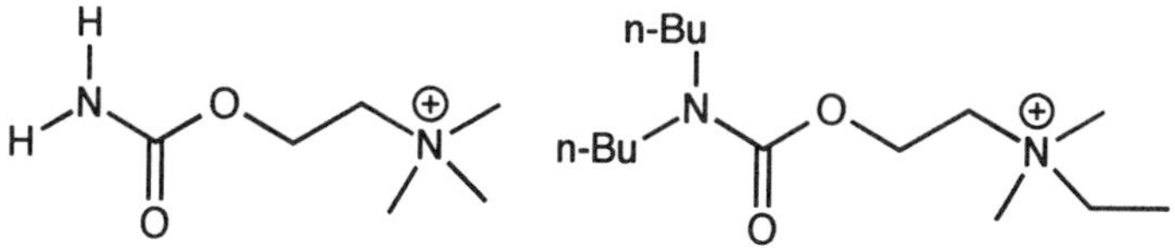

Fig. 12.17 Carbachol (left) and dibutoline (right).

In morphine (agonist), the replacement of the N-methyl group by a more bulky radical such as N-allyl, N-cyclopropylmethyl or N-cyclobutylmethyl leads to powerful antagonists of the opiate receptors (see Chapter 17: Unsaturated Groups).

Introduction of bulkiness in a cationic head does not always cause a change from agonist to antagonist. Thus the analogue N-propylapomorphine is a more powerful dopaminergic agonist than the apomorphine itself.

E.   Conclusion

Variations in homologous series often relate to the search for optimal lipophilicity. In the cyclo-polymethylenic series, conformational problems may also be a factor. For difunctional polymethylenic derivatives, intercharge distances and, possibly, elements of symmetry (see Chapters 15 and 26) can take over. Whereas the activity profile is generally preserved during homology changes, very large differences in potency can be found, that confound the old adage 'methyl, ethyl, propyl, butyl, futile'.

V. VINYLOGUES AND BENZOLOGUES

The vinylogy principle was first formulated by Claisen in 1926,[24] who observed for formylacetone acidic properties similar to that of acetic acid. The vinyl goup plays the role of an electron-conducting channel between the carbonyl and the hydroxyl group. The same effect explains the acidity of ascorbic acid (Fig. 12.18).

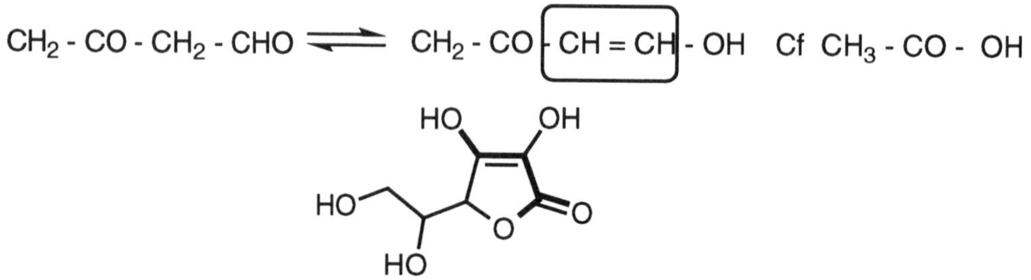

$$CH_2 - CO - CH_2 - CHO \rightleftharpoons CH_2 - CO \boxed{- CH = CH} - OH \quad Cf \; CH_3 - CO - OH$$

Fig. 12.18   Formylacetone (enolic form) and vitamin C are comparable in acidity to carboxylic acids.

Today the vinylogy principle is explained by the mesomeric effect and it applies to all conjugated systems: imine and ethynyl groups, phenyl rings, aromatic heterocycles (Fig. 12.19). For a review of the chemical aspects of the vinylogy principle, see Krishnamurthy.[25]

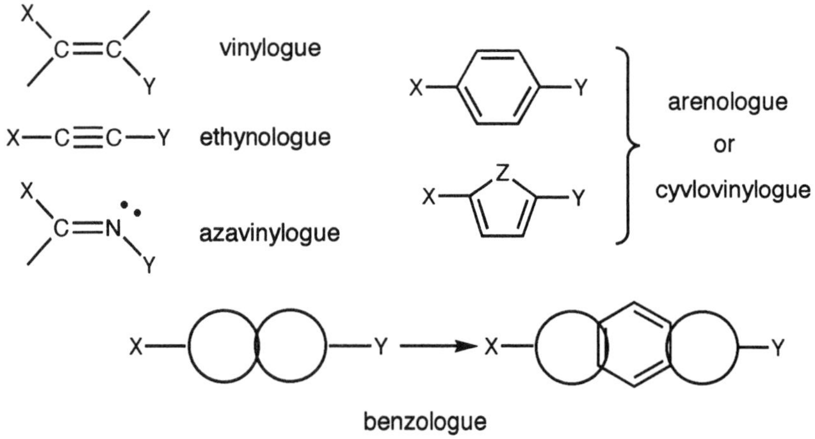

Fig. 12.19   Vinylogy and its extensions.

A. Applications of the vinylogy principle

Although numerous applications of the vinylogy concept are found in the medicinal chemistry literature, only a very few of them are of practical interest, mainly because the preparation of vinylogues usually leads to compounds that are more sensitive to metabolic degradation and more toxic (reactivity of the conjugated double bond) than the parent drug, without being more active.

1. *Authentic vinylogues*

The vinylogues of phenylbutazone,[26] and of pethidine (C. G. Wermuth, unpublished results) have the same type of activity as the parent drug, but the duration of action, especially for the pethidine analogue, is notably shorter than that of the original molecule (Fig. 12.20). This is probably due to an easier metabolic degradation of the styryl double bond.

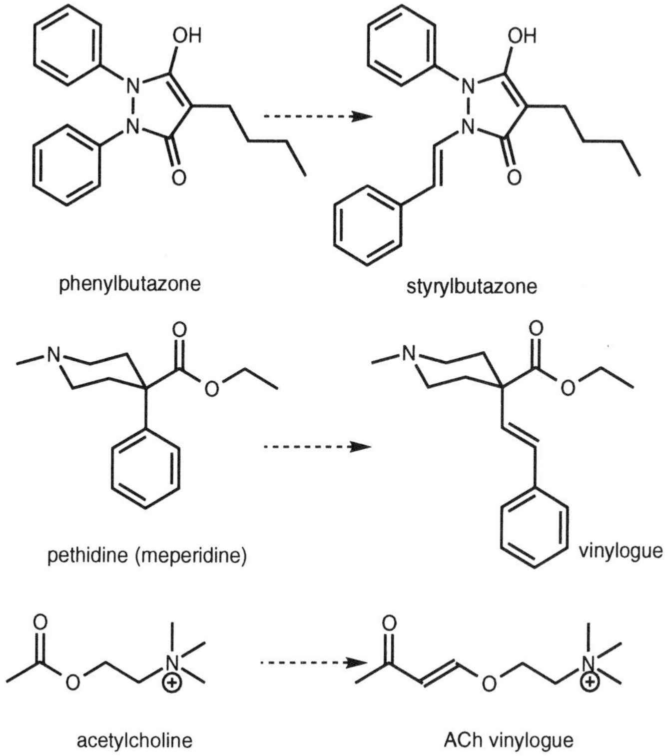

Fig. 12.20 Vinylogues of phenylbutazone, pethidine and acetylcholine.

In preparing the vinylogue of acetylcholine (Fig. 12.20), Tenconi and Barzaghi[27] succeeded in separating the nicotinic from the muscarinic activity (Table 12.4).

Wright *et al.*[28] described a series of hydroxamic acid vinylogues acting as dual inhibitors of 5-lipoxygenase (5-LO; $IC_{50} = 0.15 \times 10^{-6}$ M) and of interleukin-1β (IL-1β) biosynthesis ($IC_{50} = 2.8 \times 10^{-6}$ M) which might be useful as antiinflammatory drugs (Fig. 12.21). For such

Table 12.4 Cholinergic profile of the vinylogue of acetylcholine.[27]

Compound	Nicotinic activity	Muscarinic activity	Sensitivity to ACh-esterase
ACh	+	+	Sensitive
Vinylogue	+	Insensitive	Insensitive

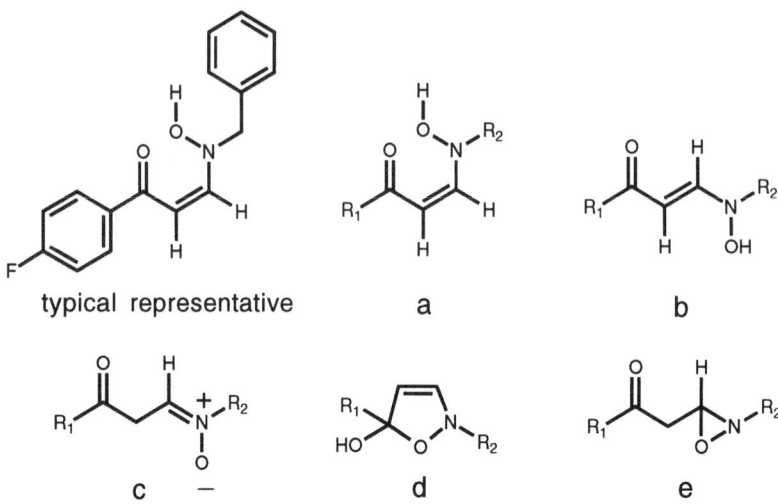

Fig. 12.21   Hydroxamic acid vinylogues and their various isomeric forms.[27]

compounds several possible isomeric and tautomeric forms can be considered. These include the (*E*) and (*Z*) geometrical isomers (a and b), as well as the tautomers nitrone (c), 5-hydroxyisoxazolidine (d), and oxaziridine (e). Examination of the ^{1}H and ^{13}C NMR spectra of the vinylogues revealed that each of the tautomeric possibilities is present in solution in varying proportions. The relative proportion of each isomer was found to be dependent upon the solvent, the pH, and its chemical structure.

2.   Ethynologues

Some ethynologues of biologically active compounds were prepared by Dunoguès and his group, but unfortunately they did not describe their biological activity: aspirin ethynologue,[29] nicotinamide and isoniazide ethynologues,[30] chalcones ethynologues[31].

3.   Azavinylogues

As a rule, simple azavinylogues are unstable compounds, owing to the ready hydrolysis of the imino bond. However, the particular case of *O*-alkylated oximes (X—CH=N—O—Y; with Y = R or Ar) can be interesting insofar as the oximic imino bond was shown to be biostable.[32] Preparing azavinylogues of β-blocking agents (Fig. 12.22) led to some active compounds.[33-35] The proposal was made that the stable oxime C=NOCH$_2$ could mimic a portion of an aromatic ring, thus simulating an aryl or an aryloxymethylene group.[36]

Reduction of the imino bond results in a decrease but not loss of activity and ether derivatives retain activity.[35] The tricyclic oxime β-blocker IPS 339 showed high selectivity for β$_2$-receptors.[33,34] Noxiptyline (Agedal®, Bayer) is the oximic equivalent of amitriptyline (for review see Hoffmeister;[32,37] for crystal structure see Bandoli[38]).

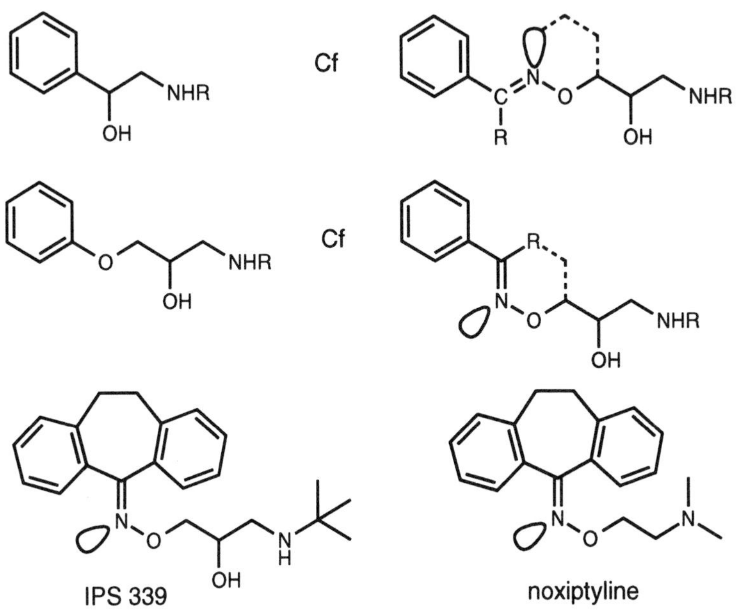

Fig. 12.22   Oxime ethers as azavinylogues.

4. Cyclovinylogues

These vinylogues have the advantage of being more stable towards *in vivo* metabolism. In addition, they allow molecular variations with *ortho*, *meta* and *para* positional isomers. Thus, for cyclovinylogues of procaine the highest local anaesthetic activity was found with the *meta* derivative, which also showed the best dissociation between local anaesthetic and antiarrhythmic activity (Table 12.5).[39]

Similar results were observed with cyclovinylogues of lidocaine.[40] For other references, see Valenti.[41] Compound TA-1801 (ethyl 2-(4-chlorophenyl)-5-(2-furyl)-4-oxazoleacetate),[42] can to some extent be considered as an arenologue of clofibrate (Fig. 12.23).

Table 12.5   Cyclovinylogues of procainamide, relative activity with regard to procainamide.[39]

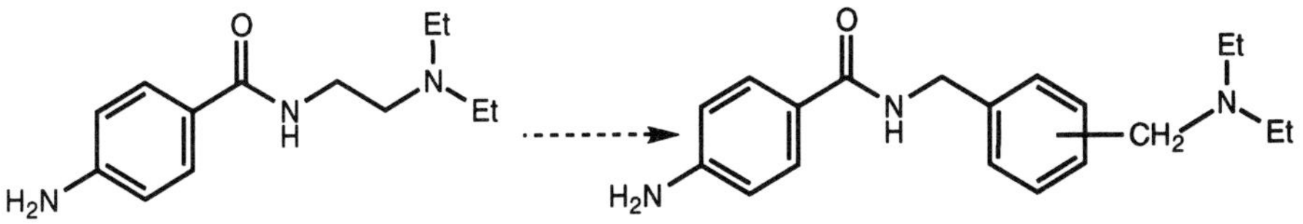

Compound	Local anaesthetic power	Antiarrhythmic activity
Procainamide	1	1
Ortho cyclovinylogue	~ 0	0.17
Meta cyclovinylogue	47	0
Para cyclovinylogue	35	0

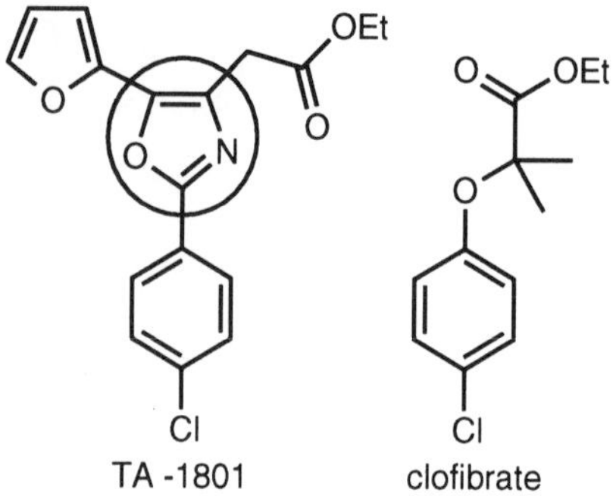

Fig. 12.23   TA-1801, an arenologue of clofibrate.[41]

Pyrroline-3-ones were used as peptidic bond surrogates by Hirshman and his group[43] In such compounds, thanks to vinylogy, the carbonyl and the amino group show the same chemical reactivity as that of a secondary amide (Fig. 12.24).

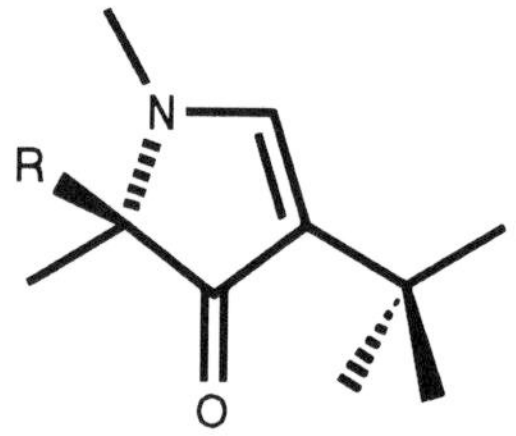

Fig. 12.24   The vinylogous relationship between the carbonyl and the amino group in pyrroline-3-ones confers on them the reactivity of secondary amides.[42]

5. Benzologues

Linear and angular benzologues of guanine[44] and adenine[45–47] were published without any indication of biological activity (Fig. 12.25). A review article on chemistry and biochemistry of benzologues was published by Leonard and Hiremath.[48] More recently, linear and angular benzologues of xanthines showed submicromolar affinities for rat brain A_1 and A_2 adenosine receptors[49] and benzologues of quinolone antibacterials maintained high antimicrobial activity.[50]

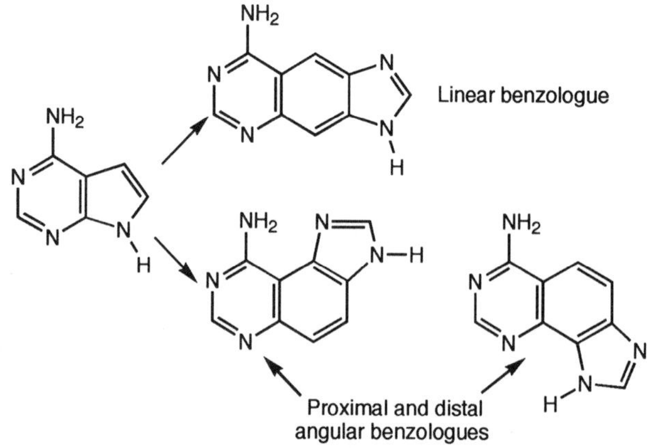

Fig. 12.25   Linear and angular adenine benzologues.

B. Comments

Owing to important changes in geometry vinylogues often have unpredictable activity. For this reason vinylogues play a minor role in medicinal chemistry. In addition, their metabolic vulnerability or their increased toxicity may represent a significant drawback.

However, the vinylogy principle is sometimes applied to the design of bioisosteres. Thus, the guanidino group of the benzimidazole fenbendazole[51] can be compared to its vinylogue[52] in the corresponding imidazo[1,2-*a*]pyridine (Fig. 12.26). Both compounds are anthelminthics of similar potency.

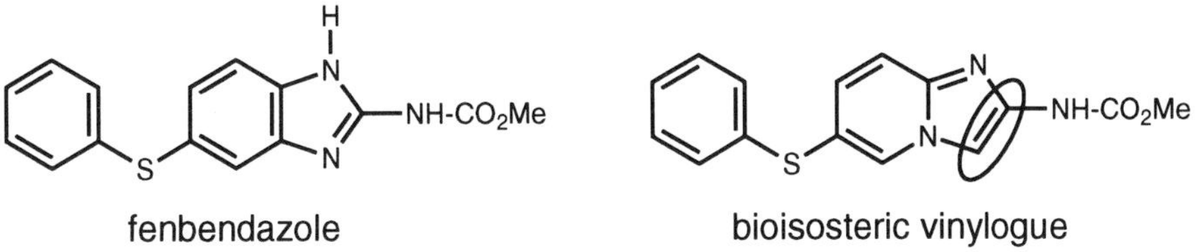

Fig. 12.26 Application of the vinylogy principle to the design of a fenbendazole bioisostere.[51]

The vinylogy principle can account for unexpected chemical reactivity that is not always recognized at first glance (Fig. 12.27). So, for example, the basicity of the N1 nitrogen is strengthened in compound CGS 8216 thanks to the vinylogous influence of the quinoline nitrogen. For a similar reason the carbonyl group of benzopiperidones or of 3-acyl-indoles behaves chemically more like an amidic carbonyl than a ketonic one. In 2-methoxy-*p*-benzoquinone the reactivity of the methoxy group is that of a carboxylic ester, rendering it susceptible to attack by secondary amines.

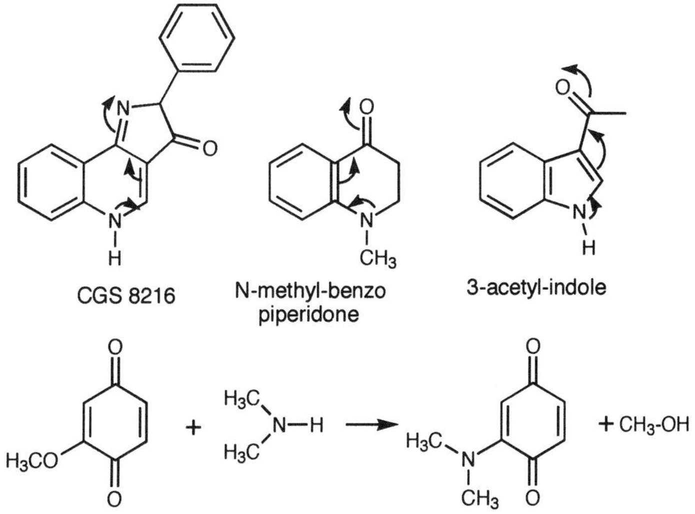

Fig. 12.27 Unexpected chemical reactivities attributable to vinylogy.

REFERENCES

1. Gerhardt, C. (1853) Principes de la classification sériaire. In *Traite de Chimie Organique*, pp. 121–142. Firmin Didot Frères, Paris.

2. Ward, J. S., Merritt, L., Klimkowski, V. J. *et al.* (1992) Novel functional M_1 selective muscarinic agonists. 2. Synthesis and structure–activity relationships of 3-pyrazinyl-1,2,5,6-tetrahydro-1-methylpyridines. Construction of a molecular model for the M_1 pharmacophore. *J. Med. Chem.* **35**: 4011–4019.

3. Cook, L., Ternai, B. and Ghosh, P. (1987) Inhibition of human sputum elastase by substituted 2-pyrones. *J. Med. Chem.* **30**: 1017–1023.

4. Thorsett, E. D. (1986) Conformationally restricted inhibitors of angiotensin converting enzyme. In Combet-Farnoux, C. (ed.) *Actualités de Chimie Thérapeutique,* pp. 257–268. Société de Chimie Thérapeutique, Chatenay-Malabry.

5. Eden, J. M., Higginbottom, M., Hill, D. R., Horwell, D. C., Hunter, J. C., Martin, K., Pritchard, M. C., Rahman, S. S., Richardson, R. S. and Roiberts, E. (1993) Rationally designed 'dipeptoid' analogues of cholecystokinin (CCK): N-terminal structure-affinity relationships of α-methyltryptophan derivatives. *Eur. J. Med. Chem.* **28**: 37–45.

6. Cheronis, J. C., Whalley, E. T., Nguyen, K. T., Eubanks, S. R., Allen, L. G., Duggan, M. J., Loy, S. D., Bonham, K. A. and Blodgett, J. K. (1992) A new class of bradykinin antagonists: synthesis and *in vitro* activity of bissuccinimidoalkane peptide dimers. *J. Med. Chem.* **35**: 1563–1572.

7. Wang, W. and Lown, J. W. (1992) Anti-HIV-I activity of linked lexitropsins. *J. Med. Chem.* **35**: 2890–2897.

8. Press, J. B., Wright Jr, W. B., Chan, P. S., Haug, M. F., Marsico, J. W. and Tomcufcik, A. S. (1987) Thromboxane synthetase inhibitors and antihypertensive agents. 3. N-[(1H-Imidazol-1-yl)alkyl]heteroaryl amides as potent enzyme inhibitors. *J. Med. Chem.* **30**: 1036–1040.

9. Nicolai, E., Goyard, J., Benchetrit, T., Teulon, J. M., Caussade, F., Virone, A., Delchambre, C. and Cloarec, A. (1992) Synthesis and structure–activity relationships of novel benzimidazole and imidazo[4,5-*b*]pyridine acid derivatives as thromboxane A_2 receptor antagonists. *J. Med. Chem.* **36**: 1175–1187.

10. Ginos, J. Z., Stevens, J. M. and Nichols, D. E. (1979) Structure–activity relationships of N-substituted dopamine and 2-Amino-6,7-dihydroxy-1,2,3,4-tetrahydronaphthalene analogues: behavioral effects in lesioned and reserpinized mice. *J. Med. Chem.* **22**: 1323–1329.

11. Godfroid, J.-J., Broquet, C., Jouquey, S. *et al.* (1987) Structure–activity relationship in PAF-acether. 3. Hydrophobic contribution to agonistic activity. *J. Med. Chem.* **30**: 792–797.

12. Bustard, T. M. (1974) Optimization of alkyl modifications by Fibonacci search. *J. Med. Chem.* **17**: 777–778.

13. Santora, N. J. and Auyang, K. (1975) Non-computer approach to structure–activity study. An expanded Fibonacci search applied to structurally diverse types of compounds. *J. Med. Chem.* **18**: 959–963.

14. Martin, Y. C. (1987) *Quantitative Drug Design, a Critical Introduction,* pp 257–261. Marcel Dekker, New York.

15. Koelzer, P. P. and Wehr, K. H. (1958) Beziehungen zwischen chemischer Konstitution un pharmakologischer Wirkung bei mehreren Klassen neuren Lokalanaesthetica. *Arzneimittel-Forsch.* **8**: 544–550.

16. Funcke, A. B. H., Ernsting, M. J. E., Rekker, R. F. and Nauta, W. T. (1953) Untersuchungen über Spasmolytica. 1. Mandelsäureester. *Arzneimittel-Forsch.* **3**: 503–506.

17. Wermuth, C. G., Bourguignon, J.-J., Schlewer G. *et al.* (1987) Synthesis and structure–activity relationships of a series of aminopyridazine derivatives of γ-aminobutyric acid acting as selective $GABA_A$ antagonists. *J. Med. Chem.* **30**: 239–249.

18. Magidson, O. J. and Strukow, I. T. (1933) Die Derivate des 8-Aminochinolins als Antimalariapräparate. Mitteilung II: Der Einfluß der Länge der Kette in Stellung 8. *Arch. Pharm.* **271**: 569–580.

19. Raison, C. G. and Standen, O. D. (1995) The schistosomicidal activity of symmetrical diaminodiphenoxyalkanes. *Br. J. Pharmacol.* **10**: 191–199.

20. Fairley, T. A., Tidwell, R. R., Donkor, I., Naiman, N. A., Ohemeng, K. A., Lombardy, R. J.,

Bentley, J. A. and Cory, M. (1993) Structure, DNA minor groove binding, and base pair specificity of alkyl- and aryl-linked bis(amidinobenzimidazoles) and bis(amidinoindoles). *J. Med. Chem.* **36**: 1746–1753.

21. Herron, D. K., Goodson, T., Bollinger, N. G., Swanson-Bean, D., Wright, I. G., Staten, G. S., Thompson, A. S., Froelich, L. L. and Jackson, W. T. (1992) Leukotriene B4 receptor antagonists: the LY 255 283 series of hydroxyacetophenones. *J. Med. Chem.* **35**: 1818–1828.

22. Pattison, F. L. M. (1959) *Toxic Aliphatic Fluorine Compounds*. Elsevier, Amsterdam.

23. Ariëns, E. J. (1964) *Molecular Pharmacology*, vol. 1. Academic Press, New York.

24. Claisen, L. (1926) Zu den *O*-Alkylderivaten des Benzoyl-acetons und den aus ihnen entstehenden Isooxazolen. *Ber. dtsch. chem. Ges.* **59**: 144–153.

25. Krishnamurthy, S. (1982) The principle of vinylogy. *J. Chem. Educ.* **59**: 543–547.

26. Yamamoto, H. and Kaneko, S.-I. (1970) Synthesis of 1-phenyl-2-styryl-3,5-dioxopyrazolidines as antiinflammatory agents. *J. Med. Chem.* **13**: 292–295.

27. Tenconi, F. and Barzaghi, F. (1964) Attivita nicotinica di vinil-analoghi di esteri della colina. *Boll. Chim. Pharmaceut.* **103**: 569–575.

28. Wright, S. W., Harris, R. R., Kerr, J. S. *et al.* (1962) Synthesis, chemical, and biological properties of vinylogous hydroxamic acids: dual inhibitors of 5-lipoxygenase and IL-1 biosynthesis. *J. Med. Chem.* **35**: 4061–4068.

29. Babin, P., Bourgeois, P. and Dunoguès, J. (1976) Synthèse de l'éthynologue de l'acide acétylsalicylique. *C. R. Acad. Sci. (Paris)* **283**: 149–152.

30. Babin, P., Cassagne, A., Dunoguès, J., Duboudin, F. and Lapouyade, P. (1981) Ethynologues du nicotinamide et de l'isoniazide. *J. Heterocyclic Chem.* **18**: 519–523.

31. Babin, P., Lapouyade, P. and Dunoguès, J. (1982) Synthesis of chalcone ethynologues with a pharmacological objective. *Can. J. Chem.* **60**: 379–382.

32. Hoffmeister, F. (1969) Zur Frage pharmakologisch-klinischer Wirkungsbeziehungen bei Antidepressiva, dargestellt am Beispiel von Noxiptilin. *Arzneimittel-Forsch.* **19**: 458–467.

33. Leclerc, G., Mann, A., Wermuth, C. G., Bieth, N. and Schwartz, J. (1977) Synthesis and β-adrenergic blocking activity of a novel class of aromatic oxime ethers. *J. Med. Chem.* **20**: 1657–1662.

34. Imbs, J. L., Miesch, F., Schwartz, J., Velly, J., Leclerc, G., Mann, A. and Wermuth, C. G. (1977) A potent new β$_2$-adrenoceptor blocking agent. *Brit. J. Pharmacol.* 357–362.

35. Leclerc, G., Bieth, N. and Schwartz, J. (1980) Synthesis and β-adrenergic blocking activity of new aliphatic oxime ethers. *J. Med. Chem.* **23**: 620–624.

36. Macchia, B., Balsamo, A., Lapucci, A., Martinelli, A., Macchia, F., Bresci, M. C., Fantoni, B. and Martinotti, E. (1985) An interdisciplinary approach to the design of new structures active at the β-adrenergic receptor. Aliphatic oxime ether derivatives. *J. Med. Chem.* **28**: 153–160.

37. Aichinger, G., Behner, O., Hoffmeister, F. and Schütz, S. (1969) Basische tricyclische Oximinoäther und ihre pharmakologischen Eigenschaften. *Arzneimittel-Forsch.* **19**: 838–845.

38. Bandoli, G. and Nicolini, M. (1983) Crystal structure of the antidepressant noxiptyline hydrochloride (5-dimethylaminoethyloximino-5H-dibenzo[a,d]-cyclohepta-1,4-diene hydrochloride). *J. Crystallogr. Spectrosc. Res.* **13**: 191–199.

39. Valenti, P., Mazzotti, M., Rampa, A. and Magistretti, M. J. (1982) Cyclovinylogues of procainamide. *Arch. Pharm.* **315**: 1003–1007.

40. Valenti, P., Montanari, P., Da Re, P., Soldani, G. and Bertelli, A. (1980) Synthesis and pharmacological properties of three lidocaine cyclovinylogues. *Arch. Pharm.* **313**: 280–284.

41. Valenti, P., Montanari, P., Fabbri, G., Giovannini, L. and Giacomelli, A. (1985) Cyclo-vinylogues of some antimuscarinic drugs. *Arch. Pharm.* **318**: 222–224.

42. Mooriya, T., Seki, M., Takabe, S., Matsumoto, K., Takashima, K. and Mori, T. (1987) Compound TA-1801 [ethyl 2-(4-chlorophenyl)-5-(2-furyl)-4-oxazoleacetate]. *J. Pharm. Sci.* **76**: S164.

43. Smith III, A. B., Keenan, T. P., Holcomb, R. C., Sprengeler, P. A., Guzman, M. C., Wood, J. L., Caroll, P. J. and Hirschmann, R. (1992) Design, synthesis and crystal structure of a pyrrolinone-based peptidomimetic possessing the conformation of a β-strand: potential application to the design of novel inhibitors of proteolytic enzymes. *J. Am. Chem. Soc.* **114**: 10672–10674.

44. Cottis, S. G., Clarke, P. B. and Tieckelmann, H. (1965) Pyrazolo[3,4-b]pyridines and pyrazolo[3',4':6,5]pyrido[2,3-d]pyrimidines. *J. Heterocycl. Chem.* **2**: 192–201.

45. Leonard, N. J., Morrice, A. G. and Sprecker, M. A. (1975) Linear benzoadenine. A stretched-out analog of adenine. *J. Org. Chem.* **40**: 356–363.

46. Morrice, A. G., Sprecker, M. A. and Leonard, N. J. (1975) The angular benzoadenines. 9-Aminoimidazo[4,5-f]quinazoline and 6-aminoimidazo[4,5-h]quinazoline. *J. Org. Chem.* **40**: 363–366.

47. Leonard, N. J., Sprecker, M. A. and Morrice, A. G. (1976) Defined dimensional changes in enzyme substrates and cofactors. Synthesis of lin-benzoadenosine and enzymatic evaluation of derivatives of the benzopurines. *J. Am. Chem. Soc.* **98**: 3987–3994.

48. Leonard, N. J. and Hiremath, S. P. (1986) Dimensional probes of binding and activity. *Tetrahedron* **42**: 1917–1961.

49. Schneller, S. W., Ibay, A. C., Christ, W. J. and Bruns, R. F. (1989) Linear and proximal benzo-separated alkylated xanthines as adenosine-receptor antagonists. *J. Med. Chem.* **32**: 2247–2254.

50. Jordis, U., Sauter, F., Rudolf, M. and Cai, G. (1988) Synthesen neuer Chinolon-Chemotherapeutika 1: Pyridochinoline und Pyridophenanthroline als 'lin-benzo-Nalidixinsäure'-Derivate. *Monatsh. Chem.* **119**: 761–780.

51. Averkin, E. A., Beard, C. C., Dvorak, C. A. *et al.* (1972) Methyl 5(6)-phenylsulfinyl-2-benzimidazolecarbamate, a new, potent anthelmintic. *J. Med. Chem.* **15**: 1164–1166.

52. Bochis, R. J., Dybas, R. A., Eskola, P. *et al.* (1978) Methyl 6-(phenylsulfinyl)imidazo[1,2-a]pyridine-2-carbamate, a potent, new anthelmintic. *J. Med. Chem.* **21**: 235–237.

13

Molecular Variations Based on Isosteric Replacements

CAMILLE G. WERMUTH

Si ce n'est toi c'est donc ton frère
If it isn't you, then it's your brother
Jean de La Fontaine (1621–1695) *Le loup et l'agneau*

THE PRACTICE OF MEDICINAL CHEMISTRY
ISBN 0-12-744640-0

The replacement in an active molecule of an atom or a group of atoms by another one presenting a comparable electronic and steric arrangement is based on the concept of *isosterism*. The term isosterism was introduced in 1919 by the physicist Langmuir[1] who was mainly interested in the physicochemical relationships of isosteric molecules. When, in addition to their physicochemical analogy, compounds share some common biological properties, the term *bioisosterism*, introduced by Friedman in 1951,[2] is used, even if the physicochemical resemblance is only vague.

I. HISTORY: DEVELOPMENT OF THE ISOSTERISM CONCEPT

The development of the concept of isosterism has its roots in the attempts to extend to entire molecules the knowledge acquired for elements, namely that two elements possesssing an identical peripheral electronic distribution also possess similar chemical properties.

A. The molecular number

Allen, in 1918, defined the *molecular number* of a compound in a similar way to the atomic number:

$$N = aN_1 + bN_2 + cN_3 + \cdots + zN_i$$

where

N = molecular number,
$N_1, N_2, N_3, \ldots N_i$ = respective atomic numbers of each element of the molecule,
$a, b, \ldots z$ = number of each element present in the molecule.

Compare ammonium and sodium cations as an example. The atomic number of nitrogen is 7 and that of hydrogen is 1. Thus the molecular number of the ammonium cation can be calculated and compared to that of the sodium ion:

	Atomic number	*Molecular number*
NH_4^+	$7 + (4 \times 1)$	11
Na^+	11	11

Possessing the same molecular number, the ammonium cation should resemble the sodium cation. This is roughly true. More generally, two compounds with identical molecular numbers present at least some similar physical properties (e.g. specific heat).

B.   The isosterism concept

Independently from Allen, Langmuir in 1919[1] defined the concept of isosterism:

> Comolecules are thus isosteric if they contain the same number and arrangement of electrons. The comolecules of isosteres must, therefore, contain the same number of atoms. The essential differences between isosteres are confined to the charges on the nuclei of the constituent atoms.

Langmuir cites a list of 21 kinds of isosteres such as

$$O^{2-}, F^-, Ne, Na^+, Mg^{2+}, Al^{3+} \quad \text{or} \quad ClO_4^-, SO_4^{2-}, PO_4^{3-}$$

The first example clearly demonstrates that isosterism does not inevitably imply 'isoelectric' structures (having the same total electric charge), but it becomes evident that isoelectronic isosteres show the closest analogies:

$$C{=}O \text{ and } N{=}N \quad CO_2 \text{ and } NO_2 \quad N{=}N{=}N^- \text{ and } N{=}C{=}O^-$$

In the field of organic chemistry, Langmuir predicted the analogy between diazomethane and ketene, which was only discovered later.

$$\text{>}C{=}\overset{+}{N}{=}\overset{\overset{..}{}}{N} \quad \text{cf.} \quad \text{>}C{=}\overset{..}{N}{=}\overset{..}{O}$$

C.   The notion of pseudoatoms and Grimm's hydride displacement law

Later, in 1925, Grimm formulated the 'hydride displacement law',[3-5] according to which the addition of hydrogen to an atom confers on the aggregate the properties of the atom of next highest atomic number. An isoelectronic relationship exists among such aggregates, which were named *pseudoatoms*. Thus, when a proton is 'added' to the O^{2-} ion in the nuclear sense, an isotope of fluorine is obtained (Fig. 13.1).

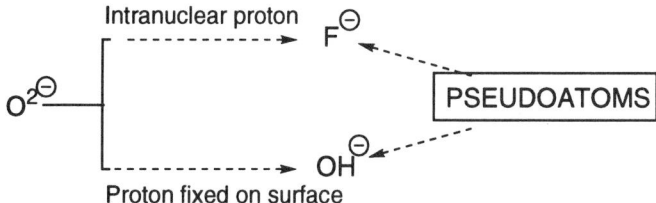

Fig. 13.1   The notion of pseudoatoms.

When the same proton is introduced at the peripheral electronic level, a 'pseudo-F', in other words an OH^-, is created. In this context, the H^+ ion, having penetrated the electronic shell of the oxygen, is assumed to be masked by the greater atom and to exert only negligible effect towards the outside. The fluoride anion F^- and the hydroxyl anion OH^- therefore show some analogies. The generalization of the pseudoatom concept represents the so-called 'hydride displacement law' proposed in a tabular form by Grimm.[3,4]. In each vertical column (Table 13.1), the original atom is followed by its isosteric pseudoatoms.

Table 13.1 Hydride displacement law: in each vertical column the atom is followed by its pseudoatoms.[3-5]

		Number of electrons			
6	7	8	9	10	11
C^{4-}	N^{3-}	$-O-$	$-F$	Ne	Na^+
	CH^{3-}	$-NH-$	$-OH$	FH	
		$-CH_2-$	$-NH_2$	OH_2	
			$-CH_3$	NH_3	OH_3^+
				CH_4	NH_4^+

D.   Erlenmeyer's expansion of the isosterism concept

Starting in 1932, Erlenmeyer published a series of detailed studies on the isosterism concept, and particularly about its first applications to biological problems.[6] Erlenmeyer proposed his own definition of isosteres as elements, molecules or ions in which the peripheral layers of electrons may be considered identical.[7] Erlenmeyer also proposed three expansions of the isosterism concept as follows:

1. To the whole group of elements present in a given column of the periodic table. Thus, silicon becomes isosteric to carbon, sulphur to oxygen, and so on.
2. To the pseudoatoms, with the aim of including groups that at a first glance seem totally different but which, in practice, possess rather similar properties. This is the case for the pseudohalogens, for example (Cl $\cong$ CN $\cong$ SCN, etc.)
3. To the ring equivalents: The equivalence between —CH=CH— and —S— explaining the well-known analogy between benzene and thiophene (Table 13.2).

Table 13.2 The sulphur atom is approximately equivalent to an ethylenic group (size, mass, capacity to provide an aromatic lone pair)

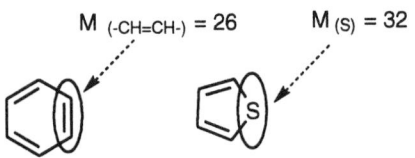

$M_{(-CH=CH-)} = 26$ $M_{(S)} = 32$

Compound	BP°C	Isostere	BP°C
Benzene	80°	Thiophene	84°
Methylbenzene	110°	2-Methylthiophene	113°
Chlorobenzene	132°	2-Chlorothiophene	130°
Acetylbenzene	200°	2-Acetylthiophene	214°

E.   Isosterism criteria, present conceptions

The main criterion for isosterism is that two isosteric molecules must present similar, if not identical, volumes and shapes. Ideally, isosteric compounds should be isomorphic and able to co-crystallize. Among the other physical properties that isosteric compounds usually share are boiling point, density, viscosity and thermal conductivity. However, certain properties must be different: dipolar moments, polarity, polarization, size and shape (e.g. in comparing F^- and OH^-, the size and the shape of H cannot be totally neglected). After all, the external orbitals may be hybridized differently.

In conclusion, it became evident to physicists that the concept of isosterism, developed before quantum-mechanical theories, could not provide at the molecular level the same results as those that the periodic classification had provided for the elements, namely a correlation between electronic structure and physical and chemical properties. In the field of medicinal chemistry, the isosterism concept, taken in its broadest sense, has proved to be a research tool of the utmost importance. The main reason for this is that isosteres are often much more alike in their biological than in their physical and chemical properties. An illustrative example is found in the comparison of oxazolidine-diones and hydantoins, which possess different chemical reactivities but present a similar antiepileptic profile (Fig. 13.2).

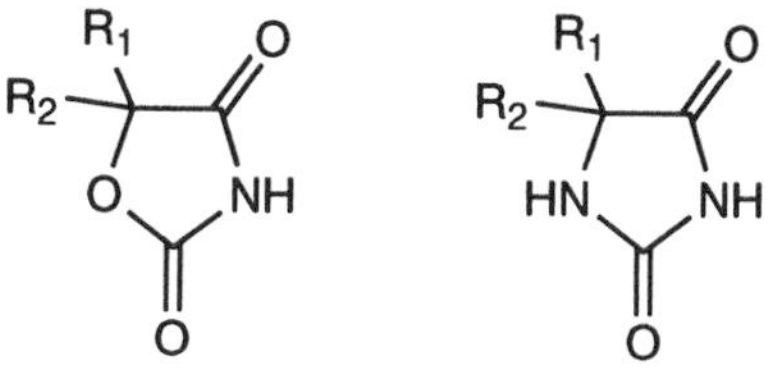

Fig. 13.2   5,5′-Disubstituted oxazolidine-diones (I) and hydantoins (II) show similar antiepileptic profiles.

F.   The bioisosterism concept — Friedman's and Thornber's definitions

Recognizing the usefulness of the isosterism concept in the design of biologically active molecules, Friedman[2] proposed to call *bio*isosteres compounds 'which fit the broadest definition of isosteres and have the same type of biological activity'. This definition received rapid acceptance and is now commonly used. Moreover, Friedman considers that isosteres that exhibit opposite properties (antagonists) have also to be considered as bioisosteres, since usually they interact with the same recognition site. This is the case for *p*-aminobenzoic acid and *p*-aminobenzene sulfonamide and also for glutamic acid and its phosphonic analogues.

The use of the term isosterism has largely been taken beyond its original meaning when employed in medicinal chemistry, and Thornber[8] proposes a loose and flexible definition of the term bioisostere: 'Bioisosteres are groups or molecules which have chemical and physical similarities producing broadly similar biological effects'.

The term nonclassical isosterism is often used interchangeably with the term bioisosterism, for example, when one has to deal with isosteres that do not possess the same number of atoms but which have in common some key parameter of importance for the activity in a given series. Thus, the two GABAergic agonists isoguvacine and THIP (Fig. 13.3) possess similar pharmacological properties to GABA itself. The key parameters in these compounds are the acidic ($pK_a \approx 4$) and the basic (protonated nitrogen) functions with an intercharge distance of $\approx 5.1\,\text{Å}$.

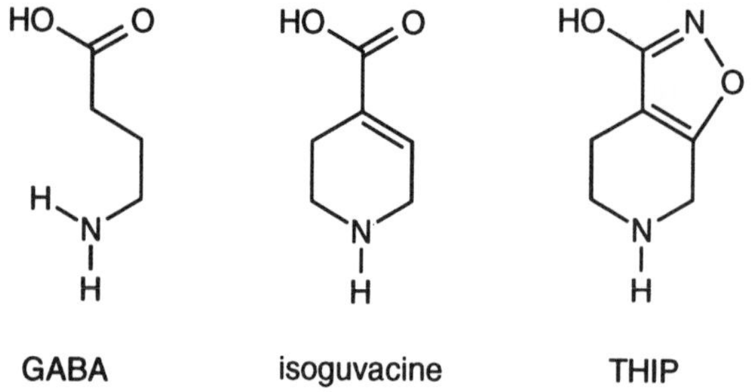

GABA   isoguvacine   THIP

Fig. 13.3   An example of bioisosterism, or nonclassical isosterism GABA, isoguvacine and THIP are all agonists at the GABA$_A$ receptor. The 3-hydroxyisoxazole ring has a comparable acidity to that of a carboxylic acid function.[9]

II.   CURRENTLY ENCOUNTERED ISOSTERIC AND BIOISOSTERIC MODIFICATIONS

As the distinction between isosteres and bioisosteres is of rather academic interest, it is preferred, in this chapter, to treat both categories together. Consequently, divalent series such as O$=$, HN$=$, and H$_2$C$=$ can be discussed together with S$=$ for example. However, the correct nomenclature will be used as much as possible, keeping in mind, nevertheless, that 'isosteric replacement' embraces both true isosteres and bioisosteres.

A.   Replacement of univalent atoms and groups

Halogens (particularly chlorine) can be replaced by other electron-attracting functions such as trifluoromethyl or cyano groups. In the antibiotic chloramphenicol, both the chlorine atoms of the dichloroacetic moiety and of the *p*-nitrophenyl group yielded productive isosteric replacements (Table 13.3). Many other examples of univalent atom or group replacements are found in the chapters dealing with substituent effects (Chapter 17) and with quantitative structure–activity relationships (Chapter 19).

Table 13.3   Isosteric replacements in the amphenicol family.

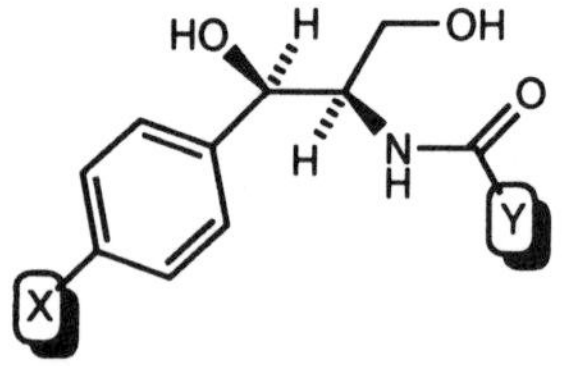

Compound	X	Y
Chloramphenicol	$-NO_2$	$-CH-Cl_2$
Thiamphenicol	CH_3-SO_2-	$-CH-Cl_2$
Cetophenicol	CH_3-CO-	$-CH-Cl_2$
Azidamphenicol	$-NO_2$	$-CH-N_3$

B.   Interchange of divalent atoms and groups

A first series of frequently interchanged divalent atoms or groups is represented by O, S, NH and CH_2, and many interesting examples are found in the literature. In a study on meperidine analogues (Table 13.4) potent analgesic compounds were found for X = O, NH, and CH_2.[10] Surprisingly, the sulfur analogue showed only moderate activity. As an *in vivo* test was used to assess the activity, the weaker effect may be attributable to a faster metabolism (sulfoxide or sulfone formation?).

Table 13.4   Meperidine analogues.[10]

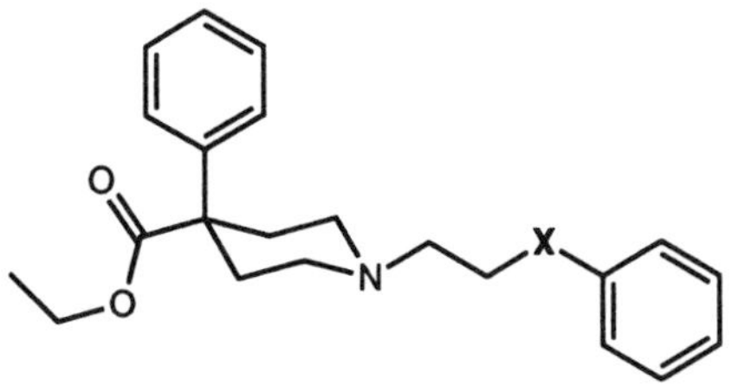

X	Analgesic potency (meperidine = 1)
O	12
NH	80
CH_2	20
S	1.5

Similar changes can be applied to cyclic series, for example to a series such as piperidine–morpholine–thiomorpholine–piperazine, or in introducing oxygen or sulfur atoms into cyclic ketoprofen analogues.[11]

Table 13.5   Physostigmines (left) and carbaisosteres (right).[12]

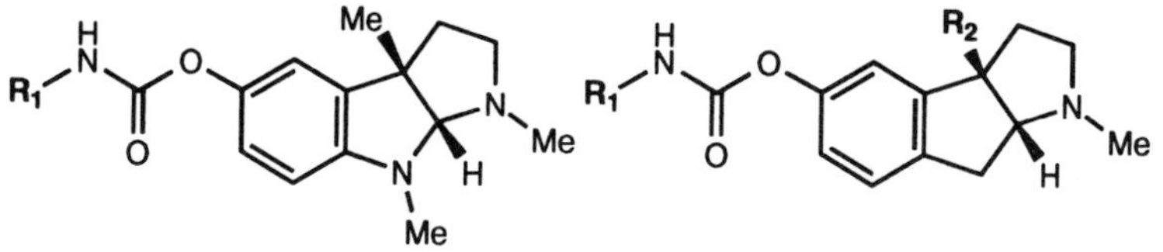

Compound	R_1	R_2	IC_{50} (nM)	LD_{50} (mg/kg)
(−)-Physostigmine	CH_3	CH_3	128	0.88
(−)-Heptyl physostigmine	n-C_7H_{13}	CH_3	110	24
(±)-Carba-isostere 1	n-C_7H_{13}	CH_3	114	21
(−)-Carba-isostere 2a	n-C_7H_{13}	C_2H_5	36	6
(+)-Carba-isostere 2b	n-C_7H_{13}	C_2H_5	211	18

With the objective of designing a more stable analogue of the acetylcholinesterase inhibitor alkaloid physostigmine, Chen *et al.*[12] prepared some 8-carba isosteres of physostigmine (Table 13.5). The authors envisaged that replacing the *N*-methyl group at N8 of the physostigmine nucleus by a methylene group would increase its chemical and metabolic stability, thanks to the change of the less stable aminal group to a more stable amino group.

The carba isosteres are as potent or more potent than the corresponding physostigmines. In addition, the (−)-enantiomers, which possess the same absolute configuration at C3a and C8a as that of physostigmine are generally 6 to 12 times more potent in inhibiting acetylcholinesterase than the corresponding (+)-enantiomers.

C. Interchange of trivalent atoms and groups

The substitution of −CH= by −N= in aromatic rings has been one of the most successful applications of classical isosterism (see following section on ring equivalents). Aminopyrine and its isostere are about equally active as antipyretics[13] (Fig. 13.4). Similar interchanges are found in proceeding from desipramine to nortriptyline and protriptyline (Fig. 13.4) or among the antihistaminics, when comparing ethylenediamine derived compounds to the diarylpropylamines (Fig. 13.4).

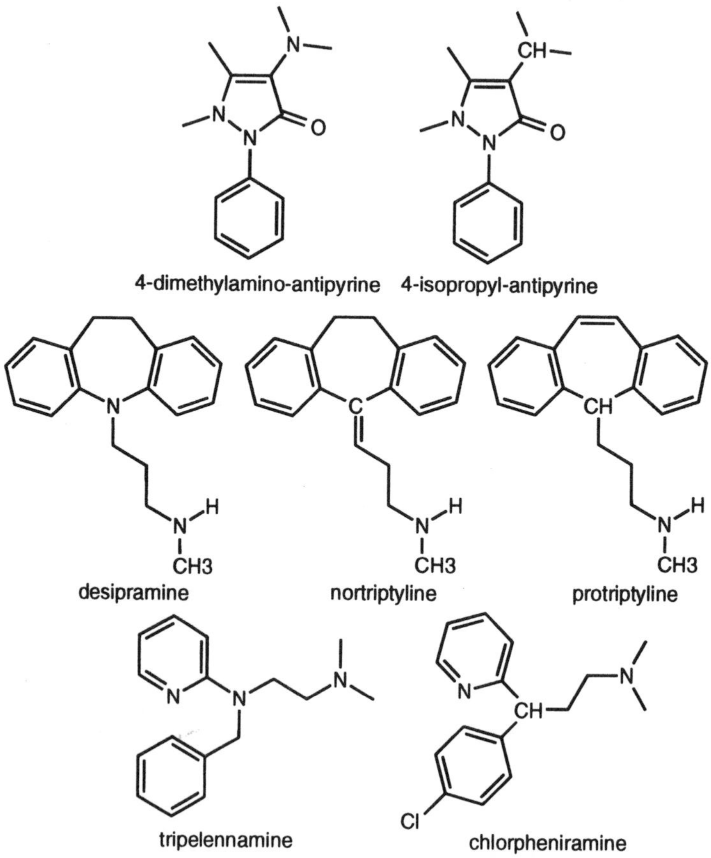

Fig. 13.4 Interchange of trivalent atoms and groups.

D.   Ring equivalents

The substitution of $-CH=$ by $-N=$ or $-CH=CH-$ by $-S-$ in aromatic rings has been one of the most successful applications of classical isosterism. Early examples are found in the sulfonamide antibacterials with the development of sulfapyridine, sulfapyrimidine, sulfathiazole, etc. (Fig. 13.5).

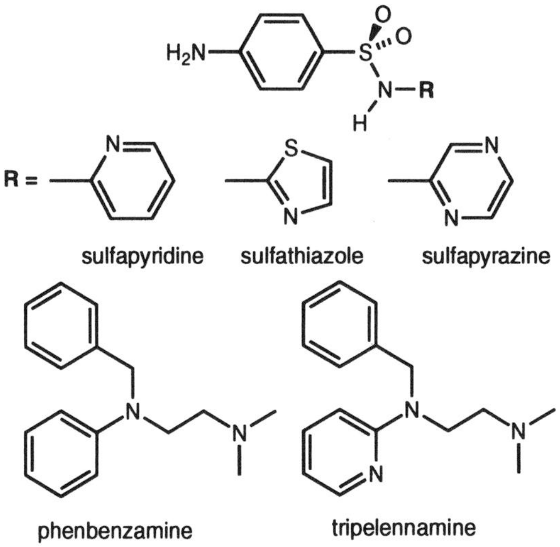

Fig. 13.5   Classical ring equivalents.

Other examples are found in the neuroleptic or antidepressant tricyclics, in the benzodiazepine tranquillizers and antiepileptics, and in the development of semisynthetic penicillins and cephalosporins with broader spectra of activity and greater stability towards β-lactamases.

In all these cases no *essential* activity difference is found between the original drug and its isostere. However, it can happen that the procedure fails. Binder *et al.*[14] for example, reported that thieno[2,3-*d*]isoxazole-3-methanesulfonamide, the thiophene analogue of the anticonvulsant drug zonisamide (Fig. 13.6),[15] was practically inactive against pentetrazole- or electric shock-induced convulsions in mice, even at high doses.

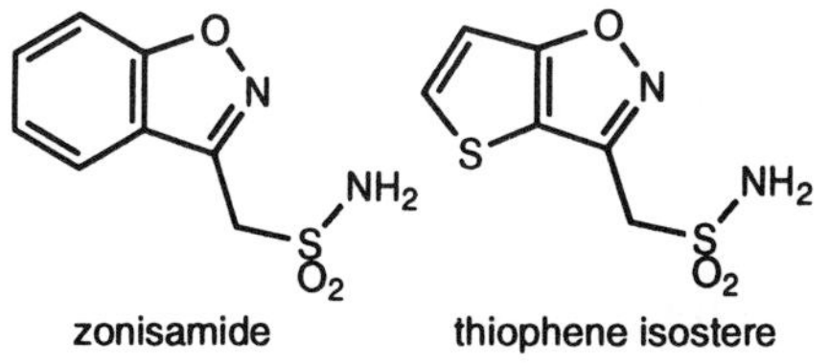

Fig. 13.6   The thiophene isostere of zonisamide is practically inactive as an anticonvulsant.

The concept of ring equivalents has been generalized to any possible heterocyclic system and represents a huge number of possible variations. Table 13.6 lists some less well-known studies on ring equivalents in aromatic series.

Table 13.6 Ring equivalents.

Original ring	Bioisostere	Activity	Reference
1-Phenylpyrazolone	1-Phenyltriazolone	Analgesic	Gold-Aubert et al.[16]
1,2,4-Triazole	1,3-Thiazole imidazole	Antiviral	Alonzo et al.[17]
Indole	Indazole	5-HT3 antagonists	Fludzinski et al.[18]
3,4-Dialkoxyphenyl	Indole	Phosphodiesterase inhibitors	Blaskó et al.[19]
3,4-Dialkoxyphenyl	Indole	GABA uptake inhibitors	Kardos et al.[20]
Quinoline-2-carboxylate	Indole-2-carboxylate	Glycine antagonists	Salituro et al.[21]
o-Nitrophenyl	Furoxane	Calcium antagonist	Calvino et al.[22]
spiro-Hydantoin	spiro-Hydroxyacetic acid unit	Aldose reductase inhibitor	Lipinski et al.[23]

Another particularly impressive example of ring bioisosterism is found in the development of the antiulcer H_2-receptor histamine antagonists in which the initial imidazole ring was changed to various other 'equivalents' such as a furan, a thiazole and finally a phenyl ring (Fig. 13.7). A detailed and very interesting account of the discovery and the development of these compounds is found in Ganellin and Roberts' book.[24]

One of the major problems when dealing with isosteric or bioisosteric replacements in *heterocyclic systems* is the selection of the *a priori* most promising candidate among several dozens of possible rings. A simple clue can be the knowledge and the comparison of the boiling points of the basic heterocycles. Thus, in the search for an ideal surrogate of the pyridazine ring, the comparison of the boiling points of seven possible ring candidates (Fig. 13.8), led us to reject the isomeric pyrimidine ring and to select the 1,2,4-triazine and the 1,3,4-thiadiazole rings.[25] Effectively, the observed biological activities were at least partially in accordance with the boiling point selection criteria (Table 13.7). On the reserpine ptosis and the 5-HT potentiation tests, the closest activities result from the replacement of the pyridazine ring (BP=208°C) by the 1,3,4,-thiadiazole (BP=204–205°C) or the 1,2,4-triazine (BP=200°C) ring. The pyrazine- and the pyrimidine-derived analogues are clearly less active on these two tests. The attenuation of the turning behaviour, after unilateral intrastriatal injection of the compounds in 6-hydroxydopamine-lesioned mice, reflects the dopaminergic properties of the molecules. Apparently these properties are insensitive to the bioisosteric variations.

A possible interpretation of these results could be the fact that in the heterocyclic series the boiling point is correlated to the dipolar moment of the molecule and that, for two heterocyclic rings having the same aromatic geometry, the similarity of the dipolar moments may represent the dominant feature.

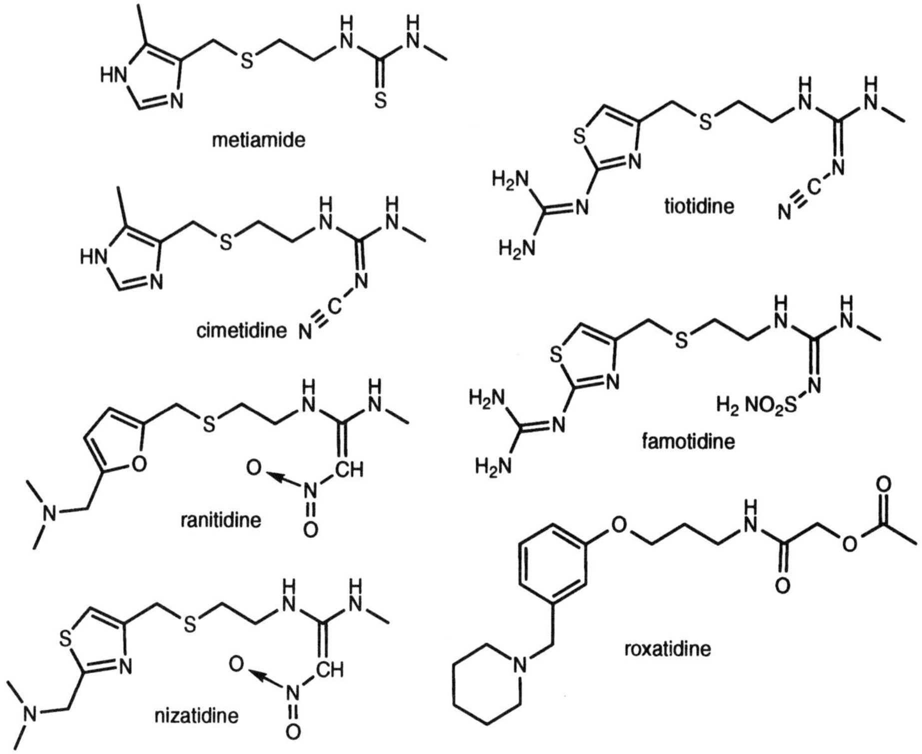

metiamide

tiotidine

cimetidine

famotidine

ranitidine

roxatidine

nizatidine

Fig. 13.7 Antiulcer H₂-receptor histamine antagonists: evolution of structures in the course of the time. Note the progressive use of a furan, a thiazole, and finally a phenyl ring in place of the original imidazole ring.

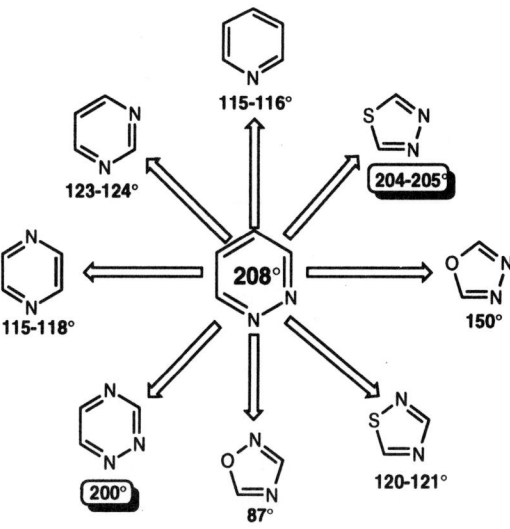

115–116°

123–124°

204–205°

115–118°

208°

150°

200°

87°

120–121°

Fig. 13.8 Structure and boiling points of pyridazine isosteres.

Table 13.7   Cyclic equivalents of the pyridazine ring.[25]

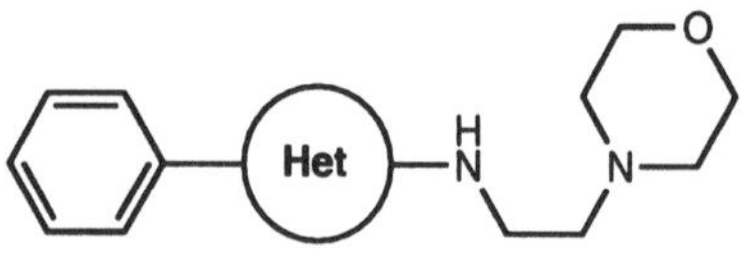

Central heterocycle	Reserpine ptosis (ED_{50})	5-HT potentiation (ED_{50})	Turning (minimal effective dose)
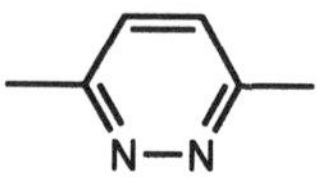	6	3.7	0.5
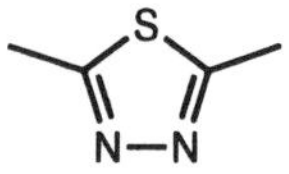	4.5	6	0.1
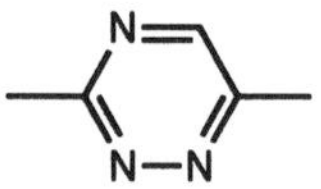	>10	6	2
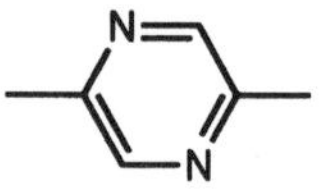	24	30	0.1
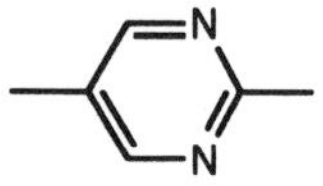	>100	>50	2

Better bioisosteric design possibilities are provided by quantum chemical calculations. Mallamo *et al.*[26] made use of electrostatic potential surface maps complementarity in defining sulfonyl heterocycles bioisosteric to the steroidal antiandrogenic drug zanoterone (Fig. 13.9). Striking differences in the electrostatic potential surfaces accounted for the observed variability in the furan (active) and the thiophene (inactive) analogues of zanoterone (which contains a pyrazole ring). Good androgen receptor affinity was then anticipated—and effectively found—for the oxazole and the thiazole analogues of zanoterone.

The apparent failure of the isosterism concept for the inactive thiophene, inverted furan and pyrimidine is thus interpretable on a rational basis.

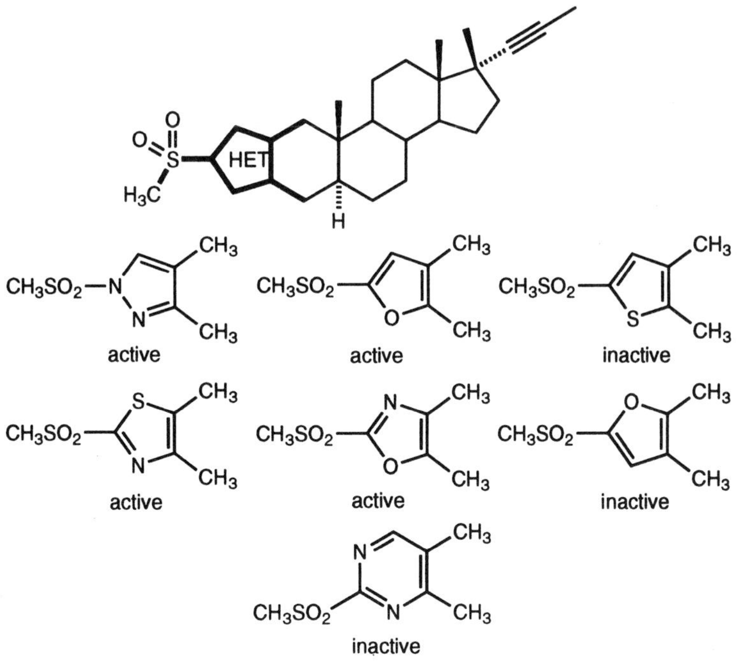

Fig. 13.9 Zanoterone isosteres.[26]

E. Groups with similar polar effects

1. Surrogates of the carboxylic acid function

The carboxylic function of active compounds has been changed to direct derivatives such as hydroxamic acids (R—CO—NH—OH), acylcyanamides (R—CO—NH—CN) and acylsulfonamides (R—CO—NH—SO$_2$—R′; to planar acidic heterocycles such as tetrazoles, hydroxyisoxazoles, etc. or even to nonplanar sulfur- or phosphorus-derived acidic functions (Table 13.8).

Direct derivatives comprise hydroxamic acids[37–41], acylcyanamides[28,42] and acylsulfonamides[35] in which an acidic NH group replaces the acidic OH group. These bioisosteres are mainly of academic interest. Exception are the anti-inflammatory hydroxamates bufexamac,[37] ibuproxam,[38] and oxametacin[39,43] (Fig. 13.10). While ibuproxam is metabolized to ibuprofen (CONHOH → COOH) in man,[44] oxametacin is metabolically stable in man and is a true bioisostere rather than a prodrug.[45,46]

Among the planar acidic heterocycles the main representatives are tetrazoles and 3-hydroxyisoxazoles. The medicinal chemistry of tetrazoles has been reviewed[47] and recent examples are found in various domains.[21,29,30,48] Tetrazole surrogates have the broadest field of applications, they can increase potency,[29,30] improve bioavailability[48,49] or bring some selectivity (the GABA tetrazole analogue inhibits GABA-transaminase, but not succinic semialdehyde dehydrogenase.[50] However, in some instances tetrazole analogues are poorly active.[51]

Hydroxyisoxazoles and other cognate heterocyclic phenols encompassing an acidity range

Table 13.8 Carboxylic acid isosteres.

Structure	Name	Properties	Reference
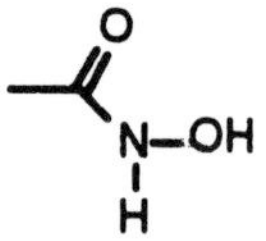	Hydroxamic acids	High chelating power	Almquist et al.[27]
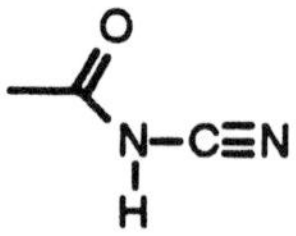	Acyl-cyanamides	Mainly academic interest	von Kohler et al.[28] Shirota et al.
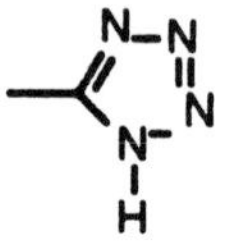	Tetrazoles	Very popular Great number of publications. Recent in use. pK_a = 6.6 to 7.2	Bovy et al.[29] Marshall et al.[30]
(X = O or S)	Mercaptoazoles + sulfinylazoles + sulfonylazoles Isoxazoles Isothiazoles	Phosphonate isosteres pK_a mercapto: 8.2–11.5 pK_a sulfinyl: 5.2–9.8 pK_a sulfonyl: 4.8–8.7 GABA and glutamic acid analogues	Chen et al.[12] Krogsgaard-Larsen et al.[9] Krogsgaard-Larsen[31]
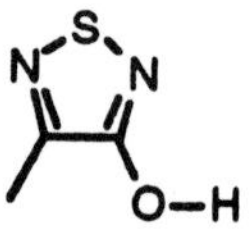	Hydroxythiadiazole	Isoxazole isostere $pK_a \sim 5$	Lunn et al.[32]
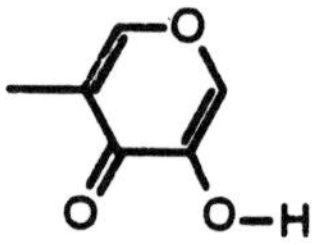	Hydroxychromes	Kojic acid derivatives: as GABA agonists	Atkinson et al.[33]
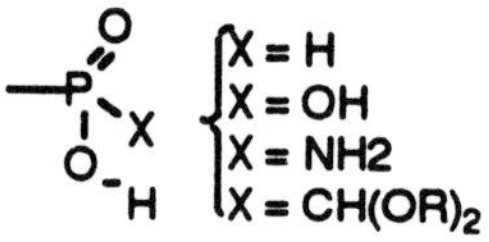 X = H, X = OH, X = NH2, X = CH(OR)$_2$	Phosphinates Phosphonates Phosphonamides	Many examples in the glutamate antagonist series and in the GABA$_B$ antagonists	Froestl et al[34]
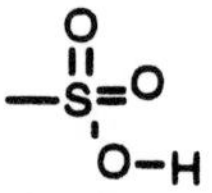	Sulphonates	Sulphonic analogues of GABA and glutamic acid	Rosowsky et al. (1984)
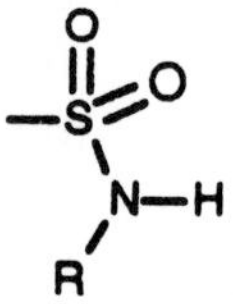	Sulphonamides	Weak acids, used rather as equivalents of phenolic hydroxyls: catecholamine analogues	von Kohler et al.[28]
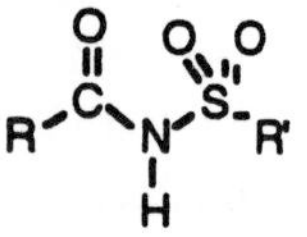	Acylsulphonamides	Glycine GABA β-alanine antiatherosclerotics $pK_a \sim 4,5$	Drummond and Johnson[35] Albright et al.[36]

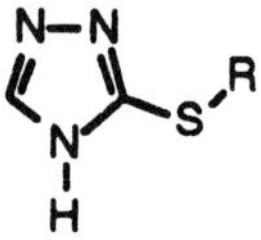

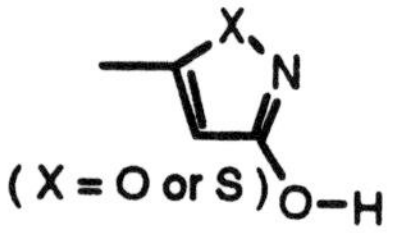

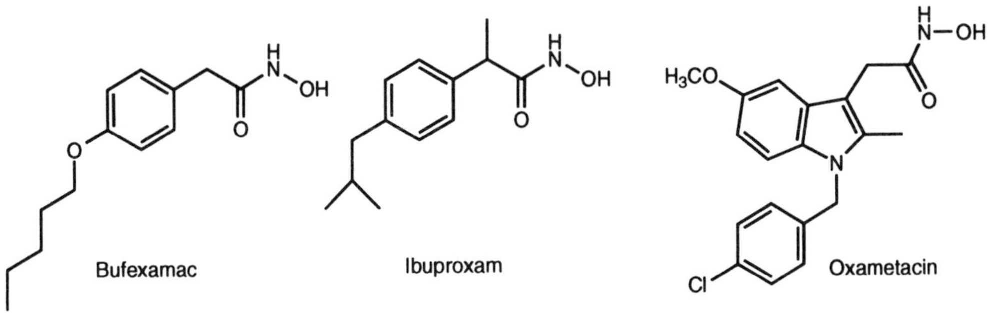

Fig. 13.10 Hydroxamate isosteres of anti-inflammatory drugs.

from 3.0 to 7.1 were incorporated in GABA agonists, antagonists and uptake inhibitors.[52,53] The experience gained with 3-hydroxyisoxazoles in the GABA field was also transferable to glutamate receptor ligands and led to selective antagonists for glutamic acid receptor subtypes.[54]

Other interesting but less studied heterocyclic surrogates are 3,5-dioxo-1,2,4-oxadiazolidine,[55] 3-hydroxy-1,2,5-thiadiazoles[32] and 3-hydroxy-γ-pyrones.[33,56]

Non planar sulfur- or phosphorous-derived acidic functions: The most extensive use of phosphonates was made in the design of amino acid neurotransmitter antagonists such as glutamate[57] and GABA$_B$ antagonists.[34]

In a series of CCK antagonists derived from the nonpeptide CCK-B selective antagonist CI-988, Drysdale *et al.*[58] prepared a series of carboxylate surrogates spanning a pK_a range of <1 (sulfonic acid) to >9.5 (thio-1,2,4-triazole). The affinity and the selectivity of the compounds were rationalized by consideration of the pK_a values, charge distribution, and geometry of the respective acid mimics (Table 13.9).

Diaminocyclobutenedione, was proposed by Kinney *et al.*[59] as an original surrogate of the α-amino carboxylic acid function (Fig. 13.11).

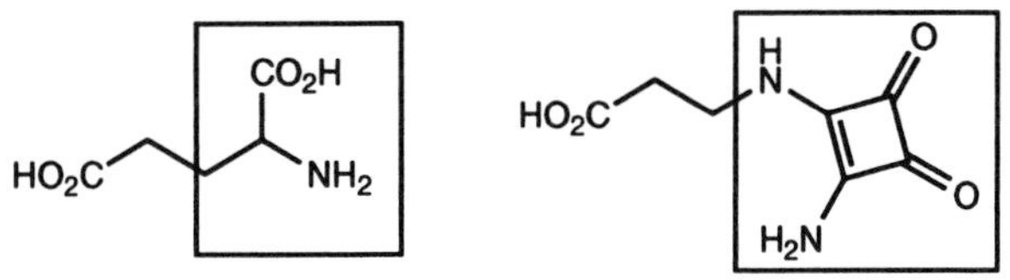

Fig. 13.11 3,4-Diamino-3-cyclobutene-1,2-dione as surrogate of the α-amino carboxylic acid function.[59]

2. Surrogates of the ester function

The change from ester to amide (procaine→procainamide) was already illustrated above as an example of classical isosterism. Similarly, the lactone ring of the muscarinic agonist pilocarpine was changed into various, still active, isosteres such as the corresponding thiolactone, lactam, lactol, and thiolactol.[60] A series of aspirin isosteres has been prepared by replacing the carboxylic ether oxygen successively by a nitrogen, sulfur or carbon isosteric equivalent.[61] None of the isosteric compounds showed any activity. This result is readily understood since the particular role of aspirin as an acylating agent of the enzyme cyclooxygenase has been demonstrated.[62]

Table 13.9   Exploration of the carboxyl isomerism possibilities in a series of CCK antagonists[58]

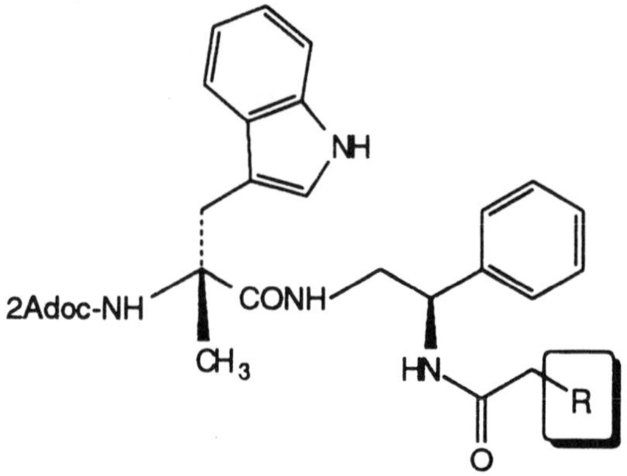

R	IC$_{50}$ (nM) CCK-B	IC$_{50}$ (nM) CCK-A	A/B ratio	pK_a
$-CH_2-COOH$	1.7	4500	2500	5.6

Charge-distributed monoanionic acid mimics

R	IC$_{50}$ (nM) CCK-B	IC$_{50}$ (nM) CCK-A	A/B ratio	pK_a
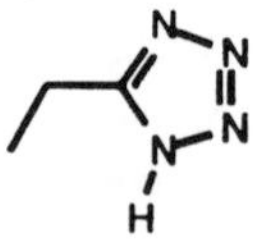	6.0	970	160	5.4
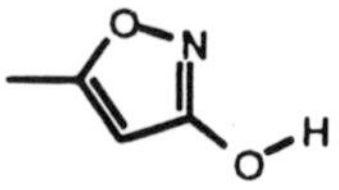	2.6	1700	650	6.5
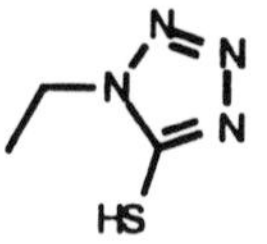	2.4	620	260	4.3
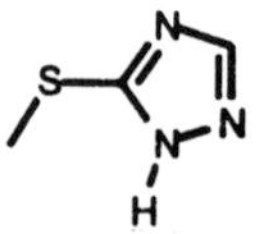	2.5	680	270	>9.5
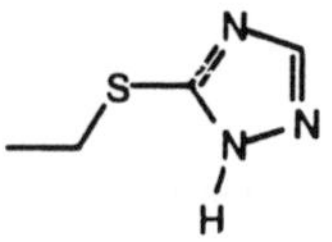	16	850	53	>9.5
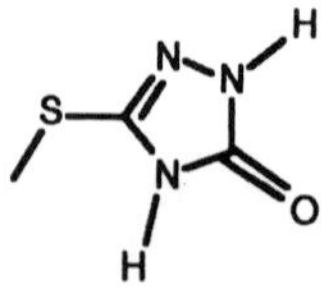	4.3	660	150	7.7
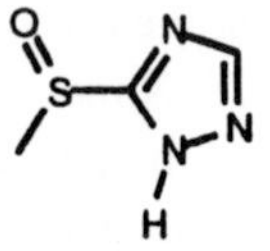	1.7	940	550	7.0

Table 13.9 — *Continued*

R	IC$_{50}$ (nM) CCK-B	IC$_{50}$ (nM) CCK-A	A/B ratio	pK_a
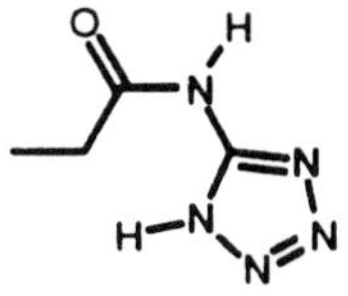	6.3	1300	200	5.2
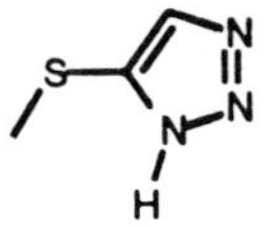	18	600	33	>8.2
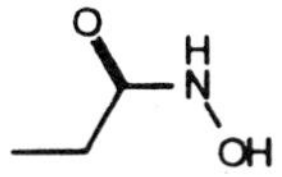	14	1300	93	>9.5

Point-charge monoanionic acid mimics

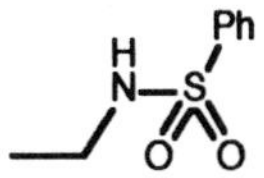	70	300	4.3	>9.5
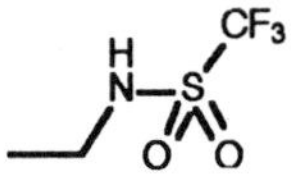	77	680	9	7.9
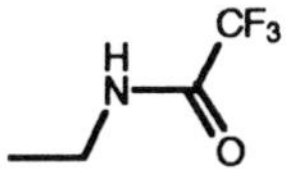	110	790	7	>9.5
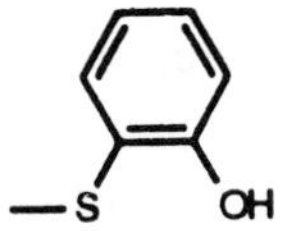	80	510	6.4	>9.5
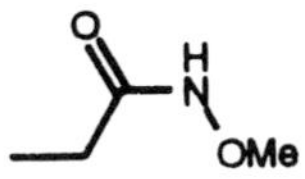	21	1500	71	>9.5

Tetrahedral acid mimics

P(O)(OH)$_2$	27	5200	190	3.4; 7.7
CH$_2$—P(O)(OH)$_2$	23	2700	120	3.4; 7.8
P(O)(OH)(OEt)	12	480	40	6.5
P(O)(OH)Me	12	1700	140	3.8
CH$_2$—P(O)(OH)Me	23	4400	190	3.7
CH$_2$—SO$_3$Na	1.3	1010	780	—

In addition to these classical changes, much use was made of 1,2,4-oxadiazoles or 1,2,4,-thiadiazoles as carboxylic ester surrogates in series of benzodiazepine and muscarinic[63,64] receptor ligands (Fig. 13.12). For muscarinic agonists, numerous successful attempts to replace the oxadiazole ring by other heterocyclic ring systems have been published.[65-67] By substituting in pilocarpine the lactonic ester function by its carbamate equivalent, a much more stable analogue was obtained (See Chapter 38).

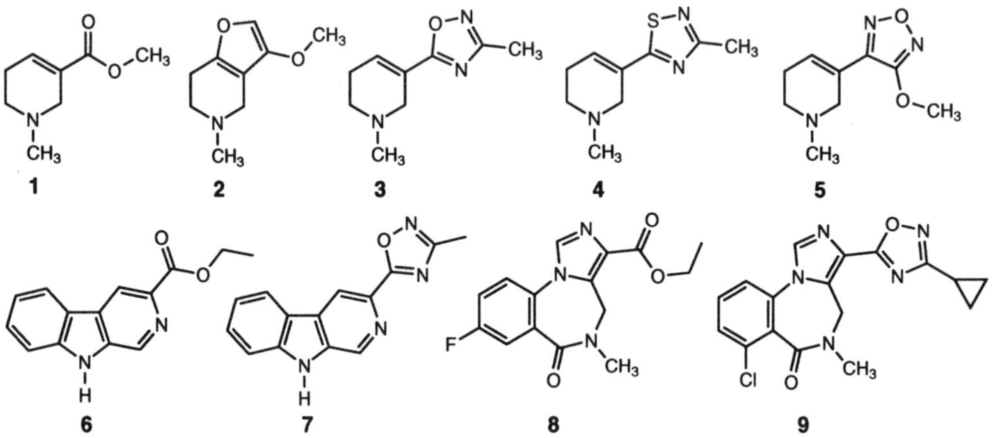

Fig. 13.12   1,2,4-Oxadiazoles and related five-membered heterocycles as ester surrogates.

The change in (−)-cocaine of the carbomethoxy substituent into carbethoxyisoxazole doubles the potency in [³H]mazindol binding and [³H]dopamine uptake. Astonishingly, the replacement of the carbomethoxy group by a chlorovinyl moiety produces a comparable gain in potency, thus arguing against the involvement of the carbomethoxy group in H-bonding[68] (Fig. 13.13).

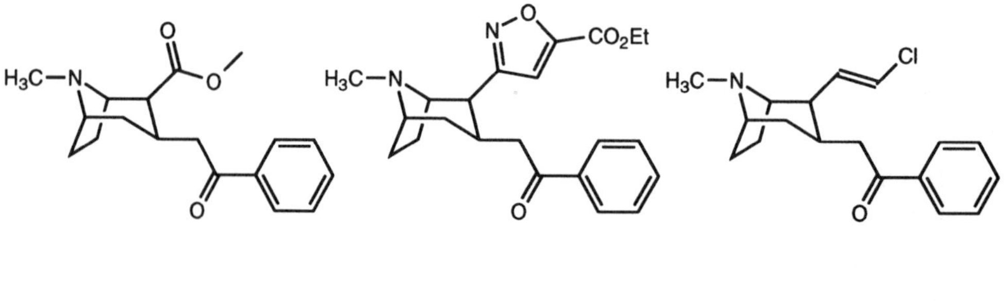

Fig. 13.13   Replacement in (−)-cocaine of the carbomethoxy group by a carbethoxyisoxazole and a chlorovinyl moiety.

Another rather unusual example of ester isosterism is the replacement of the ether oxygen by a fluoronitrogen (Fig. 13.14a) as mentioned by Lipinski.[69] Other uncommon examples are found in the replacement of the ester function of acetylcholine by exo–endo amidinic functions of 3-aminopyridazines in muscarinic agonists (Fig. 13.14b)[70] and of the carbomethoxy group of α-yohimbine (rauwolscine) by an *N*-methylsulphonamide function (Fig. 13.14c).[71]

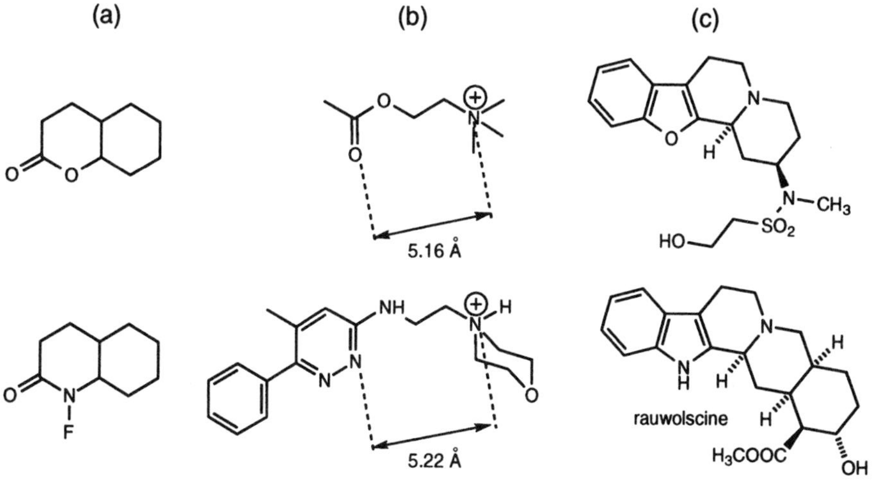

Fig. 13.14 (a) Replacement of ester ether oxygen by a fluoronitrogen. (b) Exo–endo amidine in place of a carboxylic ester functionality. (c) *N*-Methylsulphonamide analogue of α-yohimbine (rauwolscine).

3. Amides and peptides

Carboxamides are usually converted to sulphonamides as illustrated by the synthesis of the hypoglycaemic sulphonyl isostere of glybenclamide.[72] The isosteric replacements for peptidic bonds have been summarized by Spatola[73] and by Fauchère.[74] The most used and well-established modifications are *N*-methylation; configuration change (D-configuration at Cα); formation of a retroamide or an α-azapeptide; use of aminoisobutyric or dehydroamino acids; replacement of the amidic bond by an ester (depsipeptide), ketomethylene, hydroxyethylene or thioamide functional group; carba replacement of the amidic carbonyl, and use of an olefinic double bond (Fig. 13.15).

More unusual isosteric replacements for the peptidic bond were recently proposed. Among these, hydroxyethylureas served in the design of a novel class of potent HIV-1 protease inhibitors, diacylcyclopropanes in the design of novel renin inhibitors, and pyrroline-3-ones for various proteolytic enzyme inhibitors.[75,76] Vinyl fluorides can probably be considered as representing the closest possible bioisosteres of the peptide bond. The synthetic methods available allow, by an appropriate selection of the precursors, the preparation of analogues of dipeptidic combinations of amino acids bearing no other functionalities in their side-chains, e.g. Gly, Ala, Val, Phe, Pro.[77] Vinyl fluorides have been used in the design of bioisosteres of Substance P[76] and of the analgesic dipeptide 2,6,-dimethyl-L-tyrosyl-D-alanine-phenylpropionamide.[78]

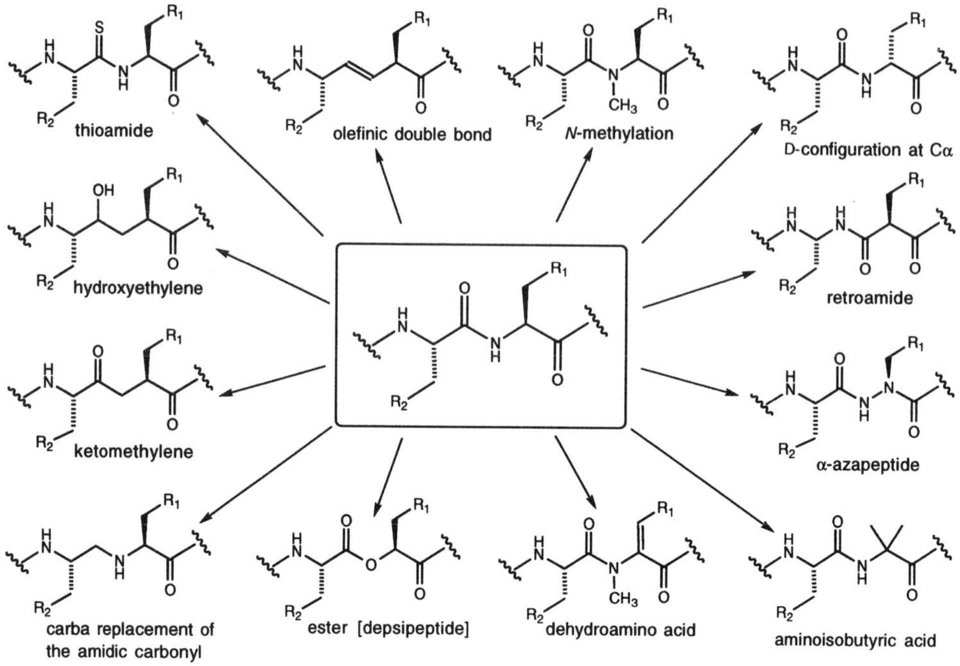

Fig. 13.15   Well-established isosteric replacements for peptidic bonds.[73,74]

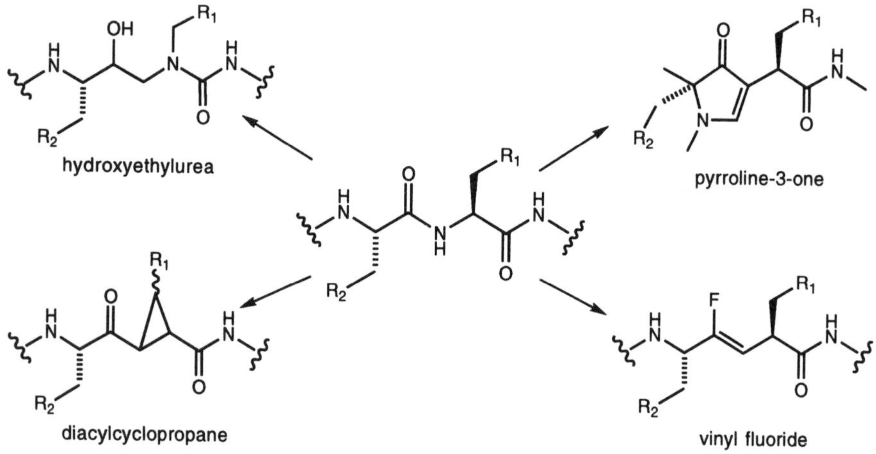

Fig. 13.16   Unusual isosteric replacements for peptidic bonds.

4.   Urea and thiourea equivalents

In the histaminic H_2 receptor antagonist series, the classical urea–thiourea–guanidine progression was successfully completed by the use of the N-nitro- and N-cyanoguanidines and, later, by 1,1-diamino-2-nitroethylene groups[24] (Fig. 13.17). Cyano amidines and carbamoyl amidines were also used,[79] and structure–activity relationship patterns were rationalized in terms of dipole moment orientation of related bioisosteric groups.[80]

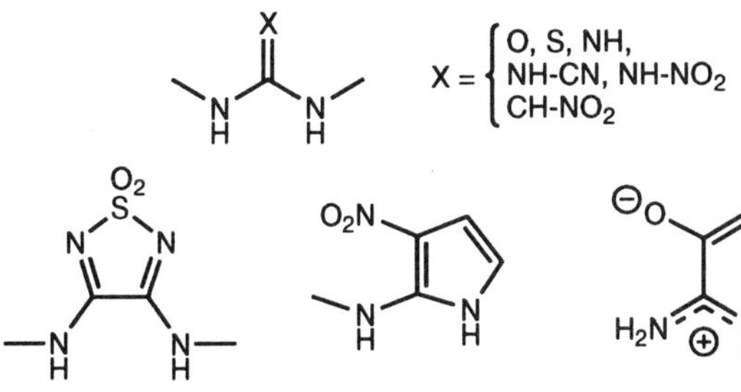

Fig. 13.17 Urea and thiourea equivalents.

Among more exotic surrogates, the 3,4-diamino thiadiazole dioxide moiety was proposed as a weakly acidic urea equivalent[81] as well as exo–endo amidinic heterocyles bearing an electron-attracting function in the α position[82,83] (Fig. 13.17).

F. Reversal of functional groups

The reversal of the peptidic functional groups is often used in peptide chemistry. The retropeptides obtained are generally more resistant to enzymatic attacks (Fig. 13.15).[74,84] But the strategy of functional inversion can also be applied to nonpeptidic compounds. A historical example is the change from orthoform to neo-orthoform (orthocaine; Fig. 13.18). The unwanted side-effects, often encountered with aromatic *p*-amino substituted compounds ('*para* effects', essentially of allergic origin) are abolished in the *m*-amino isomer, whereas the local anaesthetic activity is maintained. Similarly the '*meta*' isomer of benoxinate has a local anesthetic activity identical to that of benoxinate itself.[85]

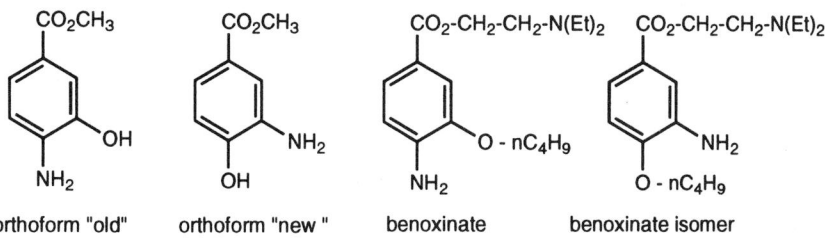

Fig. 13.18 Positional isomery in local anaesthetics.[85]

The inversion of the ester function of meperidine leads to 1-methyl-4-phenyl-4-propionoxy piperidine (Fig. 13.19) which is five times more potent as an analgesic drug than meperidine and represents the model compound of the series of inverted esters.[10]

The change from indomethacin to clometacin, although representing a clean example of functional group reversal, causes more profound alterations than that shown in the previous examples. At a first glance, this change can even seem too drastic, however, in turning the molecule of clometacin by 180°, the resemblance with the parent molecule becomes evident. Indomethacin is mainly used as a nonsteroidal anti-inflammatory agent and occasionally as an analgesic; clometacin, on the other hand, is usually recommended as an analgesic and shows weak anti-inflammatory properties.

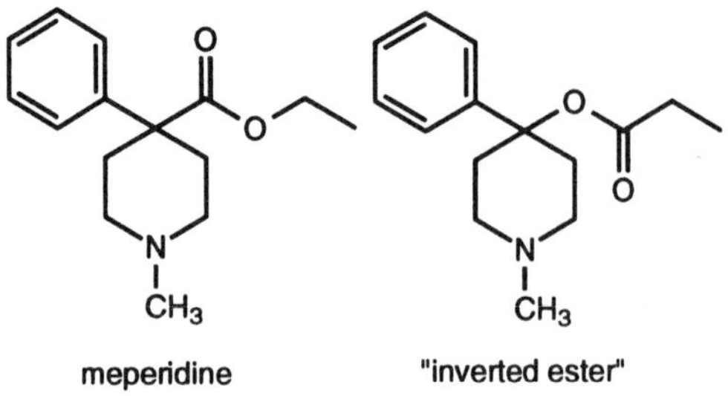

Fig. 13.19 Meperidine and the corresponding inverted ester.[10]

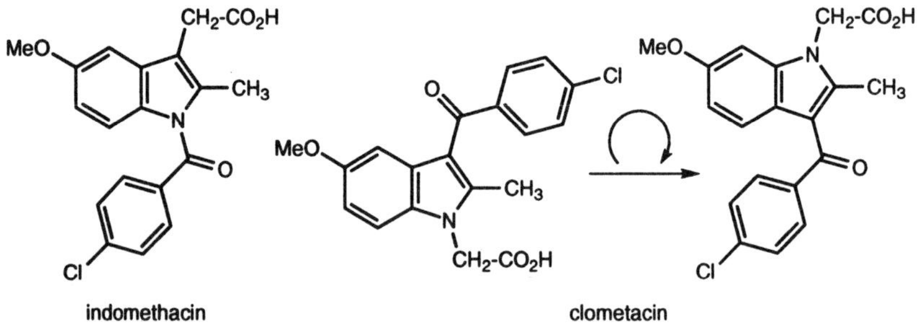

Fig. 13.20 Functional inversion applied to indomethacin.

III. ANALYSIS OF MODIFICATIONS RESULTING FROM ISOSTERISM

It is rare that the replacement of a part of a molecule by an isosteric or bioisosteric group leads to a *strictly identical* active principle. In practice, that is not even sought, and one prefers that the new compound produces a change compared with the parent molecule. In general the isosteric replacement, even though it represents a subtle structural change, results in a modified profile: some properties of the parent molecule will remain unaltered, others will be changed. Bioisosterism will be productive if it increases the potency, the selectivity and the bioavailability, or decreases the toxicity and undesirable effects of the compound. In proceeding to isosteric modifications one will focus *predominantly* on a given parameter (structural, electronic, hydrophilic) but it is all but impossible not to alter several parameters simultaneously.

A. Structural parameters

These will be important when the portion of the molecule involved in the isosteric change serves to maintain other functions in a particular geometry. This is the case for tricyclic psychotropic drugs (Fig. 13.21). In the two antidepressants (imipramine and maprotiline), the bioisosterism is geometrical insofar as the dihedral angle α formed by the two benzo rings is comparable:

α=65° for the dibenzazepine and α=55° for the dibenzocycloheptadiene.[86] This angle is only 25° for the neuroleptic phenothiazines and the thioxanthenes. In these examples the part of the molecule modified by isomerism is not involved in the interaction with the receptor. It serves only to position correctly the other elements of the molecule.

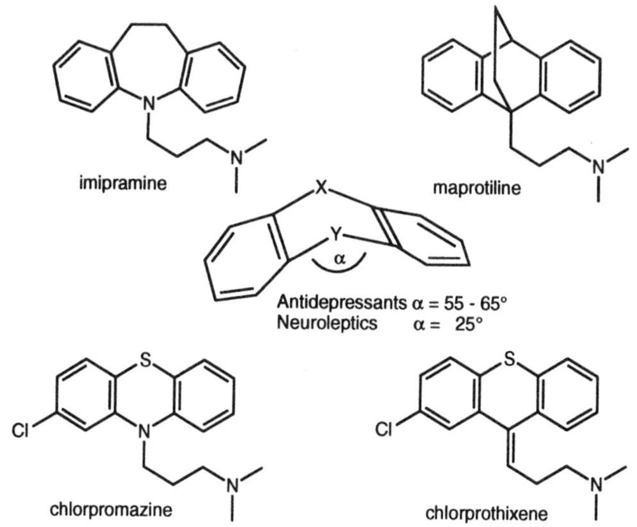

Fig. 13.21 The tricyclic antidepressants (imipramine and maprotiline) are characterized by an dihedral angle of 55–65° between the two benzo rings; this angle is only 25° for the tricyclic neuroleptics (chlorpromazine, chlorprothixene).[86]

B. Electronic parameters

Electronic parameters govern the nature and the quality of ligand–receptor or ligand–enzyme interactions. The relevant parameters will be inductive or mesomeric effects, polarizability, pK_a, capacity to form hydrogen bonds, etc. Despite their very different substituents in the *meta* position, the two epinephrine analogues (Fig. 13.22) exert comparable biological effects: they are both β-adrenergic agonists. In fact the key parameter resides in the very close pK_a values.[87]

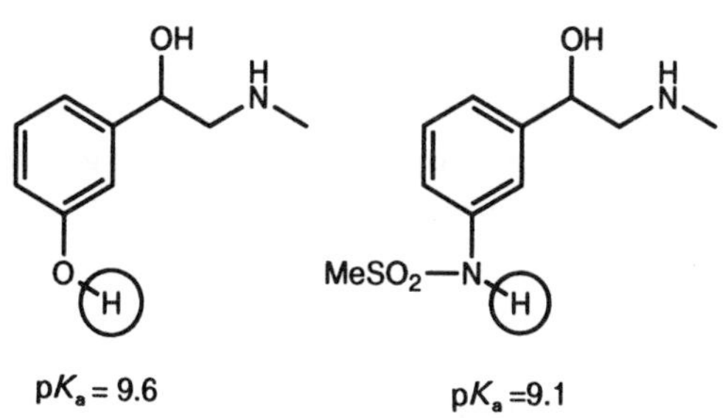

Fig. 13.22 An example of bioisosterism, or nonclassical isosterism; the methylsulphonamide substituent has comparable acidity to the phenolic hydroxyl group.[76]

C.   Solubility parameters

When the functional group involved in the isosteric change plays a role in the absorption, the distribution or the excretion of the active molecule, the hydrophilic–lipophilic parameters become important. Imagine in an active molecule the replacement of $-CF_3$ by $-CN$ (Fig. 13.23). The electron-attracting effects of the two groups will be comparable, but the molecule with the cyano function will clearly be more hydrophilic. This loss in lipophilicity can then be corrected in attaching elsewhere on the molecule a propyl, isopropyl or cyclopropyl group.

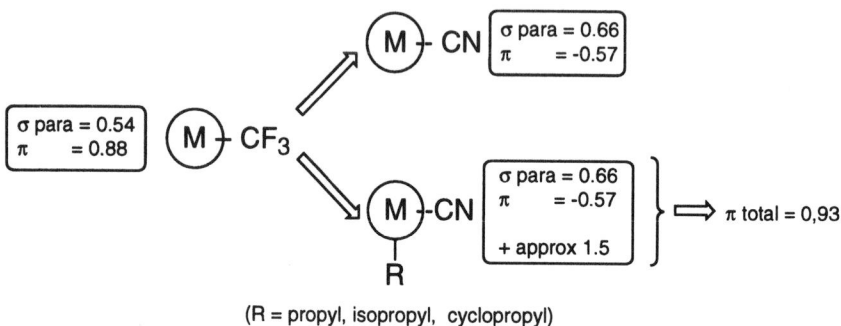

(R = propyl, isopropyl, cyclopropyl)

Fig. 13.23 The loss in lipophilicity resulting from the bioisosteric exchange of a CF_3 for a CN has to be compensated by the equivalent of a three-carbon residue.

IV.   ANOMALIES IN ISOSTERISM

In this section, two applications of the bioisosterism concept that show unusual behaviours of commonly encountered atoms or groups are discussed.

A.   Fluorine–hydrogen isosterism

There is an anomaly in the fact that fluorine does not resemble other halogens, notably chlorine, and that, on the other hand, it often mimics an atom of hydrogen.[88]

(a) Steric aspects.   The fluorine atom is considerably smaller than the rest of the halogen atoms. Seen from the steric point of view, it resembles hydrogen more than chlorine (Table 13.10). Effectively fluoro derivatives differ from the other halogenated derivatives because with carbon fluorine forms particularly stable bonds and, in contrast to other halogens, is only rarely ionized or displaced. Because it is both chemically inert and of small size, organic fluorine is often compared to hydrogen.

This relates in particular to the incorporation by living organisms of fluoroacetic acid in place of acetic[89] acid or of 5-fluoronicotinic acid and 5-fluorouracil as antimetabolites (see Chapter 17, the section on halogens). This 'fraudulent' incorporation leads to lethal syntheses.[90] This is generally not the case with the corresponding chlorinated, brominated or iodinated analogues.

Table 13.10 Fluorine–hydrogen isosterism. Observe the comparable sizes of the two atoms, whereas chlorine is close to the methyl and trifluoromethyl.

Parameter	H	F	Cl	CH$_3$	CF$_3$
Atomic radius	0.29	0.64	0.99	-	-
Van der Waals radius	1.2	1.35	1.80	≈2	≈2
Molecular refractivity	1.03	0.92	6.03	5.65	5.02
Electronic effect (*para* σ)[a]	0.00	0.06	0.23	−0.17	0.54
Resonance effect (𝕽)[a]	0.00	−0.34	−0.15	−0.13	0.19
Electronic effect (σ*)[b]	–	3.08	2.68	0.00	2.85

[a]For aromatic systems, [b]for aliphatic systems

(b) Electronic aspects. Fluorine is the most electronegative of the halogens (Table 13.10) and forms particularly stable bonds with carbon atoms. This chemical inertia explains why fluoro derivatives are more resistant to metabolic degradation (Fig. 13.24). Thus for the β-haloalkylamines (nitrogen mustards), the alkylating activity is lost when chlorine or bromine are replaced by fluorine or by hydrogen.[91]

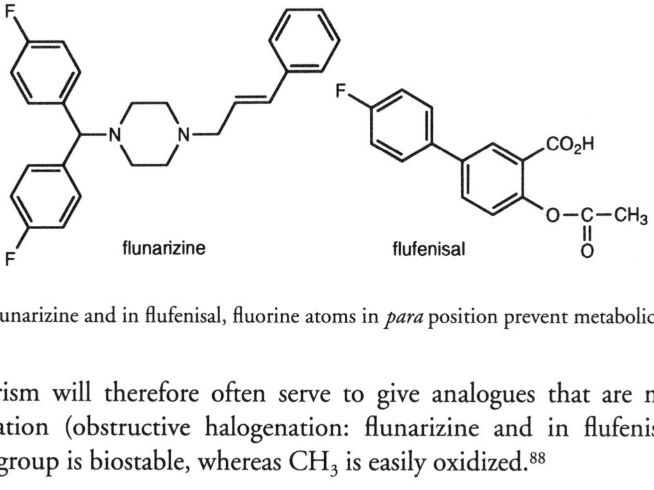

Fig. 13.24 In flunarizine and in flufenisal, fluorine atoms in *para* position prevent metabolic hydroxylation.

H ↔ F isosterism will therefore often serve to give analogues that are more resistant to metabolic degradation (obstructive halogenation: flunarizine and in flufenisal, Fig. 13.24). Similarly the CF$_3$ group is biostable, whereas CH$_3$ is easily oxidized.[88]

(c) Absence of d orbitals. Another difference between fluorine and the other halogens comes from the absence of a d orbital for fluorine, and thus its incapacity to participate in resonance effects with a donor of electrons p (Fig. 13.25). This explains why *p*-fluorophenol is slightly less acidic than phenol, while for other *p*-halogenated phenols the acidity changes in parallel with the atomic number (Table 13.11).[88]

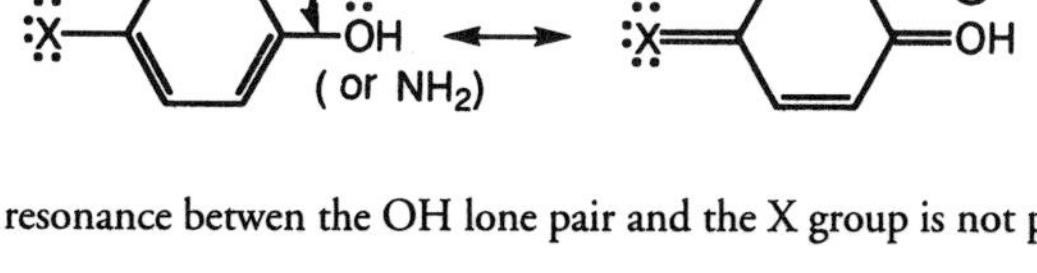

Fig. 13.25 The resonance betwen the OH lone pair and the X group is not possible if X = F.

Table 13.11 Dissociation constants of *para*-halogenated phenols.[88]

Compound	Dissociation constant $K_a \times 10^{-10}$
Phenol	0.32
p-Fluorophenol	0.26
p-Chlorophenol	1.32
p-Bromophenol	1.55
p-Iodophenol	2.19

(d) Case study. A good example of continous variation of activity in halogenated compounds is provided by a series of antihistaminic drugs related to tripelennamine (Fig. 13.26, X = H). Apparently we are dealing here with a classical isosteric series: F, Cl, Br, I, but sensitive to steric hindrance in the *para* position. Probably what happens *in vivo* is *p*-hydroxylation of the benzene ring. The best candidate becomes then the *p*-fluoro compound, since it is not bulkier than the unsubstituted compound while being biostable.

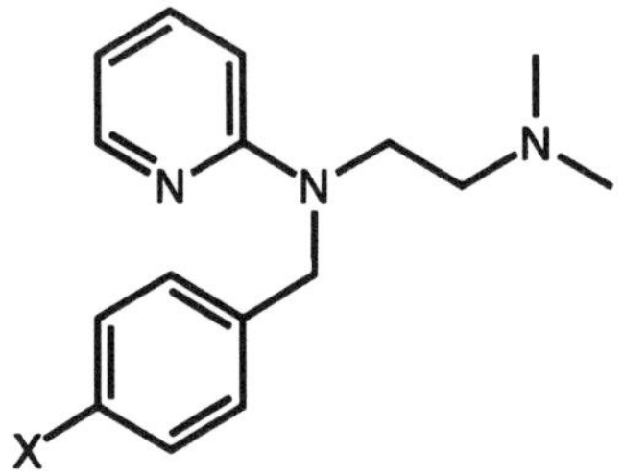

X	Activity
H	1
F	3-4
Cl	2-3
Br	1
I	0.3-0.5

Fig. 13.26 Variation of activity in a series of antihistaminic compounds as a function of the halogated *para*-substituent.[81]

B. Exchange of ether oxygen and methylene group

Ether oxygen atoms and methylene groups possess similar tetrahedral structure and should normally be isosteric. In fact the $O \leftrightarrow CH_2$ isosterism very often yields anomalous results and brought Friedman[2] to the interesting observation 'that the omission of the ether oxygen changes biological activity much less in some cases than the replacement by the isosteric methylene group' (Fig. 13.27). In the meperidine series, for example, the change from the *N*-phenoxypropyl derivative to the isosteric phenoxybutyl decreases the analgesic potency by a factor of 10, whereas the omission of the ether oxygen yields a slightly more potent compound.[10] A list of seven other examples is given by Schatz in the second edition of Burger's *Medicinal Chemistry*.[93]

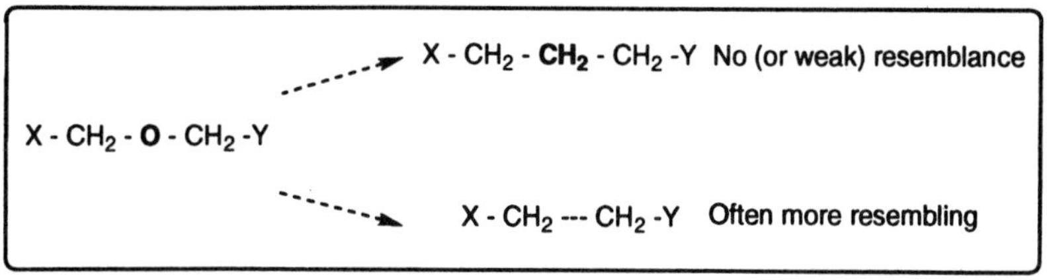

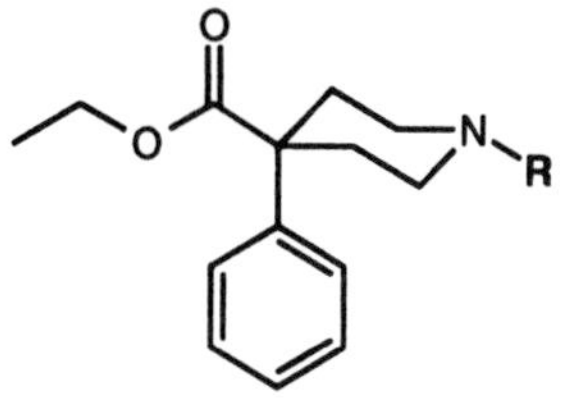

R =	Analgesic Potency (meperidine = 1)
$-(CH_2)_3-O-C_6H_5$	15
$-(CH_2)_3-CH_2\cdot C_6H_5$	1.5
$-(CH_2)_3-C_6H_5$	20

Fig. 13.27 Friedman's ether oxygen–methylene group paradox.[2]

The explanation for this anomalous behaviour may be that the omission of the ether oxygen yields a closer compound in terms of lipophilicity than its replacement by a methylene. An example that can be compared to Friedman's paradox is found in the resemblance of the phenylethyl type β-blockers (e.g. dichloroisoprenaline, sotalol) to the phenoxypropanol type (e.g. practolol, acebutolol).

V. MINOR METALLOIDS — TOXIC ISOSTERES

In this section we describe some 'exotic' applications of the bioisostery concept involving the utilization of unusual elements such as silicon, boron and selenium.

A. Carbon–silicon bioisosterism

Silicon is directly below carbon in the periodic table and the incorporation of silicon in place of carbon in biologically active substances has been a temptation for many organic chemists. However, the extent of this isosterism remains limited. For reviews on the subject, see Fessenden and Fessenden,[94] Tacke and Zilch[95,96] and Ricci *et al.*[97]

Silicon is more electropositive than carbon (and even more so if compared to oxygen and nitrogen) and the covalent silicon–carbon bonds in the sp^3 hybridization state are 20% longer than the corresponding carbon–carbon bond. Compared to their carbon bioisosteres, silicon-containing molecules are more sensitive to hydrolysis and to nucleophilic attack in general. Given the chemical reactivity of silicon, carbon–silicon isosterism is generally practised only if the silicon is present in the centre of a quaternary structure, as is the case for substances collected in Fig. 13.28. Among these, *m*-trimethylsilylphenyl *N*-methylcarbamate and *m*-trimethylsilyl-α-trifluoroacetophenone (zifrosilone) are acetylcholinesterase inhibitors,[98–100] sila-meprobamate is a CNS depressant,[101] sila-pridinol is an anticholinergic,[102] flusilazole is a fungicide for agricultural use,[103] and (+)-RP 71,602 is a potent and selective 5-HT$_{2A}$ antagonist.[104]

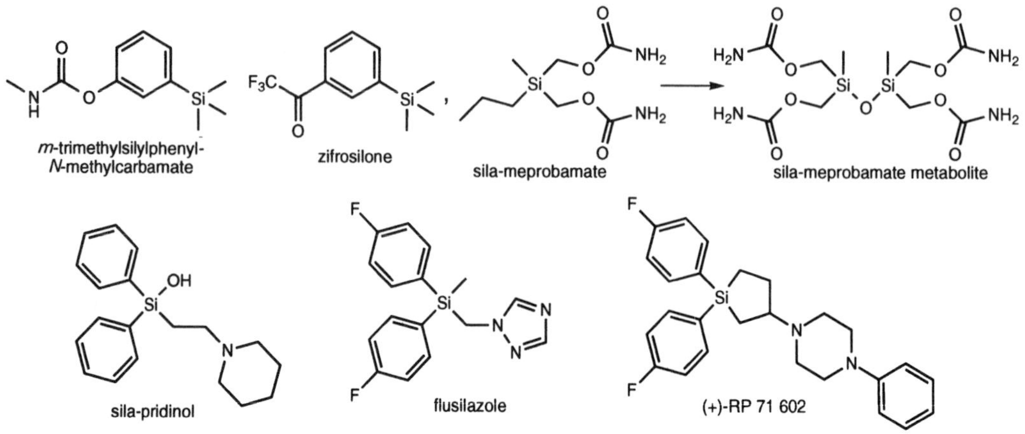

Fig. 13.28 Organosilicon active substances.

But even when located in the centre of a quaternary structure, the silicon atom can easily be attacked. Thus, 1-chloro-1-sila-bicyclo(2,2,1)heptane can still be hydrolysed by an attack on the vacant d orbital;[105] this attack is *lateral* and therefore possible even in the cases where the corresponding carbon derivative would have been inert towards S$_N$2 reaction (Fig. 13.29). This sensitivity towards lateral attacks explains the four times shorter duration of action of sila-meprobamate compared to its carbon isostere on a model of tranquillizing activity in mice (rotarod test, potentiation of hexobarbital-induced sleep; intraperitoneal injection).[101] On the other hand, when given orally, sila-meprobamate is practically inactive. One of the first metabolites formed has been characterized as being a disiloxane[106] (Fig. 13.28). For the two phenyltrimethylsilyl-derived AChE inhibitors, the rather positively charged trimethylsilyl group mimics the trimethylammonium function present in acetylcholine. For these compounds, metabolic oxidation does not take place on the silicon but on one of methyl groups (Si—CH$_3$→Si—CH$_2$—OH).[99]

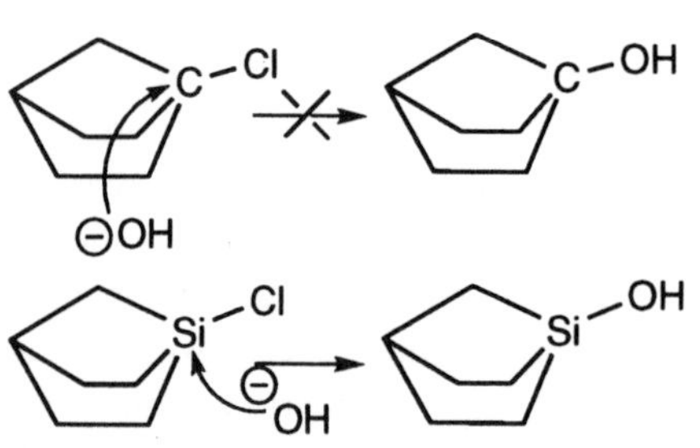

Fig. 13.29 Owing to the presence of a vacant d orbital, a lateral attack can substitute for dorsal attack in organosilicon derivatives.[94]

B. Carbon–boron isosterism

Organoboron derivatives, even more than organosilicon compounds, are sensitive to hydrolytic degradation that always leads to the final formation of boric acid. But boric acid has teratogenic properties in chickens. It produces the same malformations as those produced by a riboflavin (vitamin B_2) deficiency and the administration of riboflavin prevents these toxic effects.[107,108] The mechanism by which boric acid produces a deficiency in riboflavin is not known. In man the chronic utilization of boron derivatives results in cases of borism (dry skin, cutaneous eruptions, gastric troubles).[109]

Few medicines based on boron are known; in general boric acid or a boronic acid serve to esterify an α-diol or an *o*-diphenol. This is the case for the emetic antimony borotartrates of the ancient pharmacopoeias; for the injectable catecholamine solutions; for tolboxane,[110] which is close to meprobamate and was commercially available as a tranquillizer some decades ago; and also for the phenylboronic esters of chloramphenicol.[111] Boromycin was the first natural product containing boron. It is a complex between boric acid and a polyhydroxylated tetradentate macrocycle.[112] Some boronic analogues of amino acids were prepared as chymotrypsin and elastase inhibitors.[113] The most important medical use of derivatives of boron derivatives is the treatment of some tumours by neutron capture therapy,[114–116] the problem here being to ensure a sufficient concentration of the product in the tumour being treated.

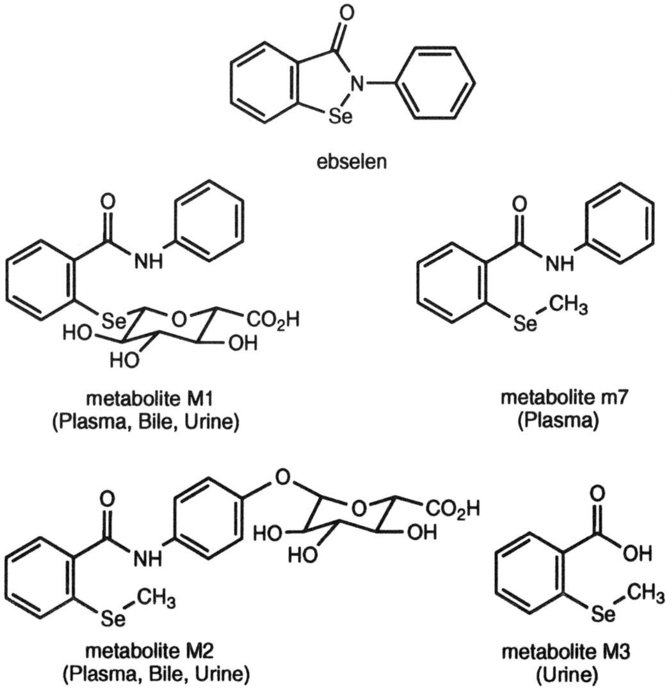

Fig. 13.30   Ebselen and its main metabolites.[119]

C. Bioisosterism involving selenium

Selenium and its derivatives are highly toxic and with the exception of ^{75}Se derivatives that serve diagnostic purposes (e.g. ^{75}Se-selenomethionine, used as a radioactive imaging agent in pancreatic scanning), there is no chemically defined seleno-organic drug on the market. Klayman reviewed a large number of selenium derivatives as chemotherapeutic agents in 1973.[117] Selenium bioisosteres of sulphur compounds are mainly used as research tools (e.g. bis(2-chloroethyl) selenide as selenium bioisostere of the classical sulphur mustards[118]). Selenocysteine is present in the catalytic site of mammalian glutathione peroxidase and this explains the importance of selenium as an essential trace element.

The only selenium-containing drug candidate is *ebselen* (Fig. 13.30), which owes its antioxidant and anti-inflammatory properties to its interference with the selenoenzyme glutathione peroxidase.[120] Because of its strongly bound selenium moiety, only metabolites of low toxicity are formed.[119]

REFERENCES

1. Langmuir, I. (1919) Isomorphism, isosterism and covalence. *J. Am. Chem. Soc.* **41**: 1543–1559.
2. Friedman, H. L. (1951) Influence of isosteric replacements upon biological activity. In *Symposium on Chemical-Biological Correlation*. National Research Council Publication, Washington D.C.
3. Grimm, H. G. (1925) Über Bau und Grösse der Nichtmetallhydride. *Z. Elektrochem.* **31**: 474–480.
4. Grimm, H. G. (1929) The system of chemical compounds from the viewpoint of atom research, several problems of experimental research. Part I. *Naturwissenschaften* **17**: 535–540.
5. Grimm, H. G. (1929) The system of chemical compounds from the viewpoint of atom research, several problems of experimental research. Part II. *Naturwissenschaften* **17**: 557–564.
6. Erlenmeyer, H. and Leo, M. (1932) Über Pseudoatome. *Helv. Chim. Acta* **15**: 1171–1186.
7. Erlenmeyer, H. (1948) Les composés isostères et le problème de la ressemblance en chimie. *Bull. Soc. Chim. Biol.* **30**: 792–805.
8. Thornber, C. W. (1979) Isosterism and molecular modification in drug design. *Chem. Soc. Rev.* **8**: 563–580.
9. Krogsgaard-Larsen, P., Hjeds, H., Falch, E., Jørgensen, F. S. and Nielsen, L. (1988) Recent advances in GABA agonists, antagonists and uptake inhibitors: structure–activity relationships and therapeutic potential. In Testa, B. (ed.) *Advances in Drug Research*, pp. 381–456. Academic Press, London.
10. Janssen, P. A. J. and Van der Eycken, C. A. M. (1968) The chemical anatomy of potent morphine-like analgesics. In Burger, A. (ed.) *Drugs Affecting the Central Nervous System*, pp. 25–60. Marcel Dekker, New York.
11. Boyle, E. A., Mangan, F. R., Markwell, R. E., Smith, S. A., Thompson, M. J., Ward, R. W. and Wyman, P. A. (1986) 7-Aroyl-2,3-dihydrobenzo[*b*]furan-3-carboxylic acids and 7-benzoyl-2,3-dihydrobenzo{*b*]thiophene-3-carboxylic acids as analgesic agents. *J. Med. Chem.* **29**: 894–898.
12. Chen, Y. L., Nielsen, J., Hedberg, K. D. A., Jones, S., Russo, L., Johnson, J., Ives, J. and Liston, D. (1992) Syntheses, resolution, and structure–activity relationships of potent acetylcholinesterase inhibitors: 898 carbaphysostigmine analogues. *J. Med. Chem.* **35**: 1429–1434.
13. Erlenmeyer, H. and Willi, E. (1935) Zusammenhänge zwischen Konstitution und Wirkung bei Pyrazolonderivaten. *Helv. Chim. Acta* **18**: 740–743.
14. Binder, D., Noe, C. R., Holzer, W. and Baumann, K. (1987) Thiophen als Strukturelement Physiologisch Aktiver Substanzen, 16. Thienoisoxazole Durch Substitution am Oximstickstoff. *Arch. Pharm.* **320**: 837–843.
15. Uno, H., Kurokawa, M., Masuda and Nishimura, H. (1979) Studies on 3-substituted 1,2-benzisoxazole derivatives. 6. Syntheses of 3-(sulfamoylmethyl)-1,2-benzisoxazole derivatives and their anticonvulsant activities. *J. Med. Chem.* **22**: 180–183.

16. Gold-Aubert, P., Melkonian, D. and Toribio, L. (1964) Synthèses de nouvelles phényl-1-triazoline-1,2,4-ones-5 substituées en 3 et 4. *Helv. Chim. Acta* **47**: 2068–2071.

17. Alonso, R., Andrès, J. I., Garcia-Lopez, M. -T., de las Heras, F. G., Herranz, R., Alarcòn, B. and Carrasco, L. (1985) Synthesis and antiviral evaluation of nucleosides of 5-methylimidazole-4-carboxamide. *J. Med. Chem.* **28**: 834–838.

18. Fludzinski, P., Evrard, D. A., Bloomquist, W. E. and Lacefield, W. B. (1987) Indazoles as indole bioisosteres: synthesis and evaluation of the tropanyl ester and amide of indazole-3-carboxylate as antagonists to the serotonin 5HT$_3$ receptor. *J. Med. Chem.* **30**: 1535–1537.

19. Blaskó, G., Major, E., Blaskó, G., Rózsa, I. and Szántay, C. (1986) Pyrimido(1,6-*a*]pyrido(3,4-*b*] indoles as new platelet inhibiting agents. *Eur. J. Med. Chem.* **21**: 91–95.

20. Kardos, J., Blaskó, G., Simonyi, M. and Szántay, C. (1985) Octahydroindolo[2,3-a]quinolizin-2-one, a novel structure for γ-aminobutyric acid (GABA) uptake inhibition. *Eur. J. Med. Chem.* **21**: 151–154.

21. Salituro, F. G., Harrison, B. L., Baron, B. M., Nyce, P. L., Stewart, K. T., Kehne, J. H., White, H. S. and McDonald, I. (1992) 3-(2-Carboxyindol-3-yl)propionic acid-based antagonists of the *N*-methyl-D-aspartic receptor associated glycine binding site. *J. Med. Chem.* **35**: 1791–1799.

22. Calvino, R., Stilo, A. D., Fruttero, R., Gasco, A. M., Sorba, G. and Gasco, A. (1993) Pharmacochemistry of the furoxan ring: recent developments. *Il Farmaco* **48**: 321–334.

23. Lipinski, C. A., Aldinger, C. E., Beyer, T. A., Bordner, J., Burdi, D. F., Bussolotti, D. L., Inskeep, P. B. and Siegel, T. W. (1992) Hydantoin isosteres. *In vivo* active spiro hydroxy acetic aldose reductase inhibitors. *J. Med. Chem.* **35**: 2169–2177.

24. Ganellin, C. R. (1993) Discovery of cimetidine, ranitidine and other H$_2$-receptor histamine antagonists. In Ganellin, C. R. and Roberts, S. M. (eds) *Medicinal Chemistry — The Role of Organic Chemistry in Drug Research*, pp. 227–255. Academic Press, London.

25. Morin, I. (1991) 3-Aryl as-triazines: bioisostérie avec les 6-aryl pyridazines 1991. PhD thesis, Université Louis Pasteur, Strasbourg.

26. Mallamo, J. P., Pilling, G. M., Wetzel, J. R., Kowalczik, P. J., Bell, M. R., Kullnig, R. K., Batzold, F. H., Juniewiecz, P. E., Winnecker, R. C. and Luss, H. R. (1992) Antiandrogenic steroidal sulfonyl heterocycles. Utility of electrostatic complementarity in defining bioisosteric sulfonyl heterocycles. *J. Med. Chem.* **35**: 1663–1670.

27. Almquist, R. G., Chao, W. R. and Jennings-White, C. (1985) Synthesis and biological activity of carboxylic acid replacement analogues of the potent angiotensin converting enzyme inhibitor 5(S)-benzamido-4-oxo-6-phenylhexanoyl-L-proline. *J. Med. Chem.* **28**: 1067–1071.

28. Kohler, H. V., Eichler, B. and Salewski, R. (1970) Untersuchungen zum sauerstoffanalogen Charakter der C(CN)$_2$ -und NCN-gruppen. *Z. Anorg. Chem.* **379**: 183–192.

29. Bovy, P. R., Reitz, D. B., Collins, J. T., Chamberlain, T. S., Olins, G. M., Corpus, V. M., McMahon, E. G., Palomo, M. A., Koepke, J. P., McGraw, D. E. and Gaw, G. J. (1993) Nonpeptide angiotensin II antagonists: *N*-phenyl-1-*H*-pyrrole derivatives are angiotensin II receptor antagonists. *J. Med. Chem.* **36**: 101–110.

30. Marshall, W. S., Goodson, T., Cullinan, G. J., Swanson-Bean, D., Haisch, K. D., Rinkema, L. E. and Fleisch, J. H. (1987) Leukotriene receptor antagonists. I. Synthesis and structure–activity relationships of alkoxyacetophenone derivatives. *J. Med. Chem.* **30**: 682–689.

31. Krogsgaard-Larsen, P. (1990) In Hansch, C., Sammes, P. G., Taylor, J. B. and Emmet, J. C. (eds), *Comprehensive Medicinal Chemistry*, pp. 493–537. Pergamon Press, Oxford.

32. Lunn, W. H. W., Schoepp, D. D., Lodge, D., True, R. A. and Millar, J. D. (1992) LY262466, DL-2-amino-3-(4-hydroxy-1,2,5-thiazol-3-yl) propanoic acid hydrochloride, a novel and selective agonist at the AMPA excitatory amino acid receptor. In *XIIth International Symposium on Medicinal Chemistry*. Basel, Switzerland, September 13–17.

33. Atkinson, J. G., Girard, Y., Rokach, J., Rooney, C. S., McFarlane, C. S., Rackham, A. and Share, N. N. (1979) Kojic amine-A novel γ-aminobutyric acid analogue. *J. Med. Chem.* **22**:90–106.

34. Froestl, W., Furet, P., Hall, R. G., Mickel, S. J., Strub, D., Sprecher, G. v., Baumann, P. A., Bernasconi, R., Brugger, F., Felner, A., Gentsch, C., Hauser, K., Jaeckel, J., Karlsson, G., Klebs, K., Maître, L., Marescaux, C., Moser, P., Pozza, M. F. and Rihs, G. (1993) GABA$_B$ antagonists: novel CNS-active compounds. In Testa, B., Kyburz, E., Fuhrer, W. and Giger, R. (eds) *Perspectives in Medicinal Chemistry*, pp. 259–272. VHC, Weinheim.

35. Drummond, J. T. and Johnson, G. (1988) Convenient procedure for the preparation of alkyl end aryl substituted N-(aminoalkylacyl)sulfonamides. *Tetrahedron Lett.* **29**: 1653–1656.

36. Albright, J. D., DeVries, V. G., Du, M. D., Largis, E. E., Miner, T. G., Reich, M. F. and Shepherd, R. G. (1983) Potential antiatherosclerotic agents. 3. Substituted benzoic and non benzoic analogues of cetabon. *J. Med. Chem.* **26**: 1393–1411.

37. Buu-Hoï, N. P., Lambelin, G., Lepoivre, C., Gillet, C., Gautier, M. and Thiriaux, J. (1965) Un nouvel agent antiinflammatoire de structure non stéroïdique: l'acide p-butoxyphénylacéthydroxamique. *C. R. Acad. Sci. (Paris)* **261**: 2259–2262.

38. Orzalesi, G. and Selleri, R. (1974) Pharmaceutical 2-(4-isobutylphenyl) propionohydroxamic acid. German Patent 2 400 531 (24 July 1974; to Societa Italo-Britannica L. Manetti & H. Roberts e C.) *Chem. Abstr.* **81**: 120272i.

39. De Martiis, F., Corsico, N., Franzone, J. S. and Tamietto, T. (1975) Valutazione farmaco-tossicologica di un nuovo agente antifiammatorio non steroideo: l'acido indoxamico. *Boll. Chim. Farm.* **114**: 319–333.

40. Summers, J. B., Masdiyasni, H., Holms, J. H., Ratajczik, J. D., Dyer, R. D. and Carter, G. W. (1987) Hydroxamic acid inhibitors of 5-lipoxygenase. *J. Med. Chem.* **30**: 574–580.

41. Bergeron, R. J., Liu, Z. -R., McManis, J. S. and Wiegand, J. (1992) Structural alterations in desferrioxamine compatible with iron clearance in animals. *J. Med. Chem.* **35**: 4739–4744.

42. Kwon, C. -H., Nagasawa, H. T., DeMaster, E. G. and Shirota, F. N. (1986) Acyl, N-protected α-aminoacyl, and peptidyl derivatives as prodrug forms of the alcohol deterrent agent cyanamide. *J. Med. Chem.* **29**: 1922–1929.

43. De Martiis, F., Franzone, J. S. and Tamietto, T. (1975) Sintesi e proprieta antiflogistiche di alcuni acidici indolil-acetoidrossammici. *Bol. Chim. Farm.* **114**: 309–318.

44. Orzalesi, G., Mari, F., Bertol, E., Selleri, R. and Pisaturo, G. (1980) Anti-inflammatory agents: determination of ibuproxam and its metabolite in humans. *Arzneim.-Forsch.* **30**: 1607–1609.

45. Demay, F. and De Sy, J. (1982) A new non-steroidal anti-inflammatory drug (NSAID) in current rheumatologic practice (oxamethacin). *Curr. Ther. Res.* **31**: 113–118.

46. Vergin, H. v., Ferber, H., Brunner, F. and Kukovetz, W. R. (1981) Pharmakokinetik und Biotransformation von Oxametacin bei gesunden Probanden. *Arzneim.-Forsch* **31**: 513–518.

47. Singh, H., Chawla, A. S., Kapoor, V. K., Paul, D. and Malhotra, R. K. (1980) Medicinal chemistry of tetrazoles. In Ellis, G. P. and West, G. B. (eds) *Progress in Medicinal Chemistry*, pp. 151–183. Elsevier, Amsterdam.

48. Ashton, W. T., Cantone, C. L., Chang, L. L., Hutchins, S. M., Strelitz, R., MacCross, M., Chang, R. S. L., Lotti, V. J., Faust, K. A., Chen, T. -B., Bunting, P., Schorn, T. W., Sivlighn, S. D. and Siegl, P. K. S. (1993) Nonpeptide angiotensin II antagonists derived from 4H-1,2,4-triazoles and 3H-imidazo[1,2-b][1,2,4]triazoles. *J. Med. Chem.* **36**: 591–609.

49. Marshall, W. S., Goodson, T., Cullinan, G. J., Swanson-Bean, D., Haisch, K. D., Rinkema, L. E. and Fleisch, J. H. (1987) Leukotriene receptor antagonists. 1. Synthesis and structure–activity relationships of alkoxyacetophenone derivatives. *J. Med. Chem.* **30**: 682–689.

50. Kraus, J. L. (1983) Isosterism and molecular modification in drug design: tetrazole analogue of GABA: Effects on enzymes of the gamma-aminobutyrate system. *Pharmacol. Res. Commun.* **15**: 183–189.

51. Schlewer, G., Wermuth, C. G. and Chambon, J. -P. (1984) Analogues tétrazoliques d'agents GABA-mimétiques. *Eur. J. Med. Chem.* **19**: 181–186.

52. Krogsgaard-Larsen, P., Rodolskov-Christiansen, T. (1979) GABA agonists. Synthesis and structure–activity studies on analogues of isoguvacine and THIP. *Eur. J. Med. Chem.* **14**: 157–164.

53. Krogsgaard-Larsen, P. (1981) γ-Aminobutyric acid agonists, antagonists, and uptake inhibitors. Design and therapeutic aspects. *J. Med. Chem.* **24**: 1377–1383.

54. Krogsgaard-Larsen, P., Ferkany, J. W., Nielsen, E. O., Madsen, U., Ebert, B., Johansen, J. S., Diemer, S. H., Bruhn, T., Beattie, D. T. and Curtis, D. R. (1991) Novel class of amino acid antagonists at non-N-methyl-D-aspartic acid excitatory amino acid receptors. Synthesis, *in vitro* and *in vivo* pharmacology, and neuroprotection. *J. Med. Chem.* **34**: 123–130.

55. Kraus, J. L. (1983) Isosterism and molecular modification in drug design: new n-dipropylacetate analogs as inhibitors of succinic semi aldehyde dehydrogenase. *Pharmacol. Res. Commun.* **15**: 119–129.

56. Lichtenthaler, F. W. and Heidel, P. (1969) Intermediates in the formation of γ-pyrones from hexose derivatives: a simple synthesis of kojic acid and hydroxymaltol. *Angew. Chem. Int. Ed.* **8**: 978–979.

57. Watkins, J. C., Krogsgaard-Larsen, P. and Honoré, T. (1990) Structure–activity relationships in the development of excitatory amino acid receptor agonists and competitive antagonists. *Trends Pharm. Sci.* **11**: 25–33.

58. Drysdale, M. J., Pritchard, M. C. and Horwell, D. C. (1992) Rationally designed 'dipeptoid' analogues of CCK. Acid mimics of the potent and selective non peptide CCK-B receptor antagonist CI-988. *J. Med. Chem.* **35**: 2573–2581.

59. Kinney, W. A., Lee, N. E., Garrison, D. T., Podlesny, Jr., E. J., Simmonds, J. T., Bramlet, D., Notvest, R. R., Kowal, D. M. and Tasse, R. P. (1992) Bioisosteric replacement of the α-amino carboxylic functionality in 2-amino-5-phosphonopentanoic acid yields unique 3,4-diamino-3-cyclobutene-1,2-dione containing NMDA antagonists. *J. Med. Chem.* **35**: 4720–4726.

60. Shapiro, G., Floersheim, P. Boelsterli, J., Amstutz, R., Bolliger, G., Gammenthaler, H., Gmelin, G., Supavilai, P. and Walkinshaw, M. (1992) Muscarinic activity of the thiolactone, lactam, lactol, and thiolactol analogues of pilocarpine and a hypothetical model for the binding of agonists to the m_1 receptor. *J. Med. Chem.* **35**: 15–27.

61. Thompkins, L. and Lee, K. H. (1975) Comparison of analgesic effects of isosteric variations of salicylic acid and aspirin (acetylsalicylic acid). *J. Pharm. Sci.* **64**: 760–763.

62. Roth, G. J., Stanford, N., Majerus, P. W. (1975) Acetylation of prostaglandine synthase by aspirin. *Proc. Nat. Acad. Sci., USA* **72**: 3073–3076.

63. Saunders, J., Cassidy, M., Freedman, S. B., Harley, E. A., Iversen, L. L., Kneen, C., MacLeod, A. M., Merchant, K., Snow, R. J. and Baker, R. (1990) Novel quinuclidine-based ligands for the muscarinic cholinergic receptor. *J. Med. Chem.* **33**: 1128–1138.

64. Sauerberg, P., Kindtler, J. W., Nielsen, L., Sheardown, M. J. and Honoré, T. (1991) Muscarinic cholinergic agonists and antagonists of the 3-(3-alkyl-1,2,4-oxadiazol-5-yl)-1,2,5,6-tetra-hydropyridine type. Synthesis and structure–activity relationships. *J. Med. Chem.* **34**: 687–692.

65. Sauerberg, P., Olesen, P. H., Nielsen, S., Treppendahl, S. M. J. S., Honoré, T., Mitch, C. H., Ward, J. S., Pike, A. J., Bymaster, F. P., Sawyer, B. D. and Shannon, H. E. (1992) Novel functional M_1 selective muscarinic agonists. Synthesis and structure–activity relationships of 3-(1,2,5-thiadiazolyl)-1,2,5,6-tetrahydro-1-methylpyridines. *J. Med. Chem.* **35**: 2274–2263.

66. Wadsworth, H. J., Jenkins, S. M., Orlek, B. S., Cassidy, F., Clark, M. S. G., Brown, F., Riley, G. J., Graves, D., Hawkins, J. and Naylor, C. (1992) Synthesis and muscarinic activities of quinuclidin-3-yltriazole and -tetrazole derivatives. *J. Med. Chem.* **35**: 1280–1290.

67. Street, L. J., Baker, R., Book, T., Reeve, A. J., Saunders, J., Willson, T., Marwood, R. S., Patel, S. and Freedman, S. B. (1992) Synthesis and muscarinic activity of quinuclidinyl- and (1-azanorbornyl)pyrazine derivatives. *J. Med. Chem.* **35**: 295–305.

68. Kozikowski, A. P., Roberti, M., Xiang, L., Bergmann, J. S., Callahan, P. M., Cunningham, K. A. and Johnson, K. M. (1993) Structure–activity relationship studies of cocaine: replacement of the C-2 ester group by vinyl argues against H-bonding and provides an esterase-resistant, high-affinity cocaine analogue. *J. Med. Chem.* **35**: 4764–4766.

69. Lipinski, C. A. (1986) Bioisosterism in drug design. In Bailey, D. M. (ed.) *Anual Reports in Medicinal Chemistry*, pp. 283–291. Academic Press, San Diego.

70. Wermuth, C. G. (1993) Aminopyridazines — an alternate route to potent muscarinic agonists with no cholinergic syndrome. *Il Farmaco* **48**: 253–274.

71. Huff, J. R., Anderson, P. S., Baldwin, J. J., Clineschmidt, B. V., Guare, J. P., Lotti, V. J., Pettibone, D. J., Randall, W. C. and Vacca, J. P. (1985) N-(1,3,4,6,7,12b-hexahydro-2H-benzo[b]furo[2,3-a]quinolizin-2-yl)-N-methyl-2-hydroxyethane-sulfonamide: a potent and selective α_2-adrenoreceptor antagonist. *J. Med. Chem.* **28**: 1756–1759.

72. Fournier, J. -P., Moreau, R. C., Narcisse, G. and Choay, P. (1982) Synthèse et propriétés pharmacologiques de sulfonylurées isostères du glibenclamide. *Eur. J. Med. Chem.* **17**: 81–84.

73. Spatola, A. F. (1983) Peptide backbone modifications: structure–activity analysis of peptides containing amide bond surrogates. In Weinstein, B. (ed.) *Chemistry and Biochemistry of Amino Acids, Peptides and Proteins*, pp. 267–357. Marcel Dekker, New York.

74. Fauchère, J. -L. (1986) Elements for the rational design of peptide drugs. In Testa, B. (ed.) *Advances in Drug Research*, pp. 29–69. Academic Press, London.

75. Smith III, A. B., Holcomb, R. C., Guzman, M. C., Keenan, T. P., Sprengeler, P. A. and Hirschmann, R. (1993) An effective synthesis of scalemic 3,5,5-trisubstituted pyrrolin-4-ones. *Tetrahedron Lett.* **34**: 63–66.

76. Smith III, A. B., Keenan, T. P., Holcomb, R. C., Sprengeler, P. A., Guzman, M. C., Wood, J. L., Carroll, P. J. and Hirschmann, R. (1992) Design, synthesis and crystal structure of a pyrrolinone-based peptidomimetic possessing the conformation of a β-strand: potential application to the design of novel inhibitors of proteolytic enzymes. *J. Amer. Chem. Soc.* **114**: 10672–10674.

77. Allmendinger, T., Felder, E. and Hungerbuehler, E. (1991) Fluoroolefin dipeptide isosteres. In Weldi, J. T. (ed.) *Selective Fluorination in Organic and Bioorganic Chemistry*, pp. 186–195. American Chemical Society, Washington.

78. Chandrakumar, N. S., Yonan, P. K., Stapelfeld, A., Svage, M., Rorbacher, E., Contreras, P. C. and Hammond, D. (1992) Preparation and opioid activity of analogues of the analgesis dipeptide 2,6-dimethyl-l-tyrosyl-*N*-(3-phenylpropyl)-D-alanylamide. *J. Med. Chem.* **35**: 223–233.

79. Yanagisawa, I., Hirata, Y. and Ishii, Y. (1984) Histamine H$_2$ receptor antagonists. 1. Synthesis of *N*-cyano and *N*-carbamoyl amidine derivatives and their biological activities. *J. Med. Chem.* **27**: 849–857.

80. Young, R. C., Durant, G. J., Emmet, J. C., Ganellin, C. R., Graham, M. J., Mitchell, R. C., Prain, H. D. and Roantree, M. L. (1986) Dipole moment in relation to H$_2$ receptor antagonist activity for cimetidine analogues. *J. Med. Chem.* **29**: 44–49.

81. Lumma Jr, W. C., Anderson, P. S., Baldwin, J. J., Bolhofer, W. A., Habecker, C. N., Hirshfield, J. M., Pietruszkewicz, A. M., Randall, W. C., Torchiana, M. L., Britcher, S. F., Clineschmidt, B. V., Denny, G. H., Hirschmann, R., Hoffman, J. M., Phillips, B. T. and Streeter, K. B. (1982) Inhibitors of gastric acid secretion: 3,4-diamino-1,2,5-thiadiazole 1-oxides and 1,1-dioxides as urea equivalents in a series of histamine H$_2$-receptor antagonists. *J. Med. Chem.* **25**: 207–210.

82. Young, R. C., Ganellin, C. R., Graham, M. J. and Grant, E. H. (1982) The dipole moments of 1,3-dimethylthiourea, 1,3-dimethyl-2-cyanoguanidine and 1,1-bis-methylamino-2-nitroethene in aqueous solution. *Tetrahedron* **38**: 1493–1497.

83. Young, R. C., Ganellin, C. R., Graham, M. J., Roantree, M. J. and Grant, E. H. (1985) The dielectric properties of seven polar amidine-containing compounds of biological interest. *Tetrahedron Lett.* **26**: 1897–1900.

84. Plattner, J. J. and Norbeck, D. W. (1990) Obstacles to drug development from peptide leads. In Clark, C. R. and Moos, W. H. (eds) *Drug Discovery Technologies*, pp. 92–126. Ellis Horwood Limited, New York.

85. Büchi, J., Stünzi, E., Flury, M., Hirt, R., Labhart, P. and Ragaz, L. (1951) Über lokalanästhetisch wirksame basische Ester und Amide verschiedener Alkoxy-amino-benzoesäuren. *Helv. Chim. Acta* **34**: 1002–1013.

86. Wilhelm, M. (1975) The chemistry of polycyclic psycho-active drugs: serendipity or systematic investigation? *Pharm. J.* **214**: 414–416.

87. Larson, A. A. and Lish, P. M. (1964) A new bio-isostere: alkylsulphonamido-phenethanolamines. *Nature (London)* **203**: 1283–1285.

88. Chenoweth, M. B. and McCarthy, L. P. (1963) On the mechanism of the pharmacophoric effect of halogenation. *Pharmacol. Rev.* **15**: 673–707.

89. Goldman, P. (1969) The carbon–florine bond in compounds of biological interest. *Science* **164**: 1123–1130.

90. Peters, R. A. (1963) *Biochemical Lesions and Lethal Synthesis*. Pergamon Press, Oxford.

91. Chapman, N. B., James, J. W., Graham, J. D. P. and Lewis, G. P. (1952) Chemical reactivity and pharmacological activity among 2-haloethylamine derivatives with a naphtylmethyl group. *Chem. Ind. (London)* 805–807.

92. Vaughan, J. R. J., Anderson, G. W., Clapp, R. C., Clark, J. H., English, J. P., Howard, K. L., Marson, H. W., Sutherland, L. H. and Denton, J. J. (1949) Antihistamine agents. IV. Halogenated N,N-dimethyl-N′-benzyl-N-(2-pyridyl)-ethylenediamines. *J. Org. Chem.* **14**: 228–234.

93. Schatz, V. B. (1963) Isosterism and bioisosterism. In Burger, A. (ed.) *Medicinal Chemistry*, pp. 72–88. Interscience Publishers, Inc., New York.

94. Fessenden, R. J. and Fessenden, J. S. (1967) The biological properties of silicon compounds. In Harper, N. J. and Simmonds, A. B. (eds), *Advances in Drug Research*, pp. 95–132. Academic Press, London.

95. Tacke, R. and Zilch, H. (1986) Drug-design by sila-substitution and microbial transformations of organosilicon compounds: some recent results. *L'Actualité Chimique*, 75–82.

96. Tacke, R. and Zilch, H. (1986) Sila-substitution — a useful strategy for drug design? *Endeavour, New Series* **10**: 191–197.

97. Ricci, A., Seconi, G. and Taddei, M. (1989) Bioorganosilicon chemistry: trends and perspectives. *Chimica Oggi-Chemistry Today* 7: 15–21.
98. Metcalf, R. L. and Fukuto, T. R. (1965) Silicon-containing carbamate insecticides. *J. Econ. Entomol.* **58**: 1151.
99. Anonymous Zifrosilone. *Drugs Fut.* **19**: 854–855.
100. Hornsperger, J. -M., Collard, N. -N., Heydt, J. G., Giacobini, E., Funes, S., Dow, J. and Schirlin, D. (1994) Trimethysilylated trifluoromethyl ketones, a novel class of acetylcholinesterase inhibitors: biochemical and pharmacological profile of MDL 73,745. *Biochem. Soc. Transactions* 22: 758–763.
101. Fessendon, R. J. and Coon, M. D. (1965) Silicon-substituted medicinal agents. Silacarbamates related to meprobamate. *J. Med. Chem.* **8**: 604–608.
102. Tacke, R. (1980) Sila-pharmaka, XIX. Sila-pridinol und Pridinol: Darstellung und Eigenschaften sowie Strukturen im kristallinen und gelösten Zustand. *Chem. Ber.* **113**: 1962–1980.
103. Moberg, W. K. (1985) Synthesis of flusilazole. US patent 4 510 136 to DuPont.
104. Damour, D. M. B., Dutruc-Rosset, G., Doble, A., Piot, O. and Mignani, S. (1994) 1,1-Diphenyl-3-dialkylamino-1-silacyclopentane derivatives: a new class of potent and selective 5-HT$_{2A}$ antagonists. *Bioorg. Med. Chem. Lett.* 4: 415–420.
105. Sommer, L. H., Bennet, O. F., Campbell, P. G. and Weyenberg, D. R. (1957) Stereochemistry of hydride ion displacement from silicon. Enhanced rates at bridgehead and 4-ring silicon atoms. *J. Am. Chem. Soc.* **79**: 3295–3296.
106. Fessenden, R. J. and Ahlfors, C. (1967) The metabolic fate of some silicon-containing carbamates. *J. Med. Chem.* **10**: 810–812.
107. Landauer, W. (1954) On the chemical production of developmental abnormalities and of phenocopies in chicken embryos. *J. Cell. Comp. Physiol.* **43**(1): 261–305.
108. Landauer, W. and Clark, E. M. (1964) On the role of riboflavin in the teratogenic activity of boric acid. *J. Exptl. Zool.* **156**: 307–312.
109. Browning, E. (1969) *Toxicity of Industrial Metals.* Second Edition ed., pp. 90–97. Appleton-Century-Crofts, New York.
110. Caujolle, Pham-Huu-Chan (1968) Structure chimique et activité spasmolytique des organoboriques. *Arch. Int. Pharmacodyn. Ther.* **172**: 467–474.
111. Mubarak, S. I. M., Stanford, J. B. and Sugden, J. K. (1984) Some aspects of the antimicrobial and chemical properties of phenyl boronate esters of chloramphenicol. *Drug Dev. Ind. Pharm.* **10**: 1131–1160.
112. Dünitz, J. D., Hawley, D. M., Miklos, D., White, D. N. J., Berlin, Y., Marusik, R. and Prelog, V. (1971) Structure of boromycin. *Helv. Chim. Acta* **54**: 1709–1713.
113. Kinder, D. H. and Katzenellenbogen, J. A. (1985) Acylamino boronic acids and difluoroborane analogues of amino acids: potent inhibitors of chymotrypsine and elastase. *J. Med. Chem.* **28**: 1917–1925.
114. Alam, F., Soloway, A. H., Bapat, B. V., Barth, R. F. and Adams, D. M. (1989) Boron compounds for neutron capture therapy. *Basic Life Sci.* **50**: 107–111.
115. Kahl, S. B., Joel, D. D., Finkel, G. C., Micca, P. L., Nawrocky, M. M. and Coderre, J. A. (1989) A carboranyl porphyrin for boron neutron capture therapy of brain tumours. *Basic Life Sci.* **50**: 193–203.
116. Gabel, D. (1989) Tumor-seeking for boron neutron capture therapy: synthesis and biodistribution. *Basic Life Sci.* **50**: 233–241.
117. Klayman, D. L., Günther, W. H. H. (1973) *Organic Selenium Compounds: Their Chemistry and Biology.* Wiley-Interscience, New York.
118. Kang, S.-I. and Spears, C. P. (1987) Linear free energy relationships and cytotoxicities of para-substituted 2-haloethyl aryl selenides and bis(-chloroethyl) selenides. *J. Med. Chem.* **30**: 597–602.
119. Fischer, H., Terlinden, R., Löhr, J. P. and Römer, A. (1988) A novel biologically active selenoorganic compound. VIII. Biotransformation of ebselen. *Xenobiotica* **18**: 1347–1359.
120. Parnham, M. J. and Graf, E. (1987) Seleno-organic compounds and the therapy of hydroperoxide-linked pathological conditions. *Biochem. Pharmacol.* **36**: 3095–3102.

14

Ring Transformations

CAMILLE G. WERMUTH

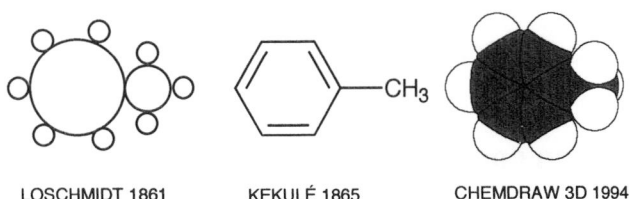

LOSCHMIDT 1861   KEKULÉ 1865   CHEMDRAW 3D 1994

The Loschmidt formula for the toluene ring system[1]

THE PRACTICE OF MEDICINAL CHEMISTRY
ISBN 0-12-744640-0

I.   INTRODUCTION

When active molecules contain cyclic systems, these can be opened, expanded, contracted, modified in many other ways, or even abolished. Conversely, noncyclic molecules can be cyclized or attached to, or included in, ring systems.

In the daily practice of medicinal chemistry, three kinds of approaches are currently used. The first approach does not affect the global complexity of the cyclic system and yields generally close analogues (or 'me-too' compounds) of the original active principle. For this we propose the term *analogical approach*. It consists of ring–chain transformations, ring contractions or expansions, and various other ring transformations. The second strategy, called the *disjunctive approach*[2] aims at the progressive simplification of the original active principle (which is often a natural compound). The objective is to extract information about the minimal structure that is required for activity. Finally, the *conjunctive approach*[2] is based on the creation or addition of supplementary rings. The objective is to constrain an originally flexible compound and to impose precise conformations and configurations. The preparation of such molecules is of prime importance in the exploration of ligand–receptor interaction and for molecular modelling studies.

II.   ANALOGICAL APPROACHES

A.   Analogy by ring opening: open-chain analogues

Open-ring analogues of cyclic active principles (open drugs, open-chain analogues) can be designed and synthesized. The usefulness of such compounds is rather questionable, and it appears that most of them were prepared for me-too purposes. Two possibilities can be envisaged:

(a)   The open analogue is again cyclized after oxidation or dehydration by a metabolic enzyme. We deal here with potential rings, which represent nothing more than metabolic precursors of the active species

(b)   The open analogue does not cyclize *in vivo* but can present some conformational analogy with the ring-containing active principle. These kinds of analogues are known as *pseudocycles*.

1.   *Potential rings:* in vivo *return to the cyclic derivative*

Compounds generating the active form after *in vivo* cyclization are in fact prodrugs and will be discussed in a more detailed manner in Chapters 31 and 32.

A historical example is the antimalarial drug proguanil[3] (Fig. 14.1). It was observed that this compound is inactive *in vitro* cultures of *Plasmodium gallinaceum*, but that the serum of animals treated with proguanil is active in these cultures. It was concluded that the actual active principle was a metabolite,[5] which was subsequently identified as cycloguanil.[4] In tropical medicine, proguanil is preferred to cycloguanil, the latter compound being too rapidly eliminated by the kidney.

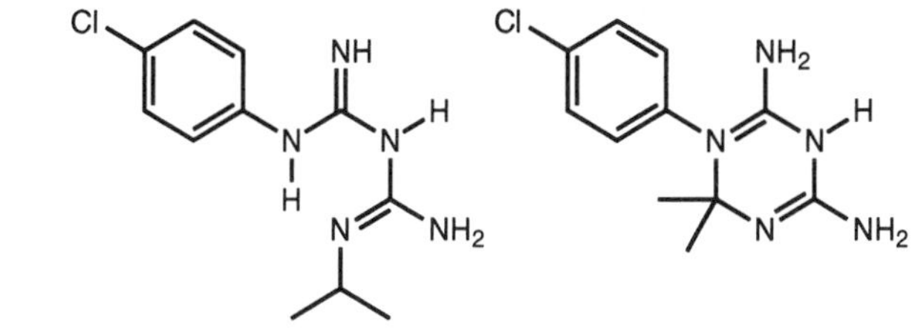

proguanil   cycloguanil

Fig. 14.1 Cycloguanil is the active metabolite of proguanil.[4]

Potassium canrenoate is a water-soluble prodrug and can be administered parenterally (Fig. 14.2). It has no intrinsic activity, but it can exert its diuretic activity (as an aldosterone antagonist) because of its interconversion with canrenone. Canrenone is itself the major metabolite of spironolactone.[6]

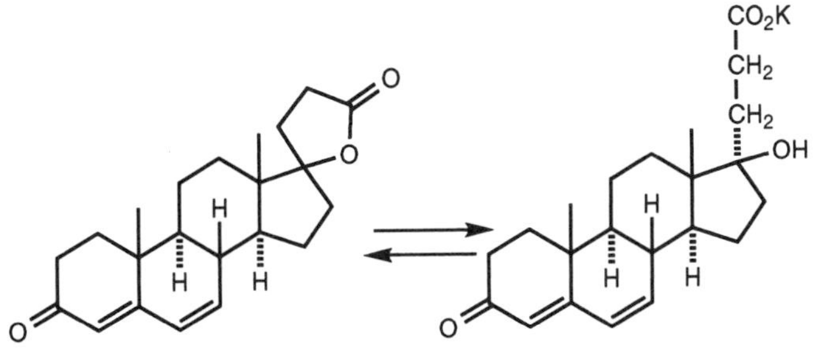

canrenone   potassium canrenoate

Fig. 14.2 *In vivo* the inactive potassium canrenoate cyclizes to canrenone.[6]

2. Irreversible compounds: pseudocycles

The open analogue is assumed to present a similar conformation to that of the cyclic one. Before denoting something a pseudocycle it must be ascertained by NMR or X-ray crystallography that it really mimics the ring-closed analogue.

(a) Diethylstilbestrol. It is currently accepted that the theory of pseudocycles was elaborated to account for the estrogenic activity of compounds such as bisdehydrodoisynolic acid, allenestrol and diethylstilbestrol (Fig. 14.3). The similarity with the natural hormone estradiol is striking. Nevertheless, it is highly probable that for receptor binding, the general shape of the molecules, and the distances separating the functional groups are more important than their degree of cyclization.[7]

(b) Clonidine. Open analogues of the centrally acting hypotensive agent clonidine (Fig. 14.4) have a similar activity profile but with a 30 to 100-fold loss in potency.[8] Surprisingly seco-clonidine, which is the closest analogue of clonidine, was found to be less active than the corresponding monomethyl derivative.

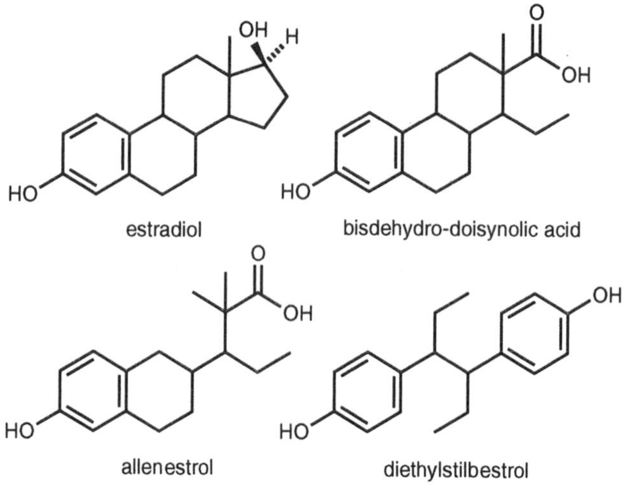

Fig. 14.3   Open analogues of estradiol.

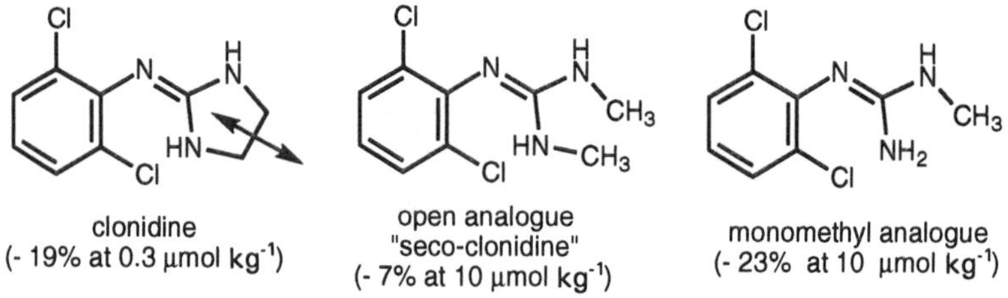

Fig. 14.4   Open analogues of clonidine (the hypotensive activity is expressed as variation of the arterial bood pressure 30 min after intravenous injection in pentobarbital-anaesthezised rats).[8]

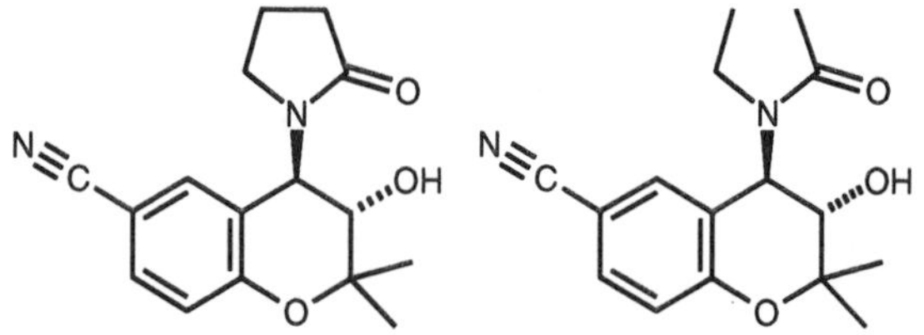

	cromakalim	open chain analogue
Dose (p.o.) (mg kg^{-1})	0.3	1.0
Max. decrease in blood pressure (%)	39±4	22±5

Fig. 14.5   Cromakalim and its open-chain analogue.[9]

(c) Cromakalim.   A more recent example is the open chain analogue of cromakalim, which was prepared as a more flexible pyrrolidone replacement (Fig. 14.5). It retains about a third of the potency of cromakalim.[9]

(d) Tetrahydrofolic acid.   Open-chain analogues of 5,6,7,8-tetrahydrofolic acid were prepared by researchers from Burroughs Wellcome.[10] None of the ring-opened analogues was as potent as the ring-closed lead structure in inhibiting tumour cell growth.

B.   Analogy by ring closure

Cyclizing open structures or creating an additional ring system in a given structure represents one of the useful methods in the search for biologically active conformations. The end result is a more constrained molecule, with an imposed conformation. The inconvenience is that additional isomeric centres may be introduced and that the selected cyclization mode might not lead to the active conformation adopted by the open-chain drug.

(a) Mevinolin and compactin.   An example of reversible ring closure is found with mevinolin and compactin, which are both potent inhibitors of hydroxymethylglutaryl-coenzyme A reductase (HMG-CoA reductase), the rate-determing enzyme in the *de novo* biosynthesis of cholesterol. *In vivo* these ring-closed derivatives (Fig. 14.6) are hydrolysed to the open chain 3,5-dihydroxyvaleric acid form that mimics the structure of the proposed intermediate in the reduction of HMG-CoA by HMG-CoA reductase.[11]

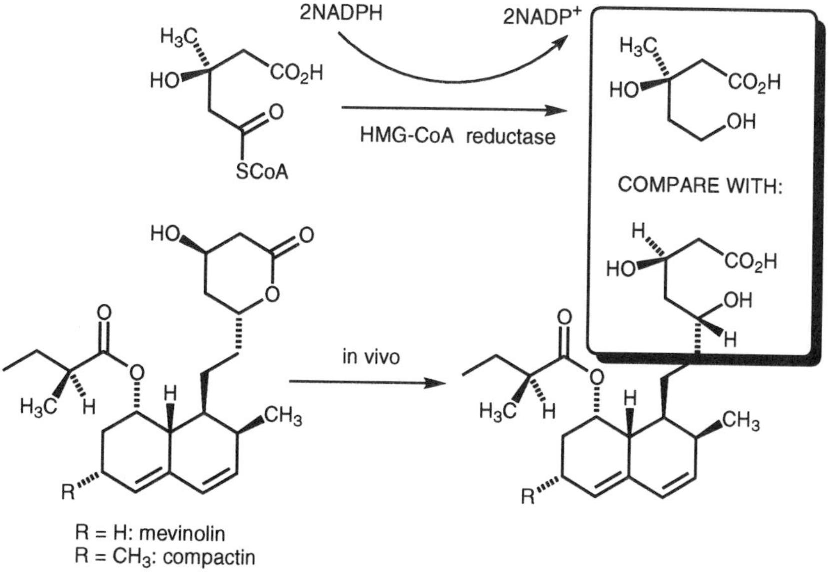

Fig. 14.6   The chemically stable lactones mevinolin and compactin represent the ring-closed form of the *in vivo* active parent.

(b) Arylpropionic analgesic and anti-inflammatory drugs. The potent analgesic benzoylindane carboxylic acid, TAI-901,[12] is the cyclized analogue of the well-known anti-inflammatory analgesic agent ketoprofen (Fig. 14.7). The corresponding heterocyclic analogues were also prepared.[13] The compounds show potent analgesic activities with low gastric irritation.

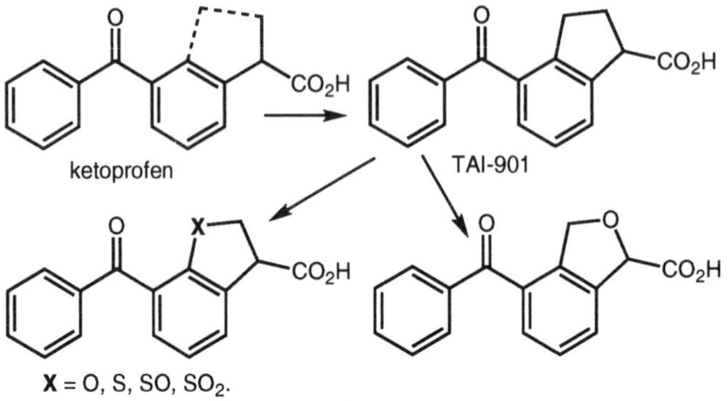

Fig. 14.7   Ring-closed me-too's of ketoprofen.

(c) The sulpiride side-chain.   Among the numerous benzamide drugs developed by the Delagrange scientists, some have diethylaminoethyl side-chains (e.g. tiapride), whereas others, such as sulpiride, have N-ethylpyrrolidinylmethyl side-chains that can be considered as the corresponding ring-closed analogues (Fig. 14.8). Both compounds are dopaminergic antagonists with neurotropic and antiemetic activity. Note that the ring closure creates an asymmetric centre; the commercial form is the racemate, the slightly more active isomer being the (S)-$(-)$-sulpiride.[16] An additional constraining factor results from the establishment of a hydrogen bond between the amidic N—H hydrogen and the methoxy oxygen.[14] A conformationally restricted remoxipride analogue in which the intramolecular hydrogen bond is replaced by a covalent bond (Fig. 14.8) is equipotent in D_2-receptor preparations.[15]

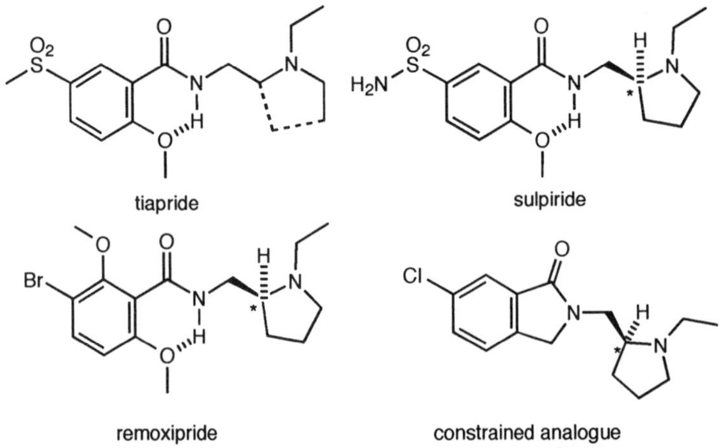

Fig. 14.8   The typical sulpiride side-chain results formally from a ring closure of the diethylaminoethyl side-chain of earlier prepared derivatives such as tiapride. Observe the intramolecular hydrogen bond that creates a pseudocycle[14] and which can be mimicked by a covalent analogue.[15]

(d) Cyclized dopamine: the ADTNs. The 2-amino-5,6-dihydroxy- and the 2-amino-6,7-dihydroxy-1,2,3,4-tetrahydronaphtalenes are cyclized analogues of dopamine, corresponding to the α- and the β-rotamer respectively (Fig. 14.9). As the cyclization generates a chiral centre, four different ADTNs are possible, showing differential affinities for the dopamine receptors.[17] An extensive study of the aminotetralins and analogues containing additional rings (octahydrobenz[g]quinolines) and compounds resulting from ring enlargements was published by Seiler *et al.*[18]

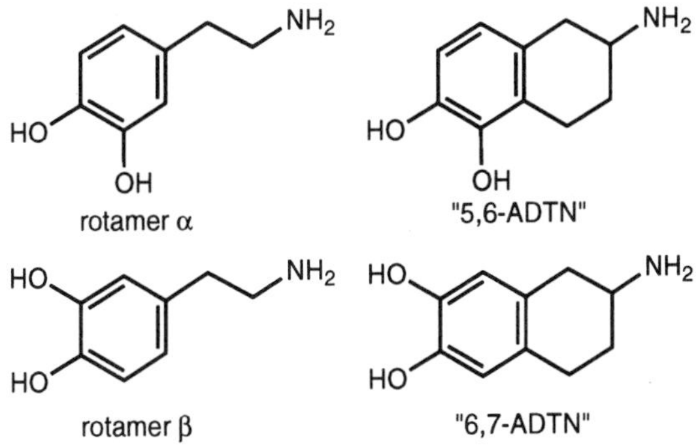

Fig. 14.9 Ring-closed analogues of the two rotamers of dopamine.

(e) GABAergic agonists. The transition from GABA to *trans*-4-aminocrotonic acid, followed by cyclization into isoguvacine, and finally into THIP (Fig. 14.10), achieves simultaneously the rigidification of the flexible GABA molecule and the production of THIP, a metabolically stable and still potent GABA agonist.[19]

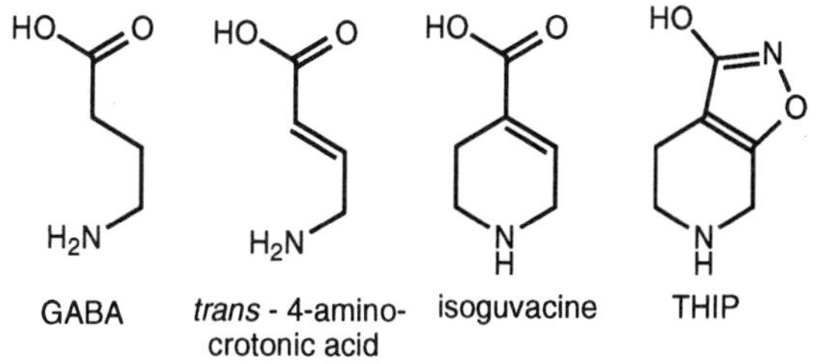

Fig. 14.10 GABAergic agonists.[19]

Starting from the structural information contained in the solid state form of the potent GABA$_B$ agonist baclofen, regarded as a possible bioactive conformation, Mann *et al.*[20] rigidified the baclofen structure by means of methylene, ethylene or propylene units (Fig. 14.11). Surprisingly the ethylene-bridged analogue (Fig. 14.11; *n* = 2; 1-(aminomethyl)-5-chloro-2,3-dihydro-1*H*-indene-1-acetic acid), which can be considered as representing the optimal mimic of the solid-state conformation of baclofen, was found to be inactive. This finding suggests that the ethylene bridge occupies an area of bulk intolerance, or that the solid-state conformation of

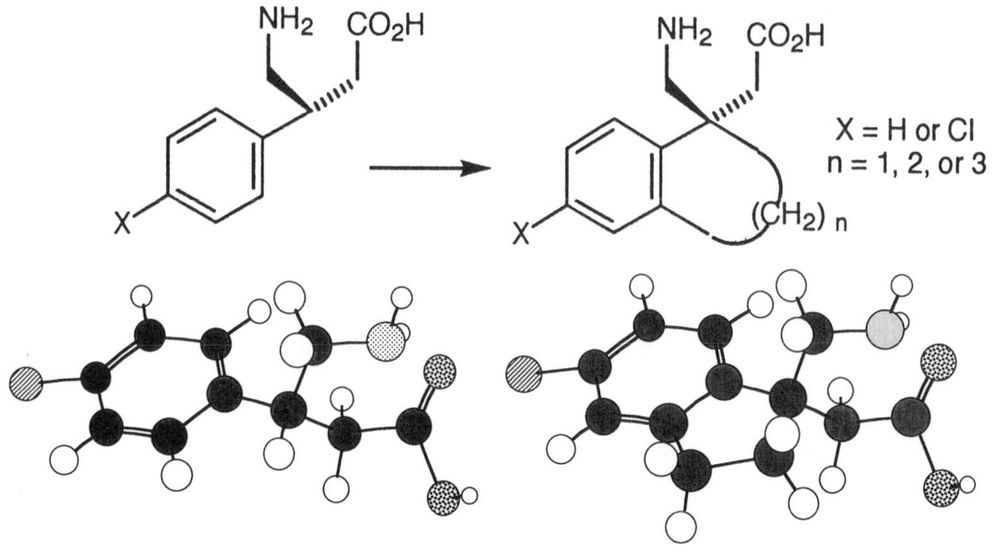

Fig. 14.11 Baclofen in the solid-state conformation (left) and the corresponding ethylene-bridged analogue (right).[20]

baclofen does not correspond to its bioactive conformation, or that a certain degree of conformational flexibility is required for binding to and activation of GABA$_B$ receptors.

(f) Ring-closed analogue of nicotine. The following example illustrates a very intriguing result. With natural (S)-(−)-nicotine,[21] the ring-closure strategy yielded a compound that possesses the same pharmacological profile as nicotine but which totally fails to compete for [^{3}H]nicotine binding (Fig. 14.12). The conformationally restricted (+)-*cis*-2,3,3a,4,5,9b-hexahydro-1-methyl-1*H*-pyrrolo-[3,2-*h*]isoquinoline has the 3aR,9bS configuration as determined by X-ray crystallography and corresponds thus to (S)-(−)-nicotine. *In vivo* this compound demonstrates a pharmacological profile similar to that of (S)-(−)-nicotine with an ED$_{50}$ of 7.13 μM/kg for the inhibition of spontaneous activity and 7.45 mM/kg for antinociception (tail flick test) compared to 4.44 and 4.81 mM/kg respectively, for (S)-(−)-nicotine. However the failure of mecamylamine (a well-established nicotinic antagonist) to antagonize the effects of the bridged analogue and the absence of competition for [^{3}H]nicotine binding suggest that either it binds to an as-yet-unidentified nicotinic receptor or that it represents a novel class of non-nicotinic analgesics.

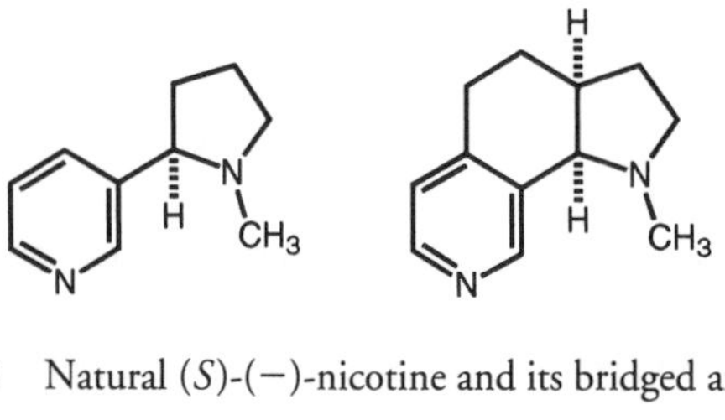

Fig.14.12 Natural (S)-(−)-nicotine and its bridged analogue[21].

(g) Cyclic analogues of β-blockers. Classical β-blockers possess a number of pharmacological properties, e.g. β-blocking, quinidine-like, local anaesthetic and hypotensive. With the hope of achieving some specificity, Basil *et al.*[22] considered the possibility of synthesizing ring-closed analogues (Fig. 14.13). One of the compounds prepared, 3,4-dihydro-3-hydroxy-6-methyl-1,5-benzoxazocine was a potent β-blocker. This activity is unlikely to be due to hydrolysis to the open-chain derivative since the corresponding primary amine, formed by hydrolysis of the benzoxazocine ring has less than 0.25 the activity of the latter. On the other hand, it is difficult to reconcile the benzoxazocine configuration with the structural requirements associated with the occupation of β-receptors.

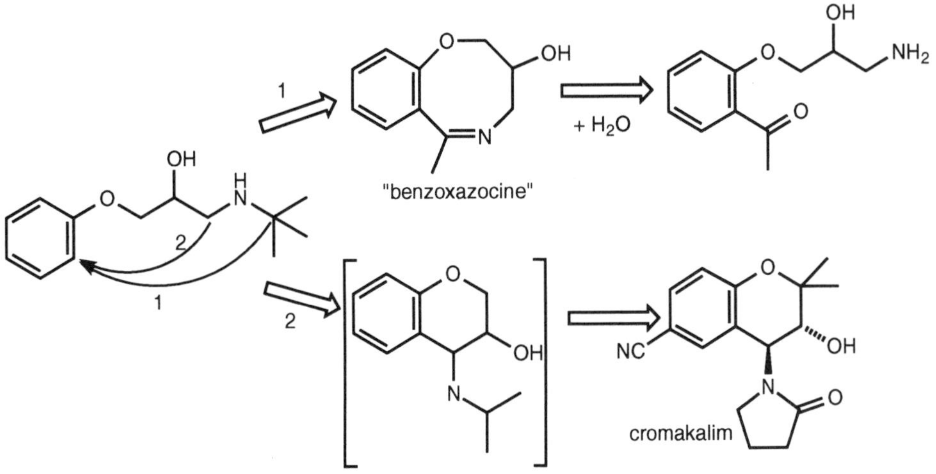

Fig. 14.13 Cyclized analogues of β-blocking phenylpropanolamines.[22,24]

Later studies by Evans *et al.*[23,24] also envisaged the synthesis of cyclized analogues of the phenylpropanolamine type of β-blockers. The authors hoped that by restricting the conformation (by cyclizing the carbon atom bearing the terminal amino group to the aromatic ring, see Fig. 14.13), β-blocking activity would be lost but antihypertensive activity might be retained. This turned out to be true in animal tests and in double-blind clinical studies, so the potassium channel activator cromakalim was developed.[24]

(h) Cyclized diphenhydramine. Nefopam (Fig. 14.14) is the representative of a new class of centrally acting skeletal muscle relaxants, also possessing a benzoxazocine structure.[25] Formally nefopam is a cyclized analogue of orphenadrine and diphenhydramine. In contrast to the parent molecules, nefopam has no antihistaminic activity, retaining only the muscle relaxant effects. Clinically nefopam is used as muscle relaxant, but also — and this was not originally anticipated — it is an antidepressant and an analgesic. These clinical indications can be explained by the interference of nefopam with serotonergic transmission. More precisely, studies of the separated stereoisomers of nefopam explain its serotonin uptake properties and suggest that descending serotonergic pathways are involved in its antinociceptive activity.[26]

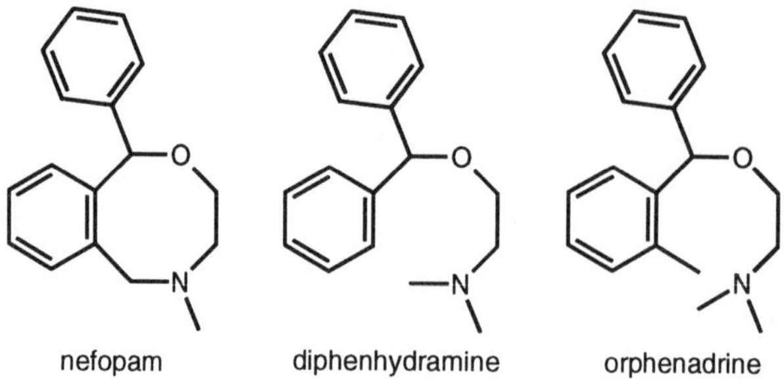

Fig. 14.14   Nefopam is a cyclized analogue of orphenadrine and diphenhydramine.[25]

(i) Ring variations around phenylbutazone. The anti-inflammatory drug phenylbutazone ((**1**), Fig. 14.15) led to many me-too copies, such as the ring-opened analogue bumadizon (**2**) (Ca^{2+} salt = Eumotol®[27]) or the ring-closed analogue apazone (**3**) (Prolixan®[28]). The cinnoline derivative (**4**)[29] results again from a ring closure and served as model for the design of its open counterpart, the styrylbutazone (**5**).[30] The quinolinyl-3,5-dioxopyrazolidine (**6**)[31] represents another interesting ring variation with a 7-chloroquinoline moiety in the butazone portion.

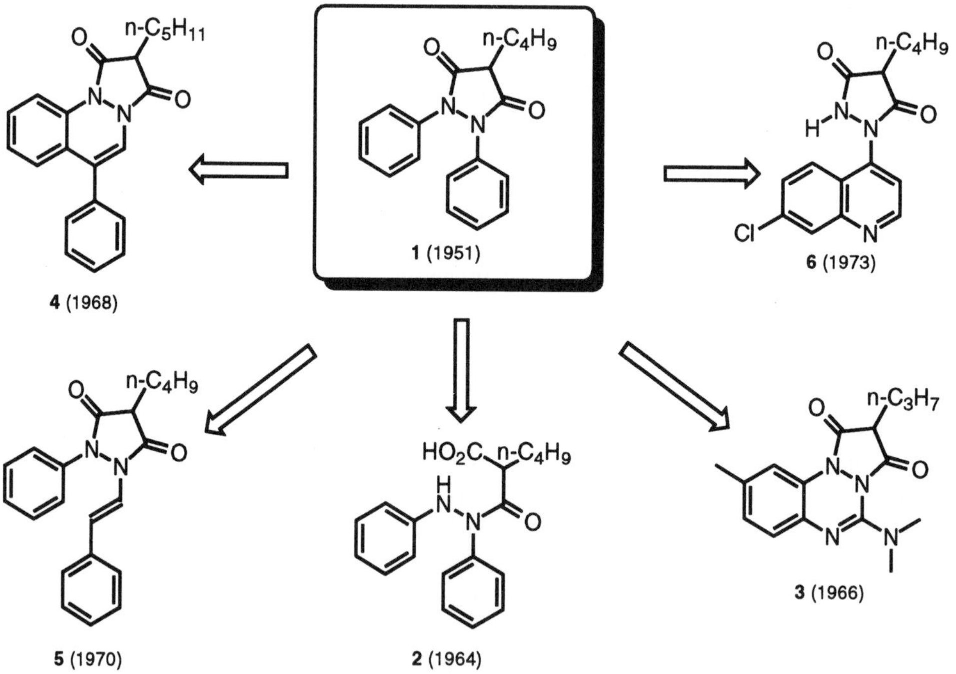

Fig. 14.15   Successive ring openings and closures in phenylbutazone-derived anti-inflammatory drugs.

C.   Other analogies

Applied to ring systems, the following molecular modifications seem to be conducted mainly with the objective of by-passing patent protections and to allow the synthesis of me-too products.

1.   *Ring enlargement and ring contraction*

Ring enlargement and ring contraction can be considered as homologous variations in the cyclic series and have already been mentioned in Chapter 12. We show in Fig. 14.16 two additional examples taken from the barbituric and from the opiate series, respectively. In the case of the change of the barbiturics to hydantoins, the contraction is accompanied by the loss of a carbonyl group (Fig. 14.17). Nevertheless potent antiepileptics are found in both series. Oxotremorine and its ring-opened analogue oxo-2 (Fig. 14.18) are partial muscarinic agonists producing large guanine nucleotide shifts in the heart (32 and 23, respectively), suggesting strong M_2 agonist-like effects.[32]

The corresponding piperidinic analogue oxo-pip,[33] with a predicted antagonist [³H]QNB/[³H]CD ratio of 2.2, produced only a weak shift (5.0) in the concentration–response curve with the addition of the stable guanine nucleotide analogue.[32] Thus the change from a pyrrolidine to a piperidine ring is able to change a partial agonist into an antagonist.

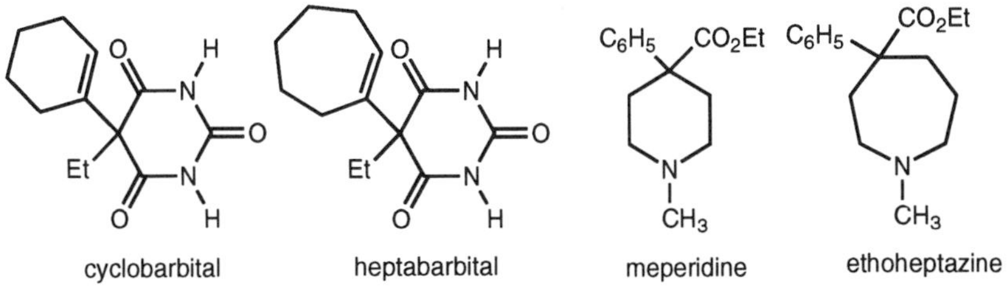

cyclobarbital   heptabarbital   meperidine   ethoheptazine

Fig. 14.16   Six-membered rings exchanged for seven-membered rings.

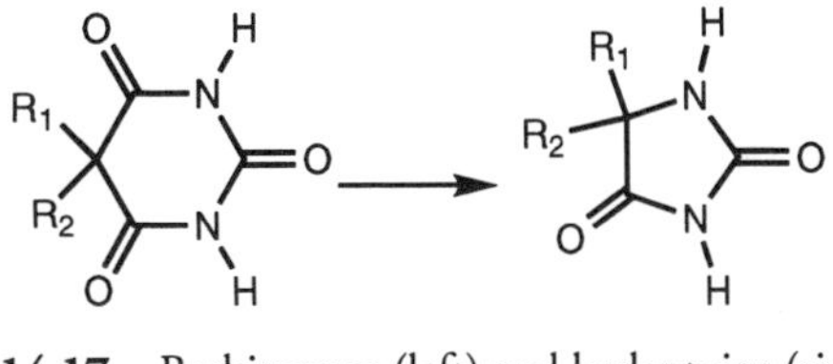

Fig. 14.17   Barbiturates (left) and hydantoins (right).

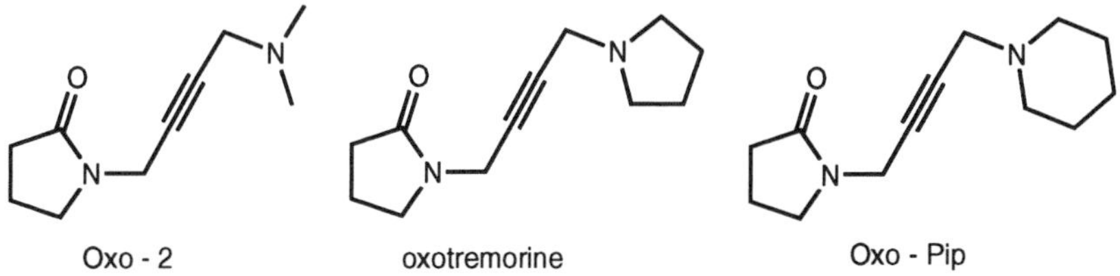

Oxo - 2   oxotremorine   Oxo - Pip

Fig. 14.18   Oxotremorine yields ring-opened and ring-extended analogues.[32]

2.   *Reorganization of ring systems*

The four molecular variations described below represent more 'exotic' approaches to the design and manipulation of the original ring systems. They may bring useful alternatives, allowing escape from overcrowded avenues of research.

(a) Transforming simple rings into spiro *derivatives or into bi- or tricyclic systems.* A first example is in the guanethidine analogues.[34] As the original guanethidine patents covered ring sizes varying from five-membered to ten-membered rings, a possible way around them was the design of isolipophilic *spiro* systems (Dausse compounds a and b[35,36], Fig. 14.19). Another possibility, originating from Takeda scientists, involves the use of an azethidine surrogate for the ethylenediamine chain.[37] Finally, polycyclic systems can replace the octahydroazocine ring, as illustrated by the bicyclic compounds c and d from Dausse[38] or by the tricyclic compound from Lumière Laboratories.[39,40] Many other imaginative solutions were proposed; they are well reviewed by Mull and Maxwell.[34]

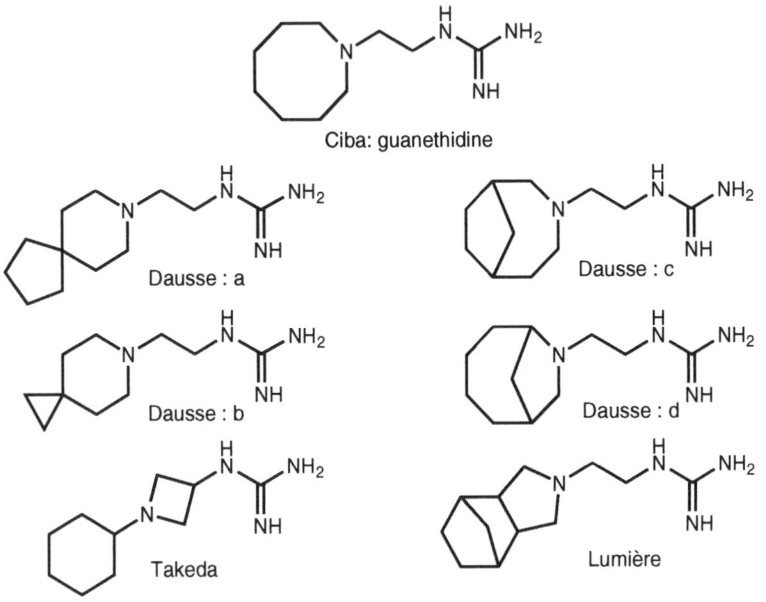

Fig. 14.19   Alternative possibilities in the design of guanethidine analogues.

(b) Splitting benzo compounds ('benzo cracking').   Dissociation of a fused ring system (Fig. 14.20), particularly by splitting a benzo compound, can sometimes improve its solubility but only alter slightly its pharmacokinetic profile and its long-term toxicity.

(c) Restructuring ring systems.   Among the above-mentioned molecular variations on ring systems, some can be used *simultaneously*. Thus the splitting of the benzimidazole heterocycle in the anthelmintic thiabendazole and the concomitant association of the two five-membered rings yields tetramisole (Fig. 14.21). One of the two enantiomers of tetramisole, the L-(−)-form, or levamisole, is also a potent anthelmintic.

The change from the D_1-selective dopaminergic agonist DPTI (4-(3,4-dihydroxyphenyl)-1,2,3,4-tetrahydroisoquinoline) to the equally D_1-selective compound SKF 38 393 is a combination of benzo cracking, a new benzo fusion and ring enlargement (Fig. 14.18). As a result, the compounds still resemble each other and both are recognized by the dopamine D_1-receptor.[18]

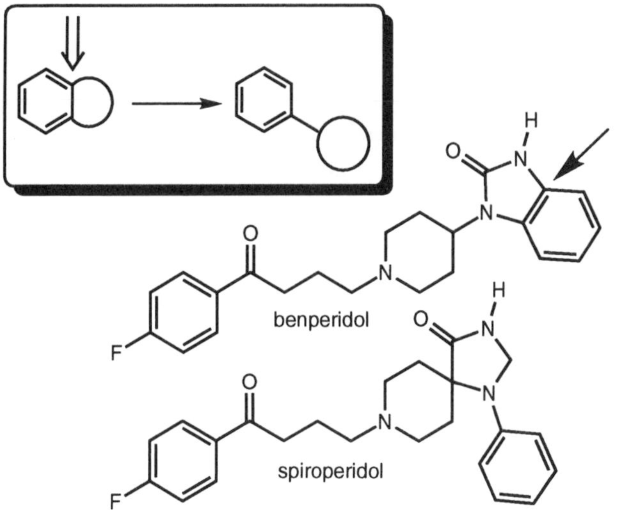

Fig. 14.20   Splitting of fused rings often yields drugs with similar activity, sometimes with improved solubility and/or less toxicity.

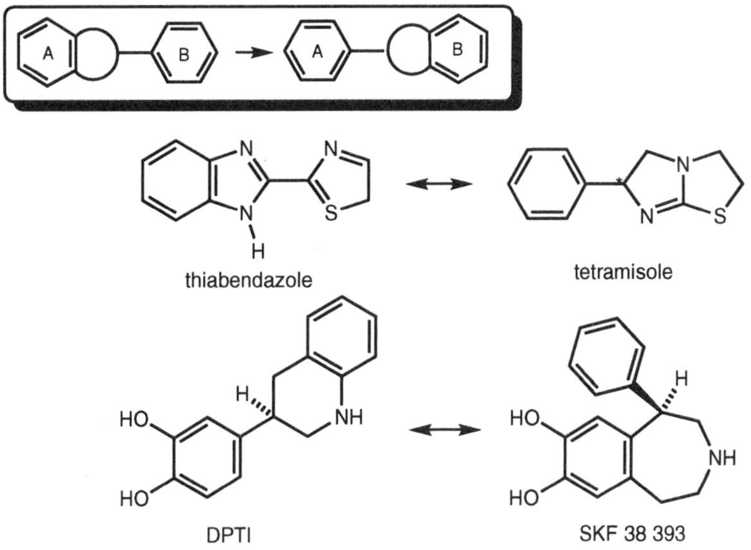

Fig. 14.21   Restructured ring systems.

(d) Ring dissociation.   The natural compound khellin generated two families of cardioactive drugs: on one side the benzopyrones, illustrated by the 3-methyl-chromone[41] and chromonar (carbochromen); on the other side the benzofurans, illustrated by amiodarone (Fig. 14.22). Both families possess antiarrhythmic and antianginal properties.

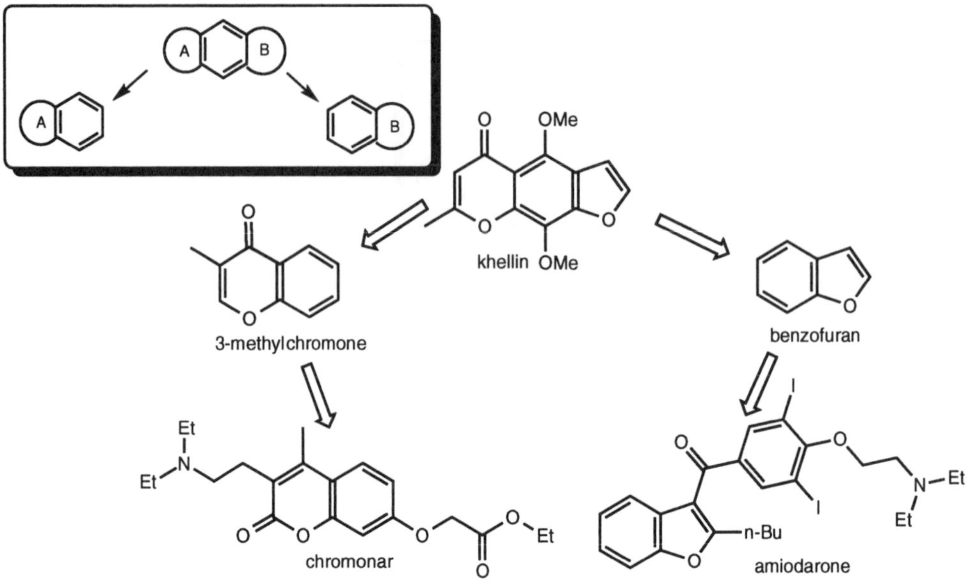

Fig. 14.22 Cardioactive drugs obtained by dissociation of the khellin molecule into benzopyrones and benzofurans.

III. DISJUNCTIVE APPROACHES

Starting from a polycyclic structure (which is often of natural origin), the chemist proceeds to progressive simplifications of the molecule ('molecular striptease'). Sometimes very simple reasoning guides the medicinal chemist and the final compound has only a remote resemblance to the model compound. Such an exercise led to the transformation of the natural compound asperlicin to a totally synthetic simplified benzodiazepine derivative (see Fig. 14.26).

(a) Cocaine-derived local anaesthetics. Figure 14.23 illustrates how simplified synthetic copies of cocaine were designed. The change from cocaine to procaine retains the local anaesthetic effects without the narcotic properties.

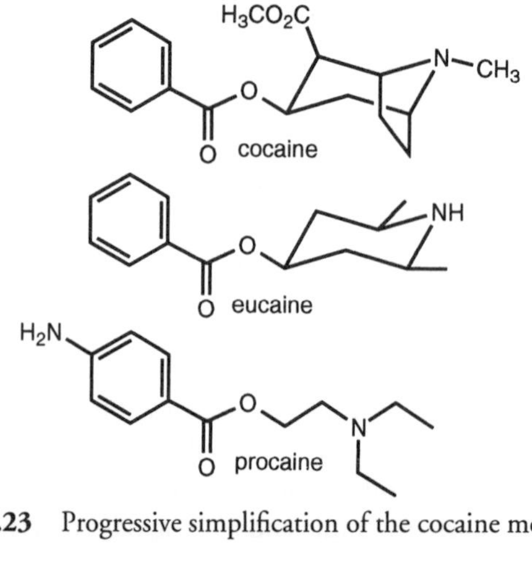

Fig. 14.23 Progressive simplification of the cocaine molecule.

(b) Morphinic analgesics.   Probably more than a thousand more or less simplified analogues of the alkaloid morphine have been investigated.[42] Many of them were inactive, but it was rapidly recognized that the phenylpiperidine unit was crucial for the central analgesic properties (Fig. 14.24). In contrast to what was observed for cocaine, however, no clear discrimination between the analgesic and the narcotic properties could be achieved.

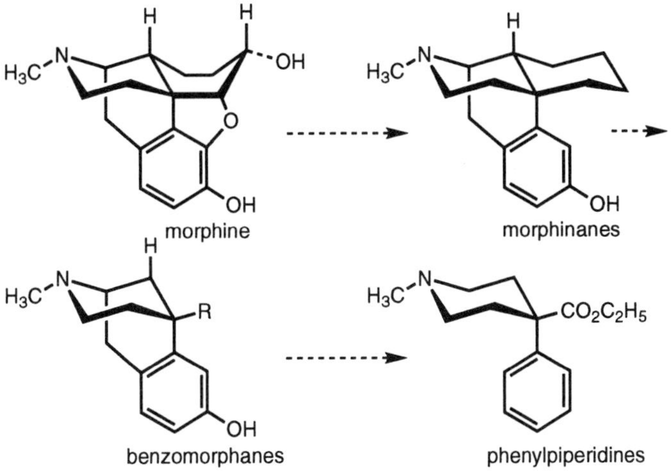

Fig. 14.24   Progressive simplification of the morphine molecule.

(c) Dopamine autoreceptor agonists.   The discovery of 3-(3-hydroxyphenyl)-*N-n*-propyl piperidine ((±)-3-PPP), a centrally acting dopamine receptor agonist with selectivity for dopaminergic autoreceptors,[43] offers a potential alternative to neuroleptics in the treatment of schizrenia. The structure of (±)-3-PPP (Fig. 14.25) can be considered as resulting from a

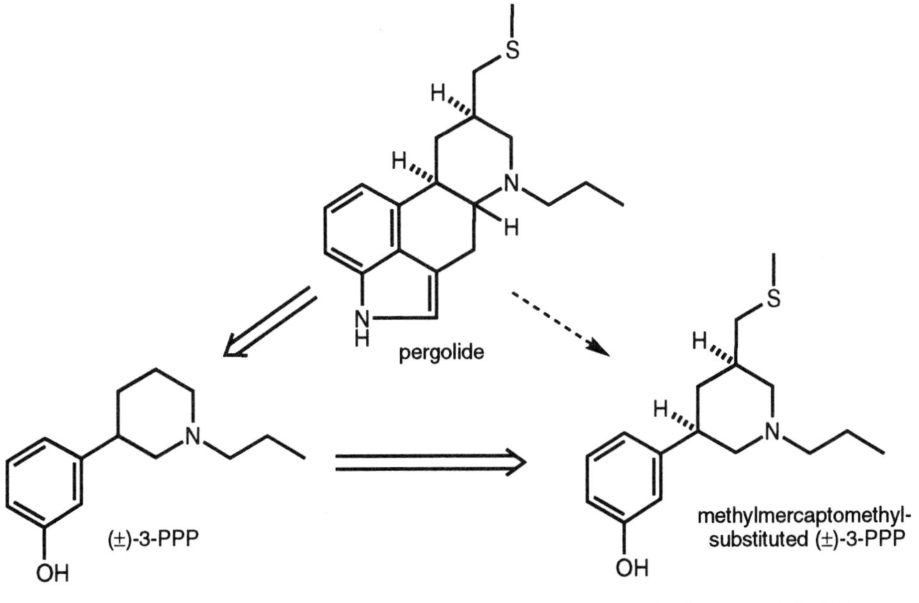

Fig. 14.25   3-PPP is a result of the disjunctive approach applied to pergolide.[43,44]

disjunctive approach applied to pergolide.[45,46] Surprisingly, an increase in the pergolide-like character of 3-PPP, through incorporation of a methylmercaptomethyl group, did not improve the potency.[44]

(d) CCK antagonists.   After the discovery of the potent CCK antagonistic activity of the natural compound asperlicin,[47] scientists from the Merck group first prepared some simple semisynthetic derivatives.[48] Then, recognizing in asperlicin the elements of a benzodiazepinone and a tetrahydroindole, they followed the hunch that these elements alone might confer some CCK antagonistic activity.[49] This reasoning proved to be valid (Fig. 14.26).

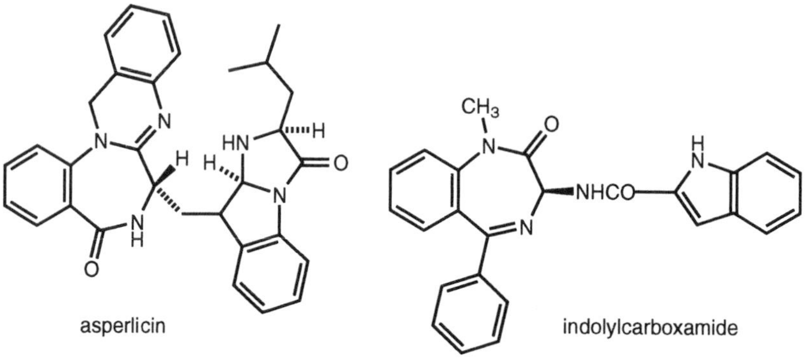

Fig. 14.26   Productive disjunction of the asperlicin molecule.[49]

IV.   CONJUNCTIVE APPROACHES

As already mentioned at the beginning of this chapter, the purpose of the conjunctive method lies in the design of compounds structurally more complex than the lead compound. In practice this is generally achieved in creating and/or adding supplementary ring systems to constrain the molecule and to impose specific conformations.

A.   Dopaminergic antagonists

Starting from the flexible haloperidol molecule, Humber and colleagues[50] designed the rigid (+)-butaclamol that contains three clearly defined stereocentres (Fig. 14.27). The same stereochemical requirements as in (+)-butaclamol are found in compound Ro 14-8625 prepared by Imhof *et al.*[51]

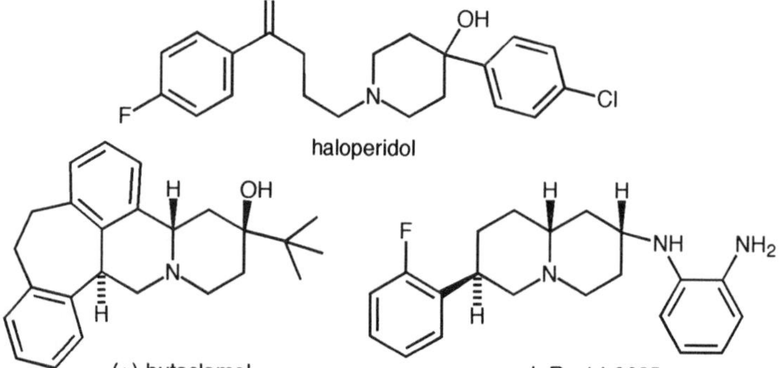

Fig. 14.27   The conjunctive method applied to the design of haloperidol-derived dopaminergic antagonists.

B. Glutamate NMDA and AMPA receptor antagonists

The progressive change of glutamic acid to D-AP5,[52] to the piperidine analogue CGS 19755[53] and finally to the tetrahydroisoquinoline PD 134705,[54] led to NMDA receptor antagonists. Similarly, rigidification into the perhydroquinolines (**7**), (**8**) and (**9**)[55] (Fig. 14.28) illustrates another application of the conjunctive approach that led to potent AMPA antagonists. In addition to the elements enhancing structural rigidity, these latter compounds contain three new chiral centres.

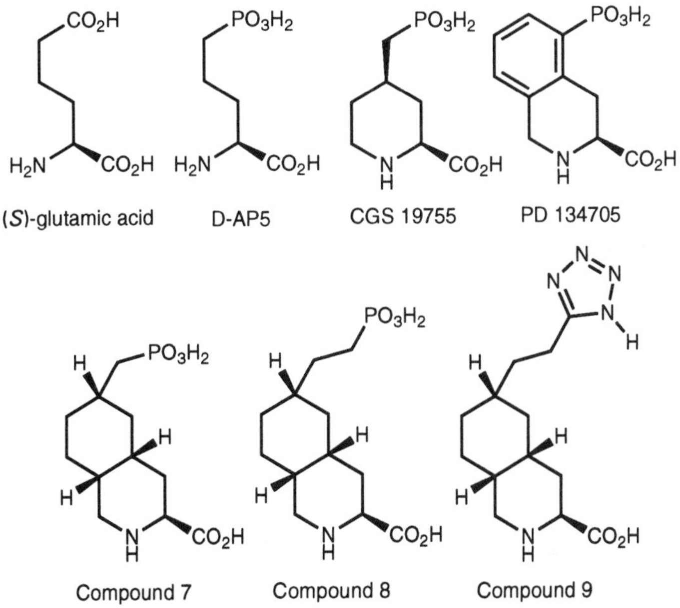

Fig. 14.28 The conjunctive method applied to the design of NMDA and AMPA receptor antagonists.

Since the development in 1980 of norfloxacin[56] as a useful antibacterial agent, a large number of analogues have been synthesized. Among them, the conjunctive approach led to highly potent tetracyclic analogues[57] (Fig. 14.29).

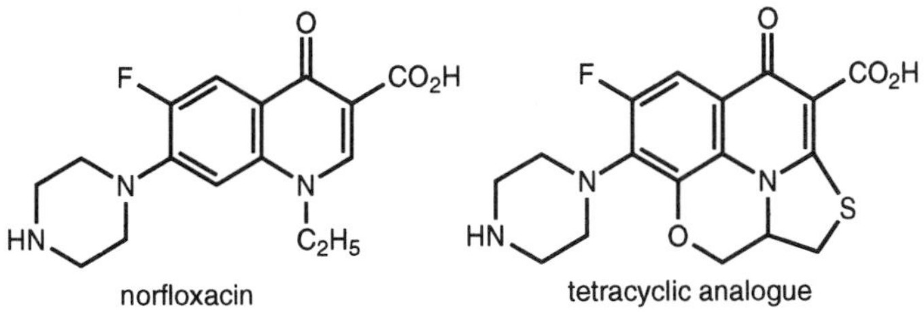

Fig. 14.29 Norfloxacin and its tetracyclic analogue.[56]

A number annelated analogues of the 5-HT$_3$ antagonist ondansetron were investigated (Fig. 14.30) in a similar way. Among them, cilansetron (n = 1) was found to be about ten times more potent without loss in selectivity.[58]

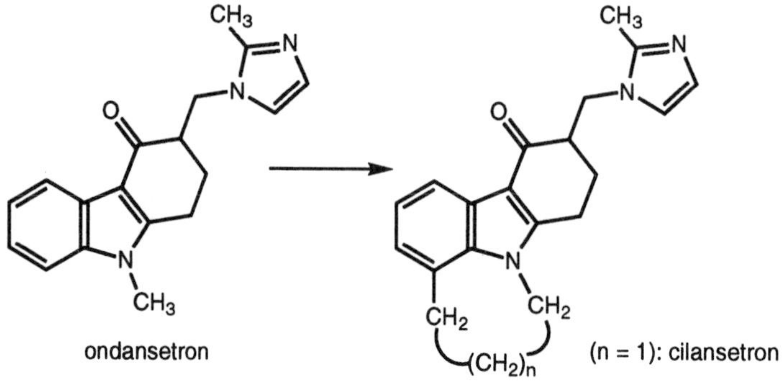

Fig. 14.30 Cilansetron, an annelated analogue of ondansetron.[58]

The well-known angiotensin converting enzyme (ACE) inhibitor captopril has a relatively simple structure and therefore represents an excellent starting material for the conjunctive approaches (Fig. 14.31). Modelling studies based on a template structure constructed from the superposition of the energy-minimized benzo-fused ACE inhibitors shown in Fig. 14.31 suggested the synthesis of the 13-membered heterocyclic lactam analogue.[59]

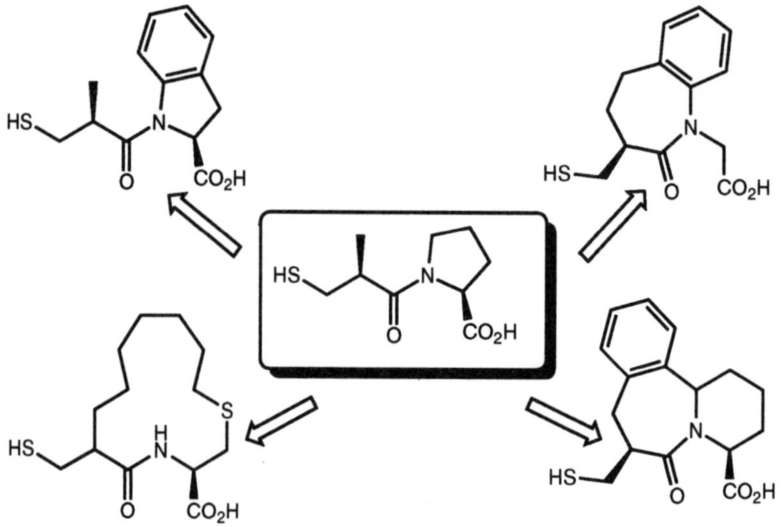

Fig. 14.31 Angiotensin converting enzyme inhibitors derived from captopril.

V.   CONCLUSION

As seen earlier, molecular variations involving the study of homologous series or the application of the vinylogy concept induce relatively minor changes in the pharmacological profile and rather result in optimizing the potency. However, modifying ring systems — ring–chain transformation, ring contractions and expansions, reorganization of cyclic systems — represents a highly efficient approach in the exploration of the requirements governing drug–receptor interactions and sometimes even provides novel drug candidates.

REFERENCES

1. Loschmidt, J. (1861) *Chemische Studien. I. A. Constitutions-Formeln der Organischen Chemie in Geographischer Darstellung. B. Das Mariotte'sche Gesetz.* Carol Gerold's Sohen Wien [Reprinted in 1989 by Aldrich Chemical Company, Inc., Milwaukee, Aldruch catalogue number Z-18,567-0, Wien].
2. Schueller, F. W. (1960) *Chemobiodynamics and Drug Design.* MacGraw-Hill, New York.
3. Curd, F. H. S., Davey, D. G. and Rose, F. L. (1945) Studies on synthetic antimalarial drugs—X. Some biguanide derivatives as new types of antimalarial substances with both therapeutic and causal prophylactic activity. *Ann. Trop. Med.* **39**: 208–214.
4. Crowther, A. F. and Levi, A. A. (1953) Proguanyl — the isolation of a metabolite with high antimalarial activity. *Br. J. Pharmacol.* **8**: 93–101.
5. Hawking, F. and Perry, W. L. M. (1948) Activation of paludrine. *Br. J. Pharmacol.* **3**: 320–331.
6. Weiner, I. M. (1990) Drugs affecting renal function and electrolyte metabolism. In Goodman-Gilman, A., Rall, T. W., Nies, A. S. and Taylor, P. (eds) *Goodman and Gilman's The Pharmacological Basis of Therapeutics*, pp. 708–731. Pergamon Press, New York.
7. Buzetta, B. and Hospital, M. (1978) Relations structure–activité. In Cohen, Y. (ed.) *Pharmacologie Moléculaire*, pp. 27–36. Masson, Paris.
8. Rouot, B., Leclerc, G., Wermuth, C. G., Miesch, F. and Schwartz, J. (1978) Synthèse et essais pharmacologiques d'arylguanidines, analogues ouverts de la clonidine. *Eur. J. Med. Chem.* **13**: 337–342.
9. Ashwood, V. A., Cassidy, F., Coldwell, M. C., Evans, J. M., Hamilton, T. C., Howlett, D. R., Smith, D. M. and Stemp, G. (1990) Synthesis and antihypertensive activity of 4-(substituted-carbonylamino)-2H-1-benzopyrans. *J. Med. Chem.* **33**: 2667–2672.
10. Bigham, E. C., Hodson, S. T., Mallory, W. R., Wilson, D., Duch, D. S., Smith, G. K. and Foreign, R. (1992) Synthesis and biological activity of open-chain analogues of 5,6,7,8-tetrahydrofolic acid — potential antitumor agents. *J. Med. Chem.* **35**: 1399–1410.
11. Nakamura, C. E. and Abeles, R. H. (1985) Mode of interaction of β-hydroxy-β-methylglutaryl-coenzyme A reductase with strong binding inhibitors: compactin and related compounds. *Biochemistry* **24**: 1364–1376.
12. Kawai, K., Tamura, S., Morimoto, S., Ishii, H. and Kuzuna, S. (1982) Pharmacology of 4-benzoyl-1-indancarboxylic acid (TAI-901) and 4-(4-methylbenzoyl)-1-indancarboxylic acid (TAI-908). *Arzneimittel-Forsch.* **32**: 113–117.
13. Boyle, E. A., Mangan, F. R., Markwell, R. E., Smith, S. A., Thomson, M. J., Ward, R. W. and Wyman, P. A. (1986) 7-Aroyl-2,3-dihydrobenzo[*b*]furan-3-carboxylic acids and 7-benzoyl-2,3-dihydrobenzo[*b*]thiophene-3-carboxylic acids as analgesic agents. *J. Med. Chem.* **29**: 894–898.
14. Waterbeemd van de, H. and Testa, B. (1983) Theoretical conformational studies of some dopamine antagonistic benzamide drugs: 3-pyrrolidyl- and 4-piperidyl derivatives. *J. Med. Chem.* **26**: 203–207.
15. Norman, M. H., Kelley, J. L. and Hollingsworth, E. B. (1993) Conformationally restricted analogues of remoxipride as potential antipsychotic agents. *J. Med. Chem.* **36**: 3417–3423.
16. Jenner, P., Clow, A., Reavill, C., Theodoru, A. and Marsden, C. D. (1980) Stereoselective actions of substituted benzamide drugs on cerebral dopamine mechanisms. *J. Pharm Pharmacol.* **32**: 39–44.

17. Cannon, J. G., Lee, T., Goldman, H. D., Costall, B. and Naylor, R. J. (1977) Central dopamine agonist properties of some 2-aminotetralin derivatives after peripheral and intracerebral administration. *J. Med. Chem.* **20**: 1111–1116.

18. Seiler, M. P., Bölsterli, J. J., Floersheim, P., Hagenbach, A., Markstein, R., Pfäffli, P., Widmer, A. and Wüthrich, H. (1993) Recognition at dopamine receptor subtypes. In Testa, B., Kyburz, E., Fuhrer, W. and Giger, G. (eds) *Perspectives in Medicinal Chemistry*, pp. 221–237. Verlag Helvetica Chemica Acta and VCH, Basel and Weinheim.

19. Krogsgaard-Larsen, P., Hjeds, H., Falch, E., Jørgensen, F. S. and Nielsen, L. (1988) Recent advances in GABA agonists, antagonists and uptake inhibitors: structure–activity relationships and therapeutic potential. In Testa, B. (ed.) *Advances in Drug Research*, pp. 381–456. Academic Press, London.

20. Mann, A., Boulanger, T., Brandau, B., Durant, F., Evrard, G., Heaulme, M., Desaulles, E. and Wermuth, C. G. (1991) Synthesis and biochemical evaluation of baclofen analogues locked in the baclofen solid-state conformation. *J. Med. Chem.* **34**: 1307–1313.

21. Glassco, W., Suchocki, J., George, C., Martin, B. R. and May, E. L. (1993) Synthesis, optical resolution, absolute configuration, and preliminary pharmacology of (+)- and (−)-*cis*-2,3,3a,4,5,9b-hexahydro-1-methyl-1*H*-pyrrolo-[3,2-*h*]isoquinoline, a structural analog of nicotine. *J. Med. Chem.* **36**: 3381–3385.

22. Basil, B., Coffee, E. C. J., Gell, D. L., Maxwell, D. R., Sheffield, D. J. and Wooldridge, K. R. H. (1970) A new class of sympathetic β-receptor blocking agents. 3,4-Dihydro-3-hydroxy-1,5-benzoxazocines. *J. Med. Chem.* **13**: 403–406.

23. Evans, J. M., Fake, C. S., Hamilton, T. C., Poyser, R. H. and Watts, E. A. (1983) Synthesis and antihypertensive activity of substituted *trans*-4-amino-3,4-dihydro-2,2-dimethyl-2*H*-1-benzopyran-3-ols. *J. Med. Chem.* **26**: 1582–1589.

24. Stemp, G. and Evans, J. M. (1993) Discovery and development of cromokalim and related potassium channel activators. In Ganellin, C. R. and Roberts, S. M. (eds) *Medicinal Chemistry*, pp. 141–162. Academic Press, London.

25. Heel, R. C., Brogden, R. N., Pakes, G. E., Speight, T. M. and Avery, G. S. (1980) Nefopam: a review of its pharmacological properties and therapeutic efficacy. *Drugs* **19**: 249–267.

26. Glaser, R. and Donnel, D. (1989) Stereoisomer diferentiation for the analgesic drug nefopam hydrochloride using modelling studies of serotonin uptake area. *J. Pharm. Sci.* **78**: 87–90.

27. Pfister, R., Sallmann, A. and Hammerschmidt, W. (1969) Substituted malonic acid hydrazides. US patent 3 455 999 (July 15, 1969 to Geigy Chemical Corporation).

28. Mixich, G. (1968) Zum chemischen verhalten des antiphlogisticums "Azapropazon" (Mi 85) = 3-dimethylamino-7-methyl-1,2-(*n*-propylmalonyl)-1,2-dihydro-1,2,4-benzotriazin. *Helv. Chim. Acta* **51**: 532–538.

29. Jahn, U. and Wagner-Jauregg, T. (1968) Vergleich von Zwei neuen Klassen Antiphlogisticher Substanzen im Collier-Test. *Arzneimittel-Forsch.* **18**: 120–121.

30. Yamamoto, H. and Kaneko, S. -I. (1970) Synthesis of 1-phenyl-2-styryl-3,5-dioxopyrazolidines as antiinflammatory agents. *J. Med. Chem.* **13**: 292–295.

31. Wermuth, C. G. and Choay, J. (1973) Nouveaux dérivés de la pyrazolidine, leur procédé de fabrication et médicaments contenant ces nouveaux dérivés. French patent 2 244 513 (July 12, 1973 to Choay, S. A.).

32. Trybulski, E. J., Zhang, J., Kramss, R. H. and Mangano, R. M. (1993) The synthesis and biochemical pharmacology of enantiomerically pure methylated oxotremorine derivatives. *J. Med. Chem.* **36**: 3533–3541.

33. Ringdahl, B. and Jenden, D. J. (1983) Pharmacological properties of oxotremorine and its analogues. *Life Sci.* **32**: 2401–2413.

34. Mull, R. P. and Maxwell, R. A. (1967) Guanethidine and related adrenergic neuronal blocking agents. In Schlittler, E. (ed.) *Antihypertensive Agents*, pp. 115–149. Academic Press, New York.

35. Giudicelli, R., Najer, H. and Lefèvre, F. (1965) Comparaison des durées d'action du *N*-β-guanidino-éthyl-aza-6 spiro[2,5]octane (LD 3598) et de la guanéthidine. *Compt. Rend. Acad. Sci.* **260**: 726–729.

36. Najer, H., Giudicelli, R. and Sette, J. (1964) Guanidines douées d'action antihypertensive, 4e mémoire: *N*-β-guanidinoéthyl azaspiro alcanes (1ère partie). *Bull Soc. Chim. France* 2572–2581.

37. Toda, N., Usui, H. and Shimamoto, K. (1972) Modification by AZ-55, guanethidine and bretylium of responses of atria and aortic strips to transmural stimulation. *Jpn. J. Pharmacol.* **22**: 125–135.

38. Najer, H., Giudicelli, R. and Sette, J. (1962) Guanidines douées d'activité antihypertensive, 3e mémoire: N-β-guanidinoéthyl azabicyclo alcanes. *Bull. Soc. Chim. France* 1593–1597.

39. Anonymous. (1964) New basic derivatives of 6,9-endomethylene-3-azabicyclo[4.3.0]nonane. British patent 972 088 (Feb. 19, 1962 to Laboratoire Lumière, S. A.).

40. Anonymous. (1964) New basic derivatives of 6,9-endoxo-3-azabicyclo[4.3.0]nonane. British patent 973 533 (Feb. 21, 1962 to Laboratoire Lumière, S. A.).

41. Jongebreur, G. (1952) Relation between the chemical constitution and the pharmacological action, especially on the coronary vessels of the heart, of some synthesized pyrones and khellin. *Arch. Int. Pharmacodynamie* **90**: 384–411.

42. Janssen, P. A. J. and Van der Eycken, C. A. M. (1968) The chemical anatomy of potent morphine-like analgesics. In Burger, A. (ed.) *Drugs Affecting the Central Nervous System*, pp. 25–60. Marcel Dekker, New York.

43. Hjorth, S., Carlsson, A., Wikström, H., Lindberg, P., Sanchez, D., Hacksell, U., Arvidsson, L. -E., Svensson, U. and Nilsson, J. L. G. (1981) 3-PPP, a new centrally acting DA-receptor agonist with selectivity for autoreceptors. *Life Sci.* **28**: 1225–1238.

44. Kelly, T. R., Howard, H. R., Koe, K. and Sarges, R. (1985) Synthesis and dopamine autoreceptor activity of a 5-(methylmercapto)methyl-substituted derivative of (±)-3-PPP (3-(3-hydroxyphenyl)-1-n-propylpiperidine). *J. Med. Chem.* **28**: 1368–1371.

45. Fuller, R. W., Clemens, J. A., Kornfeld, E. C., Snoddy, H. D., Smalstig, E. B. and Bach, N. J. (1979) Effects of (8β)-8-[(methylthio) methyl]-6-propylergoline on dopaminergic function and brain dopamine turnover in rats. *Life Sci.* **24**: 375–382.

46. Bach, N. J., Kornfeld, E. C., Jones, N. D., Chaney, M. O., Dorman, D. E., Paschal, J. W., Clemens, J. A. and Smalstig, E. B. (1980) Bicyclic and tricyclic ergoline partial structures. Rigid 3-(2-aminoethyl)pyrazoles as dopamine agonists. *J. Med. Chem.* **23**: 481–491.

47. Chang, R. S. L. and Lotti, V. Y. (1986) Biochemical and pharmacological characterization of an extremely potent and selective nonpeptide CCK antagonist. *Proc. Natl. Acad. Sci. USA* **83**: 4923–4926.

48. Bock, M. G., DiPardo, R. M., Rittle, K. E., Evans, B. E., Freidinger, R. M., Veber, D. F., Chang, R. S. L., Chen, T.-B., Keegan, M. E. and Lotti, V. J. (1986) Cholecystokinin antagonists. Synthesis of asperlicin analogues with improved potency and water solubility. *J. Med. Chem.* **29**: 1941–1945.

49. Evans, B. E., Rittle, K. E., Bock, M. G. *et al.* (1988) Methods for drug discovery: development of potent, selective, orally effective cholecystokin antagonists. *J. Med. Chem.* **31**: 2235–2246.

50. Bruderlein, F. T., Humber, L. G. and Voith, K. (1975) Neuroleptic agents of the benzocycloheptapyridoisoquinoline series. 1. Syntheses and stereochemical and structural requirements for activity of butaclamol and related compounds. *J. Med. Chem.* **18**: 185–191.

51. Imhof, R., Kyburz, E. and Daly, J. J. (1984) Design, synthesis, and X-ray data of novel potential antipsychotic agents. Substituted 7-phenylquinolizidines: stereospecific, neuroleptic, and antinociceptive properties. *J. Med. Chem.* **27**: 165–175.

52. Evans, R. H., Francis, A. A., Jones, A. W., Smith, D. A. S. and Watkins, J. C. (1982) The effects of a series of ω-phosphonic α-carboxylic amino acids on electrically evoked and excitant amino acid-induced responses in isolated spinal cord preparations. *Br. J. Pharmacol.* **75**: 65–75.

53. Hutchinson, A. J., Williams, M., Angst, C. *et al.* (1989) 4-(Phosphonoalkyl) and 4-(phosphonoalkenyl)-2-piperidinecarboxylic acids: synthesis, activity at N-methyl-D-aspartic acid receptors, and anticonvulsant activity. *J. Med. Chem.* **32**: 2171–2178.

54. Humblet, C., Johnson, G., Malone, T. and Ortwine, D. F. (1990) Design, synthesis and molecular modelling of phosphonoalkyl-substituted tetrahydroisoquinolines as competitive NMDA antagonists. In *Proceedings of the XIth International Symposium on Medicinal Chemistry*, Jerusalem, Israel.

55. Ornstein, P. L., Arnold, M. D., Augenstein, N. K., Lodge, D., Leander, J. D. and Schoepp, D. D. (1993) (3SR,4aRS,6RS,8aRS)-6-[2-(1H-Tetrazol-5-yl)ethyl]decahydroisoquinoline-3-carboxylic acid: a structurally novel, systematically active, competitive AMPA receptor antagonist. *J. Med. Chem.* **36**: 2046–2048.

56. Koga, H., Itoh, A., Murayama, S., Suzue, S. and Irikura, T. (1980) Structure–activity relationships of antibacterial 6,7- and 7,8-disubstituted 1-alkyl-1,4-dihydro-4-oxoquinoline-3-carboxylic acids. *J. Med. Chem.* **23**: 1358–1363.

57. Jinbo, Y., Taguchi, M., Inoue, Y., Kondo, H., Miyasaka, T., Tsujishita, H., Sakamoto, F. and Tsukamoto, G. (1993) Synthesis and antibacterial activity of a new series of tetracyclic pyridone carboxylic acids. 2. *J. Med. Chem.* **36**: 3148–3153.

58. Wijngaarde van, I., Hamminga, D., Hes, R. V., Standaar, P. J., Tipker, J., Tulp, M. T. M., Mol, F., Olivier, B. and Jonge de, A. (1993) Development of high-affinity 5-HT3 receptor antagonists. Structure–affinity relationships of novel 1,7-annelated indole derivatives. 1. *J. Med. Chem.* **36**: 3693–3699.

59. Stanton, J. L., Sperbeck, D. M., Trapani, A. J., Cote, D., Sakane, Y., Berry, C. J. and Ghai, R. D. (1993) Heterocyclic lactam derivatives as dual angiotensin converting enzyme and neutral endopeptidase 24.11 inhibitors. *J. Med. Chem.* **36**: 3829–3833.

15

Identical and Nonidentical Twin Drugs

JEAN-JACQUES BOURGUIGNON

> *There is in living organisms, human beings and societies a balance*
> *between these main two forces, between creative asymmetry,*
> *imagination, or revolution and cooperative symmetry logic or order;*
> *between Dionysios and Apollon*
> Jean-Pierre Changeux

THE PRACTICE OF MEDICINAL CHEMISTRY
ISBN 0-12-744640-0

I.   INTRODUCTION

The present chapter deals with *twin drugs*, which means drugs containing two pharmacophoric groups combined *covalently* in a single molecule. This definition excludes the combination of two drugs in one salt such as procaine penicillin.[1] Twin drugs may result from the combination of two identical moieties (identical twin drugs), or from the combination of two different drug entities (nonidentical twin drugs). The first strategy consists of molecular variations based on duplication, while the second one results from associative synthesis (Fig. 15.1).

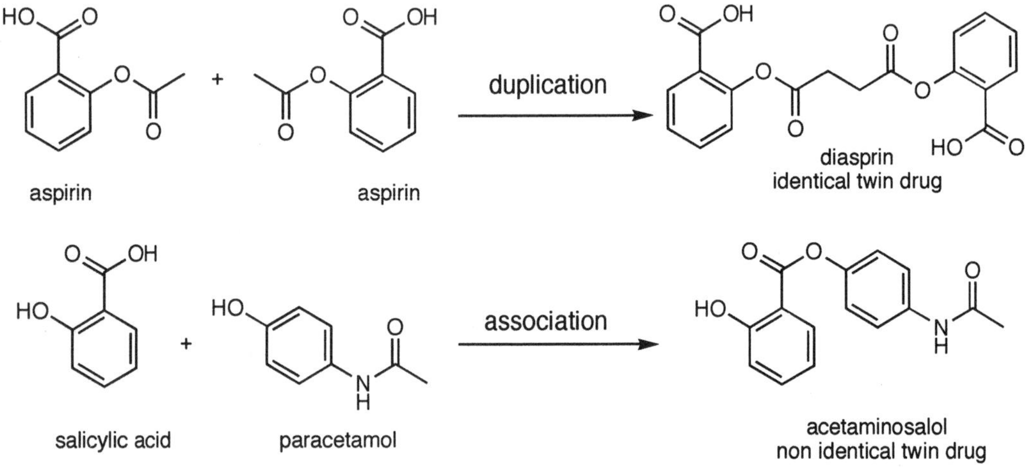

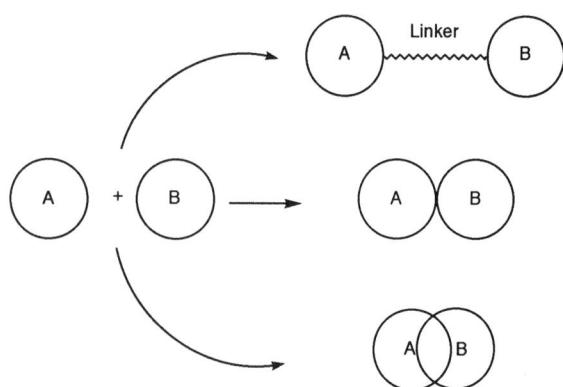

Fig. 15.1   Identical and non identical analgesic twin drugs.

The two drug entities have to be located at the most appropriate distance for interaction with the specific binding sites. They can be linked by a spacer group, placed close together (no linker), or even overlap (Fig. 15.2). Sometimes the spacer group can establish additional interactions, thus increasing the affinity for a specific target.

Fig. 15.2   Various modes of combining two moieties in twin drugs. A = B, identical twin drugs; A ≠ B, non-identical twin drugs.

Concerning the mode of association of the two drug entities, and referring to polymer chemistry nomenclature, each molecule can be formally represented with a head (H) and a tail (T), and thus may offer different modes of connection (Fig. 15.3).

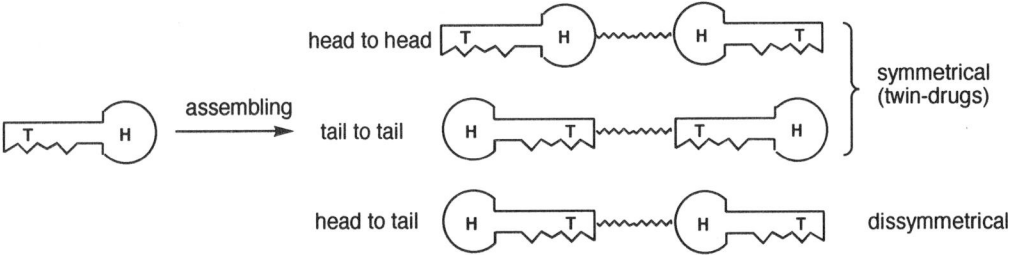

Fig. 15.3 Modes of connection of the two components in identical twin drugs.

Another aspect that has to be considered when designing twin drugs relates to their metabolic fate. Two possibilities can be envisaged: (1) The twin drug regenerates its constituents *in vivo*; it has then to be considered as a prodrug, the duplication procedure having only improved the pharmacokinetic or the pharmaceutic properties; (2) The twin drug is not split *in vivo*; the rationale of this procedure is not always obvious. It suggests the existence of a symmetrical architecture in the target macromolecule, as there is the possibility of occupying an additional binding site. This site is not necessarily involved in triggering the biological response but can entail an increase in affinity.

The majority of the identical twin drugs described in the literature are symmetrical and bind to a single target macromolecule. The two pharmacophoric moieties, or functional groups, are identical, and are linked in a symmetrical fashion involving head-to-head or tail-to-tail association modes (Fig. 15.4). However head-to-tail connected twin drugs are not uncommon as illustrated by salicyl salicylate and amentoflavone (Fig. 15.4).

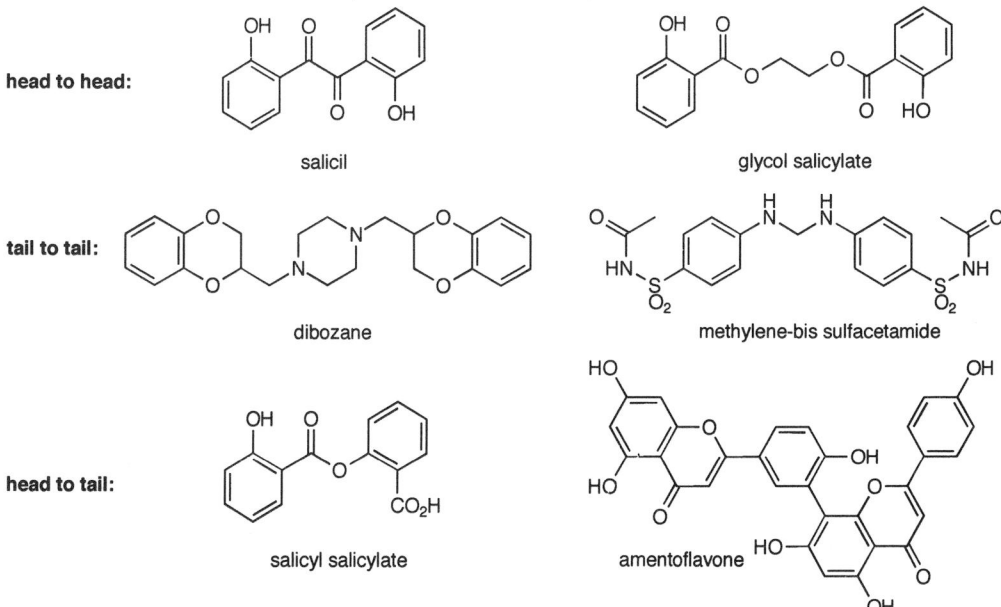

Fig. 15.4 Association modes for identical twin drugs.

In nonidentical twin drugs the two pharmacophoric groups bind to different biological targets and thus elicit different pharmacological responses. Such drugs are also termed *dual-acting drugs* or hybrids, and their design was called the *symbiotic approach* by Baldwin *et al.*[2] Two strategies govern this approach (Fig. 15.5). The first combines, in a kind of chimera, two nonidentical pharmacophoric moieties into structurally allowed areas of the molecule so as to build a hybrid drug (associative synthesis). The second strategy starts with a lead compound found to exhibit already both activities (intrinsically dual-acting drug), and proceeds to its optimization. The starting dual acting lead compounds can be selected by computerized matching of biological profiles.[2]

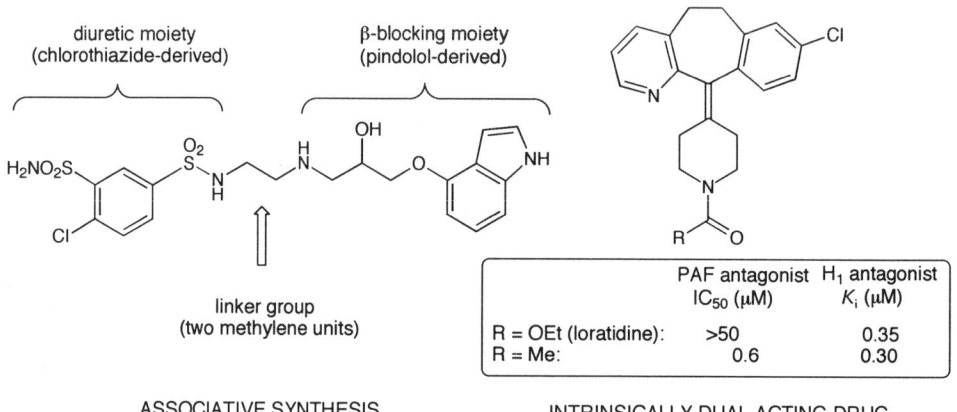

	PAF antagonist IC$_{50}$ (µM)	H$_1$ antagonist K$_i$ (µM)
R = OEt (loratidine):	>50	0.35
R = Me:	0.6	0.30

Fig. 15.5   Twin drugs acting at two different targets: they can result from the combination of two different drugs[3] or from a unique molecule intrinsically combining two activities.[4]

The main advantage of the symbiotic approach over the concomitant administration of two separated drugs resides in the pharmacokinetics. When a mixture of two drugs is administered, each pharmacological activity depends on individual absorption, metabolism, and excretion profiles, whereas the hybrid presents its own pharmacokinetic profile with some expected improvement in its *in vivo* efficacy. In particular, the twin drug must express both activities in an appropriate balance. A *stoichiometric* association of diazepam (2–20 mg/day) with aspirin (200–2000 mg/day) would be nonsense. Another conceptual aspect is that, even when a compound shows equal affinities for two different receptors, it cannot interact *simultaneously* with both of them.

II.   IDENTICAL TWIN DRUGS

A.   Symmetry in natural compounds

Nature is efficient in producing compounds with a high degree of symmetry. It is now claimed that symmetry-involving forces including electromagnetic forces are important in biology, particularly for the assembly of macromolecules. In addition, the ordering of water in organized systems and the symmetry of interactions may play important roles in biological processes.[5-7] As typical examples to be given here, DNA, by means of its symmetrical double-stranded structure, determines the cell's morphology and function. The aggregation of insulin monomers to hexamers in the presence of zinc affords a macromolecular complex with high degree of symmetry[8] (C_3 symmetry). These well-organized macromolecular systems constitute binding sites for smaller molecules including water and ions.

Symmetrical natural compounds present generally a C_2 symmetry axis, examples are the alkaloids lobelanine, sparteine, carzinophilin A or isochondrodendrine, the antibiotic actinomycin C, the anticoagulant dicumarol and the antispermatogenic gossypol[1,9] (Fig. 15.6). Gossypol, a bisphenolic compound isolated from cottonseed oil, interferes with oestradiol and is used in China for its direct antispermatogenic activity. It suffers, however, from considerable side-effects.

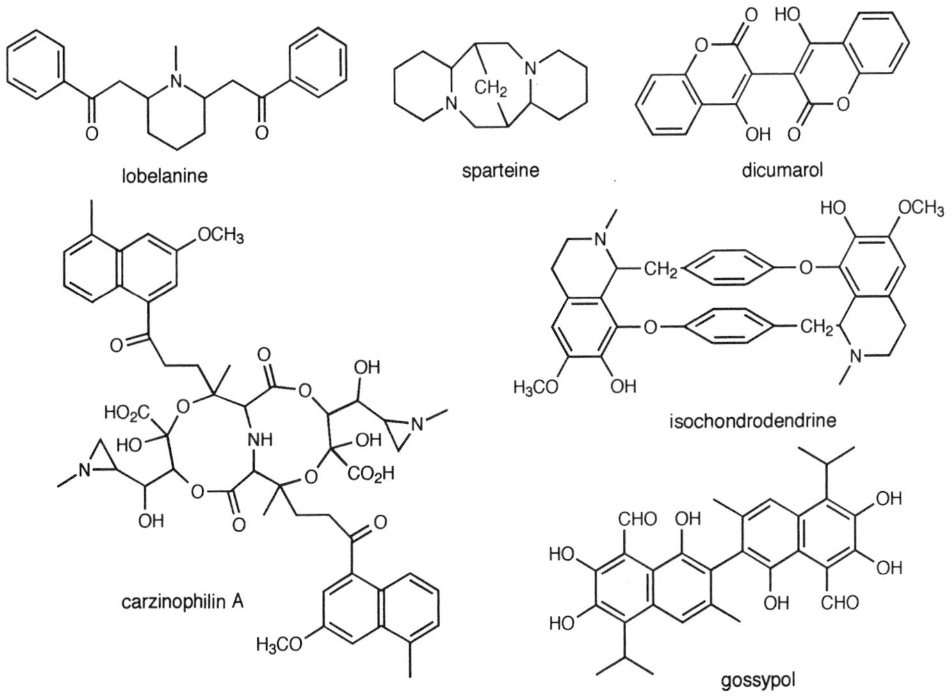

Fig. 15.6 Symmetrical natural compounds presenting a C_2 symmetry axis.

However, some examples of C_3 symmetrical compounds are known. Valinomycin, a cyclic peptide lactone antibiotic, is a highly selective K$^+$-carrier. It consists of a cyclic trimer of the tetrapeptide L-valine, D-α-hydroxyisovaleric acid (Hyi), D-valine and L-lactate (Fig. 15.7). The C_3 symmetrical growth-promoting agent enterobactin is a cyclic lactonic N-acylated serine trimer.

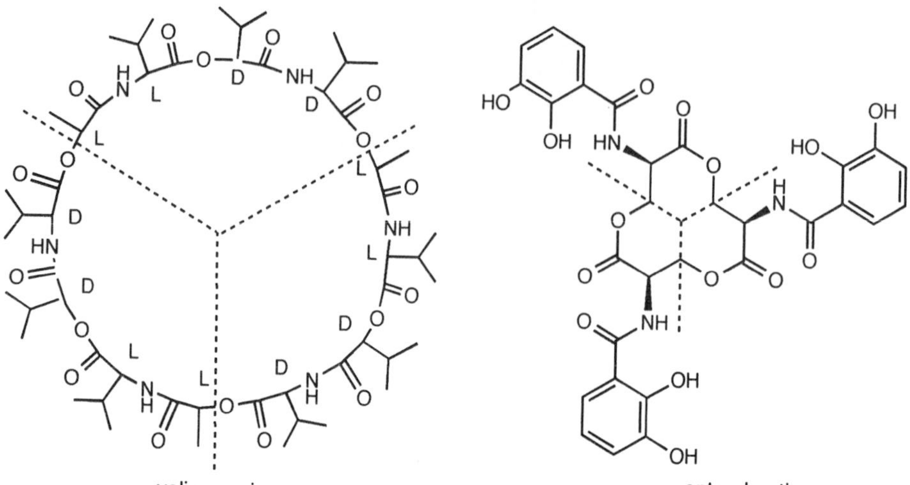

valinomycin   enterobactin

Fig. 15.7   Valinomycin and enterobactin: two natural antibiotics presenting a C_3 symmetry axis.

B.   Twin drugs acting on receptors

Identical twin drugs have shown increasing potencies and/or modified selectivity profiles as receptor ligands when compared to their corresponding single drug.

1.   Ligands of biogenic amine receptors

Several receptors of biogenic amines (catecholamines), quaternary ammoniums (acetylcholine, PAF-acether), and peptides (angiotensin, endothelin) belong to the well-known class of G-protein-coupled receptors. They present one subunit with seven transmembrane spanning domains, three extracellular and three intracellular loops, which are coupled to G-proteins. Duplication of drugs within this series of ligands has been efficient in several cases.

(a) Adrenergic receptors.   The development of polyamine disulphides such as APC or benextramine (Fig. 15.8) allowed the hypothesis of symmetrical properties of α-adrenergic receptors.[10] Among the α-adrenergic antagonists, duplication of the benzodioxane piperoxan led to dibozane.[1] Several β$_1$-selective adrenoreceptor antagonists have been designed by duplication of the well-known propanolamine structure, oxprenolol.[1.1] Similarly the vasodilator coralgil presents a symmetrical structure that results from the appropriate duplication of a parent compound.[1]

(b) Muscarinic acetylcholine receptors.   Methoctramine (Fig. 15.9) is a useful probe for characterizing acetylcholine muscarinic receptor subtypes where it appears as a selective M$_2$-antagonist (pA_2 = 7.8; guinea-pig left atrium[12]). Interestingly, benextramine (Fig. 15.8), the closely related structural analogue of methoctramine, shows high affinity for two other G-protein-coupled receptors (α-adrenergic receptor, neuropeptide Y receptor). In other words, starting from a common pattern, symmetrical twin drugs acting as antagonists at different G-protein-coupled receptors, have been designed. The replacement of the 2-methoxybenzyl group

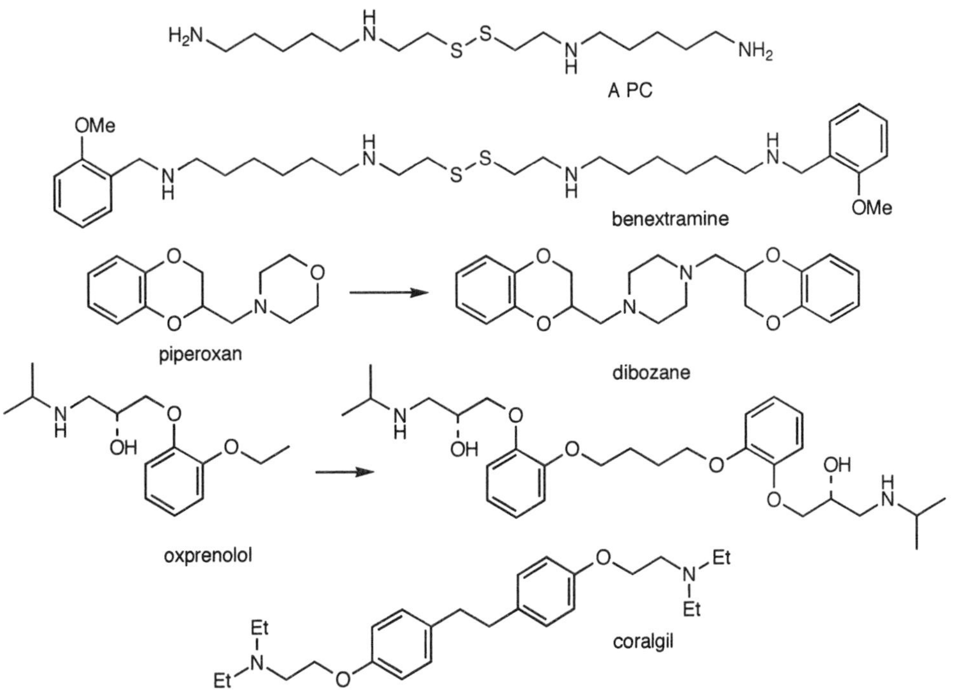

Fig. 15.8 Adrenergic ligands.

in methoctramine by the hydrophobic tricyclic moiety of pirenzepine leads to a very potent M_2-antagonist with a pA_2 of 9.14, whereas pirenzepine is known as a selective M_1-antagonist. Thus, duplication of pirenzepine leads to a potent antagonist with a reversed M_2/M_1 selectivity profile.[12] Similarly duplication of N-(3-dimethylaminopropyl)phthalimide leads to N,N'-dimethyl-N,N'-[3-(2-phthalimido)propyl-1,6-hexanediamine (Fig. 15.9), that is also a potent and selective M_2 antagonist ($K_i = 18$ nM).[13]

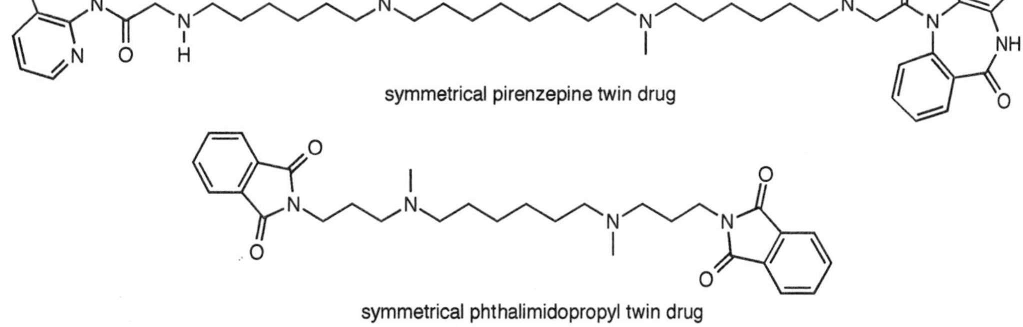

Fig. 15.9 Ligands of the muscarinic acetylcholine receptor.

(c) PAF-acether receptors.   Several natural products such as veraguensin[14] were found to inhibit the binding of the platelet-activating factor (PAF) to its specific receptor site (IC$_{50}$ 1.1 µM). Starting from veraguensin, further investigation led to the design of the more potent symmetrical compound L 652 731 2 (IC$_{50}$ = 19 nM; Fig. 15.10), or the unsymmetrical analogue L 659 989 3 (IC$_{50}$ =1 nM). Other symmetrical PAF-antagonists have been prepared starting from piperazine as symmetrical core[15,16] (Fig.15.10).

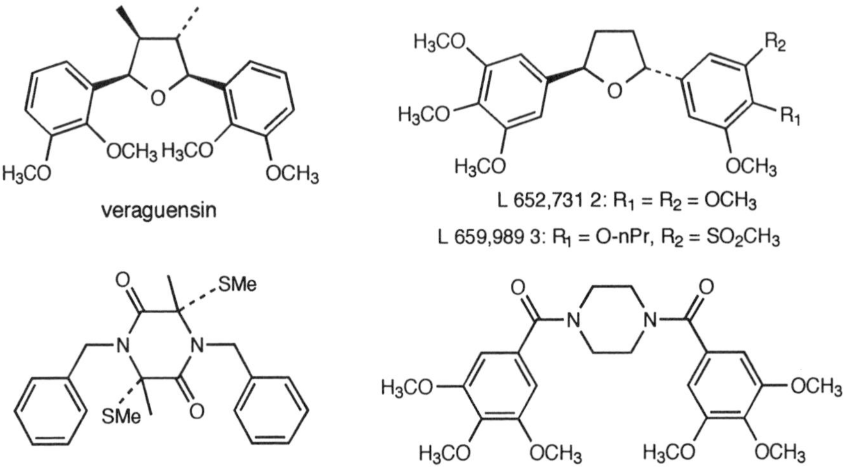

Fig. 15.10   PAF-acether antagonists.

2.   Ligands of peptide receptors

Several studies have previously reported that dimerization of peptidergic receptor ligands can result in an increase in affinity, potency, and/or metabolic resistance (see references 8–15 in ref. 17) A systematic study of dimerization of cysteine-containing bradykinin peptidic analogues by means of various bismaleidoalkane linkers led to compounds with a 10- to 50-fold higher *in vitro* activity.[17] Initial screening efforts directed toward the discovery of small molecules possessing bradykinin receptor activity identified symmetrical bis-cationic phosphonium salts as lead compounds.[18] They are fairly potent ligands of the bradykinin receptors (K_i = 3 µM). However, the distance separating the positively charged salts was determined to be approximately 10 Å. This distance is in good agreement with that found between guanidinium cations of Arg(1) and Arg(9) in an energetically stable conformation of bradykinin.

Several covalently linked insulin dimers have been used for the study of the relationship between the binding of insulin to its receptor and subsequent events in insulin action mediated by a specific protein kinase.[19]

In attempts to demonstrate that opioid receptors can be crosslinked, opioid-peptides, opiate alkaloids and benzomorphans have been dimerized (see references 1–9 in ref. 20) In several cases the resulting compounds have shown significant increases in potencies when compared to their monomeric counterparts. The increase in potency, correlated with affinity for specific classes of opioid receptors, depends on the length of the spacer group (see Fig. 15.11). Thus, the optimal

ENKEPHALIN TWIN DRUGS	IC$_{50}$, nM	
	δ	μ
H-Tyr-D-Ala-Gly-Phe-NH$_2$	33	3
H-Tyr-D-Ala-Gly-Phe-NH | (CH$_2$)$_n$ | H-Tyr-D-Ala-Gly-Phe-NH	n = 2 n = 12	1.7 1.1	1.8 96

norbinaltorphimine

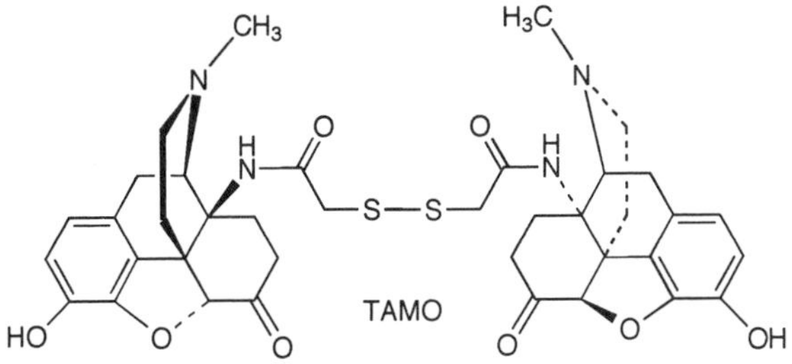

TAMO

Fig. 15.11   Dimeric ligands for opioid receptors.

length of opioid twin drugs spacers highlights specific membrane organization, differing from one opioid receptor to the other.[21,22]

Dimeric enkephalines have shown better analgesic properties than their monomeric counterparts.[2] Norbinaltorphimine (Fig. 15.11), a dimeric morphine derivative, is a selective antagonist for the κ opioid receptor and is widely used as a pharmacological tool in opioid research.[23] The design of this compound was based originally on the assumption that bridging of two opioid pharmacophores might constitute a means conferring selectivity (see references 3–5 in ref. 23) The authors suggest that the selectivity for κ receptors arises as a consequence of the second half of the molecule, which facilitates its interaction with a typical subsite of the κ receptor. Interestingly another structurally related compound, the C$_2$-symmetrical dithiobisdihydromorphinone (TAMO) binds covalently to the μ opioid receptor with long-term antagonistic properties.[24]

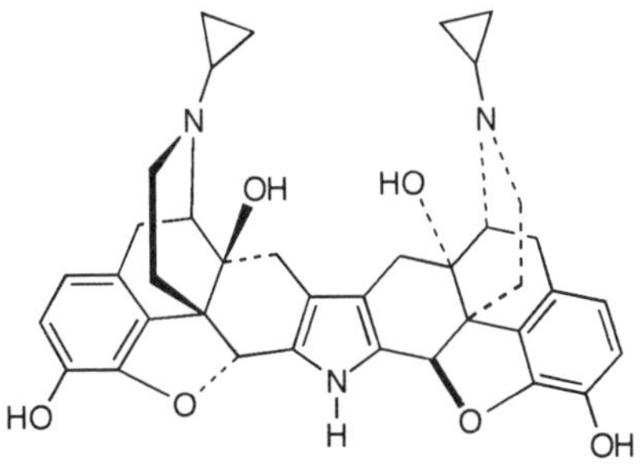

Benextramine (BTX) produces a long-acting antagonism of neuropeptide Y (NPY)-induced pressor activity, and irreversibly inhibits [³H]NPY binding to a subpopulation of neuropeptide Y binding sites in rat membranes.[25]

3.   Other examples of identical twin drugs as receptor ligands

The Ca^{2+} channel antagonist nifedipine, a typical representative of 1,4-dihydropyridines, has been used to explore the topographic relationship between 1,4-dihydropyridine binding sites within the voltage-dependent Ca^{2+} channel complex. A series of 1-n-alkane-diylbis-1,4-dihydropyridines were synthesized and tested on [³H]nitrendipine binding. Compared to the highly potent nitrendipine (IC$_{50}$ = 0.2 nM), the symmetrical bis-dihydropyridine BDHP is about ten times as potent[26] (Fig. 15.12).

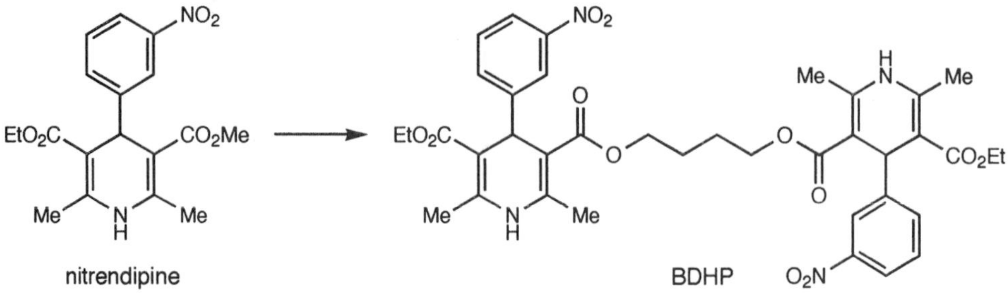

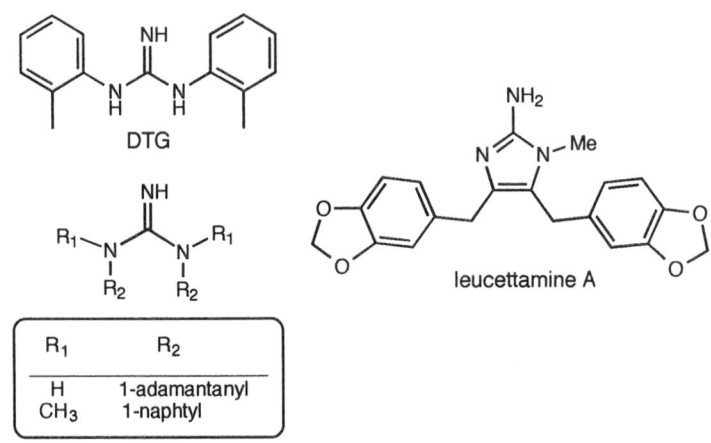

Fig. 15.12   Duplication of nitrendipine, a Ca^{2+} channel antagonist.

Ditolylguanidine (DTG, Fig. 15.13) is a selective and potent ligand for the brain σ binding site, and presents original behavioural properties when compared with opioid and phencyclidine (PCP)-like drugs.[27] Other analogues (R = adamantanyl, naphtyl) bind potently to PCP receptors, and are promising as neuroprotective agents.[28] The N-methyl derivative of the 2-aminoimidazole alkaloid leucettamine A, isolated from marine sponge, is a pure antagonist of leukotriene B_4 (LTB4) receptors ($K_i = 1.3\,\mu M$).[29]

R_1	R_2
H	1-adamantanyl
CH_3	1-naphtyl

Fig. 15.13   Other examples of symmetrical receptor ligands.

C.   Twin drugs as enzyme inhibitors

Kinetic manifestations of molecular symmetry changes have been analysed and have highlighted an effective regulation of enzyme activity.[30] Moreover the symmetrical arrangement of the enzyme into homodimers or tetramers lies the active site of the enzyme in a highly symmetrical fashion. To the symmetrical binding site of the enzyme will correspond generally symmetrical inhibitors (identical twin drugs).

1.   HIV-enzyme inhibitors

Different targets essential for viral replication have been selected in the search for new leads as anti-HIV (human immunodeficiency virus) compounds. One of them is the HIV reverse transcriptase (RT). The type 1 and type 2 RT are heterodimers consisting of two chains, which share a high degree of homology in their amino acid sequences. Numerous inhibitors of the HIV RT are known (Fig. 15.14), but they are unable to treat AIDS. The bisnaphthalene trisulfonic acid derivative suramin is a well-known potent inhibitor of HIV-1 RT, and was used as a lead for the search of novel anti-HIV drugs.[31] SAR analysis led to suramin monomeric derivatives with comparable *in vitro* potencies. Most striking, however, is the influence of the palmitoyl functional group in this series of compounds in conferring activity against both HIV-1 and HIV-2 RT.

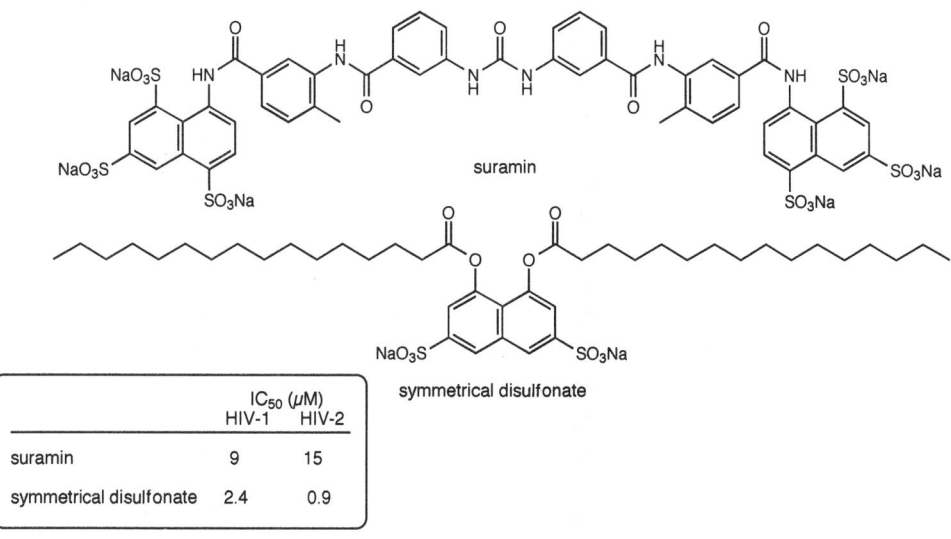

	IC$_{50}$ (µM)	
	HIV-1	HIV-2
suramin	9	15
symmetrical disulfonate	2.4	0.9

Fig. 15.14   HIV reverse transcriptase inhibitors.

The other important enzyme for viral replication is the HIV protease (HIV PR).[32] In just a few years, because of its obvious therapeutic interest, this enzyme has become one of the best-characterized enzymes. More than 170 structures of HIV PR and its complexes with various inhibitors have been solved by protein crystallography techniques.[32,33] It is a homodimeric aspartic protease. In Chapter 19, Fig. 19.21 clearly shows the symmetrical nature of the crystallized enzyme. The conserved active-site residues (Asp,[25] Thr[26] and Gly[27] from both monomers) are located in loops, and form a symmetrical and highly hydrogen-bonded arrangement.[32] However, from a mechanistic point of view, the reaction, which involves a water molecule, is not symmetrical because one of the two Asp residues is protonated and then establishes an H-bond with a specific amide oxygen of the substrate (see Fig. 15.15). The other is ionized and can ionize the water molecule, which hydrolyses properly the amide function between the tyrosyl and prolyl residues.[34]

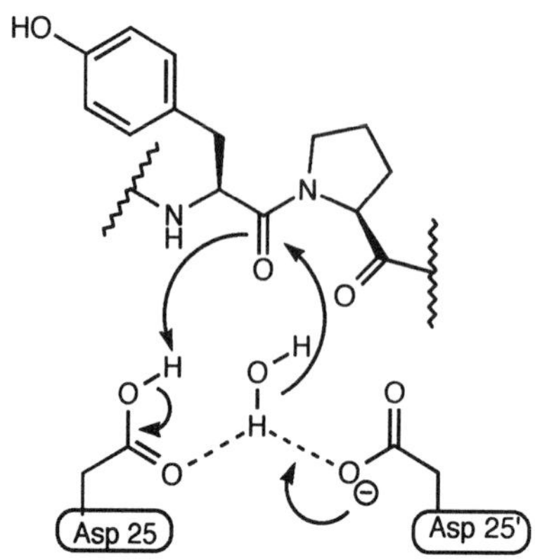

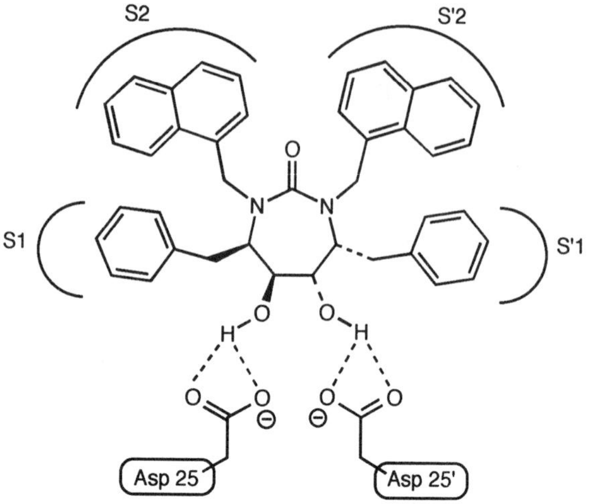

Fig. 15.15   The Asp-assisted hydrolysis of Tyr-Pro by HIV protease is a dissymmetrical process, whereas the inhibition of the enzyme by compound XK 263 implies a C_2 symmetrical complex.

Because retroviral proteases are symmetrical homodimers, efforts were directed toward inhibitors that would embody the predicted characteristic of the enzyme active site. The design should satisfy a major constraint: for a productive and symmetrical interaction between the inhibitor and enzyme to occur, their C_2 axes should coincide. The design of inhibitors of HIV PR has led to symmetrical compounds, which can be divided into two groups (i): pseudosymmetrical compounds, which contain asymmetric atoms in close proximity to the inhibitor two-fold axis; (ii) fully C_2-symmetrical inhibitors. The first symmetrical inhibitors were described by Erickson *et al.*[35] The most active compound was the pseudosymmetrical alcohol A 74 704 (Fig. 15.16). A series of C_2 symmetrical diols were also described. The chirality of alcohols does not influence the affinity of these compounds.[36] The cyclic urea XK 263[32] (Fig. 15.15) showed about the same potency as the diol A 75 925.

From the screening program on penicillin derivatives, followed by design and synthesis of lead compounds, emerged the final product GR-116624X[32,37] (Fig. 15.16), a C_2 symmetrical diamide. They also effectively blocked the cytopathic effect of HIV-1 in cellular assays.

2.   Identical twin drugs as protein kinase inhibitors

The structure of the native insulin receptor was established as a disulphide-linked heterotetramer β–α–α–β. However, it is more appropriate to regard the insulin receptor as a homodimer of two α–β units. It was found that the β-subunit possessed intrinsic tyrosine-specific protein kinase activity which requires β–β interaction.[8] Therefore, tyrosine protein kinase active sites are symmetrically located in the receptor complex. It is not surprising to find many other examples of protein kinase inhibitors showing the same symmetrical characteristics.

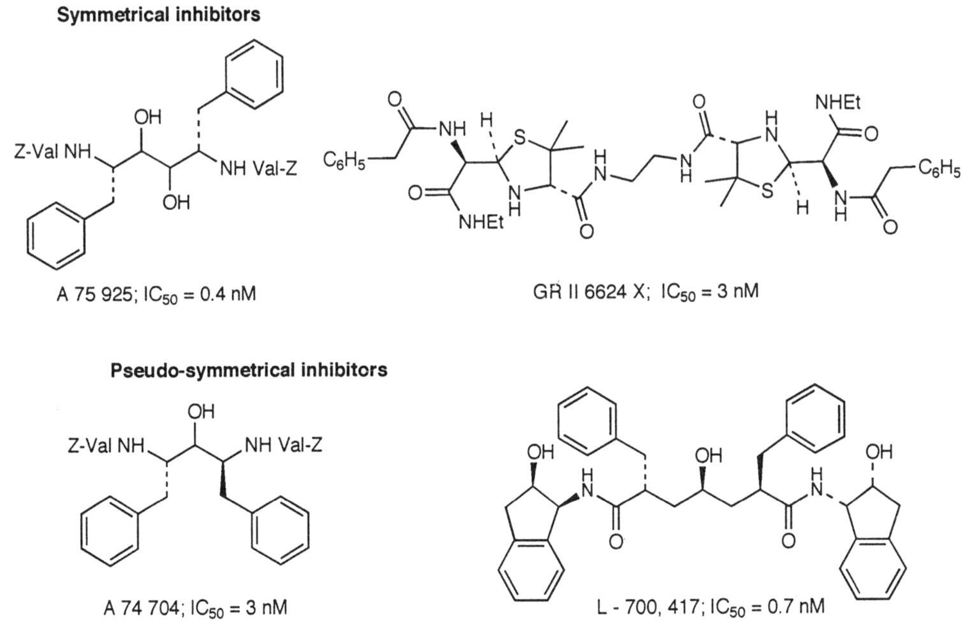

Symmetrical inhibitors

A 75 925; IC_{50} = 0.4 nM   GR II 6624 X; IC_{50} = 3 nM

Pseudo-symmetrical inhibitors

A 74 704; IC_{50} = 3 nM   L - 700, 417; IC_{50} = 0.7 nM

Fig. 15.16   Symmetrical and pseudosymmetrical HIV protease inhibitors.

The protein kinase C (PKC) isoenzyme family plays a pivotal role in the signal transduction pathways of hormones, neurotransmitters and other endogenous substances. Activation of PKC following receptor occupation leads to catalytic transfer of γ-phosphate of ATP to serine or threonine in proteins. Thus PKC appears as a modulator of mechanisms of cell proliferation and gene expression. The microbial alkaloid staurosporine is a potent PKC-inhibitor (IC_{50} = 9 nM), but is nonselective and inhibits many other PKs. Using its structure as a guide, the staurosporine aglycon (Fig. 15.17) was found to exhibit an IC_{50} of 300 nM, but with an improved selectivity profile compared to the native alkaloid.[38] Starting from this parent compound, dianilinophthalimides and diindolyl maleimides were prepared. They are potent PK inhibitors, but with some interesting reverse selectivity profile, when considering epidermal growth factor (EGF) receptor protein kinase and PKC. Thus the IC_{50} values (nM) for the EGF receptor protein kinase and for the protein kinase C, are respectively 0.3/80 for the dianilinophthalimides, and >80/0.2 for the diindolyl maleimides.

The *trans*-stilbene piceatannol, a known antileukaemic principle in the seeds of *Euphorbia lagascae*, inhibits protein tyrosine kinase (PTK).[39] It was chosen as a lead compound for further SAR analysis, and the fully symmetrical 5-hydroxy isomer was found four times more potent as a PTK inhibitor than piceatannol. In recent years tyrphostins were described as PTK inhibitors. When compared with the reference monomer A 46, the bistyrphostin was found to be 150 times more potent in protein tyrosine kinase assays (Fig. 15.17).[40]

Other natural polycyclic compounds like hypericin proved to be PKC inhibitors, and present generally high degrees of symmetry.[41] All these compounds might be useful as chemotherapeutic agents for human cancer, immune and metabolic disorders.

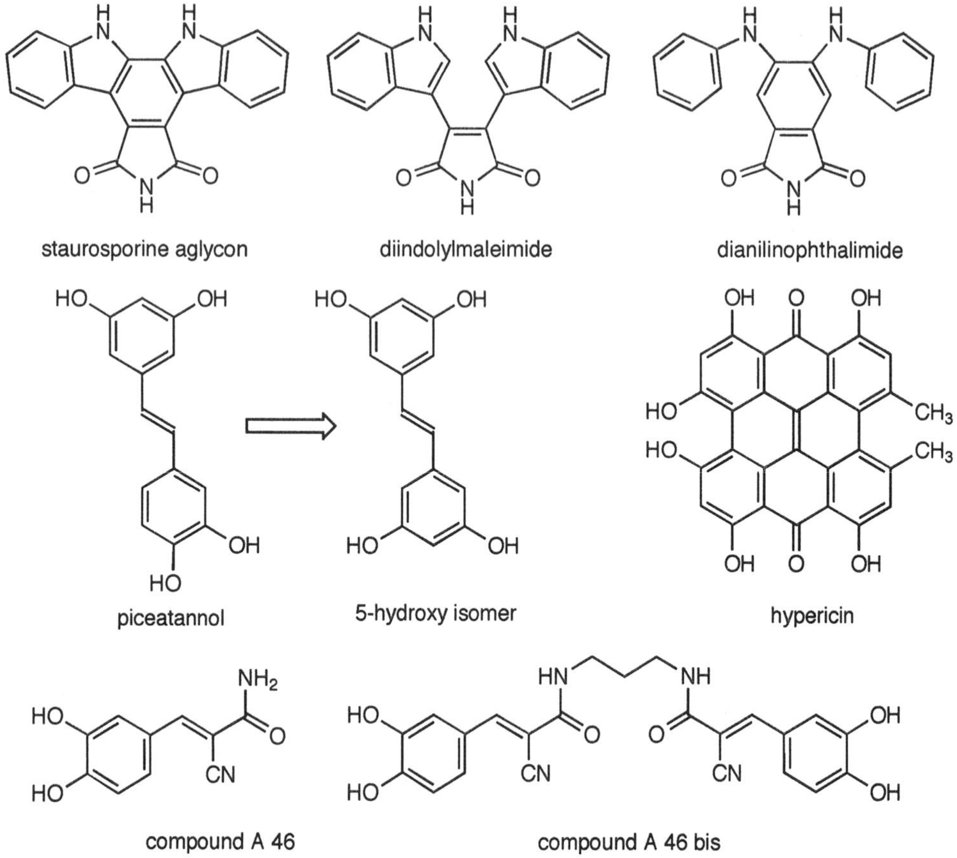

Fig. 15.17   Protein kinase inhibitors.

3.   *Other identical twin drugs as enzyme inhibitors*

Collagen is deposited during life-threatening fibroses. Inhibition of prolyl hydrolase may have some therapeutic interest as this enzyme is involved in collagen biosynthesis. The 2,2'-bipyridine bearing in a symmetrical manner two carboxylates is the most potent inhibitor (IC_{50} = 0.2 μM) of this enzyme yet reported.[42] The strong beneficial effect of drug duplication observed here may result in a binding mode at a single binding site in each catalytic subunit. The symmetrical diacid MDL 201 404 (Fig. 15.18) inhibits human neutrophil elastase.[43] This compound is also effective in animal models of inflammation and has been selected as a clinical candidate.

Bridged dinucleosides are competitive inhibitors of rat liver adenosine kinases.[44] In particular, the bisadenosine dodecane showed an IC_{50} of 75 nM.

A series of symmetrical ureas have been described as inhibitors of acyl-CoA cholesterol acyltransferase (ACAT).[45] The best compound (YM 17E), (IC_{50} = 44 nM) is currently under further development as possible anticholesterolaemic drug.

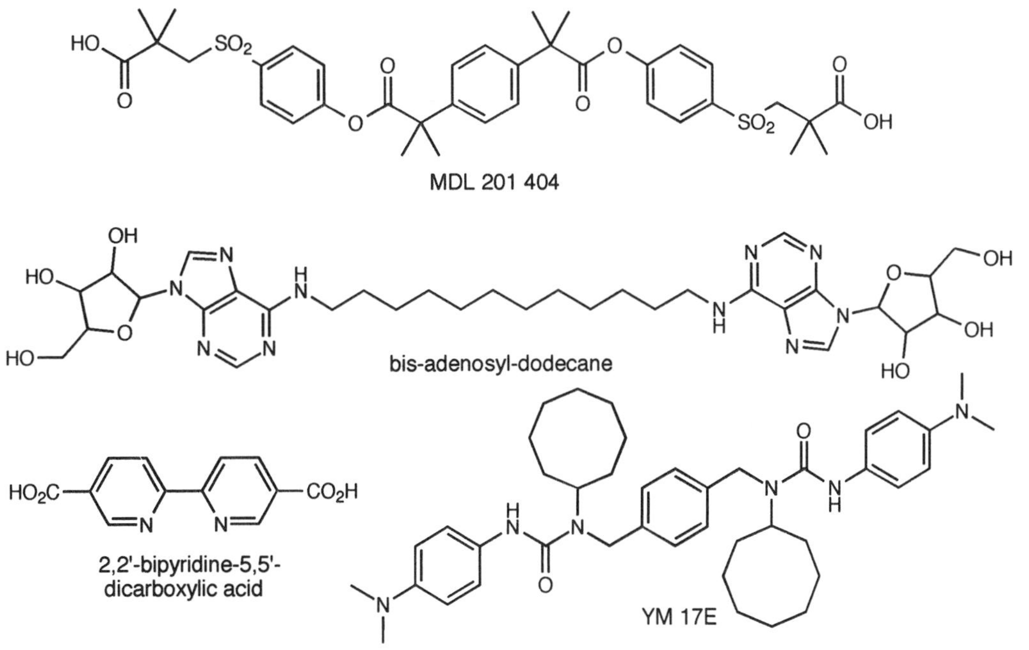

Fig. 15.18 Identical twin drugs as various enzyme inhibitors.

Benzamidine is a competitive inhibitor of many trypsin-like serine proteases including factor Xa. A series of bisbenzamidines were shown to be potent inhibitors of factor Xa[46] (Fig. 15.19). Modification of the linker between the two amidino groups (DABE, K_i = 570 nM) and introduction of an accessory binding site through a carbonyl group yielded a highly potent inhibitor of bovine Xa (BABCH, K_i = 13 nM). Unfortunately, this compound also inhibits other enzymes belonging to the same family (trypsin, urokinase and plasmin).

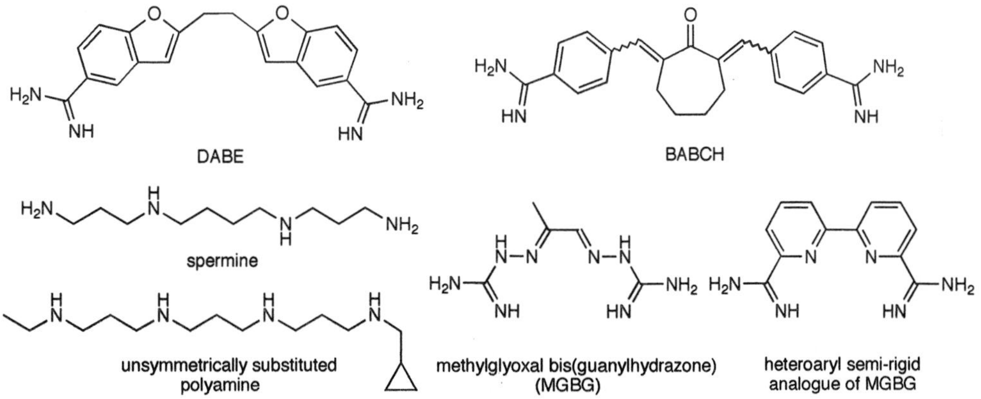

Fig. 15.19 Diamidines, polyamines and methylglyoxal bis(guanyl hydrazone).

The enzymes involved in the polyamine metabolic pathway have recently been the subject of intensive study, and a number of specific inhibitors have been designed as potential antitumour and antiparasitic agents.[47] The diamine putrescine and the polyamines spermidine and spermine play an important role in cell growth. Spermidine-spermine-N_1-acetyltransferase (SSAT) is a rate-limiting step in polyamine catabolism. In contrast to the symmetrical character of substrates (spermine), unsymmetrically substituted polyamine analogues are effective inhibitors of SSAT, and exhibit promising antitumour activity against cultured human lung cancer cells.

S-adenosylmethionine decarboxylase (SAMDC) is another rate-limiting enzyme of polyamine biosynthesis. Its activity is controlled by endogenous polyamines. Interest in SAMDC as a therapeutic target started with the antileukaemic bisguanylhydrazone derivative, an inhibitor of SAMDC (IC_{50} = 1 µM). Analogues were synthesized in order to improve both its potency and its selectivity toward other enzymes.[48] The semirigid fully symmetrical bipyridine analogue was found the most potent (IC_{50} = 6 nM), and selective within this series.

D.   Twin drugs acting as DNA ligands

The DNA molecule is the primary target of many antitumour agents. Among the binding modes of drugs to DNA, both intercalative and nonintercalative mechanisms have been described. It has long been known that small molecules that bind to DNA can distort its structure. For efficient binding by intercalation they require in their structure planar polycyclic systems. However, because of the symmetrical arrangement of the helical double strand, symmetry is also found in the structure of DNA ligands.

Polycyclic systems bearing symmetrical polyamine side-chains, in particular, can interact, as polycations, with the phosphate groups of DNA. The discovery of anthracycline antibiotics led to the synthesis of less toxic symmetrical anthraquinone derivatives (mitoxantrone, ametantrone) that bear aminoethylaminoethanol groups.[49] Two anthracene derivatives,[50] bisantrene and its bis-N,N-dimethylaminoethylaminobenzyl (DAEAB) analogue show the same general structure and mechanism of action (Fig. 15.20).

Pentamidine and the bisamidinobenzimidazoles bind to the minor groove of DNA and show higher affinity for AT-rich regions than for GC base pairs.[51] Compounds with an even number of methylenes connecting benzimidazole rings have a higher affinity for DNA than those with an odd number of methylenes.

A series of 1,4-bis(ethyl)piperazine-derived twin drugs were recently designed as RNA major-groove-binding cations.[52] The piperazine dione NSC 135 758 binds covalently and in a symmetrical manner to DNA.[53] The naturally occurring quinoxaline antitumour antibiotic echinomycin contains two identical chromophores attached symmetrically to a depsipeptide ring (Ser-Ala-Cys-Val)$_2$. As shown by X-ray crystallography, it yields a stable complex with the DNA tetramers d(ACGT)$_2$ and d(TCGA)$_2$.[54] In a similar fashion, the octapeptide YSPTSPSY corresponds mainly to the heptad repeat unit of RNA polymerase II, and interacts with DNA by bisintercalation.[55]

Netropsin and distamycin are prototypical representatives of selective binding agents to the DNA minor groove. They present in their structure N-methylpyrrole carboxamide repeating units. Bisnetropsins linked by various flexible or rigid linkers have been described. The compounds containing rigid fumaryl or p-phenylene dicarbonyl linkers exhibited the highest antiviral and anticancer properties.[56]

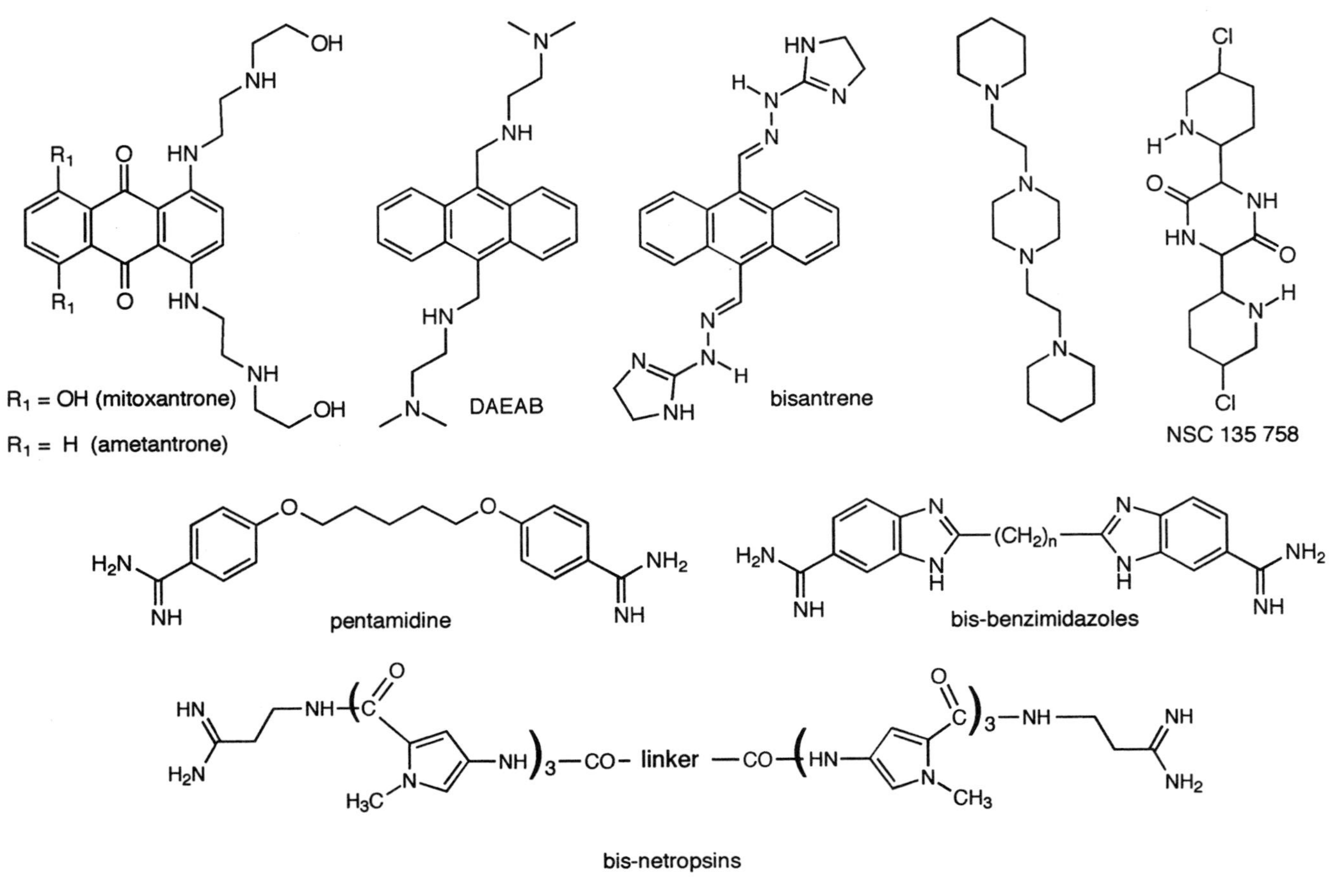

Fig. 15.20 DNA intercalating agents.

E. Other identical twin drugs of pharmacological interest

1. *Twin drugs as surface-active antibacterial agents*

Among the classical twin drugs developed in the past, several were described as efficient surface-active antibacterial agents. The stability of biological membranes is involved in the functioning of cells, including bacteria and fungi. Hence any agent that disrupts the membrane or interferes with its integrity, particularly its symmetry, may cause irreversible damage to the cell. Ionophoric antibiotics can function as 'cage' carriers of an ion through the lipid membrane (for example, valinomycin). Another antibiotic, gramicidin A, a 15-amino-acid peptide, can form a head-to-head helix, spanning the total width of the cell membrane, and can then constitute a transmembrane channel for the bacteria with consequent bacteriostatic properties.

Chlorhexidine (Fig. 15.21) is a very effective antiseptic drug with low toxicity in mammalians. Chlorhexidine is used in disinfectant soaps and is active at low concentrations ($1\,\text{mg}\,l^{-1}$). Hexachlorophene, a twin drug of 2,4,5-trichlorophenol, is used as bactericide and veterinary flukicide. It is more potent and less toxic than the corresponding monomer.[1] Well-known symmetrical compounds such as dioxin (TCDD: tetrachlorodibenzodioxin, a contaminant produced during the 2,4,5-trichlorophenol manufacture) or the herbicide paraquat, are highly toxic. Their toxicity, generally as a consequence of their high metabolic resistance, has been associated by authors with their lipophilicity combined with a high level of symmetry in their structure. The widespread environmental contaminant 2,4,5-2',4',5'-hexachlorobiphenyl is accumulated within the lung and kidney of animals.[57]

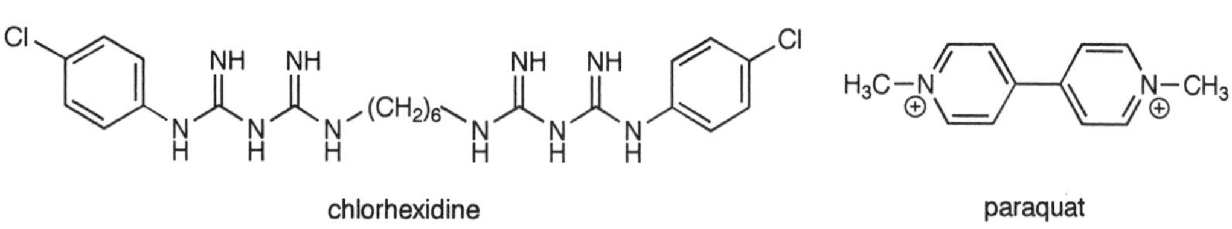

Fig. 15.21 Surface-active antibacterial agents and insecticides.

2. *Other CNS-active twin drugs*

Beyond the CNS twin drugs discussed above, meprobamate (Fig. 15.22) has been developed for its anxiolytic and antiepileptic properties. Here the functional unit is an unsubstituted carbamate, and the linker represents a lipophilic group (4,4-dimethylheptyl). Disulfiram is used to treat alcoholism. Diethyl dithiocarbamate, the major metabolite of disulfiram has been

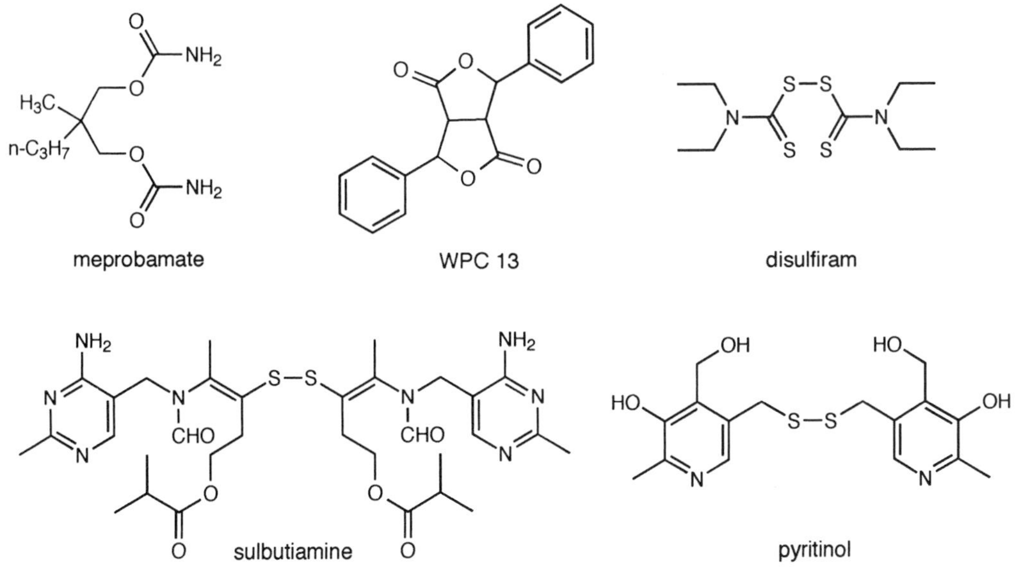

Fig. 15.22   Additional CNS-acting twin drugs and symmetrical compounds.

recently shown to block dopamine β-hydroxylase, and may be the reason for the hypotensive effects characteristic of the disulfiram-mediated modulation of ethanol metabolism.[58]

A head-to-head dimer, the bislactone lignan WPC-13, enhances cerebral metabolism.[59] Sulbutiamine and pyritinol are disulfide twin drugs of vitamin B_1 and B_6, respectively (Fig. 15.22). Chronic administration of sulbutiamine (the O,O'-diisobutyrate of thiamine disulfide) is claimed to improve long-term memory formation in mice.[59] Pyritinol has no vitamine B_6 activity, but is used as nootropic to improve disturbed glucose metabolism, dementia and cerebrovascular injuries.[59]

3.   Other identical twin drugs

The antioxidant probucol (Fig. 15.23) lowers the cholesterol level in blood. Ethambutol shows tuberculostatic properties. Cromolyn, a chromone heterocycle, is useful in the inhalation

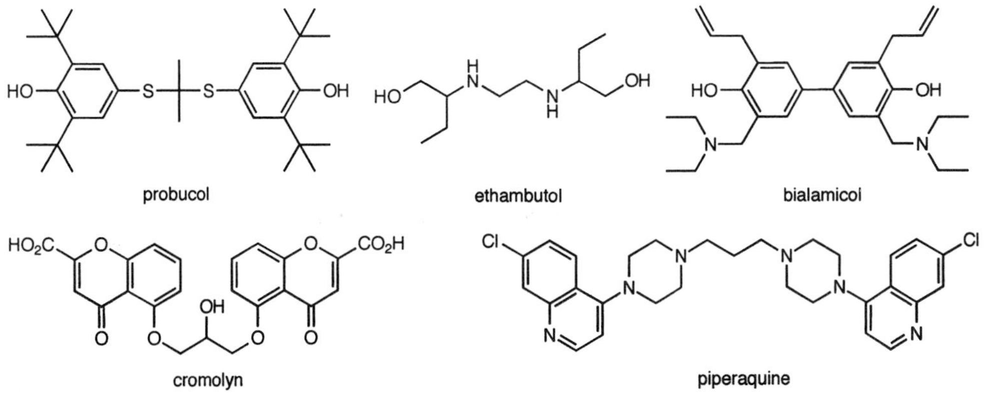

Fig. 15.23   Various identical twin drugs.

treatment of bronchial asthma and dicumarol is a potent anticoagulant compound. Natural phenolic compounds such as mallotojaponin[60] were shown to possess antiherpetic properties. Highly lipophilic (aralkyl)-bis(carbamoyl)piperidines[61] constitute an attractive group of compounds known to inhibit ADP-induced platelet aggregation.

Based on the observation that several bisquinolines such as piperaquine[62] have notable activity and longer duration of action against chloroquine-resistant malaria, a series of derivatives were tested *in vitro* against *Plasmodium falciparum* and *in vivo* against *Plasmodium berghei.* The activity profile of these compounds was strongly dependent upon the nature of the connecting bridge between the quinoline rings (optimum for $n = 2$). Some of them showed promising results. Other symmetrical polyamines such as bialamicol and bis(benzyl)polyamines have shown efficient antimalarial properties against *Plasmodium falciparum.*[63] Pentamidine and other bis(benzamidine) derivatives, constitute an important class of antiprotozoal (*Trypanosoma, Leishmania*) agents.[64]

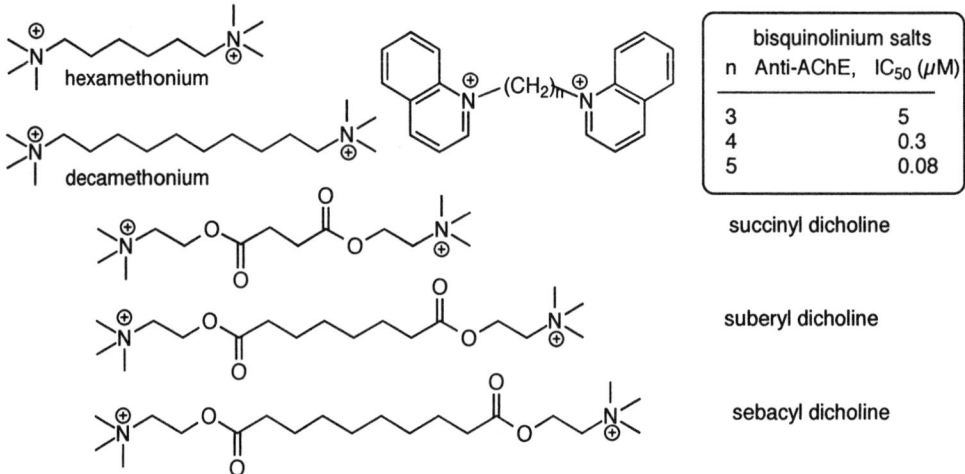

	bisquinolinium salts	
n	Anti-AChE,	IC_{50} (μM)
3		5
4		0.3
5		0.08

Fig. 15.24   Cholinergic twin drugs.

The search for cationic cholinergic agents has led to numerous twin drugs. The bis-quaternary ammonium salts hexamethonium ($n = 6$) and decamethonium ($n = 10$) are potent blockers in ganglia and in the neuromuscular junction, respectively (Fig. 15.24). Other neuromuscular blocking agents such as succinyl ($n = 2$), suberyl ($n = 6$) and sebacoyl dicholines ($n = 8$) can be regarded as pure ACh twin drugs. The bisquinolinium salts present anti-AChE activities depending upon the length of the linker.

III.   NONIDENTICAL TWIN DRUGS: DUAL-ACTING DRUGS

Dual-acting drugs exert their dual action on two different receptors, or on two binding sites of a single receptor, on two enzymes, or on both a receptor and an enzyme. Other studies describe combinations of a molecular hypothesis (identification of a target) with a physiological hypothesis.

A. Hybrid molecules as ligands of two different receptors

Receptors of biogenic amines including noradrenaline, serotonin, dopamine and histamine possess physical and biochemical similarities. They interact with a G-protein, initiating a cascade of events leading to a physiological change. In terms of molecular recognition, all the ligands of the G-protein-coupled receptors possess in their structure a basic nitrogen, protonated at pH 7.4, able to establish coulombic interaction with the carboxylate anion of a typical Asp systematically located in the third transmembranar helix. Moreover, additional binding sites involving residues in the vicinity of the Asp lead to increasing affinity with some selectivity profile towards different types (5-HT, D, NA, ACh, etc.) and subtypes (5-HT_{1A}–5-HT_{1B}, 5-HT_2, 5-HT_4) within the 5HT-receptors. In most cases, according to Ariens's theory, introduction of bulky, lipophilic groups turns agonists into antagonists. Because pharmacophores of all these ligands are similar, the control of their selectivity constitutes an important challenge for medicinal chemists. However, for therapeutic purposes, it may be of interest to synthesize hybrid drugs that bind potently to different G-protein-coupled receptors, and, even more, with an agonist, antagonist or mixed agonist/antagonist profile.

In cardiovascular research labetalol (Fig. 15.25) lowers blood pressure by blocking α- as well as β-adrenoreceptors.[65] In the structure of D2343, both β-agonistic and α-antagonistic adrenoreceptor characteristics are combined.[66]

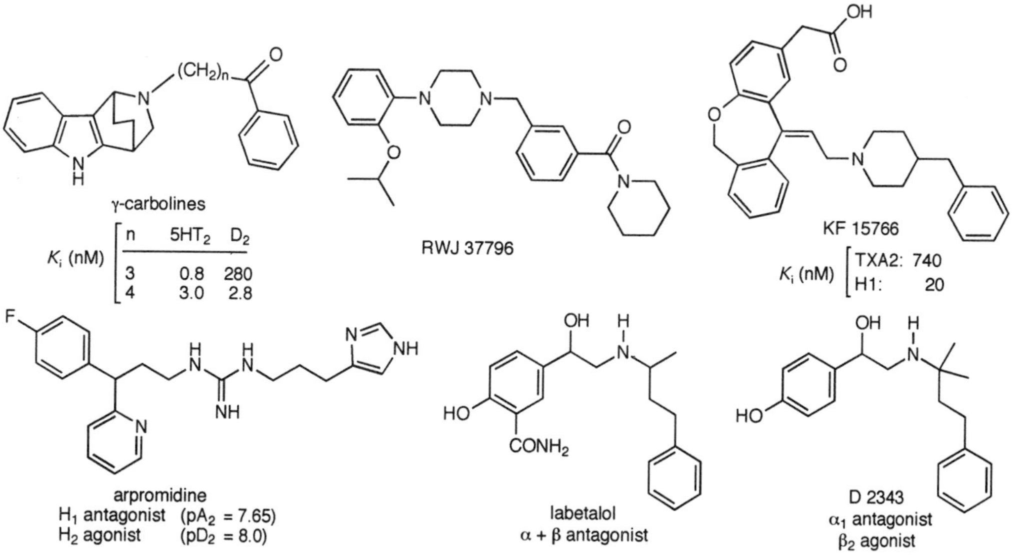

Fig. 15.25 Dual binding ligands on G-protein-coupled receptors.

Dysfunction of dopaminergic and serotoninergic systems is involved in the pathology of a number of psychiatric disorders. Among the various pharmacological properties of the 5-HT_2 antagonist ritanserin, coadministration of this compound with classical neuroleptics in the treatment of schizophrenic patients reduces the incidence of extrapyramidal symptoms. Thus it has been proposed to combine in a same molecule 5-HT_2 receptor and D_2 receptor antagonistic properties using pharmacophore models.[67] Bridged γ-carbolines initially reported as σ receptor ligands, associate potent affinities for 5-HT_2 and moderate affinity for D_2 receptors. Increasing the length of the linker within the corresponding homologous series ($n = 3 \rightarrow 4$), afforded a novel compound with equipotent, nanomolar affinity for both 5-HT$_2$ and D$_2$ receptors.[68] Recently, more complex hybrid molecules have been described. The novel arylpiperazine RWJ-37796 is an antipsychotic with low extrapyramidal effects and presents high affinities (K_i < 4 nM) for D$_2$/D$_3$/5-HT$_{1A}$/α$_{1A}$-adrenergic receptors.[69]

Anti-allergic drugs have been developed by combining in the same molecule histamine H$_1$ antagonistic and H$_2$ agonistic properties.[70] The H$_1$-antihistaminic drug loratidine (Fig. 15.5) presents weak PAF-antagonistic properties. Taking into account the physiological importance of PAF in asthma, it was of therapeutic potential interest to antagonize by a single molecule the action of both mediators. N-Acyl substitution clearly reverses the relative H$_1$/PAF affinity balance for this series of compounds as shown in Fig. 15.5.[4]

Thromboxane A$_2$ (TXA$_2$) is also implicated in the pathophysiological conditions of asthma. Therefore efforts have been made to design TXA$_2$ receptor antagonists. The symbiotic approach led to the recent discovery of dibenzoxepin derivatives with both histamine H$_1$ and TXA$_2$ dual antagonizing activity. In particular, compound KF 15766 (Fig. 15.25) shows good oral activity in several models of asthma and possesses a large safety margin.[71]

Peptide receptors today constitute a large research area, in which the concept of dual-acting drugs can be applied. In this perspective, characterization of high sequence homologies of various endogenous peptides and proteins, or identification of similar amino acid residues involved in molecular recognition processes with their specific receptors, may help to build the pharmacological hypothesis. Thus, the cholecystokinin (CCK) octapeptide analogue SNF 9007 binds to CCK and opioid delta receptors, and constitutes an original pharmacological tool.[72] The hormone angiotensin II (AT) is involved in vascular smooth muscle contraction and release of other endogenous substances. The AT$_1$ and AT$_2$ receptors are present in varying proportions in many tissues and organs. Thus, balanced dual-affinity AT$_1$ and AT$_2$ antagonists may constitute efficient pharmacological tools.[73] In a similar manner bis(succinimido)hexane peptide dimers of bradykinin with combined B$_1$ and B$_2$ receptor subtype antagonist activity may be useful in the treatment of inflammatory disorders.[74]

Dual-acting drugs can also result from the combination of ligands belonging to completely distinct pharmacophores. They are usually designed starting from a purely physiological hypothesis. An illustration is given by binary drugs derived from substance P and adenosine receptor ligands. As activation of these two receptors produces the same effect (e.g. hypotension and analgesia), it was of therapeutic interest to combine in a single compound antagonists acting on these receptors. This was achieved by linking together a 8-arylxanthine (A$_1$ receptor antagonist) and the substance P terminal pentapeptide (Fig. 15.26). The affinities obtained with

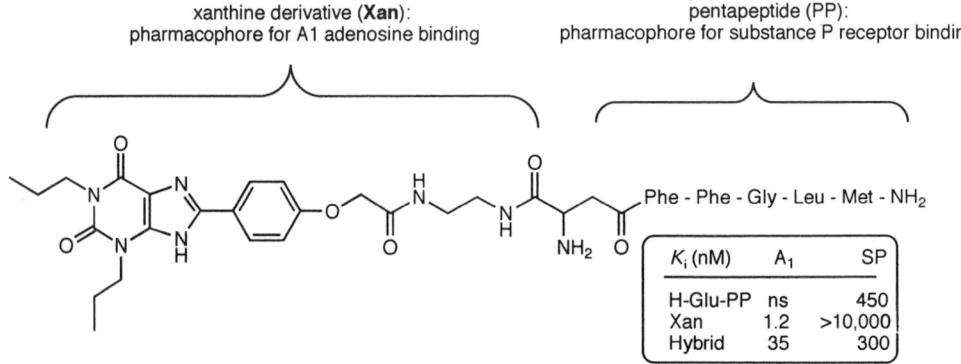

K_i (nM)	A$_1$	SP
H-Glu-PP	ns	450
Xan	1.2	>10,000
Hybrid	35	300

Fig. 15.26 Example of a hybrid acting on two different receptors.

the resulting twin drug are of similar magnitude for both receptors.[75] As postulated earlier for opiate receptors,[76] it was suggested that the A_1 and the SP receptors are located in proximity on the same membrane and that the twin drug is able to interact simultaneously with both of them.

Activators of protein kinase C such as phospholipids or diacylglycerol interact with the regulatory domain, while both ATP and protein substrate interact with the catalytic domain. Most of the different protein kinase C inhibitors are known to bind on only one of these binding sites. However, novel protein kinase C inhibitors were designed as compounds able to interact simultaneously with two of these four binding sites according to the bisubstrate concept. It is noteworthy that, using this approach, the combination of two substrates required by the enzyme to form a single molecule leads to partially additive binding energies, but also a significant entropic contribution. Thus, the association of isoquinoline 5-sulfonamide, as an ATP mimetic, to a polyarginine heptapeptide (Fig. 15.27), as substrate mimetic by means of a flexible aminoethyl-β-alanine spacer leads to a potent mixed protein kinase C and protein kinase A inhibitor.[77]

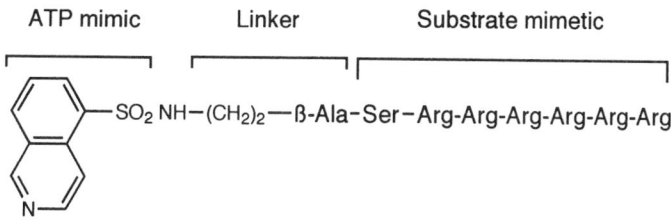

Fig. 15.27   Bisubstrate approach applied to the design of PK inhibitors.

In a similar fashion, biscations such as decamethonium (Fig. 15.24) inhibit AChE with one cation bound to the active site (ACh cation binding) and one cation bound to the peripheral site of the enzyme.[78] In this case the symmetrical structure of the inhibitor does not allow us to hypothesize any symmetrical character of the enzymatic structure.

B.   Hybrids as inhibitors of two different enzymes

As observed with receptors, enzymatic systems can be subdivided into enzyme families, and each enzymatic type presents several isoforms. Thus, for pharmacological and therapeutic purposes, it may be of interest to combine in a same molecule structural characteristics for inhibition of two different isoenzymes, two enzymes belonging to the same family, or two enzymes for which inhibitors show pharmacophore similarities.

Cyclooxygenase (CO) and 5-lipoxygenase (5-LO) are enzymes that catalyse the rate-limiting steps in the biosynthesis of prostaglandins and leukotrienes. Thus, dual inhibitors of both CO and 5-LO are being studied as anti-inflammatory agents with an improved safety profile in comparison to nonsteroidal anti-inflammatory drugs. The thiazolone CI-1004, for example, (Fig. 15.28) was identified as a nonulcerogenic, water-soluble and orally active anti-inflammatory agent.[79] Minaprine (Fig. 15.28) is an atypical antidepressant drug that enhances both serotonergic and dopaminergic transmission.[80] These effects are partially caused by monoamine oxidase inhibition.[81] In contrast to tricyclic antidepressants, minaprine is devoid of cholinolytic effects and, even more, presents cholinomimetic properties.[82] These may result from its muscarinic M_1-agonist profile but also from its weak inhibition of acetylcholinesterase.[83] Thus, minaprine represents an original lead in the search of new dual-acting drugs for the treatment of cholinergic deficits involved in senile dementia of the Alzheimer type.[84–86] Steroids have been used as a basic frame for synthesizing dual inhibitors of type 1 and 2 steroid 5α-reductases,[87] or of cholesterol biosynthesis.[88]

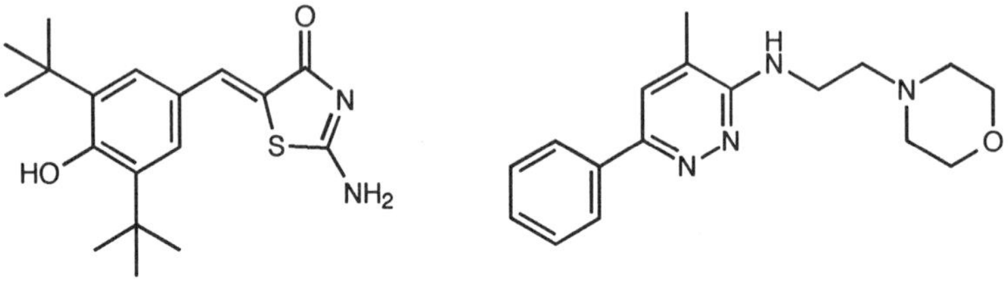

CI - 1004   minaprine

Fig. 15-28   Hybrids acting on two different enzymes.

In order to prevent the degradation of endogenous or synthetic peptides, the search of inhibitors of peptidases and proteases constitutes another important challenge. Because the same peptide may serve as a common substrate for different degrading enzymes, efforts were made recently in the design of multipeptidase inhibitors. Neurotensin (NT) and neuromedin N(NN) appear to act at a common receptor, probably because they have a common C-terminal sequence involved in molecular recognition processes with the receptor. Structural modifications of this C-terminal part led to a potent inhibitor of several metallopeptidases including different endopeptidases with potential analgesic properties.[89]

The inactivation of the endogenous opioid peptide enkephalin is one of the physiological roles of neutral endopeptidase (NEP). A large number of NEP inhibitors have been synthesized and are presently undergoing clinical trials. It has been suggested that simultaneous inhibition of ACE and NEP might be advantageous in the treatment of congestive heart failure or

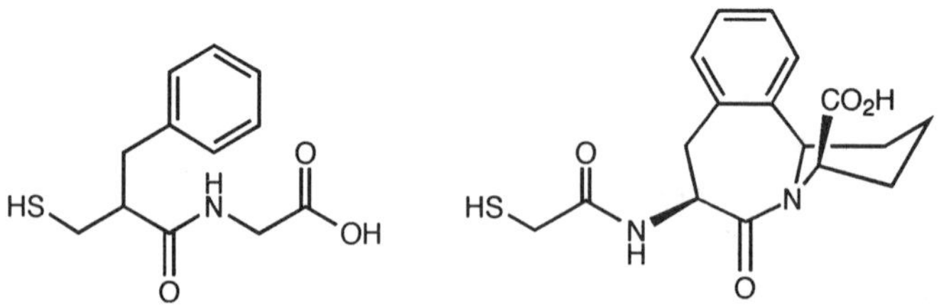

thiorphan   benzazepinone

K_i (nM)		ACE	NEP
	thiorphan	130	2
	benzazepinone	2	5

Fig. 15.29   Dual-acting enzyme inhibitors of zinc metallopeptidases.

hypertension. Because these two mechanistically related metallopeptidases possess some subsite and substrate similarities, it was possible to design a dual NEP-ACE inhibitor. Thiorphan, the well-known inhibitor of enkephalinase (NEP) has dual NEP-ACE inhibiting properties, but it is hundred times less potent as an ACE inhibitor than as NEP inhibitor (Fig. 15.29). NEP cleaves the Phe–Leu bond in Leu-enkephalin. Recently a rigid benzazepinone was designed as PheLeu mimetic. Introduction on benzazepinone of the typical mercaptoacetyl moiety needed for NEP inhibition afforded a potent dual NEP-ACE inhibitor.[90]

C. Hybrids acting at one receptor and one enzyme

Hybrid molecules acting simultaneously on a receptor and on an enzyme may produce potent synergistic effects. A recent illustration is given by the example of dibenzoxepin derivatives interfering with thromboxane A_2 (TXA$_2$), a powerful inducer of platelet aggregation and vascular smooth-muscle contraction. Efforts were undertaken to control the actions of TXA$_2$ either in inhibiting the biosynthesis of TXA$_2$ (TXA$_2$ synthase (TXS) inhibitors) or in blocking the action of TXA$_2$ at the receptor (TXA$_2$ receptor antagonists). As a result of pharmacological and clinical observations, it emerged that TXS-inhibiting and TXA$_2$-antagonistic properties can be combined in a single molecule. The dibenzoxepin shown in Fig. 15.30 exhibits the dual action in *ex vivo* experiments and presents significant protective effects in a rat acute renal failure model.[91]

Depending upon the physiological hypothesis, both targets may belong to different systems. Thus, TXS inhibition and dihydropyridine calcium antagonistic properties led to novel compounds such as FEC 24 265 with a more favourable *in vivo* pharmacological profile, particularly in pathologies where both enhanced TXA$_2$ synthesis and cellular Ca^{2+} overload are involved.[92]

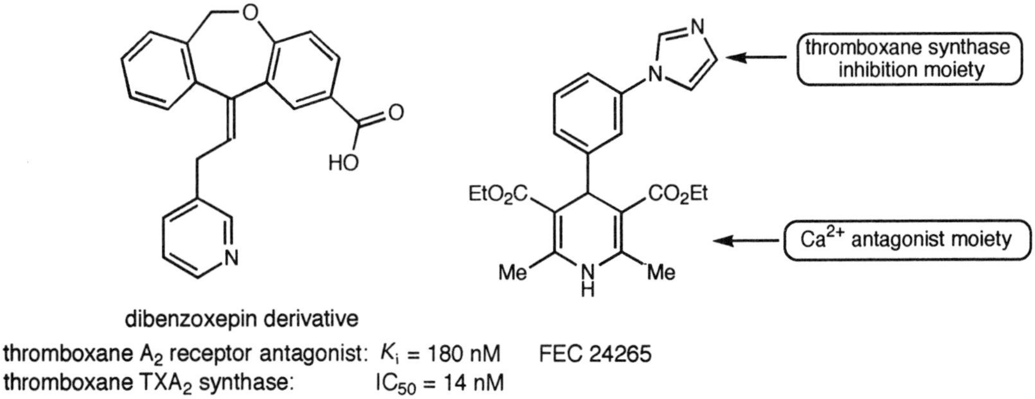

dibenzoxepin derivative
thromboxane A$_2$ receptor antagonist: K_i = 180 nM   FEC 24265
thromboxane TXA$_2$ synthase: IC_{50} = 14 nM

Fig. 15.30   Hybrids acting at one receptor and at one enzyme.

D. Other examples of dual-acting drugs

No single drug has proved to be entirely satisfactory in the long-term treatment of essential hypertension. Combined treatment is necessary to evoke an optimal result and a β-blocker–diuretic combination is widely used as first-line therapy for hypertension management.

Thus, an antihypertensive drug having both β-blocker and moderate diuretic properties in the same molecule would be of great interest. The advantage of such a compound over a classical combination results from a balanced dual activity during the course of drug action, as the single entity would be adsorbed, metabolized and excreted at a typical rate for a given subject. Few attempts to synthesize hybrid molecules by combining the structures of a β-adrenoreceptor antagonist and a diuretic are described, probably owing to the difficulty of accommodating the individual sets of optimal structural requirements for the two activities in a single molecule. The example given in Fig. 15.31 was achieved by replacing the conventional alkyl substituent at the side-chain nitrogen atom of a β-blocker by a 2-chlorobenzene sulfonamide moiety, conferring diuretic properties on the hybrid. The choice of an ethyl group as a linker between the two pharmacophoric groups maintained both pharmacological profiles.[3,66] In an analogous manner, the association of a β-blocker with a diphenylalkylamino moiety results in a unique nonsympathomimetic[93] and nonglycoside positive inotropic agent for the treatment of CHF. In prizidilol a typical hydrazino pyridazine core is combined with propanolol, leading to a dual vasodilator/β-blocker.[66] In another association the aryloxypropanolamine group is linked to capsaicin, a natural compound with cardiotonic properties.[94] A new dihydropyridine calcium-channel antagonist containing a nitrate ester side-chain has been shown to exhibit original antihypertensive properties.[95]

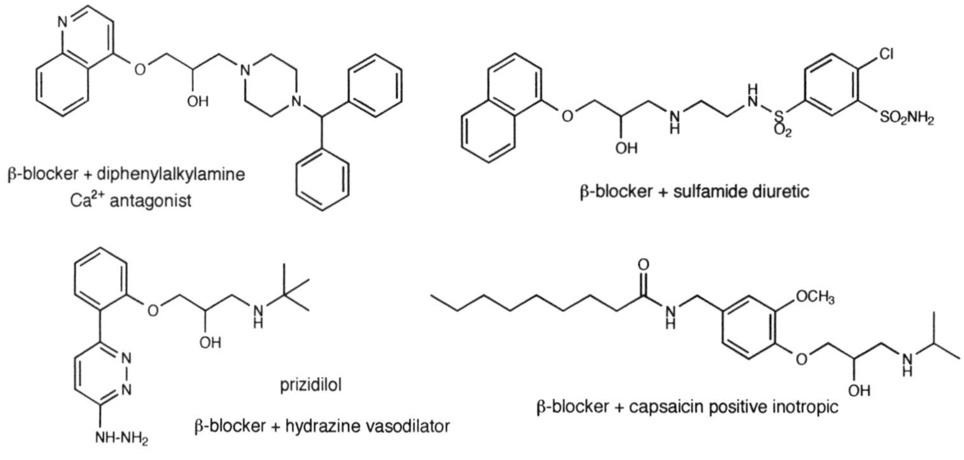

β-blocker + diphenylalkylamine
Ca²⁺ antagonist

β-blocker + sulfamide diuretic

prizidilol
β-blocker + hydrazine vasodilator

β-blocker + capsaicin positive inotropic

Fig. 15.31   Dual-acting drugs derived from β-blockers.

Hybrid antibiotics combining structural features of chloramphenicol, sparsomycin and puromycin have been synthesized[96] (Fig. 15.32). Other dual-acting antibacterial drugs linking quinolones to cephalosporin demonstrated potent activity against a broad spectrum of Gram-positive and Gram-negative bacteria including β-lactam-resistant strain.[97]

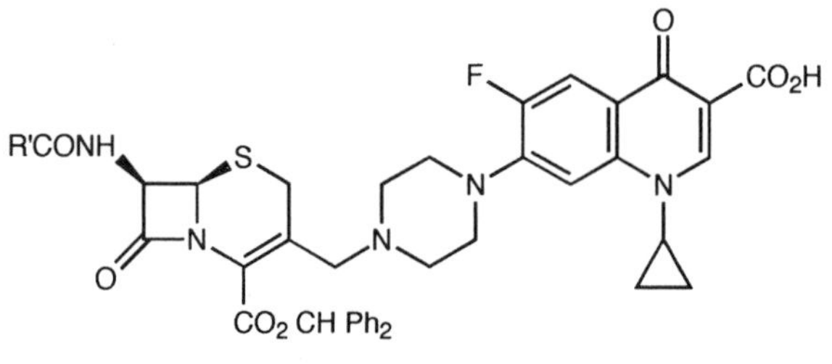

Fig. 15.32   Dual-acting quinolone-linked cephalosporins as antibacterials.

IV. CONCLUSION

The principle of combining two pharmacophoric groups in a single molecule can be extended to other classes of drugs such as pro-drugs (see Chapters 31 and 32), molecular chameleons,[98] and ligand-bearing metal complexes.[99] Peptidic hormones can be considered as dual-acting drugs, with specific amino acid residues needed for molecular recognition by the receptor ('message') and others responsible for the transport and access to the receptor ('address'[100]).

Twin drugs combining two structural components in a single molecule have been described in numerous domains of medicinal chemistry. Historically they resulted from empirical structural modifications, but today rational design of dual-binding ligands may involve the knowledge of the structure of the protein that contains these binding sites. Protein X-ray crystallography has in several cases revealed a high degree of symmetry resulting from the existence of dimeric (C-2), trimeric (C-3) or tetrameric protein assemblies. This finding has to be associated with the increasing potency of identical twin drugs, which can simultaneously fit to the symmetrical binding sites of the protein complex. Recent studies dealing with the design of HIV proteases strongly support this hypothesis. However, combining in the same molecule two nonidentical pharmacophore components can lead to a new compound, which may not bind simultaneously to each considered binding site. Recent findings in molecular pharmacology, molecular biology, enzymology and physiology will help to select pertinent pairs of targets involved in different pathologies. For therapeutic purposes the earlier search for selective drugs is replaced today by the design of nonselective drugs, but with control of their selectivity profile, using 'the dual acting drug' concept.

The design of dual-acting drugs is promising but is much more difficult than the conventional design of a compound with a single activity. Some limitations will be discussed briefly:[2,66]

(1) Combining two pharmacophore components in a single molecule may lead to an inactive compound. A typical example is the combination of the vasodilator nifedipine with a β-blocker, which led to a hybrid devoid of any of the expected pharmacological activities. This example emphasizes the importance of a good knowledge of SAR data within each pharmacophore (types of interaction, steric hindrance-sensitive regions, local hydrophilic and hydrophobic areas), and the choice of the linker (nature and position of the linkage). However, in some cases, two respective SARs may prove mutually exclusive.

(2) The hybrid may show the desired pharmacological profile, but the attempt may fail because of the appearance of unforseen toxicological problems.

(3) The balanced potency of dual-acting drugs has to be carefully evaluated. Design of agonist/antagonist hybrids has to take into consideration that drugs with antagonistic activity on receptors usually have to be given in concentrations significantly less than those needed for agonists (affinities in the nanomolar and micromolar range, respectively). In a similar manner, design of hybrids combining a receptor ligand and an enzyme inhibitor should take into account both efficacies and particularly the kinetic properties of the considered enzyme.

The approach is nevertheless workable, and successful attempts have been obtained in cardiovascular research, particularly for the treatment of hypertension. The gastrointestinal system represents another interesting field of application for dual-acting drugs. Only a few hybrids are at present used clinically for the central nervous system. However, the approach seems to be applicable to the treatment of diseases that require restoration of the dopaminergic or cholinergic balance.

In spite of the limitations, numerous recent articles deal with the design of twin drugs acting in various systems. The most illustrative of them have been reported in this chapter, and account for the increasing interest of the twin drug approach in drug design.

REFERENCES

1. Ariëns, E. J. (1971) Drug design — a general introduction. In Ariëns, E. J. (ed.) *Drug Design*, pp. 1–270. Academic Press, New York.
2. Baldwin, J. J., Lumma, W. C., Lundell, G. F., Ponticello, G. S., Raab, A. W., Engelhardt, E. L., Hirschmann, R., Sweet, C. S. and Scriabine, A. (1979) Symbiotic approach to drug design: antihypertensive β-adrenergic blocking agents. *J. Med. Chem.* **22:** 1284–1290.
3. Cecchetti, V., Fravolini, A., Schiaffella, F., Tabarrini, O., Bruni, G. and Segre, G. (1993) *o*-Chlorobenzenesulfonamidic derivatives of (aryloxy)propanolamines as β-blocking/diuretic agents. *J. Med. Chem.* **36:** 157–161.
4. Piwinski, J. J., Wong, J. K., Green, M. J., Ganguly, A. K., Billah, M. M., West, Jr. R.E. and Kreutner, W. (1991) Dual antagonists of platelet activating factor and histamine. Identification of structural requirements for dual activity of *N*-acyl-4-(5,6-dihydro-11*H*-benzo[5,6]cyclohepta-[1,2-*b*]pyridin-11-ylene)piperidines. *J. Med. Chem.* **34:** 457–461.
5. Changeux, J. P. (1969) Remarks on the symmetry and cooperative properties of biological membranes. In Engström, A. and Strandberg, B. (eds) *Symmetry and Function of Biological Systems at the Macromolecular Level*, pp. 235–256. Almqvist and Wiksell, Stockholm.
6. Blundell, T., Sewell, T. and Turnbell, B. (1981) Symmetry in the structure and organization of proteins. In Dodson, G., Glusker, J. P. and Sayre, D. (eds) *Struct. Stud. Mol. Biol. Interest*, pp. 390–403. Oxford University Press, London.
7. Garay, A. S. (1979) Broken symmetries in physics and their relevance in chemistry and biology. *Stud. Phys. Theor. Chem.* **7:** *(Origins Opt. Act. Nat.)*: 245–257.
8. Siddle, K. (1992) The insulin receptor. In Burgen, A. and Barnard, E. A. (eds) *Receptor Subunits and Complexes*, pp. 261–351. Cambridge University Press, Cambridge.
9. Bell, M. R., Batzold, F. H. and Winneker, R. C. (1986) Chemical control of fertility. In Bailey, D. M. (ed.) *Annual Reports in Medicinal Chemistry*, pp. 169–177. Academic Press, San Diego.
10. Melchiorre, C. (1981) Tetramine disulfides: a new tool in α-adrenergic pharmacology. *Tr. Pharmacol. Sci.* **2:** 209–211.
11. Kierstead, R. W., Faraone, A., Mennona, F., Mullin, J., Guthrie, R. W. and Crowley, H. (1983) Beta-1-selective adrenoceptor antagonists. Blocking activity of a series of binary (aryloxy) propanolamines. *J. Med. Chem.* **26:** 1561–1569.
12. Melchiorre, C., Bolognesi, M. L., Chiarini, A., Minarini, A. and Spampinato, S. (1993) Synthesis and biological activity of some methoctramine-related tetraamines bearing a 11-acetyl-5,11-dihydro-6*H*-pyrido[2,3-*b*][1,4]-benzodiazepin-6-one moiety as antimuscarinics: a second generation of highly selective M$_2$ muscarinic receptor antagonists. *J. Med. Chem.* **36:** 3734–3737.
13. Hudkins, R. L., Stubbins, J. F., DeHaven-Hudkins, D. L. and Yamamura, H. I. (1991) M2 receptor activity of *N,N'*-dimethyl *N,N'*-bis[3-(2-phthalimido)propyl] 1,6-hexanediamine dihydrochloride. *Abstr. Pap. Am. Chem. Soc. (202 Meet., Pt. 1, MEDI 140).*
14. Biftu, T., Chabala, J. C., Acton, J., Beattle, T., Brooker, D. and Bugianesi, R. (1988) Synthesis and structure–activity relationship of 2,5-diaryltetrahydrofurans as PAF antagonists. *Prostaglandins* **35:** 846.
15. Shimazaki, N., Shima, I., Hemmi, K., Tsurumi, Y. and Hashimoto, M. (1987) Diketopiperazine derivatives, a new series of platelet-activating factor inhibitors. *Chem. Pharm. Bull.* **35:** 3527–3530.
16. Lamouri, A., Heymans, F., Tavet, F., Dive, G., Batt, J. P., Blavet, N., Braquet, P. and Godfroid, J.-P. (1993) Design and modeling of new platelet-activating factor antagonists. 1. Synthesis and

biological activity of 1,4-bis(3′,4′,5′-trimethoxybenzoyl)-2-[[(substituted carbonyl and carbamoyl)oxy]methyl]piperazines. *J. Med. Chem.* **36**: 990–1000.

17. Cheronis, J. C., Whalley, E. T., Nguyen, K. T., Eubanks, S. R., Allen, L. G., Duggan, M. J., Loy, S. D., Bonham, K. A. and Blodgett, J. K. (1992) A new class of bradykinin antagonists: synthesis and *in vitro* activity of bissuccinimidoalkane peptide dimers. *J. Med. Chem.* **35**: 1563–1572.

18. Salvino, J. M., Seoane, P. R., Douty, B. D., Awad, M. A., Dolle, R. E., Houck, W. T., Faunce, D. M. and Sawutz, D. G. (1993) Design of potent non-peptide competitive antagonists of the human bradykinin B₂ receptor. *J. Med. Chem.* **36**: 2583–2584.

19. Roth, R. A., Cassell, D. J., Morgan, D. O., Tatnell, M. A., Jones, R. H., Schüttler, A. and Brandenburg, D. Effects of covalently linked insulin dimers on receptor kinase activity and receptor down regulation. *FEBS Lett.* **170**: 360–364.

20. Costa, T., Wüster, M., Herz, A., Shimohigashi, Y., Chen, H. -C. and Rodbard, D. (1985) Receptor binding and biological activity of bivalent enkephalins. *Biochem. Pharmacol.* **34**: 25–30.

21. Shimohigashi, Y., Costa, T., Chen, H.-C. and Rodbart, D. (1982) Dimeric tetrapeptide enkephalins display extraordinary selectivity for the δ opiate receptor. *Nature.* **297**: 333–335.

22. Shimohigashi, Y., Ogasawara, T., Koshizaka, T., Waki, M., Kato, T., Izumyia, N., Kurono, M. and Yagi, K. (1987) Interaction of dimers of inactive enkephalins fragments with μ opiate receptors. *Biochem. Biophys. Res. Commun.* **145**: 1109–1115.

23. Lin, C.-E., Takemori, A. E. and Portoghese, P. S. (1993) Synthesis and κ-opioid antagonist selectivity of a norbinaltorphimine congener. Identification of the address moiety required for κ-antagonist activity. *J. Med. Chem.* **36**: 2412–2415.

24. Archer, S., Seyed-Mozaffari, A., Jiang, Q. and Bidlack, J. M. (1994) 14α,14′β-[Dithiobis[2-oxo-2,1-ethanediyl)imino]]bis(7,8-dihydromorphinone) and 14α,14′β-[dithiobis[2-oxo-2,1-ethanediyl)imino]]bis[7,8-dihydro-*N*-(cyclopropyl-methyl) normorphinone]: chemistry and opioid binding properties. *J. Med. Chem.* **37**: 1578–1585.

25. Doughty, M. B., Chaurasia, C. S. and Li, K. (1993) Benextramine–neuropeptide Y receptor interactions: contributions of the benzylic moieties to [³H]neuropeptide Y displacement activity. *J. Med. Chem.* **36**: 272–279.

26. Joslyn, A. F., Luchowski, E. and Triggle, D. J. (1988) Dimeric 1,4-dihydropyridines as calcium channel antagonists. *J. Med. Chem.* **31**: 1489–1492.

27. Holtzman, S. G. (1989) Opioid and phencyclidine-like discriminative effects of ditolylguanidine, a selective *sigma* ligand. *J. Pharmacol. Exp. Ther.* **248**: 1054–1062.

28. Goldin, S. M., Katragadda, S., Hu, L. Y., Reddy, N. L., Fischer, J. B., Knapp, A. G. and Margolin, L. D. (1993) Preparation of substituted guanidines and derivatives as modulators of neurotransmitter release and novel methodology for identifying neurotransmitter release blockers. PCT Int. Appl. WO 92 14697 (Sept. 1992, to Cambridge Neuroscience, Inc.) [*Chem. Abstr.* **118**: 80645g].

29. Chan, G. W., Mong, S., Hemling, M. E., Freyer, A. J., Offen, P. H. and DeBrosse, C. W. (1993) New leukotriene B₄ receptor antagonist: leucettamine A and related imidazole alkaloids from the marine sponge *Leucetta microraphis. J. Nat. Prod.* **56**: 116–121.

30. Saifullin, S. R. and Kurganov, B. I. (1991) Kinetic manifestations of molecular symmetry changes in oligomeric enzymes in adsorptive systems. *J. Chem. Biochem. Kinet.* **1**: 77–84. [*Chem. Abstr.* **116**: 123912v.]

31. Tan, G. T., Wickramasinghe, A., Verma, S., Singh, R., Hughes, S. H., Pezzuto, J. M., Baba, M. and Mohan, P. (1992) Potential anti-AIDS naphtalenesulfonic acid derivatives. Synthesis and inhibition of HIV-1 induced cytopathogenesis and HIV-1 and HIV-2 reverse transcriptase activity. *J. Med. Chem.* **35**: 4846–4853.

32. Appelt, K. (1993) Crystal structures of HIV-1 protease-inhibitor complexes. *Persp. Drug Discov. Des.* **1**: 23–48.

33. Bone, R., Vacca, J. P., Anderson, P. S. and Holloway, M. K. (1991) X-ray crystal structure of the HIV protease complex with L-700,417, an inhibitor with pseudo C₂ symmetry. *J. Am. Chem. Soc.* **113**: 9382–9384.

34. Hyland, L. J., Tomaszek, Jr. T. A., Roberts, G. D. *et al.* (1991) Human immunodeficiency virus-1 protease. 1. Initial velocity studies and kinetic characterization of reaction intermediates by ¹⁸O isotope exchange. *Biochemistry.* **30**: 8441–8453.

35. Erickson, J. W., Neidhardt, D. J., VanDrie, J. *et al.* (1990) Design, activity, and 2.8 angström crystal structure of a C₂ symmetric inhibitor complexed to HIV-1 protease. *Science.* **249**: 527–533.

36. Kempf, D. J., Codacovi, L., Wang, X. C. *et al.* (1993) Symmetry-based inhibitors of HIV protease. Structure–activity studies of acylated 2,4-diamino-1,5-diphenyl-3-hydroxypentane and 2,5-diamino-1,6-diphenylhexane-3,4-diol. *J. Med. Chem.* **36**: 320–330.

37. Wonacott, A., Cooke, R., Hayes, F. R., Hann, M. M., Jhoti, H., McMeekin, P., Mistry, A., Murray-Rust, P., Singh, O. M. P. and Weir, M. P. (1993) A series of penicillin-derived C_2 symmetric inhibitors of HIV-1 proteinase: structural and modeling studies. *J. Med. Chem.* **36**: 3113–3119.

38. Trinks, U., Buchdunger, E., Furet, P. *et al.* (1994) Dianilinophthalimides: potent and selective, ATP-competitive inhibitors of the EGF-receptor protein tyrosine kinase. *J. Med. Chem.* **37**: 1015–1027.

39. Thakkar, K., Geahlen, R. L. and Cushman, M. (1993) Synthesis and protein-tyrosine kinase inhibitory activity of polyhydroxylated stilbene analogues of piceatannol. *J. Med. Chem.* **36**: 2950–2955.

40. Levitzki, A. and Gilon, C. Tyrphostins as molecular tools and potential antiproliferative drugs. *Trends Pharmacol. Sci.* **12**: 171–174.

41. Takahashi, I., Nakanishi, S., Kobayashi, E., Nakano, H., Suzuki, K. and Tamaoki, T. (1989) Hypericin and pseudohypericin specifically inhibit protein kinase C: possible relation to their antiretroviral activity. *Biochem. Biophys. Res. Commun.* **165**: 1207–1212.

42. Hales, N. J. and Beattie, J. F. (1993) Novel inhibitors of prolyl 4-hydroxylase. 5. The intriguing structure–activity relationship seen with 2,2′-bipyridine and its 5,5′-dicarboxylic acid derivatives. *J. Med. Chem.* **36**: 3853–3858.

43. Oleksyszyn, J. and Kirschenheuter, G. P. (1993) Aromatic esters of phenyldialkanoates as inhibitors of human neutrophil elastase. US Patent 5 216 022 (1 June, 1993, to Cortech, Inc.). [*Chem. Abstr.* **119**: 225690a.]

44. Agathocleous, D. C., Page, P. C. B., Cosstick, R., Galpin, I. J., McLennan, A. G. and Prescott, M. (1990) Synthesis of bridged nucleosides. *Tetrahedron.* **46**: 2047–2058.

45. Ito, N., Yasunaga, T., Iizumi, Y. and Araki, T. (1990) Bis(ureidoalkyl)benzenes for inhibition of acylcoenzyme A cholesterol transferase (ACAT). European Patent Application EP 325 397 (26 July, 1989, to Yamanouchi Pharmaceutical Co., Ltd.). [*Chem. Abstr.* **112**: 55271a.]

46. Mao, S. -S. (1993) Factor Xa inhibitors. *Perspect. Drug Disc. Des.* **1**: 423–430.

47. Saab, N. H., West, E. E., Bieszk, N. C., Preuss, C. V., Mank, A. R., Casero, Jr, R. A. and Woster, P. M. (1993) Synthesis and evaluation of unsymmetrically substituted polyamine analogues as modulators of human spermidine/spermine-N^1-acetyltransferase (SSAT) and as potential antitumor agents. *J. Med. Chem.* **36**: 2998–3004.

48. Stanek, J., Caravatti, G., Capraro, H.-G., Furet, P., Mett, H., Schneider, P. and Regenass, U. (1993) *S*-Adenosylmethionine decarboxylase inhibitors. new aryl and heteroaryl analogues of methylglyoxal bis(guanylhydrazone). *J. Med. Chem.* **36**: 46–54.

49. Stefanska, B., Dzieduszycka, M., Martelli, S., Tarasiuk, J., Bontemps-Gracz, M. and Borowski, E. (1993) 6-[(Aminoalkyl)amino]-substituted 7*H*-benzo[*e*]perimidin-7-ones as novel antineoplastic agents. Synthesis and biological evaluation. *J. Med. Chem.* **36**: 38–41.

50. Wunz, T. P., Dorr, R. T., Alberts, D. S., Tunget, C. L., Einspahr, J., Milton, S. and Remers, W. (1987) New antitumor agents containing the anthracene nucleus. *J. Med. Chem.* **30**: 1313–1321.

51. Fairley, T. A., Tidwell, R. R., Donkor, I., Naiman, N. A., Ohemeng, K. A., Lombardy, R. J., Bentley, J. A. and Cory, M. (1993) Structure, DNA minor groove binding, and base pair specificity of alkyl- and aryl-linked bis(amidinobenzimidazoles) and bis(amidinoindoles). *J. Med. Chem.* **36**: 1746–1753.

52. McConnaughie, A. W., Spychala, J., Zhao, M., Boykin, D. and Wilson, W. D. (1994) Design and synthesis of RNA-specific groove-binding cations: implications for antiviral drug design. *J. Med. Chem.* **37**: 1063–1069.

53. Skibo, E. B., Islam, I., Heileman, M. J. and Schulz, W. G. (1994) Structure-activity studies of benzimidazole-based DNA-cleaving agents. Comparison of benzimidazole, pyrrolobenzimidazole, and tetrahydropyridobenzimidazole analogues. *J. Med. Chem.* **37**: 78–92.

54. Gallego, J., Ortiz, R. A. and Gago, F. (1993) A molecular dynamics study of the bis-intercalation complexes of echinomycin with d(ACGT)$_2$ and d(TCGA)$_2$: rationale for sequence-specific Hoogsteen base pairing. *J. Med. Chem.* **36**: 1548–1561.

55. Harding, M. M. (1992) NMR studies on YSPTSPSY: implications for the design of DNA bisintercalators. *J. Med. Chem.* **35**: 4658–4664.

56. Rao, K. E., Krowicki, K., Balzarini, J., De Clerq, E., Newman, R. A. and Lown, J. W. (1991) Novel linked antiviral and antitumor agents related to netropsin-2: Synthesis and biological evaluation. In Combet-Farnoux, C., (ed) *Actualités de Chimie Thérapeutique*. pp. 21–42. Société de Chimie Thérapeutique, Chatenay, Malabry.

57. Brandt, I., Lund, J., Bergman, A., Klasson-Wheler, E., Poellinger, L. and Gustafsson, J. -A. (1985) Target cells for the polychlorinated biphenyl metabolite 4,4'-bis(methylsulfonyl)-2,2',5,5'-tetrachlorobiphenyl in lung and kidney. *Drug Metab. Dispos.* **13:** 490–494.

58. Rall, T. W. (1990) Hypnotics and sedatives; ethanol. In Goodman-Gilman, A., Rall, T. W., Nies, A. S. and Taylor, P. (eds) *Goodman and Gilman's The Pharmacological Basis of Therapeutics*, 8th edn, pp. 345–382. Pergamon Press, New York.

59. Fröstl, W. and Maître, L. (1989) The families of cognition enhancers. *Pharmacopsychiatr.* **22:** (Supplement) 54–100.

60. Arisawa, M., Fujita, A., Hayashi, T., Hayashi, K., Ochiai, H. and Morita, N. (1990) Cytotoxic and antiherpetic activity of phloroglucinol derivatives from *Mallotus japonicus* (Euphorbiaceae). *Chem. Pharm. Bull.* **38:** 1624–1626.

61. Feng, Z., Gollamudi, R., Dillingham, E. O., Bond, S. E., Lyman, B. A., Purcell, W. P., Hill, R. J. and Korfmacher, W. A. (1992) Molecular determinants of the platelet aggregation inhibitory activity of carbamoylpiperidines. *J. Med. Chem.* **35:** 2952–2958.

62. Vennerström, J. L., Ellis, W. Y., Ager Jr, A. L., Anderson, S. L., Gerena, L. and Milhous, W. K. (1992) Bisquinolines. 1. *N,N*-Bis(7-chloroquinolin-4-yl) alkanediamines with potential against chloroquine-resistant malaria. *J. Med. Chem.* **35:** 2129–2134.

63. Edwards, M. L., Stemerick, D. M., Bitonti, A. J., Dumont, J. A., McCann, P. P., Bey, P. and Sjoerdsma, A. (1991) Antimalarial polyamine analogues. *J. Med. Chem.* **34:** 569–574.

64. Ulrich, P. and Cerami, A. (1984) Trypanocidal 1,3-arylene diketone bis(guanylhydrazone)s. Structure–activity relationship among substituted and heterocyclic analogues. *J. Med. Chem.* **27:** 35–40.

65. Brittain, R. T., Drew, G. M. and Levy, G. P. (1980) The α- and β-adrenoceptor blocking potencies of labetalol and its individual stereoisomers. *Br. J. Pharmacol.* **69:** 282P–283P.

66. Nicolaus, B. J. R. (1983) Symbiotic approach to drug design. In Gross, F. (ed.) *Decision Making in Drug Research*, pp. 173–186. Raven Press, New York.

67. Andersen, K., Liljefors, T., Gundertofte, K., Perregaard, J. and Bogeso, K. P. (1994) Development of a receptor-interaction model for serotonin 5-HT$_2$ receptor antagonists. Predicting selectivity with respect to dopamine D$_2$ receptors. *J. Med. Chem.* **37:** 950–962.

68. Mewshaw, R. E., Silverman, L. S., Mathew, R. M. *et al.* (1993) Bridged γ-carbolines and derivatives possessing selective and combined affinity for 5-HT$_2$ and D$_2$ receptors. *J. Med. Chem.* **36:** 1488–1495.

69. Reitz, A. B., Bennett, D. J., Blum, P. S., Codd, E. E., Maryanoff, C. A., Ortegon, M. E., Renzi, M. J., Scott, M. K., Shank, R. P. and Vaught, J. L. (1994) A new arylpiperazine antipsychotic with high D$_2$/D$_3$/5-HT$_{1A}$/α_{1A}-adrenergic affinity and low potential for extrapyramidal effects. *J. Med. Chem.* **37:** 1060–1062.

70. Buschauer, A. (1989) Synthesis and *in vitro* pharmacology of arpromidine and related phenyl(pyridylalkyl)guanidines, a potential new class of positive inotropic drugs. *J. Med. Chem.* **32:** 1963–1970.

71. Ohshima, E., Takami, H., Harakawa, H. *et al.* (1993) Dibenz[*b,e*]oxepin derivatives: novel antiallergic agents possessing thromboxane A$_2$ and histamine H$_1$ dual antagonizing activity 1. *J. Med. Chem.* **36:** 417–420.

72. Rao, R. K., Levenson, S., Fang, S. -N., Hruby, V. J., Yamamura, H. I. and Porreca, F. (1994) Characterisation of SNF 9007, a novel cholecystokinin/opioid ligand in mouse ileum *in vitro*: evidence for involvement of cholecystokinin$_A$ and cholecystokinin$_B$ receptors in regulation of ion transport. *J. Pharmacol. Exp. Ther.* **268:** 1003–1009.

73. De Laszlo, S. E., Quagliato, C. S., Greenlee, W. J. *et al.* (1993) A potent, orally active, balanced affinity angiotensin II AT$_1$ antagonist and AT$_2$ binding inhibitor. *J. Med. Chem.* **36:** 3207–3210.

74. Cheronis, J. C., Whalley, E. T., Allen, L. G., Loy, S. D., Elder, M. W., Duggan, M. J., Gross, K. L. and Blodgett, J. K. (1994) Design, synthesis, and *in vitro* activity of bis(succinimido)hexane peptide heterodimers with combined B$_1$ and B$_2$ antagonist activity. *J. Med. Chem.* **37:** 348–355.

75. Jacobson, K. A., Lipkowski, A. W., Moody, T. W., Padgett, W., Pijl, E., Kirk, K. L. and Daly, J. W. (1987) Binary drugs: conjugates of purines and a peptide that binds to both adenosine and substance P. *J. Med. Chem.* **30:** 1529–1532.

76. Portoghese, P. S., Larson, D. L., Yim, C. B., Sayre, L. M., Ronsisvalle, G., Lipkowski, A. W., Takermori, A. E., Rice, K. R. and Tam, S. W. (1985) Stereostructure–activity relationship of opioid agonist and antagonist bivalent ligands. Evidence for bridging between opioid receptors. *J. Med. Chem.* **28:** 1140–1141.

77. Ricouart, A., Gesquière, J. C., Tartar, A. and Sergheraert, C. (1991) Design of potent protein kinase inhibitors using the bisubstrate approach. *J. Med. Chem.* **34:** 73–78.

78. Taylor, P. and Lappi, S. (1975) Interaction of fluorescence probes with acetycholinesterase. The site and specificity of propidium binding. *Biochemistry.* **14:** 1989–1997.

79. Unangst, P. C., Connor, D. T., Cetenko, W. A., Sorenson, R. J., Kostlan, C. R., Sircar, J. C., Wright, C. D., Schrier, D. J. and Dyer, R. D. (1994) Synthesis and biological evaluation of 5-[[3,5-bis(1,1-dimethylethyl)-4-hydroxyphenyl]methylene] oxazoles, -thiazoles, and imidazoles: novel dual 5-lipoxygenase and cyclooxygenase inhibitors with antiinflammatory activity. *J. Med. Chem.* **37:** 322–328.

80. Wermuth, C. G., Schlewer, G., Bourguignon, J.-J., Maghioros, G., Bouchet, M.-J., Moire, C., Kan, J.-P., Worms, P. and Bizière, K (1989) 3-Aminopryridazine derivatives with atypical antidepressant, serotonergic, and dopaminergic activities. *J. Med. Chem.* **32:** 528–537.

81. Bizière, K., Kan, J.-P., Soulihac, J., Muyard, J.-P. and Roncucci, R. (1982) Pharmacological evaluation of minaprine dihydrochloride, a new psychotropic drug. *Arzneimittel-Forsch.* **32:** 824–831.

82. Worms, P., Kan, J. P., Steinberg, R., Terranova, J.-P., Pério, A. and Bizière, K. (1989) Cholinomimetic properties of minaprine. *Naunyn-Schmiedeberg's Arch. Pharmacol.* **340:** 411–418.

83. Garattini, S., Forloni, G. L., Tirelli, S., Ladinsky, H. and Consolo, S. (1984) Neurochemical effects of minaprine, a novel psychotropic drug, on the central cholinergic system of the rat. *Psychopharmacology.* **82:** 210–214.

84. Wermuth, C. G., Bourguignon, J. J., Hoffmann, R., Boigegrain, R., Brodin, R., Kan, J. P. and Soubrié, P. (1992) SR 46559 A and related aminopyridazines are potent muscarinic agonists with no cholinergic syndrome. *Bioorg. Med. Chem. Lett.* **2:** 833–838.

85. Schumacher, C., Steinberg, R., Kan, J. P., Michaud, J. C., Bourguignon, J. J., Wermuth, C. G., Feltz, P., Worms, P. and Bizière, K. (1989) Pharmacological characterization of the aminopyridazine SR 95639A, a selective M_1 muscarinic agonist. *Eur. J. Pharmacol.* **166:** 139–147.

86. Kan, J. P., Steinberg, R., Oury-Donat, F. *et al.* (1993) SR 46559A: a novel and potent muscarinic compound with no cholinergic syndrome. *Psychopharmacology.* **112:** 219–227.

87. Frye, S. V., Haffner, C. D., Maloney, P. R. *et al.* (1993) 6-Azasteroids: potent dual inhibitors of human type 1 and 2 steroid 5α-reductase. *J. Med. Chem.* **36:** 4313–4315.

88. Frye, L. L., Cusack, K. P. and Leonard, D. A. (1993) 32-Methyl-32-oxy-lanosterols: dual-action inhibitors of cholesterol biosynthesis. *J. Med. Chem.* **36:** 410–416.

89. Doulut, S., Dubuc, I., Rodriguez, M. *et al.* (1993) Synthesis and analgesic effects of *N*-[3-[(hydroxyamino)carbonyl]-1-oxo-2(*R*)-benzylpropyl]-L-isoleucyl-L-leucine, a new potent inhibitor of multiple neurotensin/neuromedin N degrading enzymes. *J. Med. Chem.* **36:** 1369–1379.

90. Flynn, G. A., Beight, D. W., Mehdi, S., Koehl, G. R., Giroux, E. L., French, J. F., Hake, P. W. and Dage, R. C. (1993) Application of a conformationally restricted Phe-Leu dipeptide mimetic to the design of a combined inhibitor of angiotensin I-converting enzyme and neutral endopeptidase 24.11. *J. Med. Chem.* **36:** 2420–2423.

91. Ohshima, E., Sato, H., Obase, H., Miki, I., Ishii, A., Kawakage, M., Shirakura, S., Karasawa, A. and Kubo, K. (1993) Dibenzoxepin derivatives: thromboxane A_2 synthase inhibition and thromboxane A_2 receptor antagonism combined in one molecule. *J. Med. Chem.* **36:** 1613–1618.

92. Cozzi, P., Carganico, G., Fusar, D., Grossoni, M., Menichincheri, M., Pinciroli, V., Tonani, R., Vaghi, F. and Salvati, P. (1993) Imidazol-1-yl and pyridin-3-yl derivatives of 4-phenyl-1,4-dihydropyridines combining Ca⁺⁺ antagonism and thromboxane A_2 synthase inhibition. *J. Med. Chem.* **36:** 2964–2972.

93. Sircar, I., Haleen, S. J. and Burke, S. E. (1992) Synthesis and biological activity of 4-(diphenylmethyl)-α-[(4-quinolinyloxy)methyl]-1-piperazineethanol and related compounds. *J. Med. Chem.* **35:** 4442–4449.

94. Chen, I. -J., Yeh, J. -L., Liou, S. -J. and Shen, A. -Y. (1994) Guaiacoxypropanolamine derivatives of capsaicin: a new family of β-adrenoceptor blockers with intrinsic cardiotonic properties. *J. Med. Chem.* **37:** 938–943.

95. Ogawa, T., Nakazato, A., Tsuchida, K. and Hatayama, K. (1993) Synthesis and antihypertensive activities of new 1,4-dihydropyridine derivatives containing a nitrooxy moiety at the 3-ester position. *Chem. Pharm. Bull.* **41:** 108–116.

96. Zemlicka, J., Fernandez-Moyano, M. C., Ariatti, M., Zurenko, G. E., Grady, J. E. and Ballesta, J. P. G. (1993) Hybrids of antibiotics inhibiting protein synthesis. Synthesis and biological activity. *J. Med. Chem.* **36:** 1239–1244.

97. Albrecht, H. A., Beskid, G., Christenson, J. G., Deitcher, K. H., Georgopapadakou, N. H., Keith, D. D., Konzelmann, F. M., Pruess, D. L. and Wei, C. C. (1994) Dual-action cephalosporins incorporating a 3′-tertiary-amine-linked quinolone. *J. Med. Chem.* **37:** 400–407.

98. Carrupt, P. -A., Testa, B., Bechalany, A., El Tayar, N., Descas, P. and Perrissoud, P. (1991) Morphine-6-glucuronide and morphine-3-glucuronide as molecular chameleons with unexpected lipophilicity. In Silipo, C. and Vittoria, A. (eds) *QSAR: Rational Approaches to the Design of Bioactive Compounds*, pp. 541–544. Elsevier Science Publishers, B.V., Amsterdam.

99. Chi, D. Y., O'Neil, J. P., Anderson, C. J., Welch, M. J. and Katzenellenbogen, J. A. (1994) Homodimeric and heterodimeric bis(amino thiol) oxometal complexes with rhenium(V) and technetium(V). Control of heterodimeric complex formation and an approach to metal complexes and mimic steroid hormones. *J. Med. Chem.* **37:** 928–937.

100. Portoghese, P. S., Sultana, M. and Takemori, A. E. (1989) Design of peptidomimetic δ opioid receptor antagonists using the message-address concept. *J. Med. Chem.* **33:** 1714–1720.

16

Application Strategies for Primary Structure–Activity Relationship Exploration

CAMILLE G. WERMUTH

Le bon sens est la chose du monde la mieux partagée:
car chacun pense en être si bien pourvu, que ceux même qui
sont les plus difficiles à contenter en tout autre chose,
n'ont point coutume d'en désirer plus qu'ils n'en ont.

Good sense is the worldly thing which is best shared:
for everyone thinks they are so well provided with it,
that even those who are the most difficult to satisfy in every other matter,
are not in the habit of desiring more of it than they already have.
René Descartes (1596–1650)[1]

THE PRACTICE OF MEDICINAL CHEMISTRY
ISBN 0-12-744640-0

When confronted with a new lead structure or when, for patent reasons, it is necessary to enlarge the protection perimeter around newly discovered structures, the medicinal chemist may be daunted by the immensity of the task. The aim of the present chapter is to provide some guidelines and strategies for rendering easier and more efficacious the decision on which compounds to prepare and which ones to reject. The proposed guidelines derive essentially from common-sense reasoning, a feature that may explain why they are often forgotten. In addition to his personal experience, the author was inspired by the articles of Messer,[2] Cavalla,[3] Craig[4] and Austel.[5]

I. GENERAL STRATEGIES

Before considering the different possibilities for molecular variation presented in the previous chapters (homology, isostery, ring system modifications and synthesis of twin drugs, etc.), one has to decide what kind of general strategy should be applied. Depending on the lead structure's size and on its degree of complexity, the strategy may involve a simplification (disjunctive approach), conservation of the same level of complexity (analogical approach) or enlargement through additional elements (conjunctive approach).

Simplification of the original lead compound is especially appropriate for natural substances. This approach, known as the *disjunctive approach*[6] (see Chapter 14) consists in a molecular dissection that deletes functions, structural elements or cycles. Classic examples of disjunctive approaches are found in the pruning of physostigmine to yield neostigmine (Fig. 16.1) and in the change from somatostatin to a simplified hexapeptide (see Chapter 20).[7] Other examples of disjunctive approaches are collected in Table 16.1. The main result of the methodology is the identification of the portions of the molecule that are essential for the expected biological activity and those that are not.

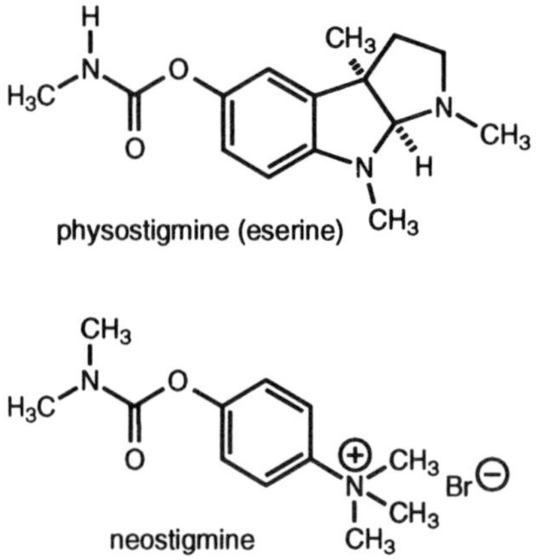

Fig. 16.1 Neostigmine is the result of disjunctive approach applied to physostigmine.

Table 16.1 Drugs resulting from disjunctive manipulations.

Lead	Derivative
Cocaine	Procaine
Tubocurarine	Decamethonium
Morphine	Morphinanes
	Benzomorphanes
	Phenylpiperidines
Atebrine	Chloroquine
Asperlicin	Benzodiazepine analogue
Phylloquinone (vitamine K_1)	Menadione (vitamine K_3)
Triamterene	Amiloride
Cimetidine	Roxatidine
Somatostatin	Simplified peptide
Bothrops jaraca venin	Teprotide Captopril

Table 16.2 Drug analogues possessing a similar size to the model compound.

Initial drug	Analogue
Chlorpromazine	Thioridazine
Imipramine	Amitryptyline
Propranolol	Pindolol
Furosemide	Bumetamide
Enalapril	Perindopril
Cimetidine	Ranitidine
Pravastatin	Fluindostatin

Conservation of the lead compound's degree of complexity proceeds usually through isosteric exchanges or functional inversions and can be considered as being the *analogical approach*[8] (Table 16.2).

Finally, when additional moieties are grafted on to the molecule, one speaks of *conjunctive approaches*.[6] These can also consist in the attachment of additional structural elements, as in the association of two separate drugs (associative synthesis, nonsymmetrical twin drugs, the symbiotic approach[9]) or in the duplication of the parent drug (symmetrical twin drugs).

The change of the $GABA_B$ receptor agonist CGP 27 492 to the $GABA_B$ receptor antagonist CGP 54 062 (Fig. 16.2) represents a typical example of the conjunctive approach resulting from the attachment of additional structural elements.[10] A similar case is provided by the design of the H_2-receptor agonist impromidine.[11]

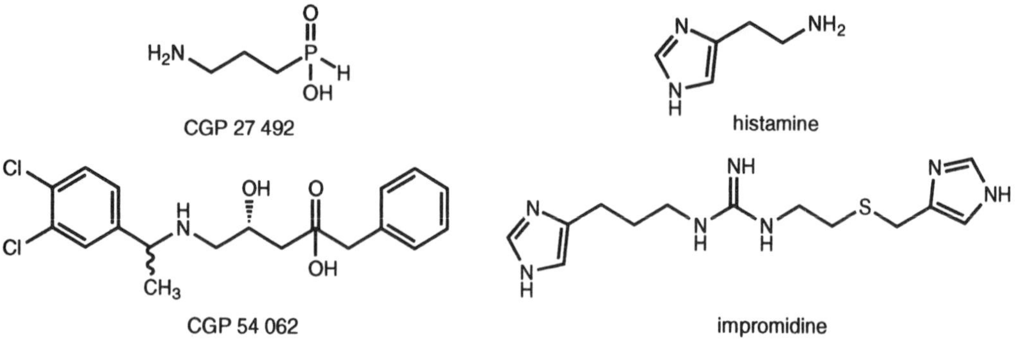

Fig. 16.2 Conjunctive approach in drug design. The attachment of two benzylic groups and a hydroxyl in *S*-configuration changes a GABA$_B$ receptor agonist into a GABA$_B$ antagonist[10]. Similarly the H$_2$-histaminergic agonist impromidine is the result of a conjunctive approach applied to histamine.[11]

Examples of drugs resulting from *associative synthesis* (nonsymmetrical twin drugs) and of *duplication* of the parent drug (symmetrical twin drugs) are listed in Tables 16.3 and 16.4. A more detailed study is presented in Chapters 15 and 26.

Table 16.3 Nonsymmetrical twin drugs.

Drug 1	Drug 2	Twin drug
Caffeine	Amphetamine	Fenethylline
Aspirin	Paracetamol	Benorylate
Clofibric acid	Nicotinic acid	Etofibrate
Hydrazinopyridazine	β-Blocker	Prizidilol
Pindolol	Captopril	BW-B385C[12]

Table 16.4 Symmetrical twin drugs.

Drug	Activity
Bialamicol	Antiamoebic
Ethambucol	Tuberculostatic
Probucol	Antihyperlipoproteinaemic
Thiamin disulphide	Vitamin
Dicumarol	Anticoagulant
Netropsin	DNA binding agent
Succinylcholine	Skeletal muscle relaxant

II. MOLECULAR DESIGN STRATEGY

Each time one has to deal with a new lead compound, the first important step of the drug design procedure is to apply systematically the molecular variation methodologies presented as primary exploration of structure–activity relationships in Chapters 12 to 15. It is therefore

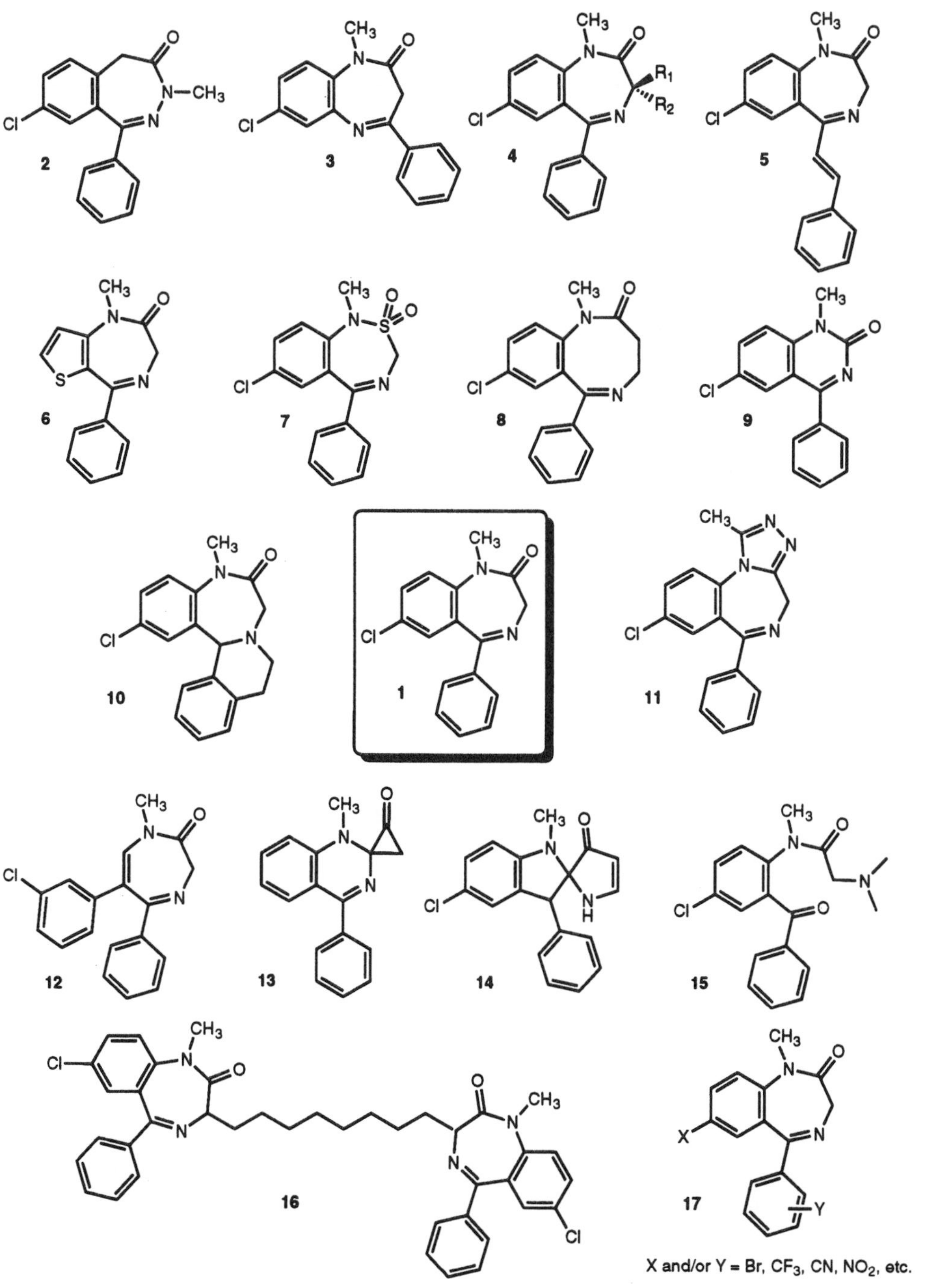

Fig. 16.3 Molecular variations applied to diazepam (**1**). Compounds (**2**) and (**3**) are positional isomers; optical isomerism is introduced in (**4**). Compound (**5**) is a vinylogue (vinylogy is also used for to render amidic the carbonyl of (**14**), (**6**) and (**7**) are isosteres. Compounds (**8**) to (**15**) result from various ring modifications: enlargement (**8**), contraction (**9**), introduction of additional rings (**10** and **11**), benzo splitting (**12**), use of spiro systems (**13** and **14**), and in ring opening (**15**). Compound (**16**) is a symmetrical twin drug and compound (**17**) underlines that many substituent variations can be used. The structures presented do not strictly correspond to existing molecules.

highly recommended to grab a sheet of paper or to plug in the computer and to draw all the possible structural analogues of the lead. For this purpose, all the possibilities offered by the molecular variation methodology should be freely used: the reader is encouraged to apply successively isomeric, homologous, vinylogous and, of course, isosteric replacements; and also try functional exchanges, ring modifications, symmetrical and nonsymmetrical twin drugs, and so on. This strategy allows one, starting from a given lead compound, to envisage an extremely high number of structural variations in a purely formal manner. Applied systematically, it turns out to be very useful because it makes one think and because it generates new ideas.

The richness of this purely formal procedure is illustrated in Fig. 16.3, where it is applied to the well-known anxiolytic diazepam. In combining the different individual modifications, a bewildering number of structures can be envisaged! Even when applied to a known structure such as a benzodiazepine, the *systematic* application of the strategy allows identification of unknown analogues and generates interesting new ideas (Fig. 16.3). However, a disadvantage of this procedure is that others can also follow the same reasoning and end up with the same ideas. It is therefore recommended to use this approach preferentially with leads that are your own.

III. APPLICATION RULES

It would certainly be tiresome and beyond the possibilities of a medicinal chemistry team to be forced to prepare all the compounds imagined by means of 'paper' chemistry. The following rules aim to codify precisely the use of all the strategies and to increase their efficacy by establishing priorities and selection rules.

A. Rule 1: The minor modifications rule

This rule[8] can be defined as giving priority to the design of analogues that are close to the lead structure and that result from only minor changes. Minor changes are achieved by very simple organic reactions such as hydrogenations, hydroxylations, methylations, acetylations, racemate resolutions, changes in substituents and isosteric replacements. The modification can produce either an increase in potency or an increase in selectivity or even sometimes the suppression of unwanted side-effects (Table 16.5).

The minor modifications rule, even supported by prestigious results, is largely unrecognized. Making use of ordinary chemistry, it is not always accepted with enthusiasm by organic chemists. The very simple reactions that are involved do not add much to their fame and they are more fascinated by the challenge of a total synthesis, especially of a natural substance bearing many chiral centres. Seen from a practical point of view, priority has nevertheless to be given to this principle. Its simplicity of implementation, and especially the spectacular results that it brings, militate in its favour.

B. Rule 2: The biological logic rule

The second rule of application rests on the earliest possible utilization of biochemical data. Indeed, even when a medicinal chemist ignores all of the biochemistry of the substance that she

Table 16.5 Minor modifications.

Original compound	Modified compound	Result[a]
Ergotamine	Dihydroergotamine	Increase in potency as α-adrenergic antagonist decrease in toxicity
Chlorothiazide	Hydrochlorothiazide	20-fold increase in potency
Chloroquine	Hydroxychloroquine	Decrease in toxicity
Morphine	Codeine	Change in activity profile (analgesic → antitussive)
Carbachol	Bethanechol	Increase in selectivity (exclusively muscarinic)
Imipramine	Desmethylimipramine	Change in activity profile (noradrenergic → serotonergic)
Tolbutamide	Chlorpropamide	Longer duration of action (5–7 h → 24–48 h)
Racemic amphetamine	Dexamphetamine	Fewer cardiovascular side-effects

[a]Taken from ref. 13.

studies, she learns to consider the former from the biochemical angle that will provide a good number of subjects to think about and may sometimes allow anticipation of the behaviour of the molecule. In particular, biological activity may be rationalized if it stems from the chemical or physicochemical properties of the series.

Very general properties can be foreseen in so far as functions or moieties present in the structure can suggest interference with a biological system; for example, hydrazines or hydroxylamines and pyridoxal-containing coenzymes, complexing agents and metallic coenzymes, electron donors or acceptors and oxido-reduction coenzymes, tensioactive amphiphilic substances and production of haemolysis in erythrocytes. In a more precise manner, the alkylating properties of compounds such as the nitrogen mustards, the nitrosoureas and the mitomycins, or the cross-linking properties of *cis*-platinum derivatives relate to their anticancer activity. The activity of anthracyclines, ellipticine and the anthracene-diones has been shown to be due to to intercalation in the double helix of DNA. The anticoccidial polyether ionophores are potent complexing agents for mono- and divalent cations.

The biological action of a compound is also readily explicable if it mimics a natural substrate or mediator. This is the case for enzymes with inhibitors (angiotensin I and captopril), suicide substrates (GABA and vigabatrin), antimetabolites (*p*-aminobenzoic acid and *p*-aminobenzenesuphonamide) and for receptors with agonists (acetylcholine and muscarine), antagonists (GABA and gabazine) and uptake inhibitors (GABA and nipecotic acid). The analogy with the endogenous substance can be sometimes very vague, as seen with quaternary ammonium compounds that all present more or less affinity for the cholinergic receptors, or with purines, which are often recognized by the phosphodiesterases.

The pathways of drug metabolism follow some general rules (see Chapters 28 and 29) and the metabolites of a given substance can, at least qualitatively, be imagined in advance. As a consequence, various measures can be taken to favour or, conversely, to slow down the biodegradation. Some chemical groupings are more prone than others to yield unwanted toxic metabolites (see Chapter 30). Among the best known are the aromatic nitro and amino compounds, the bromoarenes, the hydrazines and the hydroxylamines, and the polyhalogenated aliphatic or aromatic compounds. Finally, if the active principle is an acid or a base, the choice of the salifying counterion also has to follow some selection criteria (see Chapter 34). Oxalates and nitrates, for example, are not very popular, whereas hydrochlorides represent a satisfactory compromise.

C.   Rule 3: The structural logic rule

This rule implies that, as soon as some structural data are available (intercharge distances, *E-* or *Z*-conformations, axial or equatorial substituent orientations, misoriented substituents, etc.), they have to be fed back into drug design. When dealing with enzymes or receptors of unknown structure, one route to such information consists in comparing already known active compounds, recognized by the same molecular target, and to deduce the important stereoelectronic features associated with potency and selectivity. This approach is referred to as pharmacophore identification or receptor mapping (see Chapters 19 and 22). Initially presented by Marshall *et al.*,[14] it has some predictive merit[15,16] and at least avoids unnecessary syntheses of *a priori* inactive compounds. In practice the most efficient methods consist of steady comings and goings between synthetic and computer chemistry in order to achieve the ideal interplay between intuition and computer assistance.

A structural guide is also available for drugs designed to bind to the neurotransmitters of the central nervous system. On the basis of a comparison of the crystal structures of recognized representative compounds from each of eight major CNS active drug classes, Andrews and Lloyd[17,18] identified a common structural basis, essentially characterized by an aromatic plane distant about 5 Å from a nitrogen moiety. The explanation for this finding resides in the biochemical origin of the neurotransmitters.[16] Most of them are of the arylethylamine type, as a result of the decarboxylation of aromatic amino acids such as dopa or histidine.

Another example is given by acetylcholine which can be considered as bioisosteric with GABA, this property explains the observation that a compound such as the $GABA_A$ receptor antagonist bicuculline is recognized by both the $GABA_A$ and the nicotinic receptors.[16]

D.   Rule 4: The right substituent choice

Half of all the existing drugs contain easily substituted aromatic rings. The replacement, in such rings, of a hydrogen by a substituent (alkyl, halogen, hydroxyl, nitro, cyano, alkoxy, amino, carboxylate) can dramatically modify the intensity, the duration, and perhaps even the nature of the pharmacological effect (see Chapters 17, 18 and 19). It therefore becomes of prime importance to proceed to the optimal choice of substituents so as to explore with the smallest set possible the three-dimensional space formed by lipophilic, electronic and steric parameter coordinates (Fig. 16.4).

The right substituent choice minimizes the number of test compounds that have to be synthesized to explore a significant volume of the space. This represents a three-dimensional extension of the Craig plot discussed by Craig[4] and by Austel[5] and reproduced in Chapter 19.

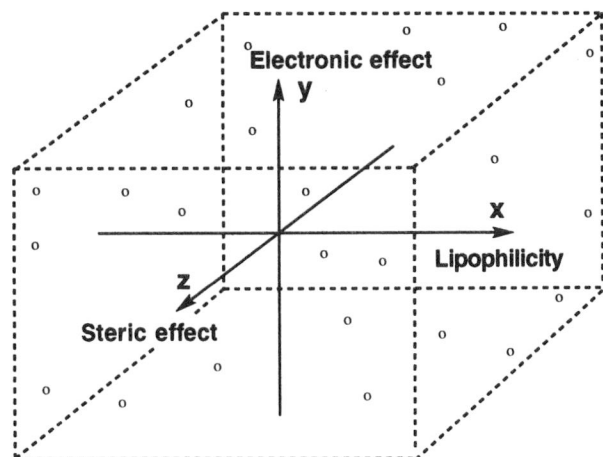

Fig. 16.4 Three-dimensional space formed by lipophilic, electronic and steric coordinates.

E. Rule 5: The easy organic synthesis (EOS) rule

Synthesis of new compounds is a costly and lengthy process, and therefore any measure able to render it more efficacious is welcome. Thus for example, when the decision is taken to prepare a given set of compounds, why not first prepare those whose synthesis is the easiest? In the same line of thought, why not prepare first compounds for which intermediates are commercially available?

A particular recommendation is to synthesize heterocycles. In statistics established in 1982 on 1522 drug molecules, Kleemann and Engel[19] highlighted the fact that, among the synthetic drugs, 62% contained at least one heterocyclic ring, the percentage within natural compounds being even higher (77%). Indeed, heterocycles present many advantages: (1) They allow the insertion of elements capable of giving interactions that the carbocycles do not give. (2) They allow a greater number of combinations. It therefore becomes easier to be original. (3) They represent rigid analogues of endogenous substances that themselves are often nitrogenous metabolites of amino acids. (4) Often their facile synthesis permits the preparation of large series.[20] One of the major problems when dealing with isosteric or bioisosteric replacements in heterocyclic systems is the selection of the *a priori* most promising candidate among several dozens of possible rings. A simple clue, which reflects the dipolar moment, can be given by knowledge and comparison of the boiling points of the basic heterocycles (see Chapter 13).

F. Rule 6: Eliminate the chiral centres

Although optical isomerism will be discussed in Chapter 21, some practical considerations on chiral molecules are appropriate here. Nowadays it is well accepted that racemates and both enantiomers usually represent three different pharmacological entities and that it requires extensive pharmacological, toxicological and clinical pharmacological research before it can be decided whether it is advantageous to use racemates or enantiomers in clinical practice.

According to Soudijn,[21] these research efforts could be reduced to about one-third if drugs without centres or planes of asymmetry could be developed with the same or higher affinity. Effectively, *asymmetry is far from being an absolute requisite for activity.* The alkaloid morphine possesses five chiral centres; on the other hand its synthetic derivative fentanyl is devoid of any asymmetric centre but nonetheless belongs to the most potent analgesics known. In some instances the chiral centres can be at least partially eliminated. This is the case for the synthetic analogues of the HMG-CoA reductase inhibitor mevinolin. Mevinolin itself (Fig. 16.5) has seven asymmetric centres, but SAR studies rapidly revealed that the five chiral centres contained in the hexahydronaphthalene are unnecessary for HMG-CoA inhibition. The second generation of mevinolin analogues, illustrated in Fig. 16.5 by the compound HR 780, retains only two of the initial seven chiral centres.[22]

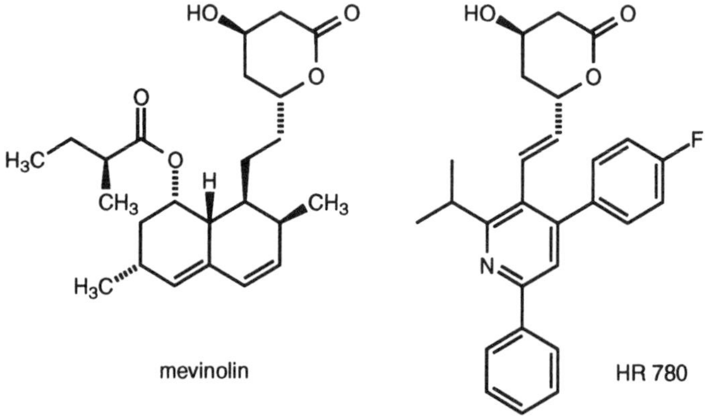

Fig. 16.5 Deletion of five out of seven chiral centres still yields highly potent mevinolin analogues.[22]

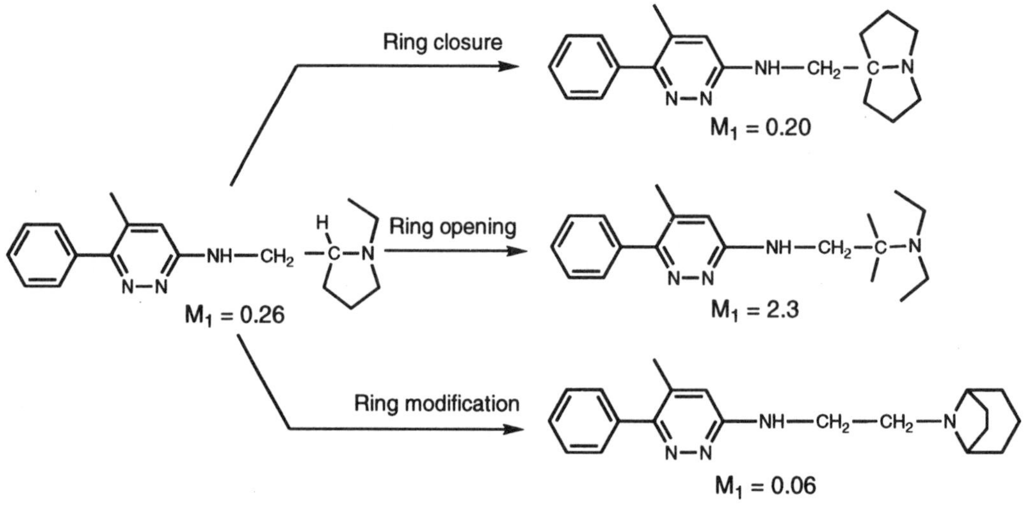

Fig. 16.6 Introducing symmetry and thus abolishing a chiral centre (affinity values for M_1 receptor preparations expressed as micromoles).

Usually chiral centres are eliminated in creating symmetry. Thus, in a series of muscarinic agonists derived from 3-aminopyridazines, one of the most favourable side-chains was the racemic 2-N-ethylpyrrolidinylmethyl chain, that is the side-chain of sulpiride (Fig. 16.6). The 5-methyl-6-phenylpyridazine bearing this basic chain at its 3-amino function presented a 0.26 micromolar affinity for M_1-muscarinic receptor preparations.[23] After resolution of the racemate, the corresponding enantiomers showed only a 6-fold difference in M_1 affinity. It was therefore decided to eliminate the chiral center by introducing symmetry either by ring opening or by ring closure, or even by replacing the 2-N-ethylpyrrolidinylmethyl unit by the nonchiral tropane ring. The structures so modified show affinities similar to that of the corresponding chiral molecule.[23]

When one nevertheless has to deal with chiral centres, why not first prepare the racemic compound and start with an enantioselective synthesis only if an interesting activity is found? This latter point is tricky, because many people believe that two enantiomers might happen to antagonize each other. They refer to the numerous examples published in the literature.[21,24–26] In reality, two optical isomers *are never antagonists at comparable dosages*. This comes from the space-relationship required for the interaction with the receptor site, which is only slightly altered by passing from S- to R-forms, or vice-versa. If one of the enantiomers achieves the optimal fit to the receptor site in exchanging the highest number of noncovalent linkages, the others only gives rise to weaker interactions, even under the most favourable conditions (Fig. 16.7).

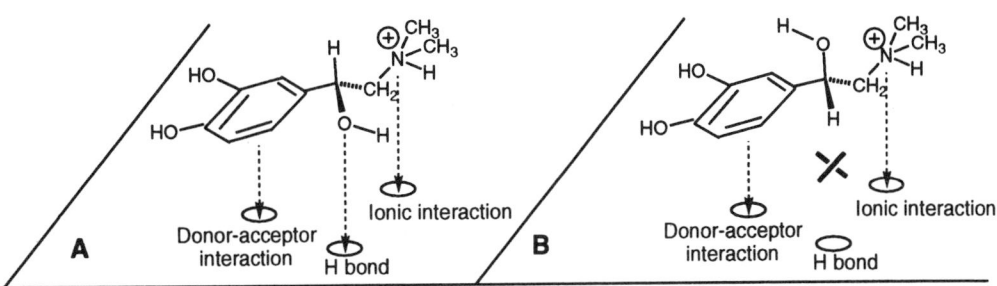

Fig. 16.7   Interaction capacities of the natural R-(+)-epinephrine and its S(−) antipode. Assuming for simplicity that the natural R-(+)-epinephrine establishes a three-point interaction with its receptor (A) the combination of the donor–acceptor interaction, the hydrogen bond and the ionic interaction will generate energies of the order 12–17 kcal mol⁻¹, which corresponds to binding constants of 10⁻⁹ to 10⁻¹² M.[27] The less active isomer, S-(+)-epinephrine, may establish only a two-point contact (B). The loss of the hydrogen bond interaction represents to approximately 3 kcal mol⁻¹; this isomer should therefore possess an approximately 100-fold lower affinity. Experience confirms this estimate. If we consider less abstract models it becomes apparent that the less potent enantiomer also is able to develop three intermolecular bonds to the receptor, provided it approaches the receptor in a different manner. However, the probability of this alternative binding mode triggering the same biological response is close to nil.

From a practical point of view, this absence of *stoichiometric* antagonism entails two consequences: (a) if a racemic mixture does not show any activity, it is useless to carry out the separation of the two enantiomers; (b) a racemic mixture usually has the average potency of both constituents; thus, the maximal benefit one can achieve in resolving racemic mixtures is an increase of the activity to twice of that of the racemate.

G. Rule 7: The pharmacological logic rule

We insisted in Chapter 4 on the fact that a correctly performed pharmacological study must satisfy certain criteria (relationship between dose and effect, presentation of the coinfidence limits, comparison with a reference compound, determination of the time of the peak action). On the chemical side it is also extremely important to provide the pharmacologists with reference compounds published by competitor laboratories. Even if it is felt tedious and time consuming to resynthesize an already described compound, the operation is always worthwhile and sometimes surprising. How often a good-looking published molecule for which attractive activities are claimed loses much of its charm once it is reinvestigated by one's own team! Another point that may contribute to increasing the credibility of your work is the so-called *a contrario* probe. In other words, when your own structure–activity relationship studies allow identification of the molecular features associated with high activity, proceed, of course, to the synthesis of the most interesting representatives, but also prepare at least one compound that, according to your results, should be inactive.

REFERENCES

1. Descartes, R. (1972) Discours de la méthode, 1ére partie, 1637. In Robinet, A. (ed.), *Les Nouveaux Classiques Larousse*, p. 27. Librairie Larousse, Paris.
2. Messer, M. (1984) Traditional or pragmatic research. In Jolles, G. and Wooddridge, K. R. M. (eds) *Drug Design: Fact or Fantasy?* pp. 217–224. Academic Press, London.
3. Cavalla, J. F. (1983) Drug design valuable for refining an active drug. In Gross, F. (ed.) *Decision Making in Drug Research*, pp. 165–172. Raven Press, New York.
4. Craig, P. N. (1980) Guidelines for drug and analog design. In Wolffe, M. E. (ed.) *The Basis of Medicinal Chemistry*, pp. 331–348. Wiley-Interscience, New York.
5. Austel, V. (1984) Features and problems in practical drug design. In Charton, M. and Motoc, I. (eds) *Steric Effects in Drug Design*, pp. 8–19. Lange and Springer, Berlin.
6. Schueller, F. W. (1960) *Chemobiodynamics and Drug Design.* McGrawHill, New York.
7. Freidinger, R. M. and Veber, D. F. (1984) Design of novel cyclic hexapeptide somatostatin analogs from a model of the bioactive conformation. In Vida, J. A. and Gordon, M. (eds) *Conformationally Directed Drug Design*, pp. 169–187. American Chemical Society, Washington DC.
8. Wermuth, C. G. (1966) Modifications chimiques des médicaments en vue de l'amélioration de leur action. *Agressologie*, **7**: 213–219.
9. Nicolaus, B. J. R. (1983) *Symbiotic approach to drug design.* In Gross, F. (ed.) *Decision Making in Drug Research*, pp. 173–186. Raven Press, New York.
10. Froestl, W., Furet, P., Hall, R. G. *et al.* (1993) $GABA_B$ antagonists: novel CNS-active compounds. In Testa, B., Kyburz, E., Fuhrer, W. and Giger, R. (eds) *Perspectives in Medicinal Chemistry*, pp. 259–272. VHC, Weinheim.
11. Durant, G. J., Duncan, W. A. M., Ganellin, C. R., Parsons, M. E., Blakemore, R. C. and Rasmussen, A. C. (1978) Impromidine (SK&F 92 676) is a very potent and specific agonist for histamine H_2 receptors. *Nature*, **276**: 403–405.
12. Hardy, G. W. and Allan, G. (1988) BW-B3895C. *Drugs Fut.* **13**: 204–206.
13. Goodman-Gilman, A., Rall, T. W., Nies, A. S. and Taylor, P. (eds) (1990) *Goodman and Gilman's The Pharmacological Basis of Therapeutics*, 8th edn. Pergamon Press, New York.
14. Marshall, G. R., Barry, C. D., Bosshard, H. E., Dammkoehler, R.A. and Dunn, D. A. (1979) The conformational parameter in drug design: the active analog approach. In Olson, E. C. and Christoffersen, R. E. (eds) *Computer-assisted Drug Design*, pp. 205–226. American Chemical Society, Washington DC.
15. Marshall, G. R. and Cramer III, D. R. (1988) Three-dimensional structure–activity relationships. *Trends Pharmacol. Sci.* **9**: 285–289.

16. Wermuth, C. G. and Langer, T. (1993) Pharmacophore identification. In Kubinyi, H. (ed.) *3D QSAR in Drug Design — Theory, Methods, and Applications,* pp. 117–136. ESCOM, Leiden.
17. Andrews, P. R. and Lloyd, E. J. (1983) A common structural basis for c.n.s. drug action. *J. Pharm. Pharmacol.* **35**: 516–518.
18. Lloyd, E. J. and Andrews, P. R. (1986) A common structural model for central nervous system drugs and their receptors. *J. Med. Chem.* **29**: 453–462.
19. Kleemann, A. and Engel, J. (1982) *Pharmazeutische Wirkstoffe-Synthese, Patente, Anwendungen* (Preface). Georg Thieme Verlag, Stuttgart.
20. Messer, S. (1982) Personal communication. Rhône-Poulenc Recherches, Centre de Recherches Nicolas Grillet.
21. Soudijn, W. (1983) Advantages and disadvantages in the application of bioactive racemates or specific isomers as drugs. In Ariëns, E. J., Soudijn, W. and Timmermans, P. B. M. W. M. (eds) *Stereochemistry and Biological Activity of Drugs,* pp. 89–102. Blackwell Scientific Publications, Oxford.
22. Baader, E., Bartmann, W., Beck, G. *et al.* (1990) Rational approaches to enzyme inhibitors: new HMG-CoA reductase inhibitors. In Claassen, V. (ed.) *Trends in Drug Research,* pp. 49–71. Elsevier, Amsterdam.
23. Wermuth, C. G. (1993) Aminopyridazines—an alternative route to potent muscarinic agonists with no cholinergic syndrome. *Il Farmaco* **48**: 253–274.
24. Towart, R., Wehninger, E. and Meyer, H. (1981) Effects of unsymmetrical ester substituted 1,4-dihydropyridine derivatives and their optical isomers on contraction of smooth muscle. *Naunyn-Schmiedeberg's Arch. Pharmacol.* **317**: 183–185.
25. Lotti, V. J. and Taylor, D. A. (1982) α_2-Adrenergic agonist and antagonist activity of the respective (−)- and (+)-enantiomers of 6-ethyl-9-oxaergoline. *Eur. J. Pharmacol.* **85**: 211–215.
26. Hof, R. P., Rüegg, U. T., Hof, A. and Vogel, A. (1985) Stereoselectivity at the calcium channel: opposite action of the enantiomers of a 1,4-dihydropyridine. *J. Cardiovasc. Pharmacol.* **7**: 689–693.
27. Farmer, P. S. and Ariëns, E. J. (1982) Speculations on the design of nonpeptidic peptidomimetics. *Trends Pharmacol. Sci.* **3**: 362–365.

PART IV

Substituents and Functions: Qualitative and Quantitative Aspects of Structure–Activity Relationships

17

Specific Substituent Effects

CAMILLE G. WERMUTH

*Fifty percent of the currently used drugs contain at least one
aromatic ring that can be matter of substitution*
John Taylor[1]

THE PRACTICE OF MEDICINAL CHEMISTRY
ISBN 0-12-744640-0

I. INTRODUCTION

The replacement, in an active molecule, of a hydrogen atom by a substituent (alkyl, halogen, hydroxyl, nitro, cyano, alkoxy, amino, carboxylate, etc.) can deeply modify the potency, the duration, and perhaps even the nature of the pharmacological effect. Structure–activity relationship studies implying substituent modifications therefore represent common practice in medicinal chemistry, all the more since half of the existing drugs contain easily substituted aromatic rings. The perturbations brought by the substituent can affect various parameters of a drug molecule such as its *partition coefficient, electronic density, conformation, bioavailability, pharmacokinetics,* and, finally its capacity to establish *direct interactions* between the substituent and the receptor or the enzyme.

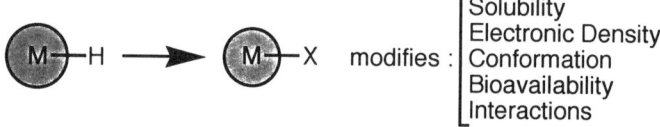

In reality it is impossible to modify only one alone of these five parameters. Thus, for example, the replacement of a hydrogen atom by a methyl group will simultaneously affect the five parameters listed above. Nevertheless, through a careful selection of the appropriate substituent, it is possible to vary one of the parameters in a *dominant* manner.

To illustrate the repercussions on the biological activity resulting from substituent effects, we will study successively the effects of methyl groups, of unsaturated groups, and of halogen substitution. Hydroxy groups, thiols and finally acidic or basic functions will be discussed more briefly.

II.   METHYL GROUPS

In this section we show how a methyl group, so often considered chemically inert, is able to alter deeply the pharmacological properties of a molecule. We will envisage successively effects on the solubility, conformational effects, electronic effects and effects on the bioavailability and the pharmacokinetics. In a final paragraph we will present some possibilities for replacing the methyl group by related groups and extend the study to some larger alkyl groups.

A.   Effects on solubility

As a rule, the attachment of one or several methyl groups on an active molecule renders it more lipophilic and therefore less soluble in water. However, in some particular cases, the attachment results in an increase of the water solubility by mechanisms such as increase of hydrophobic bonding possibilities or diminution of the crystal lattice energy.

1.   Increase of lipophilicity

Normally one expects that methyl groups increase the lipophilicity. Indeed, the partition coefficient P between n-octanol and water is $P = 490$ for toluene, compared to $P = 135$ for benzene.[2] Similarly one will find (for the system olive oil–water) $P = 83$ and $P = 360$ for acetamide and propionamide, or $P = 15$ and $P = 44$ for urea and N-methylurea, respectively.[3] More generally, the passage of (M)—H to (M)—CH$_3$ gives place to a positive increment of 0.52 in Hansch constant calculations (Chapter 19).

2.   Hydrophobic interactions

There are exceptions to the above rule: grafting one or several methyl groups can render the molecule more compact (more 'globular'). A good example is provided by aliphatic alcohols.[4] As expected, one observes that the increase in lipophilicity when passing from n-butanol to n-pentanol is accompanied by a decrease of the water solubility. However, 2-pentanol, and even more neopentanol, although possessing one methyl more than n-butanol, are *less* lipophilic, which means *more* soluble in water (Table 17.1).

Table 17.1   Solubility in water at 20°C of n-butanol (**1**), n-pentanol (**2**), 2-pentanol (**3**) and neopentanol (**4**).[4]

Compound	Solubility (g/100g H$_2$O)
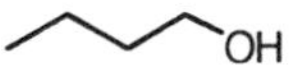 **1** OH	8.2
2 OH	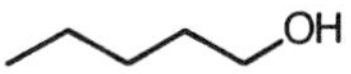 2.4
3 OH	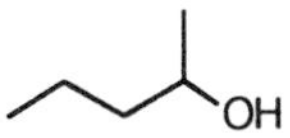 4.9
4 OH	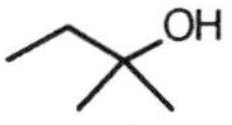 12.2

How do we explain this anomaly? It has to be attributed simply to an *entropic effect.*[5] In aqueous solution the particle is imprisoned in a tridimensional network (a cluster) of structured water molecules. On the other hand, a smaller number of structured water molecules is needed to create a cluster around a compact molecule than around an extended one (Fig. 17.1). This new structural arrangement is energetically favourable. For the same reason, molecules having some basic side-chains linked to an aromatic ring are more soluble than anticipated. In these derivatives, the chain folds in such a manner (Fig. 17.2) that the cationic head becomes placed under the aromatic ring and can establish a typical donor–acceptor interaction with the π cloud of the aromatic ring ('folding effect').[6]

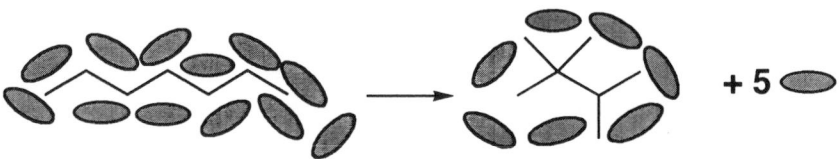

Fig. 17.1   Fewer structured water molecules are needed to envelope a compact molecule (2,2,3-trimethylbutane) than an extended one (*n*-heptane).

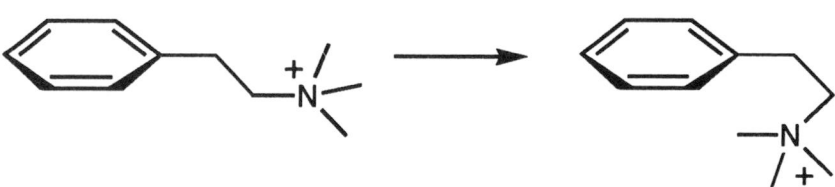

Fig. 17.2   Aralkylamines salts are more water-soluble than expected because they can adopt a folded, more compact, conformation that favours solvation.[6]

3.   Crystal lattice cohesion

A greater water solubility can also result from a decrease of the crystal lattice energy, the methyl groups hindering the various intermolecular interactions (hydrogen bonds, dipole–dipole bonds, etc.). In the antibacterial sulfonamide series, the substitution of the pyrimidine ring of sulfadiazine by one, then two, methyl groups causes an increase in solubility (Table 17.2).[7] *A priori*, one would expect that the methyl substituted derivatives would be less soluble, for the double reason that they show increased lipophilicity and that they are less dissociated than the parent molecule. Indeed, the inductive character of the methyl groups disfavours ionization and the nonionized form of a molecule is always less soluble than the corresponding ionized form. Despite this unfavourable electronic effect, sulfamidine is approximately 5 times more soluble than sulfadiazine. Similarly, the grafting of only one methyl group to the herbicide simazine provides atrazine, which is 14 times more soluble in water (Fig. 17.3).[8]

Table 17.2   Increased water solubility caused by insertion of methyl groups.[7]

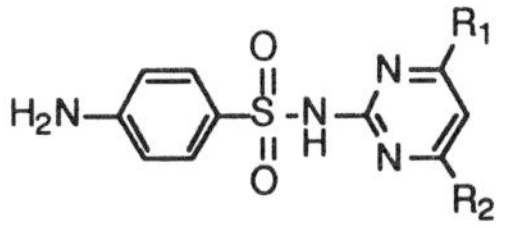

R_1	R_2	Drug	pK (acidic)	Percentage ionized at pH 5.2	Solubility, pH 5.2, 37°C (M)
H	H	Sulfadiazine	6.5	3.9	0.0005
CH_3	H	Sulfamerazine	7.1	1.4	0.0013
CH_3	CH_3	Sulfamidine	7.4	0.7	0.0024

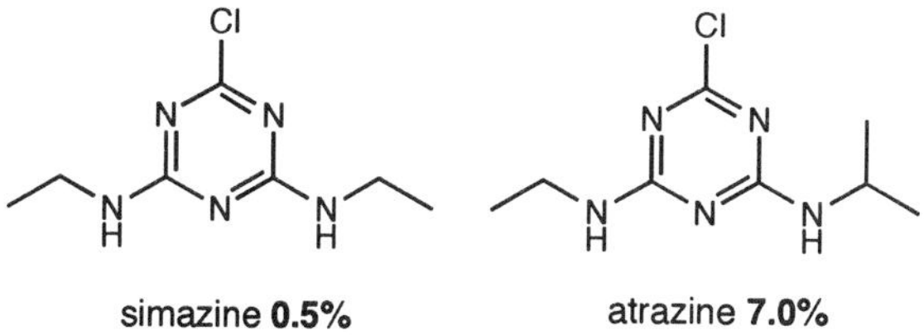

simazine **0.5%**   atrazine **7.0%**

Fig. 17.3   Comparison of the water solubility at 25°C of simazine and atrazin.[8]

B.   Conformational effects

The steric hindrance generated by a methyl group can create constraints and impose particular conformations that may be favourable or unfavourable for ligand–receptor interactions.

Harms and Nauta have studied the effects of methyl substitution on the aromatic ring of the spasmolytic *diphenhydramine*.[9] The presence of a methyl in *para* position corresponds to a 3.7-fold increase in antihistaminic activity compared to the nonsubstituted derivative (Fig. 17.4). Conversely, the presence of a methyl in *ortho* position inactivates the molecule (1/5 of the activity of the nonsubstituted derivative).

diphenhydramine   ortho-Me diphenhydramine   phenindamine

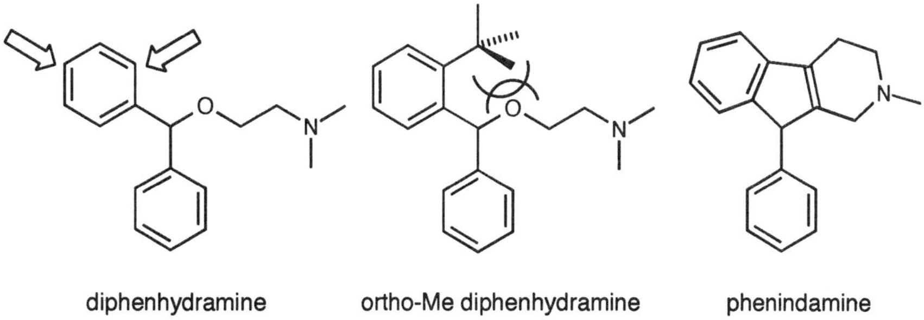

Fig. 17.4   The presence on diphenhydramine of an *ortho*-methyl group prevents the side-chain adopting the favourable coplanar conformation as found in phenindamine.[9]

The explanation proposed by the authors is as follows: the methyl group in *ortho* position prevents the side-chain from adopting the usual 'antihistaminic' conformation such as found in phenindamine, for example. Curiously the *ortho–ortho'*-disubstituted analogue of diphenhydramine shows local anaesthetic properties (40 time those of diphenhydramine).

In steroids the two angular methyl groups in positions 18 and 19 stand on the surface and form a screen above the β face (Fig. 17.5). This entails selective attacks on the rear face (α face) of the molecule.[10] In addition, the presence of the methyl in position 18 imposes a preferential conformation to the methylketone chain placed in position 17.[10]

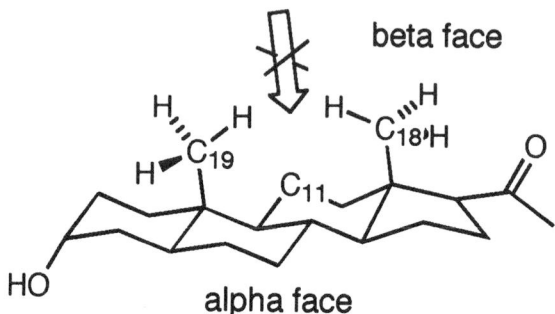

Fig. 17.5   The two angular methyl groups in positions 18 and 19 of the steroidal skeleton protect the carbon-11 from β face attacks.[10]

The antihypertensive imidazoline *clonidine* (Fig. 17.6; $R_1 = R_2 = Cl$) and its analogues activate specific receptors of the central nervous system. The maximal activity in this series is always observed when *both* the ortho positions are substituted ($R_1 = R_2 =$ methyl, chlorine or ethyl, etc.). This situation implies a restrained rotation of the atropisomery type and the impossibility of the two cycles lying in a coplanar situation. Correspondingly, the geometry of the molecule becomes close to that of the norepinephrine.[11]

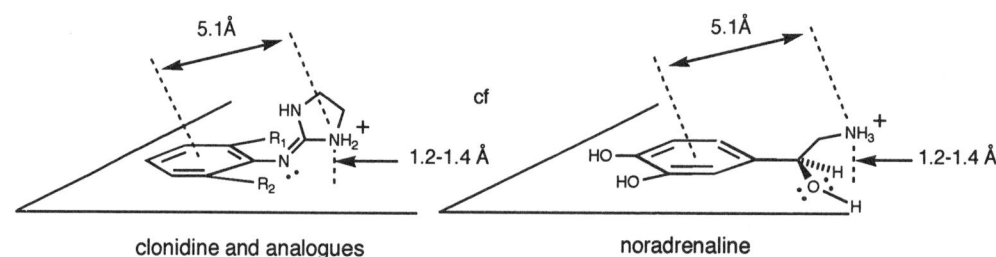

Fig. 17.6   The restricted rotation resulting from *ortho-* and *ortho'*-substitution imposes a quasiperpendicular orientation of the imidazolinic ring towards the phenyl ring.[11]

Leuprotide, deslorelin, and *nafarelin* are synthetic analogues of luteinizing hormone-releasing hormone (LHRH; pGlu-His-Trp-Ser-Tyr-Gly-Leu-Arg-Pro-GlyNH₂). They possess agonist properties and are currently used in the treatment of prostate cancer, endometriosis, precocious puberty, and other indications that are testosterone- or estrogen-dependent. In separately substituting each peptide bond of these analogues with *N*-methyl groups, various interesting results were observed.[12]

(1)   The introduction of an *N*-methyl group in the peptide's backbone at position 7 favours the bioactive conformation, i.e. a β-turn extending from residues 5 to 8 of the peptide. Thus, the *N*-Me-Leu[7] analogue of nafarelin (pGlu-His-Trp-Ser-Tyr-D2Nal-Leu-Arg-Pro-Gly-GlyNH$_2$; D2Nal = D-3-(2-naphtyl)alanine), is *20 times more potent* than nafarelin.

(2)   The other *N*-methyl analogues are generally less active than the nonmethylated compounds.

(3)   For some of the compounds, *N*-methylation resulted in a conversion of LHRH agonists to antagonists.

(4)   *N*-Methylation also improved the pharmacokinetics, mainly in increasing the stability against enzymatic degradation (see below, Section II.D).

C.   Electronic effects

The methyl group and, more generally all alkyl groups, are the only substituents acting by an inductive electron-donating effect. All the other groups are electron donors by mesomeric effects. This means that the methyl and the alkyls are electron donors in any environment, while a basic group, dimethylaminoethyl for example, will be a mesomeric donor in basic or neutral medium, but will become strongly electron-attracting by protonation in the gastric medium (pH ~2). Table 17.3, taken from Chu[13] presents some numerical values for substituents commonly met in medicinal chemistry. Hansch's π constant accounts for the contribution of lipophilicity, Hammet's σ constants reflect the electronic effects, and the molecular refraction (MR) is related to the volume of the substituent. The table illustrates clearly the dramatic change in Hammet's σ limit when passing from a free amino group (σ = −0.66) to a protonated one (σ = +0.60).

Table 17.3   Some common substituent constants. (Taken from Chu.[13])

Group	π	σ	MR
H	0.00	0.00	1.03
CH$_3$	0.56	−0.17	5.65
CF$_3$	0.88	0.54	5.02
Cl	0.71	0.23	6.03
OH	−0.67	−0.37	2.85
OCH$_3$	−0.02	−0.27	7.87
NH$_2$	−1.23	−0.66	5.42
NH$_3^+$	–	0.60	–
NO$_2$	−0.28	0.78	7.36
CN	−0.57	0.66	6.33
CO$_2$H	−0.32	0.45	6.93
COCH$_3$	−0.55	0.50	11.18

A practical consequence is that it is always judicious to include a methyl (or an alkyl) group in a SAR study. Thus, in any series of R-substituted molecules, when one wants to vary R, the methyl group is generally chosen as the representative of an electron donating group, the second substituent being chosen from the electron attractors (Cl, CN, NO$_2$, CF$_3$, etc.).

Compared to methycaine (Fig. 17.7), the 4-methyl derivative is more active *in vivo*, thanks to the inductive electron-donating effect of its methyl group. This latter exerts two synergic effects.[14] The first results in lesser reactivity of the ester carbonyl, retarding the ester group hydrolysis. The second effect is increased capacity of the carbonyl group to form hydrogen bonds, and therefore to achieve better interaction with the receptor.

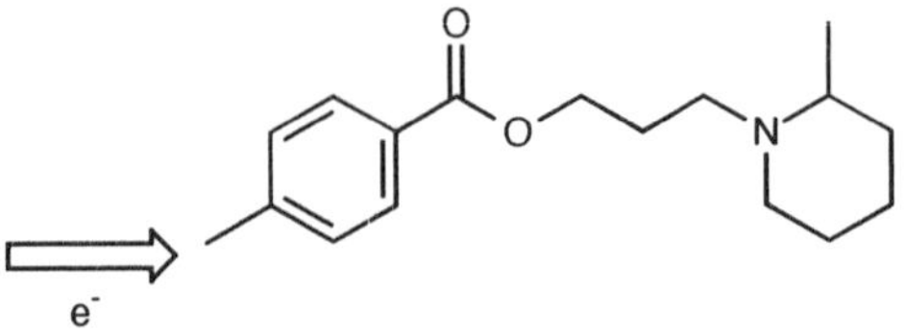

Fig. 17.7   Stabilization of the ester function thanks to an inductive effect of the *p*-methyl group.[14]

The pharmacological profile of histamine is profoundly altered by methylation. Thus 2-methylhistamine is active in stimulating the guinea-pig ileum (H$_1$ site) with 17% of the histamine potency (Fig. 17.8), but is only slightly active as a stimulant of gastric secretion in the rat (H$_2$ site). The reversed type of selectivity is shown, to a remarkable degree, by 4-methylhistamine, which has only 0.2% of the potency of histamine on the ileum yet nearly half the potency of histamine as a stimulant of gastric secretion. Thus a 200-fold discrimination towards the H$_2$ receptor is achieved.[15]

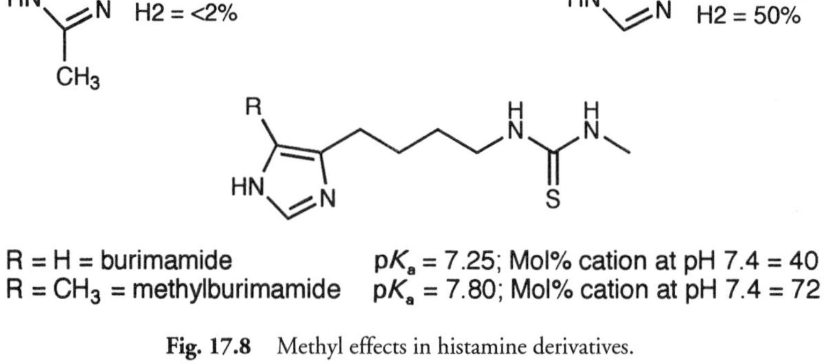

R = H = burimamide   pK$_a$ = 7.25; Mol% cation at pH 7.4 = 40
R = CH$_3$ = methylburimamide   pK$_a$ = 7.80; Mol% cation at pH 7.4 = 72

Fig. 17.8   Methyl effects in histamine derivatives.

The electron-donating effect of methyl groups is also reflected by the pK$_a$ values of burimamide compared to that of methylburimamide (Fig. 17.8).[16]

Phenanthrene itself is not carcinogenic, whereas 5,6-dimethyl-phenanthrene is highly carcinogenic. Methyl groups in positions 5 and 6 increase the electronic density around the carbon atoms 9 and 10 ('K region'). This activation allows the formation of an epoxide under biological conditions (Fig. 17.9). Such epoxides, like other carcinogens, are alkylating agents.

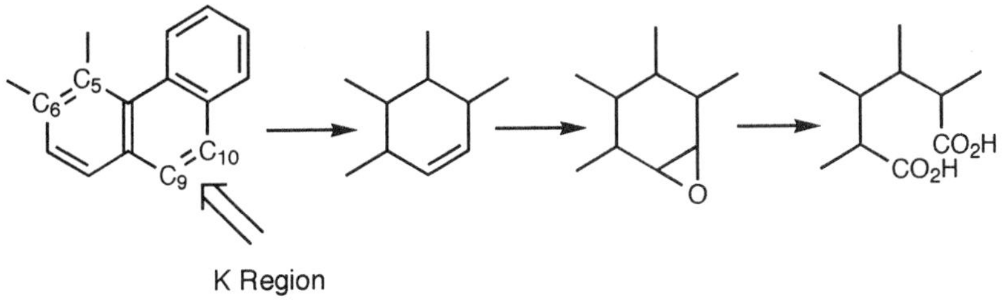

K Region

Fig. 17.9 Activation of the K region in 5,6-dimethylphenanthrene by an inductive effect of the methyl groups in positions 5 and 6.[17]

The activation of the double bond also explains the formation of ring-opened compounds that one finds in animals, bound to the plasmatic proteins, after administration of polycyclic hydrocarbons.[17]

D. Effects on metabolism

Seen from the metabolic point of view the methyl group plays a particularly important role. There are three possibilities: (a) the methyl group is oxidized, (b) the methyl group is transported, (c) the methyl group is not (or is only slightly) attacked and can then serve as blocking group.

1. Oxidation of the methyl group

The oxidation of the methyl group usually continues up to the carboxyl stage (Fig. 17.10). This is observed for camphor, for 2-methylpyridine and for the drugs tolbutamide and alpidem, explaining the relatively short half-lives of these latter compounds.

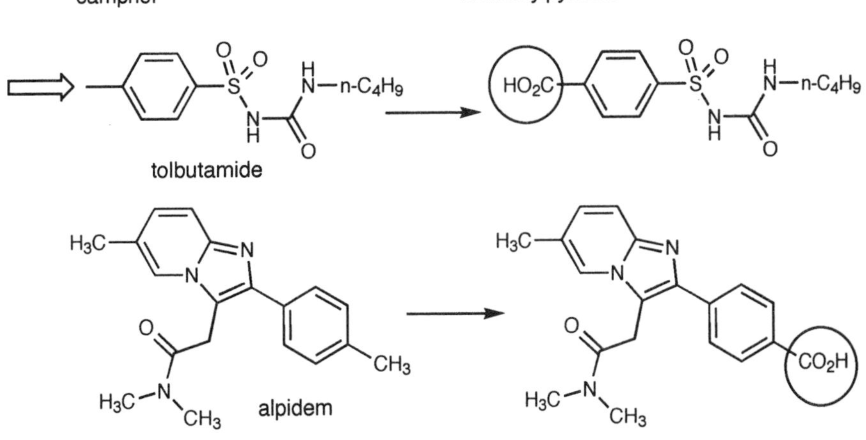

camphor

2-methylpyridine

tolbutamide

alpidem

Fig. 17.10 Examples of oxidation of methyl to carboxyl groups.

The attachment of a methyl group, especially on aromatic rings, often represents a good means of detoxification. It is rapidly oxidized to an inactive and easy-to-eliminate carboxylic group. When the grafted chains are longer than methyl, the attack takes place preferentially at the benzylic position or at position $\omega - 1$ (Fig. 17.11).

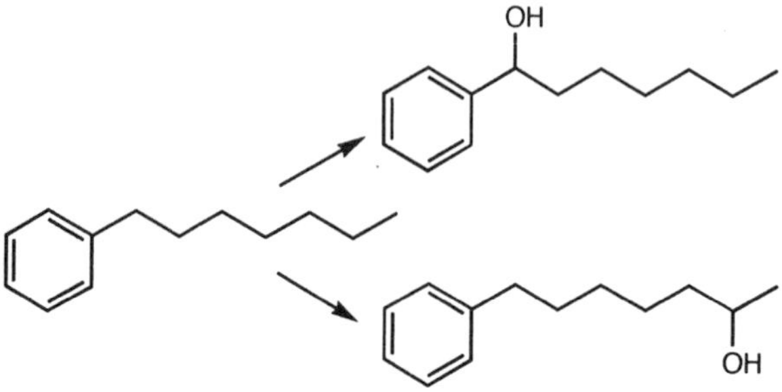

Fig. 17.11 Privileged oxidative attacks of long chains.

Angular methyl groups of steroids are usually resistant to metabolic oxidation, probably owing to local steric hindrance.

2. The methyl group is transported

A methyl group, when grafted on a nitrogen or sulfur atom, can transform these into 'onium' able to act as methyl donor. In living organisms the usual suppliers of methyl groups are choline and methionine. Methionine is first activated *in vivo* by combination with adenosine to yield *S*-adenosylmethionine (SAM; Fig. 17.12).

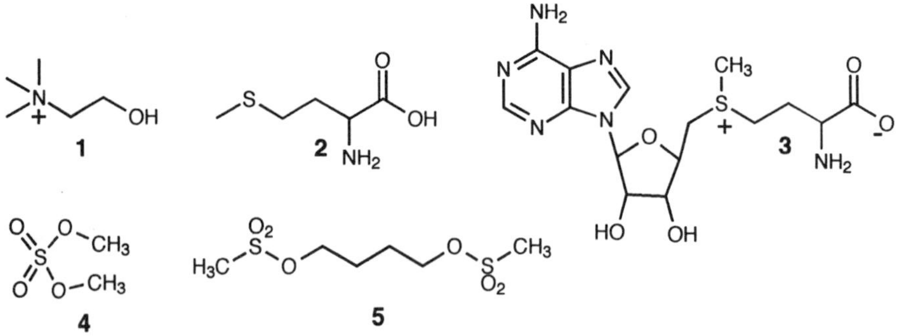

Fig. 17.12 Methyl donors and alkylating compounds choline (**1**), methionine (**2**), *S*-adenosylmethionine (**3**), dimethyl sulfate (**4**) and butane-1,4-diol bis(methane sulfonate) (**5**) (busulfan).

More generally, any *S*- or *N*-methylated drug can *a priori* constitute a methyl donor. On the other hand, when the methyl (or alkyl) group is linked to a good leaving group, as found for alkyl sulfates or sulfonates, alkylating reagents are produced and there exists a huge risk of carcinogenicity.

3. The methyl group serves to block a reactive function

A reactive function, such as an active hydrogen belonging to a hydroxyl, thiol or amino, can be masked by methylation. Methyl groups can serve to protect even carbon atoms from metabolic hydroxylation.

The ene–diol function is essential to the antioxidant properties of vitamin C; it is therefore not surprising that its methylation leads to an inactive compound (Fig. 17.13).

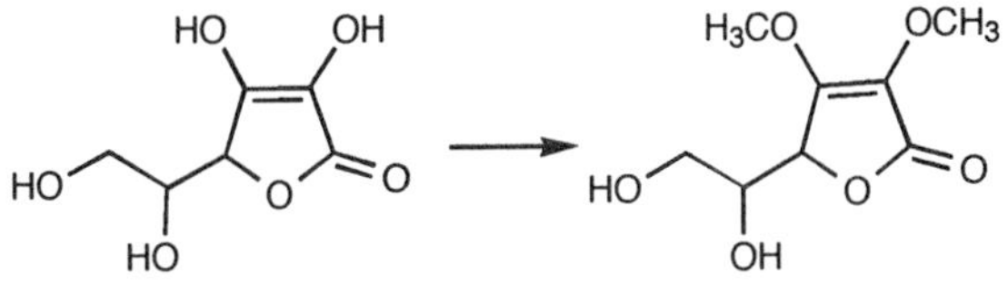

Fig. 17.13 The methylation of the ene–diol function of ascorbic acid leads to a chemically stable but pharmacologically inactive compound.

Ethylenebis(dithiocarbamic acid) (nabam) is a fungicide. Through bioactivation it gives birth to an alkylating diisothiocyanate able to block the reactive thiol functions of parasitic fungi. *N*-Methylation of nabam inactivates the compound because it prevents its transformation into diisothiocyanate [18] (Fig. 17.14).

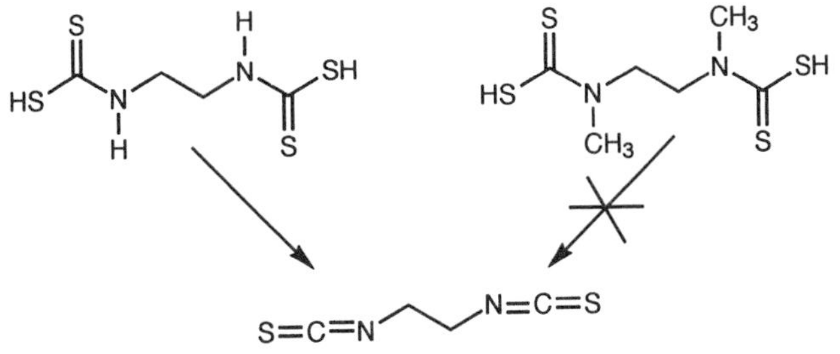

Fig. 17.14   *N*-Methylation of ethylenebis(dithiocarbamic acid).

As such, the endogenous peptides, methionine- and leucine enkephalin are inactive by the oral route. Starting from Met-enkephalin, Roemer *et al.* prepared a less vulnerable analogue of methionine enkephalin (Tyr-D-Ala-Gly-*N*-Me-Phe-Met(*O*)-ol), with prolonged parenteral and oral analgesic activity.[19] As depicted in Fig. 17.15, several modifications were needed: replacement of glycine by the nonnatural D-alanine, *N*-methylation of the Gly-Phe amide bond, oxidation of methionine to the sulfoxide, and reduction of the C-terminus to the alcohol.

For other examples of drug development starting from peptide leads, see the excellent reviews of Plattner and Norbeck[20] and of Fauchère.[21]

Tetramethylbenzidine, is a safe substitute for benzidine. For many years' benzidine has been used as a sensitive and specific reagent for the detection of blood. However, its extreme carcinogenicity, due to the metabolite 3,3'-dihydroxybenzidine (Fig. 17.16), has curtailed its use. In the search of a safe substitute, tetramethylbenzidine (3,3',5,5'-tetramethylbenzidine) was selected. With this compound *ortho*-hydroxylation is impossible, and it does not produce

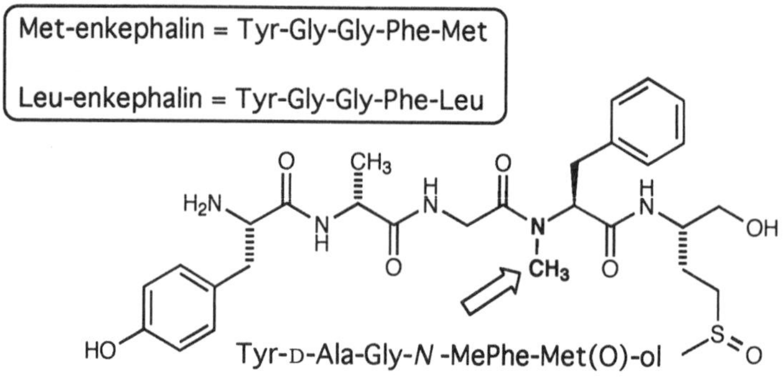

Met-enkephalin = Tyr-Gly-Gly-Phe-Met

Leu-enkephalin = Tyr-Gly-Gly-Phe-Leu

Tyr-D-Ala-Gly-N-MePhe-Met(O)-ol

Fig. 17.15   Less vulnerable analogue of Met-enkephalin.[19]

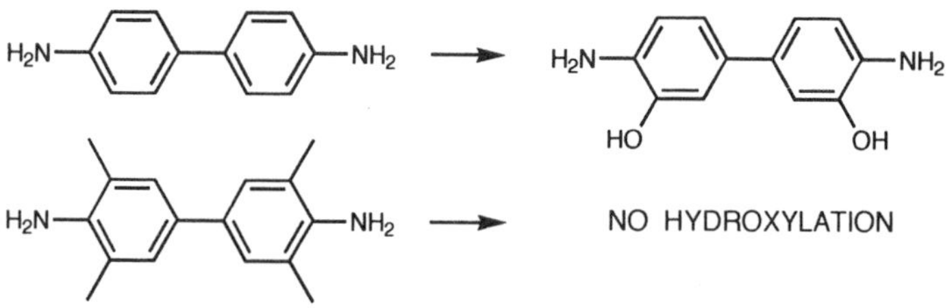

NO HYDROXYLATION

Fig. 17.16   Protection by methyl groups of aromatic carbon hydroxylation.[22]

tumours. On the other hand, it proved to be as sensitive as benzidine in routine clinical tests for detection of occult blood in urine or faeces.[22] Comparable reasoning guided the synthesis of mono- or disubstituted analogues of paracetamol. Methyl or higher alkyl groups in *ortho* position (with regard to the phenolic hydroxyl) yielded safer analgesics showing less hepatotoxicity.[23]

In steroids the 6α position (e.g. prednisolone, Fig. 17.17) normally hydroxylated. Attachment of a methyl in this position prevents this hydroxylation. Halogens (particularly fluorine) serve even better because they are completely insensitive to oxidative attacks.

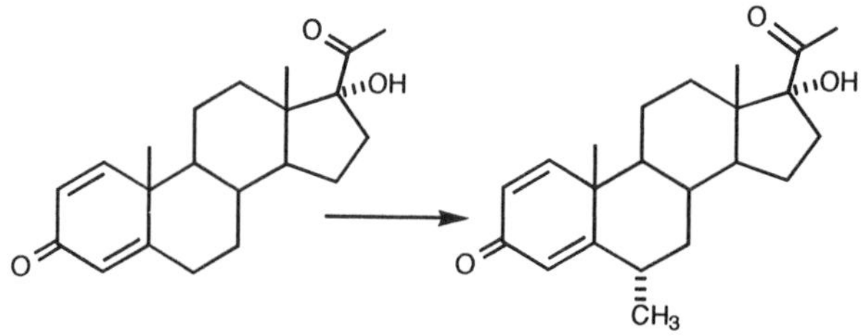

Fig. 17.17   Protection of prednisolone against metabolic hydroxylations.

E. Extensions — cognate groups

The methyl group is the prototype of a saturated aliphatic substituent with lipophilic and electron-donor inductive effect. In some instances it can advantageously be replaced by related groups bringing symmetry or increased lipophilicity or an increased inductive effect. We rehearse some possibilities below.

1. Numerical values

The values reported in Table 17.4, taken from Tute,[24] allow the comparison of some characteristic alkyl groups. Note the comparable bulkiness (E values) of the isopropyl and cyclopentyl groups, while the *t*-butyl group is far more voluminous. Furthermore, it is remarkable that the electron-donor effect of the cyclopentyl group is superior to that of the cyclohexyl group.

Table 17.4   Lipophilic, steric, and electronic descriptors for some current aliphatic rests.[24]

Group	π	σ	E
Methyl	0.50	−0.07	0.00
Isopropyl	1.30	−0.19	−1.08
Cyclopropyl	1.20[a]	−0.30[b]	–
Cyclobutyl	1.80	−0.20	−0.67
Tertiobutyl	1.98	−0.30	−2.46
Cyclopentyl	2.14	−0.20	−1.12
Cyclohexyl	2.51	−0.15	−1.40

[a]Taken from Hansch and Anderson.[27]
[b]Taken from Martin.[28]

2. gem-*Dimethyl* and spiro-*cyclopropyl*

gem-Dimethyl and *spiro*-cyclopropyl groups are useful for rendering a carbon atom quaternary and therefore resistant to metabolic attack. They can also constitute means of introducing symmetry into a chiral centre. The *spiro*-cyclopropyl moiety has been used to synthesize a more lipophilic analogue of glycine (Fig. 17.18).[25]

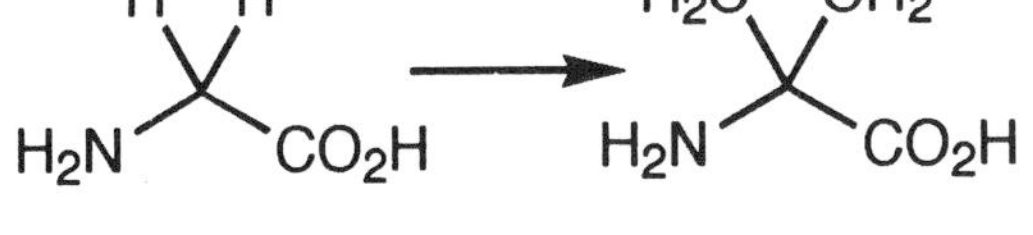

Fig. 17.18   *spiro*-Cyclopropyl glycine derivative with agonist properties for the glycine receptor.[25]

3. Isopropyl and cyclopropyl

The cyclopropyl group is less bulky than the isopropyl group for a maximal electron-donor effect. For a review of cyclopropane derivatives in medicinal chemistry, see Cussac *et al.*[26]

4.   The cyclopentyl group

The cyclopentyl group creates the maximal inductive effect for a relatively reasonable bulkiness. It is often a good filling for a hydrophobic pocket, as illustrated for the cAMP phosphodiesterase inhibitor rolipram. The inhibitory activity towards type IV cAMP-phosphodiesterase is increased ten times when the *meta*-methoxy group is replaced by a *meta*-cyclopentyl group (rolipram) (Fig. 17.19).[27] Presumably the cyclopentyl group optimally fills a hydrophobic pocket of the active site of the enzyme.

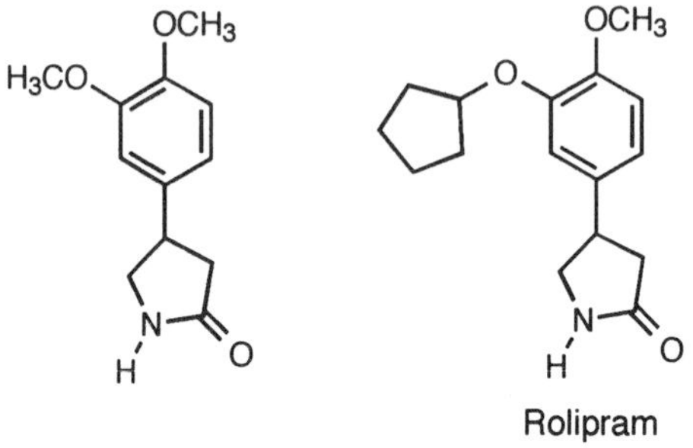

Fig. 17.19   Structures of rolipram and of its dimethoxy analogue.[29]

The cyclopentyl group has also proved advantageous in replacing a *gem*-dimethyl in a series of inhibitors of acyl-CoA-cholesterol acyltransferase, which is an enzyme involved in the absorption of alimentary cholesterol (Fig. 17.20).[28]

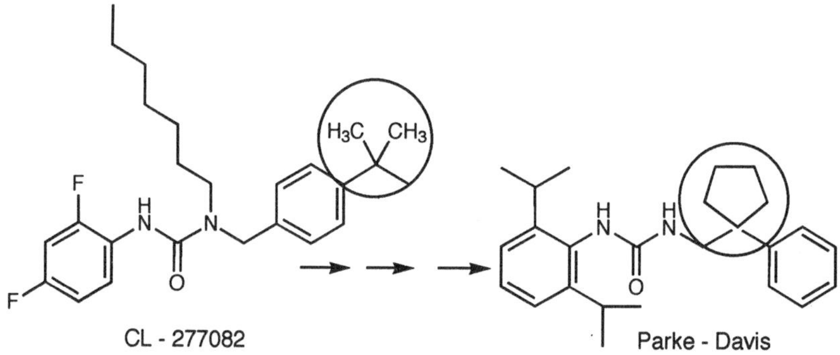

Fig. 17.20   Replacement of a *gem*-dimethyl by a cyclopentyl group.[30]

III.   EFFECTS OF UNSATURATED GROUPS

The introduction of an unsaturated group (vinyl, ethynyl, allyl, etc.) in a drug molecule generally entails one or several of the following consequences.[29,30]

(1)   Increase of the narcotic power and the toxicity in comparison with the corresponding saturated compound. Ethylene, acetylene, trichlorethylene, divinyl oxide and, by extension, cyclopropane (in which the incomplete overlap of the σ orbitals can be compared to π orbitals) are examples of unsaturated narcotics.

(2) The possibility of the existence of geometrical isomery.
(3) The existence of electronic effects: the unsaturated groups behave as electron attractors through inductive effects. Furthermore direct interactions of donor–acceptor type are possible owing to the π electron cloud surrounding multiple bonds.
(4) The possibility of activation through conjugation: the association of several unsaturated functions in conjugated positions (dienes, enynes, enones, enolides, polyunsaturated derivatives) renders the corresponding molecules very reactive. It particularly facilitates the addition of biological nucleophiles and notably of thiols.
(5) Facilitation of metabolism. The unsaturated element often constitutes the vulnerable site of the molecule, which will be attacked first (for example, by formation of an epoxide that evolves into a diol which, in turn, can undergo oxidative cleavage), but this is not always the case.

With regard to classification, we will distinguish four series of unsaturated derivatives: the *vinyl* series, the *allyl* series, the *acetylenic* series, and the *ring unsaturated derivatives* that are bioisosteric to aromatic rings.

A. VINYL SERIES

Beside active substances containing actual vinyl groups, this series comprises molecules containing substituted vinyl groups as well as cyclopropyl groups.

1. Vinyl groups

Vinyl groups are not extensively used in medicinal chemistry. Divinyl oxide is an excellent general anaesthetic but it polymerizes easily and forms peroxides. Stabilization of the compound is usually achieved by addition of 0.01% of its weight of *N*-phenyl α-naphtylamine. On the other hand, compounds such as kainic acid, vinylbital, quinine, 17α-vinyltestosterone, compound SKF 100047, and vigabatrin (Fig. 17.21) are perfectly stable vinyl dervatives.

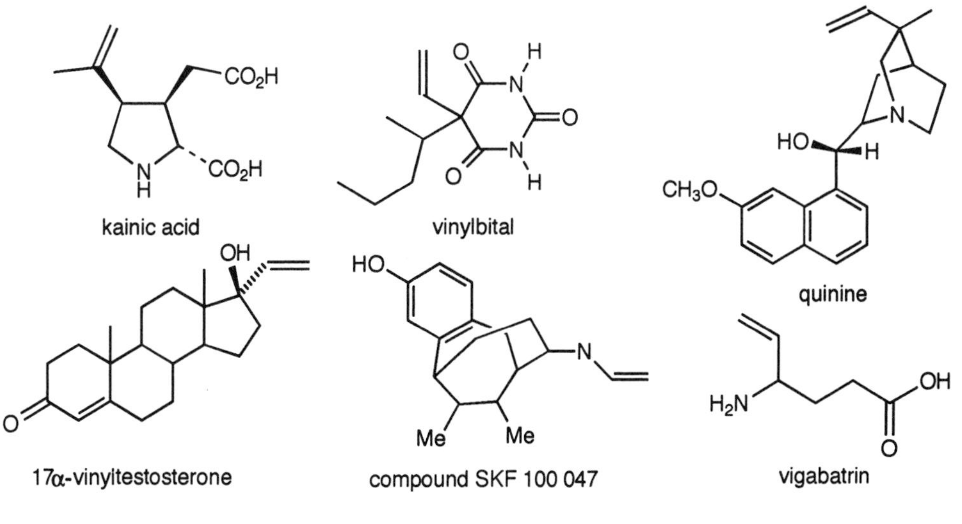

kainic acid

vinylbital

quinine

17α-vinyltestosterone

compound SKF 100 047

vigabatrin

Fig. 17.21 Drugs containing a vinyl group.

Synthetic or natural vinylic epoxides (kapurimycin A_3) produce radical-induced DNA cleavage, even in the presence of the protecting glutathionyl radicals. This property may constitute a starting point for the treatment of radiotherapy-resistant tumours for which the resistance is due to a local increase of the glutathione level.[31]

Substituted vinyl derivatives comprise unsaturated barbiturates such as vinbarbital, the acetylcholinesterase inhibitor huperzine A2, and various antifungal imlidazoles bearing *gem-* and *vic*-dialkylvinyl groups[32] (Fig. 17.22). Some chlorovinyl derivatives were proposed as morphinic antagonists (see Fig. 17.25). For the α-styryl carbinol-derived antifungal agents DuP 860 and DuP 991, oxidation into vinyl epoxides has been observed in solubilized systems (water and propylene glycol, or glycerol, or poly(ethylene glycol) 400).[33]

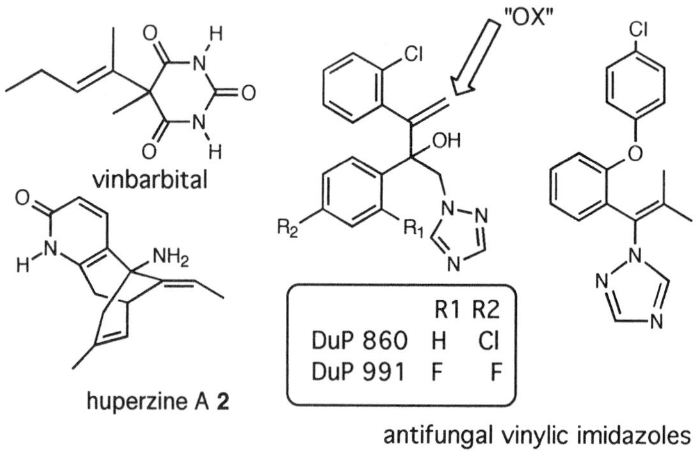

	R1	R2
DuP 860	H	Cl
DuP 991	F	F

vinbarbital

huperzine A 2

antifungal vinylic imidazoles

Fig. 17.22 Substituted vinyl derivatives are less sensitive to epoxidation than unsubstituted ones such as the compounds DuP 860 and DuP 991.

2. Cyclopropyl groups

Cyclopropyl rings can constitute interesting substitutes for vinyl groups when these are too fragile or when they give place to unwanted isomeries or tautomeries. Thus tranylcypromine, an antidepressant acting by inhibition of the monoamine oxidases, is a stable compound, while its ethylenic analogue is not (Fig. 17.23). A supplementary advantage in the use of cyclopropyl analogues comes from their fixed stereochemistry: there is no spontaneous conversion from *cis* to *trans* isomers as is frequently observed with ethylenic derivatives.

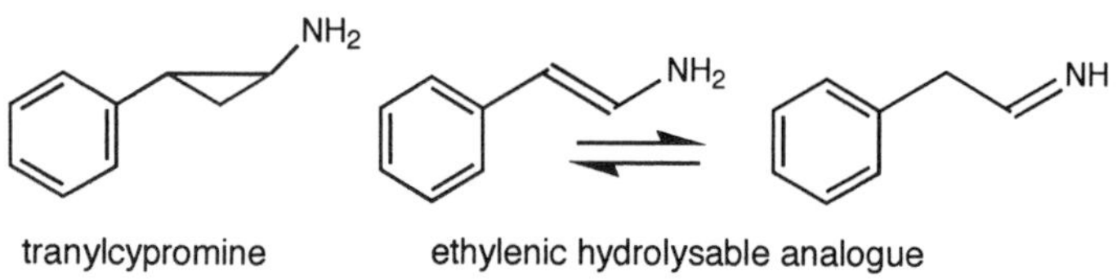

tranylcypromine   ethylenic hydrolysable analogue

Fig. 17.23 Tranylcypromine represents a stable substitute of the enamine aminostyrene.

B.   Allylic series

All allylic derivatives are relatively hepatotoxic and irritant. Allylic alcohol itself serves to create experimental hepatic lesions that allow testing of hepatoprotective drugs. We consider three categories of allylic derivatives: C-allyl derivatives, N-allyl derivatives, and O- and S-allyl derivatives, which often possess alkylating properties.

1.   C-Allyl derivatives

These present the double advantage of being lipophilic (rapid onset) and giving fast biodegradation (short duration of action). However, they often conserve the intrinsic hepatotoxicity the of the allyl group.[34] Allobarbital is a sedative-hypnotic that is no longer used; allylestrenol acts as a pure progestative hormone, and alprenolol is a β-blocker (Fig. 17.24).

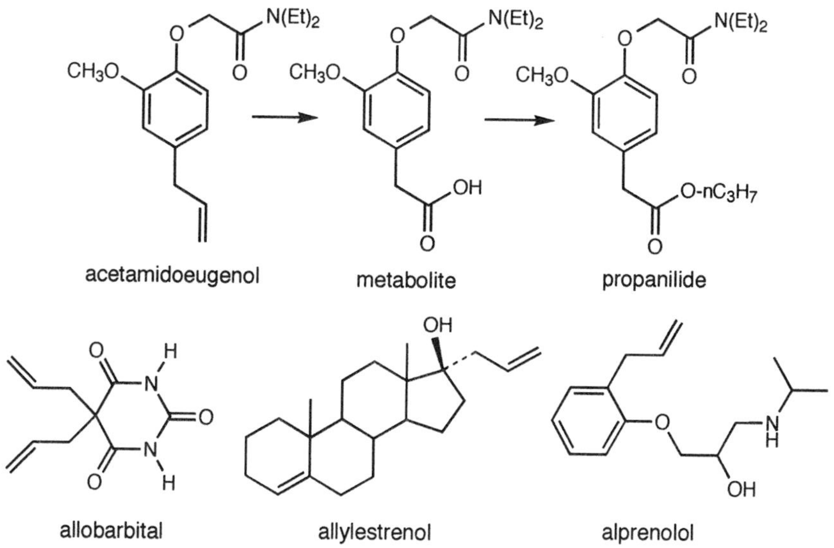

| acetamidoeugenol | metabolite | propanilide |

| allobarbital | allylestrenol | alprenolol |

Fig. 17.24   C-Allyl derivatives.

Acetamidoeugenol is an intravenous anaesthetic of ultrashort duration of action; it has been withdrawn because it provokes irritations and lesions of the vascular wall. Acetamidoeugenol is oxidized very rapidly *in vivo* to the corresponding arylacetic acid. This observation was the basis of the synthesis of another intravenous short-acting anaesthetic: propanilide (Fig. 17.24).[35]

2.   N-Allyl derivatives

The replacement in morphine, and in some of its simplified analogues, of the N-methyl group by an N-allyl group (and subsequently by some related groups)[36] has constituted a decisive step in the study of opiate analgesics. Indeed, this modification achieved for the first time the conversion of morphinic receptor agonists into the corresponding antagonists (Fig. 17.25).

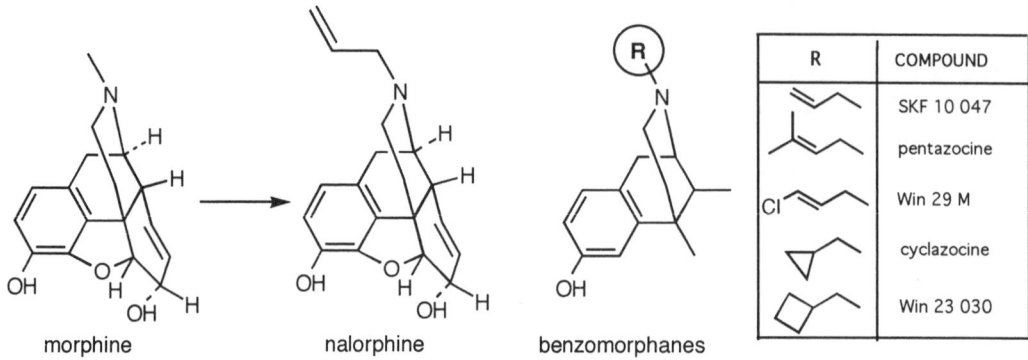

Fig. 17.25   Nalorphine and cognate derivatives.[38]

Aloxidone and albutoine are anticonvulsivant *N*-allyl derivatives of hydantoin and thiohydantoin (Fig. 17.26). The dibenzazepine azapetine is an α-adrenergic blocking agent used as a peripheral vasodilator.

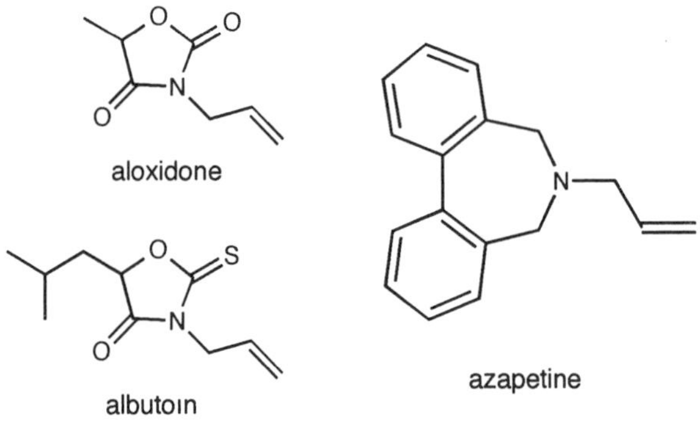

aloxidone

albutoin

azapetine

Fig. 17.26   *N*-Allyl derivatives of hydantoin, thiohydantoin and dibenzazepine.

3.   O- and S-Allyl derivatives

Several of these compounds figure in the *Merck Index*. The β-blocking oxprenolol, the arylacetic analgesic–anti-inflammatory drug aclofenac and the fungicide enilconazole are *O*-allyl derivatives. Penicillin O and penicillin S are both *S*-allyl derivatives.

Alkylating allyl derivatives.   When the allyl group bears a good leaving group, it easily generates the allylic cation. This cation is stabilized by mesomery, and is an excellent electrophile. Many natural compounds can release allylic alcohols. A first example is found in allicin, the antibacterial principle of garlic, which results from the action of alliinase on alliin (Fig. 17.27). Several varieties of senecio (*Senecio vulgaris* L., Compositae, *Senecio platyphyllus*, etc.) contain alkaloids derived from pyrrolizidine: senecionine, seneciphylline, etc. These substances provoke hepatic cancers, notably in cattle. Here, too, the alkylating properties are ascribed to the allylic structure (Fig. 17.27).[37] It is reasonable also to implicate the formation of allylic carbamates in mitomycins A, B and C, which are antimitotic drugs used in cancer therapy. Presumably the allyl function is created by an elimination reaction involving the departure of an acetalic hydroxy or methoxy group (Fig. 17.27).

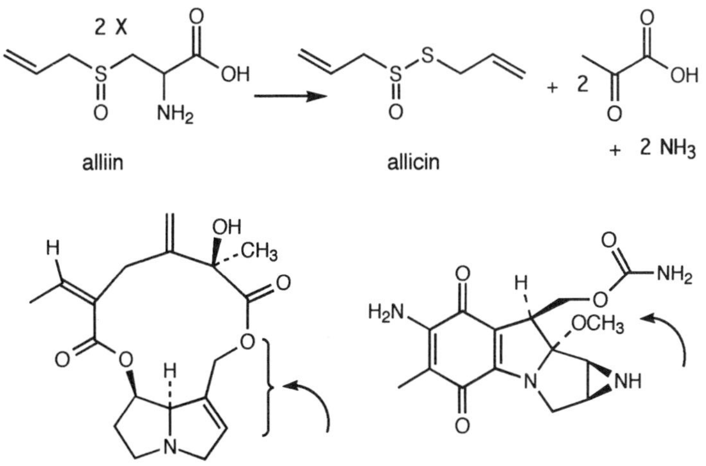

Fig. 17.27   Alkylating allylic derivatives.

C.   Acetylenic series

Acetylenic groups are used for their electronic effects, as equivalents of aromatic rings and to impose structural constraints.

1.   *Electronic effects*

The acetylene function exerts an electron-attracting effect. This effect can be reinforced by substitution of the acetylenic hydrogen. Ethynyl compounds are essentially found among the light sedative-hypnotic drugs (CNS-depressing effect of the unsaturated derivatives) and in steroid series, where their fixation in position 17α provides orally active steroids (Fig. 17.28).

  In the sedative-hypnotic series, most of the acetylenic alcohols are used as carbamic esters: meparfynol, ethinamate, etc. The bromoethynyl moiety confers an acidity comparable to that induced by a trichloromethyl group. Bromoethynylcyclohexanol is sufficiently acidic to form salts; its bismuth salt was used for a while as an antisyphilitic drug under the name of biarsamide. In the steroid series the metabolism of the ethynyl group can lead (by hydration of the triple bond) to 17α-methylketones.

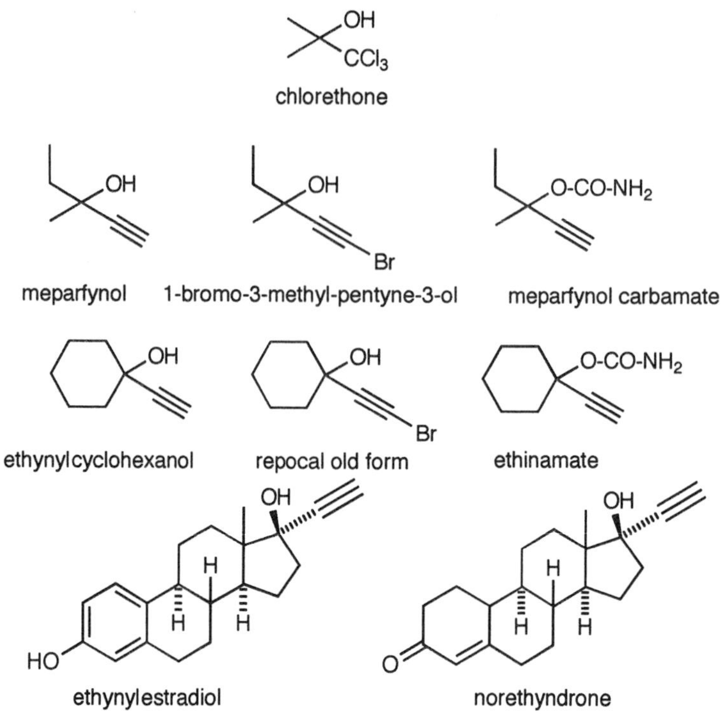

chlorethone

meparfynol   1-bromo-3-methyl-pentyne-3-ol   meparfynol carbamate

ethynylcyclohexanol   repocal old form   ethinamate

ethynylestradiol   norethyndrone

Fig. 17.28   Ethynylated drugs.

2.   Aromatic ring equivalents

Thanks to their π electron clouds and to their small volume, ethynyl groups can sometimes function as bioisosteres of aromatic rings and give similar donor–acceptor interactions. However, such acetylenic analogues are more rapidly metabolized. Sodium methohexital, for example (Fig. 17.29), is used as an injectable barbituric for very short anaesthesia. The obsolete antitussive drug Labazyl® is an analogue of the reversed pethidines in which the phenyl ring has been replaced by a propargyl group.

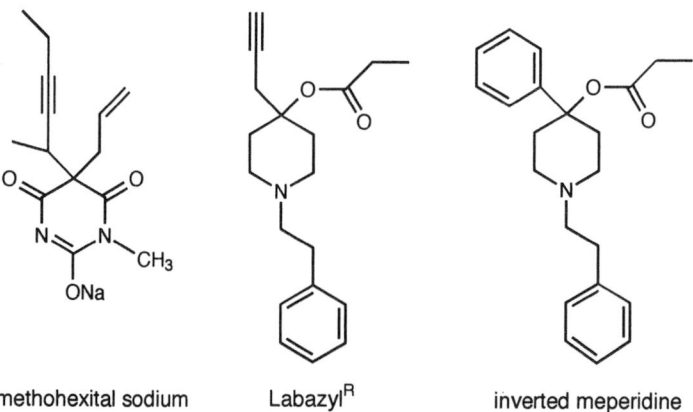

methohexital sodium   Labazyl^R   inverted meperidine

Fig. 17.29   Acetylenic rests as aromatic ring equivalents.

3.   *Structural constraints*

In inserting an acetylenic function between two carbon atoms, one achieves a structure with four 'on-line' atoms representing a rigid entity with a distance of 4.2 Å between the two extreme atoms (Fig. 17.30). This kind of arrangement is found in the cholinergic agonist oxotremorine and in the GABA analogue 4-aminotetrolic acid. This latter compound is recognized, like GABA itself, by the enzyme GABA-transaminase for which it acts as an inhibitor[38] (Fig. 17.30).

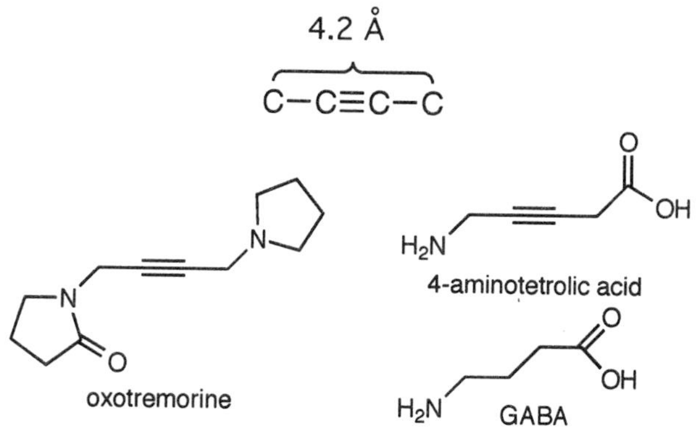

Fig. 17.30   Rigidity and extension imposed by a triple bond.

D.   **Cyclenic equivalents of the phenyl ring**

The cyclohexenyl ring and, to a lesser extent the cyclopentenyl and cycloheptenyl rings can sometimes replace a phenyl ring. This is the case for the barbiturics cyclobarbital and heptabarbital, which are entirely comparable to phenobarbital. From the metabolic point of view, the cyclohexenyl ring is oxidized in a position α to the double bond to produce the corresponding cyclohexenone (Fig. 17.31).

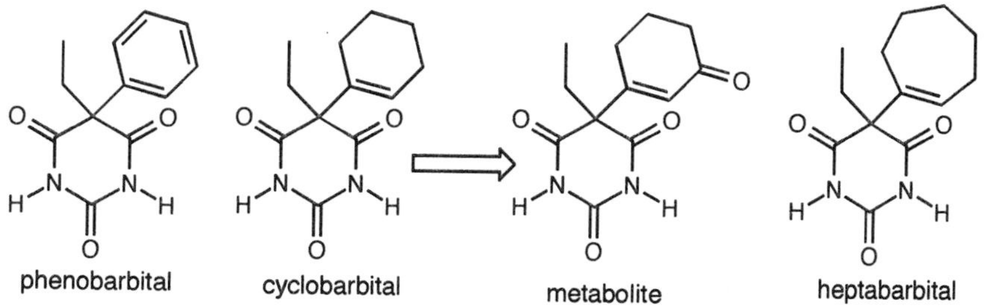

Fig. 17.31   Cyclenic equivalents of the phenyl ring.

Another example is given by the benzodiazepine series, where tetrazepam can be compared to diazepam. However, in this case there is a slight difference in the activity profile: tetrazepam is less sedative, hypnotic and anticonvulsant than diazepam; on the other hand it has greater muscle relaxant and analgesic effects, which indicates its use in visceral and articular pain. From the chemical point of view, the cyclohexenic double bond is introduced in a rather unexpected manner by means of a radicalar rearrangement of an *N*-chloroamide[39] (Fig. 17.32).

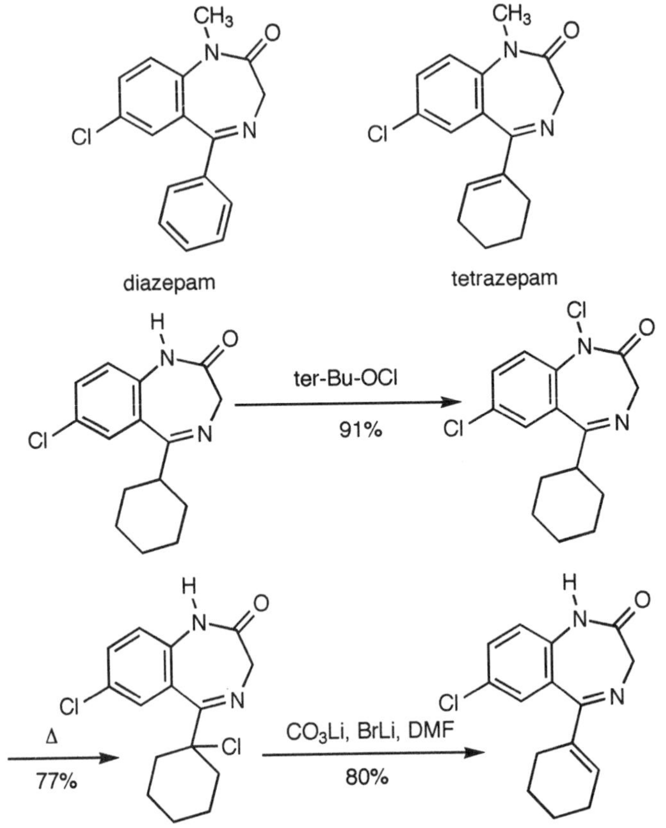

Fig. 17.32   Cyclenic equivalents in the benzodiazepine series.

IV. EFFECTS OF HALOGENATION

Currently, one drug out of three is a halogenated derivative and halogens are found in drugs belonging to practically all therapeutic classes. That has not always been the case; indeed, in the past medicines were mostly of natural origin and natural-substance chemistry is relatively scarce in halogenated substances. Halogen-containing drugs entered usage only after 1820. The first organic halogenated drugs were mainly used for their depressive action on the central nervous system: production of general anaesthesia with chloroform; sedation or hypnosis with chloral and bromural. From the twentieth century on, a regular growth of the number of halogenated drugs is observed; this became explosive after the end of the Second World War. Even halogenated drugs from natural origin became available, such as chlortetracycline or chloramphenicol, and substances from marine origin or from fermentation broths.

A.   The importance of the halogens in the exploration of structure–activity relationships

1.   Steric effects

The obstruction of a molecule by halogen substitution can impose certain conformations or mask certain functions. In the case of clonidine the bulky halogen atoms prevent free rotation and maintain the planes of the aromatic rings in positions perpendicular to each other (Fig. 17.33A).[11]

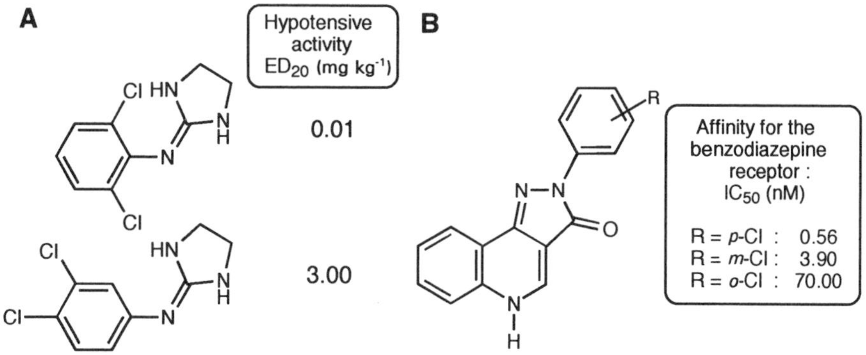

Fig. 17.33   (A) The *ortho–ortho'* substitution in clonidine maintains the planes of the aromatic rings in a perpendicular position to each other. (B): The *ortho*-chloro isomer of the benzodiazepine ligand CGS-9896 has a 125-fold lower affinity than the parent molecule.

In a series of benzodiazepine receptor ligands derived from CGS-9896, strong steric effects are described by Fryer *et al.* (Fig. 17.33B).[40] Indeed, the *ortho* and *para* isomers can be considered as having the same lipophilicity and very similar electronic effects. Thus, the reduction of binding affinity of the *ortho*-chloro compound is attributed to the steric effect.

2.   Electronic effects

The electronic effects of the halogens are ascribed to their inductive electron-attracting properties. These are maximal for chlorine and bromine, less marked for iodine, and very weak for fluorine. The mesomeric donor effect of the halogen atoms is usually not involved in biological media. The influences of halogens on the potency of monoamine oxidase inhibition and on dopamine uptake blockade *in vitro* are shown in Fig. 17.34. The choice of the optimal substituent allows noticeable gains in potency compared to the parent molecule.[41,42]

Progressive mono- and disubstitution of benzodiazepinones related to diazepam enhances the affinity for the mitochondrial benzodiazepine receptor (MBR) by a factor of 233 (Fig. 17.35).

N-Acylation of L-tryptophan benzyl esters, followed by replacement of the 3,5-dimethyl groups by their trifluoromethyl analogues, achieved an almost thousandfold increase in potency in a series of substance P receptor antagonists (Fig. 17.36).[43]

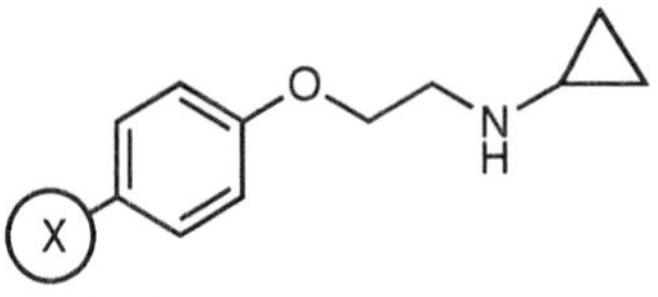

Monoamine Oxidase Inhibition: IC_{50} (nM)

X = H :	1200
X = Br :	200
X = CF_3 :	100
X = SO_2CF_3 :	27

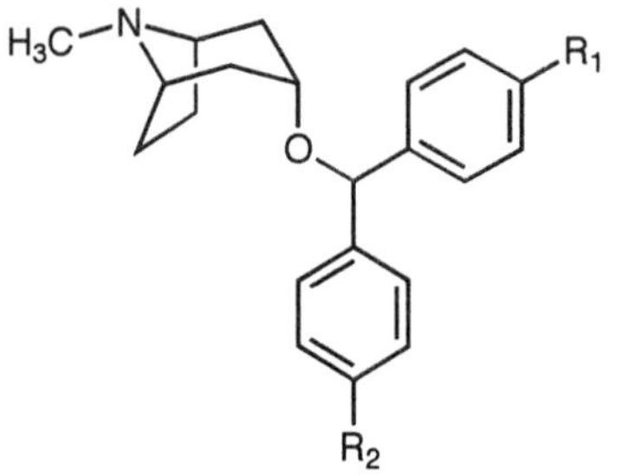

$[^3H]$ Dopamine Uptake: IC_{50} (nM)

$R_1 = R_2 = CH_3O$:	2876
$R_1 = H$, $R_2 = Cl$:	115
$R_1 = R_2 = Cl$:	75

Fig. 17.34   Influence of halogenated subsituents on monoamine-oxidase inhibition potency *in vitro*.

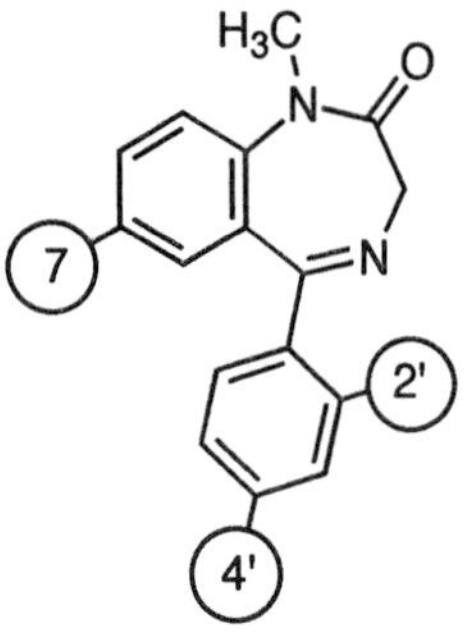

Code Number	Substitution Pattern 2'	4'	7	IC_{50} nM MBR
Ro 5-3464	H	H	H	700
Ro 5-5115	H	Cl	H	54
Diazepam	H	H	Cl	72
Ro 5-6900	Cl	H	Cl	11
Ro 5-4864	H	Cl	Cl	3

Fig. 17.35   Chlorine effects in the benzodiazepine series.[45]

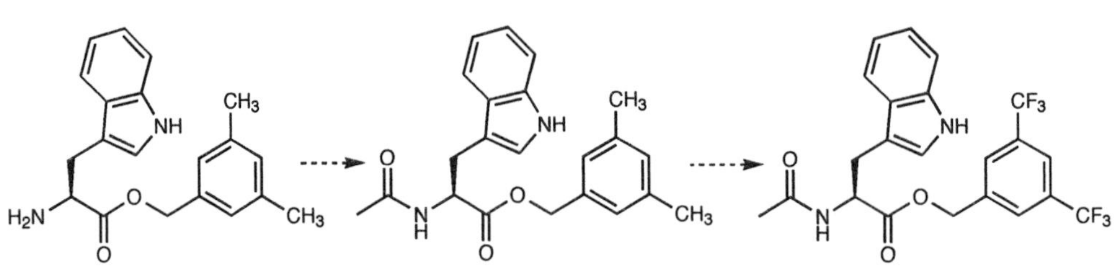

1533   67   1.6

Fig. 17.36   Successive *N*-acetylation and $CH_3 \rightarrow CF_3$ replacement yield a 958-fold increase in affinity.[46] Figures represent human NK_1 receptor binding: IC_{50} (nM).

3. *Hydrophobic effects*

The predominantly lipophilic influence of halogen substitution is seen in the classical cases of the halocarbon anaesthetics, the halogenophenol antiseptics and the halogenated insecticides (Fig. 17.32). For these compounds there is a direct correlation between biological activity and certain physicochemical parameters such as partition coefficient, surface tension or vapour pressure. The accumulation of halogen atoms favours the passage of the biomembranes and access to the CNS.

$CHCl_3$, $CHBr_3$, CCl_3CHOH

CF_3 - CHBrCl (halothane)

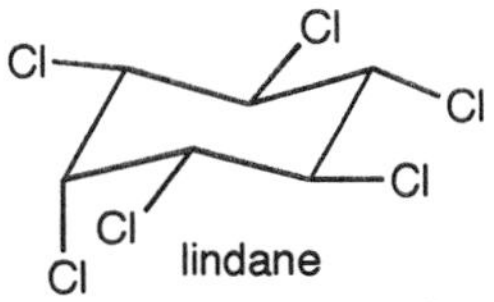

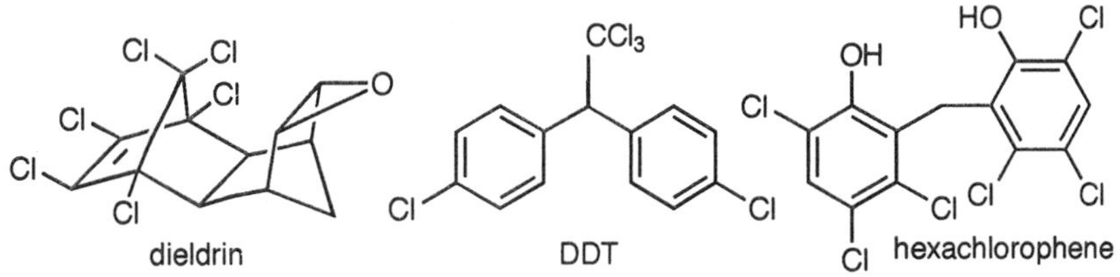

Fig. 17.37 Compounds in which the halogens play an essentially lipophilic role.

4. *Reactivity of the halogens*

All C–halogen bonds, except C—F are weaker than C—H (Table 17.5).

Table 17.5 Atomic radii and characteristics of carbon–halogen bonds. (Taken from Buu-Hoi.[47])

Atomic radius (Å)	Bond[a]	Interatomic distance (Å)	Bond strength (kcal mol^{-1})
H: 0.29	C—H	1.14	93
F: 0.64	C—F	1.45	114
Cl: 0.99	C—Cl	1.74	72
Br: 1.14	C—Br	1.90	59
I: 1.33	C—I	2.12	45

[a] In aliphatic series.

5. *Usefulness of the halogens and of cognate functions*

Depending upon their physical properties and their reactivity, the derivatives of fluorine, chlorine, bromine and iodine present various degrees of usefulness (Table 17.6).

(1) The most used halogens in medicinal chemistry are chlorine and fluorine attached to a nonactivated carbon atom. Fluorine presents the advantage of its small bulkiness (van

Table 17.6 Some substituent constants for halogens and equivalent functions. (Taken from Chu.[13])

Group	π	σ	MR	F	R
H	0.00	0.00	1.03	0.00	0.00
F	0.14	0.06	0.92	0.43	−0.34
Cl	0.71	0.23	6.03	0.41	−0.15
Br	0.86	0.23	8.88	0.44	−0.17
I	1.12	0.18	13.94	0.40	0.19
CF_3	0.88	0.54	5.02	0.38	0.19
CH_3	0.56	−0.17	5.65	−0.04	−0.13
CN	−0.57	0.66	6.33	0.51	0.19
SO_2CF_3	0.55	0.93	12.86	0.73	0.26
SCF_3	1.44	0.50	13.81	0.35	0.18
SCN	0.41	0.52	13.40	0.36	0.19

der Waals radius comparable to that of hydrogen). It is used essentially to block metabolically sensitive positions of a molecule.

The CF_3 group is comparable in size to chlorine and can advantageously replace it when it is placed in an activated position (e.g. R—CO—Cl → R—CO—CF$_3$). A chlorine substituent produces *simultaneously* an increase in lipophilicity, an electron attracting effect and a metabolic obstruction.

(2) In certain active molecules the role of the fluorine or chlorine atoms is not apparent at first glance. Thus, for example, two compounds chemically as different as *m*-trifluoromethylphenylethylamine and 5-hydroxytryptamine show many pharmacological analogies. In this case the explanation lies in the similitude of the electrostatic potential maps (Fig. 17.38). Conversely, two closely related pyrazoloquinolines, compounds CGS 8216 and its *para*-chloro analogue CGS 9896, present totally opposed activity profiles on the same benzodiazepine receptor.[45] A dramatic effect resulting from chlorine substitution is also found in the change from β-phenyl-GABA to β-(*p*-chlorophenyl)-GABA.[46]

(3) Bromine has fewer applications than either fluorine or chlorine, and is most often incorporated as a bromoaryl. The drawback of bromine is that it generates alkylating reactive intermediates more easily than do chlorine or fluorine (see Chapter 30) and therefore, in long-term treatment, it can confer toxic potentialities to the molecule that bears it.

(4) Iodine as a substituent group is the least used of the halogens because the weakness of the carbon–iodine bond means that iodide ions may be released and this can trigger either acute hypersensitivity reactions (larynx oedema, cutaneous haemorrhages, fever, arthralgies, etc.) or chronic reactions ('iodism'). However, iodine is indispensable to the treatment of certain thyroidal deficiencies and also has some other specific uses: covalent iodine derivatives serve as radiological contrast media and iodine-131 (half-life 8 days) is used as radioactive tracing agent.

(5) Extensions — cognate groups: Chlorine, trifluoromethyl, cyano or azido groups are more or less bioisosteres. Other possible candidates are SCN, SCF$_3$, SO$_2$CF$_3$ and CH=CF$_2$ (see Chapter 13).

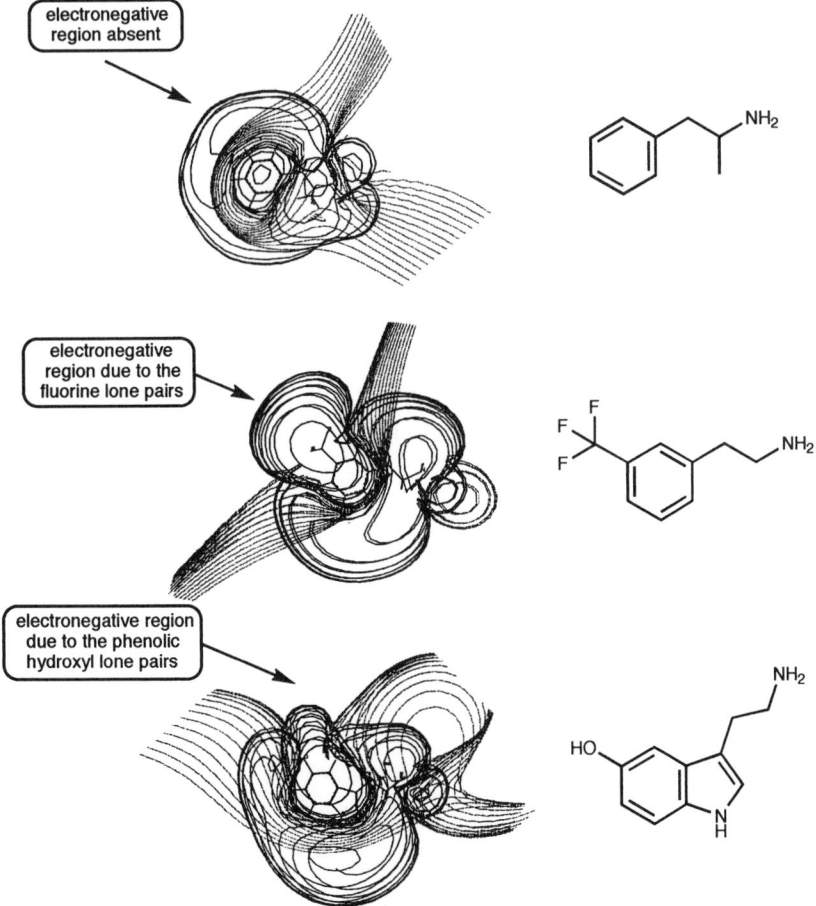

Fig. 17.38 Electrostatic potential maps.

V. EFFECTS OF HYDROXYLATION

The substitution of OH for H affects biological activity profoundly, as in the conversion of ethane to ethanol or benzene to phenol. Simple alcohols have narcotic properties and simple phenols bacteriostatic properties. Polyfunctional compounds can act as chelating or complexing agents.

A. Effects on solubility

The introduction of an alcoholic or a phenolic hydroxy group into an active molecule changes the partition coefficient towards greater hydrophilicity and renders the molecule more water-soluble. Thus, in changing benzene to phenol, or benzamide to *p*-hydroxybenzamide, the partition coefficient drops from $\log P = 2.13$ to $\log P = 1.46$ and from $\log P = 0.64$ to $\log P = 0.33$, respectively.[2] The value of the Hansch π constant for a hydroxy group is -0.67. This means that to compensate the loss in lipophilicity due to the monohydroxylation of an active compound, it is necessary to attach at an appropriate site on the molecule a chlorine atom ($\pi = 0.71$), for example.

B. Effects on the ligand–receptor interaction

For some hydroxylated drugs such as morphine, dopamine, haloperidol, γ-hydroxybutyrate, serotonin or most of the steroids, the hydroxy group is an essential element for hydrogen bonding with the receptor. For others the attachment of a hydroxy group can result in potency changes. Examples are found in hycanthone, which is 10 times more active against schistosomes than lucanthone,[47] or in hydroxylated minaprine analogues, which show a 10-fold better affinity for M_1-muscarinic receptors than the parent drugs.[48]

C. Hydroxylation and metabolism

As a rule, metabolic hydroxylation of an active compound represents a detoxication mechanism. It generally results from a first pass effect and can be followed or not by a conjugation reaction (see Chapters 29 and 30). Classical examples of drugs detoxified through hydroxylation are paracetamol, oxyphenbutazone and hydroxychloroquine. Other important reactions of hydroxy compounds, whether alcoholic or phenolic, are based on their capacity to accept activated groups through the action of group-transferring enzymes (methylation, sulfation, phosphorylation, glycosylation, etc.).

VI.   EFFECTS OF THIOL, THIOETHER AND SULFIDE GROUPS

Thiol and disulfide groups are of wide occurrence in natural products. They are found in small molecules such as lipoic acid, glutathione and thiamin, as well as in cysteine-containing peptides and proteins (hormones, enzymes, antibiotics). In all these substances, thiol and disulfide groups are clearly associated either with high chemical reactivity or with consolidation of peptide and protein architecture. Being too reactive, the thiol and the disulfide groups are normally not used in medicinal chemistry as substituents in QSAR studies. Occasionally methylthio substitution on aromatic rings is practised, but even then the thioethers obtained are very reactive. They are easily converted to sulfoxides and vice versa (see sulindac, Chapter 32).

Drugs containing thiol groups are mainly used for the strong affinity that the thiolate anion presents towards heavy metals. This is the case for thiol-containing angiotensin converting enzyme inhibitors which bind to a zinc-containing enzyme (see Chapter 6 and Ganellin and Roberts).[49]

The heavy-metal chelating properties of thiols were taken advantage of in the design of dimercaprol ('British Anti-Lewisite', BAL) as a counterpoison to the arsenical war gas lewisite (Fig. 17.39). Today dimercaprol is used to treat poisoning by compounds of gold, mercury, antimony and arsenic. The toxic nature of the heavy metals is masked and the chelate is stable enough to be excreted as such in the urine.

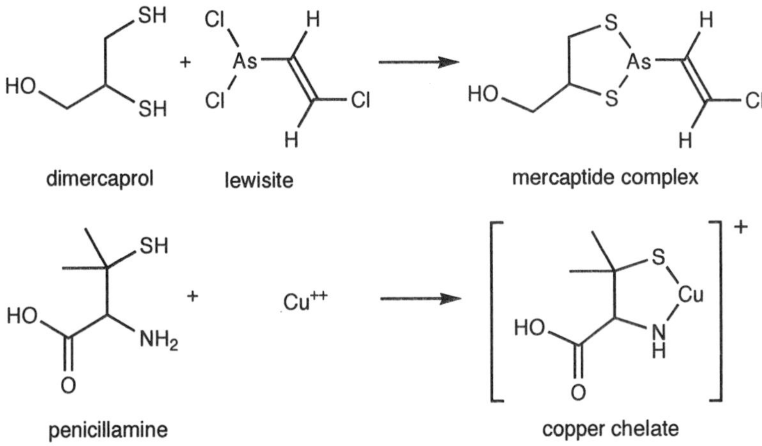

Fig. 17.39   Chelating properties of thiol derivatives.

Penicillamine (D-β,β-dimethylcysteine) is an effective chelator of copper, mecury, zinc and lead that promotes the excretion of these metals in the urine. It is used clinically in patients with Wilson's disease, with rheumatoid arthritis and with heavy-metal intoxications.[50] Ziram and ferbam are the zinc and the iron salts, respectively, of dimethyldithiocarbamic acid (Fig. 17.40). They are widely used as selective fungicides in agriculture. Pyrithione (1-hydroxy-2(1*H*)-pyridinethione), as its zinc salt (Fig. 17.40) is used in dermatology as an antiseborrhoeic.

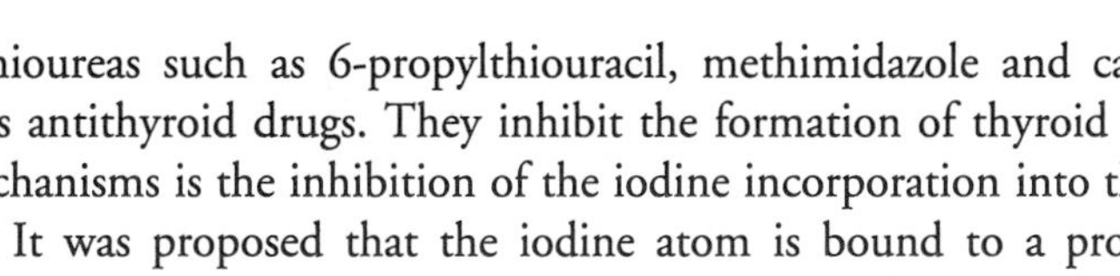

Fig.17.40   Ziram and pyrithione-zinc are chelated salts.

Heterocyclic thioureas such as 6-propylthiouracil, methimidazole and carbimidazole (Fig. 17.41) are used as antithyroid drugs. They inhibit the formation of thyroid hormones; one of the presumed mechanisms is the inhibition of the iodine incorporation into the tyrosyl residues of thyroglobulin. It was proposed that the iodine atom is bound to a protein as a sulfenyl iodide. The thioureas may act in establishing covalent —S—S— bonds and in displacing iodine as HI.[51]

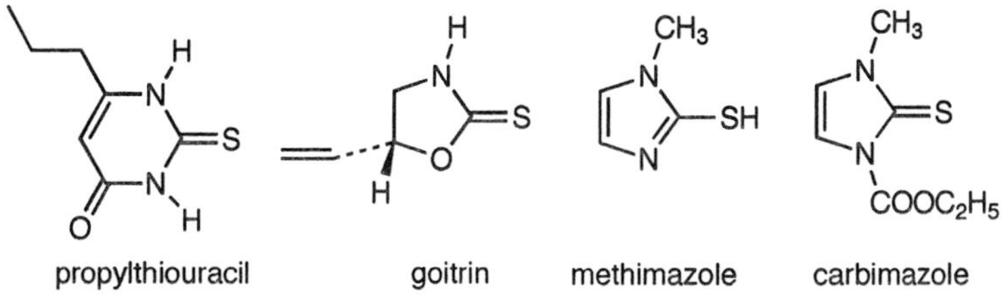

Fig. 17.41   Heterocyclic thioureas with antithyroid effects.

More generally, thiourea and its simpler aliphatic derivatives, as well as thioamides, produce goitre and have to be avoided in drug design. A natural compound, L-5-vinyl-2-thiooxazolidone (goitrin) is responsible for the goitre of cattle eating turnips or cruciferous plants.[52] Besides their affinity for metallic ions, thiol groups have other characteristics such the ability to interconvert to disulfides through redox reactions, to add to conjugated double bonds and to form complexes with the pyridine nucleotides by nucleophilic attack at the 4-position of the pyridine ring.

VII.   EFFECTS OF ACIDIC FUNCTIONS

The prototypical representatives of the group are the carboxylic acids. However, a huge number of bioisosteres such as sulfonic or phosphonic acids, tetrazoles or 3-hydroxyisoxazoles are available (see Chapter 13). In addition, functions like esters, amides, peptides, aldehydes, primary alcohols and related functions can work as prodrugs or bioprecursors (see Chapters 31 and 32).

The introduction of an acidic group into a biologically active compound that does not already contain such a group has essentially a solubilizing effect. This effect can even be enhanced through salt formation (see Chapter 34). Carboxylic acids are often highly ionized at physiological pH values and this is even more the case for sulfonic acids. As a rule, strong and highly ionized acids cannot cross the biological membranes, which are permeable only to nondissociated molecules; they are then subject to a rapid clearance from the animal body. However, once absorbed, they can establish strong ionic interactions with the basic amino acids, especially with lysine, contained in the blood serum albumin, or the enzyme and receptor proteins.

Changes in biological activity distinguish the sulfonic from the carboxylic acids. Broadly speaking, the sulfonic acids as a class are generally not biologically active. Exceptions are certain complex dyes or trypanocides (Trypan blue, suramin, etc.) and sulfonic amino acids such as taurine and hypotaurine, for which an active transport mechanism exists. For carboxylic acids the situation depends whether the carboxylic function is introduced into small or large molecules. In small molecules, the introduction of a carboxylic group fundamentally changes the biological activity. Very often the initial biological activity is destroyed and the toxicity of the parent compound is reduced. In a series of cyproheptadine analogues the replacement of a chlorine substituent on a benzo ring by a carboxylic group resulted in a 4000-fold loss in affinity for the spiperone labelled dopamine receptor.[53] Conversely, the presence of the carboxylic group can sometimes create the conditions necessary for activity (Fig. 17.42).

In large molecules, high pharmacological activity is maintained despite the presence of the carboxylic group. Examples are the anti-inflammatory arylacetic acids, the prostaglandins, cromolyn and the related antiasthmatics, and finally the β-lactam antibiotics. In these drugs the relative weight of the carboxyl is notably smaller.

With carboxyl-derived functions such as esters and amides, the initial activity of the drug, lost in introducing the carboxyl group, is often regained. Amides, ureides, hydantoins and barbiturates share CNS-depressing properties and are frequently indispensable elements of sedative, tranquillizing and anticonvulsant drugs. Nitriles as substituents are often comparable to chlorine atoms, but sometimes more toxic.

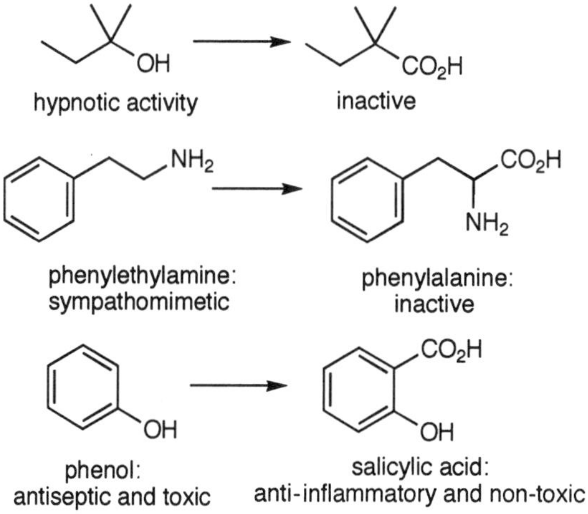

Fig. 17.42   Introduction of a carboxylic group in a small molecule can destroy the activity originally present or, conversely, create the conditions necessary for activity.

VIII.   EFFECTS OF BASIC FUNCTIONS

The basic groups met in medicinal chemistry are the amines, the amidines, the guanidines and practically all nitrogen-containing heterocycles. Basic groups are polar and one would expect that highly ionized bases (especially quaternary ammonium salts) would resemble the sulfonic acids and show limited activity owing to their mediocre membrane permeability. In practice, bases with pK_a values superior to 10 have very limited chance of reaching the CNS.

As seen for the acidic groups, the introduction of a basic group into a biologically active compound that does not already contain such a group has essentially a solubilizing effect. This effect can also be enhanced through salt formation (see Chapter 34). In drug–protein interactions the classical counteranions of organic bases are the aspartic and the glutamic carboxylates.

The biological activity of amines and basic heterocycles is immense and justifies the adage 'no biological activity without nitrogen'. Steroids, prostaglandins, and nonsteroidal anti-inflammatory drugs are, of course, exceptions. Primary amines often demonstrate less specific effect than secondary or tertiary amines. Acylation deactivates the amines strongly, as does the introduction in some other site of the molecule of a carboxylic or sulfonic group (formation of zwitterions: bipolar ions). Diamines and polyamines are usually more active than monoamines. Aromatic amines are always more hazardous than aliphatic amines and form toxic metabolites; examples are 2-naphthylamine, benzidine, aniline (see Chapter 30). They are easy to detoxicate by introducing a carboxyl group, as evidenced by the change from aniline to the nontoxic *p*-aminobenzoic acid.

REFERENCES

1. Taylor, J. (1984) The Topliss Approach — Opinion of an Industrial Scientist on QSAR Methods. Lecture given at the Louis Pasteur University at Strasbourg, March 8, 1984.
2. Rekker, R. F. and Mannhold, R. (1992) *Calculation of Drug Lipophilicity.* Verlag VCH, Weinheim, Germany.
3. Albert, A. (1979) *Selective Toxicity,* p.60. Chapman & Hall, London.
4. Ginnings, P. and Baum, R. (1937) Aqueous solubilities of the isomeric pentanols. *J. Am. Chem. Soc.* **59**: 1111–1113.
5. Nemethy, G. (1967) Hydrophobic interactions. *Angew. Chem. Int. Ed. Engl.* **6**: 195–206.
6. Hansch, C. and Anderson, S. M. (1967) The effect of intramolecular hydrophobic bonding on partition coefficients. *J. Org. Chem.* **32**: 2583–2586.
7. Gilligan, D. and Plummer, N. (1943) Comparative solubilities of sulfadiazine, sulfamerazine and sulfamethazine and their N_4-acetyl derivatives at varying pH levels. *Proc. Soc. Exp. Biol. Med.* **5**: 142–145.
8. Albert, A. (1979) *Selective Toxicity,* p. 41. Chapman & Hall, London.
9. Harms, A. F. and Nauta, W. T. (1960) The effects of alkyl substitution in drugs — I. Substituted dimethylaminoethyl benzhydryl ethers. *J. Med. Pharm. Chem.* **2**: 57–77.
10. Velluz, L. (1961) La stucture nor-stéroide. In Cheymol, J. and Hazard, R. (eds) *Actualités Pharmacologiques,* pp. 221–243. Masson & Cie, Paris.
11. Wermuth, C. G., Schwartz, J., Leclerc, G., Garnier, J. P. and Rouot, B. (1973) Communication préliminaire: conformation de la clonidine et hypothèses sur son interaction avec un récepteur α-adrénergique. *Eur. J. Med. Chem.* **8**: 115–116.
12. Haviv, F., Fitzpatrick, T. D., Swenson, R. E. *et al.* (1993) Effect of *N*-methyl substitution of the peptide bonds in luteinizing hormone-releasing hormone antagonists. *J. Med. Chem.* **36**: 363–369.
13. Chu, K. C. (1980) The quantitative analysis of structure–activity relationships. In Wolf, M. E. (ed.) *The Basis of Medicinal Chemistry/Burger's Medicinal Chemistry,* pp. 393–418. Wiley, New York.
14. McElvain, S. M. and Carney, T. P. (1946) Piperidine derivatives. XVII. Local anesthetics derived from substituted piperidinoalcohols. *J. Amer. Chem. Soc.* **68**: 2592–2600.
15. Ganellin, C. R. (1982) Cimetidine. In Bindra, J. S. and Lednicer, D. (eds) *Chronicles of Drug Discovery.* pp. 1–38. Wiley, New York.
16. Black, J. W., Durant, G. J., Emmet, J. C. and Ganellin, C. R. C. (1974) Sulphur–methylene isosterism in the development of metiamide, a new histamine H2-receptor antagonist. *Nature* **248**: 65–67.
17. Arcos, J. C. and Arcos, M. (1962) Molecular geometry and mechanisms of action of chemical carcinogens. In Jucker E. (ed.) *Progress in Drug Research,* pp. 407–581. Birkhäuser Verlag, Basel.
18. Albert, A. (1979) *Selective Toxicity,* p. 48. Chapman & Hall, London.
19. Roemer, D., Beuscher, H. H., Hill, R. C., Pless, J., Bauer, W., Cardinaux, F., Closse, A., Hauser, D. and Huguenin, R. (1977) A synthetic enkephalin analogue with prolonged parenteral and oral activity. *Nature* **268**: 547–549.
20. Plattner, J. J. and Norbeck, D. W. (1990) Obstacles to drug development from peptide leads. In Clark, C. R. and Moos, W. H. (eds) *Drug Discovery Technologies,* pp. 92–126. Ellis Horwood Limited, Chichester.
21. Fauchère, J.L. (1986) Elements for the rational design of peptide drugs. In Testa B. (ed.) *Advances in Drug Research,* pp. 29–69. Academic Press, London.
22. Holland, V. R., Saunders, B. C., Rose, F .L. and Walpole, A. L. (1974) A safer substitute for benzidine in the detection of blood. *Tetrahedron* **30**: 3299–3302.
23. Van de Straat, R., de Vries, J., Groot, E. J., Zijl, R. and Vermeulen, N. (1987) Paracetamol. 3-Monoalkyl- and 3,5-dialkyl derivatives: comparison of their hepatotoxicity in mice. *Toxicol. Appl. Pharmacol.* **89**: 183–189.
24. Tute, M. S. (1971) Principles and practice of Hansch analysis: a guide to structure–activity correlation for the medicinal chemist. In Harper, N. J. and Simmonds, A. B. (eds) *Avances in Drug Research,* pp. 1–77. Academic Press, London.
25. Nadler, V., Kloog, Y. and Sokolovsky, M. (1988) 1-Aminocyclopropane-1-carboxylic acid (ACC) mimics the effect of glycine on the NMDA receptor ion channel. *Eur. J. Pharmacol.* **157**: 115–116.

26. Cussac, M., Pierre, J. L., Boucherle, A. and Favier, F. (1975) Intérêt des dérivés du cyclopropane en Chimie Thérapeutique. *Ann. Pharm. Française* **33**: 513–529.

27. Marivet, M. C., Bourguignon, J. J., Lugnier, C., Mann, A., Stoclet, J. C. and Wermuth, C.G. (1989) Inhibition of cyclic adenosine-3′,5′-monophosphate phosphodiesterase from vascular smooth muscle by rolipram analogues. *J. Med. Chem.* **32**: 1450–1457.

28. Trivedi, B. K., Holmes, A., Stoeber, T .L., Blankley, C. J., Roark, H. W., Picard, J. A., Shaw, M. K., Essenburg, A. D., Stanfield, R. L. and Krause, B. R. (1993) Inhibitors of acyl-CoA:cholesterol acyltransferase. 4. A novel series of urea ACAT inhibitors as potential hypocholesterolemic agents. *J. Med. Chem.* **36**: 3300–3307.

29. Sexton, W. A. (ed.) (1963) *Chemical Constitution and Biological Activity*, 3rd edn, p. 103. E. & F.N. Spon, London.

30. Craig, P .N. (1980) Guidelines for drug and analog design. In Wolf, M. E. (ed.) *The Basis of Medicinal Chemistry — Burger's Medicinal Chemistry*, pp. 331–348. Wiley, New York.

31. Breen, A. P. and Murphy, J. A. (1993) Radical-induced DNA cleavage mediated by a vinyl epoxide. *J. Chem. Soc. Chem. Commun.* pp. 193–194.

32. Ogata, M., Matsumoto, H., Shimizu, S., Kida, S., Shiro, M. and Tawara, K. (1987) Synthesis and antifungal activity of new 1-vinylimidazoles. *J. Med. Chem.* **30**: 1348–1354.

33. Maurin, M. B., Addicks, W. J., Rowe, S. M. and Hogan, R. (1993) Physical chemical properties of alpha styryl carbinol antifungal agents. *Pharm. Res.* **10**: 309–312.

34. Browning, E. (1965) *Toxicity and Metabolism of Industrial Solvents*, pp. 377–381. Elsevier, New York.

35. Scholton, W. and Sy, L. (1966) Kolloid-chemische Eigenschaften eines neuen Kurznarkotikums. Teilgewicht der Mizelle und Verteilungs gleichgewicht des Wirkstoffes. *Arzneimittel-Forsch.* **16**: 679–691.

36. Milne Jr, G. M. and Johnson, M. R. (1967) Narcotic antagonists and analgesics. In Clarke, F .H. (ed.) *Annual Reports in Medicinal Chemistry*, pp. 23–32. Academic Press, New York,

37. Culvenor, C. C. J., Dann, A. T. and Dick, A. T. (1962) Alkylation as the mechanism by which the hepatotoxic pyrrolizidine alkaloids act on cell nuclei. *Nature* **195**: 570–573.

38. Beart, P .M., Uhr, M. L. and Johnston, G. A. R. (1972) Inhibition of GABA transaminase activity by 4-aminotetrolic acid. *J. Neurochem.* **19**: 1855–1861.

39. Schmitt, J. (1967) Sur un nouveau myorelaxant de la classe des benzodiazépines: le tétrazepam. *Eur. J. Med. Chem.* **2**: 254-259.

40. Fryer, R. I, Zhang, P., Rios, R., Gu, Z.-Q., Basile, A. S. and Skolnick, P (1993) Structure-activity relationship studies at the benzodiazepine receptor (BZR): a comparison of the substituent effects of pyrazoloquinolinone analogs. *J. Med. Chem.* **36**: 1669–1673.

41. Taylor, J. B. and Kennewell, P. D. (1981) *Introductory Medicinal Chemistry*, p. 89. Ellis Horwood, Chichester.

42. Newman, A. H., Allen, A. C., Izenwasser, S. and Katz, J. (1994) Novel 3α-(diphenylmethoxy)tropane analogs: potent dopamine uptake inhibitors without cocaine-like behavioral profiles. *J. Med. Chem.* **37**: 2258–2261.

43. MacLeod, A. M., Merchant, K. J., Cascieri, M. A., Sadowski, S., Ber, E., Swain, C.J. and Baker, R. (1994) *N*-Acyl-L-tryptophan benzyl esters: potent substance P receptor antagonists. *J. Med. Chem.* **36**: 2044–2045.

44. Buu-Hoi, N. P. (1961) Les dérivés organiques du fluor d'intérêt pharmacologique. In Jucker E. (ed.) *Progress in Drug Research*, pp. 9–74. Birkhäuser Verlag, Basel.

45. Gee, K. W. and Yamamura, H. I. (1982) A novel pyrazoloquinoline that interacts with brain benzodiazepine receptors: characterization of some *in vitro* and *in vivo* properties of CGS 9896. *Life Sci.* **30**: 2245–2252.

46. Bowery, N. G., Bittiger, H. and Olpe, H.-R. (eds) (1990) *GABA$_B$ Receptors in Mammalian Function*. Wiley, Chichester.

47. Rosi, D., Peruzzotti, G., Dennis, E. W., Berberian, D. A., Freele, H. and Archer, S. (1965) A new, active metabolite of 'Miracil D'. *Nature* **208**: 1005–1006.

48. Wermuth, C. G. (1993) Aminopyridazines — an alternative route to potent muscarinic agonists with no cholinergic syndrome. *Il Farmaco* **48**: 253–274.

49. Ganellin, C. R. and Roberts, S. M (1993) *Medicinal Chemistry, the Role of Organic Chemistry in Drug Research,*. 2nd edn. Academic Press, London.

50. Klaassen, C. D. (1990) Heavy metals and heavy-metal antagonists. In Goodman-Gilman, A., Rall,

T. W., Nies, A. S. and Taylor, P. (eds) *Goodman and Gilman's The Pharmacological Basis of Therapeutics*, pp. 1592–1614. Pergamon Press, New York.

51. Jirousek, L. and Pritchard, E. (1971) On the chemical iodination of tyrosine with protein sulfenyl iodide and sulfenyl periodide derivatives. *Biochim. Biophys. Acta.* **243**: 230–238.

52. Haynes Jr, R. C. (1990) Thyroid and antithyroid drugs. In Goodman-Gilman, A., Rall, T. W., Nies, A. S. and Taylor, P. (eds) *Goodman and Gilman's The Pharmacological Basis of Therapeutics*, pp. 1361–1383. Pergamon Press, New York.

53. Remy, D. C., Britcher, S. F., King, S. W. *et al.* (1983) Synthesis and receptor binding studies relevant to the neuroleptic activities of some 1-methyl-4-piperidylene-9-substituted-pyrrolo[2,1-*b*][3]benzazepine derivatives. *J. Med. Chem.* **26**: 974–980.

18

The Role of Functional Groups in Drug–Receptor Interactions

PETER R. ANDREWS

Alice remained looking thoughtfully at the mushroom for a minute, trying to make out which were the two sides of it; and, as it was perfectly round, she found this a very difficult question.
Lewis Carroll, *Alice's Adventures in Wonderland*

THE PRACTICE OF MEDICINAL CHEMISTRY
ISBN 0-12-744640-0

I. INTRODUCTION

The strength of the interaction between a drug molecule and its receptor can be determined directly from the equilibrium constant for the interaction,

$$K_d = \frac{[\text{drug}][\text{receptor}]}{[\text{complex}]} \tag{1}$$

by expressing it in terms of the corresponding free energy change:

$$\Delta G = -2.303\, RT \log K_d \tag{2}$$

Under physiological conditions ($T = 310\,\text{K}$) this is approximated (in kJ mol^{-1}) by

$$\Delta G = -5.85 \log K_d \tag{3}$$

The observed equilibrium constant thus provides a direct measurement of ΔG. For example, a drug binding with a K_d of 10^{-10} M requires $(-5.85) \times (-10) = 58.5\,\text{kJ mol}^{-1}$ to dissociate from the receptor.

The purpose of this chapter is to provide an understanding of the physical and chemical factors that contribute most significantly to the strength of drug–receptor interactions. The first part consists of a physical description of the influence of electrostatic and steric match on the various types of nonbonded drug–receptor interactions. The second part provides a more chemical interpretation, concentrating on the intrinsic strengths of individual functional group contributions to the affinity of drugs for their receptors. Finally, the relevance of these numbers to the practising medicinal chemist is discussed using inhibitors of the viral enzyme HIV-protease as typical examples.

II. THE IMPORTANCE OF THE ELECTROSTATIC AND STERIC MATCH BETWEEN DRUG AND RECEPTOR

What determines K_d? Basically, it depends on two factors. One is the electrostatic match between drug and receptor, which is primarily a function of electron density. The other is the steric match between drug and receptor, which is primarily dependent on conformation.

How do these two factors contribute to the strengths of the various bonds that make up drug–receptor interactions? In fact, most noncovalent interactions depend to some degree on both electrostatic and steric properties, but for convenience in the following discussion we will divide them into those that are primarily electrostatic and those that are primarily steric.

A.   Electrostatic interactions

Electrostatic interactions are the net result of the attractive forces between the positively charged nuclei and the negatively charged electrons of the two molecules. The attractive force between these opposite charges leads to three main bond types: charge–charge, charge–dipole and dipole–dipole interactions.

1.   Ionic bonds

The strength of any electrostatic interaction can be calculated from equation (4), where q_i and q_j are two charges separated by a distance r_{ij} in a medium of dielectric constant D. This equation applies equally to ionic interactions, where the charges q_i and q_j are integer values, or to polar interactions, in which the total energy is summed over the contributions calculated from the partial charges on all the individual atoms.

$$E = \frac{q_i q_j}{D r_{ij}} \qquad (4)$$

It follows from equation (4) that the strengths of ionic interactions are crucially dependent on the dielectric constant D of the surrounding medium. In hydrophobic environments, like the interior of a protein molecule, the dielectric constant may be as low as 4, whereas in bulk-phase water the corresponding value is 80. In other environments, intermediate values are appropriate; e.g. for interactions occurring near the surface of a protein a D value of 28 is commonly used.

It also follows from equation (4) that the strengths of ionic bonds are inversely proportional to the distance separating the two charges. However, since the strengths of other noncovalent bonds are even more sharply dependent on distance than those of ionic bonds, ionic attraction frequently dominates the initial long-range interactions between drugs and receptors.

2.   Charge–dipole and dipole–dipole interactions

Although charge–dipole and dipole–dipole interactions are weaker than ionic bonds, they are nevertheless key contributors to the overall strengths of drug–receptor interactions, since they occur in any molecule in which electronegativity differences between atoms result in significant bond, group or molecular dipole moments.

The key differences between ionic and dipolar interactions relate to their dependence on distance and orientation. For charge–dipole interactions, the strength of the interaction depends inversely on the square of the distance, while for dipole–dipole interactions it reduces with the cube of the distance separating the dipoles.

Similarly, while steric effects are of little importance in ionic interactions, stricter geometric requirements apply to dipolar interactions, which may be either attractive or repulsive depending on the orientation of the dipole moments.

3.   Inductive interactions

The formation of a drug–receptor complex is often accompanied by intramolecular and/or intermolecular redistributions of charge. In the intramolecular case this redistribution is referred to as an induced polarization, whereas a redistribution of charge between two molecules is described as a charge–transfer interaction. In either case, the resulting interactions are always attractive and strongly dependent on the distance separating the two molecules.

An interesting example of the importance of inductive interactions is the recent calculation by Bajorath *et al.* on the binding of folate and dihydrofolate to dihydrofolate reductase. This revealed a shift in net charge equivalent to half an electron from the pteridine ring to the glutamate moiety on binding to the enzyme, with the major change in density being focused on the bonds that are catalytically reduced.[1]

4. Hydrogen bonds

The most important noncovalent interactions in biological systems, hydrogen bonds, are also best described as electrostatic interactions. The approximate strength of individual hydrogen bonds can therefore be calculated from the partial charges of the atoms in the interacting groups using equation (4), which makes hydrogen bonds, like ionic bonds, important long-range recognition factors between drugs and receptors.

Unlike ionic bonds, however, hydrogen bonds are dependent to some extent on steric orientation. Thus, statistical studies[2–4] of hydrogen bonds in small-molecule crystal structures from the Cambridge Crystallographic Database show clear directional preferences, reflecting conventional hybridization concepts. On the other hand, the atomic surroundings of uncharged hydrogen-bonding groups in ligand–protein structures recorded in the Brookhaven Protein Databank showed no strong directional preferences,[5] suggesting that the energy differential favouring conventional hybridization states is small relative to other components of the interaction.

Stronger directional preferences are observed for hydrogen-bond-reinforced ionic interactions, for which analysis of protein–ligand interactions in the Brookhaven Protein Databank showed[5] that ligand carboxyl groups participate in two distinct types of binding: a close chelate-type interaction with the guanidino group of arginine, and a lateral interaction between one of the carboxyl oxygen atoms and a nitrogen atom from a variety of positively charged amino acid residues. This is consistent with the fact that the strongest hydrogen bonds are formed between groups with the greatest electrostatic character.[6,7]

B.   Steric interactions

While electrostatic interactions are the dominant interactions involving polar molecules, there are also strong interactions between nonpolar molecules, particularly at short intermolecular distances.

1. Dispersion forces

Dispersion, or London, forces are the universal forces responsible for attractive interactions between nonpolar molecules. Their occurrence is due to the fact that any atom will, at any given instant, be likely to possess a finite dipole moment as a result of the movement of electrons around the nuclei. Such fluctuating dipoles tend to induce opposite dipoles in adjacent molecules, thus resulting in a net attractive force. Although the individual interactions between pairs of atoms are relatively weak, the total contribution to binding from dispersion forces can be very significant if there is a close fit between drug and receptor. The quality of the steric match is thus the dominant factor in nonpolar interactions.

2.   *Short-range repulsive forces*

The short-range repulsive forces resulting from the overlap of the electron clouds of any two molecules increase exponentially with decreasing internuclear separation. The balance between these repulsive interactions and the dispersion forces thus determines both the minimum and the most favourable nonbonded separation between any pair of atoms. The equilibrium distance can be determined from crystal data, and is equivalent to the sum of the van der Waals radii of the two interacting atoms.

For nonpolar molecules this balance between the attractive dispersion forces and the short-range repulsive forces is generally defined in terms of the Buckingham (6-exp) potential given in equation (5) or the alternative Lennard-Jones 6-12 potential, given in equation (6):

$$E = \frac{Ae^{-Br}}{r^d} - \frac{C}{r^6} \tag{5}$$

$$E = \frac{A}{r^{12}} - \frac{C}{r^6} \tag{6}$$

3.   *Conformational energy*

While intramolecular interactions within the drug molecule are the primary factor in determining the lowest energy conformation of the unbound drug, intermolecular interactions with the receptor also have a significant effect on conformation. If the bound conformation of a flexible molecule is also its lowest energy conformation, there is no conformational energy cost involved in binding. If, on the other hand, the optimal interaction between drug and receptor requires a higher-energy conformation, this energy difference will reduce the apparent strength of the interaction between the two molecules.

C.   **The role of entropy**

1.   *Hydrophobic interactions*

When a nonpolar molecule is surrounded by water, stronger than normal water–water interactions are formed around the solute molecule to compensate for the weaker interactions between solute and water. This results in an increasingly ordered arrangement of water molecules around the solute, and thus a negative entropy of dissolution. The decrease in entropy is roughly proportional to the nonpolar surface area of the molecule. The association of two such nonpolar molecules in water reduces the total nonpolar surface area exposed to the solvent, thus reducing the amount of structured water, and therefore providing a favourable entropy of association.

As for van der Waals forces, hydrophobic interactions are individually weak (0.1 to 0.2 kJ mol^{-1} for every square angstrom of solvent-accessible hydrocarbon surface[8]), but the total contribution of hydrophobic bonds to drug–receptor interactions is substantial. Similarly, the overall strength of the hydrophobic interaction between two molecules is very dependent on the quality of the steric match between the two molecules. If this is not sufficiently close to squeeze all of the solvent from the interface, a substantial entropy penalty must be paid for each of the trapped water molecules.

2.   Rotational and translational entropy

There are also substantial entropic penalties associated with the loss of three rotational and three translational degrees of freedom of the drug molecule on binding to the receptor. Since these are replaced by six vibrational degrees of freedom in the complex, the resulting entropy change is dependent on the relative 'tightness' of the complex. For a typical ligand–protein interaction, the estimated change in free energy resulting from the loss of entropy on binding (at 310 K) ranges from 12 kJ mol^{-1} for a very weak interaction to 60 kJ mol^{-1} for a tightly bound complex.[9]

3.   Conformational entropy

In the case of flexible drug molecules there is a further entropy loss due to the conformational restriction that accompanies binding. Based on the observed entropy changes accompanying cyclization reactions, the extent of this entropy loss is estimated[10] at 5–6 kJ mol^{-1} per internal rotation, although the actual figure again depends on the overall strength of the interaction between the drug and the receptor. In the case of rigid analogues there is no such loss of conformational entropy on binding. Provided that they offer a good steric and electrostatic match to the receptor, rigid analogues should therefore have a free energy advantage relative to more flexible drugs.

III.   THE STRENGTHS OF FUNCTIONAL GROUP CONTRIBUTIONS TO DRUG–RECEPTOR INTERACTIONS

The total free energy of interaction between a drug and its receptor provides a measure of the strength of the association between the two molecules, but tells us little or nothing about the overall quality of their match. Does the observed binding reflect a composite of interactions between every part of the drug and its receptor, or is it a case of one or two strong interactions contributing sufficient energy to disguise an otherwise mediocre fit? Is the observed increase in interaction energy resulting from the addition of a new functional group consistent with what might have been anticipated? To answer these questions we need some means of estimating the individual functional group contributions to drug–receptor interactions.

A.   Measuring functional group contributions

The free energy of binding, ΔG, can be defined in terms of the binding energies for the individual functional groups that make up the drug molecule according to equation (7)

$$\Delta G = T\,\Delta S_{rt} + n_r E_r + \Sigma n_X E_X \tag{7}$$

where $T\Delta S_{rt}$ is the loss of overall rotational and translational entropy associated with binding of the drug molecule, n_r is the number of internal degrees of conformational freedom lost on binding the drug molecule, and E_r is the energy equivalent of the entropy loss associated with the loss of each degree of conformational freedom on receptor binding.

1.   Intrinsic binding energy

The final term in equation (7) is the sum of the binding energies E_X associated with each functional group X, of which there are n_X present in the drug. In the ideal case, when the specified functional group is aligned optimally and without strain with the corresponding functional group in the receptor, E_X is referred to as the intrinsic binding energy.[11] In other cases the term apparent binding energy is used.

It should be noted that each binding energy E_X is actually a combination of the various enthalpic and entropic interactions outlined above. These include the enthalpy of interaction between the functional group and its corresponding binding site on the receptor, the enthalpy changes associated with the removal of water of hydration from the functional group and its target site and the subsequent formation of bonds between the displaced water molecules, and the corresponding entropy terms associated with the displacement and subsequent bonding of water molecules.

It is apparent that these intrinsic binding energies may be regarded, at least approximately, as properties of the functional group that should be relatively independent of the groups to which the particular functional group is attached. Such intrinsic binding potentials might thus reasonably be used in an additive manner to provide an overall estimate of the drug–receptor interaction.

2.   Anchor principle

It follows from equation (7) that the binding energy, E_X, due to the interaction between the receptor and a specific functional group, X, can be estimated by comparing the binding energies for pairs of compounds that differ only in the presence or absence of the specific functional group. This approach was first applied by Page[9] who referred to it as the 'anchor principle'. It is based on the premise that the difference in binding of a drug molecule with or without the particular functional group is due to factors associated solely with that group, i.e. the binding energy E_X plus any degrees of conformational freedom lost specifically as a result of binding of group X. Other degrees of conformational freedom lost on binding and the loss of overall rotational and translational entropy associated with the remainder of the drug molecule (the anchor) are assumed to be unaffected by the presence or absence of X.

Similarly, the impact of a single amino acid substitution in the active site of an enzyme on transition state stabilization, as determined by the change in either catalytic efficiency or inhibitor binding, provides a measure of the relative binding energy of the two side-chains.

Clearly, the magnitude of the binding energies obtained using the anchor principle will vary widely with the quality of the interaction. If the functional groups are not properly aligned, as might reasonably be expected in many mutant proteins, a small or even repulsive interaction may result. Alternatively, the strength of the additional bond may be offset by a reduction in the strengths of the existing bonds. Under these circumstances the anchor principle will lead to an underestimate of the true bond strength.

3.   Average binding energy

An alternative to the pair-by-pair approach inherent in the anchor principle was developed by Andrews et al.,[12] who sought to average the contributions of individual functional groups to the observed binding energies of 200 ligand–protein interactions in aqueous solution. For this purpose, the average loss of overall rotational and translational entropy accompanying drug–receptor binding, $T\Delta S_{rt}$ in equation (7), was estimated at 58.5 kJ mol^{-1} (14 kcal mol^{-1}) at 310 K. Regression analysis against n_r (obtained by counting the number of degrees of conformational freedom in each of the 200 ligand structures) and n_X (the number of occurrences of each functional group, X, in each of the 200 ligand structures) as the independent variables was then used to obtain 'average' values of the binding energies associated with each functional group and for the loss of entropy associated with each degree of conformational freedom.

The results of this analysis showed that the loss of entropy associated with each internal rotation on receptor binding is equivalent to a reduction in the free energy of binding by an average of 3 kJ mol^{-1}, which may be compared to the estimated[10] value for the total loss of conformational freedom around a single bond of 5–6 kJ mol^{-1}. The smaller number obtained empirically implies that conformational freedom is not fully lost for all the bonds in an average drug–receptor interaction, and is consistent with experimental estimates of 1.6–3.6 kJ mol^{-1} for the entropic cost of restricting rotations in hydrocarbon chains.[13]

The corresponding binding energies obtained by the averaging process were C(sp^2 or sp^3), 3 kJ mol^{-1}; O, S, N, or halogen, 5 kJ mol^{-1}; OH and C=O, 10 and 14 kJ mol^{-1}, respectively; and CO_2^-, OPO_3^{2-}, and N$^+$, 34, 42 and 48 kJ mol^{-1}, respectively. Once again, it should be stressed that these are not intrinsic binding energies in the sense defined above. This would be the case only if each functional group in each drug in the series was optimally aligned with a corresponding functional group in the receptor. In fact, since every functional group of every drug was included in the analysis, the calculated values are averages of apparent binding energies, including those for some groups that may not interact with the receptor at all.[14] The calculated averages are thus almost certainly smaller than the corresponding intrinsic binding energies, although they follow expected trends in that charged groups lead to stronger interactions than polar groups, which in turn are stronger than nonpolar groups such as sp^2 or sp^3 carbons.

B. The methyl group and other nonpolar substituents

The initial application of the anchor principle described by Page[9] related to data on the selectivity of amino acid-tRNA synthetases, from which he estimated intrinsic binding energies for the methylene group in the range 12–14 kJ mol^{-1}. For example, the calculated binding energies (equation 3) for isoleucine (1) (Fig. 18.1) and its desmethyl analogue (2) to isoleucyl-tRNA synthetase are 29.7 and 15.9 kJ mol^{-1}, respectively, indicating that the methyl group contributes a total of 13.8 kJ mol^{-1} to the overall interaction. This estimate, having been derived

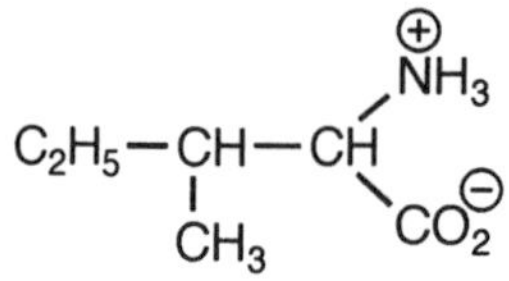

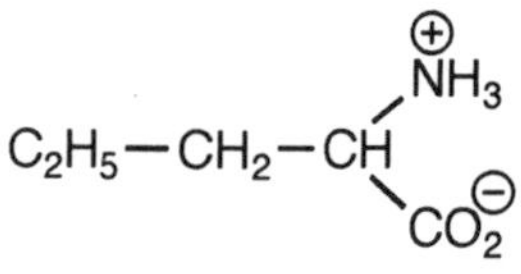

Fig. 18.1   Isoleucine (1) and desmethylisoleucine (2).

from observations on a highly selective enzyme–substrate interaction, is probably also approaching the intrinsic limit for the binding contribution of a methyl group.

There are, unfortunately, relatively few active site mutagenesis data available for mutations involving a single methyl group. The mutation of glycine to alanine in subtilisin BPN results in free energy differences of 1–3 kJ mol^{-1}, although larger changes have been observed in other enzymes.[15]

For longer hydrocarbon side-chains, the positive contribution due to dispersion forces and hydrophobic interactions tends to be offset by the loss of conformational entropy on binding. Thus, the 'average' binding energy of 3 kJ mol^{-1} obtained by Andrews *et al.* for sp^2 and sp^3 carbon groups is identical to the 'average' reduction in free energy of binding estimated for the loss of conformational freedom around a single bond.[12] Clearly, this effect will be greater in saturated hydrocarbon chains than their more conformationally constrained unsaturated or cyclic analogues.

C.   The hydroxyl group and other hydrogen bond-forming substituents

The most extensive studies of hydroxyl group contributions to drug–receptor interactions are those of Wolfenden *et al.* on the contribution of hydrogen bonds formed by hydroxyl groups in transition state analogues. In a series of 13 examples of paired ligands with and without hydroxyl groups, they used[16] the anchor principle to determine apparent binding energies for single hydroxyl groups ranging from 20 to 42 kJ mol^{-1}.

Thus, in comparing the binding of 1,6-dihydropurine ribonucleoside (**3**) (Fig. 18.2) and its 6-hydroxy derivative (**4**) to adenosine deaminase, they observed[17] K_i values for these two inhibitors of 5.4×10^{-6} M and 3×10^{-13} M respectively, reflecting a difference in binding energy of 41 kJ mol^{-1}.

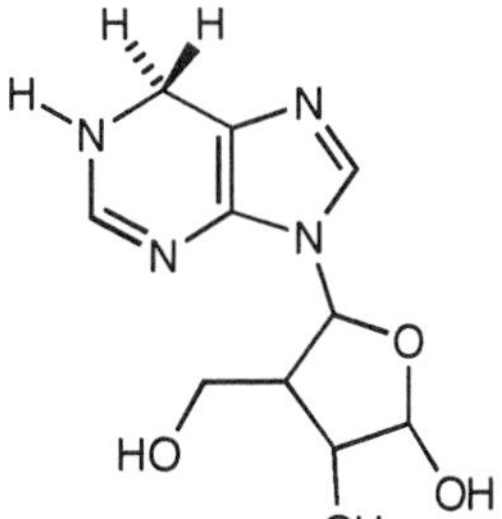

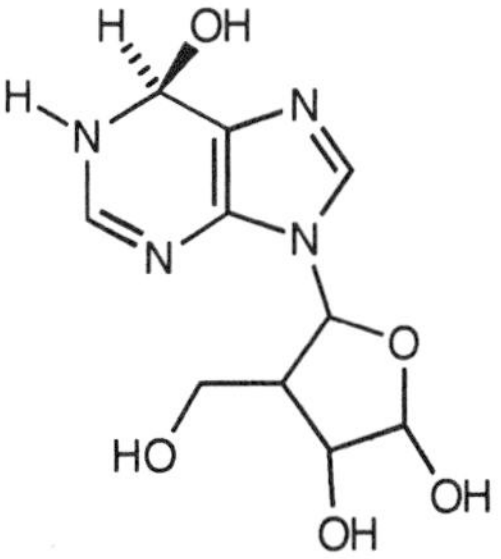

Fig. 18.2   1,6-Dihydropurine ribonucleoside (**3**) and its 6-hydroxy analogue (**4**).

As noted by Kati and Wolfenden, this remarkable affinity appears to suggest that the 6-hydroxyl group, which has very limited freedom of movement, is likely to be in almost ideal alignment with the active site, and that at least one charged active site residue is also likely to be involved in its hydrogen-bonding interaction. This conjecture has since been verified by the determination of the crystal structure[18] of the inhibitory complex between adenosine deaminase and 6-hydroxy-1,6-dihydropurine ribonucleoside, which showed that the 6-hydroxyl group interacts with a zinc atom, with a protonated histidyl residue, and with an aspartic acid residue at the enzyme's active site.

Once again, the data from active-site mutagenesis studies are less striking, but nevertheless reveal some very substantial hydrogen-bonding interactions. In Fersht's studies[19] on tyrosyl-tRNA synthetase, for example, hydrogen bonds between this enzyme and uncharged substrate groups contributed between 2 and 6 kJ mol^{-1} towards specificity, while hydrogen bonds to charged groups contributed between 15 and 19 kJ mol^{-1}, corresponding to a factor of 1000 in specificity.

These numbers are comparable to the 'average' functional group contributions determined by Andrews *et al.*, which ranged from 5 kJ mol^{-1} for uncharged H-bond acceptors (O, N, S) through 10 kJ mol^{-1} for a hydroxyl group to 14 kJ mol^{-1} for a carbonyl.

D.   Acidic and basic substituents

Application of the anchor principle to data on the selectivity of amino acid-tRNA synthetases gives[9] estimated intrinsic binding energies for the carboxyl and amino groups of 18 and >28 kJ mol^{-1}, respectively. However, since the side-chains rather than the ionic groups are the primary determinants of amino acid/tRNA synthetase specificity, these energies are likely to be underestimates.

An indication of this likelihood may be obtained using simple observations on the interactions of individual charged groups with appropriate enzymes. The phosphate ion, for example, binds alkaline phosphatase[20] with a dissociation constant of 2.3×10^{-6} M, equivalent to a ΔG value of approximately 33 kJ mol^{-1}. Taking the most conservative estimate for the loss of rotational and translational entropy associated with this interaction, 12 kJ mol^{-1} for a loosely bound complex, equation (7) then gives a lower estimate for binding of the phosphate ion of 45 kJ mol^{-1}. If the same value of $T\Delta S_{rt}$ is applied to the binding of oxalate ion to transcarboxylase,[21] for which the dissociation constant is 1.8×10^{-6} M (33 kJ mol^{-1}), equation (7) gives an apparent binding energy of 24 kJ mol^{-1} per carboxylate group after allowance for a minimal conformational entropy loss of 3 kJ mol^{-1}.

Similar results were obtained by Fersht *et al.*[19] from observed k_{cat}/K_m values in active-site mutagenesis studies. Charge–charge interactions in the tyrosyl-tRNA synthetase system ranged from 12 to 25 kJ mol^{-1} for groups interacting with the substrate pyrophosphate moiety, and up to 33 kJ mol^{-1} for the interaction between Asp78 and the substrate amino group, although in the latter case it was recognized that removal of the aspartate residue probably results in some structural reorganization in the active site.[22]

Once again, these figures are broadly consistent with the 'average' values of Andrews *et al.*,[12] which were in the range 34–48 kJ mol^{-1} for charged phosphate, amine and carboxyl groups.

IV.   PRACTICAL APPLICATIONS FOR THE MEDICINAL CHEMIST

The apparent contributions of different functional groups and/or bond types to overall binding energies derived from the various studies reviewed above are summarized in Table 18.1. Also included are corresponding values used or suggested for the overall loss of rotational and

Table 18.1   Functional group contributions to drug–receptor interactions (kJ mol^{-1}).

Functional group type	Technique employed to determine interaction energy		
	Anchor principle	Site-directed mutagenesis	'Average' energy
Nonpolar (per carbon atom)	12–14	1–3	3–6
H-bonding (uncharged)	16	2–6	5–14
H-bonding (charge-assisted)	20–42	15–19	
Charged (carboxyl, amine)	18–28+	12–25	34–48
$T\Delta S_{rt}$	12–60		58.5
E_r (internal rotation)	5–6		3

translational entropy, $T\Delta S_{rt}$, and the loss of conformational entropy resulting from restriction of free rotation, E_r.

The variations in these estimates demonstrate that they are still far from definitive, but as a rule of thumb we may state that the higher values derived using the anchor principle are the best estimates of the intrinsic binding energies of groups that are optimally aligned with matching groups in the receptor.

For 'goodness of fit' calculations, on the other hand, the optimal binding contributions determined from highly specific applications of the anchor principle are not appropriate, since the absence of detailed structural data means that the summation in equation (7) is necessarily done over all the functional groups in the drug molecule, regardless of whether or not they are directly involved in binding to the receptor. The 'average' values derived previously by Andrews et al.[12] are thus a better starting point for 'goodness of fit' calculations.

A.   Assessing a lead compound

Summation of the average contributions of individual binding groups, including allowance for conformational, rotational and translational entropy terms as shown in equation (7), provides a simple back-of-the-envelope calculation of the strength of binding which might be expected for a drug forming a typical interaction with a receptor. This figure, when compared to the observed affinity of the drug for the target receptor, then gives a direct indication of the actual quality of the electrostatic and steric match between the drug and the receptor.

1.   Binding is tighter than expected

If the observed binding of a drug to its receptor turns out to be substantially stronger than that calculated from equation (7), it is reasonable to expect that the drug structure offers a good fit to the receptor in a reasonably low-energy conformation. The structure should therefore provide an excellent starting point for the development of even more bioactive compounds.

A good example of this is biotin (**5**) (Fig. 18.3) which was the most extreme case of a positive deviation from the calculated 'average' in the the original set of 200 ligand–protein interactions studied by Andrews et al.[12]

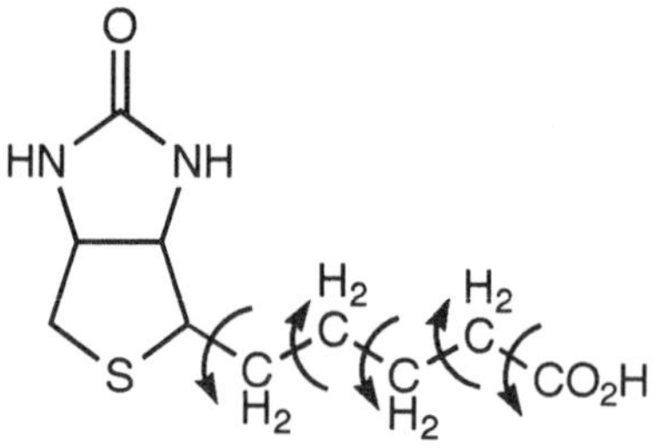

Fig. 18.3 Structure of biotin.

$$\Delta G_{av} = T\Delta S_{rt} + 5E_r + 8E_{Csp^3} + 2E_N + E_S + E_{C=O} + E_{COOH}$$
$$= -58.5 + 5(-3) + 8(3) + 2(5) + 5 + 14 + 34 = 13.5 \, kJ \, mol^{-1}$$
$$\Delta G_{obs} = -5.85 \log K_d$$
$$= -5.85 \, (-15) = 87.75 \, kJ \, mol^{-1}$$

Application of equation (7) to biotin (see above) gives an 'average' binding energy of 13.5 kJ mol^{-1}, whereas substitution into equation (3) of the experimentally observed binding constant to the protein avidin (10^{-15} mole l^{-1}) gives a binding energy of 87.75 kJ mol^{-1}. The difference of almost 75 kJ mol^{-1} implies an exceptionally good fit between biotin and the structure of the protein. It has since been established that this is indeed the case, with polarization of the biotin molecule by the protein actually leading to an ionic interaction where a neutral hydrogen-bonding interaction had been assumed.

2. Binding is looser than expected

If the observed binding is significantly weaker than anticipated on the basis of an 'average' energy calculation, the fit between the drug and the receptor is less than perfect. In some cases this will be because the match between drug and receptor is less a matter of 'hand and glove' than of 'square peg and round hole', and the only realistic option for the drug designer is to start again.

In other cases, simpler remedies may be followed:

(1) The fit may be unsatisfactory because only part of the drug is interacting with the receptor. This situation applies particularly to large drug molecules (e.g. peptide hormones), for which selective pruning of unused parts of the structure may produce simpler compounds without loss of affinity.

(2) The drug may be binding to the receptor in a comparatively high-energy conformation. In this case the design of more rigid structures that are already fixed in the desired conformation will give an increase in binding energy eqivalent to the conformational energy cost of binding the more flexible analogue.

Once again, an extreme case from the original set of 200 ligand–protein interactions studied by Andrews et al.[12] offers a simple example. Application of equation (7) to methotrexate (**6**) (Fig. 18.4) gives

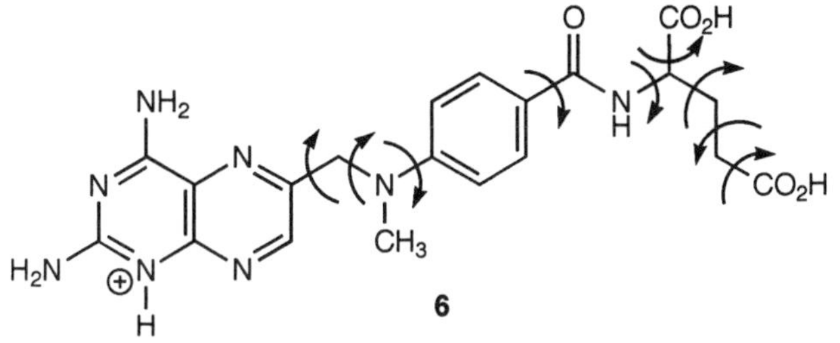

Fig. 18.4   Structure of methotrexate.

$$\Delta G_{av} = T\Delta S_{rt} + 9E_r + 5E_{Csp^3} + 12E_{Csp^2} + 7E_N + E_{C=O} + 2E_{COOH} + E_{N^+}$$
$$= -58.5 + 9(-3) + 5(3) + 12(3) + 7(5) + 14 + 2(34) + 48$$
$$= 130.5 \,\text{kJ mol}^{-1}$$
$$\Delta G_{obs} = -5.85 \log K_d$$
$$= -5.85 \,(-11) = 64.35 \,\text{kJ mol}^{-1}$$

The fact that methotrexate binds to dihydrofolate reductase some 66 kJ mol^{-1} less tightly than anticipated suggests that, despite its exceptional affinity for the enzyme ($K_d = 10^{-11}\,\text{mol}\,\text{l}^{-1}$) the drug does not offer a good overall fit to the active site of the enzyme. Again, the direct evidence of the crystal structure verifies this suggestion, with substantial parts of the structure, including one of the carboxylic acid groups, being exposed to solvent rather than utilized in binding to the enzyme.

B.   Assessing the effectiveness of substituents

Equally simple back-of-the-envelope calculations based on equation (7) can be used to predict the increase in binding energy that might be expected upon the addition of a functional group that is optimally aligned with a corresponding group in the receptor. This figure, when compared to the observed increase in affinity, gives direct feedback on whether or not the new group is actually performing the function anticipated in the design strategy.

An interesting example of how this approach can be used to assess the validity of a drug design hypothesis is provided by the receptor-based design of sialidase inhibitors as potential anti-influenza drugs.

Starting from the knowledge[23] of the structurally invariant active site of influenza A and B sialidases, von Itzstein et al. postulated[24] that substitution of the 4-hydroxyl group of the nonselective sialidase inhibitor 2-deoxy-2,3-didehydro-D-N-acetylneuraminic acid (7) (Fig. 18.5) with a positively charged substituent would fill an unoccupied pocket lined with anionic residues. Synthesis and testing of the 4-guanidino analogue (8) revealed a reduction in K_i from 10^{-6} to 10^{-10} mole l^{-1}, equivalent (from equation 18.3) to an additional binding energy of 23 kJ mol^{-1}.

Although not at the upper limit of the increments in binding energy anticipated for well-aligned ionic interactions on the basis of the data in Table 18.1, this figure is certainly consistent with the design hypothesis, as is borne out by the crystal structure of the complex.[24] This shows that the guanidino lies between two target carboxyl groups in the active site of the enzyme, although only one appears to be optimally placed for a strong interaction.

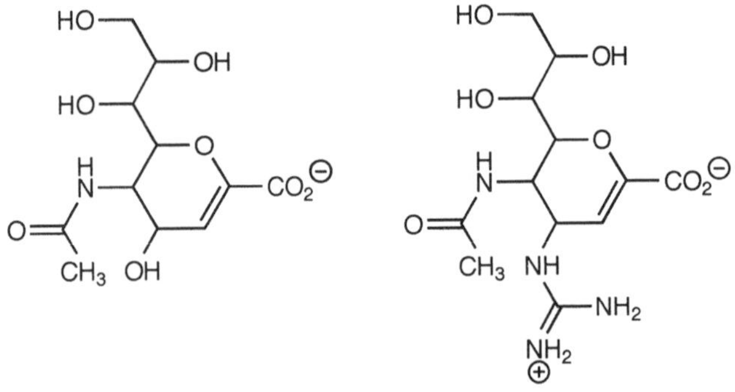

Fig. 18.5 Sialidase inhibitors: 2-deoxy-2,3-didehydro-D-N-acetylneuraminic acid (7) and its 4-guanidino analogue (8).

C. HIV-protease inhibitors: a practical example

The aspartic protease HIV-protease (HIV-PR) is an essential enzyme for the replication of human immunodeficiency virus (HIV), and is widely regarded as one of the most promising targets for the design of new drugs for the treatment of AIDS. As a result, many hundreds of inhibitor classes have already been identified, and crystal structures have been determined for at least 160 complexes of inhibitors with the enzyme.[25] HIV-PR inhibitors are thus excellent test cases for the validity or otherwise of simple 'average' binding energy calculations based on equation (7).

HIV-PR is a 99-amino-acid homodimer which uses a pair of aspartic acid carboxyl residues to cleave key peptide bonds in its polyprotein substrate. The likely nature of its interaction with a typical substrate, based on known enzyme-inhibitor structures, is summarized in Fig. 18.6.

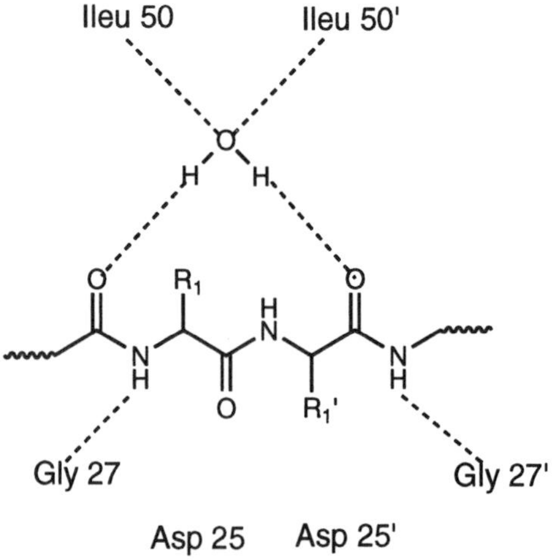

Fig. 18.6 The interaction between HIV-protease and its polyprotein substrate involves a pair of hydrogen bonds (via a buried water molecule) from substrate carbonyls of Gly 27 and Gly 27'; a pair of hydrogen bonds (via a buried water molecule) from substrate C=O groups to main-chain groups of Ile 50 and Ile 50'; and nonpolar interactions with hydrophobic residues lining the pockets that accommodate side-chains R and R'. In the transition state the carboxyl of the central (scissile) bond forms a tetrahedral hydroxy intermediate which interacts with the carboxyl groups of Asp 25 and Asp 25'.

1. *Peptidomimetic inhibitors*

Most HIV-PR inhibitor design has focused on transition state analogues, i.e. analogues based on the known sequences of peptide substrates but with the scissile bond replaced by a peptide bond isostere. Among the most effective peptide bond isosteres introduced into HIV-PR inhibitors have been the hydroxyethylene and hydroxyethylamine moieties (Fig. 18.7), in both of which the isosteric hydroxyl group is thought to mimic the tetrahedral arrangement of the amide carbonyl in the transition state by binding to the catalytically active aspartic acid carboxyl groups of HIV-PR.

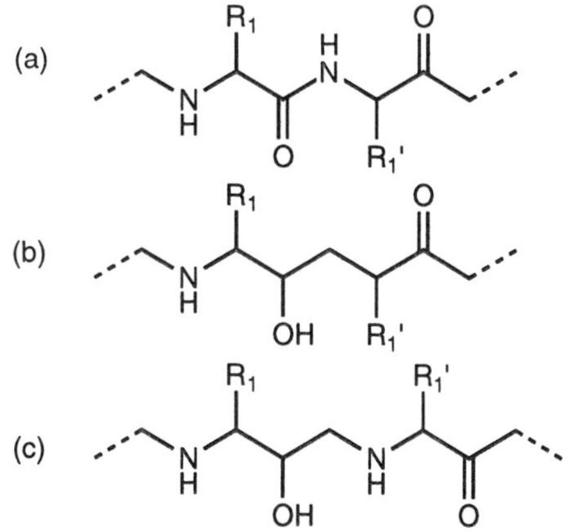

Fig. 18.7   The peptide bond (a) and its hydroxyethylene (b) and hydroxyethylamine (c) isosteres.

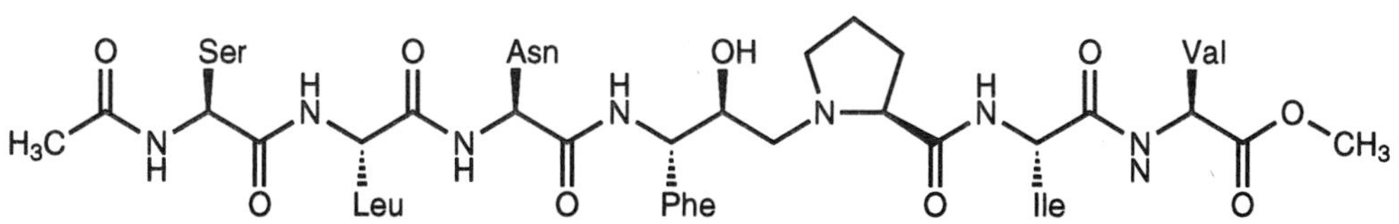

Fig. 18.8   Structure of the HIV-protease inhibitor JG-365.

A good example of this strategy is the hydroxyethylamine isostere JG-365 (**9**) (Fig. 18.8). IC$_{50}$ values[26] for inhibition of HIV-PR by JG-365 and its diastereomer are given in Table 18.2. Also listed are the corresponding binding energies calculated from equation (18.3) (using the IC$_{50}$ values as very approximate estimates of K_d) and equation (7). Following the general principles outlined above, these data lead directly to the following conclusions.

(1) The role of the hydroxyl group is confirmed by the 20-fold difference (8 kJ mol$^{-1)}$) between diastereomers, consistent with the 'average' contribution for a hydroxyl group of 11 kJ mol^{-1};

Table 18.2 Observed and calculated ('average') binding energies for JG-365 and RO-31-8959 diastereomers.

| | | | Binding energy (kJ mol^{-1}) | |
| | | IC$_{50}$ (nM) | Observed (equation 3) | Calculated (equation 7) |
	Structure[a]			
JG-365	Ac-Ser-Leu-Asn-Phe-HEA (S)-Pro-Ile-Val-OMe	3.4	50	144
	Ac-Ser-Leu-Asn-Phe-HEA (R)-Pro-Ile-Val-OMe	65	42	144
RO-31-8959	Qua-Asn-Phe-HEA(R)-Diq-NHtBu^t	<0.4	55	105
	Qua-Asn-Phe-HEA(S)-Diq-NHtBu^t	>100	41	105

[a]Qua = quinoline-2-carboxylic acid. Diq = [(4aS,8aS)-decahydroisoquinoline-3(S)-yl]carbonyloxy.

(2) Inhibition by JG-365 is substantially less than would be expected if all of its functional groups made 'average' interactions with the enzyme.

(3) It should be possible to remove a significant part of the structure of JCG-365 without loss of activity.

The validity of the last conclusion is evident in the somewhat more optimized hydroxyethylamine structure Ro-31-8959 (**10**) (Fig. 18.9), in which inhibitory activity is improved[27] and the importance of the correct orientation of the hydroxyl group is reflected in a difference in binding energy of 14 kJ mol^{-1} between the two isomers (Table 18.2). Nevertheless, the fact that the experimentally observed binding energy of the more active isomer (55 kJ mol^{-1}) is still 50 kJ mol^{-1} less than 'average' (105 kJ mol^{-1}, equation (7) suggests that further pruning of this structure should be possible without significant loss of activity.

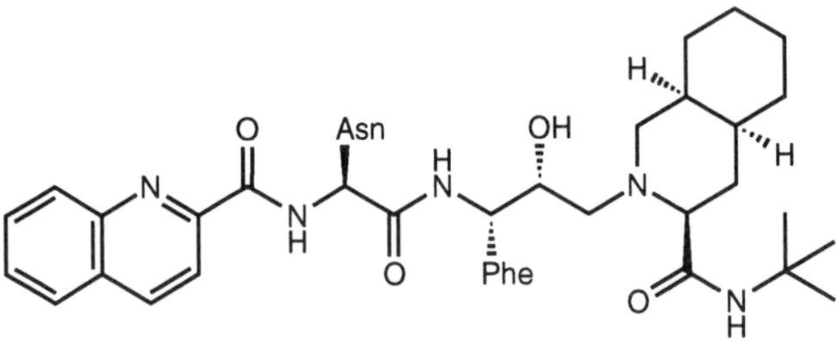

10

Fig. 18.9 Structure of the HIV-protease inhibitor Ro-31-8959.

2. Nonpeptidic inhibitors

Unfortunately, although many peptidomimetic analogues like JG-365 and Ro-31-8959 are potent and selective inhibitors of HIV-PR, they have particularly poor oral bioavailability due to rapid breakdown in the gut and bloodstream. Many laboratories have therefore employed alternative strategies in an effort to identify simpler nonpeptidic structures that might lead to better starting points for design. Some of these strategies and their outcomes are outlined below.

(a) Receptor-based lead discovery using shape-matching criteria DesJarlais *et al.*[28] used the program DOCK to search structural databases for compounds that were complementary in shape to the active site of HIV-PR. This process led to a range of possible inhibitors, of which one of the best was bromperidol, a close relative of the antipsychotic drug haloperidol (**11**) (Fig. 18.10). Subsequent testing of haloperidol showed weak inhibition (K_i = 100 μM) of the enzyme. Does this mean that haloperidol should be a good lead? Unfortunately, it does not. In fact, the observed binding energy of haloperidol (23 kJ mol^{-1}, equation (3)) is considerably less than would be expected for an 'average' interaction (67 kJ mol^{-1}, equation (7), suggesting that the fit of the drug to HIV-PR is far from optimal. This conclusion is borne out by the fact that three crystallographically observed binding modes of a closely related haloperidol derivative are all quite distinct from that initially deduced from the DOCK study.[29]

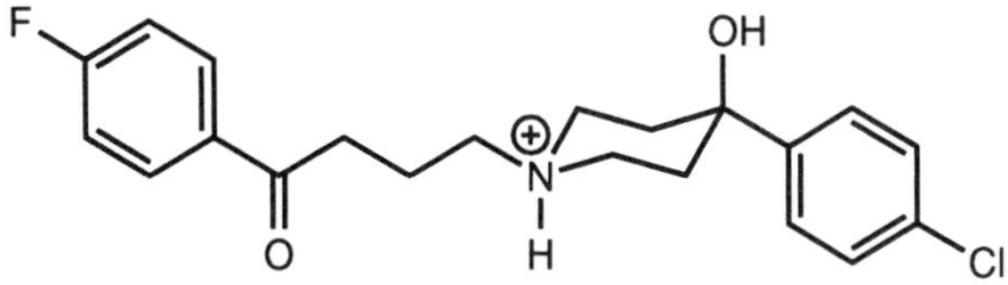

11

Fig. 18.10 Structure of the antipsychotic drug haloperidol.

(b) Receptor-based lead discovery using functional group matching criteria
X-ray crystallographic data for various peptidomimetic inhibitors binding to HIV-PR have revealed a common binding mode incorporating the following features:

(1) A central hydroxyl or diol group that binds to the catalytic aspartic acid carboxyls.
(2) Hydrogen-bond donors (generally amide NH groups) on either side of the central hydroxyl responsible for binding to main-chain carbonyls in the active site of the enzyme.
(3) Hydrophobic groups that fill the P1 and P1′ pockets of the active site of the enzyme.
(4) A buried water molecule that forms hydrogen bonds to two main-chain amide NH groups in the enzyme and two carbonyl oxygens in the inhibitor.

These constant features of the peptidomimetic inhibitors, all of which are consistent with the substrate binding mode illustrated in Fig. 18.6, clearly provide a most valuable guide to the design of nonpeptidic analogues, and numerous pharmacophore-based studies have used these data as the starting point. Of particular interest has been the prospect of incorporating the buried water molecule directly into the inhibitor structure, thus maintaining the contribution of the two hydrogen bonds mediated by the water molecule, but eliminating the entropic cost of immobilizing it in the active site of the enzyme.

This strategy was specifically adopted by Bures *et al.*,[30] who developed a pharmacophore comprising the central hydroxyl group, the adjacent hydrogen bond donors, the buried water molecule and an optional hydrophobic moiety. A systematic search of structural databases using this pharmacophore led to the discovery of a series of dibenzophenones (Table 18.3) that inhibited HIV-PR at concentrations between 10 and 100 μM.

Table 18.3 Dibenzophenone inhibitors based on a pharmacophore model derived from the binding modes of peptidomimetic inhibitors. (Adapted from ref. 25.)

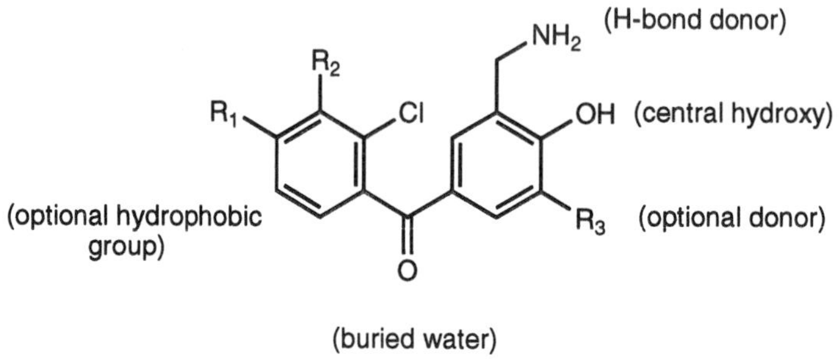

(H-bond donor) NH$_2$

OH (central hydroxy)

R$_3$ (optional donor)

(optional hydrophobic group)

(buried water)

				Binding energy (kJ mol^{-1})		
R'$_1$	R$_2$	R$_3$	IC$_{50}$ (μM)	Observed (equation 3)	Calculated (NH$_3^+$)	Calculated (NH$_2$)
OCH$_2$COOEt	Cl	CH$_2$NH$_2$	11	29	117	31
OCH$_2$COOH	Cl	CH$_2$NH$_2$	85	24	135	49
OCH$_2$COOEt	H	Cl	15	28	68	25

Comparison of experimental and 'average' binding energies for these compounds leads to the interesting question of how best to apply 'average' energy calculations. If we were to assume that the two positively charged amines formed ionic interactions with appropriate anionic groups in the active site, then the observed binding would be between 40 and 111 kJ mol^{-1} less than anticipated (Table 18.3), suggesting a less than optimal match to the active site. However, since the design hypothesis is based on the premise that only a main-chain hydrogen-bonding interaction is available to the amines, the numbers should be recalculated for neutral amine groups (5 kJ mol^{-1} rather than 48 kJ mol^{-1}). These numbers (Table 18.3) suggest that the dibenzophenone nucleus is a reasonable starting point for further optimisation, although incorporation of a charged carboxyl group in the R$_1$ substituent is clearly not the way to go!

A similar pharmacophore model, but based on a diol as the catalytic aspartate binding group, led Lam et al.[31] to a series of cyclic urea inhibitors (Table 18.4) in which the urea carbonyl takes the place of the buried water molecule. In this case, the binding of the lead diallyl compound (49 kJ mol^{-1}) is already better than might be anticipated for an 'average' interaction (38 kJ mol^{-1}), suggesting that the core structure is indeed a good match to the active site of HIV-PR. The quality of this match is confirmed by the crystal structure, which shows that the diol

Table 18.4 Simple nonpeptidic HIV-PR inhibitors based on a pharmacophore derived from peptidomimetic inhibitors.[31]

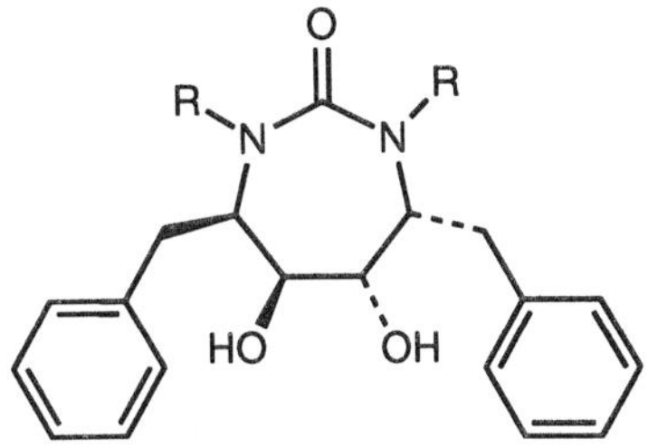

R	K_i (nM)	Binding energy (kJ mol^{-1})	
		Observed (equation 3)	Calculated (equation 7)
Allyl	4.7	49	38
Cyclopropylmethyl	2.1	51	42
β-Naphthylmethyl	0.31	56	62
p-Hydroxymethylbenzyl	0.27	56	58

oxygens are positioned to interact with the aspartyl carboxylates while the urea carbonyl forms two hydrogen bonds to main-chain amides. Further elaboration of the lead by replacement of the allyl groups shows that while the quality of the match is retained in the dicyclopropylmethyl analogue, extension of these side-chains to aromatic substituents does not enhance binding to the extent anticipated, although the data suggest that there is certainly space in the active site for further optimization of these substituents.

(c) Bioassay-based lead discovery using high-throughput screening of known chemicals   Screening of large numbers of compounds in the Parke-Davis collection against HIV-PR led[32] to the discovery of the series of pyran-2-ones shown in Table 18.5. The lead compound in this series has an experimental binding energy of 32 kJ mol^{-1} compared to a calculated 'average' value of only 14 kJ mol^{-1}, making it the best structural match to the HIV-PR active site of the various leads considered here. This is confirmed by the crystal structure of the closely related benzyl derivative, which shows that the enolic hydroxyl group binds to both aspartic carboxyls while the lactone moiety of the inhibitor takes the place of the buried water molecule, forming multiple interactions with the amide NH groups of Ile$_{50}$ and Ile$_{150}$.

Further elaboration of this lead by homologous extension of R' gives only a very slight increase in the observed binding, and the same trend is evident in the calculated ('average') binding energies. This is because the van der Waals interaction associated with each additional methylene is balanced by a corresponding loss of conformational entropy. In contrast to this observation, extension at the R position by introducing a tethered carboxyl group, although giving an order of magnitude improvement in binding, does not provide anything like the increase that would be anticipated if the carboxyl group were to interact as postulated with an arginine residue in the active site.

Table 18.5   Nonpeptidic HIV-PR inhibitors discovered by screening a known compound library.[32]

R	R'	IC_{50} (μM)	Binding energy (kJ mol^{-1})	
			Observed (equation 3)	Calculated (equation 7)
C_6H_5	C_6H_5	3.0	32	14
C_6H_5	$CH_2C_6H_5$	1.67	34	14
C_6H_5	$CH_2CH_2C_6H_5$	1.26	35	15
C_6H_5	$CH_2CH_2CH_2C_6H_5$	1.41	34	15
$C_6H_4(4\text{-}OCH_2CO_2H)$	$CH_2CH_2C_6H_5$	0.16	40	48

REFERENCES

1. Bajorath, J., Kraut, J., Li, Z., Kitson, D. H. and Hagler, A. T. (1991) Theoretical studies on the dihydrofolate reductase mechanism: electronic polarization of bound substrates. *Proc. Natl Adac. Sci. USA* **88**: 6423–6426.

2. Taylor, R., Kennard, O. and Versichel, W. (1983) Geometry of the N—H···O=C hydrogen bond. 1. Lone-pair directionality. *J. Am. Chem. Soc.* **105**: 5761–5766.

3. Taylor, R., Kennard, O. and Versichel, S. (1984) Geometry of the N—H···O=C hydrogen bond. 2. Three-center ('bifurcated') and four-center ('trifurcated') bonds. *J. Am. Chem. Soc.* **106**: 244–248.

4. Murray-Rust, P. and Glusker, J. P. (1984) Directional hudrogen bonding to sp²- and sp³-hybridized oxygen atoms and its relevance to ligand–macromolecule interactions. *J. Am. Chem. Soc.* **106**: 1018–1025.

5. Tintelnot, M. and Andrews, P. R. (1989) Goemetries of functional group interactions in enzyme–ligand complexes: guides for receptor modelling. *J. Comput.-Aided Mol. Design.* **3**: 67–84.

6. Taylor, R., Kennard, O. and Versichel, W. (1984) Geometry of the N—H···O=C hydrogen bond. 3. Hydrogen-bond distances and angles. *Acta Crystallogr.* **B40**: 280–288.

7. Gorbitz, C. H. (1989) Hydrogen-bond distances and angles in the structures of amino acids and peptides. *Acta Crystalogr.* **B45**: 390–395.

8. Sharp, K. A., Nicholls, A., Friedman, R. and Honig, B. (1991) Extracting hydrophobic free energies from experimental data: relationship to protein folding and theoretical models. *Biochemistry* **30**, 9686–9697.

9. Page, M. I. (1977) Entropy, binding energy, and enzymic catalysis. *Angew. Chem., Int. Ed. Engl.* **16**: 449–459.

10. Page, M. I. and Jencks, W. P. (1971) Entropic contributions to rate accelerations in enzymic and intramolecular reactions and the chelate effect. *Proc. Natl Acad. Sci USA* **68**: 1678–1683.

11. Jencks, W. P. (1981) On the attribution and additivity of binding energies. *Proc. Natl Acad. Sci. USA* **78**: 4046–4050.

12. Andrews, P. R., Craik, D. J. and Martin, J. L. (1984) Functional group contributions to drug-receptor interactions. *J. Med. Chem.* **27**: 1648–1657.

13. Searle, M. S. and Williams, D. H. (1992) The cost of conformational order: entropy changes in molecular associations. *J. Am. Chem. Soc.* **114**: 10690–10697.

14. Andrews, P. R, (1993) Drug–receptor intereactions. In Kubinyi, H. (ed.) *3D QSAR in Drug Design: Theory, Methods and Applications*, pp. 13–40. ESCOM, Leiden.

15. Wells, J. A. (1990) Additivity of mutational effects in proteins. *Biochemistry* **29**: 8509–8517.

16. Wolfenden, R. and Kati, W. M. (1991) Testing the limits of protein-ligand binding discrimination with transition-state analogue inhibitors. *Acc. Chem. Res.* **24**: 209–215.

17. Kati, W. M. and Wolfenden, R. (1989) Contribution of a single hydroxyl group to transition-state discrimination by adenosine deaminase: evidence for an 'entropy trap' mechanism. *Biochemistry* **28**: 7919–7927.

18. Wilson, D. K., Rudolph, F. B. and Quiocho, F. A. (1991) Atomic structure of adenosine deaminase complexed with a transition-state analog: understanding catalysis and mutations. *Science* **252**: 1278–1284.

19. Fersht, A. R., Shi, J-P., Knill-Jones, J., Lowe, D. M., Wilkinson, A. J., Blow, D. M., Brick, P., Carter, P., Waye, M. M. Y. and Winter, G. (1985) Hydrogen bonding and specificity analysed by protein engineering. *Nature* **134**, 235–238.

20. Levine, D., Reid, T. W. and Wilson, I. B. (1969) The free energy of hydrolysis of the phosphoryl-enzyme intermediate in alkaline phosphatase catalyzed reations. *Biochemistry* **8**: 2374–2380.

21. Northrop, D. B. and Wood, H. G. (1969) Transcarboxylase VII. Exchange reactions and kinetics of oxalate inhibition. *J. Biol. Chem.* **244**: 5820–5827.

22. Ward, W. H. J., Timms, D. and Fersht, A. R. (1990) Protein engineering and the study of structure–function relationships in receptors. *Trends Pharmacol. Sci.* **11**: 280–284.

23. Colman, P. M. (1989) Neuraminidase: enzyme and antigen. In Krug, R.M. (ed.) *The Influenza Virus*, pp. 175–218. Plenum Press, New York.

24. Von Itzstein, M., Wu, W-Y., Kok, G. B. *et al.* (1993) Rational design of potent sialidase-based inhibitors of influenza virus replication. *Nature* **363**: 418–423.

25. Wlodawer, A. and Erickson, J. W. (1993) Structure-based inhibitors of HIV-1 protease, *Annu. Rev. Biochem.* **62**: 543–585.

26. Rich, D. H., Sun, C-Q., Vara Prasad, J. V. N., Pathiasseril, A., Toth, M. V., Marshall, G. R., Clare, M., Mueller, R. A. and Houseman, K. (1991) Effect of hydroxyl group configuration in hydroxyethylamine dipeptide isosteres on HIV protease inhibition. Evidence for multiple binding modes. *J. Med. Chem.* **34**: 1222–1225.

27. Krohn, A., Redshaw, S., Ritchie, J.C., Graves, B. J. and Hatada, M. H. (1991) Novel binding mode of highly potent HIV-proteinase inhibitors incorporating the (R)-hydroxyethylamine isostere. *J. Med. Chem.* **34**: 3340–3342.

28. DesJarlais, R. L., Seibel, G. L., Kuntz, I. D., Furth, P. S., Alvarez, J. C., Ortiz de Montellano, P. R., DeCamp, D. L., Babé, L. M. and Craik, C. S. (1990) *Proc. Natl Acad. Sci. USA* **87**: 6644–6648.

29. Rutenber, E., Fauman, E.B., Keenan, R.J. *et al.* (1993) Structure of a non-peptide inhibitor complexed with HIV-1 protease. *J. Biol. Chem.* **268**, 21: 15343–15346.

30. Bures, M. G., Hutchins, C. W., Maus, M., Kohlbrenner, W., Kadam, S. and Erickson, J. W. (1990) *Tetahedron Comp. Methodol.* **3**: 673–680.

31. Lam, P. Y. S., Jabhav, P. K., Eyermann, C. J. *et al.* (1994) Rational design of potent, bioavailable, nonpeptide cyclic ureas as HIV protease inhibitors. *Science* **263**: 380–384.

32. Vara Prasad, J. V. N., Para, K. S., Lunney, E. A. *et al.* (1994) Novel series of achiral, low molecular weight, and potent HIV-1 protease inhibitors. *J. Am. Chem. Soc.* **116**: 6989–6990.

19

Quantitative Approaches to Structure–Activity Relationships

HAN VAN DE WATERBEEMD

Have the courage to use your own brain!
Immanuel Kant (1724–1824)

I. INTRODUCTION

The important flow of information and data on chemical compounds in a drug discovery project can be handled using appropriate chemical information data management and analysis

THE PRACTICE OF MEDICINAL CHEMISTRY
ISBN 0-12-744640-0

systems. Computer-assisted techniques are widely used to store information in databases. More recently so-called molecular spreadsheets have become available. These allow the medicinal chemist to store and visualize structural and numerical data in one single data file, which can then be used in a convenient way for structure–activity relationship (SAR) studies.

First attempts to express *quantitatively* relationships between chemical structure and bioactivity go back to the last century.[1] But only when the first computers and relevant mathematical methods became available did these approaches become more known. The credit goes to Corwin Hansch and Toshio Fujita for introducing these quantitative methods into medicinal chemistry in the 1960s.[2-4] Initially in their pioneering work Hansch and many coworkers focused their attention on the role of octanol–water partition coefficients ($\log P$) in drug transport processes. As we now know, $\log P$ is the predominant descriptor in many structure–property correlation studies. However, as we will see below, many other methods can be used to describe chemical structure in a quantitative way.

First we need some consideration of the terminology. Hansch recently called chemistry $\leftrightarrow$ life interaction studies the 'unnamed science'.[5] What was named QSAR (quantitative structure–activity relationships) is now in a state of confusion, because of the rapidly appearing multitude of new methods.[6] We have therefore proposed to call all studies aiming at broadening the understanding of correlations between intrinsic, physical and chemical or biological molecular properties, structure–property correlation (SPC) studies.[7,8] These are also called quantitative structure–property relationships (QSPR).[9] When biological properties or activities are involved, QSAR forms a subset of this.

A number of reviews have documented the history, strategy and successes of quantitative drug design, i.e. design using SPC/QSAR methods.[1-4,10-13] The impact of SPC/QSAR methods on drug discovery and lead optimization may be manifold (see Fig. 19.1).[13] Quantitative models may be derived, assisting the medicinal chemist in potency optimization and in the generation of new ideas.

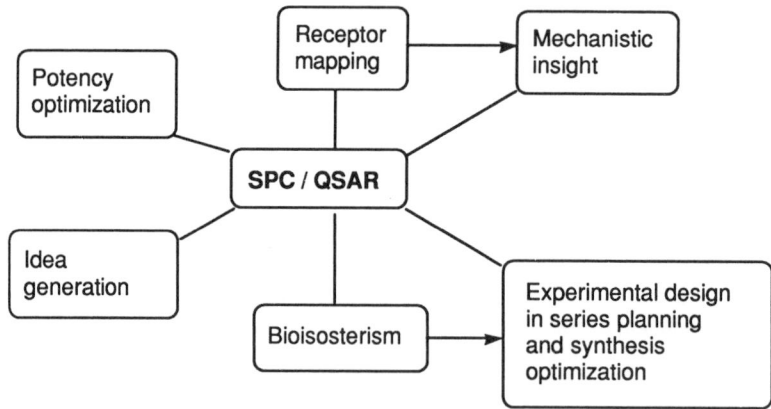

Fig. 19.1   The impact of SPC/QSAR studies on drug discovery.[13]

The elements of SPC studies are depicted In Fig. 19.2. On one side, high-quality and relevant biological data are required, while on the other relevant chemical descriptors should be defined. A further critical element is the proper choice of a model to investigate relationships between these data. If the prerequisites are met, relevant information may be extracted from the data, which can be used to obtain a better understanding of the molecular structures and possibly the mode of action at the molecular level. This information may then be used to predict the properties of new compounds.

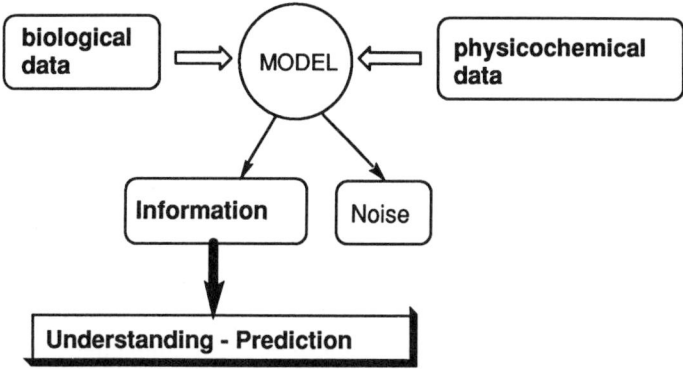

Fig. 19.2   Structure–property correlations (SPC) using different statistical data modelling techniques may provide the basis for understanding and prediction of biological activity.

The design of new compounds may be based on either a lead compound or structural information about the target, e.g. the crystal structure of an enzyme, or a combination of both. If no structural information about the target is available, the structural variation often includes variation of substituents at a particular site. The choice of proper substituents depends on synthetic feasibility and should be based on the physicochemical properties of the substituents. We therefore discuss below how these choices may be made as rationally as possible, preceded by an overview of data types of physicochemical and biological descriptors.

Next we present a number of regression methods used to find quantitative correlations or relationships between biological and physicochemical data. As well as two classical methods, the Hansch and Free–Wilson approaches, a more modern approach using partial least squares (PLS) regression is discussed. Finally, it is often of interest to investigate data sets by so-called pattern recognition methods in order to detect relationships that are not easily seen by simply inspecting the data table. These methods can be used to classify compounds into different groups.

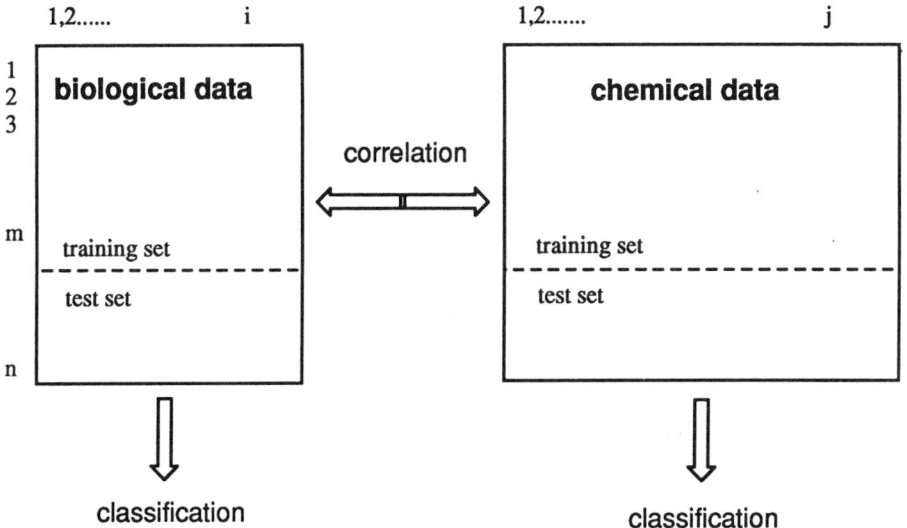

Fig. 19.3   The chemometric analysis of multivariate data tables. Two major types of studies can be defined: (1) correlation between biological and (physico)chemical data using regression techniques, and (2) classification of compounds or descriptors using pattern recognition methods.

The biological and physicochemical data relevant to a certain project may be represented as two tables and may be analysed in various ways (see Fig. 19.3). Taking biological or physicochemical data either separately or combined, pattern recognition or classification studies may be useful for detecting redundancy in the test systems or classifying the compounds in a particular way, which may be related to their specific mechanism of action. Regression or correlation studies between the biological and chemical data are of course useful to rationalize structure–activity relationships. Both kind of studies, regression or pattern recognition, are called multivariate statistical data analysis, or QSAR or SPC studies.

The starting point of an analysis should be the selection of a training or calibration set and a test or validation set. The idea is to keep some of the compounds aside for testing of the quantitative model derived with the rest of the set. Often compounds in a training set are chosen on the basis of their diversity in molecular structure. Statistical experimental design (see Section III) may be used to make more rational and well-balanced choices.

II. PHYSICOCHEMICAL AND BIOLOGICAL DESCRIPTORS

The targets of drug action may be quite diverse, including membrane-bound receptors, enzymes and DNA, for example. Biologists have developed a broad variety of biological and pharmacological test systems producing different kinds of data. Some are quite simple, e.g. IC_{50} values as a crude measure of ligand affinity, while others are more complex *in vivo* data. In the worst case results are expressed as active vs inactive, agonist vs antagonist, or as strong, medium and weak. The proper choice of a mathematical model to relate biological to chemical data depends on the quality and kind of data to be analysed. Therefore, for example, the classical Hansch approach using multiple linear regression (see below) is not suited for all purposes.

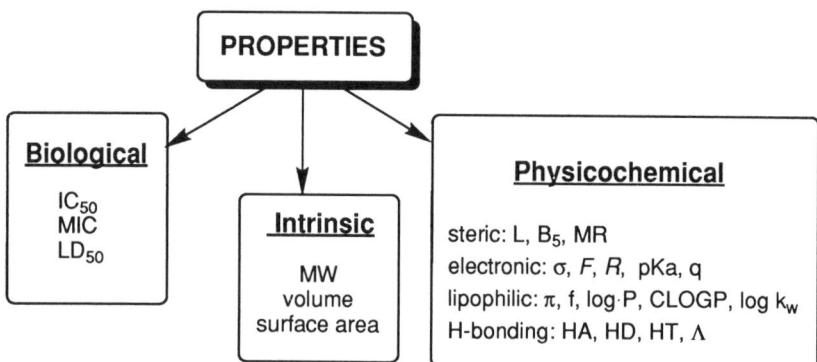

Fig. 19.4 Molecular properties can be divided into intrinsic, physicochemical and biological properties. Examples are IC_{50} (binding affinity), MIC (antibacterial minimum inhibitory concentration), LD_{50} (lethal dose), MW (molecular weight), molecular volume, surface area, L (substituent length), B_5 (substituent width), MR (molar refractivity), σ (Hammett constant), $\mathcal{F}, \mathcal{R}$ (field and resonance parameters), pK_a (ionization constants), q (atomic charges), π (Hansch constant), f (hydrophobic fragmental constant), log P (partition coefficients), log k_w (lipophilicity values from HPLC measurements), CLOGP (calculated log P values), HA (number of H-bond acceptors), HD (number of H-bond donors), HT (total H-bonding capacity), Λ (H-bond capability).

Molecular structures may be considered at different levels, each containing certain types of information.[14,15] The simplest representation is the empirical chemical formula, while a molecular electrostric potential (MEP) representation on the Van der Waals surface includes both steric and electronic information. Molecular properties can be divided into three categories (see Fig. 19.4).[7,8] Intrinsic properties are directly related to the structure without considering any interaction, such as molecular weight. When a compound interacts with a chemical or biological environment, we may define physicochemical properties, e.g. lipophilicity or ionization constants, biochemical properties, such as binding constants, and biological properties, such as activity or toxicity.

Chemical descriptors may contain structural, also called global, information, or local information for substructural parts of the molecule. A large set of chemical descriptors of molecular structures and fragments has been reported in the literature.[15] Parametrization of chemical structures or substructures is not only of great interest to SPC studies, but has much current interest in definitions of molecular similarity and diversity. This information may be used in molecular modelling studies or in combinatorial chemistry projects aiming at generating large molecular diversity in order to improve lead-finding chances. Substituent variables may be experimental or calculated, as well as pure or composite.[16] The traditional way to subdivide substituent properties is in terms of lipophilic, steric, electronic/electrostatic and H-bonding effects. These properties are usually considered in the systematic variation of a selected substitution site. More advanced methods using so-called principal properties are discussed below in Section III.C.

The lipophilicity of a compound is often considered as an important design factor since it is related to processes such as absorption, brain uptake and protein binding. Using several lines of evidence it was shown that $\log P$ values should be considered as composed of two factors (see equation 1), namely a steric and a polar contribution.[15,17]

$$\log\ P = aV - \Lambda \tag{1}$$

The molar volume V can be calculated. Thus the polarity factor Λ is obtained indirectly from $\log P$ measurements, where $\Lambda = 0$ for nonpolar compounds. Λ appears to reflect the H-bonding capacity of a compound.

The 1-octanol–water system is often taken as the reference or standard for partition coefficients. However, other partitioning systems may give useful information too. It has been recommended by Leahy and colleagues[18] to use a 'critical quartet' of solvent systems for lipophilicity measurements. They suggest that any membrane can be modelled by one of four solvents: alkane (inert), octanol (amphiprotic), chloroform (proton donor) and PGDP = propylene glycol dipelargonate (proton acceptor). It has also been found that the differences between $\log P$ values measured in two different solvent systems ($\Delta \log P$) may contain relevant information related to the H-bonding capacity of a compound.[19,20] In practice, the lipophilicities of series of compounds are often measured by reversed-phase high-performance liquid chromatography (RP-HPLC), because this technique is much more rapid than the rather tedious shake flask method used to obtain $\log P$ values. However, centrifugal partition chromatography (CPC) may be an interesting alternative for obtaining $\log P$ values.[21] Within a series of closely related compounds, $\log P$ values are correlated to $\log k_w$ values from RP-HPLC. For more diverse molecules this is often not the case. However, one should consider each lipophilicity scale as unique and reflecting, as seen above, a combination of the steric and H-bonding properties of a compound.

It should also be realized that properties such as fragment lipophilicity contributions are additive properties but may be very much dependent on the structural environment (Fig. 19.5). Some substitutions may have a more dramatic effect than expected. Radioactive labelling with

[125]I is quite common for biological studies. One should be aware, however, that aromatic iodination increases the log P of the compound by ~1 log P unit, and thus a different distribution may result. An aromatic fluoro substituent has very little effect on the lipophilicity, but mainly serves in drugs to prevent oxidative biotransformation.

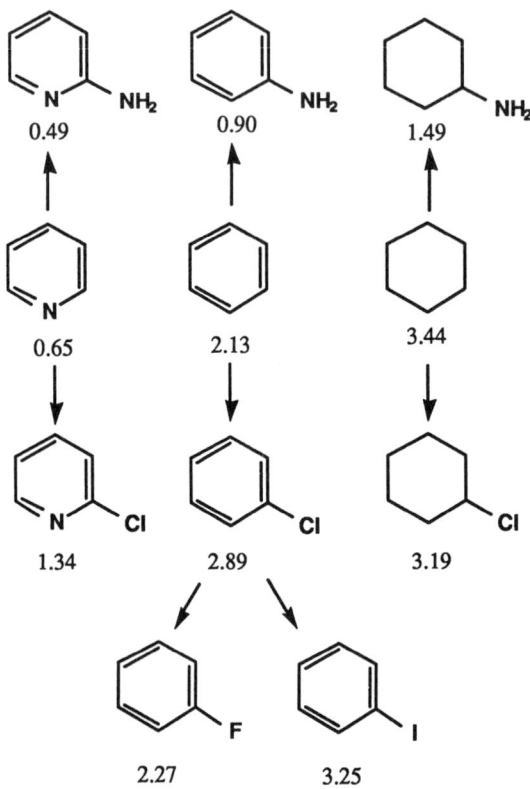

Fig. 19.5   The impact of substitution on the lipophilicity of a compound depends on its structural environment (log P values given).

III.   EXPERIMENTAL DESIGN

In medicinal chemistry optimization concerns many aspects. The optimization of the affinity for the biological target and the pharmacokinetic properties of a lead compound is the primary goal of most preclinical research projects. Secondly, optimization strategies may be applied to synthesis procedures for the minimization of cost.[22] In both cases a number of variables have to be taken into account simultaneously. Strategies that change only one variable at a time take much time and many experiments are needed. In contrast to the sequential approach, by a proper selection of a limited number of experiments the full variable space can be covered with far fewer experiments. Experimental design schemes are therefore of great help in focusing on the most informative experiments.[23,24] These techniques have been applied in two types of synthetic programmes, namely peptide design and substituent variation. We describe below how physicochemical descriptors for aromatic and aliphatic substituents may be used for substituent selection. In a similar way, relevant descriptors for amino acids may be used. It has been pointed out that only a series of compounds based on some experimental design plan is likely to produce significant QSAR equations. Therefore, careful selection of appropriate substituents and substituent variables is important.

A.   Topliss tree and Craig plot

Various strategies have been advocated to cover the physicochemical parameter space of a series of new compounds as well as possible. Hansch and Leo have used cluster analysis to define sets of aliphatic and aromatic substituents useful in the design of compounds, such that various aspects of the substituents are taken into account in a balanced way.[25]

Other familiar strategies go back to the proposals of Topliss and Craig. Both schemes are used for substituent variation at a selected site.

The Topliss substitution scheme can be used to optimize aromatic and aliphatic substituents using a fixed set of substituents. In Fig. 19.6 the Topliss procedure is depicted. It starts with the assumption that the lead compound has an unsubstituted phenyl ring. In the first step a *p*-chloro derivative is made and its activity measured. Depending on whether the activity is less than, equal to or greater than the parent, the next step is made. This consists of replacing the *p*-chloro substituent by either a methoxy or methyl group, or adding an additional chlorine substituent. This scheme applies manually the basic features of a good design plan, without statistical considerations, making it appealing to most medicinal chemists.

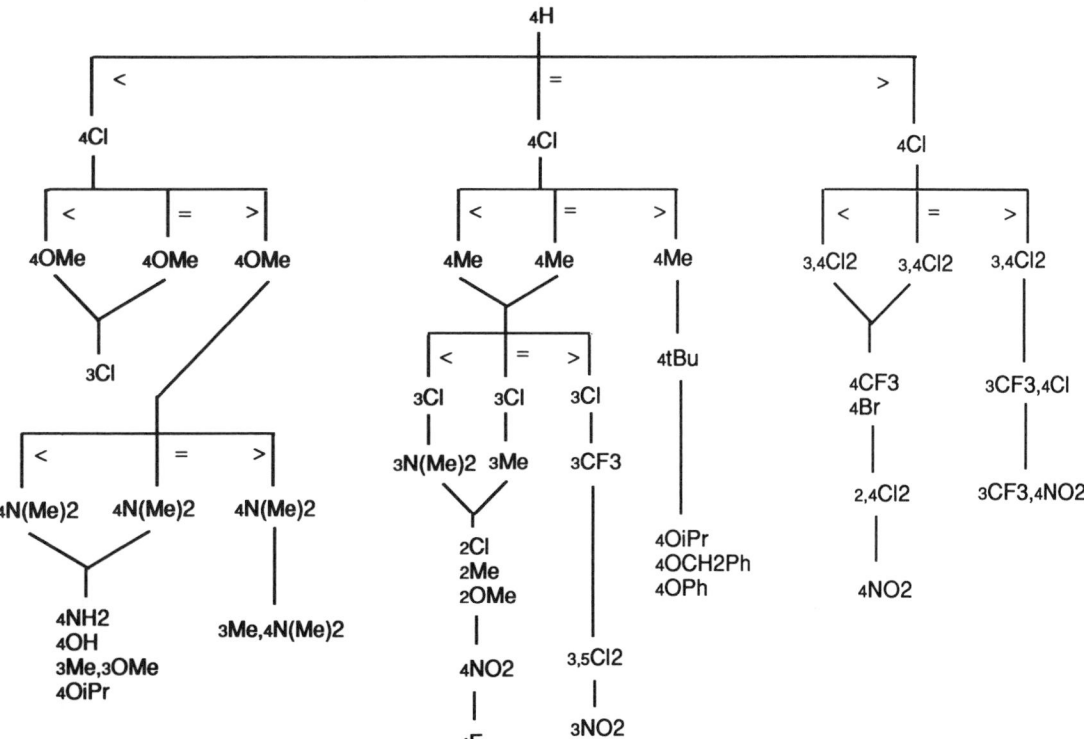

Fig. 19.6   The Topliss decision tree for the optimization of aromatic substituents: >, is more active; =, is equiactive; <, is less active than the parent compound. Descending lines indicate sequential substitutions.

A Craig plot is a two-dimensional plot of selected descriptors, e.g. Hammett σ and Hansch π values (see Fig. 19.7). From this plot substituents can be selected from each quadrant such that they vary widely in their properties, e.g. lipophilic and hydrophilic, electron donor and electron acceptor.

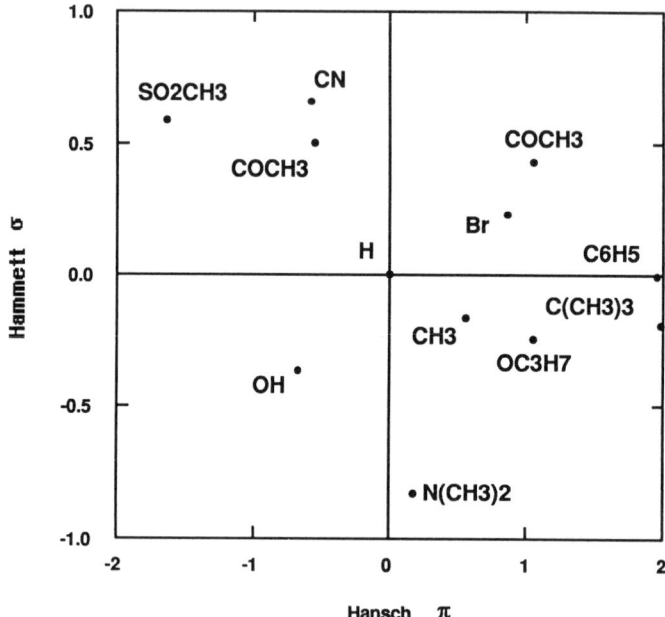

Fig. 19.7   Two-dimensional Craig plot using data in Table 19.2. Electronic properties (Hammett σ_p constants) are plotted against lipophilic (Hansch–Fujita π values) substituent properties.

A further extension would be to consider a three-dimensional Craig plot using three descriptors, e.g. reflecting steric, lipophilic and electronic properties of the substituents. In that case substituents may be chosen from the eight octants. If one wishes to consider even more descriptors, this approach becomes impractical. In that case more advanced experimental design techniques may be applied.

B.   Factorial, central composite and *D*-optimal designs

In order to limit the number of combinations, each variable may be considered at two levels, e.g. lipophilic vs hydrophilic. A two-level factorial design (FD) with k variables requires 2^k experiments. A Craig plot is an example of a 2^2 FD. Or in other words, the minimum number of compounds to be synthesized using two descriptors is four. As stated above, with many variables this number rapidly becomes impractical and fractional factorial designs (FFD) should be preferred. Using a reduction factor r, the number of experiments then becomes 2^{k-r}. This reduction factor is in practice chosen rather pragmatically, such that one has to consider 8 or 16 compounds. Further design schemes are known as central composite and *D*-optimal design. In the latter method the determinant of the variance–covariance matrix is calculated. This determinant has a maximum value for those combinations of substituents that have a maximum variance and minimum covariance in their physicochemical descriptors. The variance–covariance matrix is an important cornerstone in matrix operations used in multiple linear regression and principal component analysis, and for obtaining a correlation matrix among a set of selected variables.

C.   Principal properties of substituents

In the literature about 100 scales of substituent descriptors have been reported. In order to use this information for substituent selection, appropriate statistical methods may be used. Pattern recognition or data reduction techniques, such as principal component analysis (PCA) or cluster analysis (CA) are good choices. As explained in Section V in more detail, PCA consists of condensing or reducing the information in a data table into a few new descriptors constructed of linear combinations of the original ones. These new descriptors are called principal components or latent variables. This technique has been applied to define new descriptors for amino acids as well as for aromatic or aliphatic substituents; these are called principal properties (PPs). In the case of amino acids, the principal properties are known as z-scales, which can be used for the design of peptides.[26] An analogous approach has been used for aliphatic and aromatic substituents, using databases with 59 substituents and 121 descriptors[27] or a set of 100 substituents and 9 descriptors.[28] Recently an attempt has been made to combine both former studies to derive one unique set.[29] We selected 40 representative substituents that have a large majority of the 86 selected descriptors experimentally available. In order to avoid the prevalence of one group of variables, block weighting of variables was applied. Principal properties of 19 other substituents were obtained by projection. However, principal properties obtained in this way contain mixed information, e.g. electronic and steric.

An alternative approach is to subdivide the descriptors into four groups related to lipophilic, steric, electronic and H-bonding properties, and to apply disjoint principal component analysis to these subsets. The first two principal components of each set are called disjoint principal properties (DPPs). Thus, we derived 4×2 DPPs for 59 common substituents. Using D-optimal design criteria, a set of 12 substituents has been obtained for optimal parameter space coverage, namely CN, $COCH_3$, SO_2CH_3, OH, $N(CH_3)_2$, H, Br, CH_3, COC_6H_5, $C(CH_3)_3$, C_6H_5 and OC_3H_7. The dimethylamino group is special, since as an aliphatic substituent it might be protonated under physiological conditions. This group of substituents can be considered as a first choice in the planning of a series of compounds with substituent variations at a selected site. In our opinion these DPPs can be much better understood by organic chemists than can PPs, since they reflect the basic four familiar properties of substituents. Nevertheless, DPP values are abstract numbers not directly related to physical properties such as log P or surface area. In Table 19.1 the DPP values of this representative set of substituents are given, while in Table 19.2 some traditional lipophilic, steric and electronic descriptors are reported for the same set to illustrate the wide coverage of the properties. We are of course aware that these eight scales are no longer orthogonal to each other, because they have been obtained from four disjoint PCA calculations. However, orthogonality is not a prerequisite, provided that the data analysis method is partial least squares and not multiple linear regression (see Section IV). These DPPs can be used in the design of new compounds, as well as in SPC studies.

An illustration of the use of principal properties is a PLS (partial least squares) analysis of

Table 19.1 Disjoint principal properties (DPPs) of a representative set of organic substituents.

Substituent	Lipophilic		Steric		Electronic		H-bonding	
	l_1	l_2	s_1	s_2	e_1	e_2	h_1	h_2
H	0.00	0.00	0.00	0.00	0.00	0.00	0.00	0.00
Br	1.16	0.78	7.31	−4.29	−4.85	−3.68	0.66	−0.41
OH	−2.08	0.64	3.84	−2.07	−0.53	−5.17	4.20	1.57
CN	−1.62	0.50	6.00	−2.39	−8.48	−2.41	3.05	−0.58
COCH$_3$	−1.34	0.46	10.03	−4.15	−5.43	−0.63	3.76	−0.83
CH$_3$	1.13	0.06	5.22	−2.34	1.04	−0.69	0.01	−0.06
OC$_3$H$_7$	1.27	0.93	12.93	−0.13	−1.19	−4.45	3.45	−0.72
SO$_2$CH$_3$	−3.16	−0.05	13.83	−6.62	−8.99	−2.66	6.15	−1.91
N(CH$_3$)$_2$	−0.38	0.78	10.57	−2.64	2.69	−6.35	3.64	−0.91
C(CH$_3$)$_3$	3.85	0.18	15.31	−6.88	−0.53	3.85	−0.11	0.03
C$_6$H$_5$	3.63	0.55	16.33	−2.92	−0.76	−1.07	0.35	−0.21
COC$_6$H$_5$	0.94	0.84	19.70	−2.74	−5.32	−1.29	4.31	−1.00

l_1 and l_2, lipophilic; s_1 and s_2, steric, e_1 and e_2, electronic; h_1 and h_2, H-bonding properties.

Table 19.2 Traditional chemical descriptors of a representative set of organic substituents

Substituent	Lipophilic		Steric			Electronic	
	π(ar)	π(al)	MR	L	B$_5$	σ_p	σ_m
H	0.00	0.00	1.03	2.06	1.00	0.00	0.00
Br	0.86	0.60	8.88	3.82	1.95	0.23	0.39
OH	−0.67	−1.12	2.85	2.74	1.93	−0.37	0.12
CN	−0.57	−0.84	6.33	4.23	1.60	0.66	0.56
COCH$_3$	−0.55	−0.62	11.18	4.06	3.13	0.50	0.38
CH$_3$	0.56	0.50	5.65	2.87	2.04	−0.17	−0.17
OC$_3$H$_7$	1.05	0.45	17.06	6.05	4.42	−0.25	0.10
SO$_2$CH$_3$	−1.63	−1.50	13.49	4.11	3.17	0.59	0.52
N(CH$_3$)$_2$	0.18	−0.30	15.55	3.53	3.08	−0.83	−0.15
C(CH$_3$)$_3$	1.98	1.17	19.62	4.11	3.17	−0.20	−0.10
C$_6$H$_5$	1.96	2.15	25.36	6.28	3.11	−0.01	0.06
COC$_6$H$_5$	1.05	0.36	30.33	5.81	5.98	0.43	0.34

π(ar): Fujita–Hansch lipophilicity contribution to an aromatic ring; π(al), Fujita–Hansch lipophilicity contribution to an aliphatic chain; MR, molar refractivity (related to molar volume); L, Verloop's length descriptor in angstroms, calculated along the axis connecting the substituent to the parent; B$_5$, Verloop's width descriptor in angstroms, calculated perpendicular to L; σ_p, Hammett constant for *para* substitution; σ_m, Hammett constant for *meta* substitution.[15]

dopamine antagonistic clebopride analogues.[30] The paper describes the use of experimental design techniques to select a training set from a series of 20 synthesized and tested compounds for establishing a quantitative structure–activity relationship with good predictability. The substituents and substituent sites are given in Fig. 19.8. Five significant PPs have been derived from originally nine substituent descriptors, namely σ_m and σ_p Hammett constants, $\mathscr{F}$ and $\mathscr{R}$ Swain and Lupton field and resonance parameters, the Hansch π lipophilicity constant, MR molar refractivity, and Verloop steric parameters L, B_1 and B_5. These PPs were used in a fractional factorial design to select the training series in a PLS analysis. It was shown that with eight well-selected compounds the predictivity of the model is the same as with a model derived for all 20 compounds. This example shows that PPs indeed are good design variables and that experimental design may limit the number of compounds to be synthesized in a series to a strict minimum.

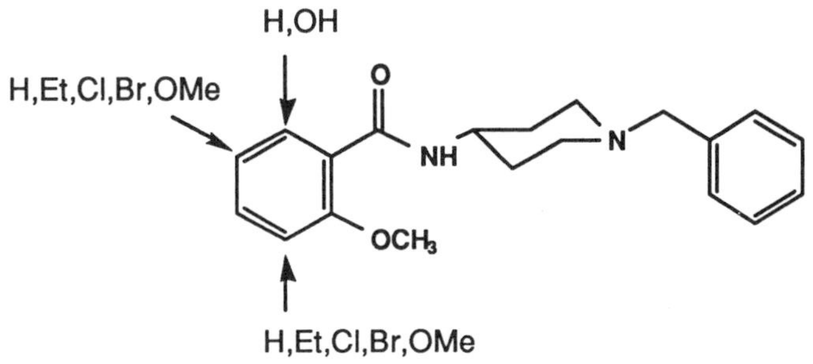

Fig. 19.8   Substituted benzamides of the clebopride type.

IV.   CORRELATION BETWEEN CHEMICAL AND BIOLOGICAL DATA

A.   The Hansch approach

In the 1960s Hansch and Fujita proposed a method for describing quantitatively relationships between biological activity and chemical descriptors.[31] This can be expressed as:

$$\text{biological activity} = f(\text{molecular or fragmental descriptors}) \tag{2}$$

The Hansch–Fujita approach is also called the linear free energy relationship (LFER) or extrathermodynamic approach, since most of the descriptors are derived from rate or equilibrium constants.

The simplest means for obtaining such a quantitative relationship is the use of multiple linear regression (MLR), available in any statistical package even for a PC. Nonlinear regression may also be used. However, as described in detail,[31] there are a number of pitfalls to this method. To avoid statistically non-significant relationships or chance correlations, one should always apply the following rules of thumb:

- the ratio of compounds to descriptors should be > 5;
- the descriptors should not be intercorrelated (interdescriptor correlation coefficient should be less than < 0.5).

A statistically more robust method that should be used instead of MLR is the partial least squares (PLS) regression method.

There are numerous examples of traditional Hansch QSAR studies in the literature. Some include large sets of descriptors while others explore just a few. If descriptor values are not readily available, indicator or dummy variables, denoting presence or absence of a certain structural feature, may be of help. This is the basis of the Free–Wilson method (see below).

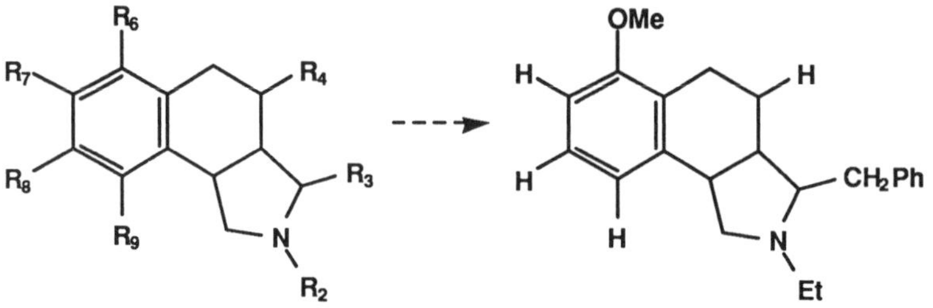

Fig. 19.9   Optimization (indicated by a dashed arrow) of substituted aminotetralin analogues by MLR.

An example is a study on substituted aminotetralin analogues designed as noradrenaline uptake inhibitors, which may serve as antidepressants[32] (Fig. 19.9). The multiple regression equation obtained is

$$\log (1/IC_{50}) = 0.31(\pm0.05)\,\pi_{R3} + 0.45(\pm0.17)\,\pi_{R9} - 0.12\,(\pm0.05)\,\pi_{R9}^2$$
$$+ 0.34(\pm0.08)\log P$$
$$+ 1.38(\pm0.20)\,I_{R9=H} - 0.22(\pm0.09)\,I_{R6=H} + 1.20(\pm0.22)\,I_{R9=OCH3} \quad (3)$$
$$+ 0.75(\pm0.21)\,I_{R6=OH} - 0.31(\pm0.14)\,I_{R2>Pr} + 0.23(\pm0.12)\,I_{R2=Et}$$
$$+ 3.09(\pm0.37)$$

$$n = 57; \; r = 0.935; \; s = 0.274; \; F = 32$$

From such equations two types of information are obtained, namely about the statistical quality and relevance, and about the chemical implications. The standard deviation of each coefficient is given in parentheses; r is the correlation coefficient, which should be between 0.85 and 1.0; s the standard deviation of the regression, which should have a value near to the experimental error in the biological dependent variable (here $\log(1/IC_{50})$); finally the F-value is a measure of the statistical significance of the regression model and is calculated as the ratio between regression and residual variances. This value should be higher than a value that can be found in a Fisher F-statistics table, and is a function of the number of degrees of freedom and the significance level.[31] In practice, r and s are the most informative statistical parameters. In SPC studies it is common to transform biological activities to their negative logarithmic form, e.g. $\log (1/IC_{50}) = - \log IC_{50} = pIC_{50}$. Thus, the most active compounds have the largest values. Among all the descriptors evaluated, only those that are relevant appear in the final equation. π_{R3} and π_{R9} are lipophilic constants for the substituents in positions 3 and 9, while $\log P$ is the overall lipophilicity of the molecule, calculated with the CLOGP program. The π_{R9}^2 term indicates that the substituent in position 9 has an optimum lipophilicity value. The other terms in the equation are indicators, e.g. $I_{R2=Et}$ takes a value of 1 when the R_2 substituent is ethyl, otherwise it is 0. This simple approach rationalizes the data and gives ideas about further possible substitutions. For example, the positive coefficient of the $\log P$ term means that increasing the lipophilicity of the compound has a positive effect on the affinity.

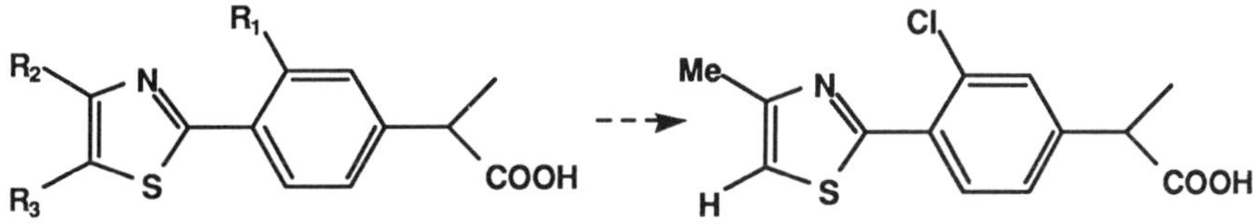

Fig. 19.10   Optimization of cyclooxygenase inhibitors by MLR.

A second example is the Hansch–Fujita analysis of cyclooxygenase inhibition.[33] The goal of the study was to understand the physicochemical background of the effect of substituents R_1, R_2 and R_3 (see Fig. 19.10) for a rational choice in the selection of compounds for further development. This detailed understanding was obtained by developing correlations for each varied position. For example, for R_1 substituted compounds, in which the thiazole ring is unsubstituted, equation (19.4) was obtained:

$$pIC_{50} = 1.08(\pm0.50)\ \pi_{R1} + 1.18\ (\pm0.97)\ \sigma_{IR1} + 5.64(\pm0.38) \tag{4}$$

$$n = 11;\ r = 0.89;\ s = 0.28;\ F = 15.81$$

In this equation, σ_I is Charton's electronic parameter for the inductive effects of the substituents. The positive coefficient indicates that electron-attracting substituents are favourable. It is demonstrated in the paper that π values are not position-independent. In addition to an intrinsic hydrophobic factor, intramolecular steric and hydrogen-bonding components are also included. This is expressed above by equation (1). The final equation including all compounds is

$$\begin{aligned} pIC_{50} &= 1.03(\pm0.42)\ \pi(R1) - 4.48(\pm1.64)\ \sigma_R(R2) - 0.86(\pm0.13)\ \Delta L(R2) \\ &+ 0.44(\pm0.27)\ \pi(R2,3) - 0.40(\pm0.26)\ \Delta L(R3) - 1.48(\pm0.52)\ I_{iso} \\ &+ 6.11(\pm0.21) \end{aligned} \tag{19.5}$$

$$n = 45;\ r = 0.95;\ s = 0.38;\ F = 54$$

This equation is statistically relevant and informative. Although six variables are used, this can be accepted since the number of compounds is sufficiently large. Furthermore, the intercorrelation between the independent variables is nonsignificant. Optimal substituents need to be lipophilic but small, since the ΔL terms have a negative coefficient. ΔL is the length of the substituent compared to a hydrogen atom. An indicator variable (I_{iso}) was assigned for compounds with the Pr^i group in the R_2 position, which appears to be detrimental to affinity for cyclooxygenase. One of the best compounds is shown in Fig. 10. Although this compound was synthesized at an early stage of the project, the analysis clarified the physicochemical background of the substituents. This can be useful to fill gaps in patent coverage or in the decision to stop a project.

B.   Free–Wilson analysis and related methods

The Free–Wilson (FW) model was proposed in 1964 at the same time as the Hansch model, but is far less used.[31,34] It uses indicator values having a value of unity for the presence of a substructural feature and zero for its absence as sole parameters in a Hansch model-like regression equation. The FW model has also been named the additivity model or the *de novo* approach. Several closely related approaches, such as the Fujita–Ban variant, offer mathematical advantages. Using this method, for example, any compound in the series may be chosen as reference., which is not the case in Free and Wilson's original formulation. The details will not be discussed here. The greatest interest of this method lies in its mixed use with Hansch analysis, as illustrated above. Thus, the combination of molecular or substructure descriptors with indicators is often the best way to proceed.

Both Hansch and Free–Wilson analysis are now considered as traditional or classical QSAR methods. Progress in chemometrics has made available a number of new statistical techniques, which are increasingly being used and will be discussed next.[35] These concern both new regression and pattern recognition techniques. Chemometrics was defined about twenty years ago as the chemical discipline that uses mathematical, statistical and related techniques to design optimal measurement procedures and experiments, and to extract maximum relevant information from chemical data. The science of chemometrics has been developed to promote applications of statistics in analytical, organic and medicinal chemistry.[6,35,36]

C.   Linear discriminant analysis (LDA)

In many biological experiments only discrete or categorical data are obtained, such as inactive/active, agonist/antagonist. In some data sets a clear separation may be found between such classes in multidimensional space. An appropriate method to describe separation between classes is linear discriminant analysis (LDA). For example, using LDA it was possible to distinguish 24 calmodulin inhibitors in three groups in terms of positive potential surface area on the side-chain, as well as the total and neutral surface areas on the ring in the inhibitor molecules.[37] This group assignment information was used to classify 29 additional inhibitors. LDA should not be considered as a technique of first choice and will therefore not be further developed here. A related method used to analyse categorical data is adaptive least squares (ALS).[37]

D.   Partial least squares (PLS)

Traditional Hansch analysis using multiple linear regression suffers from several shortcomings. One of the problems is that often one has more variables than compounds. Furthermore, there is a need to consider correlations between chemical descriptors and several biological tests simultaneously. PLS (partial least squares projections to latent structures) is a generalization of regression that is appropriate to treating these problems.[38,39] Further alternatives, such as continuum regression, are being evaluated,[40] but will not be discussed here. PLS can handle numerous and even collinear variables, and allows for a certain amount of missing data. An important part of a PLS data modelling study is the cross-validation of the results. PLS considers all independent descriptors together and calculates their modelling power, i.e. their contribution to the regression. PLS is particularly useful when many descriptors are taken into consideration. We have seen above that the alternative is MLR or PCA combined with MLR. However, experience has shown that PLS gives the most relevant and statistically significant results and should be the preferred default technique in SAR correlation studies. A nice illustration of this approach is given in the following example.

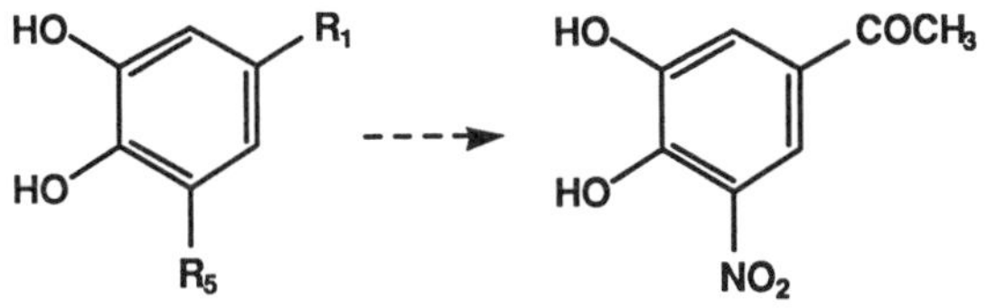

Fig. 19.11 Optimal substituent selection of soluble COMT inhibitors by PLS.

A PLS study has been performed on a series of 99 1,5-substituted-3,4-dihydroxybenzenes as catechol O-methyltransferase (COMT, EC 2.1.1.6) inhibitors[41] (Fig. 19.11). A set of 19 variables to characterize the inhibitors was considered. This is a typical situation where MLR might give incomplete results, because MLR would pick out a few variables that are correlated to the biological activity. However, there may be several good combinations of descriptors with similar statistical relevance. PLS gives a better feeling of the contribution of each of the variables considered. In this case, the best PLS model showed that inhibition activity is nonlinearly related to the size of the R5 substituent and greatly depends on the electronic nature of both R1 and R5 substituents. Electron-withdrawing substituents enhance activity.

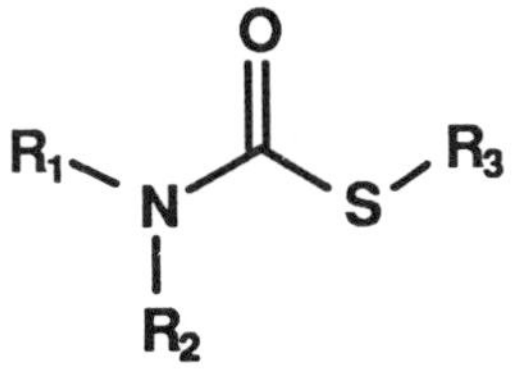

Fig. 19.12 Profile optimization using PLS for fungicidal and herbicidal thiolcarbamates

A second example concerns a PLS analysis of 83 thiolcarbamates with fungicidal and herbicidal activities[42] (Fig. 19.12). With PLS both activities, fungicidal and herbicidal, can be correlated with physicochemical properties. Remember that with the Hansch method, using MLR, only one biological variable at a time is studied. Thus, PLS can be used to optimize an activity profile. For each of the three substitution sites, a steric and a lipophilic descriptor was used. Three significant components, called t_1, t_2 and t_3, were obtained, explaining together 75.6% of the variance. Activity can now be expressed in terms of these components or latent variables, e.g.

$$\text{Fungicidal activity} = -0.482t_1 + 0.278t_2 - 0.184t_3 + 1.723 \tag{6}$$

Using this equation, the activity of 81% of the compounds in the data set is correctly predicted. In order to understand which structural parameters should be modified to improve activity, the t-values can be translated back into terms of the original variables, and then substituted into equation (6). This finally gives a MLR-like model relating biological activity to physicochemical descriptors. Insight into the data structure of the descriptors can be obtained from PLS projections plotting, for example, t_1 against t_2 (see Fig. 19.13). This information cannot be obtained using principal component analysis (PCA, see below) of the same independent variables.

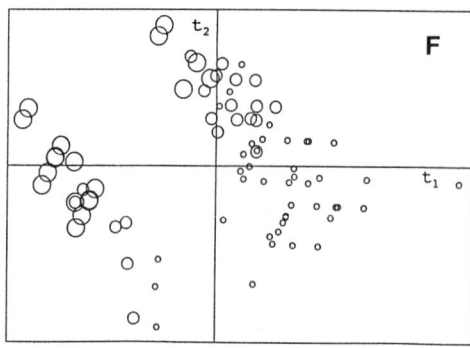

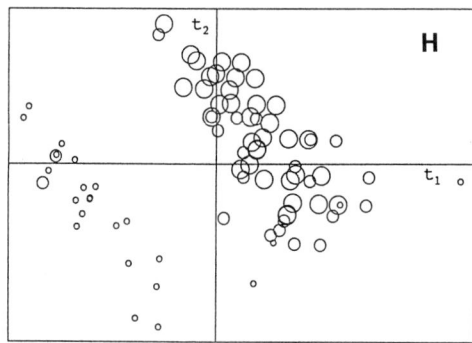

Fig. 19.13   PLS projections for thiolcarbamate data of the first latent variable t_1 against the second latent variable t_2. The size of the circles denotes the fungicidal (F) or herbicidal (H) activity.

V.   PATTERN RECOGNITION IN DATA SETS

A.   Principal component analysis (PCA)

Large data tables may hide information that is not easily detected by simple inspection of the various columns. Principal component analysis and some closely related techniques such as factor analysis (FA) and correspondence factor analysis (CFA), reduce a data matrix to new supervariables retaining a maximum of information or variance from the original data matrix. These new variables are called latent variables or principal components, and are orthogonal vectors composed of linear combinations of the original variables. This method can be used to look for potential clustering of variables or compounds, by considering chemical or biological data separately or together. When compounds cluster together in a multivariate parameter space, this means that they are 'similar' with respect to the variables considered. Thus, if we perform a PCA using biological data, clustered compounds have a similar activity profile.

The typical use of PCA is illustrated by an example from antibacterial research. In studies of the antibacterial effects of sulfones and sulfonamides in whole-cell and cell-free systems, missing data (19%) have been estimated by an iterative process using PCA.[43] However, estimation of missing values should be done with care and preferably avoided.

Using the minimal inhibitory concentration (MIC) data for nine different strains, two significant principal components could be obtained, accounting for 77.1% and 16.1%, respectively, of the data variance. The loading plot, i.e. a plot of the calculated principal components with respect to the descriptors, shows that the first component is mainly related to the seven cell-free test systems, while the second one represents the two whole-cell test results. In other words, much redundant information was obtained by measuring in nine test systems; two would have been sufficient. This separation means that the potency in each test system is governed by different physicochemical properties. The principal components can be correlated to the original variables by a procedure called principal component regression (PCR). Thus it was found that component 1 appears to be dominated by electronic factors (equation 7), while in component 2 transport (lipophilicity) properties (equation 8) play a role. The following parameters are used: Δppm(NH$_2$) is the NMR chemical shift of the amino protons relative to the unsubstituted congener; f_i is the fraction ionized at pH 7.4, and $\log k'$ is the lipophilicity measured by HPLC.

$$PC1 = -7.02(\pm 1.25)\ \Delta\text{ppm (NH}_2) + 1.81(\pm 0.42)\ f_i - 0.93(\pm 0.19) \tag{7}$$

$$PC2 = 1.40(\pm 0.52)\ \log\ k' - 3.49(\pm 1.32)\ \log(0.098 k' + 1) + 0.51(\pm 0.73) \tag{8}$$

Thus PCA may be used to extract the most relevant information from a data set. Applications of variations of PCA, such as correspondence factorial analysis and nonlinear mapping, may have small advantages with particular data sets but require expert support.

PCA can also be used for variable selection when a large number of them have to be considered. This reduced set of descriptors can then be used in a MLR or PLS analysis to find a correlation between biological and chemical data. An illustration of this procedure is the optimization of the aqueous solubility of xanthine antagonists (Fig. 19.14) by SPC/QSAR

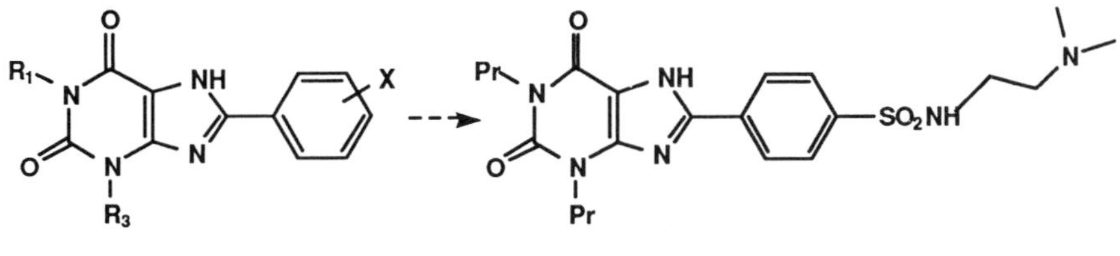

Fig. 19.14   Design of water-soluble xanthine antagonists by PCA/MLR.

methods.[44] Preprocessing of 28 parameters by PCA produced a selection of 11 significant descriptors. The final QSAR obtained by MLR was

$$PTNCYcow = -0.99(\pm 0.13)\ HACCEPT_m + 0.81(\pm 0.18)\ \pi_{R3} - 1.16(\pm 0.18)\ MR_0 \\ - 0.88(\pm 0.20)\ \sigma_0 - 1.57(\pm 0.24)\ ACID - 1.17(\pm 0.24)\ HBOND + 2.22 \tag{9}$$

$$n = 56;\ r^2 = 0.83;\ s = 0.40;\ F = 40.0$$

The quality of this equation is not excellent, but it nevertheless explains 83% of the variance. The s value should be close to the experimental error in the biological assay, here ~ 0.15. PTNCY$_{cow}$ reflects the potency of the compounds measured in a bovine membrane assay. The interpretation of this equation is as follows. An H-bond accepting group in the *meta* position of the phenyl ring (e.g. 3-NH$_2$) is unfavourable. Lipophilic groups in position R$_3$ are favourable. In the *ortho* position on the phenyl ring, large groups and H-bond acceptors (OH and OMe) are detrimental to activity, while electron-donating groups are favourable. The phenyl ring should not be substituted with carboxylic acid function. HACCEPT, ACID and HBOND are so-called indicator values, denoting absence (= 0) or presence (= 1) of a specific feature.

Since no descriptor for the *para* position in the phenyl ring appears in the equation, it was successfully attempted to improve the aqueous solubility of the compounds by introducing basic sulfonamide groups.

B.   Cluster analysis

Among the mathematical tools for investigation of patterns and clustering behaviour in data sets, two techniques are widely established, namely principal component analysis and cluster analysis. Both can be used to reduce the dimensionality of a problem. In other words, cluster analysis can be used for variable or descriptor selection from a larger set. On the other hand, cluster analysis may be used to investigate similarity among compounds. Cluster analysis is often used complementarily to PCA.

Similarity and dissimilarity among points in multidimensional space can be defined by calculating their Euclidean distance. A number of different hierarchical clustering algorithms are available, e.g. single linkage or complete linkage. The difference lies in the definition of the spatial distance between pairs of data points. The results are presented as a dendrogram, a tree-like figure in which very similar compounds or descriptors are close together. Good results are often obtained using Ward's method, which is a compromise among various clustering approaches. Clustering may still be partially due to chance and unrelated to the underlying chemical or biological meaning. Cluster significance analysis (CSA) can be used to validate cluster patterns.[45]

C.   SIMCA and related methods

It often occurs that active compounds cannot be well separated from inactive ones, e.g. in a plot of activity against a physicochemical property. Such data are called embedded or asymmetric data. Several methods have been developed to treat such data sets; the best known is the SIMCA algorithm. The SIMCA (soft independent modelling of chemical analogy) method is a tool for pattern recognition in a data set.[36] The basic idea is to build several local class models using disjoint PCA from a training data set. For new test compounds predictions can be made of the activity class to which the new compound belongs. A further development of the method is called single-class discrimination.

D.   Artificial neural networks

A number of techniques related to artificial intelligence and natural computing have been investigated in quantitative structure–activity relationships. These include learning machines[46] and rule-induction.[47] A new trend is the use of so-called natural algorithms, which are based upon principles in nature, such as natural selection in evolution. Examples are artificial neural network and genetic algorithms. Different types of neural networks have been conceived, but for QSAR studies back-propagation appears to be the most suitable approach.[48] The advantage of neural networks is that few statistical assumptions are made *a priori*. The disadvantages include the fact that no real statistical validation method has been developed. There is a danger of over-fitting of the data, resulting in poor predictions outside the training set. The results are not always easy to interpret in terms of chemistry. A certain advantage over other pattern recognition techniques such as PCA may exist in the data reduction capability of neural networks. Therefore, in conclusion should be said that this method is not mature enough to be routinely used.

VI.   VALIDATION OF STATISTICAL RESULTS BY CROSS-VALIDATION

In traditional Hansch analysis using multiple linear regression the quality of an equation is validated by a number of statistical parameters.[31] These include the correlation coefficient r, where r^2 ($\times 100\%$) is the variance explained by the equation. Furthermore, the standard deviation s of the equation should be close to the experimental error in the dependent variable, i.e. the biological data. The error in the regression coefficients should not be larger than the coefficient itself. It is preferable to report 95% confidence intervals, instead of standard errors, which are about a factor two smaller and may give too optimistic a figure.

  Modern validation techniques are called bootstrapping or cross-validation. Cross-validation (CV) evaluates a model not by how well it fits the data but by how well it predicts data. The data set consisting of n compounds is devided into groups. Leaving out one group according to a fixed or random pattern, for the reduced data set the MLR or PLS model is recalculated and the missing values are predicted. This is repeated until every compound is left out once and only once. When each time only one compound is left out, this is referred to as the leave-one-out (LOO) method. Many authors use the LOO method, although it has been shown that the leave-several-out (LSO) approach is preferable.[49] A recommendation is to divide the data set into seven groups. Using the predicted values the PRESS (predictive residual sum of squares) and SD values are obtained as

$$\text{PRESS} = \Sigma \, (\text{property}_{\text{observed}} - \text{property}_{\text{predicted}})^2 \qquad (10)$$

$$\text{SD} = \Sigma \, (\text{property}_{\text{observed}} - \text{property}_{\text{mean}})^2 \qquad (11)$$

and the cross-validated correlation coefficient is calculated as

$$Q^2 = r_{\text{cv}}^2 = (\text{SD} - \text{PRESS}) \, / \, \text{SD} \qquad (12)$$

Q^2 will always be smaller than r^2. When $Q^2 > 0.3$, a model is considered significant. Although cross-validation may seem a robust validation technique, some difficulties should not be overlooked.[31,50] Variables that do not contribute to prediction, i.e. cause noise in the model, may have detrimental effects on CV. This may particularly play a role when many variables have to be considered, such as in a 3D-QSAR CoMFA analysis (see Chapter 23). A procedure for variable selection in the case of many variables has been developed and is named GOLPE (generating optimal linear PLS estimations).[51] When compounds are strongly grouped, CV may not work well. Recent examples have shown that CV is misleading when it is applied after variable selection in stepwise MLR.[49] Thus, although cross-validation is considered as the state-of-the-art statistical validation technique, its results are only relevant when correctly applied.

VII.   PRACTICAL HINTS AND PERSPECTIVES

A manifold of chemometric statistical tools may be used to investigate quantitative structure–activity relationships or more general structure–property correlations. Some of these techniques require expert support. However, the bench chemist may successfully use a number of techniques when some basic guidelines as dicussed in this chapter are followed. The three most important methods are:

Correlation studies
- Hansch analysis using MLR
- Partial least squares (PLS) regression

Pattern recognition studies
- Principal component analysis (PCA)

Which physicochemical or structural descriptors should be used? The answer may be rather pragmatic: all those available. First of all, any experimental physicochemical property can be used, such as lipophilicity data from shake flask partitioning or measured by RP-HPLC, and ionization constants. A number of descriptors can be calculated easily, such as the molecular weight, octanol–water partition coefficients, molar refractivity, molecular volume, surface area, and the number of H-bond donating and accepting groups. Using quantum-chemical methods, a number of electronic properties may be calculated, such as partial atomic charges.

Since drugs and their targets are three-dimensional objects, it is of course appropriate to consider 3D molecular properties. This is the objective of several approaches combining statistical and modelling techniques, referred to as 3D-QSAR.[50] The comparative molecular field analysis (CoMFA) method has considerable current interest and will be discussed elsewhere in this volume (Chapter 23).

Although CAMM is more appealing to most medicinal chemists, SPC studies are of considerable interest to many projects. In many cases the two approaches complement each other well.[52,53] Nevertheless, one should be aware that in SPC as well as in modelling studies, models are being developed and used under the assumption of a single binding mode. However, X-ray studies have shown very elegantly that different binding modes may occur, even within a series of closely related structures.[54]

Molecular biology and combinatorial chemistry are contributing considerably to modern medicinal chemistry, particularly for finding new targets and lead compounds. Using parallel and traditional synthesis methods these leads will be optimized to drug candidates with desired therapeutic profiles, but also with optimal pharmacokinetic and physicochemical properties. Quantitative approaches to structure–activity relationships will continue to play a role in this optimization process. However, SPC studies are not an isolated discipline, but should be adequately integrated in preclinical research projects where the use of computer-assisted techniques, e.g. molecular modelling, 3D database searching, pharmacophore generation, *de novo* design and molecular diversity projects, has become daily practice. On the other hand, for SPC studies the experimental measurement of relevant physicochemical properties, such as aqueous solubility, ionization and complexation constants, lipophilicity and membrane transport properties, should be performed with selected compounds to guide the lead optimization process.

REFERENCES

1. Tute, M. S. (1990) History and objectives of quantitative drug design. In Hansch, C., Sammes, P. G. and Taylor, J. B. (eds) *Comprehensive Medicinal Chemistry*, vol. 4, *Quantitative Drug Design*, pp. 1–31. Pergamon Press, New York.
2. Hansch, C. (1981) The physicochemical approach to drug design and discovery (QSAR). *Drug Dev. Res.* **1**: 267–309.
3. Hansch, C. (1984) On the state of QSAR. *Drug Inf. J.* **18**: 115–122.
4. Craig, P. N. (1984) QSAR – origins and present status: a historical perspective. *Drug Inf. J.* **18**: 123–130.
5. Hansch, C. (1993) Quantitative structure–activity relationships and the unnamed science. *Acc. Chem. Res.* **26**: 147–153.
6. Hyde, R. M. and Livingstone, D. J. (1988) Perspectives in QSAR: computer chemistry and pattern recognition. *J. Computer-Aided Mol. Des.* **2**: 145–155.
7. Van de Waterbeemd, H. (1992) The history of drug research: from Hansch to the present. *Quant. Struct.–Act. Relat.* **11**: 200–204.
8. Van de Waterbeemd, H. (1993) Recent progress in QSAR-technology. *Drug Des. Discov.* **9**: 277–285.
9. Stanton, D. T., Murray, W. J. and Jurs, P. C. (1993) Comparison of QSAR and molecular similarity approaches for a structure–activity relationships study of DHFR inhibitors. *Quant. Struct.–Act. Relat.* **12**: 239–245.
10. Fujita, T. (1987) Applications of quantitative structure–activity relationships in drug design. *Acta Pharm. Jugosl.* **37**: 43–51.
11. Fujita, T. (1990) The extrathermodynamic approach to drug design. In Hansch, C., Sammes, P. G. and Taylor, J. B. (eds) *Comprehensive Medicinal Chemistry*, vol. 4, *Quantitative Drug Design*, pp. 497–560. Pergamon Press, New York.
12. Martin, Y. C. (1981) A practitioner's perspective of the role of quantitative structure–activity analysis in medicinal chemistry. *J. Med. Chem.* **24**: 229–237.
13. Topliss, J. G. (1993) Some observations on classical QSAR. *Perspect. Drug Disc. Des.* **1**: 253–268.
14. Testa, B. and Kier, L. B. (1991) The concept of molecular structure in structure–activity relationship studies and drug design. *Med. Res. Revs.* **11**: 35–48.
15. Van de Waterbeemd, H. and Testa, B. (1987) The parametrization of lipophilicity and other structural properties in drug design. *Adv. Drug Res.* **16**: 85–225.
16. Charton, M. (1991) QSAR parametrization: facts, fads and fallacies. *Newsletter International QSAR Society.* **1**: 3–6.
17. El Tayar, N., Testa, B. and Carrupt, P.A. (1992) Polar intermolecular interactions encoded in partition coefficients: an indirect estimation of hydrogen-bond parameters of polyfunctional solutes. *J. Phys. Chem.* **96**: 1455–1459.
18. Leahy, D. E., Morris, J. J., Taylor, P. J. and Wait, A. R. Membranes and their models: towards a rational choice of partitioning system (1991) In Silipo C. and Vittoria A. (eds) *QSAR: Rational Approaches to the Design of Bioactive Compounds*, pp. 75–82. Elsevier, Amsterdam.
19. Young, R. C., Mitchell, R. C., Brown, T. H., *et al.* (1988) Development of a new physicochemical model for brain penetration and its application to the design of centrally acting H_2 receptor histamine antagonists. *J. Med. Chem.* **31**: 656–671.
20. Van de Waterbeemd, H. and Kansy, M. (1992) Hydrogen-bonding capacity and brain penetration. *Chimia* **46**: 299–303.
21. El Tayar, N., Marston, A., Bechalany, A., Hostettmann, K. and Testa, B. (1989) Use of centrifugal partition chromatography for assessing partition coefficients in various solvent systems. *J. Chromatogr.* **469**: 91–99.
22. Carlson, R. and Nordahl, A., (1993) Exploring organic synthetic experimental procedures. *Topics Curr. Chem.* **166**: 1–64.
23. Sjöström, M. and Eriksson, L. (1995) Applications of statistical experimental design and PLS modelling in QSAR. In van de Waterbeemd, H. (ed.) *Methods and Principles in Medicinal Chemistry*, vol. 2. *Chemometric Methods in Molecular Design*, pp. 63–90. VCH, Weinheim.
24. Austel, V. (1995) Experimental design. In van de Waterbeemd H. (ed.) *Methods and Principles in Medicinal Chemistry*, vol. 2. *Chemometric Methods in Molecular Design*, pp. 49–62. VCH, Weinheim.

25. Hansch, C. and Leo, A. (1979) *Substituent Constants for Correlation Analysis in Chemistry and Biology.* Wiley, New York.
26. Hellberg, S., Sjöström, M., Skagerberg, B. and Wold, S. (1987) *J. Med. Chem.* **30**: 1127–1135.
27. Van de Waterbeemd, H., El Tayar, N., Carrupt, P. A. and Testa, B. (1989) Pattern recognition study of QSAR substituent descriptors. *Computer-Aided Mol. Des.* **3**: 111–132.
28. Skagerberg, B., Bonelli, D., Clementi, S., Cruciani, G. and Ebert, C. (1989) Principal properties for aromatic substituents. A multivariate approach for design in QSAR. *Quant. Struct.–Act. Relat.* **8**: 32–38.
29. van de Waterbeemd, H., Costantino, G., Clementi, S., Cruciani, G. and Valigi R. (1995) In van de Waterbeemd, H. (ed.) *Methods and Principles in Medicinal Chemistry*, vol. 2. *Chemometric Methods in Molecular Design*, pp. 103–112. VCH, Weinheim.
30. Norinder, U. and Högberg, Th. (1992) PLS-based quantitative structure–activity relationship for substituted benzamides of clebopride type. Application of experimental design in drug design. *Acta Chem. Scand.* **46**: 363–366.
31. Kubinyi, H. (1993) *QSAR: Hansch Analysis and Related Approaches.* VCH, Weinheim.
32. Kim, K. H., Basha, F., Hancock, A. and DeBernardis, J. F. (1993) Quantitative structure–activity relationships for substituted aminotetralin analogues. I: Inhibition of norepinephrine uptake. *J. Pharm. Sci.* **82**: 355–361.
33. Naito, Y., Yamaura, Y., Inoue, Y., Fukaya, C., Yokoyama, K., Nakagawa, Y. and Fujita, T. (1992) Quantitative structure–activity relationships of 2-[4-(thiazol-2-yl)phenyl]propionic acid derivatives inhibiting cyclooxygenase. *Eur. J. Med. Chem.* **27**: 645–654.
34. Kubinyi, H. (1990) The Free–Wilson method and its relationship to theextrathermodynamic approach. In Hansch, C., Sammes, P. G. and Taylor, J. B. (eds) *Comprehensive Medicinal Chemistry*, vol. 4, *Quantitative Drug Design*, pp. 589–643. Pergamon Press, New York.
35. Van de Waterbeemd, H. (ed.) (1995) *Chemometric Methods in Molecular Design.* VCH, Weinheim.
36. Dunn, W. J. and Wold, S. (1990) Pattern recognition techniques in drug design. In Hansch, C., Sammes, P. G. and Taylor, J. B. (eds) *Comprehensive Medicinal Chemistry*, vol. 4, *Quantitative Drug Design*, pp. 691–714. Pergamon Press, New York.
37. Liu, Q., Hirono, S. and Moriguchi, I. (1990) Quantitative structure–activity relationships for calmodulin inhibitors. *Chem. Pharm. Bull.* **38**: 2184–2189.
38. Cramer, R. D. (1993) Partial least squares (PLS): its strength and limitations. *Perspect. Drug Disc. Des.* **1**: 269–278.
39. Wold, S., Johansson, E. and Cocchi, M. PLS – Partial Least Squares projections to latent variables. In Kubinyi, H. (ed.) *3D QSAR in Drug Design*, pp. 523-550. Escom, Leiden.
40. Malpass, J. A., Salt. D. W., Ford, M. G., Watcyn, E. W. and Livingstone, D. J. (1994) Continuum regression. In van de Waterbeemd, H. (ed.) *Methods and Principles in Medicinal Chemistry*, vol. 3, *Advanced Computer-Assisted Techniques in Drug Discovery*, pp. 163–189. VCH, Weinheim.
41. Lotta, T., Taskinen, J., Bäckström, R. and Nissinen, E. (1992) PLS modelling of structure–activity relationships of catechol *O*-methyltransferase inhibitors. *J. Computer-Aided Mol. Des.* **6**: 253–272.
42. Miyashita, Y., Ohsako, H., Takayama, C. and Sasaki, S. (1992) Multivariate structure–activity relationships analysis of fungicidal and herbicidal thiolcarbamates using partial least squares method. *Quant. Struct.–Act. Relat.* **11**: 17-22.
43. Coats, E. A., Cordes, H.-P., Kulkarni, V. M., Richter, M., Schaper, K.-J., Wiese, M. and Seydel, J. K. (1985) Multiple regression and principal component analysis of antibacterial activities of sulfones and sulfonamides in whole cell and cell-free systems of various DDS sensitive and resistant bacterial strains. *Quant. Struct.–Act. Relat.* **3**: 99–109.
44. Hamilton, H. W., Ortwine, D. F., Worth, D. F., Badger, E. W., Bristol, J. A., Bruns, R. F., Haleen, S. J. and Steffen, R. P. (1985) Synthesis of xanthines as adenosine antagonists, a practical quantitative structure–activity relationship application. *J. Med. Chem.* **28**: 1071–1079.
45. McFarland, J. W. and Gans, D. J. (1995) Cluster significance analysis. In van de Waterbeemd, H. (ed.) *Methods and Principles in Medicinal Chemistry*, vol. 2, *Chemometric Methods in Molecular Design*, pp. 295–308. VCH, Weinheim.
46. King, R. D., Hirst, J. D. and Sternberg, M. J. E. (1993) New approaches to QSAR: neural networks and machine learning. *Perspect. Drug Discov. Des.* **1**: 279–290.
47. A-Razzak, M. and Glen, R. C. (1994) Rule induction applied to the derivation of quantitative structure–activity relationships. In van de Waterbeemd, H. (ed.) *Methods and Principles in Medicinal*

Chemistry, vol. 3, *Advanced Computer-Assisted Techniques in Drug Discovery*, pp. 319–331. VCH, Weinheim.

48. Manallack, D. T. and Livingstone, D. J. (1994) Neural networks – a tool for drug design. In van de Waterbeemd, H. (ed.) *Methods and Principles in Medicinal Chemistry*, vol. 3, *Advanced Computer-Assisted Techniques in Drug Discovery*, pp. 294–318. VCH, Weinheim.

49. Wold, S. and Eriksson, L. (1995) In van de Waterbeemd, H. (ed.) *Methods and Principles in Medicinal Chemistry*, vol. 2, *Chemometric Methods in Molecular Design*, pp. 309–318. VCH, Weinheim.

50. Kubinyi, H. (1993) (ed) *3D QSAR – Theory, Methods and Applications*, Escom, Leiden.

51. Baroni, M., Costantino, G., Cruciani, G., Riganelli, D., Valigi, R. and Clementi, S. (1993) Generating optimal linear PLS estimations (GOLPE): an advanced chemometric tool for handling 3D-QSAR problems. *Quant.Struct.–Act. Relat.* **12**: 9–20.

52. Kubinyi, H. (1990) Quantitative structure–activity relationships (QSAR) and molecular modeling in cancer research. *J.Cancer Res. Clin. Oncol.* **116**: 529–537.

53. Hansch, C. and Blaney, J. M. (1984) The new look to QSAR. In Jolles, G and Wooldridge, K. R. H. (eds) *Drug Design: Fact or Fantasy?* pp. 185–208. Academic Press, London.

54. Banner, D., Ackermann, J., Gast, A. *et. al.* (1993) Serine proteases: 3D structures, mechanisms of action and inhibitors. In Testa, B., Kyburz, E., Fuhrer, W. and Giger, R. (eds) *Perspectives in Medicinal Chemistry*, pp. 27–43. Verlag HCA, Basel and VCH, Weinheim.

PART V

Spatial Organization, Receptor Mapping and Molecular Modelling

20

Stereochemical Aspects of Drug Action I: Conformational Restriction, Steric Hindrance and Hydrophobic Collapse

PHILLIP A. HART and DANIEL H. RICH

He comes, stares, goes, lets the question resume.
He has taken whatever answer may be down to his mud-borrow gloom.
Robert Penn Warren

I. INTRODUCTION

Conformational restriction, steric hindrance and hydrophobic collapse represent important concepts that medicinal chemists utilize to optimize biological activity for a target receptor or enzyme or to gain receptor selectivity. Although these concepts were formulated independently, they are interdependent, since the lack of biological activity exhibited by synthetic analogues can, in principle, be rationalized in terms of each concept. We begin with a brief look at the origin of conformational restriction and end by illustrating how these ideas are used today.

THE PRACTICE OF MEDICINAL CHEMISTRY
ISBN 0-12-744640-0

II.   ORIGIN OF CONFORMATIONAL RESTRICTION

The importance of multiple functional groups and their spatial arrangement to effective receptor binding has been recognized for many years. The hypothesis that a fixed and specific two-dimensional distance between two oxygen functions in estrogen analogues was needed to elicit estrogenic activity[1] marks the very early thinking about the correlation of the spatial disposition of important functional groups with biological activity. It was not until the early 1950s, when our present concepts of conformational analysis were being developed,[2] that conformation was suspected to be a determinant of the spatial arrangement of functional groups. It was suggested soon thereafter that enzymes or drug receptors might prefer specific ligand conformations or distributions of conformations. Schueler hypothesized that conformational flexibility might be the important determinant for the muscarinic activity of acetylcholine, which was consistent with the attenuated activity of rigid piperidinium analogues of acetylcholine.[3-5] To rationalize how flexible ligands might bind to the muscarinic receptor more effectively than rigid counterparts, Schueler proposed that the receptor must also be flexible so as to permit better structural correlation between ligand and receptor. In contrast, Archer[6] adopted the point of view that the nicotinic and muscarinic actions of acetylcholine might be due to different conformations of the flexible ligand, which could be differentiated by conformational restriction (Archer described it as 'configurationally frozen'). He synthesized various isomers of 2-tropanyl acetate and concluded that a transoid conformation is favoured at the muscarinic receptor and that a cisoid form is favoured at the nicotinic receptor. These two studies, one emphasizing the dynamics of ligand–receptor interactions and the other the time-independent complementarity of ligand and receptor have evolved into the present. Today, the concept of rigid complementarity has led to attempts to develop 'rigid', or conformationally restricted (conformationally constrained) analogues of inherently conformationally flexible substances in order to delineate the preferred conformation that a ligand would adopt upon binding to a given receptor, which we will call the 'bioactive conformation'. In addition, conformational restriction has been applied with the expectation that very active analogues can be obtained, and as a requisite first step to simplify lead structures in the search for new drug candidates. Finally, conformational restriction is used to discover specifity among the members of multireceptor families. Throughout this chapter the reader is cautioned to recognize that even highly conformationally restricted molecules can adopt multiple, closely related conformations so that the terms *bioactive conformation* or *constrained analogue* more accurately describe an average of a limited population of closely related conformers.

III.   USE WITH SMALL LIGANDS

The principle of conformational restriction was first applied to characterize the bioactive conformation of acetylcholine acting at the muscarinic and nicotinic receptors. Conformational restriction has been applied to many other small ligands (e.g., see reviews by Martin-Smith,[7] Portoghese,[8] Mutschler and Lambrecht,[9] and Casy[10]), but the work on acetylcholine analogues exemplifies the necessary ideas and techniques required to understand the general approach, as well as its strengths and limitations, when applied to small molecules.

Acetylcholine has four bonds labelled χ_1, χ_2, χ_3 and χ_4 (see (**20.1**), Fig. 20.1), about which conformational change can take place. If one ignores the methyl group rotations and corrects for the identical conformations formed by rotations about the carbon–nitrogen bond (χ_4), a total of nine distinct acetylcholine conformations are possible. In principle, each of these conformations could have a measurably different ligand–receptor binding constant, which could be tested by synthesizing the appropriate restricted analogue. X-ray analysis of various acetylcholine crystals reveals conformational variations in the crystal depending upon the nature of the counterion.[8] Conformational analysis of acetylcholine in solution suggests that the gauche or near gauche conformation about χ_3 is the most probable one in aqueous medium, but the method is unable to specify the remaining conformational parameters for the other torsion angles.[8]

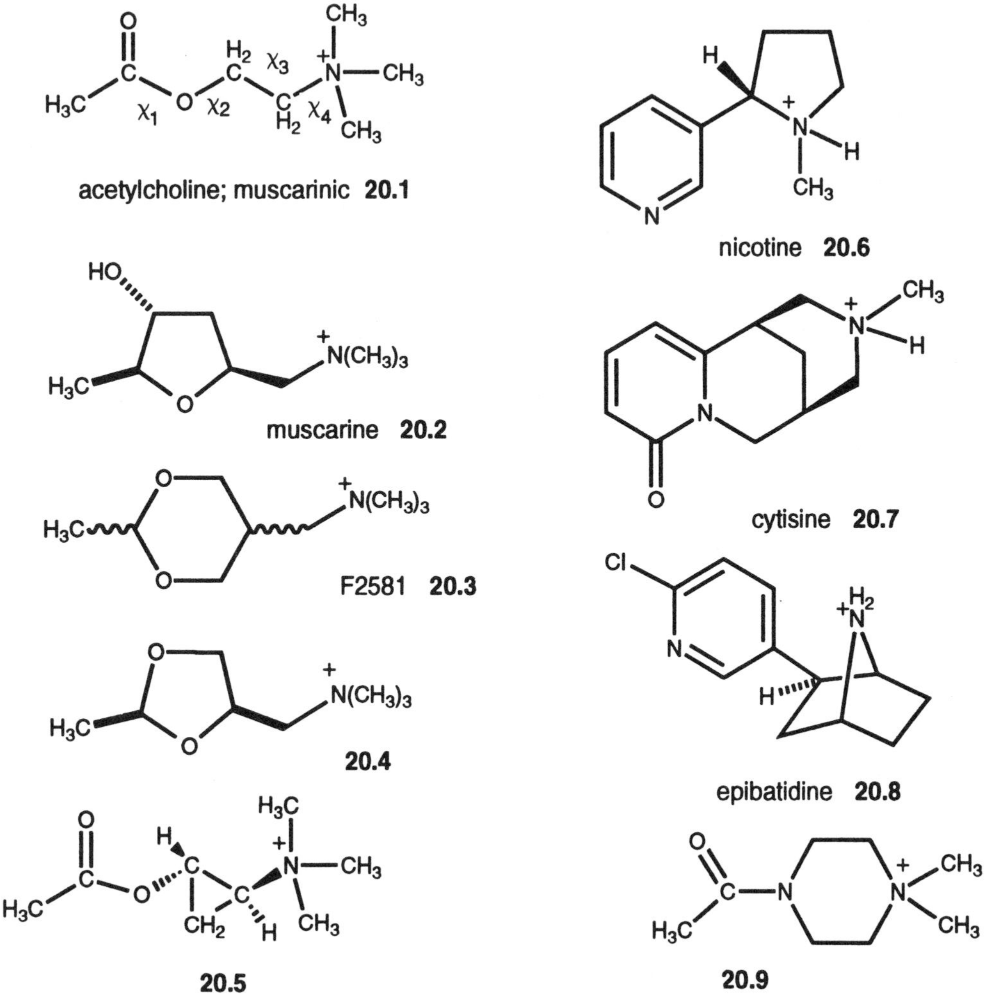

Fig. 20.1 Conformationally restricted analogues of acetylcholine.

Early work on the synthesis and bioassay of conformationally restricted acetylcholine (ACh) analogues (Fig. 20.1) suggested that *trans* rigid analogues are preferred by the muscarinic receptor.[7,8] Results pertinent to the nicotinic receptor were not conclusive. Many of the compounds (e.g. (**20.2**)–(**20.4**)) are analogues derived from muscarine. The only rigid analogue of acetylcholine to have muscarinic activity comparable to that of acetylcholine is the *trans* cyclo-propyl analogue (**20.5**),[11,12] and the corresponding *cis* cyclopropyl analogue is much less active. How does one interpret such data? Here is the first example where the interdependency of steric hindrance and conformational restriction complicate the interpretation of structure–activity data. The observed loss in biological activity for an analogue could be caused by steric hindrance between the ligand and receptor due to the added constraining atoms, or it could be caused by the inability of the ligand to attain the proper conformation for binding to the receptor. Since the added restricting atoms could cause either effect, one cannot differentiate between these two possibilities when the derivative has no biological activity. In contrast, when the synthetic analogue retains agonist activity, one can conclude that the proper conformation was realized in the ligand–receptor complex in spite of the restriction atoms.

These results illustrate the strengths and weaknesses of the conformationally restricted analogue approach. In practice, many conformationally restricted analogues must be prepared and tested to explore conformational space and to corroborate 3D models for the bioactive conformation of a small compound. Some of the active nicotinic and muscarinic agonists and antagonists studied up to 1970 are shown in Fig. 20.1. The muscarine analogues provide conformational information about the bonds, χ_1, χ_2, χ_3, in the bioactive conformation, whereas the cyclopropyl analogue (**20.5**) provides information about χ_4. Bioassay of these and related compounds shows that the nicotinic and muscarinic receptors have different structural specificities. Models for the conformations that activate each receptor were deduced by using analogues of acetylcholine in which the distances between the positive nitrogen and a hydrogen bond acceptor were constrained by the molecular structure to within certain specified distances.[13] These more or less 'rigid' structures exemplify some of the possible conformations that acetylcholine can adopt. Muscarinic activity was correlated with a conformation in which the quaternary ammonium group (or with an equivalent group such as alkyl sulfonium, —$S^+(CH_3)_2$) and an unshared pair of electrons were separated by a distance of approximately 4.4 Å. Nicotinic activity was correlated with a different conformation in which the quaternary ammonium group and the ester carbonyl group are separated by about 5.9 Å. Other authors have established similar though not identical correlations.[14,15] Recent work with epibatidine (**20.8**), the pure nicotinic agonist and central analgesic, shows that its semirigid structure is well correlated with the classical nicotinic agonist nicotine.[16–18]

Another type of conformational restriction reported recently by McGroddy[19,20] is derived from amide analogues of ACh, e.g. (**20.9**). These are selective nicotinic agonists that manifest slow *cis–trans* amide rotation that influences biological activity. The nicotinic activity of these and more constrained analogues was measured using *Torpedo* electroplaque or BC3H-1 cell-membrane or intact cells. The authors were able to differentiate the rate of initial binding (probably a function of the slow amide conformational exchange), relative antagonism (a measure of the rate of channel opening) and desensitization (a measure of the rate of ligand–receptor structural transition to a nonfunctional state). Related effects of *cis-trans* isomerization are known for tentoxin,[21] certain ACE inhibitors, and cyclosporin A (see below).

Conformationally restricted analogues of other low-molecular-mass agonists have been synthesized or discovered in attempts to characterize the bioactive conformation of the ligand. This field is vast and Fig. 20.2 shows selected examples of constrained agonist analogues of dopamine (**29.10**) vs (**20.11**),[22] GABA (**20.12**) vs (**20.13**)–(**20.14**),[23] glutamic acid (**20.15**) vs (**20.16**) and (**20.17**),[24] histamine (**20.18**) vs (**20.19**) and (**20.20**),[25] and serotonin (**20.21**) vs (**20.22**)[26] that have been discovered by application of this approach.

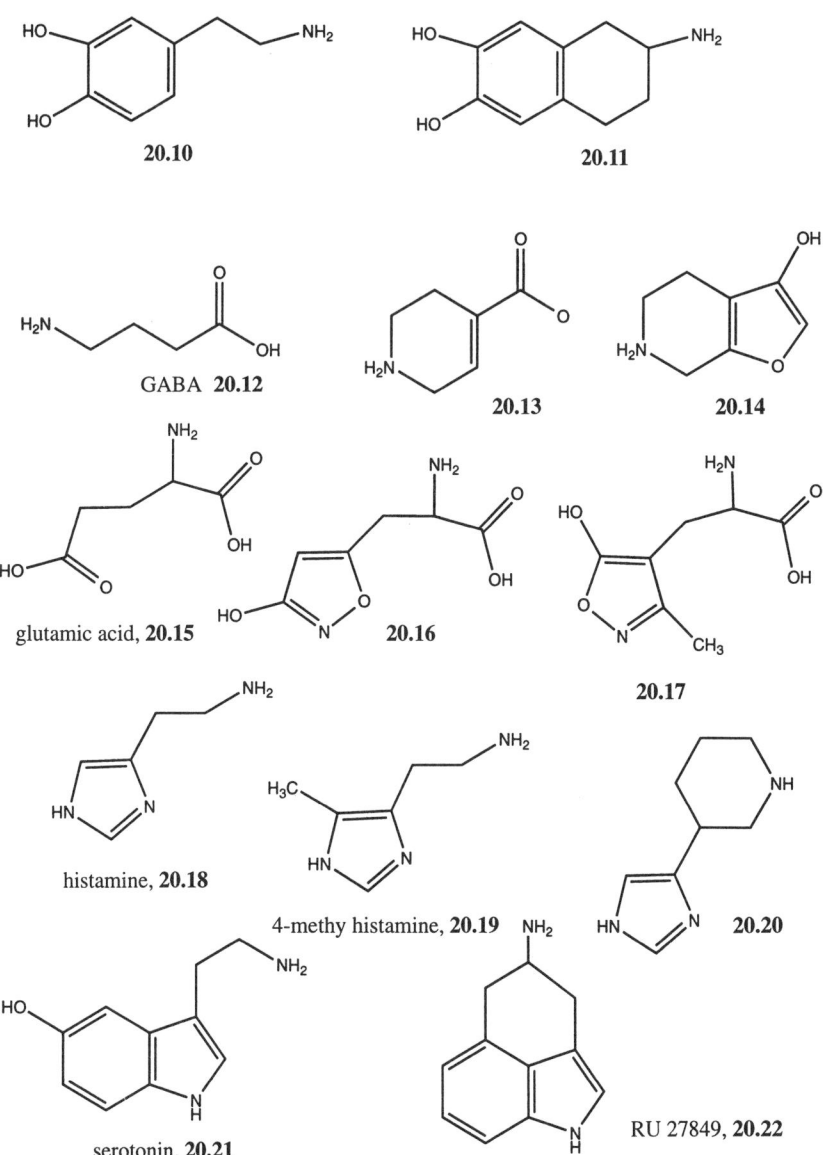

Fig. 20.2   Conformationally restricted receptor agonists.

IV.   CONFORMATIONALLY RESTRICTED RECEPTOR ANTAGONISTS

The relationship between the structures of agonists and antagonists has always fascinated medicinal chemists, and has led to a number of suggestions that some inhibitors are conformationally restricted analogues of the agonist except for the additional atoms that prevent receptor activation.[27] Recently, new methods to test whether peptide agonists and nonpeptide antagonists bind to the same atoms in a receptor have been developed by applying site-directed mutagenesis to G-protein-coupled receptors and comparing the effects of receptor mutation on agonist and antagonist binding. It appears that some peptide agonists and antagonists bind to different subsites on the protein receptor.[28] These initial results suggest that correlations of the structures of tachykinin agonists with the structures of the nonpeptide antagonists may not be valid. If these results prove to be general, they will discourage attempts to superimpose agonist and antagonist structures in other receptor systems.

V.   CONFORMATIONAL RESTRICTION OF PEPTIDES

The use of conformational restriction to probe the bioactive conformation of a molecule has been much more productive with peptides than with small molecules. For the most part, this results from the fact that small peptides have so many flexible torsion angles that enormous numbers of conformations are possible in solution. For example, a tripeptide such as thyrotropin-releasing hormone (TRH (**20.23**)) with six flexible bonds could have over 65 000 possible conformations. The number of potential conformers for larger peptides is enormous and, although modern biophysical methods, e.g. X-ray crystallography or isotope edited NMR,[29] have been used to characterize enzyme-bound conformations of peptides bound to small proteins, no biophysical method yet exists that can characterize the conformation of ligands bound to receptors. Therefore, conformational restriction remains an important and powerful method for characterizing the bioactive conformation of peptides.

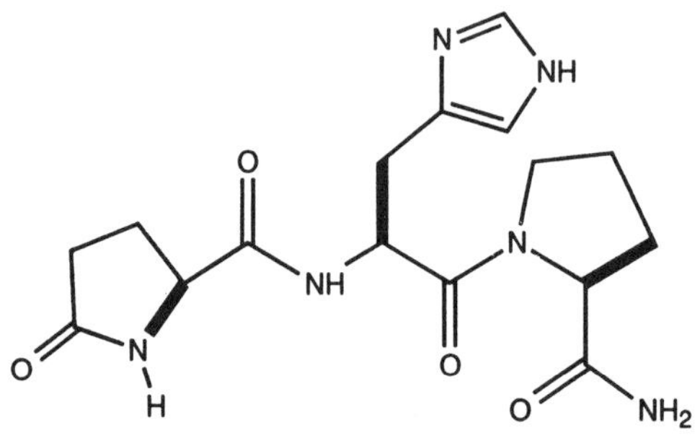

TRH, 20.23

The first successful application of conformational restriction to peptide chemistry was carried out by Veber and his associates at Merck,[30] who were trying to simplify the structure of somatostatin (Fig. 20.3 (**20.24**)) to produce an orally active derivative. Their approach was to introduce conformational restraints into the macrocyclic peptide ring system in order to reduce the number of conformations available to the analogue. Not all substitutions were expected to produce biologically active products, but those that retained activity were assumed to be able to adopt conformations close to the normal bioactive conformation. This work began from the earlier discovery by Rivier[31] that replacement of L-tryptophan in the 8-position of somatostatin by D-tryptophan produced an analogue that retained biological activity. This unusual biological result is produced when a D,L sequence (D-Trp-Lys) replaces an L,L sequence (Trp-Lys) in a peptide at a type II′ β-turn because the topography of the amino acid side-chains at these positions is essentially identical in these turns.[32] These results led Veber and associates to postulate that the amino acid sequence Phe-Trp-Lys-Thr might be part of a type II′ β-turn, and that this tetrapeptide sequence might comprise the active pharmacophore. Although this hypothesis was highly speculative for its time, it was shown to be essentially correct by applying the principle of conformational restriction (Fig. 20.3). Deletion of the N-terminal dipeptide, followed by insertion of the D-Trp at position-8, and replacement of the disulfide sulfurs with

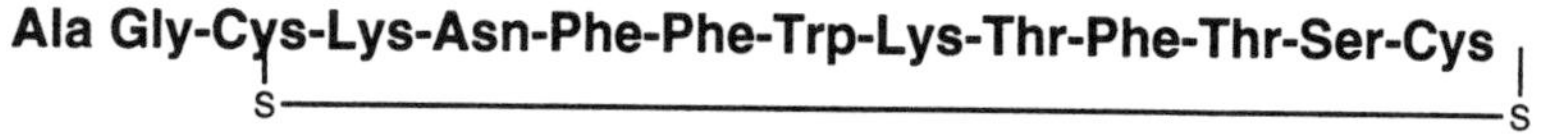

Ala Gly-Cys-Lys-Asn-Phe-Phe-Trp-Lys-Thr-Phe-Thr-Ser-Cys

Somatostatin; 20.24

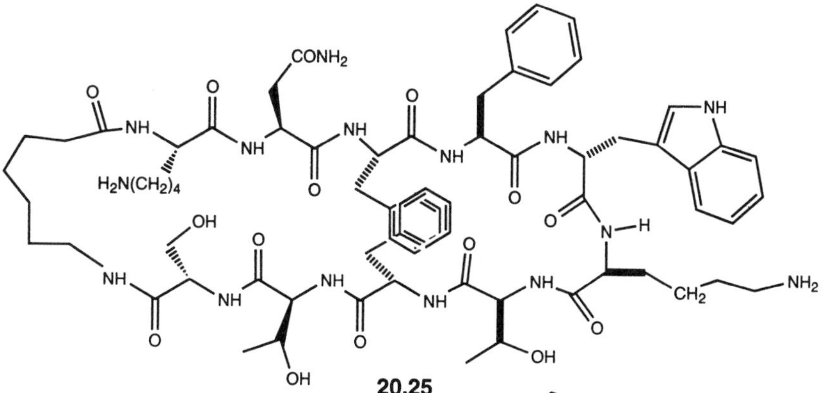

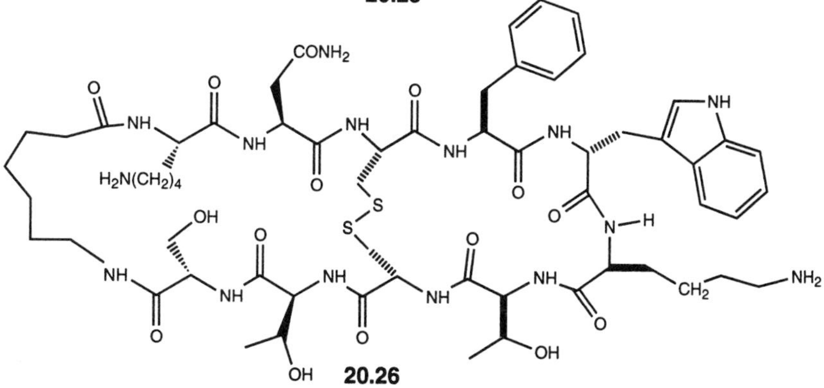

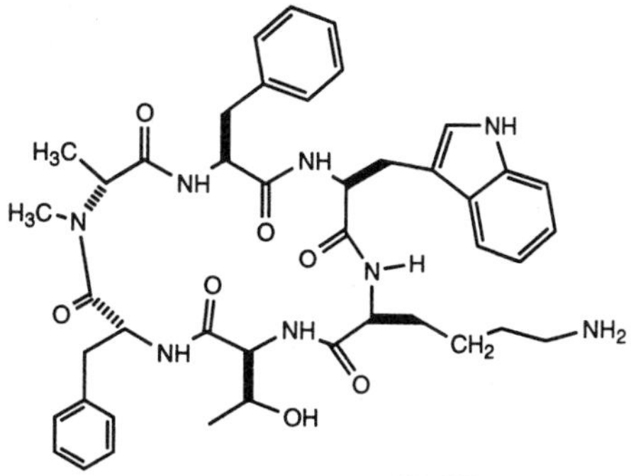

Fig. 20.3 Conformationally restricted somatostatin analogues.

carbons produced analogue (**20.25**). NMR and other data suggested that the two phenylalanine side-chains were clustered and might be replaceable by other bridging groups. This led to the analogue (**20.26**) in which a transannular disulfide bond limited the available conformations. When analogue (**20.26**) was found to retain biological activity, the disulfide units were replaced with the corresponding stable carbon derivatives, more constraints were introduced, and the process was repeated. Some analogues were designed specifically to be inactive according to the pending hypothesis, in order to provide controls. After several iterations, a biologically active cyclic hexapeptide (**29.27**) was discovered in which only 6 of the original 14 amino acids in somatostatin were needed to produce a fully active derivative. Veber also realized that the accessible surface area of the cyclic peptide was approximately the same as that of traditional drugs, e.g. benzodiazepines, and suggested that any biological activity that can be elicited by a cyclic hexapeptide or a smaller peptide could be mimicked by a nonpeptide, heterocyclic system.[33]

The work of Veber and co-workers established that valuable information about the bioactive conformation of a flexible peptide could be obtained by applying the principles of conformational restriction, and several additional examples were soon developed by following this strategy. An unusually active analogue of α-melanotropin was formed by cyclizing the more flexible precursor.[34]

Conformationally restricted enkephalin analogues e.g. (**20.28**), have been formed by cyclizing between positions 2 and 5 of enkephalin (**20.29**), and small cyclic analogues of endothelin, e.g. (**20.30**), have been discovered by applying these methods.[35]

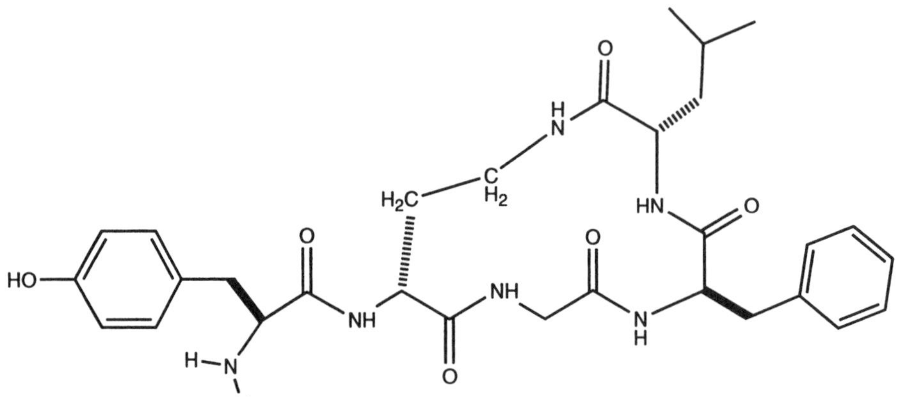

20.28

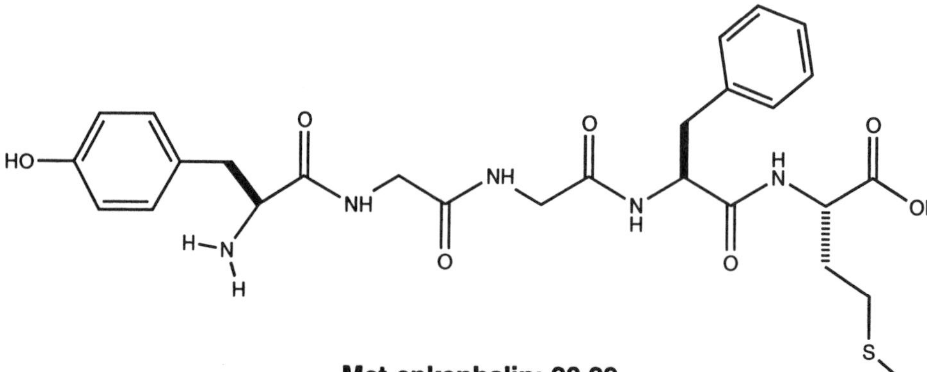

Met-enkephalin; 20.29

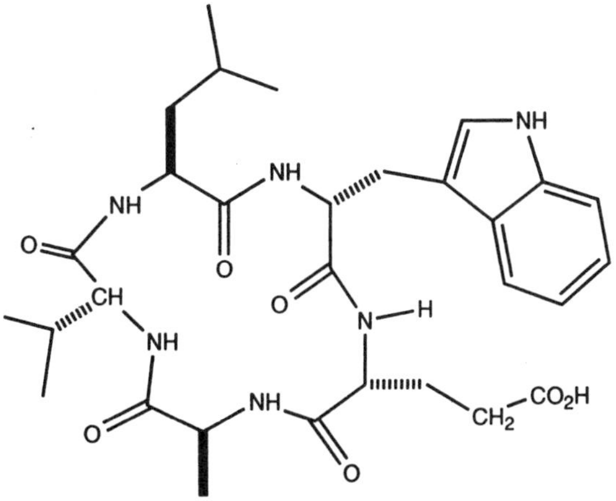

cyclo (D-Glu-Ala-D-Val-Leu-D-Trp), 20.30

Conformational restriction can be introduced into flexible peptides by a variety of methods. For example, Marshall introduced α-methylamino acid substituents into peptides as a way of decreasing the conformational space available to the resulting peptide.[36] Freidinger developed a cyclic lactam moiety (**20.31**) that stabilized β- and γ-turn structures and applied this to LH-RH (e.g. (**20.32**)) to show that β-turn about residues 6–7 was compatible with activity.[37] Conformational restriction has been applied to determine the bioactive conformation of enzyme–inhibitor systems for which no X-ray crystal structure is available. Thorsett, Wyvratt and Patchett[38] synthesized conformationally restricted bicyclic lactam derivatives of the angiotensin converting enzyme (ACE) inhibitors enalapril (**20.33**) and enalaprilat (**20.34**) (Fig. 20.4) in order to characterize torsion angles in the bioactive conformation. Analogue (**20.35**)

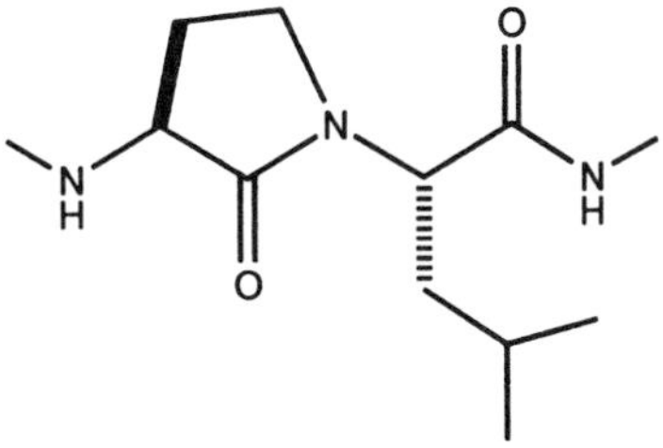

20.31

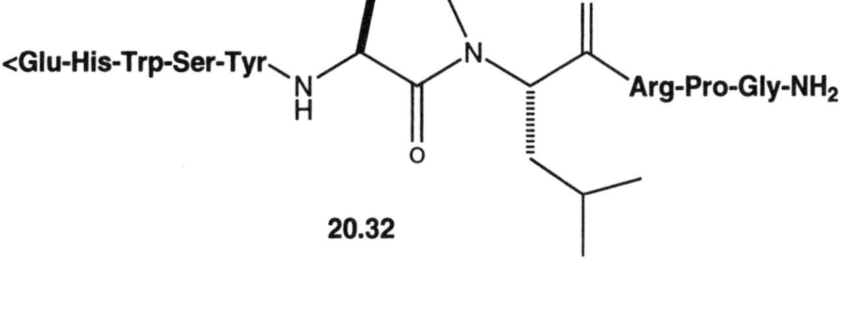

20.32

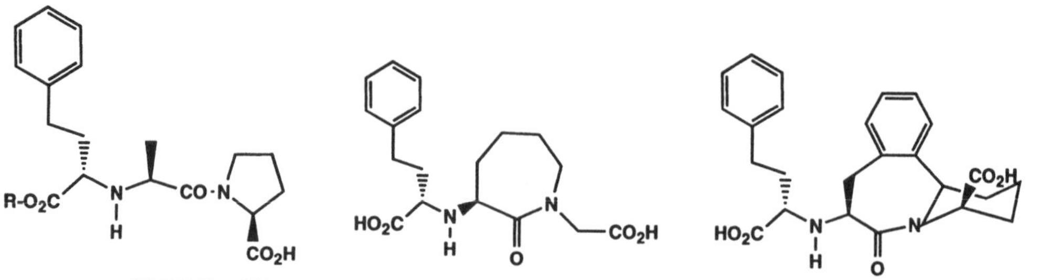

Fig. 20.4   Conformationally restricted inhibitors of angiotensin converting enzyme.

was used to constrain the torsion angle ψ. Flynn *et al.*[39] extended this principle to prepare the very tight-binding tricyclic ACE inhibitor (**20.36**). Numerous additional conformational constraints have been developed and the reader is encouraged to consult these reviews for additional examples.[40–42]

VI.   WHEN IS THE BIOACTIVE CONFORMATION FORMED?

The emergence of NMR as a method for characterizing the solution conformation of peptides was accompanied by the realization that the solution conformation might not be the same as the bioactive conformation. In the early years, the limitations in NMR technology precluded studies in highly aqueous media and only recently has it become possible to determine the enzyme-bound conformation of ligands bound to small proteins. Scepticism about the relevance of solution conformation to bioactive conformation has increased in recent years, but this is probably because many solution studies have been carried out in organic solvents, especially chloroform, because of the insolubility of organic compounds in water at the concentrations needed for NMR analysis. Except for highly conformationally restricted compounds, there is no particular reason to expect that the chloroform conformation of an organic molecule, especially one with hydrophobic groups attached via flexible tethers, should be predictive of the aqueous or bioactive conformation of that molecule. Recent developments now provide evidence that in some cases the bioactive conformation of a flexible peptide may exist to an appreciable extent in *aqueous* media prior to binding of the ligand to the protein. These observations, if general, merit careful examination because they illustrate how conformational studies should be carried out to determine the bioactive conformation of a peptide, and offer encouragement that these efforts will be productive.

Conformational restriction played an important role in the recent discovery that water induces the bioactive conformation of cyclosporin A (Sandimmune®, CsA, (**20.37**)). CsA is the drug of choice for preventing rejection of transplanted human organs and has been the subject of many synthetic, conformational and mechansim of action studies.[43] To produce immunosuppression, CsA first binds to cyclophilin A (CyP A),[44] a peptidyl prolyl *cis–trans* isomerase (PPIase),[45] to form the CsA–CyP complex, which then binds to and inhibits calcineurin (CaN), a calmodulin-dependent serine/threonine protein phosphatase,[46] thereby inhibiting interleukin-2 (IL-2) synthesis.[47]

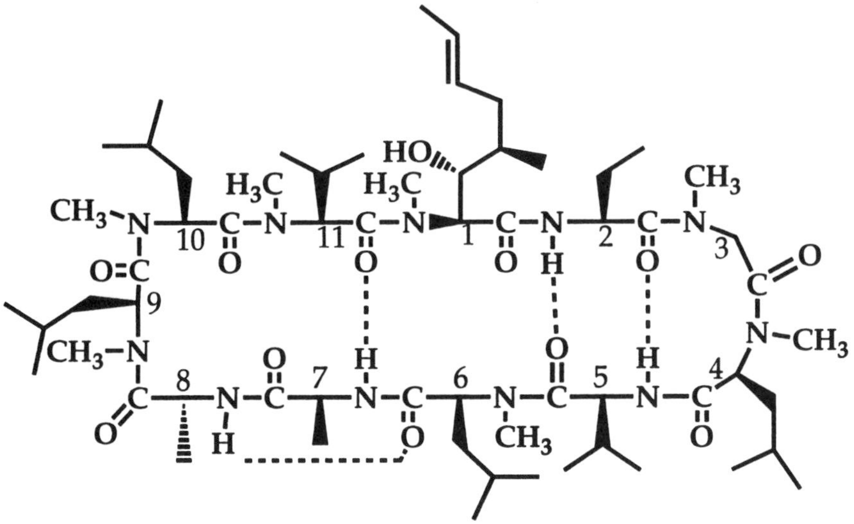

CsA, 20.37

The conformations of CsA in chloroform and when bound to cyclophilin differ dramatically. CsA adopts closely related conformations in three different crystal forms and in two different solvent systems,[48] characterized by a *cis* peptide bond between MeLeu residues 9 and 10. However, numerous attempts to prepare conformationally restricted CsA derivatives based on modifying the chloroform conformation of CsA[49] according to the strategies developed by Veber (see above) were unsuccessful. These negative results prompted a reassessment of the bioactive conformation of CsA by isotope edited NMR methods, which led to the discovery that in CsA bound to CyP the amide bond between the 9,10 residues is *trans*.[50] Complete structures of CsA bound to Cyp were reported subsequently.[51] Figure 20.5 shows stereo representations of the chloroform (**20.37c**) and the enzyme-bound (**20.37t**) conformers of CsA, and illustrates the remarkable difference in overall shape of the molecule produced by the *cis* to *trans* isomerization.

VII.   USE OF TIME-RESOLVED CONFORMATIONAL RESTRICTION. THE BIOACTIVE CONFORMATION OF CsA IS FORMED IN WATER

The dissociation constants of slowly interconverting populations of conformations can be determined when the biological response rate is faster than the rate of conformational interconversion, and in favourable cases this process can provide information about the bioactive conformation of a molecule. This principle was first demonstrated with analogues of tentoxin,[21] a phytotoxic cyclic tetrapeptide. Because certain conformers of D-MeAla-tentoxin interconvert slowly, it was possible to isolate and bioassay different conformational populations of the molecule, and to show selective inhibition of chloroplast coupling factor-1.

In a similar fashion, it has been possible to isolate different conformations of the immunosuppressive drug cyclosporin A. By preparing anhydrous THF solutions of CsA, with

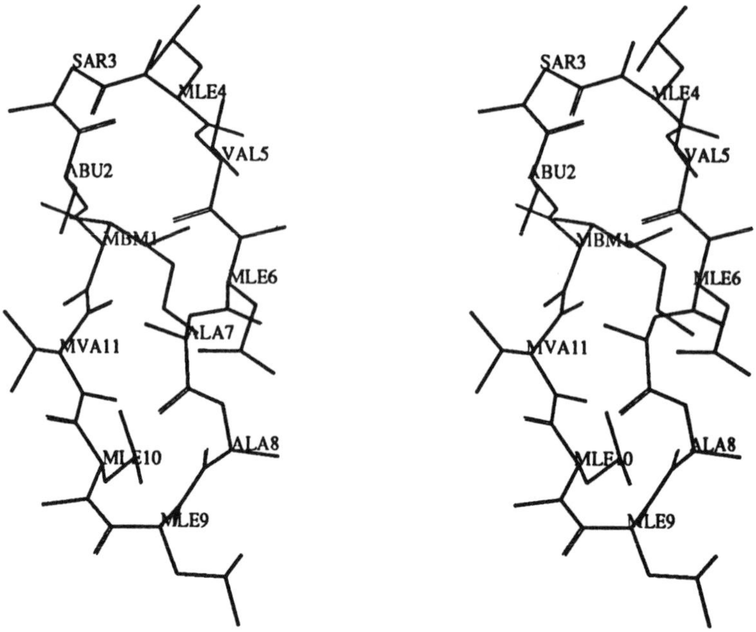

20.37c

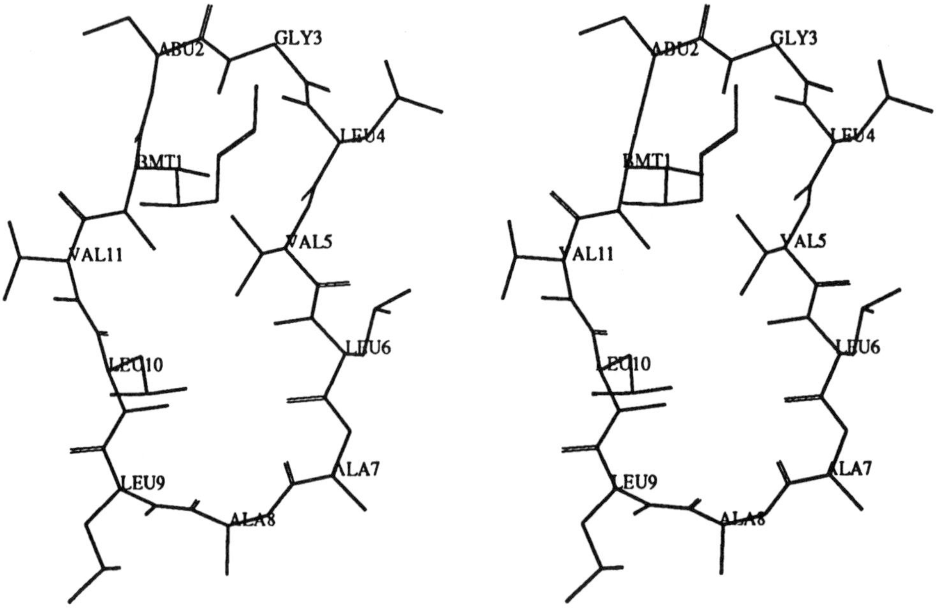

20.37t

Fig. 20.5 Relaxed stereoscopic views of chloroform (20.37c) and enzyme-bound (20.37t) conformations of cyclosporin A.

and without 0.4 M LiCl, it was possible to restrict the peptide ring system conformation in CsA to *trans* and *cis* conformers. Addition of these conformers separately to the assay buffer enabled the dissociation constants of both the *cis* and *trans* amide bond conformers in CsA for inhibition of PPIase to be determined.[52] The *trans* conformer (**20.37t**) is very active; the *cis* conformer (**20.37c**) is not, and these plus other data were used to show that CsA adopts a conformation in water that is very close to the enzyme-bound CsA conformation.[53] Recently, Wenger and co-workers at Sandoz showed by NMR experiments that a 3-substituted CsA derivative, e.g. (**20.38**) adopts a conformation in water that is essentially identical with the enzyme-bound CsA conformation.[54] Thus, formation of the bioactive conformations of CsA or (**20.38**) is driven by dissolution in water; the enzyme binds the preformed, *trans* amide conformer and does not catalyse its formation. Although multiple conformations of CsA exist in hydrogen bonding solvents, an appreciable amount of the correct conformation comparable to that of D-Ala3-CsA (**20.38**) must exist in solution prior to binding to the enzyme. This prediction, based on the

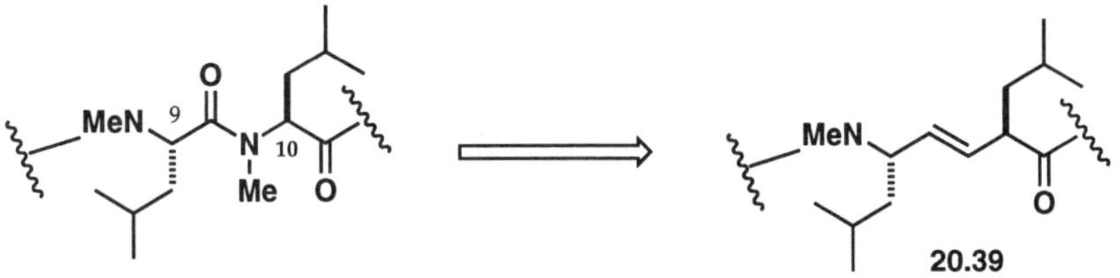

20.39

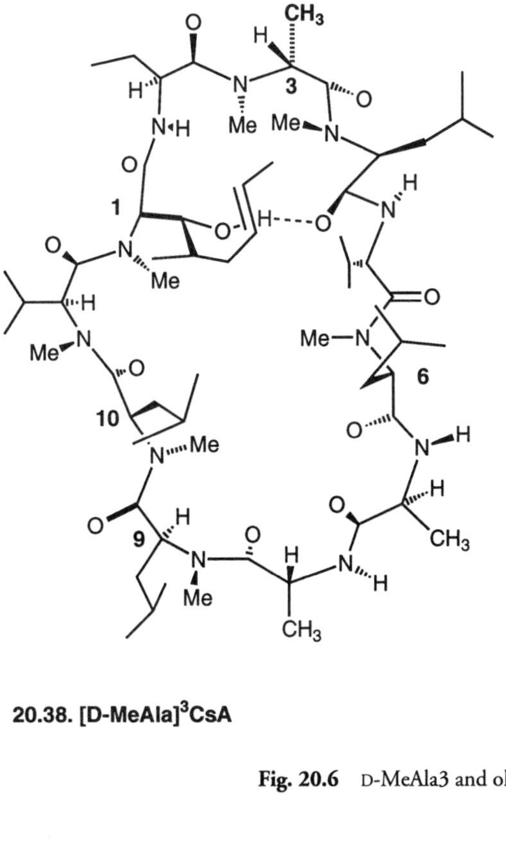

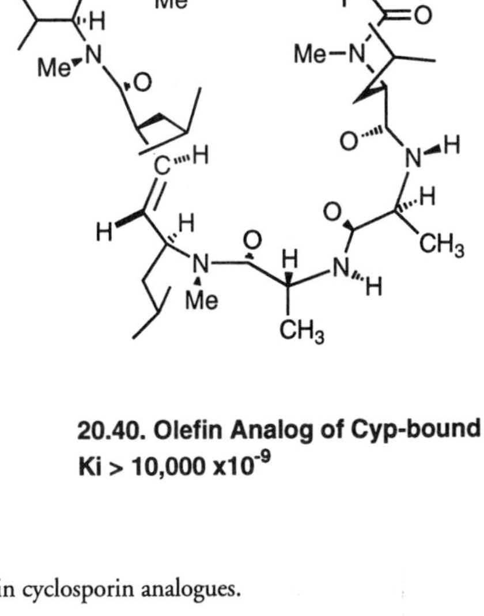

20.38. [D-MeAla]³CsA

20.40. Olefin Analog of Cyp-bound CsA
Ki > 10,000 x10⁻⁹

Fig. 20.6   D-MeAla3 and olefin cyclosporin analogues.

enzyme kinetic data, is consistent with the modest boost in activity reported for another conformationally constrained CsA derivative.[55] Interestingly, the D-MeAla-CsA derivative (**20.38**) corresponds to a CsA analogue in which one amino acid has an added single methyl group to stabilize conformational interconversions of the peptide ring system. This is an example of the α-substitution strategy proposed by Marshall.[36]

The process of constructing conformationally restricted analogues may fail for reasons other than steric hindrance or incorrect conformation. An enlightening example was encountered when the olefin isostere[56] was used in place of the *trans* amide bond in the enzyme-bound conformation of CsA. As noted previously, the amide bond between positions 9,10 in CsA switches from *cis* in organic solution to *trans* in water and in the enzyme-bound conformation. When the amide bond between MeLeu-MeLeu was replaced with the *trans* olefin isostere (**20.39**), a remarkably inactive CsA analogue (**20.40**) was formed (Fig. 20.6).[57] Although amide replacement by olefins is successful in other systems, notably in enkephalin analogues,[55] the CsA derivative had lost over four orders of magnitude in potency against cyclophilin. Subsequently, the X-ray crystal structure of CsA bound to Cyp showed that the carbonyl group in the MeLeu-MeLeu unit of CsA is hydrogen bonded to the indole NH in tryptophan-121 in cyclophilin.[58] Presumably this missing hydrogen bond is a significant factor in the loss of potency of (**20.40**), but the major point here is that conformational restriction can fail because essential groups have been deleted in the course of designing the restricted analogue.

VIII. HYDROPHOBIC COLLAPSE

The discovery that the bioactive conformation of CsA is induced by dissolution in water led to the concept of 'hydrophobic collapse' as a determinant of bioactive conformation of flexible, hydrophobic peptides and peptidemimetics in water. The medicinal chemical use of the term *hydrophobic collapse* is defined here to mean a significant conformational change in a molecule produced by dissolving the molecule in water, relative to the conformation observed for this same molecule in organic solution or *in vacuo*. With very hydrophobic molecules such as cyclosporin, it is assumed that hydrophobic clustering of side-chains plus hydrophilic interactions between the amide bonds and water help stabilize the bioactive conformation. Whether hydrophobic clustering in these conformations is purely a hydrophobic effect (see Newcomb and Gellman[59] for a case where it appears not to be) or results from a combination of multiple interactions (e.g. π–π, H-bonding; hydrophobic interactions) is not known.[60] It is safe to say that the effects of water on both pre- and post-binding conformations are critical to the pre-binding conformation of many classes of molecules and should be considered when attempting to design and interpret the biological properties of conformationally restricted analogues or peptidemimetics.

Since this concept was first proposed, several flexibile molecules have been found that adopt aqueous conformations in which hydrophobic side-chains are clustered.[61] In the cases of thrombin inhibitors and paclitaxel derivatives, hydrophobic collapse appears to induce the bioactive conformations.[62] In contrast, many receptor antagonists that bind to a variety of receptor systems are constructed from templates that should resist hydrophobic collapse.[10] The ubiquitous diphenylmethyl pharmacophoric group (**20.41**) shown in Fig. 20.7, along with some close variants, provides a hydrophobic surface that cannot self-associate owing to conformational constraints.

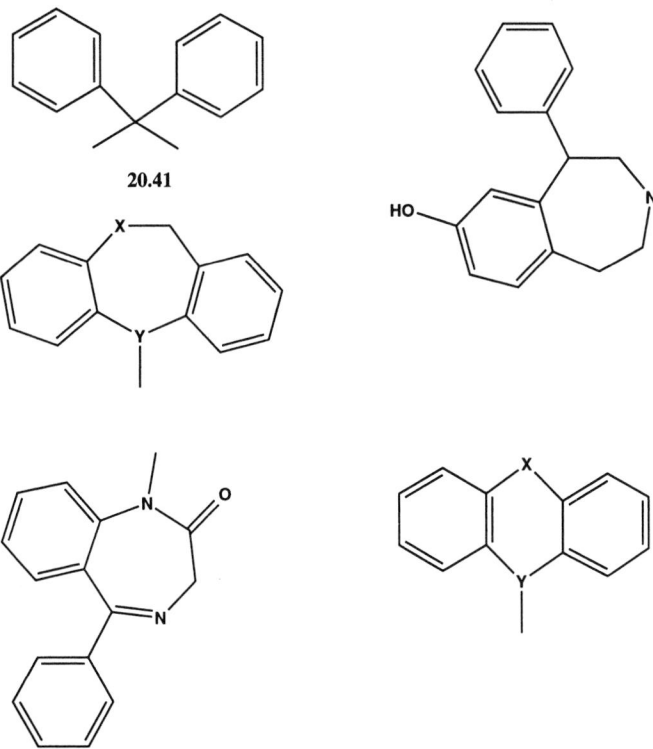

Fig. 20.7   Variations of the diphenylmethyl moiety found in drugs.

IX.   CONFORMATIONALLY CONSTRAINED RGD PEPTIDES AND DERIVATIVES

Some outstanding examples of the use of conformational restriction to characterize bioactive conformations of Arg-Gly-Asp (RGD) antagonists illustrate the present state of the art. Members of the integrin family of receptors[63] recognize and bind the peptide sequence Arg-Gly-Asp- as an important step in platelet aggregation and other physiological processes. Competitive antagonists for this process have been recognized as potential drug candidates and much effort has been directed towards identifying small ligands that might mimic the RGD peptide sequence. This drug design concept was supported by the fact that protein antagonists of integrin receptors are known that contain the RGD sequence[64] and that small peptide sequences containing the RGD moiety weakly antagonize the endogenous ligand.[65] Consequently, several groups synthesized conformationally restricted derivatives of small peptides as starting points for developing metabolically stable peptides or peptidemimetics. Ali *et al.*[66] synthesized a series of disulfide derivatives of the RGD sequence, which were designed by analogy with the somatostatin work (see above). Excellent antagonists related to (**20.42**) (Fig. 20.8) were obtained. Further constraint of the peptide system by use of the *o*-thiol benzene derivatives shown led to the novel antagonist SKF 107260 (**20.43**; Fig. 20.8), a potent, high affinity inhibitor of both platelet aggregation and binding to GPII$_B$III$_A$. Burnier's group[67] followed a similar strategy but utilized cyclic sulfides as

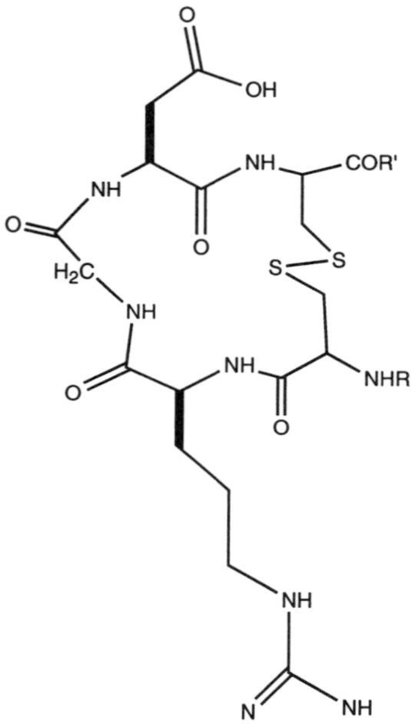

cyclo (Cys-Arg-Gly-Asp-Cys), **20.42**

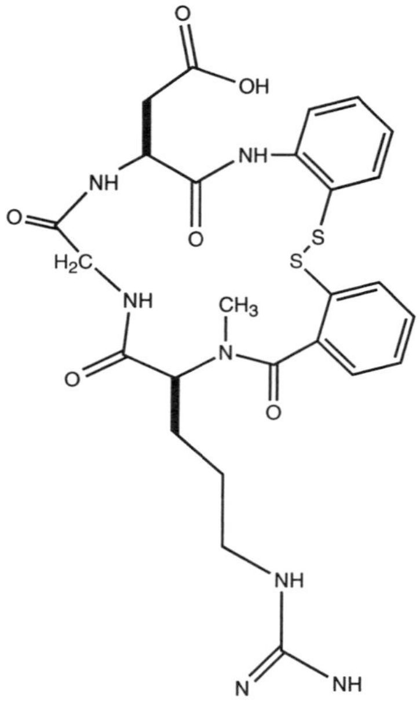

cyclo (Man-Arg-Gly-Asp-Map), **20.43**

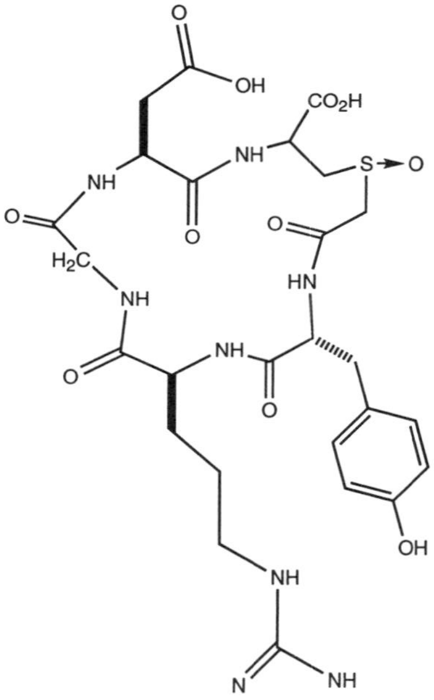

cyclo [Ac-DTyr-RGD-Cys(O)], **20.44**

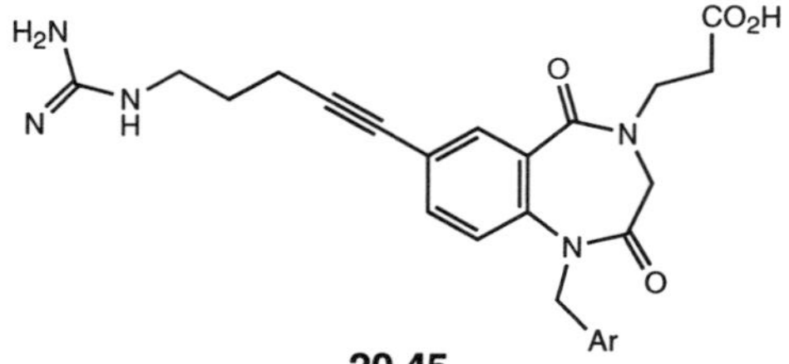

20.45

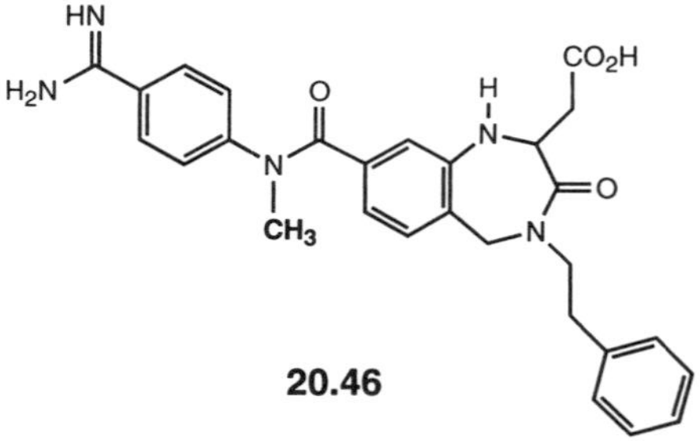

20.46

Fig. 20.8 Conformationally restricted analogues of RGD peptides.

the conformationally restricting element. These derivatives had the advantage of being rapidly synthesized by solid-phase methods. Systematic structure–activity studies with respect to the amino acid surrounding the RGD sequence and the chirality of sulfoxide derivatives led to the discovery of G-4120 (**20.44**), a potent, biologically active derivative. The conformations of both **20.43** and **20.44** in water were found to be highly constrained and prominent families of bioactive conformations could be characterized in aqueous solution by use of NMR methods and computational chemistry.[66,68] Both research teams superimposed their respective bioactive conformations, which defined the topographical orientations of the arginine and the aspartic side-chains, onto a conformationally restricted template of a class of compounds with generally suitable pharmacodynamic properties. Amazingly, both research teams employed the benzodiazepine ring system to generate two related low-molecular-mass nonpeptide RGD receptor antagonist (**20.45** and **20.46**),[69,70] which contains at least two conformational restrictions, the bicyclic heterocycle and the acetylene or carboxamide linker. The compounds shown in Fig. 20.8 represent what can be achieved by applying the principles of conformational restriction to peptides when no X-ray or NMR structural information is available for the complex between ligand and receptor. Benzodiazepines (**20.45** and **20.46**) represent peptidomimetics rationally designed *de novo* by systematically modifying a natural receptor-binding peptide. Antagonist **20.46** presents an almost perfect atom-for-atom match with the proposed bioactive conformation of the -R-6-D- pharmacophore and presents compelling evidence that true peptide mimetics can be designed by application of rational drug design.

REFERENCES

1. Schueler, F. W. (1946) Sex hormonal action and chemical constitution. *Science* **103**: 221–223.
2. Barton, D. H. R. (1950) Conformational analysis. *Experientia* **6**: 316–320.
3. Schueler, F. W. (1953) The interaction of statistical and Coulombic factors in the characterization of pharmacophoric moieties. *Arch. Int. Pharmacodyn.* **45**: 376–397.
4. Schueler, F. W. (1953) The statistical nature of the intramolecular distance factor of the muscarinic moiety. *Arch. Int.. Pharmacodyn.* **43**: 417–426.
5. Schueler, F. W. (1956) Two cyclic analogs of acetylcholine. *J. Am. Pharm. Assoc.* **4**: 197–199.
6. Archer, S., Lands, A. M. and Lewis, T. R. (1962) Isomeric 2-acetoxytropine methiodides. *J. Med. Pharm. Chem.* **5**: 423–431.
7. Martin-Smith, M., Smail, G. A. and Stenlake, J. B. (1967) The possible role of conformational isomerism in the biological actions of acetylcholine. *J. Pharm. Pharmac.* **19**: 561–589.
8. Portoghese, P. S. (1970) Relationships between stereostructure and pharmacological activities. *Annu. Rev. Pharmacol.* **10**: 51–76.
9. Mutschler, E. and Lambrecht, G. (1983) Stereoselectivity and conformation: flexible and rigid compounds. In Ariens E. J., Soudijn W. and Timmermans, P. B. M. W. M. (eds) *Stereochemistry and Biological Activity of Drugs*, pp. 63–80. Blackwell Scientific, Oxford.
10. Casy, A. F., Hassan, M. M. A. and Wu, F. C. (1971) Conformation of some acetylcholine analogs as solutes in deuterium oxide and other solvents. *J. Pharm. Sci.* **60**: 67–73.
11. Armstrong, P. D., Cannon, J. G. and Long, J. P. (1971) Conformationally rigid analogues of acetylcholine. *Nature* **220**: 56–59.
12. Cannon, J. G., Rege, A. B., Gruen, T. L. and Long, J. P. (1972) 1,2-Disubstituted cyclopropane and cyclobutane derivatives related to acetylcholine. *J. Med. Chem.* **15**: 71–75.
13. Beers, W. H. and Reich, E. (1970) Structure and activity of acetylcholine. *Nature* **228**: 917–922.
14. Chothia, C. (1970) Interaction of acetylcholine with different cholinergic nerve receptors. *Nature* **225**: 36–38.
15. Schulman, J. M., Sabio, J. L. and Disch, R. L. (1983) Recognition of cholinergic agonists by the

muscarinic receptor. 1. Acetylcholine and other agonists with the NCCOCC backbone. *J. Med. Chem.* **26**: 817–823.

16. Spande, T. F., Garraffo, H. M., Edwards, M. W., Yeh, H. J. C., Pannell, L. and Daly, J. W. (1992) Epibatidine: a novel (chloropyridyl)azabicycloheptane with potent analgesic activity from an Ecuadoran poison frog. *J. Am. Chem. Soc.* **114**: 3475–3478.

17. Qian, C., Li, T., Shen, T. Y., Libertine-Garahan, L., Eckman, J., Biftu, T. and Ip, S. (1993) Epibatidine is a nicotinic analgesic. *Eur. J. Pharm.* **250**: R13–R14.

18. Dukat, M., Damaj, M. I., Glassco, W., Dumas, D., May, E. L., Martin, B. R. and Glennon, R. A. (1994) Epibatidine: a very high affinity nicotine-receptor ligand. *Med. Chem. Res.* **4**: 131–139.

19. McGroddy, K. A. and Oswald, R. E. (1993) Solution structure and dynamics of cyclic and acyclic cholinergic agonists. *Biophys. J.* **64**: 314–324.

20. McGroddy, K. A., Carter, A. A., Tubbert, M. M. and Oswald, R. E. (1993) Analysis of cyclic and acyclic nicotinic cholinergic agonists using radioligand binding, single channel recording and nuclear magnetic resonance spectroscopy. *Biophys. J.* **64**: 325–338.

21. (a) Rich, D. H. and Bhatnagar, P. K. (1978) Isolation and conformational analysis of two conformers of D-methyl-alanine¹-tentoxin. *J. Am. Chem. Soc.,* **100**: 2218. (b) Rich, D. H., Bhatnagar, P. K., Jasensky, R. D., Steele, J. A., Uchytil, T. F. and Durbin, R. D. (1978) Two conformations of the cyclic tetrapeptide, [D-MeAla¹]-tentoxin have different biological activities. *Bioorganic Chem.* **7**: 207–214.

22. Horn, A. S. and Rogers, J. R. (1980) 2-Amino-6,7-dihydroxoytetrahydronaphthalene and the receptor-site preferred conformation of dopamine—a commentary. *J. Pharm. Pharmac.* **32**: 521–524.

23. Krogsgaard-Larsen, P. (1981) Gamma-aminobutyric acid agonists, antagonists and uptake inhibitors. Design and therapeutic aspects. *J. Med. Chem.* **24**: 1377–1383.

24. Tamura, N., Iwama, T. and Itoh, K. (1992) Synthesis and glutamate-agonistic activity of (S)-2-amino-3-(2,5-dihydro-5-oxo-3-isoxazolyl)-propanoic acid derivatives. *Chem. Pharm. Bull.* **40**: 381–386.

25. Schunack, W. (1973) Histamine analogs with cyclic sidechains. *Arch. Pharm.* **306**: 934–942.

26. Friedman, E., Meller E. and Hallock, M. (1981) Effects of conformationally-constrained analogs of serotonin on its uptake and binding in rat brain. *J. Neurochem.* **36**: 931–937.

27. Horn, A. S. and Snyder, S. H. (1971) Chlorpromazine and dopamine: conformational similarities the correlate with the antischizophrenic activity of phenothiazine drugs. *Proc. Natl. Acad. Sci. USA* **68**: 2325–2328.

28. (a) Fong, T. M., Cascieri, M. A., Yu, H., Bansal, A., Swain, C. and Strader, C. D. (1993) Amino-aromatic interaction between histidine 197 of the neurokinin-1 receptor and CP 96345. *Nature* **362**: 350–353. (b) Gether, U., Yokota, Y., Emonds-Alt, X., Breliere, J. C., Lowe, J. A., III, Snider, R. M., Nakanishi and S., Schwartz, T. W. (1993) Two nonpeptide tachykinin antagonists act through epitopes on corresponding segments of the NK1 and NK2 receptors. *Proc. Natl. Acad. Sci. USA* **90**: 6194–6198.

29. Erickson, J. W. and Fesik, S. W. (1992) Macromolecular X-ray crystallography and NMR as tools for structure-based drug design. *Ann. Rep. Med. Chem.* **27**: 271–290.

30. (a) Veber, D. F. (1979) 'Conformational considerations in the design of somatostatin analogs showing increased metabolic stability'. In Gross, E. and Meienhofer, J. (eds) *Proceedings of the Sixth American Peptide Symposium,* pp. 409–419. Pierce Chemical Co., Rockford, IL. (b) Freidinger, R. M. and Veber, D. F. (1984) Design of novel cyclic hexapeptide somatostatin analogs from a model of the bioactive conformation. In Vida, J. A., Gordon, M. (eds) *Conformationally Directed Drug Design,* pp. 169–187. American Chemical Society, Washington DC.

31. Rivier, J., Brown, M. and Vale, W. (1975) D-Trp⁸-Somatostatin: an analog of somatostatin more potent than the native molecule. *Biochem. Biophys. Res. Commun.* **65**: 746.

32. Rose, G. D., Gierasche, L. M. and Smith, J. A. (1985) Turns in peptides and proteins. *Adv. Protein. Chem.* **37**: 1.

33. Veber, D. F. (1991) Design and discovery in the development of peptide analogs. In Smith J. A. and Rivier, J. E. (eds) *Peptides: Chemistry and Biology. Proceedings of the Twelfth American Peptide Symposium, Escom,* Leiden, pp. 1–14.

34. Sawyer, T. K., Hruby, V. J., Darman, P. S. and Hadley, M. E. (1982) *Proc. Natl. Acad. Sci. USA* **79**: 1751–1755.

35. Schiller, P. W. (1984) In Udenfriend, S. and Meienhofer, J. (eds) *The Peptides: Analysis, Synthesis and*

Biology, vol. 6, pp. 219–68. Academic Press, Orlando.

36. Marshall, G. R., Gorin, F. A. and Moore, M. L. (1978) Peptide conformation and biological activity. In Clarke, F. H. (ed.) *Annual Reports in Medicinal Chemistry*, vol. 13, pp. 227–238. Academic Press, Orlando.

37. Freidinger, R. M., Veber, D. F., Perlow, D. S., Brooks, J. R. and Sapersterin, R. (1980). Bioactive conformation of luteinizing hormone releasing hormone: evidence from a conformationally constrained analog. *Science* **210**: 656–658.

38. Thorsett, E. E. (1986) *Actual. Chim. Ther.* **13**: 257. For a review on use of molecular modeling to design conformationally restricted ACE inhibitors, Hangauer, D. In Perun, T. and Probst, C. (eds) *Computer-Aided Drug Design* p. 253. Marcel Dekker, New York.

39. Flynn, G. A., Giroux, E. L. and Dage, R. C. (1987) *J. Am. Chem. Soc.* **109**: 7914.

40. Rich, D. H. (1989) Peptidase inhibitors. In Hansch, C., Sammes, P. G. and Taylor, J. B. (eds) *Comprehensive Medicinal Chemistry. The Rational Design, Mechanistic Study and Therapeutic Application of Chemical Compounds*, pp. 391–441. Pergamon Press, Oxford.

41. Wiley, R. A. and Rich, D. H. (1993) Peptidomimetics derived from natural products, *Med. Res. Rev.* **13**: 327–384.

42. Kahn, M. (1993) Peptide secondary structure mimetics: recent advances and future challenges. *SynLett* 821–826.

43. (a) Borel, J. F. (1989) Pharmacology of cyclosporine (Sandimmune®). IV. Pharmacological properties in vivo. *Pharmacol. Rev.* **41**: 259. (b) Georgiev, V. St. (1991) Immunomodulating peptides of natural and synthetic origin. *Med. Res. Rev.* **11**: 81. (c) Sigal, N. H., Dumont, F. J. (1993) Immunosuppression. In Paul, W. E. (ed.) *Fundamental Immunology,* 3rd edn. pp. 903–915. Raven Press, New York.

44. Handschumacher, R., Harding, M., Rice, J. and Drugge, R. (1984) Cyclophilin: a specific cytosolic binding protein for cyclosporin A. *Science* **226**: 544–547.

45. (a) Takahashi, N., Hayano, T. and Suzuki, M. (1989) Peptidyl-prolyl cis-trans isomerase is the cyclosporin-A-binding protein cyclophilin. *Nature* **337**: 473. (b) Fischer, G., Wittman-Liebold, B., Lang, K., Kiefhaber, T. and Schmid, F. X. (1989) Cyclophilin and peptidyl-prolyl cis-trans isomerase are probably identical proteins. *Nature* **337**: 476.

46. (a) Fruman, D. A., Klee, C. B., Bierer, B. E. and Burakoff, S. J. (1992) Calcineurin phosphatase activity in T lymphocytesis inhibited by FK506 and cyclosporin A. *Proc. Natl. Acad. Sci. USA* **89**: 3686–3690. (b) Friedman, J. and Weissman, I. (1991) Cytoplasmic candidates for immunophilin action are revealed by affinity for a new cyclophilin—one in the presence and one in the absence of CsA. *Cell* **66**: 799.

47. (a) Schreiber, S. L. and Crabtree, G. R. (1992) The mechanism of action of cyclosporin-A and FK506. *Immunol. Today* **13**: 136–142. (b) O'Keefe, S., Tamura, J., Kincaid, R. L., Tocci, M. J. and O'Neill, E. A. (1992) FK-506-sensitive and CsA-sensitive activation of the interleukin-2 promoter by calcineurin. *Nature* **357**: 692–694.

48. Loosi, H. R., Kessler, H., Oschkinat, H. P., Weber, H. P. and Petcher, T. J. (1985) *Helv. Chem. Acta* **68**: 682.

49. (a) Rich, D. H. and Goodfellow, V.: unpublished data. (b) See also Lee, J. P., Dunlap, B. and Rich, D. H. (1990) Synthesis and immunosuppressive activities of conformationally restricted cyclosporin lactam analogs. *Int. J. Peptide Protein Res.* **35**: 481–494.

50. Fesik, S. W., Gampe, R. T. Jr, Holzman, T. F., Egan, D. A., Edalji, R., Luly, J. R., Simmer, R., Helfrich, R., Kishore, V. and Rich, D. H. (1990) Isotope-edited NMR studies show cyclosporin A has a *trans* 9,10-amide bond when bound to cyclophilin. *Science* **250**: 1406–1409.

51. (a) Fesik, S. W., Gampe, R. T. Jr., Eaton, H. L. *et al.* (1991) NMR-studies of (U-C-13)cyclosporin-A bound to cyclophilin – bound conformation and portions of cyclosporin involved in binding. *Biochemistry* **30**: 6574–6583. (b) Weber, C., Wider, G., von Freyberg, B., Traber, R., Braun, W., Widmer, H. and Wüthrich, K. (1991) The NMR structure of cyclosporine-A bound to cyclophilin in aqueous-solution. *Biochemistry,* **30**: 6563–6574.

52. Kofron, J. L., Kuzmic, P., Kishore, V., Gemmecker, G., Fesik, S. W. and Rich, D. H. (1992) Lithium chloride perturbation of *cis/trans* peptide bond equilibria: effect of conformational equilibria in cyclosporin A and on the time-dependent inhibition of cyclophilin. *J. Am. Chem. Soc.* **114**: 2670–2675.

53. Rich, D. H. (1993) Effect of hydrophobic collapse on enzyme inhibitor interactions. Implications for

the design of peptidomimetics. In Testa, B., Kyburz, E., Fuhrer, W. and Giger, R. (eds) *Medicinal Chemistry 1992 – Proceedings of the XIIth International Symposium on Medicinal Chemistry*, pp. 15–25. Verlag Helvitica Chimica Acta, Basel.

54. (a) Wenger, R. M., France, J., Bovermann, G., Walliser, L., Widmer, A. and Widmer, H. (1994) The 3D structure of a cyclosporine analog in water is nearly identical to the cyclophilin-bound cyclosporine conformation. *FEBS Lett.* **340**: 255–259. (b) Altschuh, D., Vix, O., Rees, B. and Thierry, J. C. (1992) A conformation of cyclosporine-A in aqueous environment revealed by the X-ray structure of a cyclosporine–Fab complex. *Science* **256**: 92–94.

55. Alberg, D. G. and Schrieber, S. G. (1993) Structure-based design of a cyclophilin–calcineurin bridging ligand. *Science* **262**: 248–250.

56. (a) Bohnstedt, A. C., Vara Prasad, J. V. N. and Rich, D. H. (1993) Synthesis of *E*- and *Z*-alkene dipeptide isosteres. *Tetrahedron Lett.* 5217–5220. (b) Spatola, A. (1983) Peptide backbone modifications: a structure–activity analysis of peptides containing amide bond surrogates, conformational constraints, and related backbone replacements. In Weinstein, B. (ed.) *Chemistry and Biochemistry of Amino Acids, Peptides and Proteins*, vol. VII, pp. 267–357. Marcel Dekker, New York.

57. Bohnstedt, A., Flentke, G. F. and Rich, D. H: unpublished data.

58. Mikol, V., Kallen, J., Pflugl, G. and Walkinshaw, M. D. (1993) X-ray structure of a monomeric cyclophilin A–cyclosporin A crystal complex at 2.1 Å resolution. *J. Mol. Biol.* **234**: 1119–1130.

59. Newcomb, L. F. and Gellman, S. H. (1994) Aromatic stacking interactions in aqueous solution: evidence that neither classical hydrophobic effects or classical dispersion forces are important. *J. Am. Chem. Soc.* **116**: 4993–4994.

60. Tsang, K. Y., Diaz, H., Graciani, N. and Kelly, J. W. (1994) Hydrophobic cluster formation is necessary for dibenzofuran-based amino acids to function as β-sheet nucleators. *J. Am. Chem. Soc.* **116**: 3988–4005.

61. (a) Bogusky, M. J., Brady, S. F., Sisko, J. T., Nutt, R. F. and Smith, G. M. (1993) Synthesis and solution conformation of c(D-Trp-D-Cys(SO₃Na)-Pro-D-Val-Leu), a potent endothelin-A receptor antagonist. *Int. J. Peptide Protein Res.* **42**: 194–203. (b) Kemmink, J., van Mierlo, C. P. M., Scheek, R. M. and Creighton, T. E. (1993) Local structure due to an aromatic–amide interaction observed by ¹H-nuclear magnetic resonance spectroscopy in peptides related to the N terminus of bovine pancreatic trypsin inhibitor. *J. Mol. Biol.* **230**: 312–322.

62. (a) Lim, M. S. L., Johnston, E. R. and Kettner, C. A. (1993) The solution conformation of (D)Phe-Pro-containing peptides: implications on the activity of Ac-(D)Phe-Pro-boroArg-OH, a potent thrombin inhibitor. *J. Med. Chem.* **36**: 1831–1838. (b) Vander Velde, D. G., Georg, G. I., Grunewald, G. L., Gunn, C. W. and Mitscher, L. A. (1993) 'Hydrophobic collapse' of taxol and taxotere solution conformations in mixtures of water and organic solvent. *J. Am. Chem. Soc.* **115**: 11650.

63. Ruoslahti, E., Pierschbacher, M. E. (1987) New perspectives in cell adhesion: RGD and integrins. *Science* **238**: 491–497.

64. Dennis, M. K., Henzel, W. J., Pitti, R. M., Lipari, M. T., Napier, M. A., Deisher, T. A., Bunting, S. and Lazarus, R. A. (1990) Platelet glycoprotein IIb-IIIa protein antagonists from snake venom: evidence for a family of platelet-aggregation inhibitors. *Proc. Natl. Acad. Sci. USA* **87**: 2471–2475.

65. Haverstick, D. M., Cowan, J. F., Yamada, K. M. and Santoro, S. A. (1985) Inhibition of platelet adhesion to fibronectin, fibrinogen, and von Willibrand factor substrates by a synthetic tetrapeptide derived from the cell-binding domain of fibronectin. *Blood* **66**: 946–952.

66. Ali, F. E., Bennett, D. B., Calvo, R. R. *et al.* (1994) Conformationally constrained peptides and semipeptides derived from RGD as potent inhibitors of platelet fibrinogen receptor and platelet aggregation. *J. Med. Chem.* **37**: 769–780.

67. Barker, P. L., Bullens, S. and Bunting, S. (1992) Cyclic RGD peptide analogues as antiplatelet antithrombitics. *J. Med. Chem.* **35**: 2040–2048.

68. McDowell, R. S. and Gadek, T. R. (1992) Structural studies of potent constrained RGD peptides. *J. Am. Chem. Soc.* **114**: 9245–9253.

69. McDowell, R. S., Blackburn, B. K. and Gadek, T. R. *et al.* (1994) From peptide to non-peptide. 2. The *de novo* design of potent, non-peptidal inhibitors of platelet aggregation based on a benzodiazepinedione scaffold. *J. Am. Chem. Soc.* **116**: 5077–5083.

70. Bondinell, W. E., Keenan, R. M., Miller, W. H. *et al.* (1994) Design of a potent and orally active nonpeptide platelet fibrinogen receptor (GPIIb/IIIa) antagonist. *Bioorg. Med. Chem.* **2**: 897–908.

21

Stereochemical Aspects of Drug Action II: Optical Isomerism

MIKLÓS SIMONYI and GÁBOR MAKSAY

The layman talks about pairs of shoes.
Please tell when you deal with a racemate!

THE PRACTICE OF MEDICINAL CHEMISTRY
ISBN 0-12-744640-0

I.   INTRODUCTION

Life disfavours symmetry. Just look at a familiar face as it is reflected by the mirror and you immediately recognize that the apparent symmetry of the human body is nothing but a disguise. Life's dislike of symmetry is even more evident at the molecular level. Our body uses D-glucose, L-amino acids and many more molecules chosen discriminatively from the two mirror-image forms of chiral molecules. The advantage of this alertness certainly involves a kind of additional information that chiral molecules possess. A *physical* consequence of this excess information is optical activity (the ability of pure enantiomers to rotate the plane of polarized light), which has served as a fundamental analytical tool of identification for some century and a half; it also paved the way to the foundation of stereochemistry. *Chemical* consequences of chirality include differential recognition, as well as the mark of origin that some molecules display. A classic example of the latter is lactic acid; its dextrorotatory (+) form is produced by glycogenolysis during muscle activity, while laevorotatory (−) lactic acid is a microbial product in sour milk. The *biological* importance of chirality is that — owing to their chiral building blocks — constituents of living cells (proteins, carbohydrates, nucleic acids) are themselves chiral. Therefore, the agent eliciting biological functions is subject to strict structural and spatial requirements. This fact has significant consequences for the action of drugs.

A.   Plane-polarized light

Visible light is regarded as an electromagnetic wave of various wavelengths. The transmittance of normal light does not depend on the position of a refractive surface owing to electric vectors being oriented in all possible planes that contain the direction of the light ray. Scattered or reflected light, however, may have all the electric vectors in a single plane. Such plane-polarized light is obtained experimentally when ordinary light passes through a Nicol prism. Rotation of the prism causes rotation of the plane of polarization. Consequently, if another Nicol prism is placed behind the first and in a position defining the plane of polarization perpendicular to the first, no light will be transmitted by the second prism.*

B.   Optical rotation

The plane of polarized light is rotated by crystals (e.g. quartz) that have mirror image forms that cannot be superimposed on each other.[2] Pasteur found such crystals while working with sodium ammonium tartrate.[3] From the observation that a solution of each type of the crystals produced optical rotation of the same sign as the crystal itself, Pasteur concluded to the existence of nonsuperposable mirror image molecules of tartaric acid, which he called *dissymmetric*. To account for the chemical structure of organic molecules with optical isomers, van't Hoff[4] and Le Bel[5] independently challenged the proposition that these molecules are flat and inferred

---

*This trick is not only used by experimenters in the laboratory. A fraction of sunlight is plane-polarized by collisions with molecules in the atmosphere, and arrives at the earth's surface as if having passed through the first Nicol. Special cells in the compound eyes of certain insects (analogous to the second Nicol) produce a polarized-light pattern identifying the plane of polarization, which serves as a compass cue helping orientation.[1] This is how desert ants find their burrows after having caught prey in the burning heat in a landscape dotted with few landmarks. Honeybees apply the same phenomenon to navigate back to the hive.

tetrahedral orientation for the valencies of the tetravalent carbon atom. Their claim of the *asymmetry* of molecules which contain a carbon atom attached to four different substituents (thereafter termed an *asymmetric centre*) not only gained widespread acceptance but also became the most easily identifiable attribute of molecules of optically active substances. The general term for compounds having optically active form is *chiral*,[6] while an equimolar mixture of the laevorotatory and dextrorotatory *enantiomers* is the optically inactive *racemate*. There is a subtle difference between asymmetric and dissymmetric, as pointed out in the next paragraph.

C. Molecular asymmetry/dissymmetry

The concept of an asymmetric centre, or chiral centre, enabled van't Hoff and Le Bel to predict correctly the number of stereoisomers for compounds containing more than one such centre, as demonstrated by Emil Fischer's experiments[7] on sugars. In order to distinguish optical isomers, Fischer defined D (dextro) and L (laevo) configurations and assigned them to the enantiomers of glyceraldehyde (**I** and **II,** respectively). As proved later, D-glyceraldehyde, by chance,

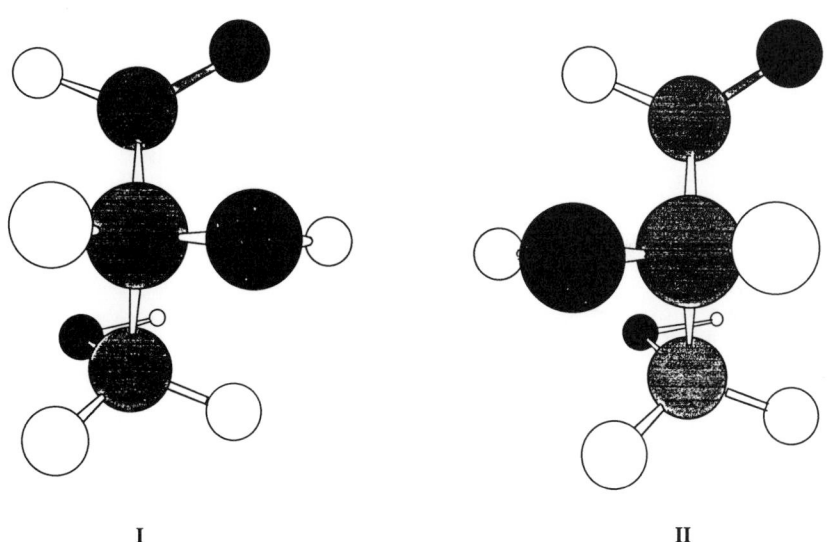

I   II

coincided with the dextrorotatory stereoisomer. A single centre of asymmetry, as in glyceraldehyde, makes the molecule both asymmetric and chiral (nonsuperposable on its mirror image), although in general these properties are not identical. Molecule **III** contains a symmetry axis around which a 180° rotation reproduces the original structure. Thus, the molecule contains a symmetry element, but is still chiral and not identical with its mirror image stereoisomer shown as **IV**. The closely related 1,3-dimethyl-*trans*-cyclobutane is not chiral, however, since it contains a centre of symmetry (**V**).

A further point is that the chiral carbon atom is neither necessary nor sufficient to make the molecule chiral. Structures **VI** and **VII** show a mirror-image pair of chiral molecules lacking any centre of asymmetry. Another example illustrates that chiral carbon atoms can be available in an achiral molecule (**VIII**) *meso*-diepoxybutane has a symmetry plane between carbons 2 and 3, hence the structure is equivalent to its mirror image.

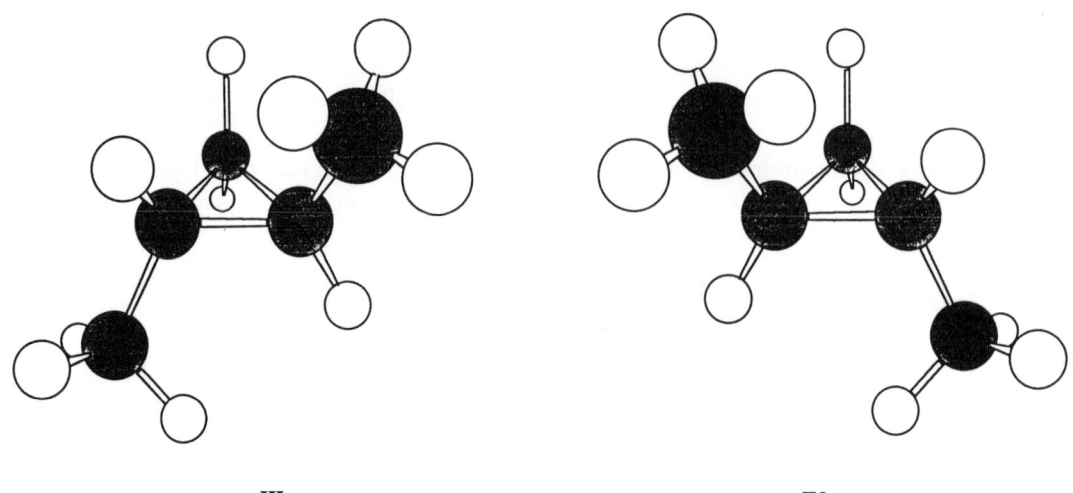

III   IV

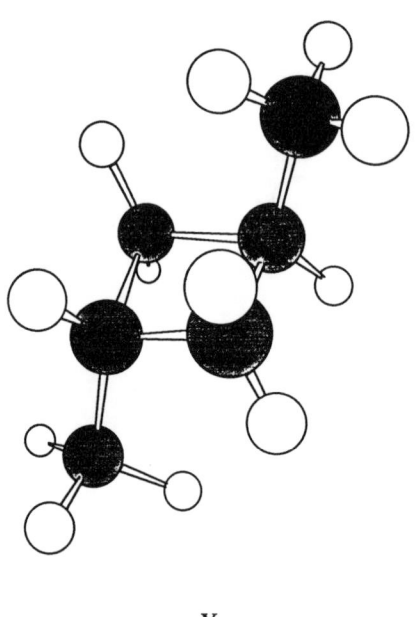

V

Asymmetric molecules lack any symmetry element, so they are chiral. A *dissymmetric* molecule, although still chiral, could have an axis of symmetry, like **III** and **IV**, but lacks the centre (unlike **V**) and the plane of symmetry (present in **VIII**), each of which would make the structure achiral. The application of the concept of chiral centres needs caution, since chirality refers to the overall geometry of the molecule (cf. **VI** and **VIII**). Still, the chiral centre was the basis of the generally accepted stereochemical notation. For molecules with a single chiral carbon atom, it is both useful and correct.

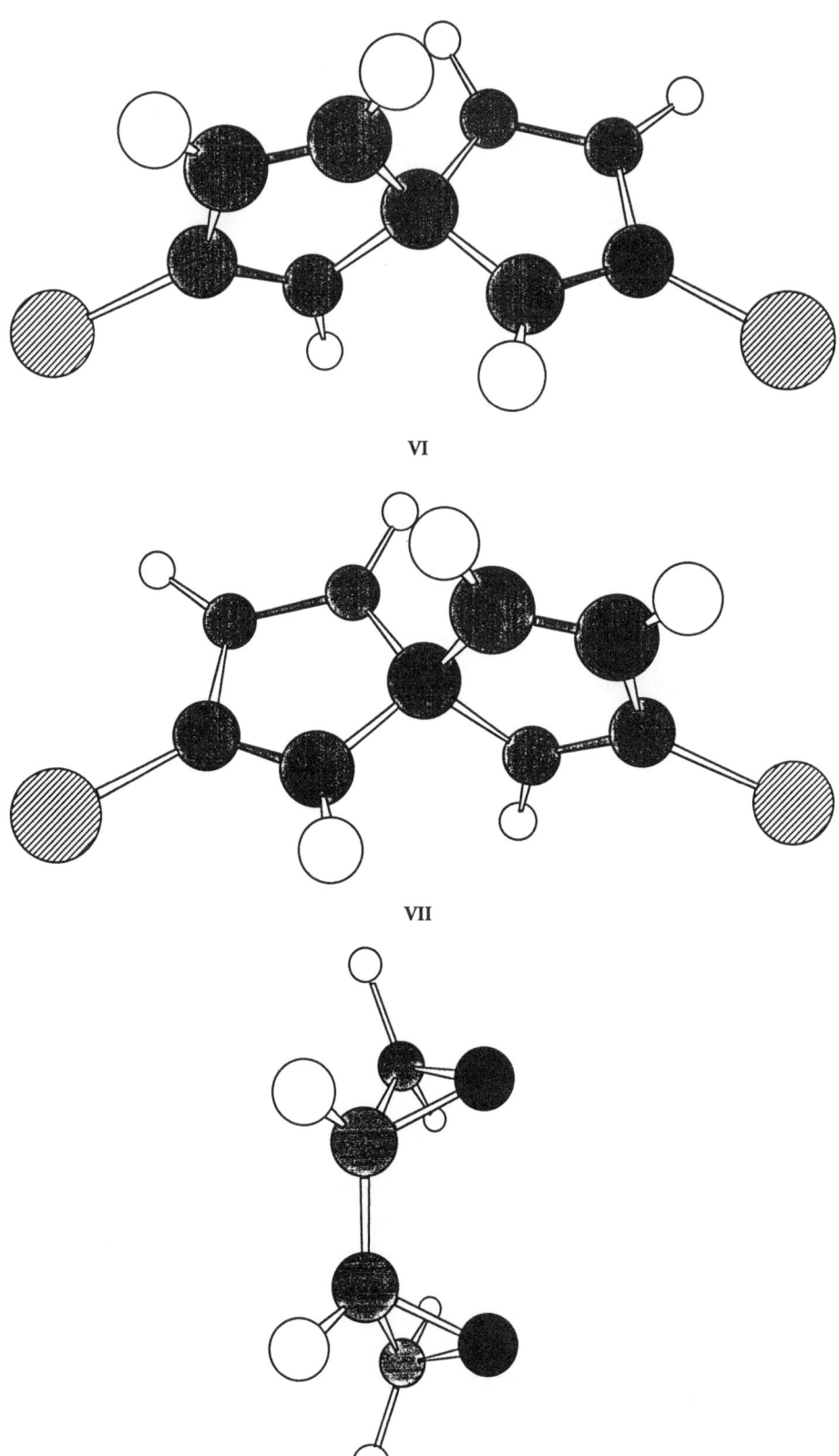

VI

VII

VIII

D. The sequence rule

Since many chiral compounds could not be related to **I** or **II,** a general definition of the absolute configuration was needed. For central asymmetry the *sequence rule* defined by Cahn, Ingold and Prelog (the CIP convention[8,9]) assigns an unequivocal order of priority (*a* > *b* > *d* > *e*) for the four different substituents around the chiral carbon atom. The centre should be viewed in such a way that the group having the lowest priority is placed at the far end from the observer (Fig. 21.1), when the remaining three groups define the direction of decreasing priority tracing either a clockwise or an anticlockwise rotation. If the structure corresponds to a clockwise sequence, the configuration is defined by the prefix (*R*)- (from *rectus*). For structures displaying a priority order corresponding to an anticlockwise sequence, the denomination is (*S*)- (from *sinister*). These prefixes define the absolute configuration of enantiomers. They are universally accepted and applied in chemistry, and IUPAC has adopted them into stereochemical nomenclature.

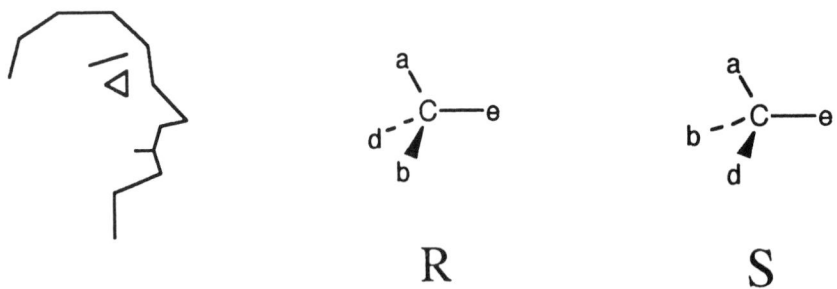

Fig. 21.1   The application of sequence rule (a>b>d>e) to define absolute configuration.

It is to be noted that most natural α-amino acids possess *S* configuration; the only exception is cystein, for which the *R* configuration is dictated by the priority rule. This is part of the reason why the D and L nomenclature is preserved, as established by Emil Fischer.

E. Helical chirality

Right-handed and left-handed helices cannot be superposed. Nonplanar cyclic molecules may be regarded as segments of a helix and, accordingly, they may have two enantiomeric forms. An important case is represented by the asymmetrically fused and substituted seven-membered ring in the family of 1,4-benzodiazepines accommodating two mirror-image conformations. These molecules may not contain any chiral centre, but are still chiral by virtue of the shape in which they exist. The energy barrier that separates the two conformers is usually not so high as to be insurmountable at room temperature, so they interconvert and are present in equal extent. Consequently, their overall assembly is optically inactive, like a racemate. Distinction of the conformers is made on the basis of a characteristic torsion angle by which they differ: the C2–C3–N4–C5 torsion angle in desmethyldiazepam is either negative (**IXa**), or positive (**IXb**). Accordingly, (**IXa**) is denoted by the *M* (minus) and (**IXb**) by the *P* (plus) prefix:

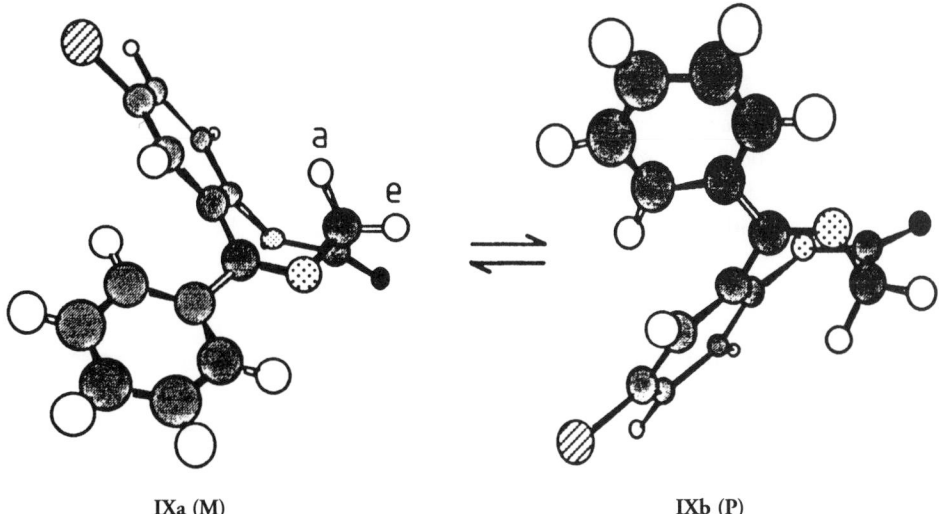

IXa (M)   IXb (P)

F. Discrimination of chiral molecules

In order to rationalize the stereoselective action of enzymes, Emil Fischer hypothesized that a substrate fits the enzyme like a key fits the lock.[10] This assumption explains stereoselectivity provided that the key (substrate) is chiral. A more detailed rationale of the relationship between steric molecular structure and biological activity was given by the idea that three critical points of the substrate have to satisfy the steric requirements of the receptor (enzyme). Easson and Stedman hypothesized[11] the action of noradrenaline to be critically dependent on the correct orientation of the side-chain hydroxyl group. This orientation is only defined if another two points around the hydroxyl-bearing carbon, e.g. the aromatic ring and the nitrogen atom, accommodate defined positions. Easson and Stedman attributed the *correct* orientation only to the R-($-$) stereoisomer (**Xa**); thus, the S-($+$) enantiomer (**Xb**) should be equipotent with dopamine (**Xc**), lacking the critical hydroxyl group. The Easson–Stedman hypothesis was proved to be quite general; it applies to both α_1- and α_2-adrenergic receptors.[12]

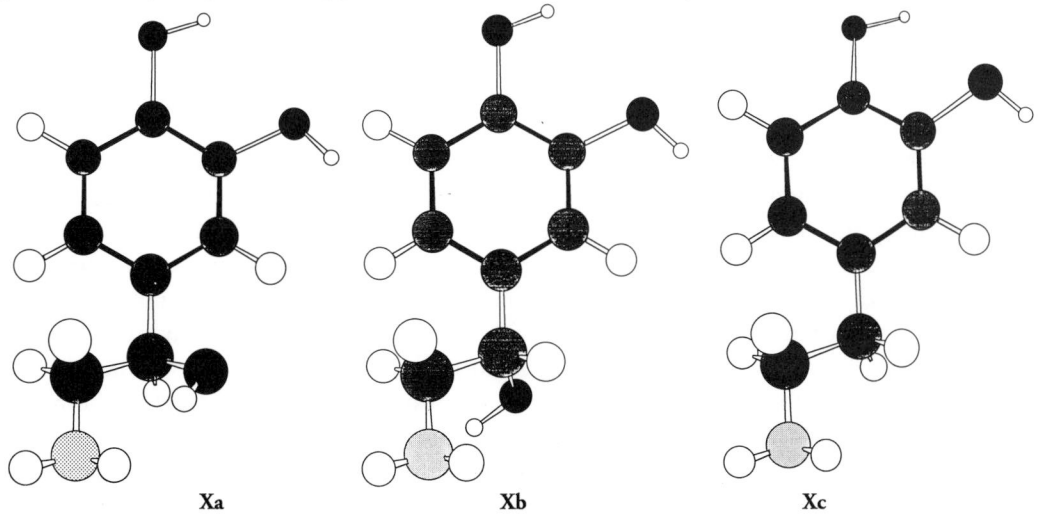

Xa   Xb   Xc

II.   DRUG–RECEPTOR INTERACTIONS

The following overview deals specifically with the stereochemistry of several aspects of drug action which will be described generally in other chapters of this book. This section addresses the key step of the action of chiral drugs on their receptors. Based on the concept of three-point attachment,[11] the initial step is a reversible binding interaction of the drug with its recognition site.

A.   Eudismic-affinity analysis

It was observed by Pfeiffer almost 40 years ago[13] that the lower the effective doses of chiral drugs the greater are the differences in the pharmacological effects of the optical isomers. Lehmann *et al.*[14] used the concept of three-point interaction[11] to find a molecular basis for the intuitive correlation observed by Pfeiffer. They introduced the terms *eutomer* and *distomer* for the more and less active enantiomers, respectively. The logarithm of the ratio of the activities of the eutomer over the distomer was called the *eudismic index* (EI). It was linearly correlated with the logarithm of the potencies of the eutomers in several homologous series of chiral agents. The slope values of several correlations, the *eudismic affinity quotients* (EAQs) were positive, in agreement with Pfeiffer's rule. Eudismic analysis has been extended to stereoisomers having more than one chiral centre.[15] Differences in the slopes (EAQ) of these *epimeric* eudismic-affinity correlations enable quantification of the relative contributions, *criticality*, of chiral centres in stereoselective recognition. The usefulness of eudismic-affinity analysis has been confirmed in several receptor binding studies of the displacing potencies (IC_{50}) of chiral agents on the specific binding of radioligands.

Several violations of Pfeiffer's rule indicate the limitations of eudismic-affinity analysis. Some of the reasons for the deviations from Pfeiffer's rule are conformational flexibility of the agents[16] and improper selection of homologous sets of compounds, as illustrated with agonists and antagonists of muscarinic acetylcholine receptors.[17]

B.   Differences in binding modes

'Wrong-way-binding', i.e. alternative binding modes, were combined with the principle of three-point interaction.[18] The following example will illustrate that even X-ray crystallographic analysis, the ultimate evidence for exact drug–receptor interactions, might be obscured by alternative binding modes. Compound (**XI**) is an antiviral agent which inhibits viral replication by preventing uncoating of certain viruses. X-ray analysis revealed that it fits along a hydrophobic canyon (pocket) of a viral protein and causes a conformational change upon binding.[19] Methylation (see the arrow to **XI**) enhanced the antiviral activity of the eutomer 20 times, while that of the distomer did not change. However, a subsequent X-ray study revealed that the methyl derivative was preferentially fitted along the binding pocket in the opposite direction.[20] That is, the effect of methyl substitution cannot be directly related to the parent compound and stereoselectivity reflects chiral discrimination at the other end of the binding pocket. Further, the removal of two methylene units from the alkyl spacer in (**XI**) returned the original orientation in binding.[20] Consequently, the binding pocket is sterically limited and the substituents and the relative distance of the similar oxazoline and isoxazole rings will determine the preferred orientation in binding. This example shows that minor structural modifications such as methyl substitution or changes in chain length might change receptor fitting and obscure eudismic-activity analysis.

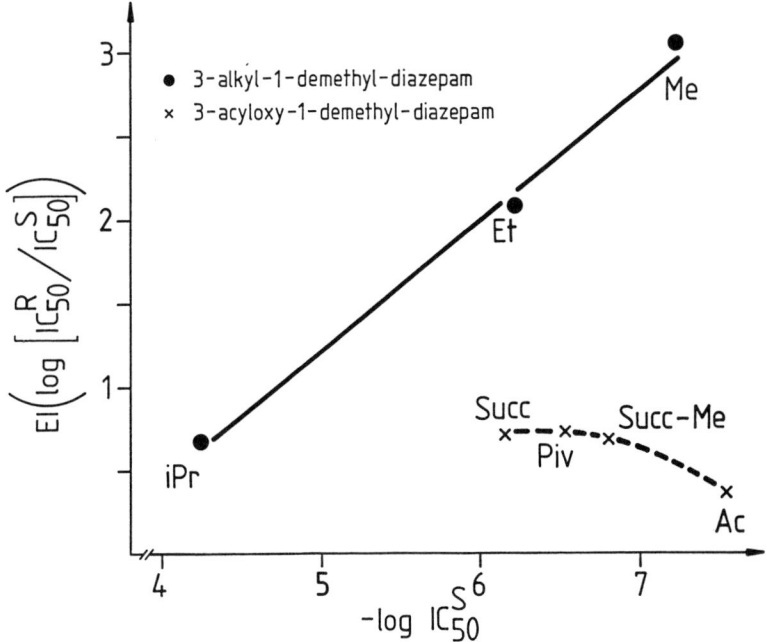

XI

Another example illustrates how can we interpret the results of eudismic-affinity analysis. One of the well-known 1,4-benzodiazepine anxiolytic drugs, desmethyldiazepam (compound (**IX**)) displays helical (i.e. conformational) chirality. It exists with concave and convex boat conformations of the diazepine ring (**IXa,b**). Its 3-alkyl and 3-acyloxy derivatives also possess central chirality. Eudismic-affinity analysis was performed on the displacing potencies of these stereoisomers for the benzodiazepine binding sites of the GABA receptor–chloride ionophore complex.[21] Figure 21.2 shows that while Pfeiffer's rule is violated by the 3-acyloxy derivatives (i.e. acetate, pivaloate, hemisuccinate and methylsuccinate esters), it is obeyed by 3-alkyl ones. That is, increasing the size of the 3-alkyl group up to isopropyl decreases displacing potencies of the (3*S*) alkyl eutomers and binding stereoselectivity simultaneously. The (3*S*) eutomer exists

Fig. 21.2   Eudismic-affinity correlations of benzodiazepine receptor binding.

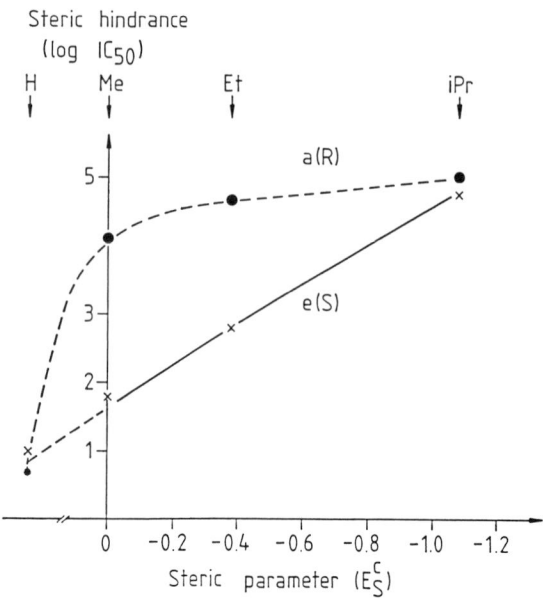

Fig. 21.3 Steric susceptibilities of axial and equatorial directions of the 3-alkyl substituents of 1-desmethyldiazepam (**IX**) for benzodiazepine receptor binding.

predominantly in its binding conformation M (**IXa**), whereas its 3-substituent is oriented in the favourable equatorial direction. The (3R) alkyl derivative is the distomer because it is hardly available in the binding conformation M where its alkyl group must accommodate to the strained pseudoaxial (*endo*) direction (see a in (**IXa**)). Consequently, the equatorial (e) and axial (a) orientations of bound 3-alkyl substituents can be assigned to the (3S) and (3R) stereoisomers, respectively. Displacing potencies are plotted in Fig. 21.3 as a function of the steric parameter E_S^c of Hancock for the alkyl groups. The curves reveal different steric susceptibilities for the equatorial versus axial orientations of 3-alkyl groups in binding of the (3S) and (3R) stereoisomers, respectively. It suggests a 'ceiling' of the receptor cavity, which hinders fitting of axial 3-alkyl substituents more than equatorial ones. Stereoselectivity is maximal for 3-methyl derivatives. It should be mentioned that equatorial and axial N-alkyl substituted atropine derivatives displayed a profile of steric hindrance similar to Fig. 21.3 for acetylcholine receptors of guinea-pig gut.[22]

The different eudismic-affinity correlation for the 3-acyloxy derivatives (Fig. 21.2) can be explained by different interactions of the carbonyloxy groups. Steric hindrance of the 3-acyloxy groups is attenuated by a binding contribution of the carbonyloxy groups. Since binding is stronger for axial 3-carbonyloxy groups, stereoselectivity declines towards the acetic esters (Ac in Fig. 21.2). The different types of binding interactions are associated with different pharmacological efficacies. The 3-acyloxy derivatives antagonized the anticonvulsant effects of benzodiazepine full agonists. Further, the (3R) distomers displayed not only lower potencies but also less agonist efficacies. There are several drugs and herbicides whose eutomers are full agonists, while the distomers are partial agonists or antagonists.[22]

The general conclusions from the example of 1,4-benzodiazepines are that (1) central chirality may often affect the binding interaction via conformational changes (i.e. helical chirality) of the ligand and (2) structural variations even within a restricted set of compounds can elicit quantitative and qualitative differences, i.e. differences in potency and efficacy, respectively, and in the binding interactions (steric hindrance for alkyl groups versus binding for carbonyloxy groups).

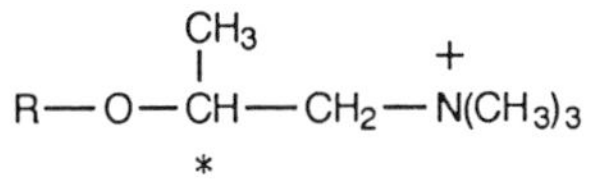

XII 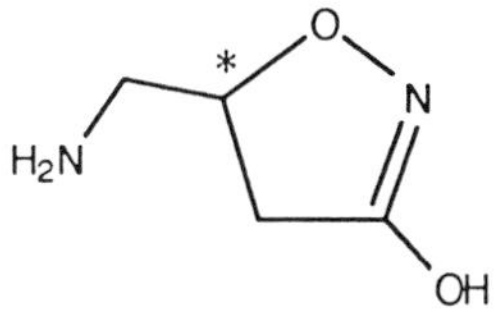   XIII

The differences in the binding modes of agonists and antagonists can be exploited in the design of selective antagonists. The attachment of proper ring systems to the agonists often leads to preferential interaction of the ligands with hydrophobic accessory sites.[22] This might decrease the importance of a chiral centre critical for agonist binding and activity. It thus leads to decreased stereoselectivity such as for the anticholinergic benzoyl esters of methylcholine (**XII**) enantiomers.[22] Analogously, receptor binding of [^{3}H]SR 95531, an arylpyridazinyl GABA$_A$ antagonist can be displaced by dihydromuscimol enantiomers (**XIII**) with lower stereoselectivity than the binding of the agonist [^{3}H]muscimol.[23] Different binding modes of agonists and antagonists are associated with different conformations, i.e. agonist and antagonist states, respectively, of their receptors. The next part will deal with conformational changes of receptors and their interactions with chiral agents.

C.   Interactions with different receptor conformations

The local anaesthetic RAC-109 (**XIV**) is a sodium channel blocker. In the resting state of the channels its blocking effect is not stereoselective. During repetitive depolarization and channel opening, the blocking potency of (−)-RAC-109, and hence the stereoselectivity, increases by more than one order of magnitude.[24] According to the modulated receptor hypothesis, stereoselectivity can be attributed to different conformations of the anaesthetic binding site corresponding to resting, activated and inactivated (desensitized) states of the sodium channels.[25] Eudismic-affinity analysis revealed that Pfeiffer's rule can be extended to several such cases. The affinities and stereoselectivities of methacholine enantiomers (R = acetyl in (**XII**) to low, high and super-high affinity states of muscarinic receptors of rat brain increased in this order.[26]

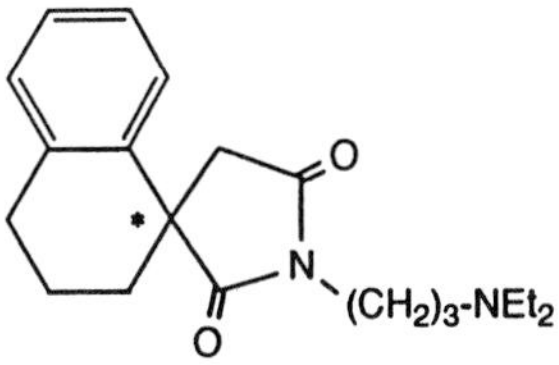

XIV 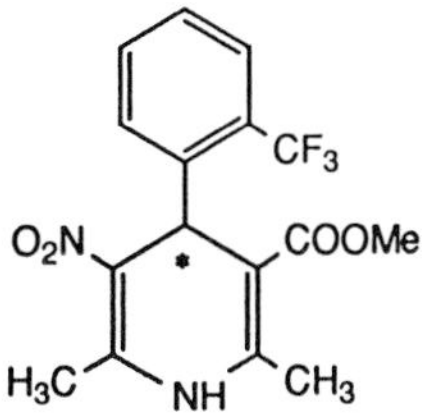   XV 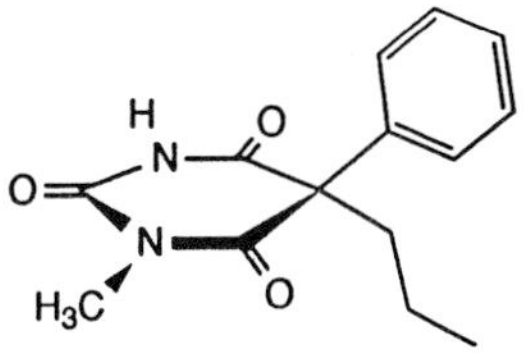   XVI

The stereoselectivity of action can be quantitative as well as qualitative. The (S) and (R) enantiomers of 1,4-dihydropyridines such as Bay K 8644 (**XV**) are activators and antagonists, respectively, at sodium[27] and L-type calcium channels.[28] The $^{36}Cl^-$ flux through GABA receptor-regulated chloride ionophores was blocked and facilitated by the convulsant (S) (+) and central depressant (R)-(−) enantiomers, respectively, of N-methyl-5-phenyl-5-propylbarbituric acid (**XVI**).[29] The binding sites of bicyclic cage convulsants such as t-butylbicyclo-phosphorothionate (TBPS) are coupled to the chloride ionophores, and different states of the ionophores are associated with different rates of [^{35}S]TBPS dissociation. The (R)-(−) enantiomer (**XVI**) elicited about ten times faster dissociation of [^{35}S]TBPS than the channel blocking (S)-(+) enantiomer.[30] The displacing potency of the eutomer, and hence the stereoselectivity, was increased by GABA (i.e. open ionophores).[31] On the other hand, desensitization of the chloride ionophores eliminated the stereoselectivity of the enantiomers of the GABA$_A$ agonist dihydromuscimol (**XIII**) to elicit $^{36}Cl^-$ flux.[32]

In summary, different channel states — closed, open and desensitized — are associated with different conformations and steric requirements of the binding sites. However, it cannot be excluded that the above enantiomers act at different sites of the same receptors.

D. Interactions with different receptors

There are promiscuous chiral agents which act on different receptors.[33] If these distinct biochemical entities share structural and functional similarities, they can be called *isoreceptors*. Eudismic-affinity analysis can also be extended to isoreceptors of different organs and species, such as for the effect and binding of methacholine enantiomers (**XII**) to muscarinic receptors of guinea-pig ileum and rat brain.[33,34] Eudismic-affinity correlations might also be used for further classification of receptor subtypes. Kappa-type opiate receptors can be selectively labelled by the benzeneacetamido agonist [^{3}H]U-69593. The stereoisomeric pairs of levorphanol–dextrorphan as well as (+)- and (−)-ethylketocyclazocine were used to displace [^{3}H]U-69593 binding to opiate receptors of guinea-pig, rat and frog brain.[35] High stereoselectivities were associated with κ_1 receptors in guinea-pig and rat brain, while low stereoselectivities might be attributed to κ_2 opiate receptors predominant in frog brain.[35]

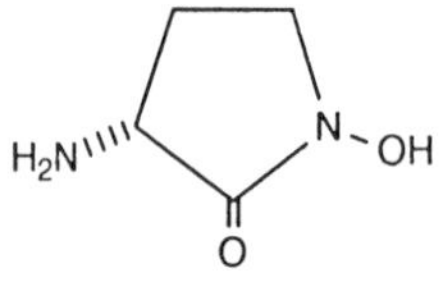

XVII 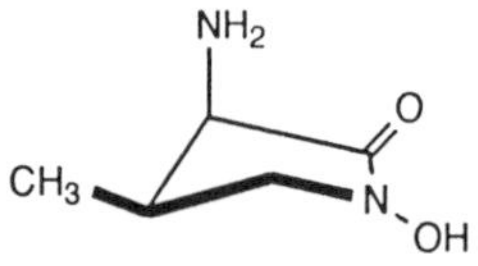   XVIII 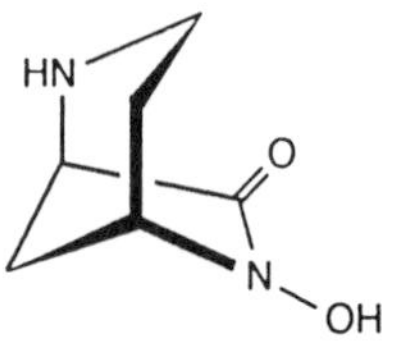   XIX

Finally, chiral agents might interact with entirely different receptors as well. (3R)-(+)-HA-966 (**XVII**) is a partial agonist at the glycine site of the N-methyl-D-aspartate-type glutamate receptors, while (3S)-HA-966 is a γ-butyrolactone-like sedative.[36] The activity of (3R)-HA-966 has been attributed to the less favoured, quasiaxial, orientation of the amino group. The binding conformation of (**XVII**) was confirmed by the increased activities of the cis-(4R)-methyl derivative (**XVIII**) and the constrained bicyclic analogue (**XIX**).[37]

The molecular action of drugs has been considered in this section according to their reversible interactions at relevant receptor sites of the living organism. It has been emphasized that the interactions of optical isomers of chiral agents are essentially different. These differences have been attributed to differences in (1) the configuration and conformation of the stereoisomers; (2) the binding modes of the stereoisomers; (3) receptor conformations elicited by the stereoisomers or by other factors; and (4) biochemically distinct sites of action.

III.   PRACTICAL ASPECTS

Apart from receptor binding, there are several practical aspects which need stereochemical consideration. The stereochemistry of drug metabolism will be considered first. Then catalytic antibodies will be described which can be used in chiral syntheses of medicinal agents. The application of chiral affinity labels will be also mentioned which can be used for the characterization of receptors.

Distinction of the enantiomers requires special chromatographic methods. Indeed, realization of enantiomeric effects became important and widely accepted only after adequate analytical methods had been developed. Now these are available in a wide variety, but are not always used, especially for pharmacological purposes. Nonselective analytical techniques decrease the value of pharmacokinetic studies because the sum of concentrations of the stereoisomers does not allow insight into their individual kinetic properties. Finally, the abundance of racemates on the drug market induced health authorities concerned with drug registration to impose enantiospecific tests of the individual enantiomers upon the process of drug development. These aspects will be dealt with in this section.

A.   Drug metabolism

The huge number of stereoselective reactions of endogenous compounds described in biochemistry textbooks is obviously beyond the scope of this chapter. As to exogenous compounds, especially drugs, enzymatic transformations of xenobiotics (catabolism) will be described in Part VI in general. It should be mentioned here that living organisms attempt to respond to the attack of xenobiotics with a great variety of nonspecific isoenzymes (e.g. hydrolases). The stereoselectivities of these enzymes are usually low owing to the low affinity of nonspecific binding, according to Pfeiffer's rule. Various biotransformations are catalysed by several isoenzymes of overlapping substrate specificities. Consequently, the sign and extent of stereoselectivities may differ among species and organs. For example, hydrolysis of the acetic ester of the anxiolytic 1,4-benzodiazepine oxazepam (the 3-hydroxyl derivative of **IX**) showed opposite stereoselectivities in brain and liver of various species, favouring the (*S*) and (*R*) enantiomers, respectively.[38] Low substrate and product stereoselectivities of cytochrome P-450-catalysed hydroxylations can be explained by these enzymes being selective for O_2 rather than for xenobiotics. In different species, opposite stereoselectivities have also often been found also for desalkylation, glucuronide conjugation, and so on, as summarized in a comprehensive review.[39] However, the dominant contribution of unique enzymatic reactions might lead to stereocontrolled reactions such as the unidirectional metabolic inversion of the enantiomers of the nonsteroidal anti-inflammatory 2-arylpropionic acids.[39–41] For examples, ibuprofen is esterified with coenzyme A by acyl-CoA synthetase, which is specific for the (*R*) acids.[40] The reactive ester is reversibly inverted by a racemase to the ester of the (S) acids and finally (S) acids are liberated by hydrolases. Racemic 2-arylpropionic acids can be thus transformed into the active (S) enantiomer, which is the anti-inflammatory drug. However, the (R) enantiomer can be considered not only as a prodrug but also a source of toxicity. (R) acids will be incorporated into hybrid triglycerides via CoA leading to a stereoselective delayed storage in adipose tissue.[41] Interestingly, the eutomers of α-phenoxypropionic acid herbicides are isosteric with the eutomers of the anti-inflammatory drugs and the distomer antagonizes herbicidal activity.[22,41] Generally, various pharmacokinetic phases might contribute to the overall stereoselectivity of drug action.

B. Catalytic antibodies

Medicinal chemists can utilize not only enzymes but also antibodies as catalysts. Catalytic antibodies can surpass catabolic enzymes in terms of versatility and stereoselectivity. This practice has been based on considerations of the transition state of enzymatic catalysis and of monoclonal antibodies. Based on the mechanism and the transition state of a reaction, one can design a transition-state analogue. We can use it as a hapten, couple it to a carrier protein, and raise monoclonal antibodies against this antigen. Some of the antibodies might catalyse the corresponding reaction like enzymes. That is why they are also called *abzymes*, by fusion with the abbreviation of antibody. Generally, the more a reaction is accelerated, the stronger the binding of its transition state will be to the enzyme/abzyme. Rate accelerations of 6×10^6 have been reached in ester hydrolysis.

The conversion of chorismate (**XXI**) into prephenate (**XXIII**) is an example of a Claisen rearrangement, a key step in the microbial biosynthesis of aromatic amino acids. Compound **XX** inhibits the rearrangement on Scheme 21.1 because it mimics the transition state **XXII**.[42] An antibody against a protein adduct (R) of hapten (**XX**) accelerated the rearrangement of (−)-chorismate (but not of its (+) stereoisomer) by more than two orders of magnitude.[42] This example might be the prototype of shape-selective, concerted reactions such as the Diels–Alder cyclization.

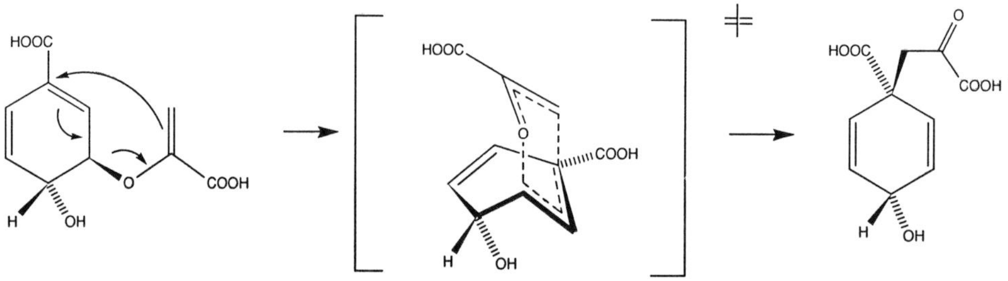

Scheme 21.1

Another example is the lipase activity of abzymes.[43] Lipases have been used as transesterification catalysts for stereoselective acylation and kinetic resolution of alcohols. The phosphonate group of antigen (**XXIV**) imparts the oxyanionic and tetrahedral features of the transition state (**XXV**) for ester hydrolysis. The antibodies against racemic (**XXIV**) were isolated and they catalysed exclusively the hydrolysis of either (*R*) or (*S*) esters (**XXV**) with great (10^3–10^5)

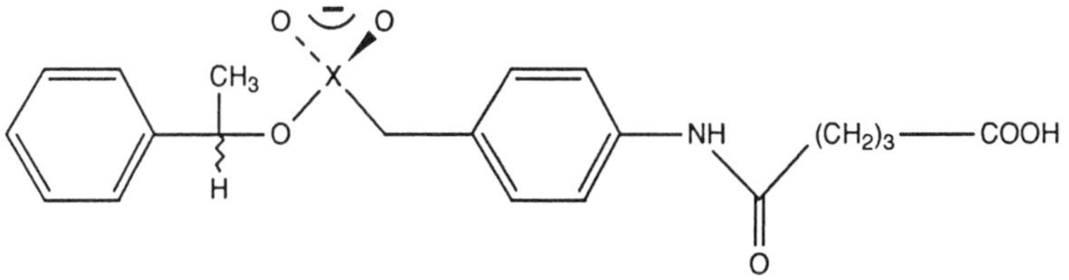

XXIV:	X = P
XXV:	X = C

accelerations.[43] Abzymes will undoubtedly facilitate stereocontrolled medicinal syntheses, such as the induction of catabolic enzymes that has been increasingly used to modulate the pharmacokinetics of drugs.

C.   Affinity labelling of receptors

Reactive groups have often been used in rational medicinal chemistry. The design of prodrugs addresses metabolic enzymes prior to the interaction with their sites of action. However, sometimes reactive derivatives are planned to modify directly the site of action or incorporate into it. These reactive derivatives may serve methodical goals in characterizing the biochemical properties of their receptors.

High-affinity reversible ligands of receptor proteins are often substituted with electrophylic groups such as isothiocyanate, which, upon binding to their receptors, might acylate a surrounding nucleophilic amino acid residue. (+)-(**XXVI**) is 100 times more potent than its (−) distomer in an antinociceptive hot-plate test. The isothiocyanate derivative (**XXVI**) was the first enantiomeric irreversible ligand of δ opioid receptors.[44] It should be noted that methyl substitution in position 3 created two chiral centres simultaneously in the symmetric parent compound. Consequently, it helped to elucidate the preferred conformation of the piperidine

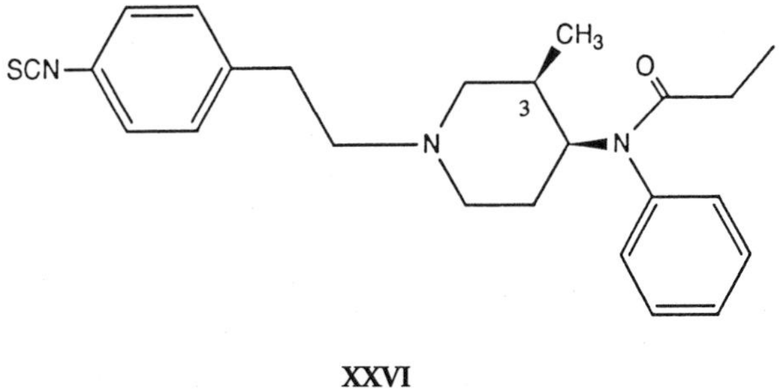

XXVI

ring in receptor binding. (+)-(**XXVI**) behaved as a partial agonist to inhibit the activity of adenylate cyclase coupled to δ opiate receptors. The distomer was 100 times less potent.[44] Such irreversible ligands can be used in radiolabelled form for the affinity labelling and isolation of receptors.

D.   Chromatographic methods

The state-of-the-art method for simultaneous determination of drug enantiomers is chromatography owing to its high sensitivity and resolving ability.[45] The 1980s onwards saw an enormous development of both liquid chromatographic instrumentation and chiral stationary phases (CSPs) on which direct chromatographic resolution of mixtures of enantiomers became possible. The idea behind the design of CSPs is to provide at least three points of interaction between the stationary phase and one of the enantiomers, with minimum of one of these interactions being stereochemically defined.[46] This is a concept closely resembling the Easson–Stedman hypothesis.[11] Although no single CSP could be expected to resolve all possible kinds of racemates, the wide variety of commercially available CSPs offer a good choice for a given problem.[47] As well as enantiomer separation leading to the determination of enantiomeric purity, the order of chromatographic elution correlates consistently with the absolute configuration within groups of related compounds, so absolute configurations can also be determined by chromatography.[48] Synthetic CSPs include helical (+)-poly(triphenymethyl methacrylate), the optical purity of which arises from the single 'propeller' structure.[49] Excellent

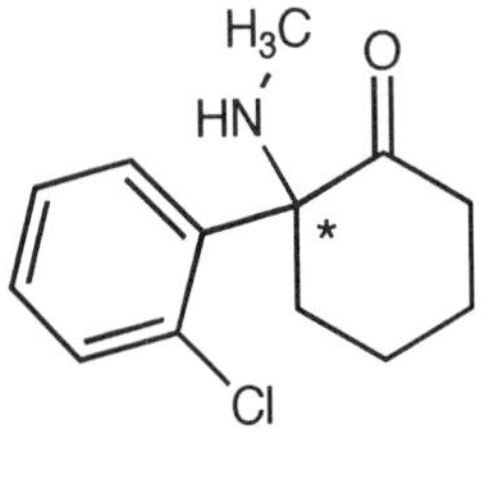

XXVII 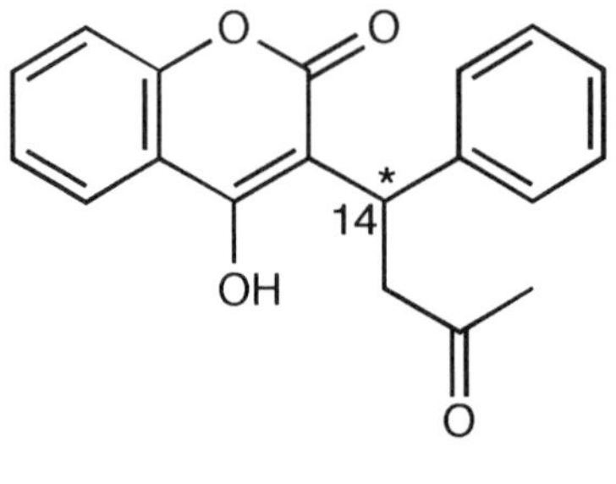   **XXVIII**

CSPs can also be obtained from natural polymers. Preparative resolution of *rac*-ketamine (**XXVII**) can be achieved on microcrystalline cellulose triacetate.[50] Cellulose tris(phenylcarbamate) was used to resolve racemic [^{14}C]warfarin (**XXVIII**) into radiolabelled enantiomers.[51] Proteins contain chiral binding sites that are highly specific even in solution. Thus, immobilized proteins could be effective CSPs. A bovine serum albumin-based HPLC column provided excellent resolution[52] for chiral sulfoxides such as **XXIX**.

Immobilized human serum albumin (HSA) can also be used for enantiomer separation, with the additional advantage of providing therapeutically relevant information. HSA contains two main binding sites allosterically coupled to each other in certain cases when two different drugs are used simultaneously[53] in the eluent. The enantioselectivity of these sites might be increased by the allosteric effect. This ligand-induced stereoselectivity is useful for the separation of

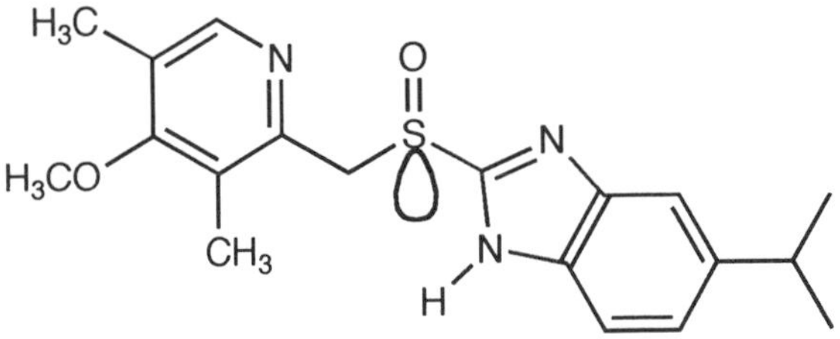

XXIX

certain racemates that otherwise would not be resolved by the same CSF.[54] Thus, the (*S*) enantiomer of warfarin (**XXX**) induces an efficient separation of lorazepam methyl ether (**XXXI**) enantiomers, which cannot be separated by the unmodified HSA column.

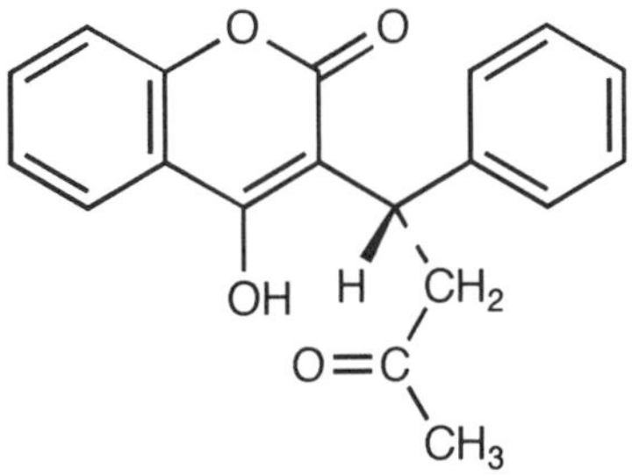

XXX

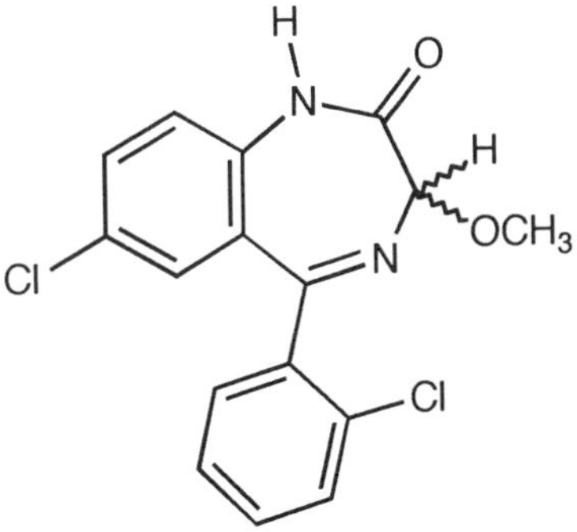

XXXI

A further protein component of human blood, α_1-acid glycoprotein, provides excellent separation for stereoisomers of vinca alkaloid analogues.[55]

Another version of enantioselective chromatography is achieved by enantiomerically pure mobile-phase additives. Cyclodextrins are known to form inclusion complexes[56] and the chiral cyclic oligosaccharide discriminates between barbiturate enantiomers. Resolution of the complexes could be achieved on standard reversed-phase HPLC columns.[57] The same technique has recently been developed for the capillary electrophoretic separation of ionic solutes.[58] Owing to the efficiency of the discrimination provided by cyclodextrin, CSPs were prepared[59] by linking cyclodextrin molecules to silica gel. Such a phase was used for the determination[60] of the composition of commercial cyclothiazide (**XXXII**), a marketed diuretic. It was shown that the drug is a mixture of *eight* stereoisomers in the form of four racemates.[60]

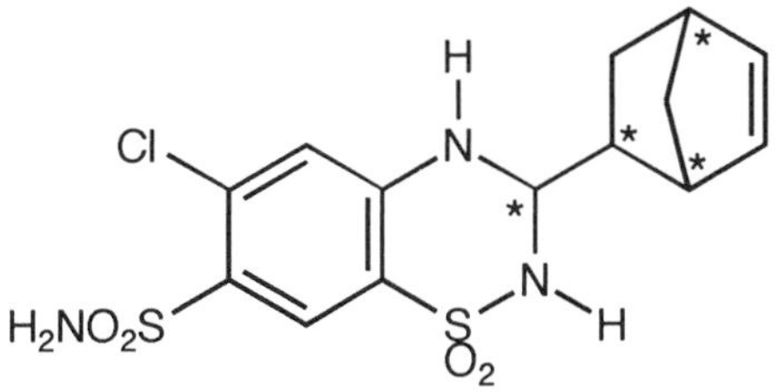

XXXII

Enantiomeric amino acids,[61] and proteins[62] have also been used as chiral additives to the chromatographic mobile phase, providing separation through enantioselective association.

The third version of the chromatographic separation of optical isomers applies chiral derivatization of the sample. Highly reactive enantiomerically pure reagents convert enantiomers of the solute into diastereoisomers that can be separated under ordinary chromatographic conditions. One such reagent is 2,3,4,6-tetra-*O*-acetyl-β-*D*-glucopyranosyl isothiocyanate (TAGIT), which reacts selectively with primary or secondary amino groups to yield thiourea derivatives. This method was successfully applied to the separation of racemic amino alcohols.[63]

E.   Pharmacokinetics

The direct importance of stereochemical factors in pharmacokinetics arises mainly from stereoselective metabolism, or elimination, as shown, for example, for propranolol,[64,65] or acenocoumarol.[66] Examples indicating enantioselective transport are rare, though not entirely absent. A recent study suggested a permeation rate of *laevo*-norgestrel across buccal and vaginal membranes almost twice as great as that of the *dextro*-enantiomer, while the two enantiomers were not discriminated by nasal or rectal membranes.[67]

An indirect, but more general, relevance stems from the realization that any confusion related to the identity of drug substances falls back to the medicinal chemist in the multidisciplinary venture of drug development. True enough, the chemist is trained to identify optical isomers, and *has* to warn the pharmacologist when racemates are involved. So any pharmacokinetic study led by specialists of medical background that applies nonstereospecific analytical methods results in the cumulative measurement of the optical isomers; the charge of *nonsense*[68] can be traced back to the general neglect of stereochemical notation (e.g. *rac-*) for racemic drugs.

A telling example[69] is given here in order to represent the problem. The oral anticoagulant warfarin is prone to altered biological effect elicited by a second drug. In a clinical study the uricosuric sulfinpyrazone (**XXXIII**) was tested for such a drug interaction. Volunteers were given this drug daily for a period of 15 days, and on day 4 they received a single oral dose of racemic warfarin. Subsequently, prothrombin time (the biological response) was measured together with analysis of warfarin level in blood plasma. Simultaneous administration of warfarin and sulfinpyrazone always produced enhanced anticoagulant effect, as compared to

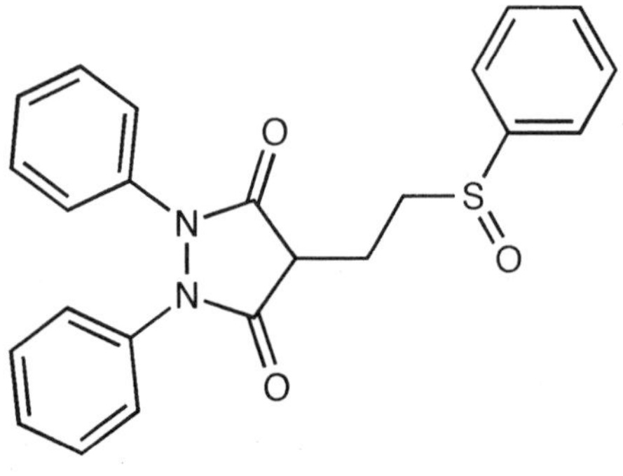

XXXIII

Table 21.1   Clinical study of the elimination half-life of warfarin.[69]

	Warfarin elimination $t_{1/2}$ (h)					
	Racemic		(R)		(S)	
	Alone	With (XXXIII)	Alone	With (XXXIII)	Alone	With (XXXIII)
Subject 1	32	44	46	18	38	49
Subject 2	65	41	87	49	25	58

warfarin administration alone. The elimination of warfarin from blood in two subjects was as shown in Table 21.1

Concentrating on the differences of elimination half-lives between the two regimes of administration, it is seen from Table 21.1 that the increased anticoagulant effect of warfarin in the presence of sulfinpyrazone is associated with a slower elimination rate, and hence increased level of total warfarin in the plasma of subject 1. The case of subject 2, however, appears to be rather confusing, because the faster elimination, and hence lower total warfarin plasma level, in the presence of sulfinpyrazone contradicts the observed higher anticoagulant effect. Enantiospecific analysis, however, explains the phenomenon, since most of the biological effect resides in (S)-warfarin (XXX), the elimination of which was slower in both subjects when sulfinpyrazone was administered simultaneously.[69] The increased elimination of (R)-warfarin confounding the interpretation arose from the stereoselective displacement by sulfinpyrazone from plasma protein binding sites[70] that showed individual variation.

Plasma protein binding can also be a source of confusion. The binding of acenocoumarol was found to represent inverse stereoselectivity to plasma protein components, indicating that the overall lack of enantioselectivity might be the result of selective molecular events of opposite sign.[71]

F.   Drug registration

In view of the implications of stereochemistry in drug action, regulatory agencies have started to update their requirements for enantiomeric and racemic drugs.[72] These concern the whole registration documentation, from analytical techniques through preclinical research to clinical trials. Although national offices may apply different measures to the problem, the general trend is that the development of a racemic drug will be an increasingly costly venture, since racemic and enantiomeric effects should be presented together. For enantiomerically pure drug applications the additional requirement will be to demonstrate enantiomeric stability. These growing burdens make at least understandable the man who declared: 'I shall now ban the synthesis of all chiral compounds in my laboratory for the future'.[73] Since nearly 50% of drugs currently on the market are chiral, such a standpoint is not a practical solution. As pointed out in Section II.B, in the design of antagonists from chiral agonists the chiral centre might become noncritical.[22] It can even be removed without a significant loss of activity, thus reducing the costs of drug development, as applied to a partial muscarinic agonist.[74]

Regulatory requirements have become even more severe ever since the thalidomide tragedy of the 1960s. Later studies revealed much higher acute toxicity for the thalidomide enantiomers than for the racemate.[75] Teratogenicity of the racemate, however, was found to be more than twice as large as that of either of the enantiomers.[75,76,77] So health authorities are justified in imposing detailed tests of stereochemical nature upon drug companies. These, however inevitably extend the gap between the medicinal chemistry laboratory and the pharmacist's counter.

IV. CONCLUSIONS

Drug molecules should always be envisaged in space in order to realize their optical isomerism of central or helical origin.

The activity of drugs is often, though not always, proportional to their stereoselectivity, as predicted by Pfeiffer's rule.

Structural and steric changes within a set of medicinal agents lead to quantitative and qualitative differences in their modes of receptor binding. The quantitative differences manifest in different efficacies of the stereoisomers (e.g. the distomer is an antagonist), while qualitative differences might be associated with a different spectrum of efficacies.

Different factors (modulatory ligands, functional states of receptors) leading to different receptor conformations also affect the stereoselectivity of drug action.

A wide range of chromatographic methods are available for both analytical and preparative separation of enantiomers.

Neglect of explicit indication of racemic composition and of enantioselective analytical techniques is the source of devalued conclusions in pharmacokinetic studies.

Owing to stereochemical implications in drug action, the development of chiral drugs is faced with additional regulatory requirements.

REFERENCES

1. Long, M. E. (1991) Secrets of animal navigation. *Natl. Geographic* **179**: 70–99.
2. Herschel, J. F. W. (1821) *Trans. Cambridge Phil. Soc.* **1**: 43.
3. Pasteur, L. (1848) *Ann. Chim. Phys.* **24**: 442.
4. van't Hoff, J. H. (1874) Voorsteil tot uitbreiding der tegenwoordig in de scheikunde gebruikte structuur-formules in de ruimte: benevens een daarmee samenhangende opmerking omtrent het verband tusschen optisch actief vermogen en chemische constitutie van organische verbingingen. *Arch. Neéland Sci. Exact Nat.* **9**: 445.
5. Le Bel, J. A. (1874) *Bull Soc. Chim. France* **22**: 337.
6. Lord Kelvin (1904) *Baltimore Lectures,* pp 618–619. Clay, London.
7. Fischer, E. (1894) *Chem. Ber.* **27**, 2985.
8. Cahn, R. S. and Ingold, C. K. (1951) Specification of configuration about quadricovalent asymmetric atoms. *J. Chem. Soc.* 612–622.
9. Cahn, R. S., Ingold, C. K. and Prelog, V. (1966) Specification of molecular chirality. *Angew. Chem. Int. Ed. Engl.* **5**: 385–415.
10. Fischer, E. (1894) Einfluss der Konfiguration auf die Wirkung der Enzyme. *Berichte* **27**: 2985–2993.
11. Easson, L. H. and Stedman, E. (1933) Studies on the relationship between chemical constitution and physiological action. V. Molecular dissimetry and physiological activity. *Biochem. J.* **27**: 1257–1266.

12. Ruffolo, R. R., Yaden, E. L. and Waddell, J. E. (1982) Stereochemical requirements of alpha-2 adrenergic receptors. *J. Pharmacol. Exp. Ther.* **222**: 645–651.

13. Pfeiffer, C. C. (1956) Optical isomerism and pharmacological action. *Sciences* **124**: 29–31.

14. Lehmann, F. P. A., Rodrigues de Miranda, J. and Ariëns, E. J. (1976) Stereoselectivity and affinity in molecular pharmacology. *Prog. Drug Res.* **20**: 101–142.

15. Lehmann, P. A. (1990) Quantitation of the criticality of chiral centers towards stereoselective recognition: epimeric eudismic analysis of 1,3-oxathiolane muscarinic agonists and antagonists. *Chirality* **2**: 211–218.

16. Barlow, R. (1990) Enantiomers: how valid is Pfeiffer's rule? *TIPS* **11**: 148–150.

17. Gualtieri, F. (1990) Pfeiffer's rule OK? *TIPS* **11**: 315–316.

18. Hamilton, C. L., Niemann, C. and Hammond, G. S. (1966) A quantitative analysis of the binding of *N*-acyl derivatives of α-amino amides by α-chymotripsin. *Proc. Natl. Acad. Sci. USA* **55**: 664–669.

19. Smith, T. J., Kremer, M. J., Luo, M., Vriend, G., Arnold, E., Kanser, G., Rossmann, M. G., McKinley, M. A., Diana, G. D. and Otto, M. J. (1986) The site of attachment in human rhinovirus 14 for antiviral agents that inhibit uncoating. *Science* **233**: 1286–1293.

20. Badger, J., Minor, I., Kremer, M. J. *et al.*. (1988) Structural analysis of a series of antiviral agents complexed with human rhinovirus 14. *Proc. Natl. Acad. Sci. USA* **85**: 3304–3308.

21. Maksay, G., Tegyey, Zs. and Simonyi, M. (1991) Central benzodiazepine receptors: In vitro efficacies and potencies of 3-substituted 1,4-benzodiazepine stereoisomers. *Mol. Pharmacol.* **39**: 725–732.

22. Ariëns, E. J. (1987) Stereochemistry in the analysis of drug action II. *Med. Res. Rev.* **7**: 367–387.

23. Maksay, G. (1990) Affinity and stereoselectivity in binding to the subsites of the GABA$_A$ receptor complex. In Simonyi M. (ed.) *Problems and Wonders of Chiral Molecules*, pp. 279–291. Akadémiai Kiadó, Budapest.

24. Yeh, J. Z. (1980) Blockade of sodium channels by stereoisomers of local anesthetics. In Fink, B. R. (ed.) *Molecular Mechanisms of Anesthesia*, pp 35–44. Raven Press, New York.

25. Kwon, Y. W. and Triggle, D. J. (1991) Chiral aspects of drug action at ion channels: a commentary on the stereoselectivity of drug actions at voltage-gated ion channels with particular reference to verapamil actions at the Ca^{2+} channel. *Chirality* **3**: 393–404.

26. Yatani, A., Kunze, D. L. and Brown, A.M. (1988) Effects of dihydropyridine calcium channel modulators on cardiac sodium channels. *Am. J. Physiol.* **254**: 140–147.

27. Birdsall, N. J. M., Hulme, E. C. and Burgen, A. (1980) The character of muscarinic receptors in different regions of the rat brain. *Proc. R. Soc. London. B* **207**: 1–12.

28. Franckowiak, G., Bechem, M., Schramm, M. and Thomas, G. (1985) The optical isomers of the 1,4-dihydropyridine Bay K 8644 show opposite effects on calcium channels. *Eur. J. Pharmac.* **114**: 223–226.

29. Allan, A. M. and Harris, R. A. (1986) Anesthetic and convulsant barbiturates alter γ-aminobutyric acid-stimulated chloride flux across brain membranes. *J. Pharmacol. Exp. Ther.* **238**: 763–768.

30. Maksay, G. and Ticku, M. K. (1985) The dissociation of [^{35}S]-*t*-butylbicyclophosphorothionate binding differentiates convulsant and depressant drugs that modulate GABAergic neurotransmission. *J. Neurochem.* **44**: 480–486.

31. Maksay, G. and Ticku, M. K. (1988) CNS depressants accelerate the dissociation of [^{35}S]TBPS binding and GABA enhances their displacing potencies. *Life Sci.* **43**: 1331–1337.

32 Kardos, J., Kovacs, I., Simon-Trompler, E. and Hajós, F. (1991) Enantioselectivity at the physiologically active GABA$_A$ receptor. *Biochem. Pharmacol.* **41**: 1141–1144.

33. Lehmann, F. P. A. (1987) A quantitative stereo-structure activity relationship analysis of the binding of promiscuous chiral ligands to different receptors. *Quant. Struct.-Act. Relat.* **6**: 57–65.

34. Aronstam, R. S., Triggle, D. J. and Eldefrawi, M. E. (1979) Structure and stereochemical requirements for muscarinic receptor binding. *Mol. Pharmacol.* **15**: 227–234.

35. Benyhe, S., Szúcs, M., Borsodi, A. and Wollemann, M. (1992) Species differences in the stereoselectivity of kappa opioid binding sites for [^{3}H]U-69593 and [^{3}H] ethylketocyclazocine. *Life Sci.* **51**: 1647–1655.

36. Singh, L., Donald, A. E., Foster, A. C. *et al.*. (1990) Enantiomers of HA-966 (3-amino-1-hydroxypyrrolid-2-one) exhibit distinct central nervous system effcts: (+)HA-966 is a selective glycine/*N*-methyl-D-aspartate receptor antagonist, but (−)-HA-966 is a potent γ-butyrolactone-like sedative. *Proc. Natl. Acad. Sci. USA* **87**: 347–351.

37. Leeson, P. D., Williams, B. J., Baker, R., Ladduwahetty, T., Moore, K. W. and Rowley, M. (1990)

Effects of five-membered ring conformation on bioreceptor recognition: identification of 3R-amino-l-hydroxy-4R-methylpyrrolidin-2-one (L-687, 414) as a potent glycine/N-methyl-D-aspartate receptor analog. *J. Chem. Soc., Chem. Commun.* 1878–1880.

38. Maksay, G., Tegyey, Zs. and Ötvös, L. (1978) Stereospecificity of esterases hydrolysing oxazepam acetate, *J. Pharm. Sci.* **67**: 1208–1210.

39. Jamali, F., Mehvar, R. and Pasutto, F. M. (1989) Enantioselective aspects of drug action and disposition. *J. Pharm. Sci.* **78**: 695–715.

40. Knights, K. M., Drew, R. and Meffin, P. M. (1988) Enantiospecific formation of fenoprofen coenzyme A thioester in vitro. *Biochem. Pharmacol.* **37**: 3539–3542.

41. Williams, K. M. (1990) Metabolic chiral inversion: ibuprofen. In Simonyi, M. (ed.) *Problems and Wonders of Chiral Molecules,* pp. 181–204. Akadémiai Kiadó; Budapest.

42. Hilvert, D., Carpenter, S. H., Nared, K. D. and Auditor, M. T. M. (1988) Catalysis of concerted reactions by antibodies: the Claisen rearrangement. *Proc. Natl. Acad. Sci. USA* **85**: 4953–4955.

43. Janda, K. D., Benkovic, S. J. and Lerner, R. A. (1989) Catalytic antibodies with lipase activity and *R* or *S* substrate selectivity. *Science* **244**: 437–440.

44. Burke, T. R., Jacobson, A. E., Rice, K. C., Silverton, J. V., Simonds, W. F., Streaty, R. A. and Klee, W. A. (1986) Probes for narcotic receptor mediated phenomena. 12. cis-(+)-methylfentanyl isothiocyanate, a potent site-directed acylating agent for δ opioid receptors. Synthesis, absolute configuration, and receptor enantioselectivity. *J. Med. Chem.* **29**: 1087–1093.

45. Hara, S. and Cazes, J. (1986) Editorial. *J. Liquid Chromatogr.* **9**, 241–242.

46. Pirkle, W. H. and House, D. W. (1979) Chiral high-pressure liquid chromatographic stationary phases. *J. Org. Chem.* **44**: 1957–1960.

47. Pirkle, W. H., Hyun, M. H. and Bank, B. (1984) A rational approach to the design of highly-effective chiral stationary phases. J. *Chromatogr.* **316**: 585–604.

48. Pirkle, W. H., Finn, J. M., Schreiner, J. L. and Hamper, B. C. (1981) A widely useful chiral stationary phase for the high performance liquid chromatography separation of enantiomers. *J. Am. Chem. Soc.* **103**: 3964–3966.

49. Okamoto, Y. and Hatada, K. (1986) Resolution of enantiomers by HPLC on optically active poly(triphenylmethyl methacrylate). *J. Liquid Chromatogr.* **9**: 369–384.

50. Blaschke, G. (1986) Chromatographic resolution of chiral drugs on polyamides and cellulose triacetate. *J. Liquid Chromatogr.* **9**: 341–368.

51. Szinai, I., Simonyi, M., Fitos, I. Tegyey, Zs. and Magyar, A. (1990) Demonstration of stereoselective disposition of warfarin enantiomers by whole-body autoradiography. *Eur. J. Drug Metab. Pharmacokinet.* **15**: 103–107.

52. Allenmark, S. (1986) Optical resolution by liquid chromatography on immobilized bovine serum albumin. *J. Liquid Chromatogr.* **9**: 425–442.

53. Fitos, I., Tegyey, Zs., Simonyi, M., Sjöholm, I., Larsson, T. and Lagercrantz, C. (1986) Stereoselective binding of 3-acetoxy and 3-hydroxy-1,4-benzodiazepine-2-ones to human serum albumin. Stereoselective allosteric interaction with warfarin enantiomers. *Biochem. Pharmacol.* **35**: 263–269.

54. Fitos, I., Visy, J., Magyar, A., Kajtár, J. and Simonyi, M. (1990) Stereoselective effect of warfarin and bilirubin on the binding of 5-(o-chlorophenyl)-1,3-dihydro-3-methyl-7-nitro-2H-1,4-benzodiazepin-2-one enantiomers to human serum albumin. *Chirality* **2**: 161–166.

55. Fitos, I., Visy, J., Simonyi, M. and Hermansson, J. (1992) Chiral high-performance liquid chromatographic separations of vinca alkaloid analogues on α_1-acid glycoprotein and human serum albumin columns. *J. Chromatogr.* **609**: 163–171.

56. Szejtli, J. (1982) *Cyclodextrins And Their Inclusion Complexes.* Akadémiai Kiadó, Budapest.

57. Sybilska, D., Żukowski, J. and Bojarski, J. (1986) Resolution of mephenytoin and some chiral barbiturates into enantiomers by reversed phase high performance liquid chromatography via β-cyclodextrin inclusion complexes. *J. Liquid Chromatogr.* **9**: 591–606.

58. Rogan, M. M., Altria, K. D. and Goodall, D. M. (1994) Enantioselective separations using capillary electrophoresis. *Chirality* **6**: 25–40.

59. Ward, T. J. and Armstrong, D.W. (1986) Improved cyclodextrin chiral phases: a comparison and review. *J. Liquid Chromatogr.* **9**: 407–423.

60. Gal, J. (1991) Excavations in drug chirality: cyclothiazide. *Chirality* **3**: 2–13.

61. Pettersson, C. and Schill, G. (1986) Separation of enantiomers in ion-pair chromatographic systems. *J. Liquid Chromatogr.* **9**: 269–290.

62. Dobashi, A., Dobashi, Y. and Hara, S. (1986) Enantioselectivity of hydrogen bond association in liquid-solid chromatography. *J. Liquid Chromatogr.* **9**: 243–267.

63. Gal, J. (1990) Chromatographic analysis of drug enantiomers: applications of 2,3,4,6-tetra-*O*-acetyl-β-D-glucopyranosyl isothiocyanate. In Simonyi, M.(ed.) *Problems and Wonders of Chiral Molecules*, pp. 137–144. Akadémiai Kiadó, Budapest,

64. Silber, B., Holford, N. H. G. and Riegelman, S. (1982) Stereoselective disposition and glucuronidation of propranolol in humans. *J. Pharm. Sci.* **71**: 699–704.

65. Weiss, Y. A., Safar, M. E., Lehner, J. P., Levenson, J. A., Simon, A. and Alexandre, J. M. (1978) (+)-Propranolol clearance, an estimation of hepatic blood flow in man. *Brit. J. Clin. Pharmacol.* **5**: 457–460.

66. Godbillon, J., Richard, J., Gerardin, H., Meinertz, T., Kasper, W. and Jahnchen, E. (1981) Pharmacokinetics of the enantiomers of acenocoumarol in man. *Br. J. Clin. Pharmacol.* **12**: 621–629.

67. Chien, Y. W. and Nair, M. (1993) Biomembrane permeation and stereochemistry. *J. Pharm. Sci.* **82**: 342–344.

68. Ariens, E. J. (1984) Stereochemistry, a basis for sophisticated nonsense in pharmacokinetics, and clinical pharmacology. *Eur. J. Clin. Pharmacol.* **26**: 663–668.

69. Trager, W. F. (1990) Coumarin anticoagulants: the influence of stereo-structure of warfarin on metabolic behaviour and as a probe of cytochrome P-450. In Simonyi, M. (ed.) *Problems and Wonders of Chiral Molecules*, pp 159–180. Akadémiai Kiadó, Budapést.

70. Toon, S. and Trager, W. F. (1984) Pharmacokinetic implications of stereoselective changes in plasma protein binding: warfarin/sulfinpyrazone. *J. Pharm. Sci.* **73**: 1671–1673.

71. Fitos, I., Visy, J., Magyar, A., Kajtár, J. and Simonyi, M. (1989) Inverse stereoselectivity in the binding of acenocoumarol to human serum albumin and αi-acid glycoprotein. *Biochem. Pharmacol.* **38**: 2259–2262.

72. Seiler, J. P. (1993) Chiral drugs — the view of the Swiss Intercantonal Office for the control of medicines. *Drug Information J.* **27**: 485–489.

73. Smith, R. L. and Caldwell, J. (1988) Racemates: towards a new year resolution? *Trends Pharmacol. Sci.* **9**: 75–77.

74. Wermuth, C. G. (1993) Aminopyridazines — an alternative route to potent muscarinic agonists with no cholinergic syndrome. *Il Farmaco* **48**: 253–274.

75. Fabro, S., Smith, R. L. and Williams, R. T. (1967) Toxicity and teratogenicity of thalidomide. *Nature,* **215**: 296.

76. Simonyi, M. (1984) On chiral drug action. *Med. Res. Rev.* **4**: 359–413.

77. A recent report indicated rapid *in vivo* interconversion of thalidomide enantiomers administered to male volunteers separately (Erikkson, T., Björkman, S., Roth, B., Fyge, Å. and Höglund, P. (1995) Stereospecific determination, chiral inversion *in vitro* and pharmacokinetics in humans of the enantiomers of thalidomide. *Chirality* **7**: 44–52). Thus, putative differences in therapeutic or adverse effects between the thalidomide enantiomers, or between enantiomeric and racemic forms, should be regarded as irrelevant.

22

Pharmacophore Identification and Receptor Mapping

HANS-DIETER HÖLTJE

One cannot guess how a model functions.
One has to look at its use and learn from that.
L. Wittgenstein (1950)

I. INTRODUCTION

It is well known that the large majority of drugs exert their action via specific binding to biomacromolecules. Above all, proteins like enzymes and receptors, but also nucleic acids serve as physiological binding partners. In all cases a very specific and unique three-dimensional structure of the drug molecule is prerequisite for a certain pharmacological activity. The initial step in the formation of drug–receptor interaction complexes is a recognition event.[1,2] The receptor has to recognize whether an approaching molecule possesses the properties necessary for binding. This characteristic three-dimensional set of structural elements is called the pharmacophore.[3] Because experimental knowledge about the particular three-dimensional

THE PRACTICE OF MEDICINAL CHEMISTRY
ISBN 0-12-744640-0

structure of receptors for most of the drugs in therapeutic use is still unavailable, corresponding hypothetical pharmacophore models are an important source for understanding drug–receptor interactions on the molecular level. In order to describe the pharmacophoric pattern correctly, the steric and the electronic features of the bioactive conformations of drug molecules have to be determined. The availability of a set of compounds from a distinct class of candidates showing a large variety in chemical structure and which interact via the same binding mechanism with the same receptor is an ideal starting point for the identification of a pharmacophore.

In course of the pharmacophore identification process, clearly two different steps have to be taken in succession. First, a conformational analysis has to be carried out. After this initial step, a common three-dimensional arrangement of functional groups is determined through a superpositioning procedure. During the second step this preliminary sterical pharmacophore model has to be checked and consolidated by electron density calculations and establishment of the corresponding molecular electrostatic potentials (MEPs).

Using programs such as GRIN/GRID or HINT, the electrostatic fields can be translated and extended to molecular interaction fields which mimic the interaction potential of the pharmacophore. Based on this three-dimensional description of the physicochemical properties, a map of suitable receptor binding sites can be constructed. This hypothetical receptor model is then used for the calculation of interaction energies between all members of the series and the receptor. The calculated binding energies should correctly reflect equivalent biological affinities.

At this point experimental structure–activity relationship data must be used to optimize and refine the pharmacophore. It is essential that as well as active substances, inactive analogues or at least congeners with low activity can also be described by the theoretical interaction energies. If this is achieved, then the receptor model can be used to predict chemical structures and biological activities of new and hitherto unknown compounds. The synthesis and subsequent confirmation of the predicted structures by pharmacological testing is the final and decisive proof for the correctness or, more precisely, the usefulness of the deduced receptor map of the pharmacophore. The derived pharmacophore model then allows conclusions regarding the structure and properties of the unknown receptor binding site.

II. METHODS

A. Conformational analysis

Some introductory remarks are necessary on ensuring that the developed pharmacophore posseses sufficient reliability. In the first place, it is important to collect a training set of at least ten structures (around fifteen or more would be better) which, as already mentioned, should represent the greatest possible structural variety in the series. In addition, the pharmacological potencies of these congeners should span a relative scale of at least 1 to 1000. These features increase the confidence level for the prediction of new structures. Another important factor which has to be considered carefully is the conformational flexibility of the drug molecules. It is extremely desirable that a semirigid, or better a rigid, highly potent congener belongs to the series to be studied. This compound may be used as template for the more flexible ones. If potent, conformationally restricted molecules are not available, the determination of the pharmacophoric conformation requires much greater effort, and the use of statistical methods such as principal component analysis (PCA) or factor analysis is imperative in order to resolve this multidimensional problem[4-6] (see Chapter 19 for further discussion).

As a first step, all molecular structures have to be generated using the computer. If possible, experimental data from X-ray crystallography, available through the Cambridge Crystallographic Data Bank,[7] are used. If structures are not included in this source, they may be constructed using fragment libraries and/or building routines offered by commercial molecular modelling software packages.[8,9] In any case, the generated geometries (bond lengths, valence, angles, etc.) have to be optimized using molecular mechanics routines before a systematic conformational search can be executed. During this search operation, rotations around all single bonds are performed in 30° or, better, 10° steps. The rotamers produced are checked using Van der Waals energy as the criterion for strong steric hindrance, and all conformers which do not pass this test are discarded.

This systematic procedure is not feasible for large systems because the amount of output data can become tremendously large. In these cases the conformational space should preferably be analysed using a molecular dynamics operation.[10] Using a random conformation, a molecular dynamics process is initiated to produce an initial dynamic structure. Then a short (e.g. 5 ps) molecular dynamics run is performed at high temperature (e.g. 900 K); subsequently the system is cooled to 300 K and molecular dynamics is continued for 10 ps. The final structure is extracted and the energy is minimized. The total cycle is repeated at least 20 times, so that 20 energy-minimized structures are produced.

Independently of the method used for conformational analysis, the conformations generated are analysed for conformational similarity and classified according to energy content, and only dissimilar conformers within a defined energy window are retained for further investigation. Depending on the molecular mechanics force field used, the window may extend from 5 to 10 kcal mol^{-1} above the absolute energy minimum.

The next task is to search for a unique common conformation of all congeners, where most if not all pharmacophoric elements of the molecules are presented superimposed. Thus we first have to define the pharmacophoric elements. This can be done best on the basis of known structure–activity relationship data. The information thus obtained facilitates enormously the subsequent superpositioning procedure, because only conformations with common positions of the important pharmacophoric elements need to be considered.

Several different superpositioning procedures are available. They comprise manual or automatic fitting by rigid-body rotation, or flexible fitting procedures where both r.m.s. (root mean square) deviation between the fitted atom pairs and conformational energies are minimized. We always use the FITIT[11] method, which has been developed in our group. This program fits each energetically accessible conformation of one molecule with each allowed conformation of a second one. The resulting fit pairs are sorted according to r.m.s. values and only fit pairs with low r.m.s. values are saved. This procedure is repeated for the complete list of molecules and in general finally yields only a small number of different pharmacophore models (Fig. 22.1).

Other methodologies for pharmacophore identification which must be mentioned are the distance geometry approach developed by Crippen[12-17] and Marshall's active analogue approach.[18,19]

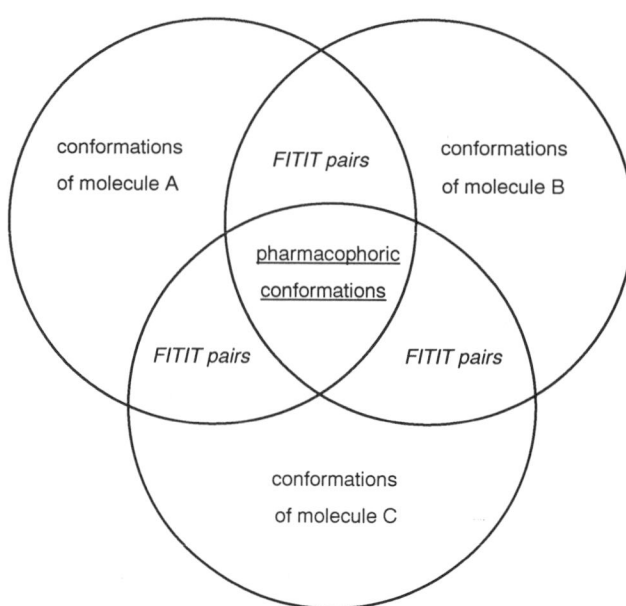

Fig. 22.1 Schematic drawing representing the FITIT procedure. The conformational space is reduced by pairwise superpositioning of energetically allowed conformations of the different chemical classes. A second superpositioning step for all selected FITIT pairs finally yields the common pharmacophoric conformations.

B. Molecular electrostatic potentials

Since the initial step in the formation of a drug–receptor interaction complex is a recognition event which is highly dependent on polar electrostatic interactions, one very easy and efficient way to test the so far purely steric pharmacophore model for significance is calculation of the molecular electrostatic potentials (MEPs)[20] for all compounds in the training set. This must of course be done for the individual pharmacophoric conformations determined.

It is well known that MEPs provide a very informative means for assessing the electronic structure of molecules; however this is extremely dependent on the method employed for the calculation of the molecular charge distribution. Two conceptually different procedural treatments of this problem are possible. Charge distributions can be determined using a topological or a quantum-chemical method. Topological methods, for example that developed by Gasteiger,[21] which is included in SYBYL, are very fast. Molecular electron densities are here calculated solely on the basis of electronegativity differences along a bond and include experimental NMR data. Only directly bonded atoms are considered and conformational aspects are completely neglected. However, if mesomeric effects are not important for the molecule investigated, the results may compare favourably with dipole moments from experimental sources. Nevertheless, it is very dangerous to use this kind of procedure without a careful check of the applicability to each individual problem.

Quantum-chemical methods, on the other hand, are divided into semiempirical and *ab initio* procedures. Semiempirical methods such as the various procedures collected in the MOPAC package (MNDO,[22a] AM1,[22b] PM3[22c]) are generally used because they are much less time consuming and may also be applied to rather large molecules. But it should be noted that these methods might lead to erroneous results for hetero atoms.[23,24] Considering the increasing computational power of workstations and the availability of mathematically optimized *ab initio* procedures (i.e. SPARTAN,[25] D-mol[26]), STO-3G, 4-31G or even 6-31G* basis set calculations for structures with the normal size of drug molecules can now be performed as standard procedure. The subsequent calculation of the MEPs should then be done on the basis of the wavefunctions[27] and not, as usually found in the commercial molecular modelling packages, using the monopole charges. The latter procedures may lead to incorrect results in regions of space close to and inside Van der Waals surfaces of molecules. Farther outside, the monopole charge-derived MEPs in general give rather reliable pictures of the electrostatic behaviour of the molecules and can be used with caution as a fast and easy accessible tool.

Regardless of the method used, it is essential to demonstrate the correctness of calculated charge densities against experimental dipole moments. Because dipole moments are conformation-dependent, this test should only be performed for rigid molecules or small and conformationally undemanding model compounds.

C.   Molecular interaction fields

So far we have taken into account only the steric and electrostatic fit of congeneric drug molecules that bind at the same receptor site. This is clearly not sufficient if one aims towards a more detailed description of the structural properties of a receptor. Besides the already mentioned characteristics, hydrophobic areas, regions of charge transfer or several types of different polar interactions can also be distinguished. A receptor map which contains three-dimensional information of this kind is very helpful in the interpretation and understanding of known experimental results but also, which is even more desirable, for the prediction of new, hitherto unknown structures.

The generation of molecular interaction fields, which are the basis for the construction of a receptor map, can be performed using a variety of programs. The most widely used are GRIN/GRID,[28] CoMFA[29] and HINT.[30,31] CoMFA is implemented in a commercial 3D QSAR program package which allows the automated treatment of large numbers of compounds under constant conditions. A prerequisite for this procedure is of course some sort of alignment for the molecules to be studied. This can be attained by determination of a pharmacophore as described earlier. However, the CoMFA method according to the authors, can itself be used for this purpose. Therefore, a typical CoMFA study starts with only a very rough alignment of the compounds, or possibly none. After calculation of interaction energies at gridded space points between the molecule of interest and a probe atom simulating, for example, hydrophobic or hydrogen bond donor properties, interaction fields can be defined. The relative three-dimensional position of these fields in the space surrounding the molecules is found with the help of statistical and chemometric methods (e.g. PLS[32]). (For detailed information about CoMFA, see Chapter 23.) After calculation of different fields, the superpositional fit for the training set can subsequently be optimized. This means that compounds with different structures which have been identified to interact with the same receptor, but cannot be superimposed using an atom-by-atom fit procedure, might nevertheless be superimposable on the basis of their corresponding molecular interaction fields.

Molecular interaction fields can also be generated using GRIN/GRID. This method is especially reliable because it is based on a very careful parametrization of the interaction terms. The parameters are founded from experimental crystallographic data; that is, the direction, type and typical strength of a particular interaction are classified according to actual crystals.

Numerous different probes are available for a graded description of the molecular properties. As in CoMFA, molecules are located in a cubic grid and interaction energies between the molecule and the probe are calculated for each grid point outside the molecular Van der Waals volume. The resulting fields may be analysed by calculation of isoenergy contours at any given energy level. Comparison of the contours for all pharmacophoric conformations and all different types of probes allows the definition of a common receptor map for a drug family.[33–35] Typical results for this kind of study are shown in Fig. 22.2 for the 5-HT$_{2a}$ antagonists[36] using an aromatic CH-probe (hydrophobic interaction) and an aliphatic OH-probe (hydrogen bond donor and acceptor interaction), respectively.

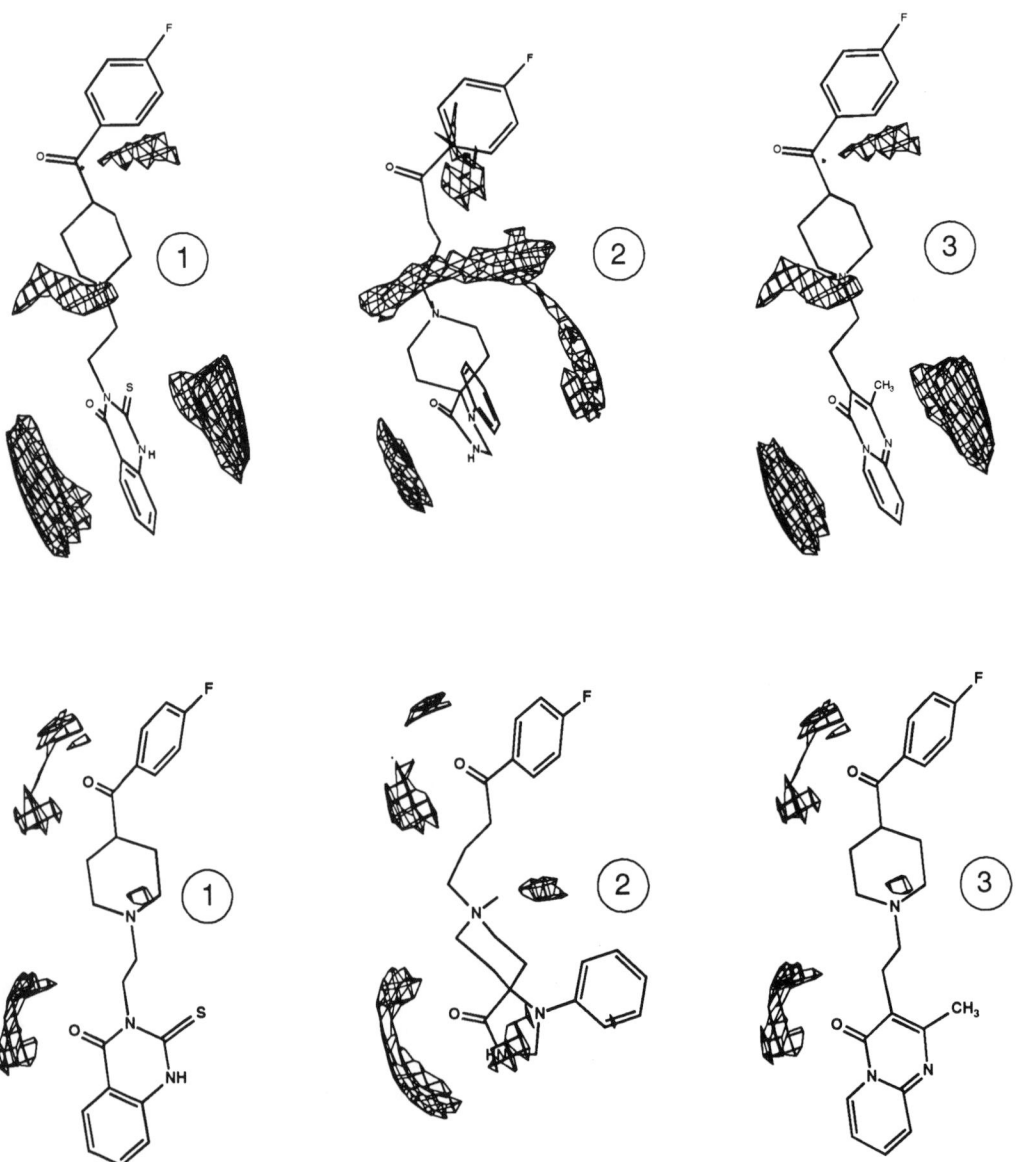

Fig. 22.2 Interaction fields calculated using GRIN/GRID: (1) altanserin; (2) pirenperone, (3) spiperone. The upper row presents hydrophobic fields calculated using an aromatic CH-probe, the contour level is $-1.55\ \mathrm{kcal\ mol^{-1}}$. The lower row shows the same molecules interacting with an OH-probe; the contour level is $-4.0\ \mathrm{kcal\ mol^{-1}}$.

The isoenergy level contours are $-1.5\,\text{kcal mol}^{-1}$ for the hydrophobic and $-4.0\,\text{kcal mol}^{-1}$ for the polar contacts.

D. Receptor mapping

The next step is then to translate this interaction field into a model of the receptor which is composed from single isolated amino acids with chemical properties that satisfy the different types of binding present in the pharmacophore. The relative three-dimensional positions of the amino acid binding sites are defined by the corresponding GRIN/GRID results. The resulting amino acid receptor model is sometimes called a pseudoreceptor.[37–39]

If experimental knowledge of the amino acid sequence of the receptor protein is absent, it may be that several different models can be constructed. The choice of one or another hypothetical receptor map is possible on the basis of calculated interaction energies and their subsequent correlation with the known binding affinities. The model producing the most significant agreement is selected for prediction purposes. Of course, the selection procedure and, coupled to this, the quality of the model are superior if structural information from molecular biochemistry can be used. This is true, for example, for the G-protein coupled receptors like the serotoninergic 5-HT_{2a} receptor.[40,41] Homology searching and sequence alignment operations have been performed intensively, so there are some ideas about selected amino acids in binding positions in the active site of the receptor[42,43] (for further information, see Chapter 25).

The next step is calculation of interaction energies and comparison with experimentally determined binding affinities. This can be done very efficiently using force field methods. For example, the DOCKING procedure and the MAXIMIN module of the SYBYL software package can be employed for optimization of interaction geometries and energy calculation. Other programs can be used equally well. As long as only relative energy differences are of interest, the results are quite reliable. However, one must be aware that the regular force field methods only describe two different types of binding forces adequately — the dispersion and the electrostatic terms.[44] The latter depends dramatically on the dielectric constant employed and it is extremely important to choose the one appropriate to the situation considered. Inside a protein environment, for example in the core of the G-protein-coupled receptor channel, the prevailing dielectric constant is assured between 3 and 5. Binding sites at protein surfaces are better treated with a value around 10. Only in special cases should the constant for vacuum conditions be used. This would be reasonable, for example, if one assumes hydrogen bonds to be of crucial importance for the binding. Since force fields naturally can only simulate the electrostatic part of hydrogen bonds and neglect the covalent part, this drawback can be roughly compensated for through an overestimation of the electrostatic interaction. We will return to the subject of energy terms which are not included in force field interaction energies in the discussion of the serotoninergic receptor model. Interaction energies are determined according to

$$IE = E_{RL} - (E_R + E_L)$$

where

IE = interaction energy;
E_{RL} = energy of the receptor–ligand complex;
E_R = energy of the isolated receptor protein;
E_L = energy of the isolated ligand.

In order to obtain comparable energy data, the interaction geometries of the complexes are generated for all the ligands in an absolutely corresponding manner. All ligands are kept in the pharmacophoric conformation and location. Hydrophobic and polar amino acids mimicking equivalent receptor binding sites are positioned according to the GRIN/GRID contours. Each individual receptor model–ligand complex is then geometry-minimized in the MAXIMIN force field. No constraints are employed. The procedure therefore simulates an induced fit between ligand and receptor which can be assumed to occur in reality. An energy cut-off of $0.01\,kcal\,mol^{-1}$ should be used.

One word of caution is necessary with respect to the experimentally derived biological activities. These should constitute pure receptor binding affinities and must stem from a single laboratory. Since the computer models simulate molecular interaction events in a highly simplified manner, the experimental data which are combined with them in a correlation equation must be as close to the molecular level as possible. It is therefore quite impermissible, and virtual nonsense, to correlate calculated interaction energies with pharmacological *in vivo* (whole animal) data, because the receptor interaction can be blurred or even completely hidden by pharmacokinetics and biotransformation of the drug molecules. Sometimes even the use of functional *in vitro* data is dangerous if a reaction cascade separates the measured event from the receptor binding interaction. If receptor map and interaction complex have been generated carefully, a rough but nevertheless correct picture of the reality may be given. But as long as the real receptor still is unknown the efficiency and meaning of the model cannot be assessed except by prediction of new substances. This should always be the ultimate test of usefulness for each hypothetically derived receptor map.

III. CASE STUDY: THE 5-HT$_{2a}$ SEROTONINERGIC RECEPTOR MAP

To portray the routes to be followed for pharmacophore identification and receptor mapping in practice, the complete suite of procedures will be demonstrated using an example from the author's laboratory.

The example to be described and discussed in detail deals with antagonists of the serotoninergic 5-HT$_{2a}$ receptor. Compounds that interact with this receptor subtype have been known for many years.[45] They can be divided into four different groups in terms of chemical structure (Fig. 22.3):

(1) butyrophenone derivatives: spiperone analogues;
(2) 4-(phenylketo)piperidines: ketanserin analogues;
(3) tricyclic compounds: cyproheptadiene analogues;
(4) irindalone analogues.

Unfortunately, this set of altogether 20 compounds does not contain any rigid molecules; but some of them are at least in parts conformationally restricted. This is true, for example, for clothiapine and irindalone as well as spiperone, while the members of the ketanserin subfamily, which contain five major rotatable bonds, show a high degree of conformational freedom.

Experimental structure activity data for the 5-HT$_{2a}$ antagonist can be summarized as follows. The pharmacological results suggest that two planar aromatic or heterocyclic ring systems

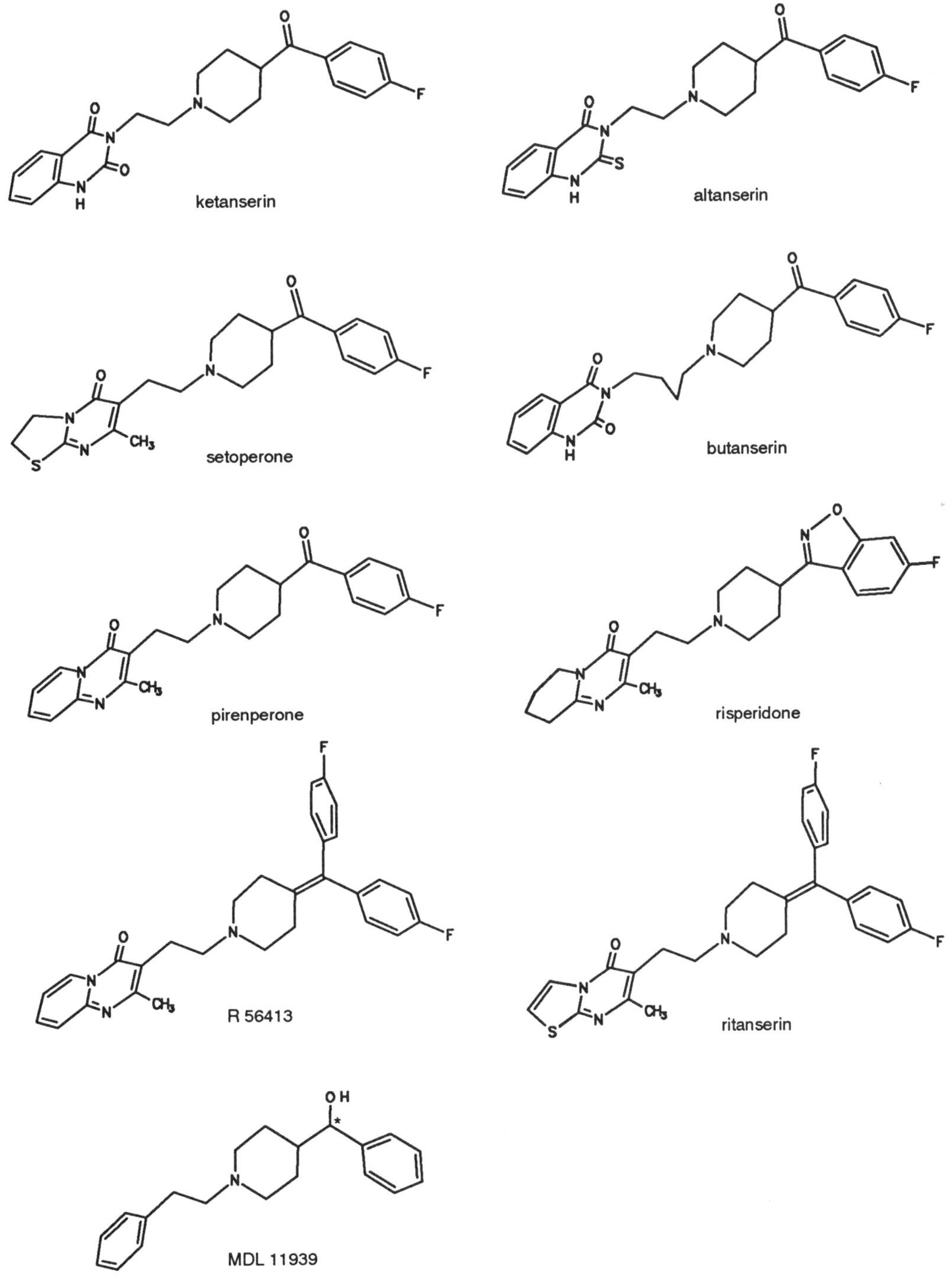

ketanserin

altanserin

setoperone

butanserin

pirenperone

risperidone

R 56413

ritanserin

MDL 11939

(a)

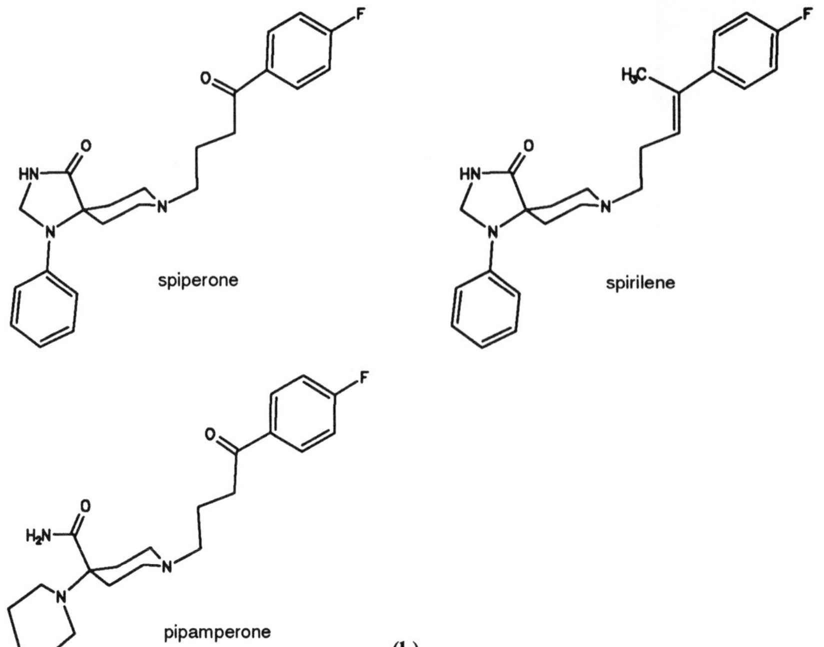

spiperone

spirilene

pipamperone

(b)

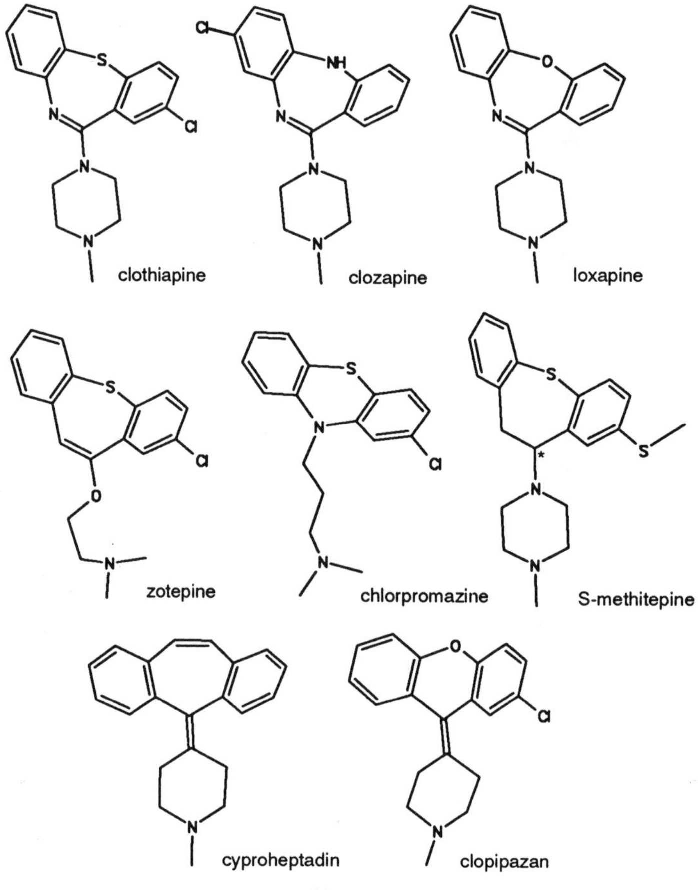

clothiapine

clozapine

loxapine

zotepine

chlorpromazine

S-methitepine

cyproheptadin

clopipazan

(c)

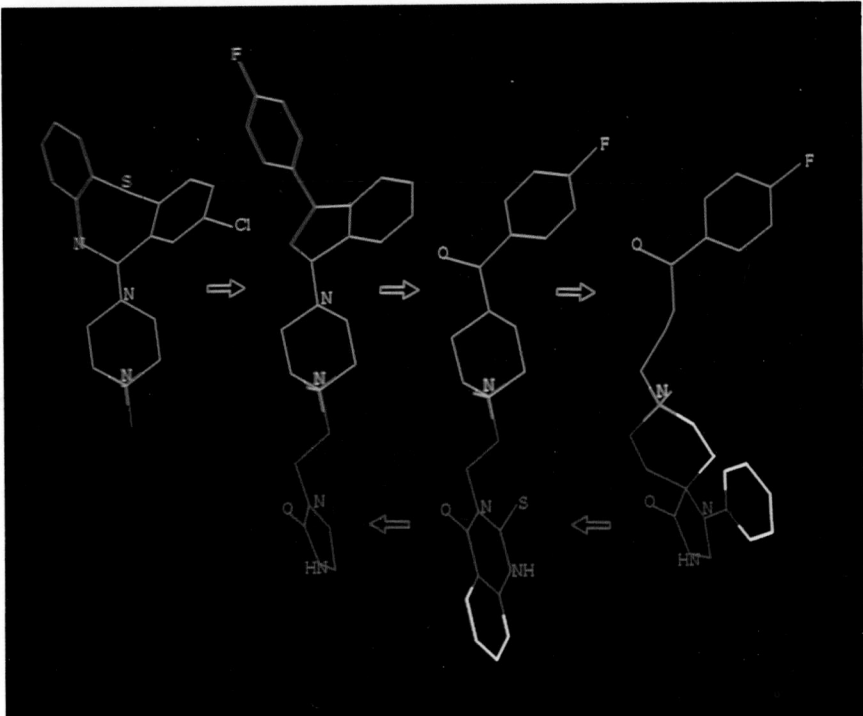

Plate 1 Schematic representation of the stepwise analogue approach. Strongly related structural elements of the different substances are colour coded.

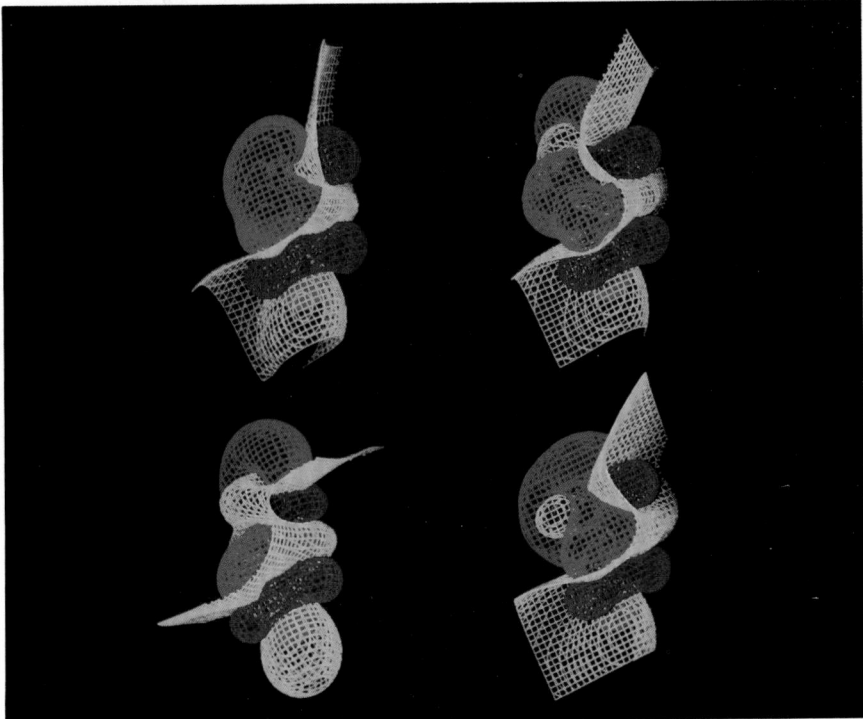

Plate 2 Molecular electrostatic potentials calculated on the basis of AM1 point charges: Top left, spiperone; top right, altanserin; bottom left, pipamperone; bottom right, butanserin. Colour code: blue = negative potential; red = positive potential; yellow = neutral potential.

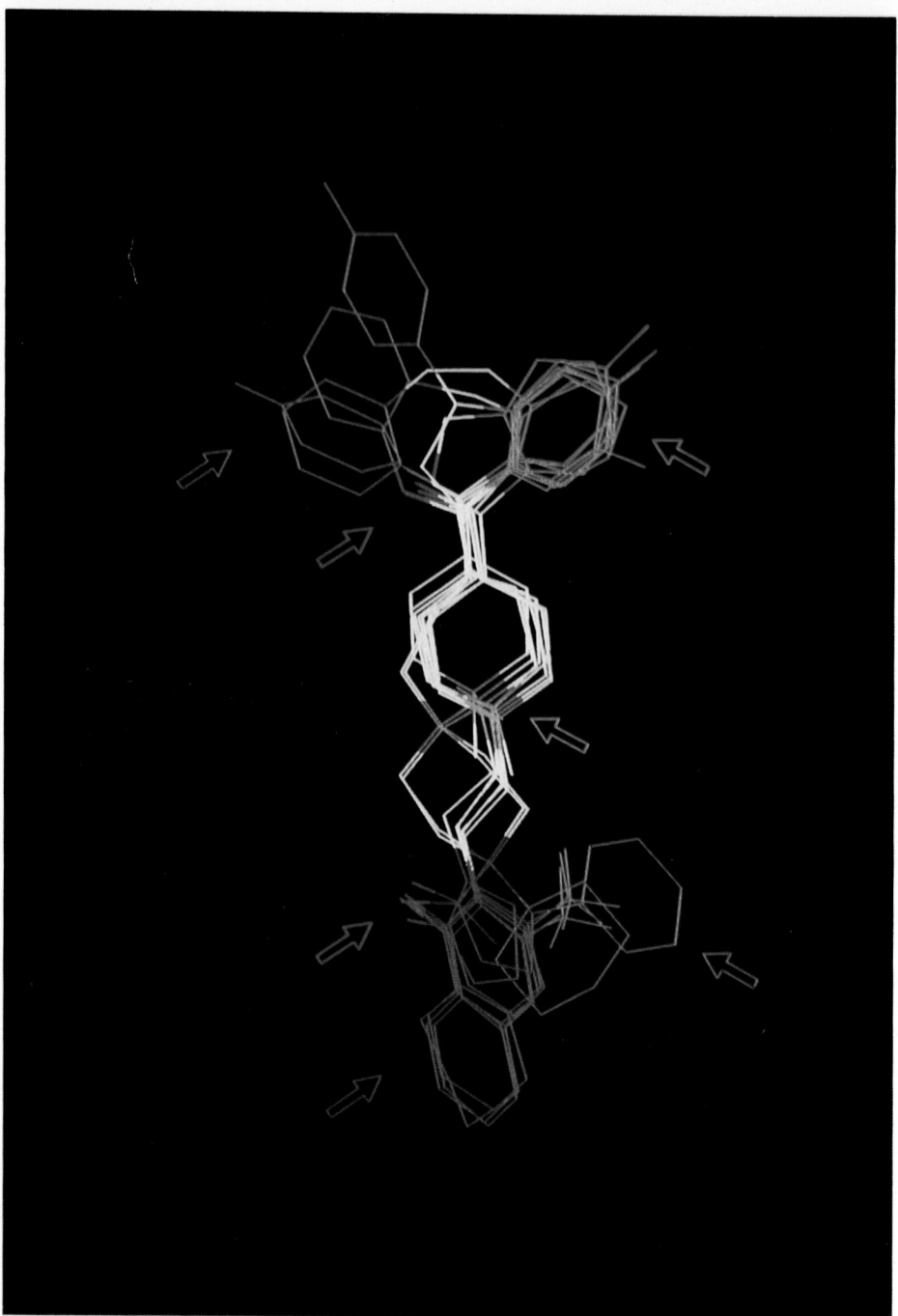

Plate 3 The 5-HT$_{2a}$-antagonistic pharmacophore. Different characteristic regions are marked by coloured arrows. Colour code: violet = hydrophobic area; green = electron-deficient aromatic system; red = electronegative heteroatoms; pink = protonated nitrogen; blue = large planar ring system (mostly heterocycles).

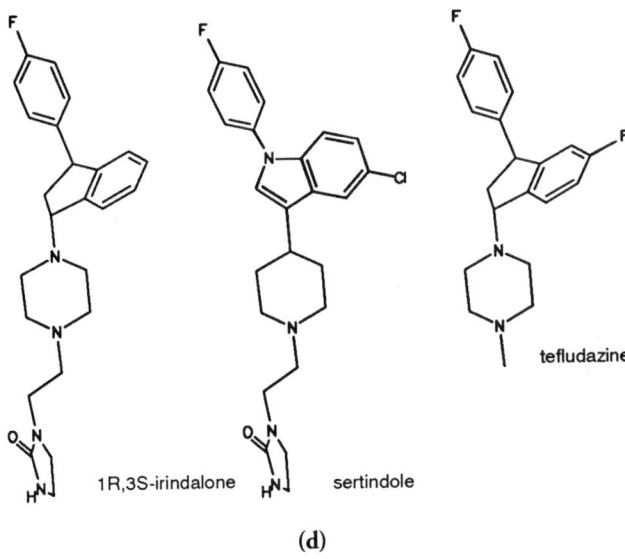

Fig. 22.3 Structural formulae of 5-HT$_{2a}$ antagonists used for pharmacophore identification: (a) ketanserin analogoues; (b) spiperone analogues; (c) cyproheptadiene analogues; (d) irindalone analogues.

separated by certain distance and connected by an aliphatic or alicyclic chain which contains a basic protonatable nitrogen seem to constitute a potent 5-HT$_{2a}$ ligand.[46,47] Additional hydrophobic substituents or a carbonyl group in the heterocyclic ring enhance the antagonistic potency[48] (Fig. 22.4).

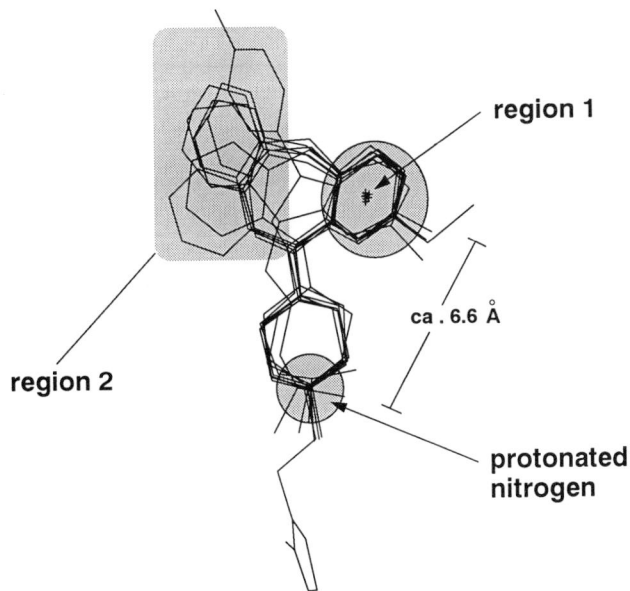

Fig. 22.4 Structure–activity relationship studies can be summarized as follows. For 5-HT$_{2a}$ affinity an aromatic centre (region 1) must be present at a distance of 6.6 Å from a protonatable nitrogen. A second hydrophobic area (region 2) close to the aromatic centre enhances receptor binding.

This knowledge was taken into account for the conformational analysis. In the case considered here, additional advantage could be drawn from the fact that various partial structural elements of the different conformationally constrained molecules can be matched with diverse regions of the highly flexible congeners. In Plate 1, comparable structural elements of the four main groups of 5-HT$_{2a}$ antagonists are colour coded and the stepwise superpositioning approach which was developed is indicated.

Next, the electronic properties for all derived pharmacophoric conformations have to be investigated. Using AM1-derived charges, we have determined and compared MEPs of all compounds. Plate 2 presents typical examples for the different groups. The high degree of similarity is evident. However, the superpositioning operation using the FITIT routine resulted in two slightly different pharmacophores. But both of them have to be treated as equally meaningful because r.m.s. values and total agreement of the MEPs within the two sets are comparably good.

In general, in a situation like this a decision on one or the other model can only be taken with consideration of the three-dimensional structure of the receptor binding site. If such information is missing, no decision is possible. However, a closer inspection of the two pharmacophores for 5-HT$_{2a}$ antagonists did bring to light one slight but significant structural divergence. In one of the two models all the protons at the pharmacophorically important cationic tertiary nitrogens are pointing in the same direction. In the other model this is not the case. Assuming that the cationic protonated nitrogen is involved in a hydrogen-bond-enforced ionic interaction with an anionic receptor binding site, the first pharmacophore model would clearly be favoured. Therefore, only this pharmacophore will be considered in the further investigation.

As described earlier, the evaluation of molecular interaction fields was performed using GRIN/GRID. The results have already been presented in Fig. 22.2. Using a variety of different

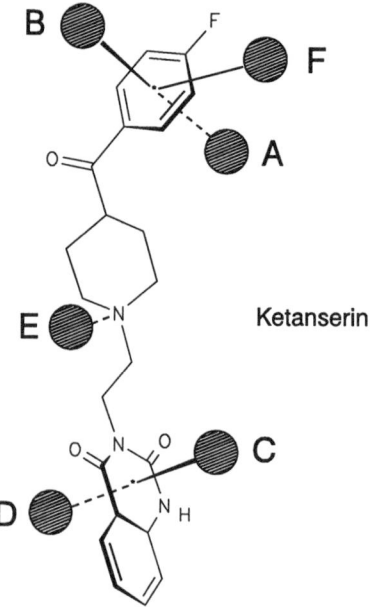

Fig. 22.5 The receptor map contains six positions for receptor contact. The map has been constructed on the basis of interaction field calculations as well as experimental structure–activity relationship data. Positions A, B, C, D and F depict hydrophobic contacts, position E is an ionic interaction.

probes, a rather detailed picture of the molecular interaction potential for 5-HT$_{2a}$ antagonists can be derived (Plate 3).

Careful inspection of Plate 3 leads almost automatically to the selection of suitable binding partners needed for the construction of the 5-HT$_{2a}$ receptor map. Hydrophobic amino acids like phenylalanine, tryptophan, valine, leucine or isoleucine should be positioned on both 'sides' of the planar cyclic systems. Opposite to the protonated nitrogen, an acidic amino acid (e.g. aspartic acid) should be used to fill the location marked by the interaction field created with a hydroxylic probe. The other regions of this field close to the two carbonyl groups found in most of the ligands should be filled with serine, threonine or tyrosine. At this point, of course, we do not know whether all the interaction possibilities discovered are in fact realized at the receptor level, and we will not be able to know this with certainty before the three-dimensional structure of the receptor protein has been elucidated. Nevertheless structure–activity relationship (SAR) studies are very helpful in deciding on the existence or absence of binding sites.

In the case under study, SAR data tell us that the carbonyl group of the fluorobenzoyl partial structural element is not essential and may be omitted without detrimental effect on the binding strength.[49] It is therefore concluded that a corresponding hydrogen-bond-donating binding site will probably not be present in the receptor. The same is true for the carbonyl element involved in the heterocyclic system. This can be deduced from the fact that ketanserin derivatives with undiminished affinity are known which instead present a thiocarbonyl[50] group or even possess a naphthyl system in place of the heterocycle.[51] In conclusion, from the three interaction sites for hydrogen-bond contacts between the ligands and the receptor protein, only the hydrogen-bond-enforced ionic interaction exerted by the protonated nitrogen will be present in the amino acid model.

One additional correction of the interaction field-derived receptor map is necessary. The serotoninergic 5-HT$_{2a}$ pharmacophore tells us that the aromatic part of the fluorobenzoyl system may be extensively substituted with hydrophobic elements and that this type of substitution leads to increasing affinity. This fact so far has not been accounted for in the receptor map, and so we have to add a third hydrophobic amino acid binding site to this region. The final receptor map then looks as shown in Fig. 22.5.

As mentioned before, the sites A through F of the map now can be occupied by different amino acids presenting the necessary chemical properties. The available biochemical information, such as amino acid sequence, bacteriorhodopsin homology, alignment studies, etc., has led us to construct the amino acid model of the 5-HT$_{2a}$ receptor presented in Fig. 22.6. Interaction energies for the complexes formed between ligands and the receptor model were calculated as described in Section II. D.

The biological data for the 5-HT$_{2a}$ ligands were taken from Elz;[52] also most of the substances were synthesized by that author. The correlation for the 15 ligands used is shown in Table 22.1 together with calculated interaction energies as well as experimental and theoretical binding affinities.

Theoretical binding affinities can be derived from the correlation equation, which is shown graphically in Fig. 22.7. The correlation seems to be quite significant. 89% of the variation in the biological data can be explained with the receptor model. On the other hand, a systematic deviation can be noticed. Some compounds (denoted by bold type in Table 22.1) are described by the model as being too weak by a constant factor of 1.0 or 1.5 orders of magnitude when compared to the experimental affinities. The inspection of the molecular formulae identifies those showing the larger deviation as fluorobenzoyl derivatives and those with smaller deviation

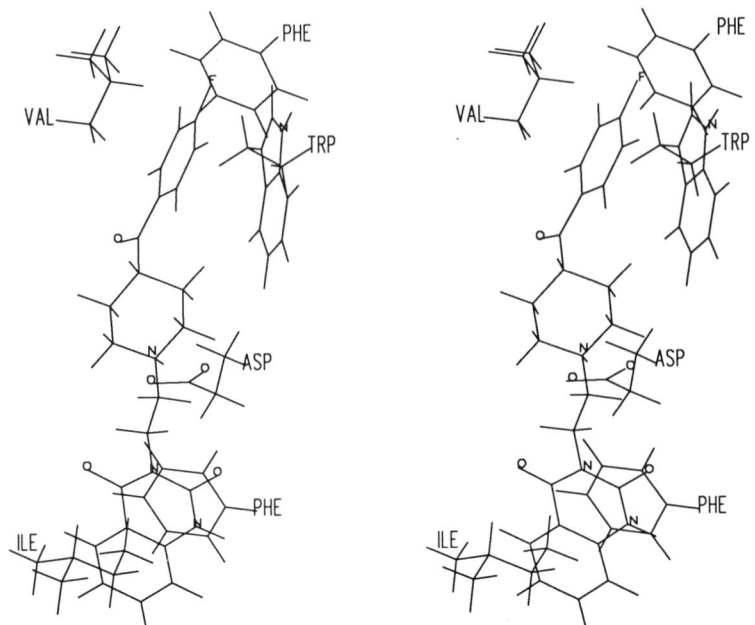

Fig. 22.6 Stereoscopic view of the 5-HT$_2$ receptor model constructed from single isolated amino acids on the basis of the receptor map (see Fig. 22.5).

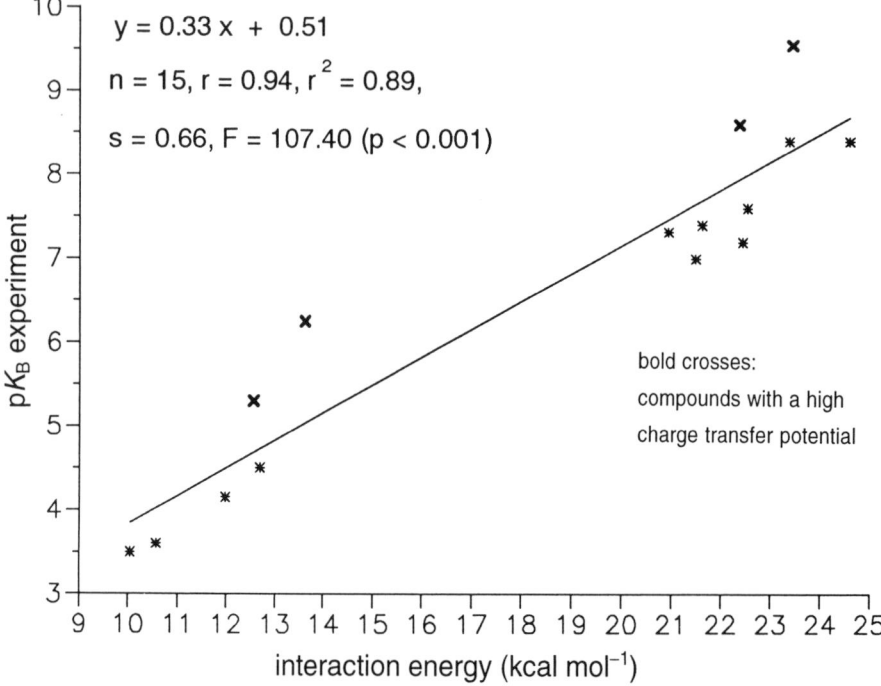

Fig. 22.7 Correlation between experimentally determined binding affinities and interaction energies calculated for complexes constructed using the receptor model. Some compounds (bold crosses) do not fit the correlation line satisfactorily.

Table 22.1   Fifteen 5-HT$_{2a}$-antagonistic substances and corresponding interaction energies calculated using the 5-HT$_{2a}$ receptor model.[a]

Compound	Interaction energy (kcal mol^{-1})	pK_B calculated	pK_B experiment
Ketanserin	23.44	7.94	9.55
EZS 15	22.38	7.60	8.60
EZS 21	22.54	7.65	7.60
EZS 32	21.62	7.35	7.40
Fluorbenzoylpiperidine (FTB)	13.62	4.73	6.25
Benzoylpiperidine (BP)	12.56	4.39	5.30
EZS 8	10.04	3.57	3.50
EZS 9	10.57	3.74	3.60
EZS 11	11.98	4.20	4.15
EZS 12	12.69	4.43	4.50
EZS 40	21.49	7.31	7.00
EZS 22	22.44	7.62	7.20
EZS 13	20.94	7.13	7.32
EZS 34	24.60	8.32	8.40
EZS 39	23.38	7.92	8.40

[a]Interaction energies are transformed into binding affinities (pK_B calculated) and compared to experimentally derived affinities (pK_B experiment).

as benzoyl derivatives. In all cases, substances which are not optimally described by the model possess an electron-deficient aromatic system. This leads to the hypothesis that for binding at the real receptor a type of interaction may be important which is not accounted for in the force field energies. According to biochemical data, the model is constructed with a tryptophan molecule as one of the binding partners of the aromatic ring system. This electron-rich amino acid could very well be involved in a charge-transfer interaction to the electron-deficient phenyl system. This type of interaction energy is not included in the force field energy. To check whether charge-transfer interactions in fact can explain the missing binding energies for the compounds mentioned, HOMO and LUMO energies were calculated for some test complexes between a truncated tryptophan (3-ethylindole) and models of the electron-deficient structures of the ligand molecules. The results are shown in Fig. 22.8.

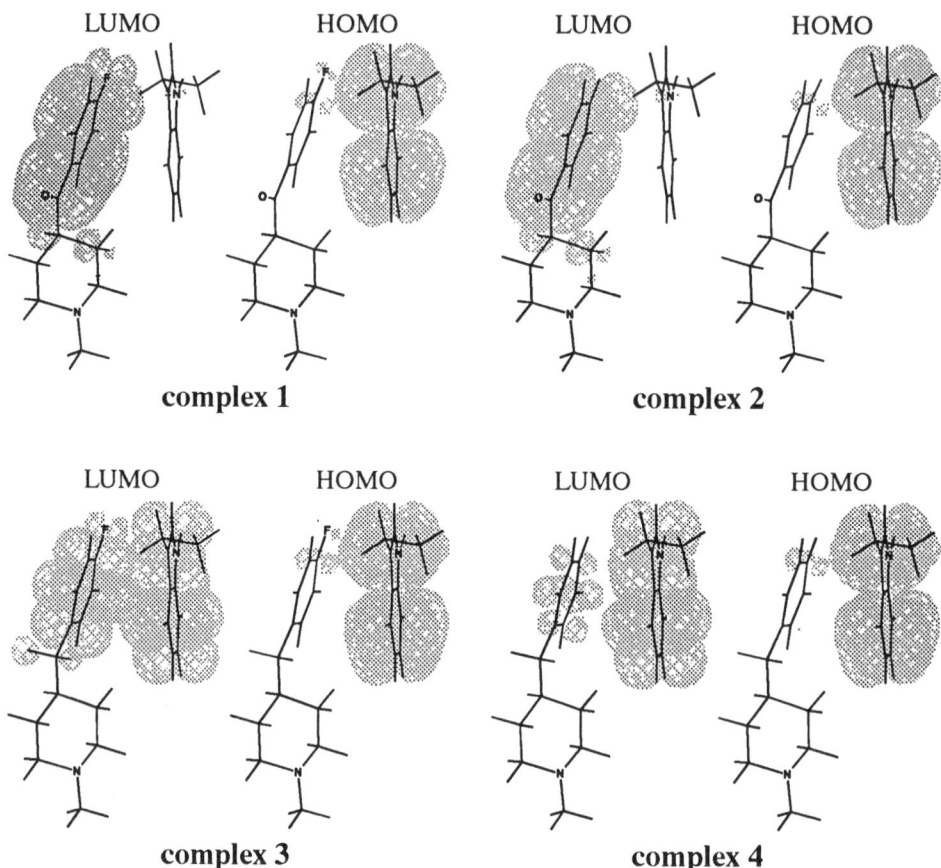

Fig. 22.8 HOMOs and LUMOs calculated using AM1 for complexes formed between ethylindole representing tryptophan and four truncated drug molecules. Charge-transfer interactions may occur in complexes 1, 2 and 3; they are impossible in complex 4.

It can clearly be seen that an electron transfer from the HOMO of electron-rich tryptophan to the LUMO of the electron-deficient partner only takes place for the fluorobenzoyl- (complex 1) and the benzoyl-*N*-methylpiperidine (complex 2) model. Only in these complexes are HOMOs and LUMOs neatly separated between the interacting molecules. In the other two cases, fluorobenzyl- (complex 3) and benzyl-*N*-methylpiperidine (complex 4), the indole system participates not only in the HOMO but also the LUMO, so that electron transfer may be drastically diminished (complex 3) or absent (complex 4). For this reason the force field interaction energies have to be corrected with a special charge-transfer correction factor for fluorobenzoyl and benzoyl derivatives. Direct combination of calculated energy values stemming from different methods is impossible, because the absolute numbers almost certainty will not match. Therefore, an adaption procedure has to be found to allow correct inclusion of the charge-transfer part into the total interaction energy. In the case reported here this could be accomplished by correlating differences between LUMO and HOMO energies of the charge-transfer complexes with experimentally derived binding affinities of the ligands. Consideration of this charge-transfer correction factor leads to a significantly improved correlation equation (see Fig. 22.9).

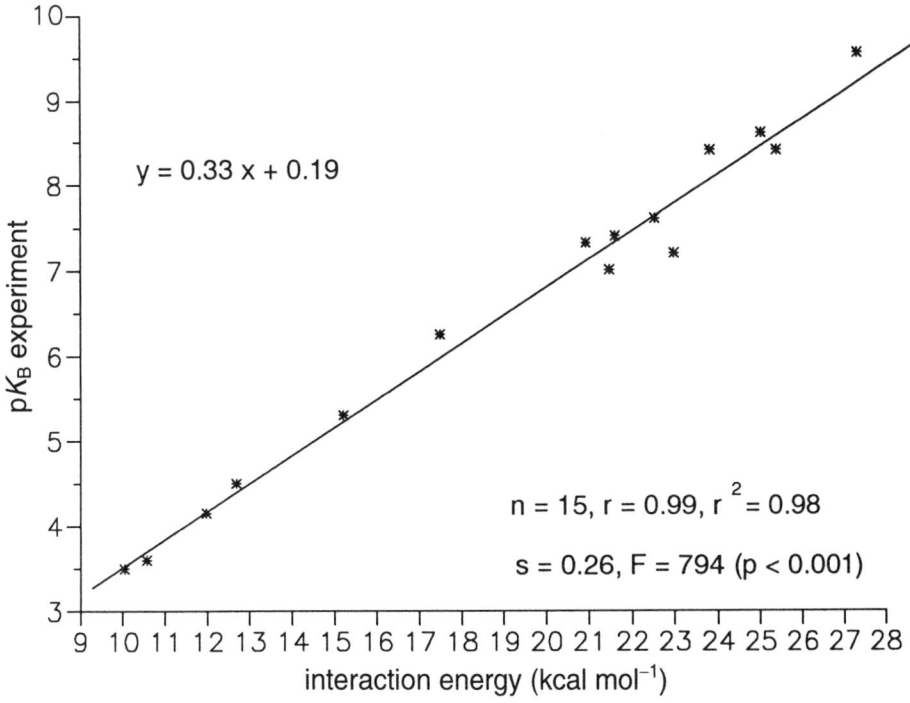

Fig. 22.9   Correlation between binding affinities and interaction energies including a charge-transfer correction term.

The F-test value is extremely high and now 98% of the variation of the biological activities for the 15 compounds in the series can be explained on the basis of the receptor model. As mentioned earlier, as long as the real receptor is unknown the efficiency and meaning of the model cannot be assessed except by prediction of new substances. Of course, the compounds must subsequently be synthesized and tested pharmacologically in order to prove or disprove the hypothesis. Based on the receptor map described, altogether ten new structures (see Table 22.2) were predicted and the respective interaction energies were calculated (including charge-transfer correction).

These energies are presented together with the predicted binding affinities collected from the correlation curve and the experimental binding affinities reported by Elz.[51] The graphical representation of the relation between predicted and experimental receptor affinities (Fig 22.10) is remarkable and shows that the developed receptor model seems to be consistent with the 'real' serotoninergic 5-HT$_{2a}$ receptor.

Table 22.2 Thirteen substances including 10 newly predicted structures and corresponding interaction energies calculated on the basis of the receptor model.[a]

Altanserin | Pirenperone | Risperidone | EZS 57 | EZS 155 (R=F) EZS 156 (R=H) | 4-Benzylpiperidine

EZS 56 | EZS 302 | EZS 300 | EZS 301 | EZS 151 (R=F) EZS 63 (R=H)

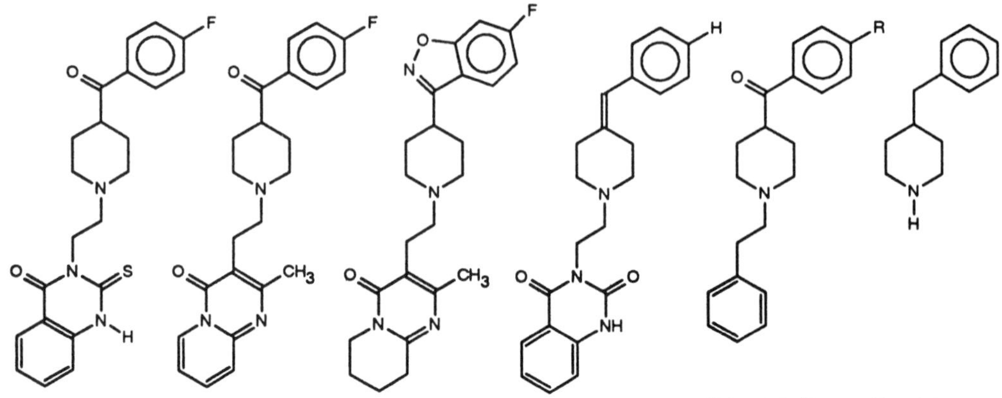

Compound	Interaction energy (kcal mol^{-1})	pK_B predicted	pK_B experiment
Altanserin	27.62	9.31	9.80
Pirenperone	27.16	9.15	9.30
Risperidone	28.69	9.66	9.70
EZS-57	22.27	7.54	7.20
EZS-155	23.91	8.08	8.50
EZS-156	21.61	7.32	8.20
EZS-302	22.09	7.48	7.70
EZS-300	23.23	7.86	7.65
EZS-301	19.37	6.58	6.25
4-Benzylpiperidine	12.64	4.36	5.00
EZS-56	25.53	8.62	8.60
EZS-151	23.64	7.99	7.40
EZS-63	21.41	7.26	7.20

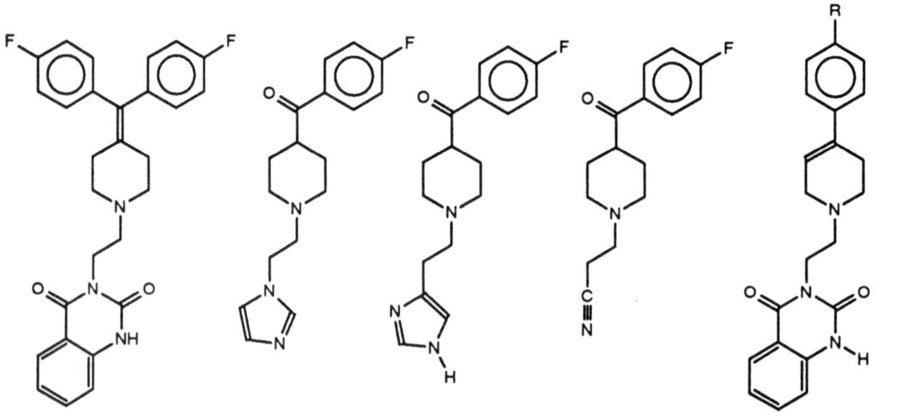

[a]Interaction energies are transformed into binding affinities (pK_B predicted) and compared to experimentally derived affinities (pK_B experiment).

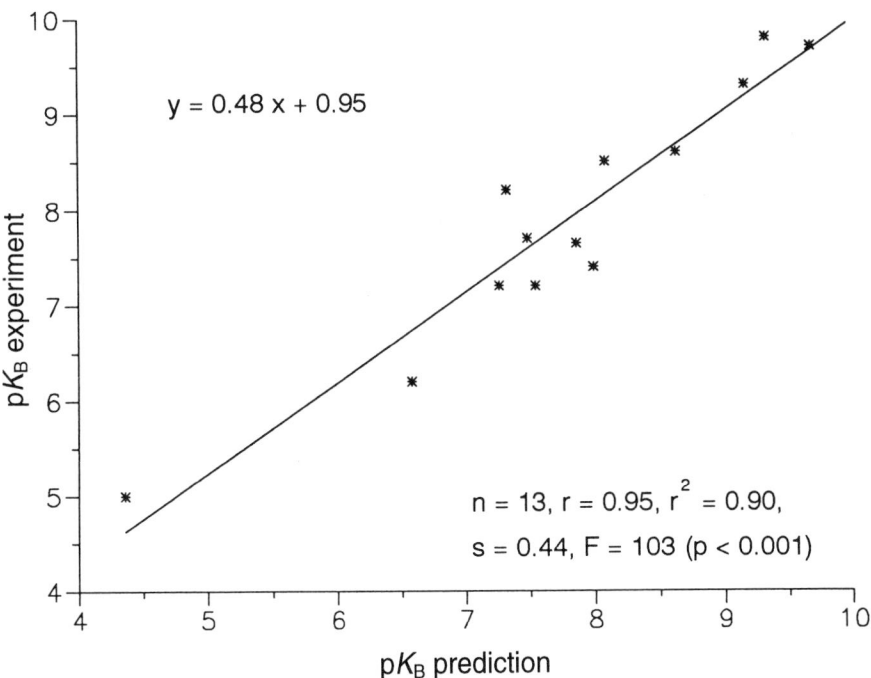

Fig. 22.10   Correlation between predicted and experimentally determined binding affinities at the 5-HT$_{2a}$ receptor for 13 antagonists including 10 newly predicted structures.

The example reported demonstrates that theoretical methods such as pharmacophore identification and receptor mapping can be successfully employed as predictive tools in medicinal chemistry.

REFERENCES

1. Kier, L. B. and Höltje, H.-D. (1975) A stochastic model of the remote recognition of preferred conformation in a drug–receptor interaction. *J. Theor. Biol.* **49**: 401–416.
2. Höltje, H.-D. (1992) Pharmacophore identification based on molecular electrostatic potentials. In Wermuth, C. G., Koga, N., Koenig, H. and Metcalf, B. (eds) *Medicinal Chemistry for the 21st Century*, pp. 181–189. Blackwell Scientific, Oxford.
3. Humblet, C. and Marshall, G. R. (1980) Pharmacophore identification and receptor mapping. *Annu. Rep. Med. Chem.* **15**: 267–276.
4. Cosentino, U., Moro, G., Pitea, D., Scolastico, S., Todeschini, R. and Scolastico, C. (1992) Pharmacophore identification by molecular modeling and chemometrics: the case of HMG-CoA reductase inhibitors. *J. Computer-Aided Mol. Design.* **6**: 47–60.
5. Belvisi, L., Brossa, S., Salimbeni, A., Scolastico, C. and Todeschini, R. (1991) Structure–activity relationship of Ca^{2+} channel blockers: a study using conformational analysis and chemometric methods. *J. Computer-Aided Mol. Design.* **5**: 571–584.
6. Cosentino, U., Moro, G., Pitea, D., Todeschino, R., Brossa, S., Gualandi, F., Scolastico, C. and Gienessi, F. (1990) Pharmacophore identification in amnesia-reversal compounds using conformational analysis and chemometric methods. *Quant. Struct.-Act. Relat.* **9**: 195–201.

7. *Cambridge Crystallographic Database*, Cambridge Crystallographic Data Centre, Cambridge, UK.

8. SYBYL, TRIPOS Associates Inc., St Louis, MO, USA.

9. INSIGHT 2, BIOSYM Technologies Inc., San Diego, CA, USA.

10. Auffinger, P. and Wipff, G. (1990) High temperature annealed molecular dynamics simulation as a tool for conformational sampling. *J. Comput. Chem.* **11**: 19–31.

11. Jendretzki, U. (1993) FITIT. Thesis, Free University of Berlin, Germany.

12. Crippen, G. M. (1977) A novel approach to calculation of conformation: distance geometry. *J. Comput. Phys.* **24**: 96–107.

13. Kuntz, I. D., Crippen, G. M. and Kollman, P.A. (1979) Applications of distance geometry to protein tertiary structure calculations. *Biopolymers* **18**: 939–957.

14. Donné-Op den Kelder, G. M. (1987) Distance geometry analysis of ligand binding to drug receptor sites. *J. Computer-Aided Mol. Des.* **1**: 257–264.

15. Ghose, A. K. and Crippen, G. M. (1985) Geometrically feasible binding modes of a flexible ligand molecule at the receptor site. *J. Comput. Chem.* **6**: 350–359.

16. Sheridan, R. P., Nilakantan, R., Dixon, J. S. and Venkataraghavan, R. J. (1986) The ensemble approach to distance geometry: application to the nicotinic pharmacophore. *J. Med. Chem.* **29**: 899–906.

17. Crippen, G. M. (1982) Prediction of new leads from a distance geometry binding site model. *Quant. Struct.-Act. Relat.* **2**: 95–100.

18. Marshall, G. R., Barry, C. D., Bosshard, H. E., Dammkoehler, R. A. and Dunn, D. A. (1979) The conformational parameter in drug design: the active analog approach. In Olson, E. C. and Christoffersen, R. E. (eds) *Computer-Assisted Drug Design. ACS Symp. Series*, vol. 112, pp. 205–226. American Chemical Society, Washington DC.

19. Marshall, G. R. (1987) Computer-aided drug design. *Annu. Rev. Pharmacol. Toxicol.* **27**: 193–213.

20. Scrocco, E. and Tomasi, J. (1978) Electronic molecular structure, reactivity and intermolecular forces: a heuristic interpretation by means of electrostatic molecular potentials. In Lödwin, P. (ed.) *Advances in Quantum Chemistry*, vol. II, pp. 115–193. Academic Press, New York.

21. Gasteiger, J. and Marsili, M. (1980) Iterative partial equalization of orbital electronegativity – a rapid access to atomic charges. *Tetrahedron* **36**: 3219–3228.

22. (a) Dewar, M. J. S. and Thiel, W. (1977) Ground states of molecules. 38. The MNDO method. Approximations and parameters. *J. Am. Chem. Soc.* **99**: 4899–4907. (1977) Ground states of molecules. 39. MNDO results for molecules containing hydrogen, carbon, nitrogen and oxygen. *J. Am. Chem. Soc.* **99**: 4907–4917. (b) Dewar, M. J. S., Zoebisch, E. G., Healy, E. F. and Stewart, J. J. P. (1985) A new general purpose quantum mechanical molecular model. *J. Am. Chem. Soc.* **107**: 3902–3909. (c) Stewart, J. J. P. (1989) Optimization of parameters for semiempirical methods I. Method. *J. Comput. Chem.* **10**: 209–220. (1989) Optimization of parameters for semiempirical methods II. Applications. *J. Comput. Chem.* **10**: 221–264.

23. Van de Waterbeemd, H., Carrupt, P. A. and Testa, B. (1986) Molecular electrostatic potential of orthopramides: implications for their interaction with the D-2 dopamine receptor. *J. Med. Chem.* **29**: 600–606.

24. Kocjan, D., Hodoscek, M. and Hadzi, D. (1986) Dopaminergic pharmacophore of ergoline and its analogs. A molecular electrostatic potential study. *J. Med. Chem.* **29**: 1418–1423.

25. SPARTAN Version 3.0, Wavefunction, Inc., Irvine, CA, USA.

26. D-mol, BIOSYM Technologies Inc., San Diego, CA, USA.

27. Alemán, C., Luque, F. J. and Orozco, M. (1993) A new scaling procedure to correct semiempirical MEP and MEP-derived properties. *J. Computer-Aided Mol. Des.* **7**: 721–742.

28. Goodford, P. J. (1985) A computational procedure for determining energetically favorable binding sites on biologically important macromolecules. *J. Med. Chem.* **28**: 849–857.

29. Cramer III, R. D., Patterson, D. E. and Bunce, J. D. (1988) Comparative molecular field analysis (CoMFA). 1. Effect of shape on binding of steroids to carrier proteins. *J. Am. Chem. Soc.* **110**: 5959–5967.

30. Kellogg, G. E., Semus, S. F. and Abraham, D. J. (1991) HINT – A new method of empirical field calculation for CoMFA. *J. Computer-Aided Mol. Des.* **5**: 545–552.

31. Kellogg, G. E., Joshi, G. S. and Abraham, D. J. (1992) New tools for modeling and understanding hydrophobicity and hydrophobic interactions. *Med. Chem. Res.* **1**: 444–453.

32. Wold, S., Johansson, E. and Cocchi, M. (1993) PLS – partial least-squares projections to latent

structures. In Kubinyi (ed.) *3D QSAR in Drug Design – Theory Methods and Applications*, ESCOM, pp. 523–550. Leiden.

33. Höltje, H.-D. and Anzali, S. (1992) Molecular modelling studies on the digitalis binding site of the Na$^+$/K$^+$-ATPase. *Die Pharmazie* **47**: 691–697.

34. Höltje, H.-D. and Dall, N. (1993) A molecular modelling study on the hormone binding site of the estrogen receptor. *Die Pharmazie* **48**: 243–249.

35. Höltje, M. and Höltje, H.-D. (1991) Molecular modelling study on the negative inotropic potencies of 1,4-dihydropyridines. *Pharm Pharmacol Lett.* **1**: 19–22.

36. Höltje, H.-D. and Jendretzki, U. (1992) Conformational analysis of 5-HT$_2$ receptor antagonists. *Pharm. Pharmacol. Lett.* **1**: 89–92.

37. Snyder, J. P., Rao, S. N., Koehler, K. F. and Pellicciari, R. (1992) Drug modeling at cell membrane receptors: the concept of pseudoreceptors. In Angeli, P., Gulini, U. and Quaglia, W. (eds) *Trends in Receptor Research*, pp. 367–403. Elsevier, Amsterdam.

38. Snyder, J. P. and Rao, S. N. (1989) Pseudoreceptors: a bridge between receptor fitting and receptor mapping in drug design. *CDA News* **4/10**: 1/13–15.

39. Rao, S. N. and Snyder, J. P. (1990) Pseudoreceptor modeling: an experiment in large scale computing. *Cray Channels*. **11**: 4–12.

40. Guan, X.-M., Peroutka, S. J. and Kobilka, B. K. (1992) Identification of a single amino acid residue responsible for the binding of a class of β-adrenergic receptor antagonists to 5-hydroxytryptamine$_{1A}$ receptors. *Mol. Pharmacol.* **41**: 695–698.

41. Kao, H.-T., Adham, N., Olsen, M. A., Weinshank, R. L., Branchek, T. A. and Hartig, P. R. (1992) Site-directed mutagenesis of a single residue changes the binding properties of the serotonin 5-HT$_2$ receptor from a human to a rat pharmacology. *FEBS Lett.* **307**: 324–328.

42. Humblet, C. and Mirzadegan, T. (1992) Models of G protein-coupled receptors. *Annu. Rep. Med. Chem.* **27**: 291–300.

43. Trumpp-Kallmeyer, S., Hoflack, J., Bruinvels, A. and Hibert, M. (1992) Modeling of G-protein-coupled receptors: application to dopamine, adrenaline, serotonin, acetylcholine, and mammalian opsin receptors. *J. Med. Chem.* **35**: 3448–3462.

44. Andrews, P. R. (1993) Drug-receptor interactions. In Kubinyi, H. (ed.) *3D QSAR in Drug Design – Theory Methods and Applications*, pp. 13–40. ESCOM, Leiden.

45. Hibert, M. F., Mir, A. K. and Fozard, J. R. (1990) Serotonin (5-HT) receptors. In Emmett, J. C. (ed.) *Comprehensive Medicinal Chemistry*, vol. 3, pp. 567–601. Pergamon Press, New York.

46. Watanabe, Y., Usui, H., Shibano, T., Tanaka, T. and Kanao, M. (1990) Syntheses of monocyclic and bicyclic 2,4(1*H*,3*H*)-pyrimidinediones and their serotonin 2 antagonist activities. *Chem. Pharm. Bull.* **38**: 2726–2732.

47. Ketanserin patent, Janssen Pharmaceutica N. V., European Patent Office. Kennis, L. E. J., Van der Aa, M. J. M., Van Heertum, A. H. M. and Jones, A. J. (1980) Nr. 0013612, Appl. Nr. 803000595.

48. Glennon, R. A. (1991) Serotonin receptor subtypes: basic and clinical aspects. In Peroutka, S. J., Venter, J. C. and Harrison, L. C. (eds) *Receptor Biochemistry and Methodology*, vol. 15, pp. 19–64. Wiley-Liss, New York.

49. Herndon, J. L., Ismaiel, A., Ingher, S. P., Teitler, M. and Glennon, R. A. (1992) Ketanserin analogues: structure–affinity relationships for 5-HT$_2$ and 5-HT$_{1C}$ serotonin receptor binding. *J. Med. Chem.* **35**: 4903–4910.

50. Bogeso, K. P., Arnt, J., Boeck, V., Christensen, A. V., Hyttel, J. and Jensen, K. G. (1988) Antihypertensive activity in a series of 1-piperazino-3-phenylindans with potent 5-HT$_2$-antagonistic activity. *J. Med. Chem.* **31**: 2247–2256.

51. Elz, S., unpublished results.

52. Elz, S. (1992) Synthesis and *in vitro* pharmacology of antiserotoninergic$_2$ ketanserin analogues and *N*-imidazolylalkyl substituted 4-(4-fluorobenzoyl)piperidine-1-carboxamidines. *XIIth International Symposium on Medicinal Chemistry*, Basel, Switzerland, poster P-128.C, abstract book, p. 349.

23

Three-Dimensional Quantitative Structure–Activity Relationships: D2 Dopamine Agonists as an Example

YVONNE CONNOLLY MARTIN and C. THOMAS LIN

A molecule would hence show strong attraction for another molecule which possessed complete
complementariness in surface configuration and distribution of active electrically charged and
hydrogen-bond forming groups, somewhat weaker attraction for those molecules with approximate
but not complete complementariness to it, and only very weak attraction for all other molecules.
L. Pauling, D. H. Campbell and D. Pressman (1943)

THE PRACTICE OF MEDICINAL CHEMISTRY
ISBN 0-12-744640-0

I. OVERVIEW OF 3D QSAR

A. Why do 3D QSAR?

A medicinal chemist is duly proud of the structure–activity information so carefully discovered and is eager to glean even more information from these data. Often the compounds are designed using computational chemistry[1] to refine a pharmacophore map — a qualitative picture of the 3D requirements for a ligand to possess a particular target bioactivity. Hence, it is attractive to examine whether computer analyses of structure–activity relationships reveal quantitative information about the 3D requirements for bioactivity of the compounds.[2,3]

3D QSAR often applies to a more diverse set of compounds than does traditional 2D QSAR. This derives from the fact that molecules are described by properties calculated directly from their 3D structures — one does not have to estimate properties from substituent constants measured on related molecules as in traditional 2D QSAR. Not only does this allow more structural diversity in the set of compounds used to derive the model, it also allows one to forecast the potency of a wider variety of compounds. Thus, a good 3D QSAR may be more general than a 2D QSAR and may help the medicinal chemist to design compounds differing more from those used to derive the model.

Notice the structural diversity of the compounds listed in Table 23.1. How would one describe the differences of physical properties of these molecules?

Of course, 3D QSAR may be ambiguous or impossible if one cannot suggest a bioactive conformation and superposition rule for the compounds.

The CoMFA method of 3D QSAR produces 3D contour plots of the locations in space at which certain properties increase or decrease biological potency.[3-8] To illustrate, Fig. 23.1 shows the contours of positive and negative steric effects of affinity for the D_2 receptor. This strong visual representation is a very attractive aid to understanding the structure–activity relationships and can help in the design of more potent compounds.

Lastly, there is a feeling that since ligands and their target biomolecules are three-dimensional, structure–activity relationships of ligands should be presented in three dimensions. To the extent that the QSAR are reliable and robust, this may be true. However, one must also understand that a poor model is a poor model whether it is in 2D or 3D. Additionally, there might be a multitude of redundant 3D models that explain the structure–activity relationships if the series as a whole does not contain enough 3D information. We will describe how to avoid self-deception when doing a 3D QSAR.

Today there are several readily available computer programs that a nonexpert can use to conduct such 3D QSAR studies. This chapter will discuss them from the viewpoint of someone who wants to derive reliable and useful models from the data but also intends to leave the details of the computer algorithms and programming to the software developers. The discussion will be illustrated by our analysis of literature D_2 agonists.

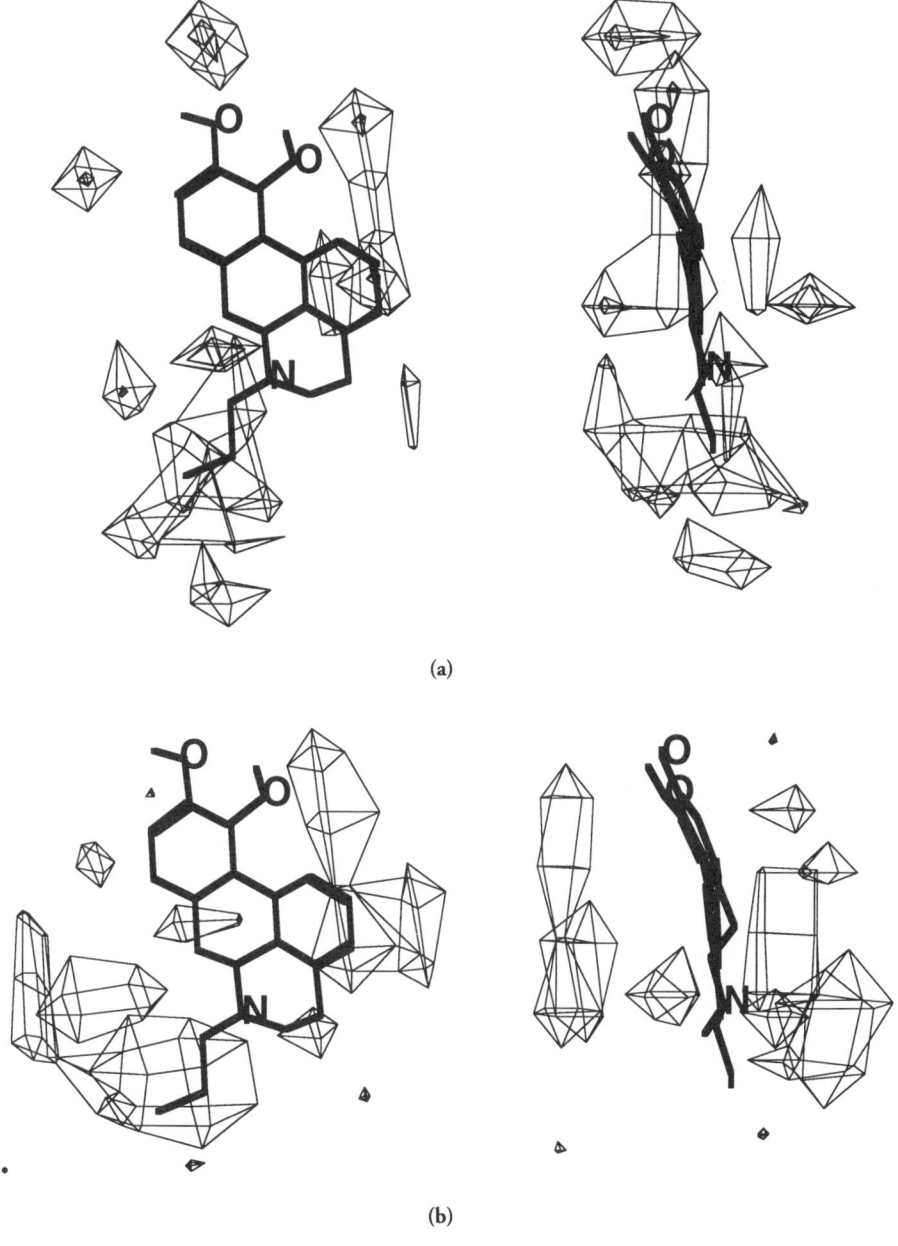

(a)

(b)

Fig. 23.1. CoMFA contours of the influence of shape on affinity for the D_2 receptor: (a) shows the regions in space where extra volume increases affinity and (b) the regions where it decreases affinity.

Table 23.1 Structures, molecular modelling results, and observed and predicted affinities of D_2 dopaminergic agonists.

Stucture	Number	Stereochemistry	X	Y	R^1	Rel. E (kcal mol^{-1})	N–O distance (Å)	pK$_i$ Obs.	pK$_i$ Fitted	pK$_i$ Cross-validated
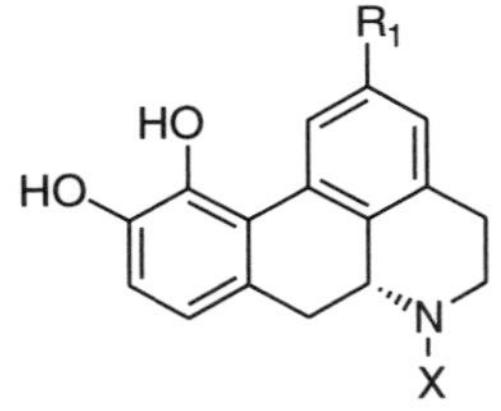	I	Shown	Pr^n	–	H	0.0	6.5	9.10	8.90	8.57
	II	Shown	Me	–	H	0.0	6.5	8.88	8.93	8.88
	III	Shown	Me	–	OH	0.0	6.5	8.66	8.87	8.99
	IV	Inverted	Me	–	H	0.8	6.5	6.00	6.04	6.63
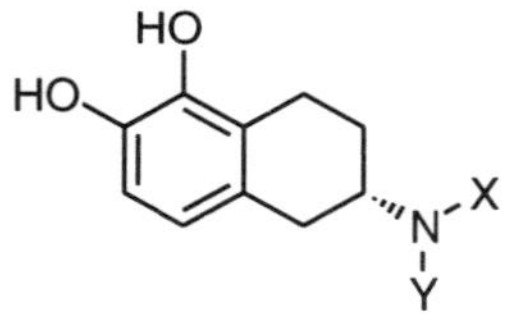	V	Shown	Pr^n	Pr^n		0.0	6.5	8.38	8.44	8.49
	VI	Shown	H	H		0.0	6.5	7.65	7.94	8.77
	VII	Inverted	Pr^n	Pr^n		1.9	6.5	7.39	7.39	7.59
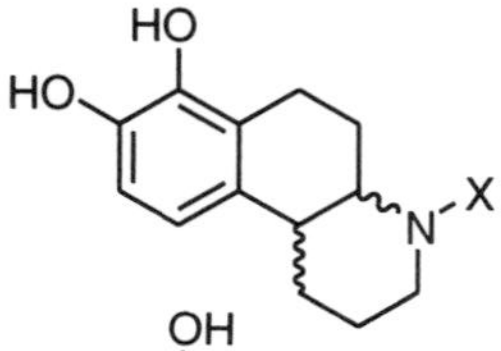	VIII	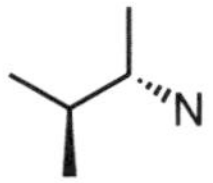	H			0.0	6.5	8.74	8.53	8.85
	IX		Et			0.0	6.5	8.40	8.38	7.68
	X	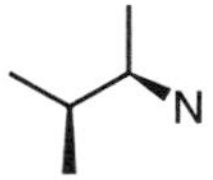	H			0.0	6.5	7.01	7.43	7.73
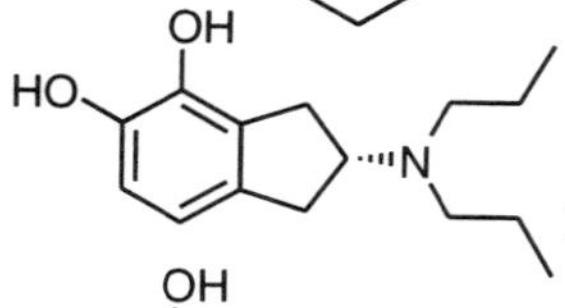	XI	Shown				0.0	5.6	7.22	6.97	6.87
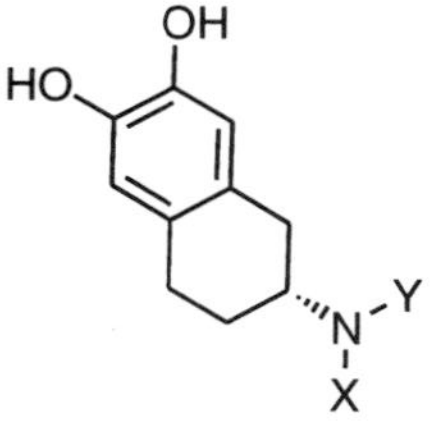	XII	Shown	H	H		0.0	7.4	8.77	8.34	7.77
	XIII	Shown	Me	Me		0.0	7.4	8.64	8.53	8.04
	XIV	Shown	Pr^n	Pr^n		0.0	7.4	7.92	8.27	8.62

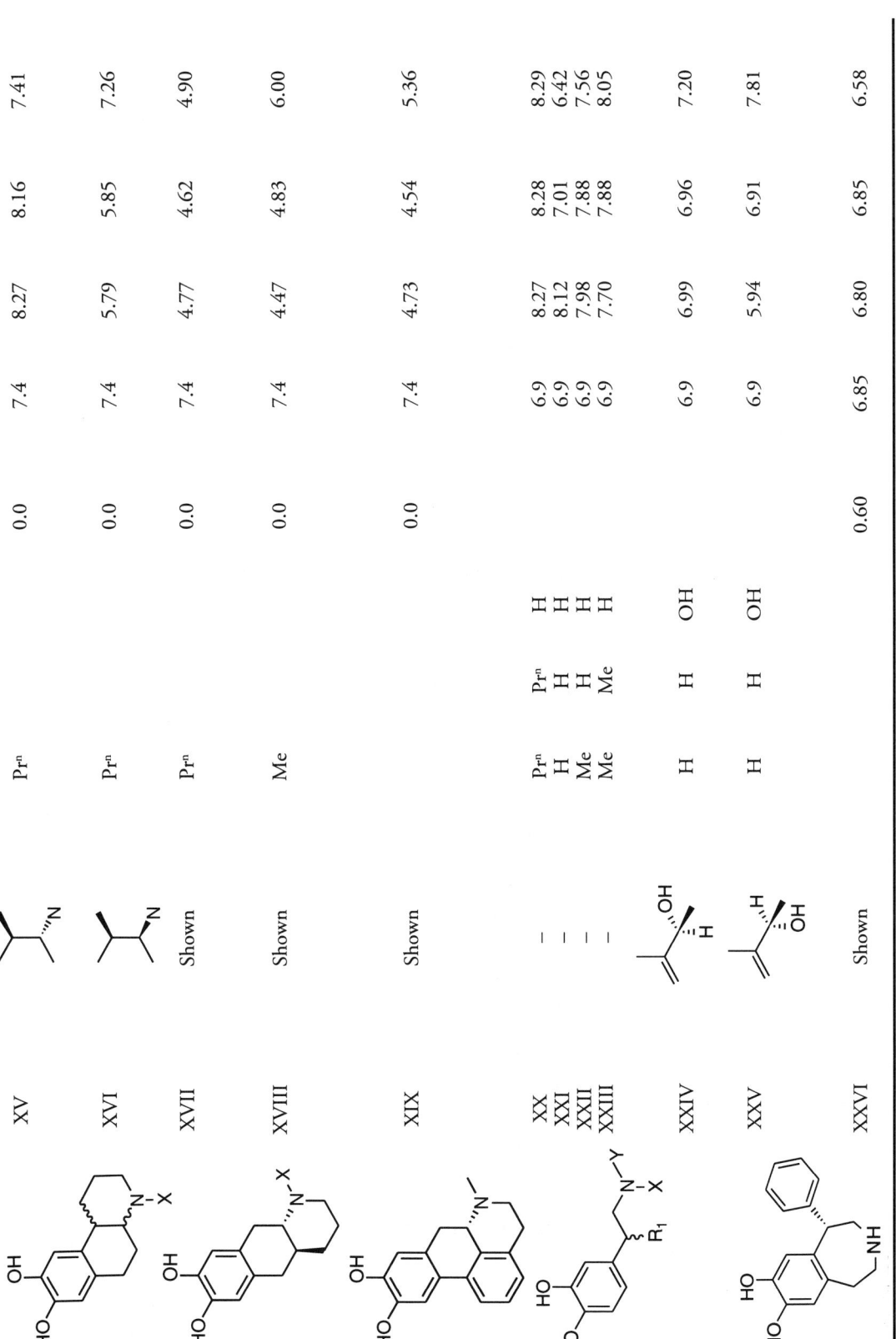

Compound	Config									
XV		Pr^n			0.0	7.4	8.27	8.16	7.41
XVI		Pr^n			0.0	7.4	5.79	5.85	7.26
XVII	Shown	Pr^n			0.0	7.4	4.77	4.62	4.90
XVIII	Shown	Me			0.0	7.4	4.47	4.83	6.00
XIX	Shown				0.0	7.4	4.73	4.54	5.36
XX	—	Pr^n	Pr^n	H		6.9	8.27	8.28	8.29
XXI	—	H	H	H		6.9	8.12	7.01	6.42
XXII	—	Me	H	H		6.9	7.98	7.88	7.56
XXIII	—	Me	Me	H		6.9	7.70	7.88	8.05
XXIV		H	H	OH		6.9	6.99	6.96	7.20
XXV		H	H	OH		6.9	5.94	6.91	7.81
XXVI	Shown				0.60	6.85	6.80	6.85	6.58

B. Overviews of commercially available 3D QSAR programs

1. Comparative molecular field analysis, CoMFA

CoMFA is the most widely used method for 3D QSAR. A recent review lists more than 90 datasets successfully analysed with CoMFA and the forecast of 297 compounds from 25 datasets not included in the analysis. The forecasts have a root-mean-square error of 0.70 logs or 0.98 kcal mol[-1].[3] Although the extensive use of CoMFA may be partly a reflection of the commercial availability of the program, the enthusiasm of the scientific community is nevertheless impressive.

A CoMFA analysis starts with traditional molecular modelling/pharmacophore mapping analysis to suggest a bioactive conformation of each molecule and ways to superimpose the molecules.[9] The logistics of this process will be discussed in a later section since they apply equally to other 3D QSAR strategies.

Once the molecules are aligned, the CoMFA analysis continues by calculating the intermolecular interaction fields surrounding each molecule. These fields are evaluated at the intersections of a 3D lattice that encloses all the molecules. In commercial CoMFA, electrostatic and steric fields are provided. The steric field of a molecule describes where in space the molecule is located. Its electrostatic field describes the influence of the partial atomic charges on the electrostatics of the surrounding space. In commercial CoMFA, explicit hydrophobic fields are not calculated.

Next, the relationships between the biological potency and the calculated fields are evaluated by the special multivariate statistical technique of partial least squares (PLS).[10] PLS is able to build a statistical model even though there are more columns of energy values than compounds because the various energy values are correlated with each other and many are unrelated to biological activity. Generally, no more than five or six linear combinations of the energy values are needed to build a model. A key aspect of the PLS analysis is the use of cross-validation — one does not merely fit the data but rather calculates many models, leaving out some of the compounds each time.[11] From this leave-n-out procedure the potencies of the omitted compounds can be forecast. Only if the forecasts are significantly better than chance is a model accepted.

Lastly, the contribution to potency of each energy value at each lattice point is calculated and contours are drawn. This final 3D visualization of the 3D QSAR results is an especially attractive feature of CoMFA since, first, it makes it easy for the investigator to evaluate how sensible the relationship is and, second, enables its use to design more potent compounds. For instance, notice that the contours in Fig. 23.1 represent the affinity-enhancing effect of adding a propyl to the nitrogen.

2. Molecular 3D similarity

3D QSAR based on 3D similarity matrices has recently been introduced.[12–14] The essence of the method is to calculate, for any 2D or 3D molecular descriptor, the similarity of each molecule with every other molecule of the dataset. For the 3D applications, the molecular modelling, choice of bioactive conformation, and superposition are the same as in CoMFA.

The similarity matrix is analysed by PLS. Because of the peculiarities of PLS, if the inputs to this analysis are the similarities between CoMFA fields of the pairs of compounds, then the procedure is very similar to a CoMFA analysis.[15] However, one difference between CoMFA and molecular similarity matrix analysis is that for the latter any measure of similarity can be used — it need not be restricted to properties at specific locations in space. A disadvantage of similarity analysis is that the user must select the properties, regions in space for fields, that are combined into one similarity number. Sterics and electrostatics are frequently combined. In contrast, the PLS analysis of CoMFA selects the relevant from irrelevant variables. Whereas CoMFA models can be expressed as contours over a reference molecule, this visualization has not been applied to molecular similarity.

Any type of molecular feature can be used to calculate the similarity of the molecules. The original applications were of electrostatic fields, but steric fields, electrostatic or steric similarities calculated by Gaussian approximations, and lipophilicity[16] have also been used.

3.   Available approaches to 3D QSAR that are not documented in the literature

The computer program CATALYST might also be available to some readers. No description of its algorithms or comparison of its performance has been reported in the refereed literature. However, it is a combination pharmacophore mapping–3D QSAR program associated with a rapid 3D searching component.[17] The user supplies the 2D structures of the molecules of interest and the program, after a day or two, replies with a hypothesis of the quantitative features required for bioactivity. Features considered include ligand hydrogen-bond donors, hydrogen-bond acceptors, ionizable basic and acidic groups, and hydrophobic groups. The evaluation of the hypotheses, the 3D QSAR, is performed by novel algorithms.

Our evaluation of the program in 1992 on a test set of 31 compounds yielded disappointing results. The forecasts of potency of an additional 30 compounds were worse than chance; the R^2 is negative, whereas CoMFA forecasts of potency from the same datasets were significantly better than chance. The model suggested by CATALYST is in contradiction of the literature[18–20] in that for dopamine the *para* O is used in the pharmacophore even though the dataset included potent *meta* monophenols. We have not re-evaluated the program since it has been revised.

Although the authors have published partial descriptions, APEX is also not documented in the refereed literature.[21,22] To run it, the user supplies all conformers of the molecules to be considered, with the corresponding partial atomic charges. The program uses a maximum 3D common substructure algorithm, such as described in DISCO below, to arrive at possible pharmacophores present in the active compounds. It scores the likelihood of a pharmacophore model on the basis of its power to discriminate between active and inactive compounds.

C.   Relationships of 2D to 3D QSAR

2D QSAR, particularly Hansch analysis, has a long track record of successful application in medicinal chemistry.[16,23,24] How can that be if molecules and their macromolecular targets are three-dimensional?

Work in our laboratory has shown that the CoMFA descriptors contain the same information as traditional Hansch descriptors and that series that are well fitted by traditional QSAR are also fitted by CoMFA.[25–31] We first examined the pK_a values of benzoic acids, the traditional Hammett σ constant, and found excellent CoMFA models using electrostatic fields calculated from point charges calculated by the semiempirical quantum-chemical program AM1. The pK_a values of imidazoles, imidazolines, phenols and anilines are also well modelled. For hydrophobic effects it was essential to include a hydrogen-bonding function as in the GRID program.[32–35]

These results emphasize the point that although the names of the molecular features used by

CoMFA and Hansch analysis might be different, both seem to capture the essence of how to describe the effect of structure modification on the ability of a compound to participate in a noncovalent interaction with a biological macromolecule.

The medicinal chemist must then decide whether 2D or 3D QSAR is appropriate for a particular research investigation. Clearly, if the intent is to design molecules with markedly different 2D backbones but the same 3D features, the work has to be done in 3D. 3D QSAR is also the method of choice when it is very difficult to estimate the descriptors for 2D QSAR.

A good 3D QSAR requires a pharmacophore hypothesis.[9] For some datasets, this can present a difficulty. A typical situation occurs if the molecules are analogues with the same type of flexibility, leading to more than one possible pharmacophore map. 3D QSAR analyses might distinguish the possibilities, but they might not.

To arrive at a unique pharmacophore map in such a case, one must synthesize (and test) active conformationally constrained analogues designed to distinguish the pharmacophore maps. For instance, we synthesized a number of compounds to establish the bioactive conformation of XXVI as a D_1 dopaminergic agonist. This work led to the identification of a novel series of potent and selective agonists.[36-38] The CoMFA built on it had excellent forecasting ability and helped set priorities for synthesis of analogues within the project.[39]

If a unique pharmacophore cannot be selected, any reasonable one can be used. The resulting 3D QSAR will strictly apply only to the type of compound used in its derivation. The problem is that once one looks at the impressive contours, it is tempting to believe that they represent actual 3D relationships between features. In fact, the contours might move in space as much as the underlying atoms from which the potentials are derived.

II.   SELECTING DATA FOR A 3D QSAR

As with any QSAR method, the first point to consider is whether the compounds have all been tested so that their relative biological potencies are directly comparable.[40] Preferably the biological tests have been done in the same laboratory under identical conditions. The biological endpoint should represent a free energy-related variable and whether it describes interactions of ligands with only one macromolecule. The biological endpoint for the D_2 agonists in Table 23.1 is the inhibition of binding of [^{3}H]spiperone, a D_2 antagonist to rat brain synaptosomes.[18]

The second consideration is whether the structure–activity information suggests that there is 3D information. If not, is one willing to settle for 3D ambiguity?

One must next consider whether the available molecular modelling methods will be successful with the particular type of compound. For instance, it might be difficult to calculate 3D descriptors for the relative ability of compounds to bind to metal sites in a protein. In other cases, optimizing the 3D structures can be a problem if molecular mechanics parameters[41-43] are not available and if semiempirical calculations[42,44,45] are not appropriate.

III.   MOLECULAR MODELLING ASPECTS

A.   Structure optimization

Even if rigid rotation around bonds is used to explore the conformers available to the compounds, 3D molecular structures are usually optimized (minimized) by either molecular mechanics or quantum-mechanical calculations. Both types of program have deficiencies; for example, each sometimes breaks or forces hydrogen bonds.

Some molecular mechanics programs may report many missing parameters that the user must establish or guess; others simply guess without warning the user.[41,43] They also sometimes incorrectly treat single bonds between two aromatic rings, as in biphenyls, aniline nitrogens and unusual substituents. Resonance interactions may not be accounted for in the calculations.

On the other hand, quantum-mechanical programs take longer to run, may fail on poor-quality input structures, and may not reproduce experimental structures as closely as a well-parametrized molecular mechanics calculation.[42,44,45] If charges from a quantum-chemical calculation are to be used in the final CoMFA, then the structure must be optimized with that program, because even minor changes in geometry can change the electron distribution. However, this final structure optimization may be done on a conformation previously optimized with molecular mechanics to be in a reasonable energy minimum.

We have found it critical to assure oneself that the program being considered accurately treats the types of molecules of interest. The easiest way to do this is to find good-quality experimental 3D structures of molecules that share features of those being studied. The Cambridge Structural Database[46] is a rich source of such information. Every substructural feature in the set of interest should be included in at least one of the test molecules. Then the possible optimization methods are applied to each of the test structures to double-check that the molecules are not unacceptably distorted from the experimental form.

We were fortunate that several crystal structures were available for D_2 agonists. Aporphines such as I–IV were particularly difficult to reproduce. For example for (II) some of the molecular mechanics programs, but not MMP2,[47] forced the biphenyl substructure to be planar with the result that the aromatic rings were bent. MMP2 also calculated reasonable lengths for the bonds of the indole ring present in such D_2 dopaminergic agonists as structure XXVII.

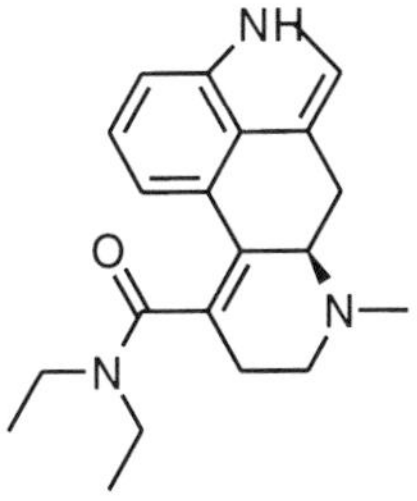

XXVII

B.   Conformational searching

This is another art for which no general rules can be stated.[48–50] The searching may be done manually, that is by constructing each of the low-energy conformers that one expects to be important. For alicyclic chains, rigid rotation can give a quick view of the accessible conformers. Some workers prefer high-temperature molecular dynamics, whereas in our laboratory we make extensive use of distance geometry, which is especially suitable for compounds that contain alicyclic rings.

Distance geometry is a special mathematical method that generates 3D structures using as input only the upper and lower bounds of the distances between each of the atoms.[49,51-53] One 3D conformation of a molecule is all that is required for input. We continue searching for new conformers until no new low-energy ones are found. This might require generating hundreds or even a thousand conformers.

No matter which method of conformational search is chosen, the final structures are refined with molecular mechanics or quantum mechanics. As with evaluating the results of an energy minimization, a conformational search is not complete until the scientist is satisfied that the generated results are sensible and comparable to experiment.

The D_2 agonists were studied a number of years ago, at which time we manually generated the various ring puckers and conformers and optimized them with MMP2.[47] (If the study were to be done today, distance geometry would be used.) Apomorphine, II, although it might look rigid, actually has at least four low-energy conformers excluding rotations of the catechols. In particular, inversion of the nitrogen gives rise to a conformer that is 0.86 kcal mol^{-1} higher in energy. The conformation in which the catechol OH groups are rotated away from the unsubstituted aromatic ring is 0.23 kcal mol^{-1} lower in energy than that in which the OH groups are rotated 180°.

Some of the strategies discussed below provide choices for the bioactive conformation based on user-supplied superposition rules. With such methods it is important to generate conformers independently to estimate the relative energy of the proposed bioactive conformation.

One need not subject every analogue to exhaustive conformational searching. Rather, those that share important conformation-determining features such as (1) ring size and (2) position and relative stereochemistry of substituents will populate the same conformational families. We typically explore the most constrained potent analogue of such a set, build all conformers of the others from those found from the first, and minimize them. In this way we have information as to the relative energy of all conformers of all the molecules. However, typically for 3D QSAR, one would choose the same conformer for all members of a series.

For the compounds in Table 23.1 we explored the conformers of II, VI, VIII, X, XI, XVIII, XXI, and XXVI and built the others from them.

C.   Calculating partial atomic charges

Partial atomic charges may be calculated by empirical methods[54] or with semiempirical or *ab initio* quantum-chemical calculations.[42,44,45,55] In our modelling of pK_a values of benzoic acids we found that charges generated with AM1[56] were superior to empirical charges and to point charges fitted from *ab initio* STO-3G[42,55] electrostatic potential surfaces. As noted above, if electrostatic effects are important in a 3D QSAR, it is important to also optimize the structure in the quantum-mechanical program.

IV.   SELECTING THE BIOACTIVE CONFORMATION, ENANTIOMER AND ALIGNMENT RULE

A.   General comments on pharmacophore mapping as a prelude to 3D QSAR

Any 3D QSAR method starts with the problem of selecting the bioactive conformation. Unless this is provided by a 3D structure of the ligand–macromolecule complex or a completely rigid potent compound, the scientist must deduce this information, perhaps aided by a computer program. The scientist must also propose how other compounds of the dataset superimpose, and frequently must also suggest the bioactive enantiomer. To do this one must first discover the pertinent information — it frequently appears in many different and sometimes obscure references. Next, one must evaluate and integrate this information. Hence it is often the case that the most difficult and subjective part of a 3D QSAR analysis is choosing the bioactive conformation, enantiomer and superposition rule.

A set of compounds well suited for pharmacophore mapping has at least one potent compound with only a few low-energy conformers and only a few features for superposition.[9] The most popular strategies emphasize first identifying those features shared by all potent molecules and subsequently analysing the less-potent ones.[57] A drop in potency of an analogue can result if it cannot fit into the binding site, if the bioactive conformation becomes a high-energy one, or if the pharmacophoric points are arranged suboptimally in three dimensions.

As noted above, for series in which all molecules have the same flexibility, no unique pharmacophore map may be possible and any one may be chosen for the QSAR.

For the D_2 dopaminergic agonists a number of conformationally constrained compounds are known, the bioactive enantiomer has been established for compounds from several different series, and extensive structure–activity investigations have revealed the groups essential for bioactivity.[19] Hence, this is an ideal set for pharmacophore mapping.

Usually one selects a relatively low-energy conformer as the bioactive one since the formation of the complex must make up for any internal energy cost of attaining the bioactive conformation. Table 23.1 lists the relative MMP2 energy of the chosen bioactive conformation for the D_2 agonists.

The problem is to quantify 'relatively' since the energy value calculated depends not only on the intrinsic accuracy of the computational method but also on how environmental effects are modelled. For instance, the calculation of the relative energies of the conformers is confounded if some of them have intramolecular hydrogen bonds, which lower the internal energy. If in forming the complex these internal hydrogen bonds have to be broken, their ground-state energy advantage is negated. Such complications are especially common in molecules that have many functional groups and are conformationally flexible, such as peptides. Similar considerations apply to intramolecular hydrophobic bonds. For a set of very flexible compounds with many functional groups, the only recourse might be simply to be certain that the proposed bioactive conformation does not contain any bad intramolecular steric contacts.

The hydrogen-bonding and electrostatic interactions that form the basis of most pharmacophores have been shown by crystallographers to be rather tolerant to deviations from ideal angles and distances.[58,59] We consider a root-mean-square fit of $1.0\,\text{Å}$ to be good and $1.5\,\text{Å}$ to be acceptable.

Ligands use hydrogen bonds and electrostatic interactions as part of the recognition of their macromolecular targets. Although the angles and distances of such interactions are not so precise as in covalent interactions, there are nevertheless well-defined optimum values of these angles and distances. Most current pharmacophore mapping studies include macromolecular 'site points' as part of the superposition rule.[60,61] Indeed, from the viewpoint of the macromolecule, it is less important where the atoms of the various ligands are located than that the requisite hydrogen bonds are made and that no bad close contacts are present. This sometimes translates into pharmacophore maps in which different ligands may approach a particular group on a protein from a number of different directions.

B. Identifying the pharmacophore points from structure–activity relationships

The superposition rule may be obvious from the structure–activity relationships of the series. For example, if deleting or mutating the properties of a particular functional group abolishes activity, one could propose that it is essential for activity, i.e. that it is part of the pharmacophore. For instance, for the D_2 agonists, it is known that removing or methylating the *meta*-OH group abolishes agonistic activity, whereas a number of *meta*-phenols are full agonists. Additionally, methylating the aromatic *N* of indoles abolishes agonistic activity.[19] Thus, we consider the *meta*-OH or indole NH to be part of the pharmacophore.

Another clue to pharmacophoric groups is found in the relative affinity of enantiomers. If inverting a chiral centre affects affinity, one might assume that the chiral atom affects the orientation of important pharmacophore features. For the dopamine agonists, inverting the stereochemistry of the carbon bearing the basic nitrogen atom decreases affinity by at least tenfold (V vs. VII). As a result of this observation plus the fact that the natural ligand is dopamine (XXI), the basic nitrogen is also proposed to be a part of the pharmacophore.

Several computer methods are available for either the identification of the bioactive conformation or the identification of both the bioactive conformation and the superposition rule. Each is based on treatment of interpoint distances. The corresponding conformations of enantiomers have identical interpoint distances; hence, the selection of the bioactive enantiomer requires additional manual deliberation. Clearly, if no molecule of known stereochemistry has been tested in the bioassay of interest, then one may be forced to accept a model that represents merely relative stereochemistry. However, if chiral compounds have been tested against the same macromolecule, that chiral information should be included in the pharmacophore map even if the observation cannot be included in the 3D QSAR.

Each of these computer methods depends on consideration of a set of structurally different potent compounds. In general, only the most potent of a set of analogues with the same conformational constraints is used, with the expectation that the others will be built by analogy once the bioactive conformation of the original is proposed. Accordingly, since V, VI, VIII, and IX are all potent compounds, we expect that the same ring pucker of the tetralin ring would be chosen. Hence, we need to include only one analogue in the original explorations. Notice that although XII has the same backbone, the arrangement of its functional groups is different and so it must be included. Deriving the pharmacophore map is easiest if the original set is selected carefully and to be the minimum size.

All the computer methods described below are commercially available and all are documented in the refereed scientific literature. None takes very long to run on a workstation. However, it might require much thought to interpret the results.

C. Approaches that suggest possible bioactive conformations given the superposition points

1. The systematic search approach

For systematic searching the user supplies a proposed superposition rule (ligand atoms and how to calculate the location of the site points) and the program returns the pharmacophore maps consistent with that rule.[57,62] If all the molecules are flexible, several pharmacophore maps may be presented. This is an advantage over a manual method, in which the user is usually satisfied to have one answer.

Systematic searching uses rigid rotation of bonds with a very fine rotation increment to generate conformers. Starting with the most constrained compound, it rotates all relevant bonds and notes the allowed distances between the pharmacophore points. The next most constrained molecule is studied next: however, special algorithms eliminate from consideration those bond rotations that lead to interpoint distances not found in the first molecule. By continuing this process the allowed distance ranges between the pharmacophore points are continually narrowed as compounds are studied. No or many pharmacophore maps may result.

For systematic searching, two other input selections are required: the choice of the lattice spacing and the lattice boundaries. These choices affect the matching of a conformer from one molecule with that from another. The most prudent action seems to be to do several runs, varying the lattice boundaries. Usually the selected conformers are energy-minimized before further use.

2.   Ensemble distance geometry

Recall that distance geometry generates conformers using only the allowed distances between each of the atoms and site points. Ensemble distance geometry extends the method by simultaneously generating conformers of all analogues for which a pharmacophore map is to be generated.[63] The user supplies the atoms or site points that correspond to each other: the program sets a 0 Å distance bound between them. It also allows atoms from different molecules to interpenetrate. Using these criteria, the program generates ensembles of superimposed molecules, one copy of each molecule in each ensemble.

In our experience, ensemble distance geometry is very useful since it is easy to use and it provides an unbiased view of the possible 3D arrangements of the pharmacophore points. However, it has two serious drawbacks. First, the structures that result from distance geometry must be optimized. Once this is done, the pharmacophoric atoms may no longer match. Second, optimization often converts many distance geometry structures to the same conformer. Although in principle a computer program could sort this out, without one it becomes a book-keeping headache to discover exactly how many 3D pharmacophore maps there are and which conformers of which molecules match each.

D.   DISCO, a program that simultaneously suggests possible superposition rules and bioactive conformations

DISCO processes user-supplied sets of conformers and provides descriptions of the pharmacophore maps for the set of molecules.[61] Usually the conformers have been processed so that the set includes only those that differ significantly, that is by at least 0.4 Å in one of the interpoint distances of interest.[64]

For every molecule the program, under user control, identifies the coordinates of the following types of points in the ligand: hydrogen-bond donor atoms, hydrogen-bond acceptor atoms, positively charged atoms, negatively charged atoms, and centres of hydrophobic rings. The locations of the complementary (macromolecular) site points are also identified as exhaustively as possible. For instance, for every OH group in an alcohol, the program places three hydrogen-bond accepting and three hydrogen-bond donating site points at idealized locations calculated from the backbone of the alcohol. Thus the user need not supply the conformers that differ in rotation of the C—OH bond.

The DISCO program then selects a reference molecule — usually that with the fewest ligand and site points and with the fewest input conformers. Using each conformer of the reference in turn, it then searches for superposition rules that form a pharmacophore map that includes every input molecule.

The user indicates how many and what types of point must be in the solution, what cut-off in relative energy of conformers should be used, and a tolerance within which each interpoint distance in the comparison conformer must match the reference. One may also identify certain compounds, such as inactive ones, as optional fits or tell the program to accept solutions that contain only some number of the active compounds. This latter feature is helpful if no pharmacophore map is found in an initial run or to explore the possibility that a larger number of points might be in common within a subset of the compounds.

A key difference between the results of DISCO and other methods is that frequently DISCO reports many pharmacophore maps. They differ in the points or the conformer of the reference used to define the map. To help the user compare these results, each map can be presented with all matching conformers of all molecules. For each superposition rule of each conformer that matches a particular map, DISCO reports the root mean square superposition value, the volume overlap with the reference, the distance tolerance, and the relative energy.

It is possible to imagine a pharmacophore map in which no atoms of the ligand superimpose even though each ligand has hydrogen-bonding and charged groups that interact with the same macromolecular sites. The macromolecule recognizes ligands one at a time on the basis of their complementarity to the binding site. Only people expect the ligands to look similar.

E.   Refining the pharmacophore map

All the previously described methods provide suggestions of the broad outlines of the possible pharmacophore maps. Even if only one is suggested, the details need to be filled in before one is ready to calculate the 3D QSAR. For instance, the above methods have probably not considered all the molecules in the dataset. Furthermore, they may have not considered the conformational degrees of freedom that do not affect the location of the pharmacophore points — for instance the conformation of the *n*-propyl substituents of compounds I, V, VII, etc. .

The final selection of the bioactive conformation and enantiomer and the superposition rule will depend on an integration of all relevant information. Some of this may not be on the same quantitative scale as the data ultimately included in the 3D QSAR. For example, chiral compounds or those with markedly different 2D structures may have been tested in a similar but not identical assay — for instance, a different species may have been the source of the tissue, a different radioligand may have been used, or perhaps the temperature or pH was changed. Alternatively, although some compounds may be so inactive that no potency value could be measured, this information might be useful in distinguishing between possible pharmacophore maps.

The possible pharmacophore maps may also be distinguished by other criteria such as the relative energy of the various bioactive conformations, how well they explain inactive analogues, how well the pharmacophore points fit (r.m.s.), and the amount of overlap of the nonpharmacophoric regions of the molecules. For all of these considerations, careful manual analysis with molecular graphics is essential. Lastly, 3D QSAR might help one distinguish between several different superposition rules.

In the consideration of the D_2 agonists, we chose apomorphine, II, as the reference compound because it is one of the highest-affinity ligands, the stereochemistry of the active enantiomer is well-established, and it has only a few low-energy conformers. Our original choice of the bioactive conformation was the minimum energy conformer, also that observed in the crystal. This choice was validated by the observation that the low-energy conformer of one of the most potent dopaminergics, VIII, was directly superimposable on the chosen conformer of apomorphine, II. Furthermore, we could not find conformers of VIII that superimpose on the next lower energy conformer of apomorphine, that in which the positions of the methyl and lone-pair (proton) are exchanged. Figure 23.2 shows these results.

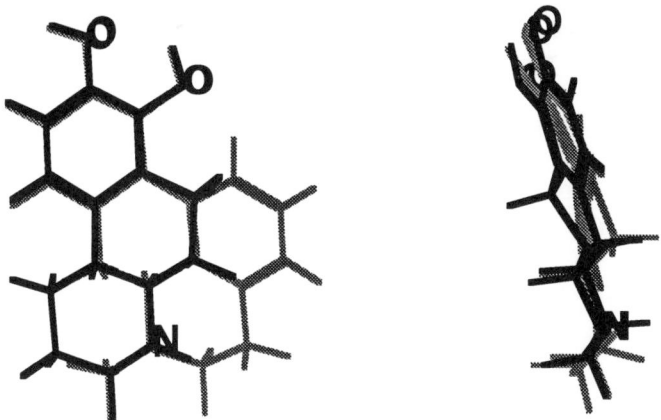

Figure 23.2.   A superposition of II (dashed lines) with VIII (solid lines).

The selection of the rotation of the catechol was facilitated by comparison of apomorphine (II) and XXVII, an indole whose bioactive enantiomer was known.[19] In comparing the conformers of apomorphine and XXVII we looked for a superposition of the hydrogen-bond donating atom, the corresponding receptor hydrogen-bond acceptor point, the basic nitrogen, and its associated receptor anionic site point. We also required that the superposition explain the chiral specificity of the compounds. Only if the *meta*-OH group is rotated as shown in Figs. 23.2 and 23.3 do the molecules superimpose well. Notice that the chiral hydrogens are on the same face. The compromise in this superposition is that the aromatic ring bearing the NH does not superimpose with that bearing the OH's. Interestingly, molecules that lack this aromatic ring are still potent D2 agonists.[18]

Once the choice of the bioactive conformation of I was made, the prototype compounds of other series were investigated. In particular, for V–IX and lll, we chose this same conformer of the 2–amino tetralin. Selection of the bioactive conformation of XV provided little choice: all the four conformers found have an N—O distance of 7.4 Å, which is 0.9 Å longer than in the reference compounds. The second lowest-energy conformer does not superimpose well since the heterocyclic ring is twisted and so the anionic site point projects at a different angle. The two remaining conformers are approximately 3 kcal mol^{-1} higher — a large amount for MMP2 energies — and they fit no better than the lowest-energy one. Similar considerations led to the choice of the low-energy conformer as the bioactive one of XVI–XVIII. The same bioactive conformation of XXVI established for D_1 activity was used for the D_2 model. It is also attractive because the unsubstituted phenyl is in a similar location in space to that in I and II.

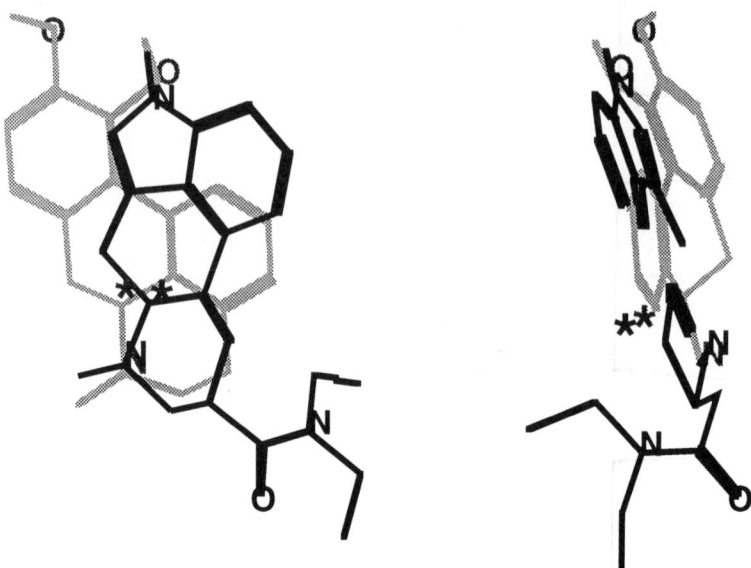

Figure 23.3. Use of XXVII To establish the rotation of the catechol OH groups in II. The chiral hydrogen atoms are indicated *.

The final alignment may be refined using a fit based on the fields of the molecules.[4] The problems with this are that the superposition is done pairwise and all lattice positions are included whether they will ultimately be found to be relevant or irrelevant to bioactivity.

V. CALCULATING THE 3D PROPERTIES

A. The spacing, location and size of the lattice for CoMFA

Once the molecules have been superimposed, one calculates their 3D properties. For CoMFA this means that a lattice is constructed such that it surrounds all the molecules, and various energy values are calculated, for each molecule, at the intersections of the lattice. The energy values are selected to describe the principal types of noncovalent forces: electrostatic, dispersion, steric repulsion, and hydrogen bonding.

How large should the lattice be? Of those considered, electrostatic forces fall off the most slowly with distance. In spite of this, the electrostatic properties at the different points are correlated both because of the nature of electrostatic forces and because, owing to the requirement for charge neutralization, increase in charge in one location is compensated for by a decrease at other locations. These factors suggest that the default lattice choice of 4 Å beyond any dimension of any molecule in the dataset is adequate for the statistical analysis. However, if the contours of a CoMFA appear to be clipped off at the boundaries of the lattice, the calculation can be repeated with a larger lattice.

What about lattice spacing? The computer program GRID uses energy values calculated on a lattice to locate on a macromolecule favourable binding sites for ligand groups.[32–35] Extensive investigations suggest that a lattice spacing of 0.33–0.50 Å is needed to reproduce experimental binding orientations. The same conclusion was reached with the program DOCK, which explores different binding orientations of a ligand within a macromolecular binding site.[65]

The usual CoMFA calculations use a 2 Å spacing. Superior results are often found using 2 Å as opposed to 1 Å spacing.[3] Why are the experiences different with CoMFA compared to GRID and DOCK? Part of the answer might lie in the intrinsic correlation between the energy values at one point with those at adjacent points. PLS can discover these correlations. Second, extensive simulation studies have shown that irrelevant data dilute the power of PLS to extract the signal[66] — it might be that closer lattice spacings, although they undoubtedly include more signal, may increase the noise disproportionally.

Sometimes it happens that CoMFA models with improved cross-validation statistics are found if the lattice is moved with respect to the compounds. Hence we routinely calculate four different CoMFA models at different lattice locations for each dataset: (1) the default; and the lattices in which all X, Y and Z lattice boundaries are incremented by an absolute value of (2) 0.5 Å, (3) 1.0 Å, and (4) 1.5 Å. If one of these lattice locations gives superior results, then the location of the boundaries is investigated further.

B. Energy field calculations

1. Steric properties

Steric properties of molecules are calculated with the normal type of Lennard–Jones potential function, which includes a large steric repulsive component that leads to positive energy values and a small steric attractive component.[34,41–43] Generally the negative, favourable, steric energies are very small and probably do not contribute to the statistics of the model.

Since positive steric energies approach $+\infty$ and there is little intrinsic difference between an energy value of $+50\,kcal\,mol^{-1}$ and one of $+51\,kcal\,mol^{-1}$, the positive steric energies are truncated at some value. Typically this is in the range of 10–$30\,kcal\,mol^{-1}$. In some cases the statistics do not deteriorate even if an energy is truncated at $1.0\,kcal\,mol^{-1}$. In these cases the steric energy values are simply indicator variables that describe whether a particular lattice point is occupied or not occupied by the particular compound.

2. Electrostatic properties

The exact calculation of electrostatic fields is more subject to differences between programs than is calculation of steric fields.[34,41–43] Fortunately for practising medicinal chemists, electrostatic contributions to potency are usually much less statistically important than are steric contributions. The reason is that electrostatic similarities are emphasized both in selecting compounds for a 3D QSAR and in the subsequent pharmacophore mapping. The remaining differences in electrostatics are often small compared to the differences in shape.

An important issue is how to treat electrostatic fields that are inside the van der Waals surface of some but not all the molecules. The problem is that if the lattice point is inside the van der Waals surface of a molecule, it is close to at least one atomic nucleus. Minute differences in the location of a lattice point with respect to the nucleus lead to extremely large variations in the electrostatic interaction energy.

In commercial CoMFA, the electrostatic energy values at these locations can be replaced by the average energy value at that location for all molecules for which this location is outside the van der Waals surface. This correction is done only if the calculation includes steric fields, since it uses the value of the steric field to establish whether the point is inside the molecule.

On the other hand, we reasoned that such locations are of little interest to a CoMFA, which is designed to use the structure–activity relationships of ligands to probe the characteristics of the macromolecular binding site. Hence, we drop these lattice points from the calculations.[25,26]

3. Hydrogen-bonding properties

Commercial CoMFA does not include an explicit term for hydrogen-bonding potential of a ligands since it is assumed that the combination of electrostatic and steric fields is enough to explain the relative hydrogen-bonding strength of substituents as well.[67] However, we have found that including or substituting a hydrogen-bonding term, as in GRID[32–35] calculations, will sometimes improve the statistics substantially. It is now possible to import fields calculated by GRID into the standard CoMFA program.

4. Hydrophobic properties

In commercial CoMFA, explicit hydrophobic fields are not calculated. Recall that hydrophobicity depends mainly on the disturbance of water structure.[68] It is empirically correlated with the size and surface area of a molecule (the amount of water displaced) and its direct interaction with water through hydrogen bonding.[68] Hence, it is possible that hydrophobicity is implicitly incorporated into the steric and electrostatic fields.

Kim studied a number of datasets for which there was a good correlation between potency and octanol–water $\log P$.[31] He found that good CoMFA models resulted if he included the hydrogen-bonding characteristics of the ligands as parametrized by the water probe. The statistics of the CoMFA models were slightly superior to those of the traditional QSARs. Steric and electrostatic fields were not sufficient to explain the data.

C. 3D similarity matrices

To perform a QSAR on molecular similarities, one calculates the similarity of every molecule in the dataset with every other molecule.[13,14] These similarities can be based on any molecular property. Usually, similarity is based on steric and electrostatic fields of the whole molecules. If the comparisons are based on molecular fields, then the considerations described in sections V.A and V.B apply here as well. However, a 0.5 Å lattice spacing seems to be preferable for the similarity of steric fields. The TSAR program offers several types of similarity calculation.[13,14]

VI. DETECTING THE RELATIONSHIP BETWEEN 3D PROPERTIES AND POTENCY USING PARTIAL LEAST SQUARES

A. General description

The statistical problem with CoMFA is that there are fewer observations than descriptors, the energy values from different fields or lattice locations. Similarity matrices have as many descriptors as compounds. Ordinary least squares, used in Hansch analysis, cannot be used for such datasets, but partial least squares (PLS), can.[10,11,69]

Ordinary least squares is built on the assumption that each of the descriptors is relevant to the response variable and is independent of all the other descriptors. In contrast, PLS assumes that some of the descriptors are irrelevant to the response variable and that the descriptors are correlated. These assumptions give PLS the power to extract a weak signal dispersed over many descriptors.

The PLS algorithm is related to principal components analysis in that PLS extracts, from the descriptor matrix, latent variables that are linear combinations of these descriptors. Thus, highly correlated descriptors would be part of the same latent variable.

PLS differs from principal components analysis in that the latent variables are extracted to explain the dependent property, the biological potency. The first latent variable (component) is that with maximum covariance with the dependent property. Each successive component maximizes the covariance with the residual unexplained dependent property within a subspace that is orthogonal to the preceding components. In the limit at which the number of components equals the number of descriptors, PLS reduces to ordinary least squares. However, usually the biological potency is explained by only a few latent variables.

B.   Validation techniques for choosing and testing the reliability of a CoMFA model

Since PLS operates on many descriptors, a realistic concern is that it would over-fit the data. For this reason PLS models are validated by leave-one-out calculations.[10] This procedure involves calculating as many models as there are data points. For each model, one of the compounds in turn is left out and its potency is predicted from the model without it. After each compound has been predicted once, an R_{cv}^2 (square of the cross-validated correlation coefficient) and $RMSE_{cv}$ (cross-validated root mean square error) are calculated from the observed and predicted potency of each compound.

The $RMSE_{cv}$ generally decreases for the first few latent variables, reaches a minimum, and then increases to indicate over-fitting of the data. The selection of the number of latent variables to include (i.e. that are important) is not as simple as including those up to the minimum $RMSE_{cv}$. If adding an additional variable decreases the $RMSE_{cv}$ by less than 5%, the simpler model is preferable because it contains most of the signal in fewer variables. In cases for which $RMSE_{cv}$ begins to decrease slowly with the addition of each latent variable, the 5% rule is usually a better criterion for the determination of the cut-off.

Table 23.2 shows the $RMSE_{cv}$ as a function of the number of latent variables for the D_2 example. Notice that for the models with steric fields only, the $RMSE_{cv}$ decreases until five latent variables are included, then it increases again. On the other hand, for the combined steric and electrostatic fields, the $RMSE_{cv}$ is substantially higher. Using the 5% reduction rule of thumb, we concluded that four latent variables of the steric fields are statistically significant. Notice also that the fitted $RMSE_{fit}$ values continue to decrease with increasing numbers of components, even though the cross-validated ones decrease and then increase again.

Clark and co-workers investigated the probability that PLS in the CoMFA context would find QSAR models that are artefacts.[66] They generated sets of random numbers to use as descriptors for a real set of biological data. They found that PLS with cross-validation, surprisingly, tends to under-fit the data. For instance, when they added a column of numbers perfectly correlated with the biological activity to a large matrix of random numbers, PLS

Table 23.2 Statistics of CoMFA models for D2 agonist affinity. (Chosen model indicated in bold.)

Number of latent variables	Steric fields only			Steric plus electrostatic fields		
	$RMSE_{cv}$	$RMSE_{fit}$	R^2_{fit}	$RMSE_{cv}$	$RMSE_{fit}$	R^2_{fit}
1	1.28	0.86	0.63	1.35	0.88	0.60
2	1.03	0.56	0.84	1.17	0.56	0.85
3	1.08	0.50	0.88	1.20	0.42	0.92
4	**0.97**	**0.45**	**0.91**	1.13	0.33	0.95
5	0.96	0.40	0.93	1.13	0.24	0.98
6	0.99	0.38	0.94	1.16	0.20	0.98
7	1.08	0.33	0.96	1.17	0.15	0.99
8	1.18	0.30	0.97	1.14	0.12	0.99
9	1.29	0.28	0.98	1.17	0.07	1.00
10	1.39	0.26	0.98	1.20	0.05	1.00

reported a lower correlation than the true one. The conclusion of their studies is that PLS is very conservative and sensitive to noise in the data.

C. Reducing the number of variables input into PLS

PLS runs faster the fewer the number of variables in the calculation. It is also sensitive to noise in the data. Hence, a CoMFA analysis generally first eliminates columns of energy values for which there is little difference between compounds. The energies in all columns are calculated in the same units, thus a simple inspection of the distribution of the variances of the columns will suggest a reasonable cut-off point. In the case of the D_2 agonists reported in Table 23.1, there were 968 columns of steric energies. This reduces to 109 columns if all columns with a standard deviation less than 2.0 kcal mol^{-1} are deleted, to 119 with 1.0 kcal mol^{-1}, to 130 with 0.5 kcal mol^{-1}, to 140 with 0.25 kcal mol^{-1} and to 148 with 0.15 kcal mol^{-1}. The calculations were done with the latter cut-off, i.e. using only the 15% of the columns with the largest variation in energy.

It is good practice to use exactly the same data for the final model calculation as for the cross-validation. If columns are deleted for the cross-validation, they should also be deleted in the final model.

D. Scaling variables

When a potential model contains both steric and electrostatic contributions, one must decide whether they need to be weighted with respect to each other. One point of view says that since the energy values are on the same scale regardless of the type of field, they should not be weighted. Another says that the two types of field must be given an equal chance to influence the statistics and so should be weighted. Since the calculations are so fast to do, there seems to be no harm in trying both approaches.

It is also possible to investigate potential QSAR descriptors that are not based on molecular fields. A popular choice is the octanol–water partition coefficient-derived $\log P$. It is essential to scale such variables or they will disappear compared to the larger-magnitude fields. One would weight each block (steric, electrostatic, and $\log P$) so that their variances were equal. Within a block each variable would be scaled to preserve the original structure.

E. The choice of the CoMFA model when more than one type of field is considered

Although the default CoMFA calculations include potential contributions of both electrostatic and steric fields, it is not necessarily true that both will be statistically significant. The only way to test this is to compare the cross-validation results of each of the fields alone and in combination. Unless the less-significant field decreases $RMSE_{cv}$ by at least 5% compared to the model without that field, there is no justification for including it in the model. Note that sometimes the contribution of a field will be reported to be rather large even though it is not statistically significant and hence should not be included in the model.

F. Interpreting CoMFA contours

One result of a CoMFA calculation is a display of the contours that show the 3D location of fields that contribute significantly to the model. Steric and electrostatic contributions are contoured separately and shown in different colours.

The steric contours are relatively easy to interpret. Positive contours show regions in space that, if occupied, increase potency: negative contours decrease potency. Since the contour plots are for visual inspection only, the contour levels can be selected in any way that enhances understanding. Thus, because they are more closely spaced, it is sometimes easier to interpret contours calculated from a model based on 1 Å spacing. For this purpose we recommend that one use the number of components suggested from the statistically better 2 Å spacing. The R^2_{fit} should agree rather closely between the 1 Å and 2 Å models.

Interpretation of the electrostatic contours is more complicated because of the electroneutrality requirement and because either positive or negative changes in electrostatics can increase potency. The electroneutrality requirement results from the fact that each molecule has a predetermined number of electrons. If a substituent withdraws electron density from one position in space, it adds electron density to another. If the series has substituents at only one position, then it may be difficult to establish which change in field is responsible for the change in potency, since both are correlated. Compounding this problem is the fact that there may be no way to know whether an increase or a decrease in electron density will increase potency. Hence, if a CoMFA shows significant electrostatic effects, the scientist must examine all the evidence to establish which is the true effect and which an artificial correlation.

G. Forecasting the potency of additional molecules

Since CoMFA models are true QSAR equations, they may be used to forecast the potency of compounds not used in their derivation. If compounds have been withheld from the analysis, because they are inactive, for example, the agreement between the observed and forecast affinities is a good test of the validity of the CoMFA. A CoMFA can also be tested to see whether it reproduces the trends in potencies measured in similar but not identical assays.

REFERENCES

1. Cohen, N. C., Blaney, J. M., Humblet, C., Gund, P. and Barry, D. C. (1990) Molecular modeling software and methods for medicinal chemistry. *J. Med. Chem.* **33**: 883–894.
2. Kubinyi, H. (ed.) (1993) *3D QSAR in Drug Design. Theory Methods and Applications*, pp. 759. Escom, Leiden.
3. Martin, Y. C., Kim, K.-H. and Lin, C. T. Comparative molecular field analysis: CoMFA. In Charton, M. (ed.) *Advances in Quantitative Structure–Property Relationships*. JAI Press, Greenwich, CT (in press).
4. Cramer III, R. D., Patterson, D. E. and Bunce, J. D. (1988) Comparative molecular field analysis (CoMFA). 1. Effect of shape on binding of steroids to carrier proteins. *J. Am. Chem. Soc.* **110**: 5959–5967.
5. Cramer III, R. D., dePriest, S. A., Patterson, D. E. and Hecht, P. (1993) The developing practice of comparative molecular field analysis. In Kubinyi, H. (ed.) *3D QSAR in Drug Design. Theory, Methods and Applications*, pp. 443–485. Escom, Leiden.
6. Cramer III, R. D., Patterson, D. E. and Bunce, J. D. (1989) Recent advances in comparative molecular field analysis (CoMFA). In Fauchère, J. L. (ed.) *QSAR: Quantitative Structure–Activity Relationships in Drug Design*, pp. 161–165. Alan R. Liss, New York.
7. Cramer III, R. D. and Wold, S. B. (1991) *Comparative Molecular Field Analysis (CoMFA)*, US Pat. 5 025 388.
8. Cramer III, R. D, Clark, M., Simeroth, P. and Patterson, D. E. (1991) Recent developments in comparative molecular field analysis (CoMFA). In Silipo, C. and Vittoria, A. (eds) *QSAR: Rational Approaches to the Design of Bioactive Compounds*, pp. 239–242. Elsevier Science, Amsterdam.
9. Martin, Y. C. (1991) Overview of concepts and methods in computer-assisted rational drug design. *Methods Enzymol.* **203**: 587–613.
10. Wold, S., Johansson, E. and Cocchi, M. (1993) PLS — Partial least-squares projections to latent structures. In Kubinyi, H. (ed.) *3D QSAR in Drug Design. Theory, Methods and Applications*, pp. 523–550. Escom, Leiden.
11. Wold, S. (1991) Validation of QSAR's. *Quant. Struct.–Act. Relat.* **10**: 191–193.
12. Burt, C. and Richards, W. G. (1990) Molecular similarity: the introduction of flexible fitting, *J. Computer-Aided Mol. Des.* **4**: 231–238.
13. Good, A. C., Peterson, S. J. and Richards, W. G. (1993) QSARS from similarity matrices — technique validation and application in the comparison of different similarity evaluation methods, *J. Med. Chem.* **36**: 2929–2937.
14. Good, A. C., So, S. S. and Richards, W. G. (1993) Structure–activity relationships from molecular similarity matrices. *J. Med. Chem.* **36**: 433–438.
15. Bush, B. L. and Nachbar, R. B. (1993) Sample-distance partial least-squares — PLS optimized for many variables, with application to CoMFA. *J. Computer-Aided Mol. Des.* **7**: 587–619.
16. Kubinyi, H. (1993) *QSAR: Hansch Analysis and Related Approaches*, vol. 1, pp. 240. VCH, Weinheim.
17. Teig, S. L. (1993) The development of meaningful 3-d search queries for drug discovery. In Collier, H. (ed.) *Recent Advances in Chemical Information II*, pp. 195–208. Royal Society of Chemistry, Cambridge.
18. Seeman, P., Watanabe, M., Grigoriadis, D., Tedesco, J. L., George, S. R., Svensson, U., Lars, J., Nilsson, G. and Neumeyer, J. L. (1985) Dopamine — D2 receptor binding sites for agonists. A tetrahedral model. *Mol. Pharm.* **28**: 391–399.
19. Cannon, J. G. (1985) Dopamine agonists: structure–activity relationships. *Progr. Drug Res.* **29**: 303–414.
20. Martin, Y. C. and Danaher, E. B. (1988) Molecular modeling of receptor–ligand interactions. In Williams, M., Glennon, R. and Timmermans, P. (eds) *Receptor Pharmacology and Function*, pp. 137–171. Dekker, NY.

21. Golender, V. and Rozenblit, A. (1983) *Logical and Combinatorial Algorithms for Drug Design.* Research Studies Press, Letchworth.

22. Golender, V. E. and Vorpagel, E. R. (1993) Computer-assisted pharmacophore identification. In Kubinyi, H. (ed.) *3D QSAR in Drug Design. Theory, Methods and Applications,* pp. 137–149. Escom, Leiden.

23. Hansch, C. (1993) Quantitative structure–activity relationships and the unnamed science. *Acc. Chem. Res.* **26**: 147–153.

24. Martin, Y. C. (1981) A practitioner's perspective on the role of quantitative structure–activity analysis in medicinal chemistry. *J. Med. Chem.* **24**: 229–237.

25. Kim, K. H. and Martin, Y. C. (1991) Direct prediction of dissociation constants (pK_a's) of clonidine-like imidazolines, 2-substituted imidazoles, and 1-methyl-2-substituted-imidazoles from 3D structures using a comparative molecular field analysis (CoMFA) approach. *J. Med. Chem.* **34**: 2056–2060.

26. Kim, K. H. and Martin, Y. C. (1991) Direct prediction of linear free energy substituent effects from 3D structures using comparative molecular field analysis. 1. Electronic effects of substituted benzoic acids. *J. Org. Chem.* **56**: 2723–2729.

27. Kim, K. H. and Martin, Y. C. (1991) Evaluation of electrostatic and steric descriptors for 3D-QSAR: the H^+ and CH_3 probes using comparative molecular field analysis (CoMFA) and the modified partial least squares method. In Silipo, C. and Vittoria, A. (eds) *QSAR: Rational Approaches to the Design of Bioactive Compounds,* pp. 151–154. Elsevier Science, Amsterdam.

28. Kim, K. H. (1991) A novel method of describing hydrophobic effects directly from 3D structures in 3D-quantitative structure–activity relationships study. *Med. Chem. Res.* **1**: 259–264.

29. Kim, K. H. (1992) Description of nonlinear dependence directly from 3D structures in 3D-quantitative structure–activity relationships. *Med. Chem. Rese.* **2**: 22–27.

30. Kim, K. H. (1993) Nonlinear dependence in comparative molecular field analysis (CoMFA). *Quant. Struct.-Act. Relat.* **7**: 71–82.

31. Kim, K. H. (1993) Comparison of classical and 3D QSAR. In Kubinyi, H. (ed.) *3D QSAR in Drug Design. Theory, Methods and Applications,* pp. 619–642. Escom, Leiden.

32. Wade, R. C., Clark, K. J. and Goodford, P. J. (1993) Further development of hydrogen bond functions for use in determining energetically favorable binding sites on molecules of known structure. 1. Ligand probe groups with the ability to form two hydrogen bonds. *J. Med. Chem.* **36**: 140–147.

33. Wade, R. C. and Goodford, P. J. (1993) Further development of hydrogen bond functions for use in determining energetically favorable binding sites on molecules of known structure. 2. Ligand probe groups with the ability to form more than two hydrogen bonds. *J. Med. Chem.* **36**: 148–156.

34. Goodford, P. (1985) A computational procedure for determining energetically favorable binding sites on biologically important macromolecules. *J. Med. Chem.* **28**: 849–857.

35. Boobbyer, D. N., Goodford, P. J., McWhinnie, P. M. and Wade, R. C. (1989) New hydrogen-bond potentials for use in determining energetically favorable binding sites on molecules of known structure. *J. Med. Chem.* **32**: 1083–1094.

36. Martin, Y. C., Kebabian, J. W., MacKenzie, R. and Schoenleber, R. (1991) Molecular modeling-based design of novel, selective, potent D1 dopamine agonists. In Silipo, C. and Vittoria, A. (eds) *QSAR: Rational Approaches to the Design of Bioactive Compounds,* pp. 469–482. Elsevier Science, Amsterdam.

37. Schoenleber, R., Michaelides, M. R., Martin, Y. C., DiDomenico, S., MacKenzie, R. G., Artman, L. D., Ackerman, M. S. and Kebabian, J. W. (1991) Design and synthesis of dopamine D1 selective antagonists. American Chemical Society Meeting, August.

38. Schoenleber, R., Martin, Y. C., Wilson, M. *et. al.* (1991) Approaches toward the rational deisgn of dopamine D1 selective agonists. American Chemical Society Meeting, August.

39. Martin, Y. C., Lin, C. T. and Wu, J. (1993) Application of CoMFA to the design and structural optimization of D1 dopaminergic agonists. In Kubinyi, H. (ed.) *3D QSAR in Drug Design. Theory, Methods and Applications,* pp. 643–660. Escom, Leiden.

40. Martin, Y. C. (1978) *Quantitative Drug Design,* pp. 425. Marcel Dekker, New York.

41. Burkert, U. and Allinger, N. L. (1982) *Molecular Mechanics,* pp. 339. American Chemical Society, Washington DC.

42. Clark, T. (1985) *A Handbook of Computational Chemistry. A Practical Guide to Chemical Structure and Energy Calculations;* pp. 332. Wiley, New York.

43. Seibel, G. L. and Kollman, P. A. (1990) Molecular mechanics and the modeling of drug structures. In Ramsden, C. A. (ed.) *Quantitative Drug Design: Comprehensive Medicinal Chemistry*, vol. 4, pp. 125–138. Pergamon, Oxford.

44. Zerner, M. C. (1991) Semiempirical molecular orbital methods. In Lipkowitz, K. B. and Boyd, D. B. (eds) *Reviews in Computational Chemistry*, vol. 1, pp. 313–360. VCH, Weinheim.

45. Stewart, J. P. (1990) Semiempirical molecular orbital methods. In Lipkowitz, K. B. and Boyd, D. B. (eds) *Reviews in Computational Chemistry*, vol. 2, pp. 45–81. VCH, Weinheim.

46. Allen, F. H., Davies, J. E., Galloy, J. J., Johnson, O., Kennard, O., Macrea, C. F., Mitchell, E. M., Mitchell, G. F., Smith, J. M. and Watson, D. G. (1991) The developments of versions 3 and 4 of the Cambridge Database System. *J. Chem. Inf. Computer Sci.* **31**: 187–204.

47. Allinger, M. L. (1987) *MMP2*. Tripos Inc., St Louis MO.

48. Bohm, H. J., Klebe, G., Lorenz, T., Mietzner, T. and Siggel, L. (1990) Different approaches to conformational analysis — a comparison of completeness, efficiency, and reliability based on the study of a 9-membered lactam. *J. Comput. Chem.* **11**: 1021–1028.

49. Blaney, J. M. and Dixon, J. S. (1991) Receptor modeling by distance geometry. *Annu. Rep. Med. Chem.* **26**: 281–285.

50. Leach, A. R. (1991) A survey of methods for searching the conformational space of small and medium-sized molecules. In Lipkowitz, K. B. and Boyd, D. B. (eds) *Reviews in Computational Chemistry*, pp. 1–55. VCH, Weinheim.

51. Blaney, J. M., Crippen, G. M., Dearing, A. and Dixon, J. S. (1990) *DGEOM — Distance Geometry, QCP590*. Quantum Chemistry Program Exchange, Indiana University, Bloomington, IN 47405.

52. Crippen, G. (1981) *Distance Geometry and Conformational Calculations*, pp. 53. Research Studies Press, Letchworth.

53. Crippen, G. M. and Havel, T. F. (1988) *Distance Geometry and Molecular Conformation*, pp. 500. Wiley, New York.

54. Gasteiger, J. and Marsili, M. (1980) Interactive partial equalization of orbital electronegativity — a rapid access to atomic charges. *Tetrahedron*, **36**: 3219–3288.

55. Hehre, W. J., Radom, L., Schleyer, P. V. R. and Pople, J. A. (1986) *Ab Initio Molecular Orbital Theory*. Wiley, New York.

56. Dewar, M. J. S., Zoebish, E. G., Healy, E. F. and Stewart, J. J. P. (1985) AM1: a new general purpose quantum mechanical molecular model. *J. Am. Chem. Soc.* **107**: 3902–3909.

57. Marshall, G. R., Barry, C. D., Bosshard, H. E., Dammkoehler, R. A. and Dunn, D. A. (1979) The conformation parameter in drug design: the active analog approach. In Olson, E. C. and Christoffersen, R. E. (eds) *Computer-Assisted Drug Design*, pp. 205–226. American Chemical Society, Washington.

58. Jeffrey, G. A. and Saenger, W. (1991) *Hydrogen Bonding in Biological Structures*, pp. 569. Springer-Verlag, Berlin.

59. Taylor, R. and Kennard, O. (1984) Hydrogen-bond geometry in organic crystals. *Acc. Chem. Res.* **17**: 320–326.

60. DePriest, S. A., Shands, E. F. B., Dammkoehler, R. A. and Marshall, G. R. (1991) 3D-QSAR: further studies on inhibitors of angiotensin-converting enzyme. In Silipo, C. and Vittoria, A. (eds) *QSAR: Rational Approaches to the Design of Bioactive Compounds*, pp. 405–414. Elsevier, Amsterdam.

61. Martin, Y. C., Bures, M. G., Danaher, E. A., DeLazzer, J., Lico, I. and Pavlik, P. A. (1993) A fast new approach to pharmacophore mapping and its application to dopaminergic and benzodiazepine agonists. *J. Computer-Aided Mol. Des.* **7**: 83–102.

62. Marshall, G. R. and Naylor, C. B. (1990) Use of molecular graphics for structural analysis of small molecules. In Ramsden, C. A. (ed.) *Quantitative Drug Design: Comprehensive Medicinal Chemistry*, vol. 4, pp. 431–458. Pergamon, Oxford.

63. Sheridan, R. P., Nilakantan, R., Dixon, J. S. and Venkataraghavan, R. (1986) The ensemble approach to distance geometry: application to the nicotinic pharmacophore. *J. Med. Chem.* **29**: 899–906.

64. Martin, Y. C. and DeLazzer, J. Family: a computer program that compares 3D structures based on interpoint distances: application to sorting hits from 3D database searching. In preparation.

65. Meng, E. C., Shoichet, B. K. and Kuntz, I. D. (1992) Automated docking with grid-based energy evaluation. *J. Comput. Chem.* **13**: 505–524.

66. Clark, M. and Cramer III, R. D. (1993) The probability of chance correlation using partial least squares (PLS). *Quant. Struct.-Act. Relat.* **12**: 137–145.

67. Dauber, P. and Hagler, A. T. (1980) Crystal packing, hydrogen bonding, and the effect of crystal forces on molecular conformation. *Acc. Chem. Res.* **13**: 105–112.

68. Taylor, P. J. (1990) Hydrophobic properties of drugs. In Ramsden, C. A. (ed.) *Quantitative Drug Design: Comprehensive Medicinal Chemistry,* vol. 4, pp. 241–294. Pergamon, Oxford.

69. Wold, S., Marten, H. and Wold, H. (1983) The multivariate calibration problem in chemistry solved by the PLS method. In Kagstrom, R. A. (ed.) *Matrix Pencils (Lecture Notes in Mathematics),* pp. 286–293. Springer-Verlag, Heidelberg.

24

The Use of X-ray Structures of Receptors and Enzymes in Drug Discovery

JEAN-MICHEL RONDEAU and HERMAN SCHREUDER

If you can look into the seeds of time,
And say which grain will grow and which will not,
Speak then to me ...
(Shakespeare, Macbeth, Act I, scene 3)[1]

THE PRACTICE OF MEDICINAL CHEMISTRY
ISBN 0-12-744640-0

I. INTRODUCTION

A. Why is protein crystallography important?

Classical methods in drug discovery, like the screening of natural products and the synthesis of large numbers of compounds, have been and are still quite successful. However, the number of compounds that need to be screened and/or synthesized before a suitable drug candidate is found is increasing steadily. Also, the requirements for efficacy and safety for a new drug to enter the market are becoming stricter every year. A potential new drug not only needs to be safe and effective but has to be better than drugs already on the market. This makes it very important for a pharmaceutical company to be first on the market with a new drug and to reduce the time needed for discovery and development as much as possible.

These challenges have prompted the pharmaceutical industry to search for more rational approaches to drug discovery in addition to the classical 'trial and error' methods.[2–9] It is essential for such rational approaches to have a thorough understanding of the drug target and/or the natural receptor–ligands or other natural effector molecules one wishes to mimic. Ideally, one would like to be able to have a look at the target molecule, to see what it looks like, how it functions etc., and subsequently use this information to design novel molecules with the desired activity or to improve existing lead compounds.

X-ray crystallography is able to provide just that. Most drug targets are proteins. Examples include receptors for hormones and neurotransmitters, specific proteases like thrombin, elastase and HIV protease, enzymes involved in bacterial cell metabolism and cell wall formation and so on.[3,10] Many of these proteins have already been crystallized and efforts to crystallize many more are under way. As will be explained in this chapter, from the X-ray diffraction pattern of these crystals crystallographers are able to calculate electron-density maps which are, in fact, images of the molecules which make up the crystals, enlarged about a hundred million times. These electron-density maps are examined using computer graphics and an atomic model is fitted (Fig. 24.1). After refinement, an atomic model is usually obtained which has an estimated mean coordinate error of 0.3–0.5 Å and which allows the investigator to examine the three-dimensional structure of the protein in great detail. Most of what is currently known about how proteins are folded has been derived from crystal structures.

X-ray crystallography is a powerful technique. There are no theoretical limits to the size of the molecules or complexes to be studied, although a practical limit is imposed by the necessity to obtain crystals of sufficient quality. Structures of protein complexes with molecular weights up to half a million daltons, and of viruses with molecular weights of several millions of daltons have been solved by X-ray crystallography.

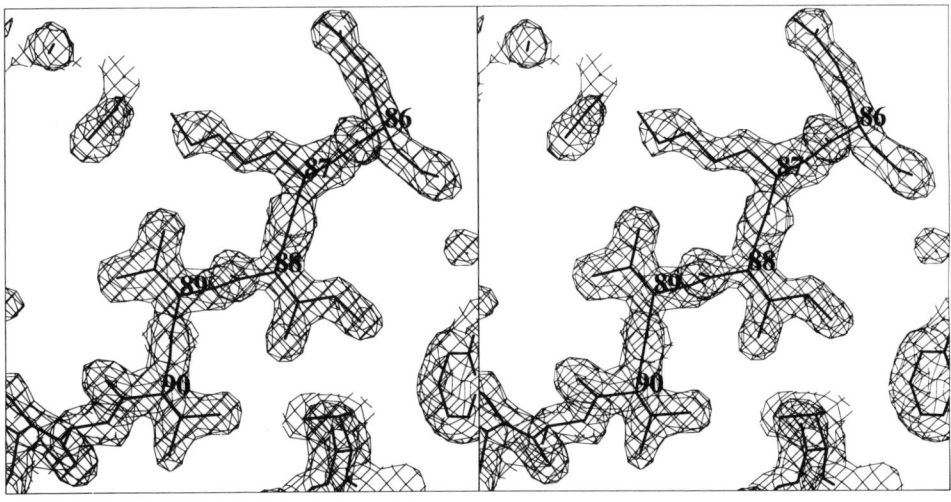

Fig. 24.1   Stereoview showing a small portion of an 1.8 Å electron-density map of porcine pancreatic elastase, contoured at 1σ (1 standard deviation) above mean. The electron-density map, drawn in thin lines, is the direct experimental result while the atomic model, drawn in thick lines, has been built into the electron-density map by the crystallographers. (To learn how to view stereoimages, see ref. 121.)

B.   What kind of information do we get from protein crystallography?

X-ray crystallographic studies can be broadly divided into the following four categories.

(1) *The determination of hitherto unknown structures.* This is still the mainstay of protein crystallography and serves as the basis for the other types of studies mentioned below.

(2) *Studies of enzymatic mechanisms.* Enzymes can often be crystallized in the presence of substrates, substrate analogues or the reaction products, which allows the identification of reactive groups in the active site (acidic and basic groups, nucleophiles, metal ions, co-factors, etc.) in close proximity to the substrate. In addition, it is often possible to obtain structural information on intermediate steps of the reaction by co-crystallization with transition-state analogues,[11] or by arresting the enzymatic reaction halfway by the use of low temperatures, inactive mutants or pH values which prevent completion of the catalytic reaction (e.g. see refs 12 and 13). This information is used, in combination with biochemical and spectroscopic data, to postulate a reaction mechanism which can be

verified, for example, by mutating putative catalytic residues or by synthesizing and testing putative transition-state analogues.

(3) *Analysis of enzyme–ligand interactions.* Small-molecule ligands like substrates, inhibitor and effector molecules are often accommodated by the crystalline protein without major changes of the crystal packing. Crystals of complexes of proteins with other macromolecules (protein, DNA, etc.) can often be obtained by co-crystallization. Crystal structures of these complexes show in great detail how the protein interacts with its ligand(s) and, in contrast to methods studying the ligand alone, shows the biologically relevant bound conformation of the ligand, information which is very important for drug design and which is often difficult to get with other methods.

(4) *Analysis of mobility and conformational changes.* This may seem impossible at first glance, since crystallography produces basically static pictures. A crystal structure represents the average of the $\sim 10^{16}$ protein molecules present in a typical crystal (space-average). It also represents the average conformation of these molecules during the 1–5 days it normally takes to collect a full diffraction pattern (time-average). However, movement of molecules in the crystal, either in the form of slightly different conformations for neighbouring molecules (static disorder) or movements with time of individual molecules (dynamic disorder), leads to a smearing of the electron density. In extreme, but not rare, cases certain flexible loops are totally invisible in the electron-density maps. Crystallographers not only refine the position of each atom in space (*xyz* coordinates), but also determine a factor which indicates how much each atom moves around in the crystal. This factor is called the temperature-factor or B-factor. Regions that are flexible in the crystal are likely to be flexible in solution and are often important for biological function. Conformational changes that are induced by ligand binding or by pH changes are studied by determining crystal structures in the absence and presence of the ligand, or at different pH values.

C.   How can protein crystallography contribute to drug discovery?

All the information mentioned above is valuable for drug design. The determination of a new protein structure often gives new insights into its biological function and the structural basis thereof. Detailed knowledge about the catalytic mechanism and the three-dimensional structure of the active site can clearly facilitate the classical approaches in rational drug design, such as the design of mechanism-based inhibitors,[14] multisubstrate analogue inhibitors[15] and transition-state analogues.[16] In addition, protein crystallography provides molecular modellers with experimental 3D models of the target which can be exploited for direct drug design.[17] Sophisticated molecular modelling tools[17] can be used to display and analyse the structural and physicochemical features of the target receptor site, which may ultimately allow the design of structurally novel lead compounds. To this end, it is important to have detailed information about conformational changes occurring upon ligand binding, as this may profoundly influence the results.

In other cases, the protein itself is viewed as a potential drug. A variety of cytokines, growth factors, growth hormones and other peptidic hormones fall into this category.[10] In general, the ultimate goal of structural analysis in this case is to facilitate the discovery of simpler, nonpeptidic molecular surrogates for the naturally occurring molecules.

In practice, the contribution of protein crystallography to drug discovery programmes may be classified into the following categories.

(1) *Elucidation of the mechanisms of drug action at the molecular level.* In some cases, protein crystallography has provided the molecular basis for the observed activity of compounds discovered either by serendipity or by (natural) product screening. For example, it showed how a series of compounds with antiviral activity against picornaviruses, notably the human common cold virus, were able to interfere with the viral disassembly step of the infection cycle.[18]

(2) *Retrospective analysis of structure–activity relationships.* X-ray structure analysis clearly facilitates the interpretation of the structure–activity data, which is sometimes far from straightforward. In particular, structure–activity relationships may be obscured by the fact that the bound conformation of a ligand is drastically different from that determined for the free molecule in solution, as happened with cyclosporin[19–25] and another immunosuppressant, FK-506.[26] Also, structural variations on a chemical lead sometimes result in different binding modes. Such changes are hard to predict. It is important in such a situation to realize quickly what is going on and to characterize fully the binding modes of what should be considered as separate series of compounds. Many such examples have been reported, including the human rhinovirus inhibitors[27] mentioned above, HIV-1 proteinase inhibitors,[28,29] haemoglobin[30] and human thrombin inhibitors.[31,32]

(3) *Structure-assisted drug design.* Protein crystallography has proved extremely valuable in guiding and accelerating further chemical elaboration of an existing lead structure.[7–9,33–40] It often allows one to identify and to discard a number of doomed drug design strategies and to focus the synthetic efforts on the most promising analogues, thus significantly reducing the total number of compounds to be synthesized before one arrives at a suitable drug candidate. Unfavourable interactions, and putative additional favourable ones, can be spotted. In this way, compounds with improved potency may be generated quickly. Furthermore, the availability of crystallographic data makes possible a detailed analysis of the bound conformation of a compound. Unfavourable high-energy conformations, when present, can be identified and ways to avoid them can be sought.[41,42] In addition, one may try to design conformationally restricted analogues, which in general show improved potency for entropic reasons.[43–48] A further advantage of enhancing the binding of an inhibitor through the introduction of conformational restraints is the potential for reducing its size.[44] When compound selectivity is an issue, protein crystallography provides a powerful means to pinpoint structural differences between structurally related enzymes or receptors which can be exploited to improve selectivity.[31,44,49–51] In general, the information gained from crystal structure analysis is not directly relevant to drug development issues such as patentability, toxicity, stability, solubility, bioavailability, formulation, and so on, but when used in combination with the appropriate expertise it allows one to predict what kind of structural modifications can be tried to improve the pharmacological properties of the compound without jeopardizing potency.[9,43] A particular example here relates to the inhibition of proteases, many of which are of pharmaceutical importance. Following recent progress in rational drug design, it is now often possible to obtain within 1 or 2 years highly potent, highly selective peptidomimetics with K_i values in the nanomolar to subnanomolar range. Unfortunately, these peptide-based molecules usually exhibit very poor pharmacological

properties. Several recent examples illustrate beautifully how protein crystallography can be used to overcome these problems by directing the design of orally active, nonpeptidic inhibitors[44,52,53] (see selected examples).

(4) *Structure-based drug design.* Structure-based drug design refers to an iterative procedure which uses the crystal structure of a target protein to design a novel lead structure, which is further elaborated during subsequent cycles of X-ray analysis, followed by design, synthesis and biological testing[2-9] (Fig. 24.2). The pioneering work on thymidylate synthase,[2,7,9,54,55] purine nucleoside phosphorylase[8,34,37-40] and more recently HIV-1 proteinase[9,56-58] illustrates the tremendous potential of this approach. While chemical expertise and intuition are still key in *de novo* structure-based drug design, more and more powerful computational approaches are being developed to guide this process.[17,59]

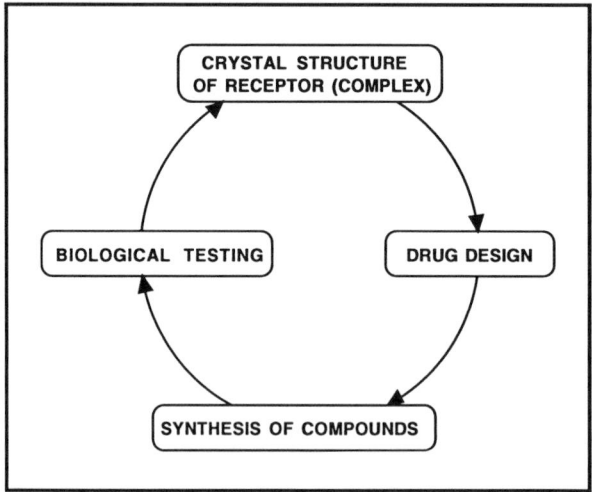

Fig. 24.2 The structure-based drug design cycle. The cycle can start either with a chemical lead, which is co-crystallized with the target protein, or with the structure of the target protein alone for *de novo* design. A number of cycles is usually necessary before one arrives at a suitable clinical candidate.

(5) In computero *drug screening.* Algorithms are emerging which allow one to carry out *'in computero'* drug screening, i.e. to search 3D chemical databases for compounds which are sterically and chemically complementary to the target receptor site, or which meet the requirement of a given pharmacophoric search model.[59-61] Although the results obtained so far with these techniques are still modest,[4,62-65] the prospects for the future are extremely promising.

II. PROTEIN CRYSTALS AND DATA COLLECTION

A. What are protein crystals?

Protein crystals, like any crystals of organic or inorganic compounds, are regular three-dimensional arrays of identical molecules or molecular complexes (Fig. 24.3). Depending on the space group, all molecules in a crystal have a limited number of unique orientations with respect to the crystal lattice. This means that the diffraction of all individual molecules adds up to yield intensities which are sufficiently strong to be measured.

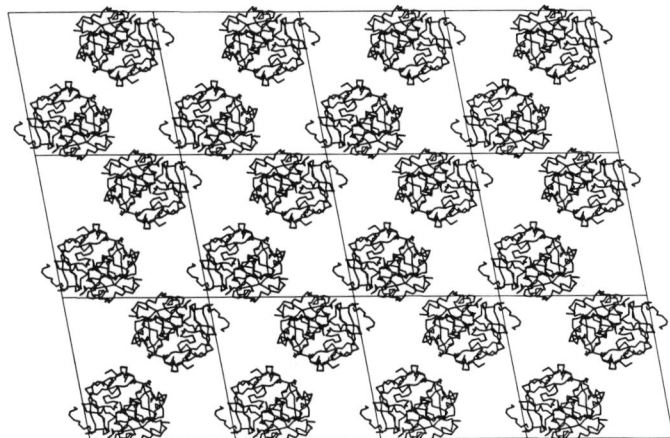

Fig. 24.3 Crystal packing of a human thrombin complex. Twelve unit cells with one layer of molecules are shown. By looking carefully, one can see that the two molecules in each unit cell are rotated 180° with respect to each other. Protein crystals used for X-ray diffraction extend into three dimensions and consist of many layers of molecules. The next layer of thrombin molecules fits into the holes in the layer shown.

B.   How do we get crystals?[66,67]

Obtaining X-ray quality crystals is often one of the most difficult parts of a structure determination, since the number of parameters which can be varied (pH, buffer, protein concentration, temperature, precipitant, additives) is enormous. An absolute requirement for successful crystallization is a sufficient quantity of pure 'crystallization grade' protein. When the crystallization conditions are unknown, one often needs as much as 200 mg of protein to find the right crystallization conditions and to produce enough crystals to solve the structure. If the crystallization conditions are already known and one is lucky, 1 mg of protein may be enough to produce a series of crystals of the same protein with different inhibitors bound. One should bear in mind, however, that published crystallization protocols are often difficult to reproduce!

Crystals are produced by slowly precipitating the protein from solution. Under the right conditions, the protein will not form an amorphous precipitate but will instead settle in a

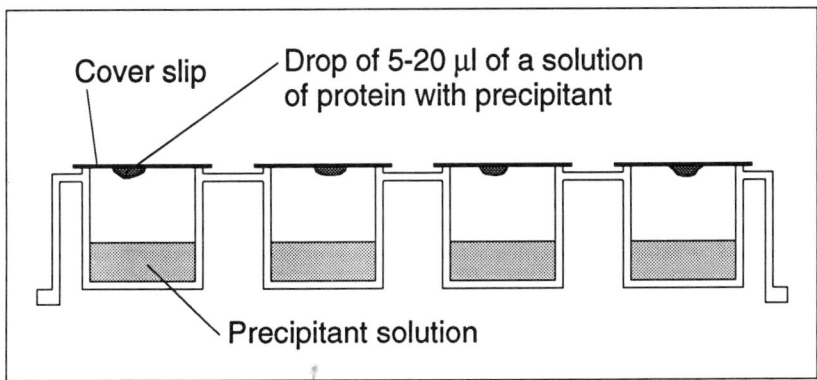

Fig. 24.4 The hanging drop crystallization setup. A drop of a solution of protein with precipitant (~5–20 μl) is suspended above a reservoir containing a much larger amount (~0.5–1.0 ml) of a more concentrated precipitant solution and the drop is allowed to equilibrate with the reservoir. Water moves from the less concentrated protein drop to the more concentrated reservoir solution via the vapour phase, causing the drop to shrink. The concentrations of protein and precipitant in the drop increase until the saturation point is reached and the protein starts to precipitate slowly. The precipitate is usually amorphous, but crystals will form in successful experiments.

well-ordered crystalline array. Methods for precipitating proteins involve dialysing away the salt, if salt is necessary to solubilize the protein, concentrating a nearly saturated protein solution by evaporation (usually in a hanging drop setup, see below) and the addition of precipitants such as poly(ethylene glycol) or ammonium sulfate. Other possibilities, which are less often used, are temperature and pH gradients. The method most often used for screening for crystallization conditions is the hanging drop method (Fig. 24.4).

C.   Preparation of crystals of protein–ligand complexes

An important part of protein crystallography which is especially relevant to drug design is the determination of protein–ligand complexes. If the ligand is a relatively small molecule, it is often possible to obtain crystals of the complex by soaking crystals of the native protein in a mother liquor containing the inhibitor. Protein crystals usually contain solvent channels which are large enough to allow the inhibitor to diffuse into the interior of the crystals. A soaking experiment requires little material (one micromole of compound is usually enough), but solubility is often a problem. The high protein content of the crystallization drop usually requires ligand concentration in the range of 0.1–1.0 mM. The problem is often overcome by dissolving the (hydrophobic) ligand in a suitable organic solvent such as dimethyl sulfoxide or acetonitrile and adding this solution to the crystallization drop to a final concentration of solvent of up to 10%. Purity may not be a problem if none of the contaminants binds to the protein. The chemical structure of the compound under study has to be known, and when chiral centres are present it is preferable to know beforehand their absolute configuration. At 2.5 Å or better resolution, it is often possible to deduce the absolute configuration from the electron-density maps. When epimerization occurs, it is in general faster than the time required to prepare the crystal and collect the data.

Soaking has some practical advantages: it is relatively fast (the soaking time ranges from a few hours to a few days); it requires minimal amounts of the ligand; and, as the crystallization conditions for the native protein are often well established, it is relatively easy to obtain large, well-diffracting crystals. However, the soaking method also has several disadvantages. Possible conformational changes induced by ligand binding may be hindered by the crystal packing and may therefore remain unobserved. The crystal lattice may be incompatible with ligand binding, causing the crystals to crack and/or dissolve upon soaking, or not to bind the ligand at all.

For this reason, if enough material is available, it is preferable to try first to obtain protein–ligand complexes via the second method: co-crystallization. For large ligands, this method is the only possibility to obtain crystals of the complex. With co-crystallization, the complex is formed in solution by adding the ligand to the protein solution, and the complex is subsequently crystallized. The advantages of this method are that, since the complex is formed in solution, conformational changes induced by the ligand are not hindered and will show up in the crystal structure. Also, the diffraction quality of the crystals is not compromised by the soaking procedure. A disadvantage is that the crystallization conditions for a complex are sometimes slightly or even completely different from the crystallization conditions for native crystals, forcing one to start from scratch to search for crystallization conditions. Another disadvantage is that it often takes several weeks to several months for a protein to crystallize and not all ligands are stable for such a long time. Also, in the context of a structure-based drug design programme, the crystallographic results should be obtained before the next round of synthesis and biological testing of compounds, and not afterwards.

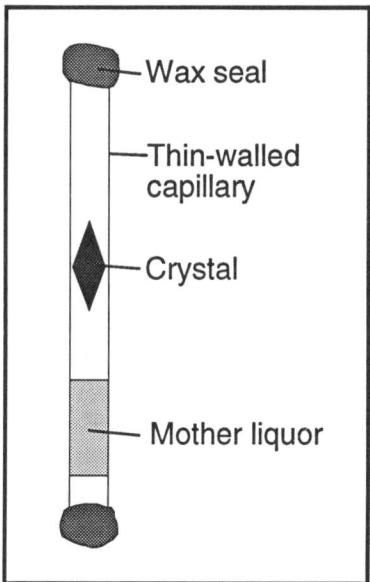

Fig. 24.5   X-ray capillary with crystal. For the diffraction experiment, the protein crystal is mounted in a special capillary to prevent it from drying out. A little mother liquor is added to maintain constant humidity.

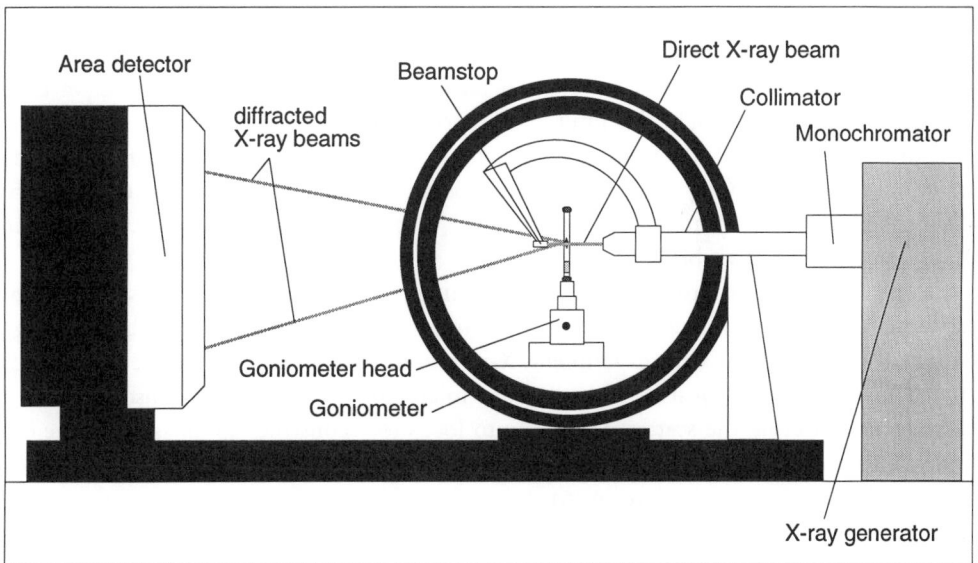

Fig. 24.6   The setup for an X-ray experiment. The X-ray generator produces a powerful beam. The monochromator selects X-rays of a single wavelength (1.54 Å for copper targets) and the collimator limits the diameter of the beam to 0.3–0.5 mm. The beam hits the crystal and some of the X-rays are diffracted by the crystal. Most X-rays pass straight through and are stopped by a small piece of lead, the beam stop. The diffracted X-rays are detected by an area detector, an imaging plate, or other detection systems. The goniometer, shown here as a large black circle, has four rotation axes and allows the crystal to be positioned in any orientation with respect to the X-ray beam.

D.   Data collection[68-72]

Protein crystals contain on average 50% solvent and, if exposed to air, they will dry out and completely disintegrate. Protein crystals are therefore mounted in sealed X-ray capillaries which contain a little mother liquor to maintain the same humidity as during crystallization (Fig. 24.5). The capillary is placed on a goniometer, a device which makes it possible to rotate the crystal in all directions, and the crystal is exposed to an intense X-ray beam (Fig. 24.6). Protein crystals are normally not larger than 0.3–0.5 mm and the diameter of the beam (0.3–0.5 mm) is chosen to match the size of the crystal so as to minimize background scattering. The crystal is slowly rotated to bring all reflections into diffracting condition.

The diffraction spots are usually recorded on electronic detectors or on detectors based on imaging plates. These detectors are able to routinely collect high-quality X-ray data sets from single crystals in 1 to 5 days. The diffraction images of these detectors are fed directly into a computer, which produces a list of reflection intensities. Ten thousand to several hundred thousand reflections are recorded per crystal, depending on the quality of the crystal and the size of the unit cell.

III.   FROM DIFFRACTION INTENSITIES TO A MOLECULAR STRUCTURE[68-72]

A.   Light microscopy and X-ray crystallography share the same basic principle

A light microscope allows us to study in great detail small objects such as insects or cell slices, but it is physically impossible to resolve any details which are smaller than half the wavelength of the light used. For blue light this limit is about 200 nm. To resolve atomic details, which are on the order of 1–5 Å (0.1–0.5 nm), electromagnetic radiation with a much shorter wavelength than light is required: X-rays. A light microscope and an X-ray setup share the same basic principle, although the practical implementation is quite different, owing to the different properties of X-rays and visible light.

In a microscope, light from a light source shines on the sample and is scattered in all directions. A set of lenses is used to reconstruct from this scattered light an enlarged image of the original sample. In an X-ray experiment, X-rays from an X-ray source hit the crystal and are scattered in all directions, just as with the light microscope. However, no lenses exist to date which are able to bring the scattered X-rays into focus to reconstruct an enlarged image of the sample. All the crystallographer can do is to record directly the scattered X-rays (the diffraction pattern) and to use computers to reconstruct an enlarged image of the sample.

B.   X-rays are scattered by electrons

Although X-rays interact only weakly with matter, they are occasionally absorbed by electrons, which start to oscillate. These oscillating electrons serve as X-ray sources which can send an X-ray photon in any direction. X-ray photons, scattered from different parts of the crystal have to

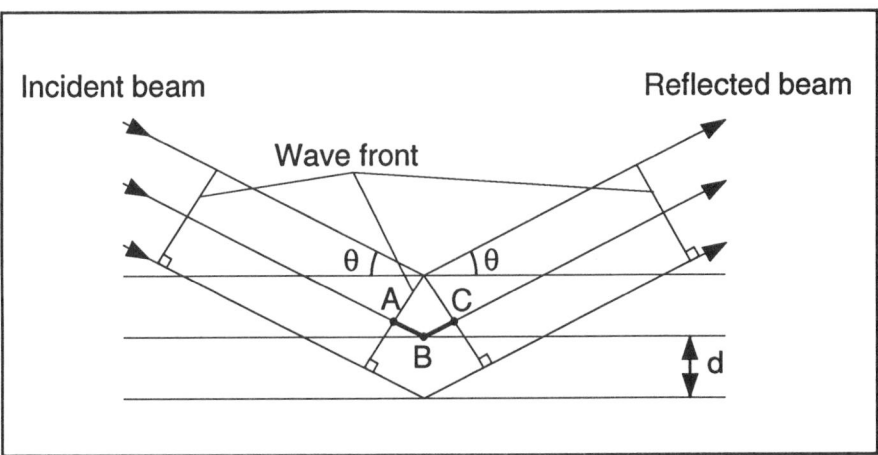

Fig. 24.7   Bragg's law. X-rays are reflected by sets of parallel planes, separated by a distance *d*, which run through the crystal. Diffraction is only observed under the following conditions. (i) The angle of the incident beam with the planes is identical to the angle of the reflected beam with the planes. This angle is indicated by θ. (ii) The path difference for beams reflected from subsequent planes (path ABC in the fig.), should equal an integer times the wavelength, such that the different beams remain in *phase*.

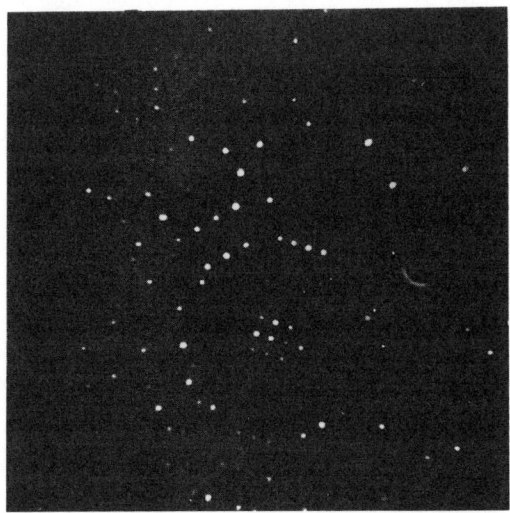

Fig. 24.8   X-ray diffraction pattern of human *myo*-inositol phosphatase recorded with a Siemens multiwire area detector. in order to collect a complete diffraction pattern, one usually needs to collect more than 1000 of these frames. The characteristic pattern of diffraction spots is caused by the fact X-rays diffracted from different unit cells in the crystal have to scatter in phase.

add up constructively in order to produce a measurable intensity. The condition under which the scattered X-rays add up constructively are laid down in Bragg's law, which treats crystals in terms of sets of parallel planes (Fig. 24.7).

Sets of planes from the different unit cells in the crystal have to scatter in phase as well. This is true only for a limited subset of planes and results in a characteristic pattern of diffraction spots (Fig. 24.8).

C.   The diffraction pattern corresponds to the Fourier transform of the crystal structure

Each diffraction spot is caused by reflection of X-rays by a particular set of planes in the crystal. If the crystal contains layers of atoms with the same spacing and orientation as a particular set of planes (if the set of planes is physically present), the corresponding diffraction spot will be strong. On the other hand, if nothing is physically present in a crystal which corresponds to a particular set of planes, the corresponding reflection will be weak. The complicated structure present in the crystal is transformed by the diffraction process into a set of diffraction spots which correspond to sets of planes (more precisely, sinusoidal density waves), just as our ear converts a complicated sound signal into a series of (sinusoidal) tones when we listen to music. This conversion of a complicated function into a series of simple sine- and cosine functions is called a Fourier transformation.

D.   The phase problem

The original function, in our case the electron density distribution in the crystal, can be regenerated with computers by performing the inverse Fourier transformation, i.e. by adding together the corresponding density waves for all reflections (see Fig. 24.9). However, in order to make this addition, we need to know not only the amplitude of the density wave but also its relative position with respect to all other density waves (the phase). The amplitude can be measured, because it is calculated from the intensity of the corresponding diffraction spot, but there is currently no way to measure the phases directly. This so-called 'phase problem' can be solved by one of the following techniques.

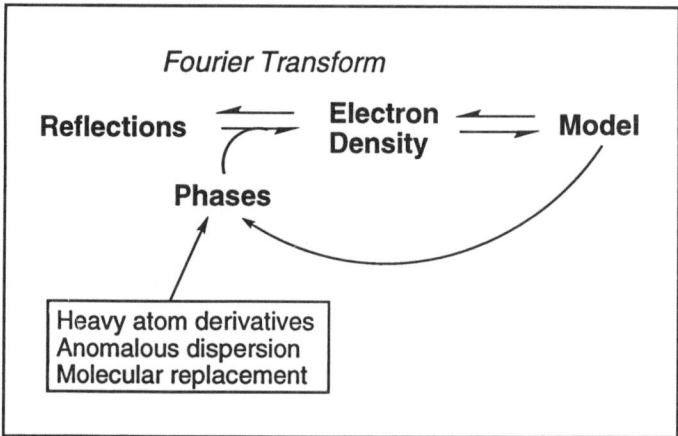

Fig. 24.9   The phase problem. The experimental data obtained in an X-ray experiment are the intensities of the reflections. By using an inverse Fourier transform, it is possible to calculate electron-density maps from these intensities. However, it is essential for this calculation to know the phase associated with each reflection. Approximate 'starting' phases can be obtained from heavy-atom derivatives, anomalous dispersion or molecular replacement (see text). More accurate phases can be derived from the refined model, once it has been obtained.

(1) *Direct methods.* These methods only work for small molecules and use phase relationships which exist between certain sets of reflections.[72]

(2) *Multiple isomorphous replacement (MIR).* This is the classical approach to structure determination of proteins of unknown fold. Crystals are soaked in solutions with salts of 'heavy' atoms (Hg, Pt, Au, etc.) under such conditions that a few of these heavy atoms attach themselves to well-defined spots on the protein molecule. The heavy-atom positions are found by analysing the differences between the native diffraction pattern and the diffraction patterns of crystals treated with heavy-atom reagents. When two or more suitable heavy-atom derivatives are found, it is possible to calculate phases and an electron density map.

(3) *Anomalous scattering.* This method makes use of the fact that some inner electrons of the heavier elements have absorption edges in the range of X-ray wavelengths. The method is used to supplement the phase information of a single heavy atom derivative, but also to obtain full phase information from proteins which are labelled with, for example, selenomethionine, a selenium-containing amino acid. The diffraction pattern is measured at different wavelengths: before, near, and after the absorption edge. This method requires a tunable X-ray source, which is only present at synchrotrons.

(4) *Molecular replacement.* When a suitable model of the unknown crystal structure is available, such a model can be used to solve the phase problem. Examples are the use of the structure of human thrombin to solve the structure of bovine thrombin, the use of the known structure of an antibody fragment to solve the structure of an unknown antibody fragment, or the use of the structure of the native enzyme to solve the structure of an inhibitor complex in a different crystal form. The model is oriented and positioned in the unit cell of the unknown crystal with the use of rotation and translation functions, and the oriented model is subsequently used to calculate phases and an electron-density map.

Method (1) can not (yet?) be used for proteins. Methods (2) and (3) can be used to solve any protein structure *de novo* and these are the methods most widely used to solve unknown protein structures. However, these approaches require testing and measuring of dozens of heavy-atom derivatives, which may still take several years in difficult cases. Method (4) is very fast; it usually takes less than a month, but it requires that the structure of a similar protein be available, which is not always the case. This method is extremely useful in solving the structures of a protein complexed with a series of inhibitors or other ligands.

E. Model building and refinement

Once an electron-density map is obtained, it is interpreted by the crystallographer. In case of a MIR map, a complete model of the protein has to be fitted to the electron density. The C^α atoms are placed first (chain tracing), and subsequently the complete main-chain and the side-chains are built. In case of molecular replacement, the model used to solve the phase problem has to be rebuilt to reflect the molecule present in the crystal. The model is usually of a similar protein and the changes involve substitution of amino acids, making insertions and deletions, changing the orientation of loops, and so on.

After (re)building, the model is refined, that is the differences between the observed diffraction amplitudes (F_o), and the diffraction amplitudes calculated from the model (F_c) are minimized, while the geometry of the model is optimized. The ratio between observations and parameters in protein crystallography is usually quite low, which makes it impossible to do a free atom refinement. It is always necessary to restrain the bond lengths, angles, etc. towards ideal values. The refinement is done by computer programs, either with least-squares methods (often referred to as energy minimization), or with molecular dynamics. Phases calculated from the refined model allow the calculation of improved electron-density maps, which are analysed by the crystallographer to again rebuild (improve) the model. Cycles of refinement and rebuilding are repeated until convergence is reached and a set of coordinates is obtained which is ready for deposition with the Protein Data Bank (PDB).[73]

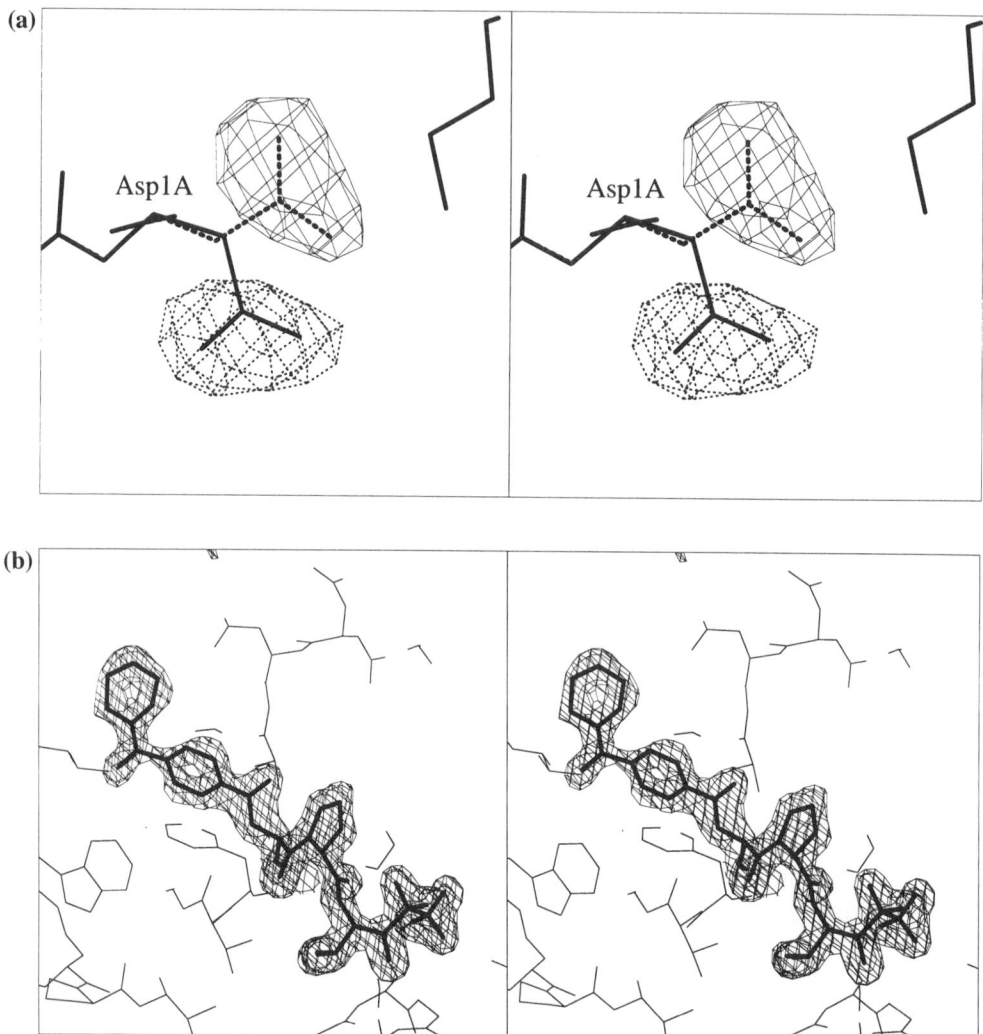

Fig. 24.10 $F_o - F_c$ difference maps. (a) Detection of errors in the model. The side-chain of Asp1A in human thrombin was deliberately moved to a wrong position and an $F_o - F_c$ difference map was calculated. The model used to calculate F_c is indicated in thick solid lines, the correct position of the side-chain is indicated in thick broken lines. Negative contours (4σ below mean) are drawn in thin broken lines and positive contours (4σ above mean) are drawn in thin solid lines. Strong negative difference density is present around the wrongly placed side-chain while strong positive density is present at the position where the side-chain should be according to the experimental data. These maps are extremely useful to spot errors in the model. (b) $F_o - F_c$ 'omit map' (see text) contoured at 3.5σ of an inhibitor bound to porcine pancreatic elastase. Protein atoms, used for calculation of F_c are indicated in thin lines, the inhibitor which has been removed from the model is drawn by thick lines. This $F_o - F_c$ density map has been calculated with a model which contains no information whatsoever about the inhibitor. The difference density shown is therefore entirely due the experimental data and can be used to verify the correctness of the placement of the inhibitor.

F. Most-used types of electron density maps

Since the direct experimental result of a crystallographic analysis is an electron-density map, and since the model is based on a (subjective) interpretation of this map, we will here discuss the types of electron density maps most often used.

(a) F_o-F_c or difference maps. These maps are obtained after subtracting the calculated structure factors (F_c) from the observed structure factors (F_o), an operation which is in a first approximation equivalent to subtracting the calculated electron density from the observed electron density. Features which are present in the 'observed' density but not in the calculated density will give peaks, while atoms present in the model (in the F_c) but not in the 'observed' electron density will result in holes (Fig. 24.10). These maps are frequently used to detect errors in the model and can also be used to obtain an unbiased electron density of a bound inhibitor, for example, by removing the inhibitor completely from the model. In this case, the resulting electron density for the inhibitor is entirely caused by the experimental data, and not by any model bias present in the phases. These maps are often referred to as 'omit maps'.

(b) $2F_o-F_c$ maps. These are the standard electron-density maps. Because of model bias, maps calculated with F_o and model phases tend to show only electron density associated with the model. As discussed above, F_o-F_c maps show everything which is in F_o but not in the model. By combining an F_o map with an F_o-F_c map, a $2F_o-F_c$ electron density map is obtained, which shows both electron density for the model and electron density for features which are not yet accounted for in the model, such as bound water molecules, carbohydrates (Fig. 24.11) and other molecules associated with the protein.

IV. USING CRYSTAL STRUCTURES: QUALITY CRITERIA

A. Errors in crystal structures

The theory of the diffraction of X-rays by crystals and of the Fourier transformation is rigorous and exact; it involves no approximations. Consequently, crystal structures have proved to be very reliable and errors are rare. However, when using a protein crystal structure, one should keep in mind that they do have certain limitations.[74,75]

The direct experimental result of a crystallographic analysis is an electron-density map, and not the atomic model everybody looks at! If errors occur in crystal structures, they most often occur at the level of the (subjective) interpretation of the electron-density maps by the crystallographer. A severe problem, especially at low resolution (lower than 3.0 Å), is the so-called model bias. To calculate an electron-density map, one needs amplitudes and phases. The amplitudes are determined experimentally, but the phases cannot be measured directly. In later stages of refinement, they are calculated from the model, which means that if the model contains errors, the phases will contain the same errors. Since phases make up at least 50% of the information which is used to calculate the electron-density maps, wrong features may still have reasonable electron density, because of these phase errors. This effect is called model bias.

Errors in crystal structures can be divided into three categories:

(a)

(b)

(c)

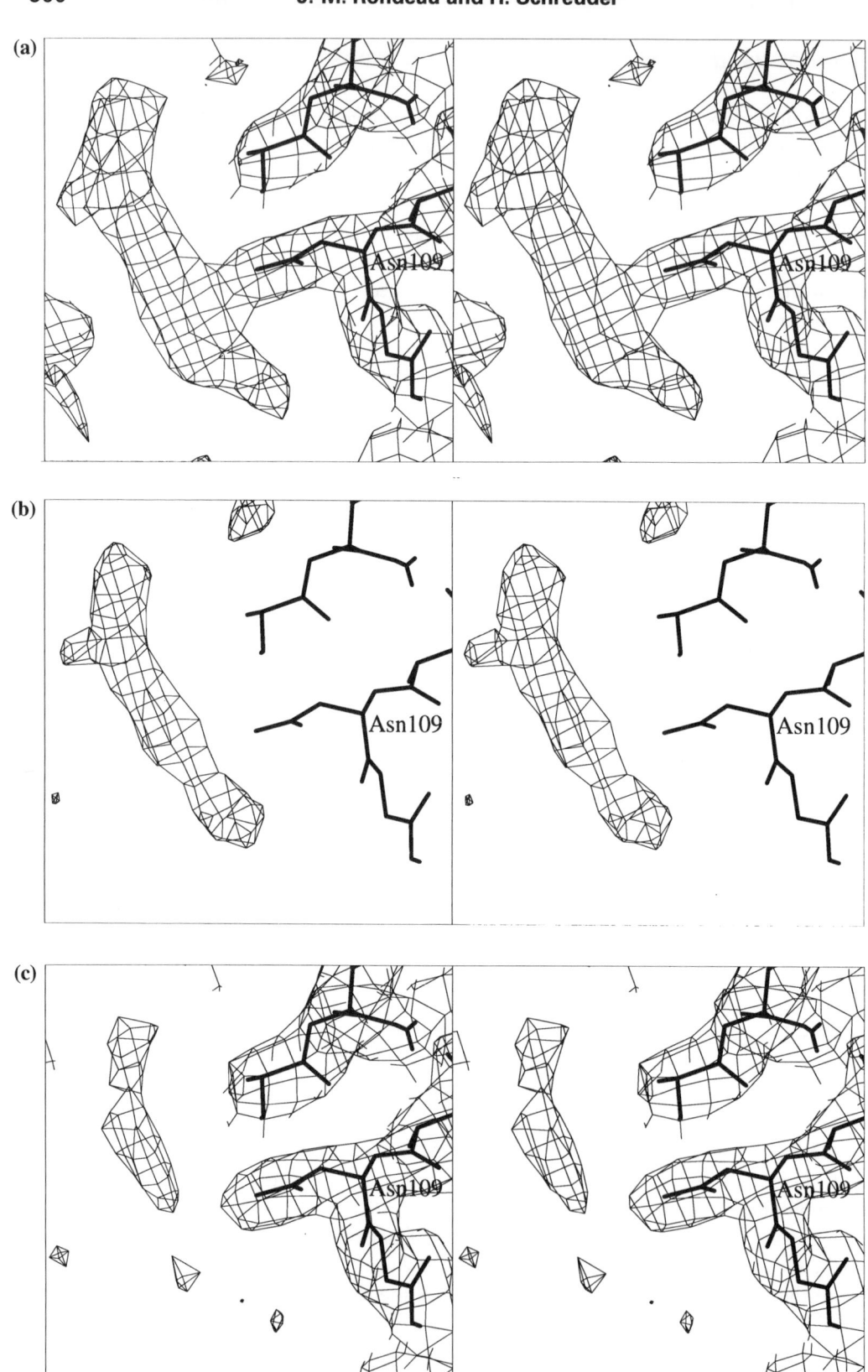

(1) *Complete garbage.* This has happened a few times in the past[74,75] but nowadays powerful software that exists to validate protein structures should be able to catch these kinds of blunders. Completely wrong structures may arise from wrong space group assignments, errors in the sign of the electron-density maps and interpretation of uninterpretable maps.

(2) *Localized errors (loops and connectivity).* Loops are often flexible and in these cases poorly defined in the electron-density maps. Crystallographers, trying to build these loops, sometimes connect wrong parts of the protein and place loops into density which does not belong to those loops. These kinds of errors occur most often with 'hot structures', when people rush to solve the structure in the shortest possible time, to stay ahead of the competition. Famous examples are the p21 ras protein[76,77] and the HIV-1 proteinase.[78–80]

(3) *Errors in main-chain dihedral angles and side-chain conformations.* When comparing structures from the same protein, independently solved by different groups, one often observes discrepancies in main-chain dihedral angles and side-chain conformations. There may be several reasons for this. Electron-density maps, especially at lower resolution ($\sim$3.0 Å or less) do not show individual atoms, but rather the overall shape of the main-chain and side-chains. From these maps, it is not always clear how to orient a peptide plane, or which side-chain conformation to choose. In addition, particular side-chains often have multiple conformations in the crystal while only a single conformation has been fitted by the crystallographer. Also, it is not possible with protein crystals to distinguish on the basis of the electron density alone between C, O and N, which means that the side-chain orientations of His, Asn and Gln are never uniquely defined by the electron density.

(4) *Other errors and limitations.* These include the assignment of bound solvent molecules and metal ions, the protonation or oxidation state of certain prosthetic groups[81] and the choice of incorrect parameters for the refinement of nonstandard groups. One should bear in mind, however, that these latter errors are usually below the accuracy of 0.3–0.5 Å of the protein structure. Protons and other light elements (Li^+, Be^{2+}) cannot be seen by protein X-ray crystallography. It is, therefore, not possible to determine the protonation state of active site residues and bound ligands with X-ray studies.

While errors of the first two categories should not happen, one cannot blame the crystallographer for errors of the third type because (i) these errors are within the error limits of the structure determination and (ii) side-chain conformations are often not wrong but merely represent one out of a number of conformations which occur in the crystal and in solution.

Fig. 24.11 The rationale behind the $2F_o - F_c$ maps. Shown is a carbohydrate attachment site at Asn109 in human leukocyte elastase. The carbohydrate chain has not been added to the model. The F_o map in (a) mainly shows the electron density of the model, owing to the model bias. Some electron density is present for the carbohydrate, but it is very weak and not connected to the Asn residue. The $F_o - F_c$ map in (b) shows only features which have not been accounted for in the model, in this case the carbohydrate moiety. The $2F_o - F_c$ map in (c) is a combination of the two and shows both density belonging to the model and strong connected density for the carbohydrate. From these figures, it is clear why crystallographers prefer a $2F_o - F_c$ map over an F_o map.

B. Quality criteria

When using crystal structures, it is important to know whether a structure is very accurate, for example allowing conclusions about the strengths of hydrogen bonds from the observed hydrogen bond length, or less accurate, which would make such conclusions quite hazardous. Below we discuss a number of parameters which crystallographers normally publish along with the description of a crystal structure, and which should allow others to judge the quality of a crystal structure.

1. Quality of the experimental data

The quality of a crystal structure cannot be better than the quality of the experimental data it is based upon. The experimental data can be judged by the following criteria.

(1) *Resolution.* This corresponds to the shortest spacing of planes (d) whose reflections have been used in map calculation and refinement (see Fig. 24.7). The smaller this spacing, the sharper and more detailed will the electron-density maps be. The resolution is probably the single most important criterion determining the quality of a crystal structure. At high resolution (better than 2.0 Å) the protein and bound water molecules are well defined and it is very unlikely that the structure will contain any serious errors. At low resolution (2.8–3.5 Å), it is usually not possible to assign bound water molecules and the crystallographer needs to be careful not to make any errors. For drug design, a resolution of 2.5 Å or better is highly desirable. However, successful structure-based drug design has been done on purine nucleoside phosphorylase at 3.2 Å.[8,34,37]

(2) *Completeness of the data.* One can calculate the total number of reflections to a certain resolution and, ideally, one would like to measure them all. However, for various reasons it is in practice often not possible to measure all reflections. If only a small fraction of the reflections is missing (~10%), and the missing reflections are weak, the electron-density maps will hardly be affected. However, if a significant fraction of the reflections is missing, this may lead to artefacts in the electron-density maps and also the problem of model bias will become more severe.

(3) *R-sym.* This is the error between multiple measurements of the same reflection and its symmetry mates. The lower the R-sym, the better. R-syms up to 10% are tolerable.

2. Quality of the model

Not only should the experimental data be of good quality, but also the model should be fitted correctly to the electron-density map. Below we list some of the most widely used criteria for judging the quality of the model.

(1) *R-factor.* This is the error between the observed amplitudes (F_o), and the amplitudes calculated from the model (F_c). Well refined structures have R-factors below 20%.

(2) *Free R-factor.* Modern refinement programs are very powerful and capable of producing reasonable refinement statistics with wrong models. In order to be sure that refinement is progressing correctly and one is not merely reducing the R-factor of a wrong model, Brünger proposed to exclude a subset of reflections from refinement and to use these reflections only for the calculation of R-factors.[82] If refinement is progressing correctly, the R-factor of the reference set of reflections will drop as well, but if the model contains

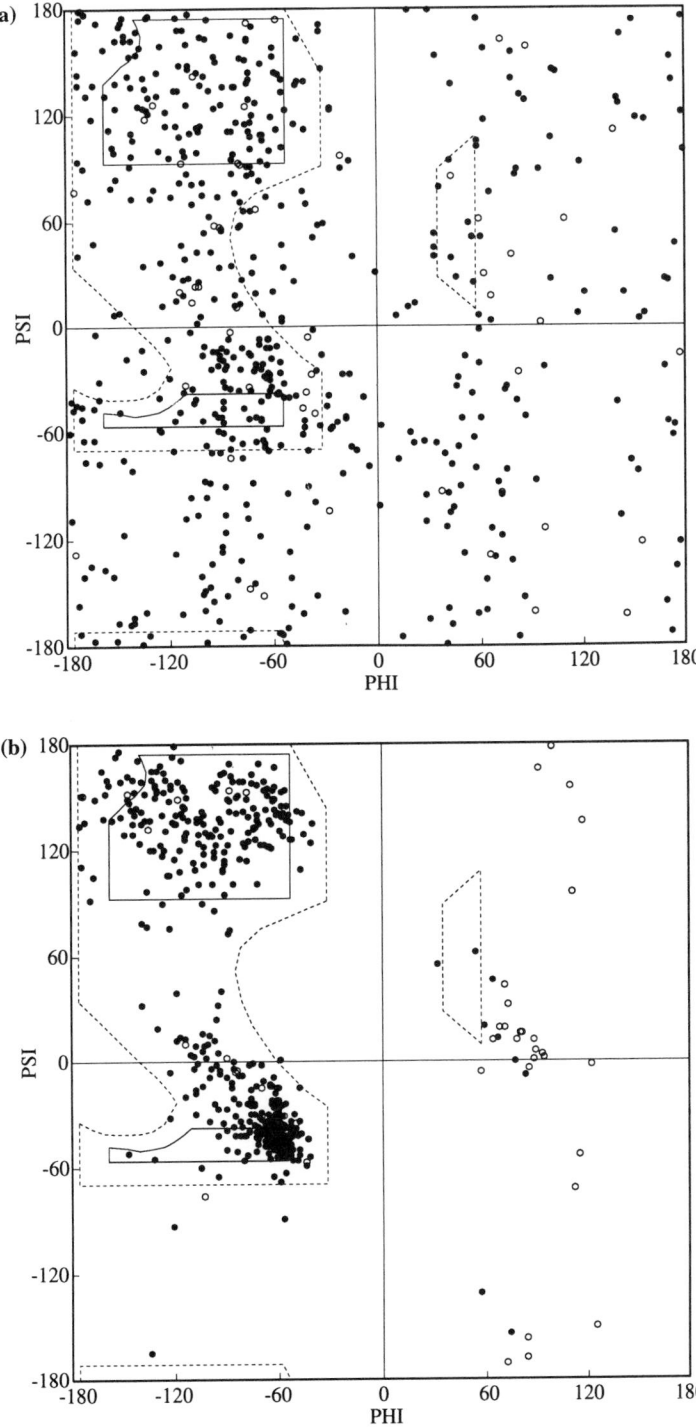

Fig. 24.12 φ,ψ plot. Open circles indicate glycine residues, filled circles indicate nonglycine residues. Residues with φ,ψ angles outside the allowed regions (indicated by broken lines) are strained. Much larger regions are allowed for glycine residues because they do not have a side-chain. When more than a few per cent of the residues have φ,ψ outside the allowed regions, one should be suspicious of errors in the structure. Panel (a) shows the φ,ψ plot of plant RuBisCo, which has been incorrectly fitted to the electron-density map.[122] Panel (b) shows the φ,ψ plot of the same protein after it has been properly fitted and refined.[123]

serious errors the *R*-factor for the reference reflections will remain essentially random (~55%). For correct structures, the free *R*-factor is generally below 35%.

(3) *Deviations from ideality of bond lengths and bond angles.* A correctly fitted model is generally not strained. Significant deviations from ideal values for bond lengths and bond angles point to problems with the crystal structure. Root-mean-square (r.m.s.) deviations from ideality should not be much larger than 0.02 Å for bond lengths, and 5° for bond angles. The bond lengths and angles are biased towards the target values which are used during refinement. *For protein crystals, it is not possible to obtain accurate unbiased values for these parameters.*

(4) *φ,ψ plot.* Because of steric hindrance, only certain combinations of the main-chain dihedral angles φ and ψ are 'allowed' (Fig. 24.12). The protein folding may force some residues to assume unallowed φ,ψ values, and this may have functional significance for active site residues.[83,84] However, if more than a few per cent of all the residues have φ,ψ values completely outside allowed regions, one should suspect errors.

C. Flexibility and temperature factors

Most proteins are flexible and many crystalline proteins contain some very flexible regions. The mobility of atoms in a crystal is expressed in terms of temperature-factors, or *B*-factors, which are optimized during refinement. The relationship between mean total displacement and *B*-factors is given in Fig. 24.13. The mean displacement of atoms with *B*-factors in excess of 60 Å² is larger than 1.5 Å. These atoms are generally poorly defined in the electron-density maps (Fig. 24.14), although in the case of static disorder these atoms may still have well-defined, albeit weak, electron density.

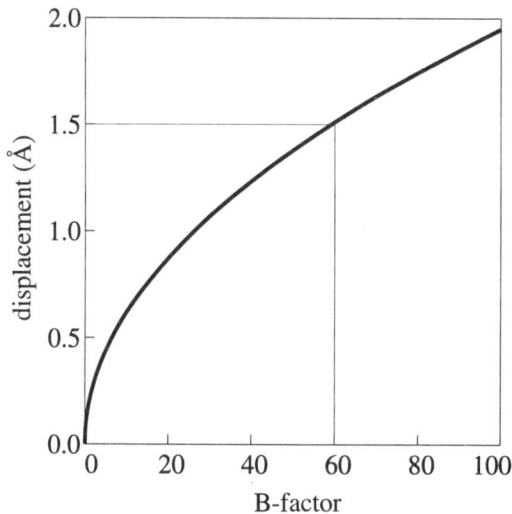

Fig. 24.13 Relationship between the total root mean square displacement and the temperature factor *B*. At temperature factors of 60 Å² and higher, the displacement becomes larger than 1.5 Å (the length of a C—C bond) and the electron density of those atoms becomes very poor (see Fig. 24.14). The formula used in the figure is derived from the relationships[124] $B = 8\pi^2 \langle u^2 \rangle$ where $\langle u^2 \rangle$ represents the displacement perpendicular to the diffracting planes. The total mean square displacement $\langle u_{Tot}^2 \rangle = 3\langle u^2 \rangle$. Hence, $\langle u_{Tot}^2 \rangle^{1/2} = (3B/8\pi^2)^{1/2}$.

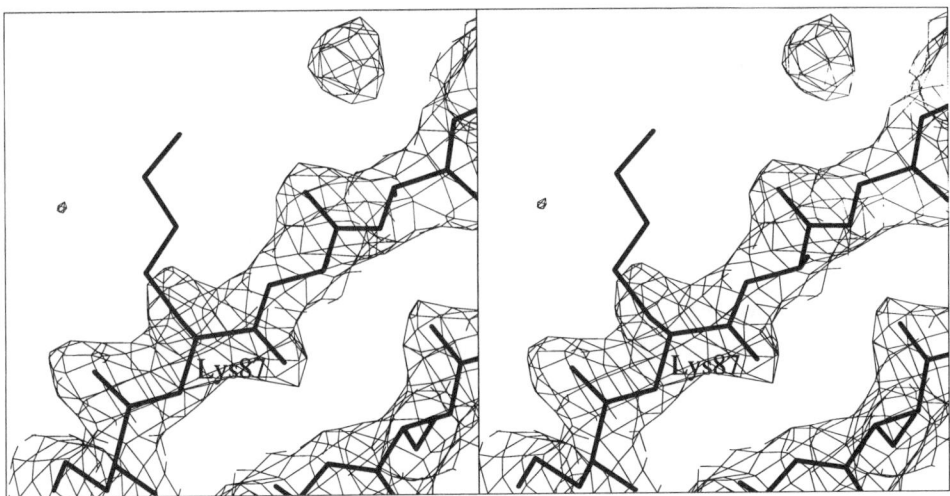

Fig. 24.14   Long and flexible side-chains (such as Arg, Lys, Glu and Gln) which are exposed to the solvent often move freely around. As a result, these side-chains have very high temperature factors and are very poorly or not at all defined in the electron-density map. Lys87, located at the surface of human thrombin, is shown as an example. One should take into account that many exposed surface residues do not have a well-defined orientation if one uses protein structures for analysis and drug design.

From the discussion above, one should not get the impression that all X-ray structures are inaccurate. On the contrary! Most X-ray structures, especially at a resolution of 2.5 Å or better, are very accurate (estimated mean coordinate errors of less than 0.5 Å) and allow researchers to look at enzymes and other proteins with unprecedented detail and clarity (see, for example, Figs 24.1 and 24.10b).

V.   SOME SELECTED EXAMPLES OF STRUCTURE-BASED DRUG DESIGN

Very early on, protein crystallography had a profound impact on drug design. The crystal structure of haemoglobin, the second protein structure to be solved, provided insights into the molecular basis of sickle cell anaemia and allowed the study of the mechanisms of action of drugs with antisickling properties.[30,85] Some general rules governing the interactions between drugs and proteins have emerged from these studies.[85] In another area, X-ray analyses of insulin led to the design of a monomeric form of the hormone which showed an improved rate of absorption.[86] However, the major contribution of protein crystallography so far relates to the design of enzyme inhibitors. Since the early days, numerous enzyme–inhibitor complexes have been studied and many more are underway. These studies have contributed a great deal to a general understanding of the basic principles underlying enzyme inhibition and they have unravelled, for many different functional classes of enzymes, the critical interactions involved in enzyme–inhibitor complexes. The know-how gained from the study of one particular enzyme also proved useful for the design of inhibitors targeting a related enzyme of unknown three-dimensional structure.[65] For instance, the discovery of captopril[87] and cilazapril,[88,89] two antihypertensive drugs acting on the angiotensin-converting enzyme (ACE), was inspired in part by crystallographic analyses of carboxypeptidase A and thermolysin. Similarly, the search for renin inhibitors has long been based on crystallographic information gleaned from fungal aspartic proteinases.[90–93] Other prominent examples of the use of protein crystallography for enzyme inhibitor design include dihydrofolate reductase,[50] α-thrombin,[31,32] elastase,[33,53,94] carbonic anhydrase,[9,41] purine nucleoside phosphorylase,[8,34,37–40] thymidylate synthase,[7,9,54,55,64] HIV-1 proteinase,[9,36,42,44,56,57,95] neutral endopeptidase 24.11[52] and, more recently, influenza neuraminidase.[96] Although the majority of current structure-based drug design programmes still deal with enzymes,[3,10] more and more effort is being put into other targets, including notably a number of proteins involved in the immune response.[10,48,97–100]

We will proceed by giving some concrete examples, selected from the recent literature, of how X-ray crystallography has aided the discovery of promising new drug candidates.

A.   Purine nucleoside phosphorylase

Purine nucleoside phosphorylase (PNP) catalyses the phosphorolysis of purine ribonucleosides and 2′-deoxyribonucleosides to the purine base and ribose- or 2-deoxyribose-α-1-phosphate. PNP is a key enzyme in the T-cell-mediated immune response. As such, it is an attractive target in a number of therapeutic areas, such as organ transplantation, T-cell-mediated autoimmune disorders and T-cell proliferative diseases. In addition, PNP appears to be responsible for the rapid inactivation of some medically important purine nucleoside analogues, including some antineoplastic agents and the antiviral drug DDI (2′,3′-dideoxyinosine). It has been the subject of a thorough and successful structure–based drug design study,[8,34,37–40,101] of which the following gives only a flavour.

1.   Why combining two improvements may sometimes be a failure

Both 8-aminoguanine and 9-deazaguanine analogues are superior inhibitors of PNP compared to the corresponding guanine analogues (Fig. 24.15). Compounds combining these two features, namely 8-amino-9-deazaguanine derivatives, were expected to be even better, but surprisingly they were not. The structural reason for this medicinal chemistry riddle was elucidated through X-ray analysis (Fig. 24.15). The N-7 position of the guanine derivatives is a hydrogen-bond acceptor, while it is a hydrogen-bond donor in the 9-deazaguanine series. Optimal hydrogen-bonding interactions between the enzyme and the 9-deazaguanine analogues are achieved through a movement of the side-chain of Asn243, which also triggers a concomitant shift in the position of Thr242. These conformational changes no longer allow the formation of a hydrogen-bond between the 8-amino substituent and the side-chain hydroxyl group of Thr242. Furthermore, an unfavourable contact with the side-chain methyl group of Thr242 is generated instead (Fig. 24.15).

2.   A chlorinated benzene ring as a replacement for a ribose moiety!

The X-ray analysis of PNP also revealed that the binding site of the ribose moiety of the substrate is essentially hydrophobic,[101] thus unravelling the hitherto unexplained potency of 9-(arylmethyl)guanine analogues. Indeed, a 'herringbone' packing interaction[102] is observed between the benzyl group of these inhibitors and two phenylalanine side-chains located in the

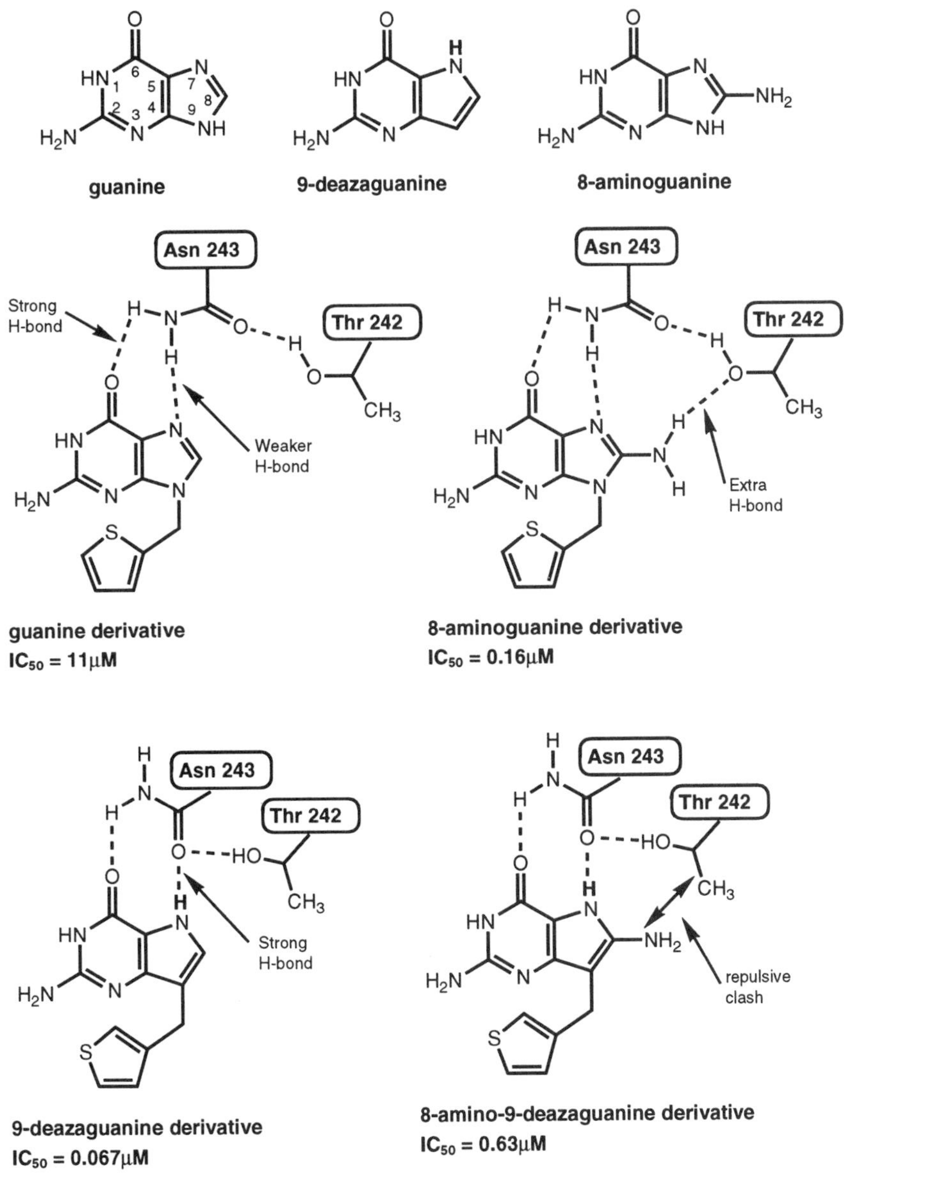

Fig. 24.15   Structure-based design of purine nucleoside phosphorylase inhibitors. For explanation, see text. (Adapted, with permission, from Montgomery, J. A. *et al.* (1993) *J. Med. Chem.* **36**: 55–69. Copyright © 1993, American Chemical Society.)

ribose binding site of PNP. The search for appropriate substituents and positions on the benzyl ring was greatly facilitated by X-ray analysis. It led to the discovery of a series of 9-(arylmethyl)-9-deazapurines that are potent, membrane-permeable inhibitors of PNP. The most potent compound in this series, (S)-9-[1-(3-chlorophenyl)-2-carboxyethyl]-9-deazaguanine has an IC$_{50}$ of 6 nM.[39] One of the compounds generated during this programme, BCX-34, is now undergoing phase II clinical trials.[8]

B.   Neutral endopeptidase 24.11

1.   Structure-based design when the structure of the target is not known

Neutral endopeptidase 24.11 (NEP) is a zinc-dependent metalloproteinase involved in the degradation of a number of peptidic transmitters.[103] In the kidney, NEP is the major enzyme responsible for the inactivation of atrial natriuretic factor (ANF), a peptidic hormone which induces natriuresis, diuresis and lowering of blood pressure.[104] The three-dimensional structure of NEP is not yet known. However, there is a wealth of structural information on a related enzyme from bacterial sources, thermolysin. Recently, potent, orally active macrocyclic NEP inhibitors were designed[52] using crystallographic data on a thermolysin complex with a phosphonamidate-based transition-state inhibitor[105] (Fig. 24.16). The crystal structure indicated that the macrocyclic structure shown in Fig. 24.16 could mimic the two leucine side-

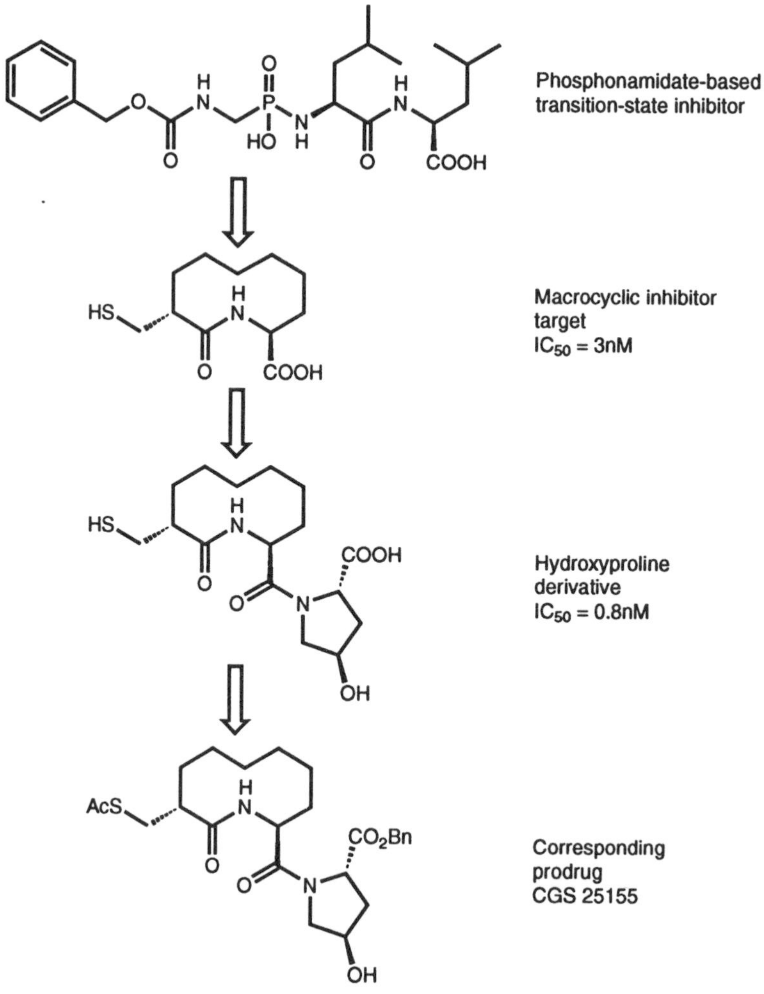

Fig. 24.16   Structure-based design of a macrocyclic inhibitor of neutral endopeptidase 24.11. For explanation, see text.

chains which were present in the original structure. In addition, it was also apparent that, in order to retain good binding affinity, the design strategy should include an internal amide moiety, a terminal carboxylate and, of course, a good zinc-binding group. The designed macrocycle was synthesized and showed an IC_{50} of 3 nM. Further chemical elaboration was aimed at extending the macrocycle with a substituent that would retain a terminal carboxylic group and at the same time allow a modification of the physicochemical properties of the compound. This led to the design of a conformationally restricted hydroxyproline derivative (Fig. 24.16). The last step of the design strategy was to mask the thiol functionality as a prodrug in order to ensure long-lasting, oral activity. It turned out that modification of the terminal carboxylate to the corresponding benzyl ester was also crucial to achieve efficacy *in vivo*. The final compound, CGS 25155, showed high selectivity for NEP and significant pharmacological effect in several *in vivo* assays[52] and was therefore selected as a clinical candidate.[52]

C. Human leukocyte elastase

1. How to convert a peptide-based lead into an orally active, nonpeptidic drug

Human leukocyte elastase (HLE) is a serine proteinase involved in inflammation and tissue degradation.[94] It is believed that suitable HLE inhibitors would be useful for the treatment of a number of disease states, such as emphysema and cystic fibrosis.[106] ICI 200 880 is a mechanism-based inhibitor of HLE which forms a stable hemiketal adduct to the active site serine Ser195 (Fig. 24.17). This compound has shown encouraging effects *in vivo* in animal models following aerosol administration. Unfortunately, it is not orally active, presumably because of its peptidic nature. Recently, orally active, nonpeptidic inhibitors of HLE were designed[53] by taking advantage of the structural information provided by the X-ray analysis of porcine pancreatic elastase in a complex with Ac-Ala-Pro-Val-trifluoromethyl ketone.[107] Careful examination of this crystal structure led to the conclusion that a substituted pyridone, 3-amino-2-oxo-1,2-dihydro-1-pyridylacetic acid, would be a suitable surrogate for the Ala-Pro portion of the parent compound (Fig. 24.17). Indeed, the designed molecule retained considerable activity against HLE (K_i = 2.8 μM).[53] Incorporation of a phenyl substituent on the pyridone ring was suggested by modelling the pyridone in the active site of the enzyme. This modification, together with the replacement of the N-acetyl group by an N-CBZ group, resulted in nanomolar potency (K_i = 4 nM). However, further structure–activity studies were necessary to achieve oral activity. First, a search for heterocycles which would retain the key features of the pyridone led to the identification of the corresponding pyrimidone derivative, which showed oral activity at 20 mg kg^{-1}. Then, it was found that the introduction of a *p*-fluoro substituent on the phenyl ring increased selectivity. Finally, a number of N-substituents were tried in an attempt to further improve oral activity. This region was targeted for chemical modification on synthetic grounds but also because modelling studies had indicated the N-terminal protecting group to be rather mobile at the enzyme surface. The unprotected 3-aminopyrimidone, despite a somewhat lower potency (K_i=101nM) *in vitro*, was found to exhibit sustained oral activity (ED_{50}=7.5 mg kg^{-1}) for more than 4 hours following oral administration, with excellent bioavailability (62% in the rat, 88% in the dog) and selectivity.[53] Thus, by combining structure–based drug design and classical structure–activity studies, a novel class of orally active, nonpeptidic HLE inhibitors was discovered.

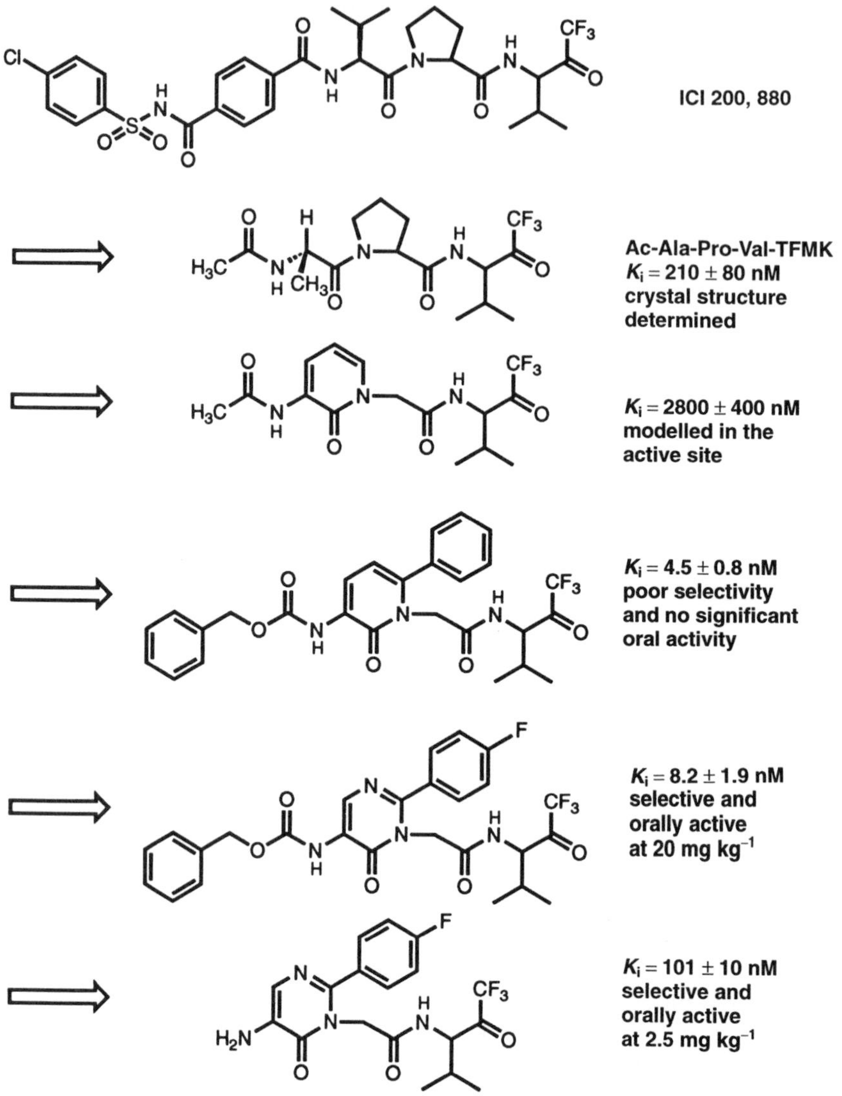

Fig. 24.17 Structure-based design of a human leukocyte elastase inhibitor. For explanation, see text.

D. Thymidylate synthase

Thymidylate synthase (TS) catalyses the methylation of deoxyuridylate to thymidylate using 5,10-methylenetetrahydrofolate (Fig. 24.18a) as a coenzyme. TS inhibitors have a potential as chemotherapeutic agents for the treatment of cancer as TS provides the sole biosynthetic source of thymidylate, a precursor in DNA biosynthesis. The design of TS inhibitors is a superb example of structure-based drug design. The reader is urged to read the original papers, which describe the work in great detail.[2,7,9,54,55]

1. When a water molecule makes the difference

Certain water molecules, especially those which interact with active site residues or participate in ligand binding, may be key players in the drug design strategy. Water-mediated hydrogen bonds and desolvation effects have a profound influence on binding, and structural mimics for active site water molecules may be included in the design of novel ligands (see the example on HIV proteinase). However, the identification of bound water molecules requires medium- to high-resolution crystallographic data (say 2.5 Å or better). The thymidylate synthase story provides a nice illustration of this point. An initial analysis at 2.8 Å resolution of TS with a bound inhibitor, the antifolate CB3717 (Fig. 24.18b), did not reveal a water molecule hydrogen-bonded to N-1 of CB3717, to the backbone carbonyl of Ala263 and the side-chain

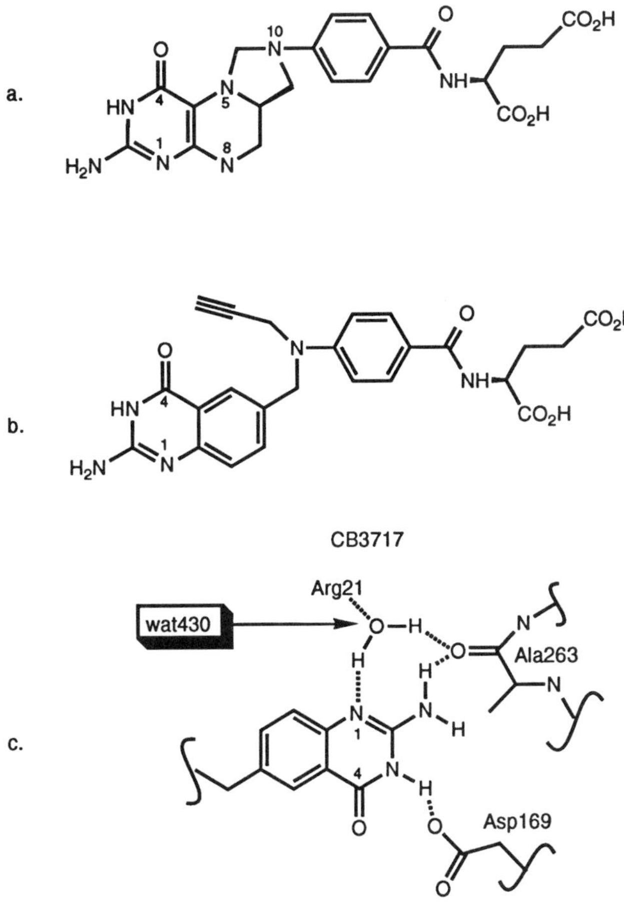

CB3717

Fig. 24.18 Structure-based design of thymidylate synthase inhibitors. (a) The coenzyme 5,10-methylenetetrahydrofolate. (b) The classical antifolate CB3717. (c) Interactions of the pteridine moiety of CB3717 with active site residues Asp169 and Ala263 and with wat430, a bound water molecule. For explanation, see text. (Adapted, with permission, from Reich, S. H. and Webber, S. E. (1993) *Perspect. Drug Dis. Des.* **1**: 371–390. Copyright © 1993, Escom Science Publishers B.V.)

guanidinium of Arg21 (Fig. 24.18c). In the meantime, analogues of CB3717 bearing a —CH in position 1 were prepared and found to be less potent than the parent compound.[7] The reason for this failure became apparent at a later stage, when 2.3 Å resolution data became available and this key water molecule (wat430) was identified.[108]

2. How to circumvent drug toxicity and mechanisms of drug resistance

The glutamate side-chain of CB3717 (Fig. 24.18b) and related compounds causes hepatic toxicity through intracellular accumulation of polyglutamylated products. In addition, glutamate-containing inhibitors require active transport to penetrate cells, which can lead to the

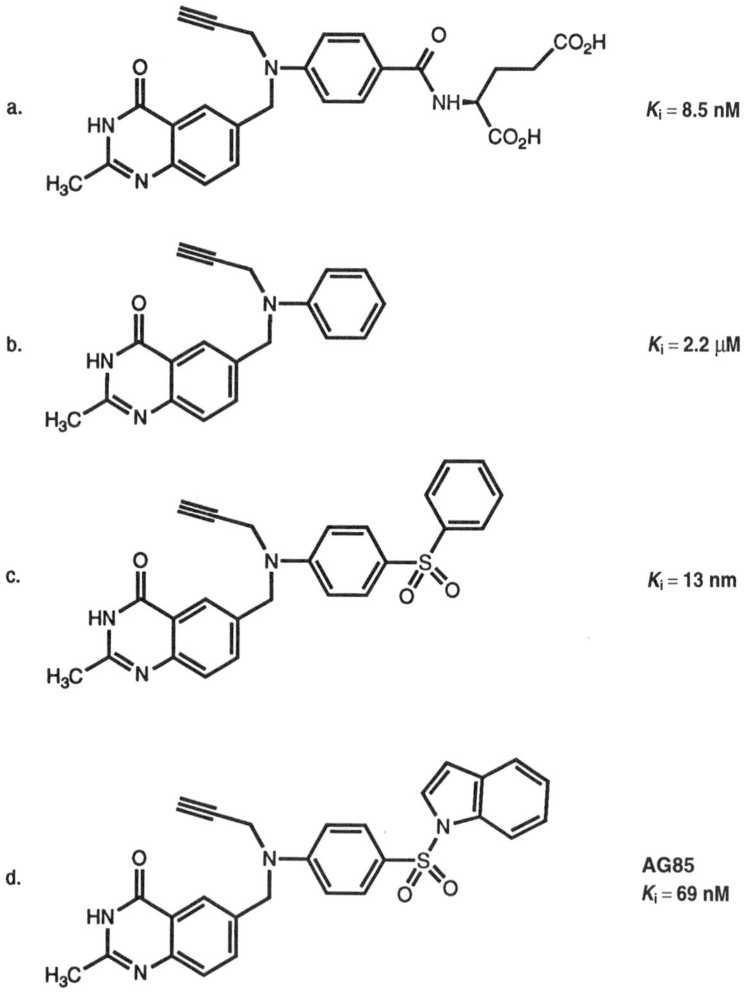

Fig. 24.19 Structure-based design of thymidylate synthase inhibitors. (a) Drug lead 2-methyl-2-desamino-N^{10}-propargyl-5,8-dideazafolic acid. (b) Derivative lacking the CO-L-glutamate moiety. (c) Designed diphenylsulfone derivative. (d) AG85, a designed N-sulfonylindole derivative selected for clinical evaluation.

development of drug resistance. Crystallographic analysis showed that the binding site of the benzoyl glutamate moiety was fairly hydrophobic and that this part of the inhibitor could be redesigned. The design was based on the 2-methyl-2-desamino derivative of CB3717, because of its greater solubility (Fig. 24.19a). This compound inhibits human TS with a K_i of 8.5 nM. Removal of the CO-L-glutamate moiety resulted in a dramatic loss of binding affinity (K_i = 2.2 μM) (Fig. 24.19b). Through iterative structure-based drug design, novel lipophilic TS inhibitors were discovered, including a series of diphenylsulfone and N-sulfonylindole derivatives[2,7] (Fig. 24.19c,d). One of the compounds designed, AG85, was selected for clinical evaluation (Fig. 24.19d).

3.   De novo *structure-based design of novel lead structures*

The discovery of structurally novel naphthostyryl-based TS inhibitors[2,9,54] represents a beautiful example of *de novo* structure-based design (Fig. 24.20). The design was based on a crystal structure of a ternary complex of TS, from which the bound inhibitor CB3717 (Fig. 24.18b) was subsequently removed for careful examination of its binding cavity. In this way, conformational changes in the binding site region triggered by substrate or cofactor binding are taken into account. In a first step, Appelt *et al.*[2] made use of the program GRID to locate, within the enzyme active site, regions interacting favourably with an aromatic CH functional probe. Naphthalene was identified as a simple chemical structure which seemed to fill the binding pocket of the pteridine moiety of CB3717. Next, hydrogen-bonding groups were added in order to retain two key interactions which had been identified in the structure with CB3717, one with wat430, a bound water molecule already mentioned above, and the other with the side-chain of Asp169 (Fig. 24.18c). A carbonyl group was therefore introduced in position 1 to accept a hydrogen bond from wat430, and an NH was placed in position 8 to donate a hydrogen bond to Asp169. This design strategy led to the naphthostyryl scaffold, a promising novel substructure[2,9,54] (Fig. 24.20). A substituent was then introduced in position 5 in order to fill up empty space in the enzyme active site. A dialkylated amine was chosen to avoid the introduction of a chiral centre and also because of ease of synthesis and further chemical modifications. Modelling of this fragment in the active site suggested the choice of a benzyl group as one of the alkyl substituents. Furthermore, it showed that position 4 of this benzene ring was suitable for the introduction of a solubilizing group. A (phenylsulfonyl)piperazine moiety was chosen because it was known from previous structure–activity studies to improve both binding and solubility.[2] The final compound was found to inhibit human TS with a K_i of 1.6 μM (Fig. 24.20). Its binding mode was analyzed by X-ray crystallography and, surprisingly, this analysis revealed that the designed hydrogen-bonded interactions were not achieved in the complex. The compound was slightly shifted with respect to its modelled position, resulting in an unfavourable interaction with the main-chain carbonyl oxygen of Ala263 and the loss of wat430. The carbonyl group of the lactam was replaced by an amino group, in an attempt to restore wat430 binding and favourable interactions with the carbonyl oxygen of Ala263, and also to strengthen the interaction with Asp169 (the amidine moiety was expected to be protonated). The resulting compound was found to inhibit human TS with a K_i of 34 nM (Fig. 24.20). This time, the X-ray analysis of the complex showed the predictions to be fully correct: wat430 had returned to its original location and the modelled hydrogen-bonding pattern was indeed observed. Replacement of the solubilizing piperazine ring by a morpholine group led to the final compound, a 2 nM inhibitor of human TS currently in clinical trials as an antitumour drug (Fig. 24.20).

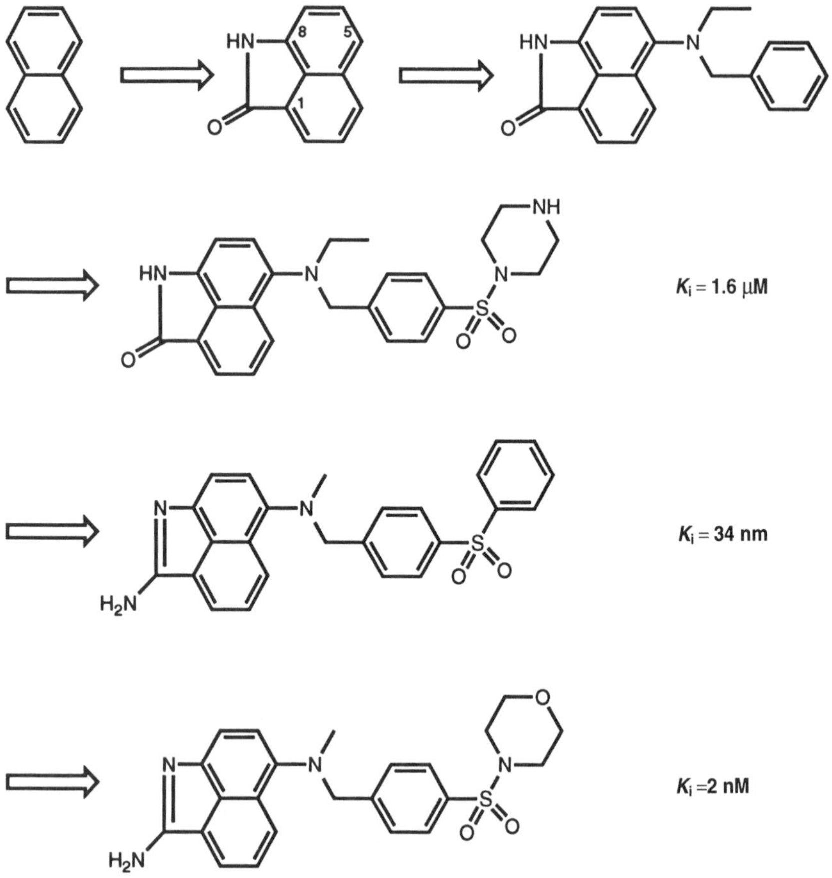

$K_i = 1.6 \ \mu M$

$K_i = 34 \ nm$

$K_i = 2 \ nM$

Fig. 24.20 Structure-based design of thymidylate synthase inhibitors: *de novo* design of a novel lead structure. See text for explanation.

E. Human immunodeficiency virus proteinase

The human immunodeficiency virus proteinase (HIV-PR) is a member of the aspartic acid proteinase family.[109] The HIV-PR is involved in the processing of the viral gag-pol polyproteins and is therefore essential for the production of new infectious HIV virions.[110] This enzyme is one of the best-characterized macromolecules from the vantage of drug design, with several hundred crystal structures determined to date.[42,95] Protein crystallography has contributed in many ways to drug discovery programmes in this field. It has revealed the three-dimensional structure of this small homodimeric enzyme (2 × 99 residues) which features a single active site with perfect 2-fold molecular symmetry.[78–80,111,112] X-ray analysis of HIV-PR–inhibitor complexes has provided the structural basis for the puzzling substrate specificity of this enzyme.[36,95,113] It has shed light on intriguing structure–activity data, notably those concerning stereochemical preferences for hydroxyethylamine-based peptidomimetics.[28,29,42,95] In several instances, protein crystallography proved useful for improving existing lead molecules.[35,36] More recently, the structural information which had accumulated over the years was used to design novel lead compounds, notably C_2-symmetric or pseudo-C_2-symmetric inhibitors[9,56,57,114] and cyclic urea derivatives.[44] Finally, HIV-PR is being used extensively as a test case to evaluate the most recent developments in the field of computational chemistry and computer-aided structure-based drug design. Interesting results have already been obtained[62,115,116] and it is likely that rational drug design in general will benefit from the massive effort put into the search for a therapeutically useful HIV-PR inhibitor.

1. Taking advantage of a strategically-located water molecule

A remarkable feature of all HIV-PR–inhibitor complexes reported so far is the presence of a tetrahedrally coordinated solvent molecule which mediates hydrogen-bonding interactions between the inhibitor and the flaps of the enzyme. This water molecule receives two hydrogen bonds from the main-chain nitrogen of Ile50 of monomer A and Ile50 of monomer B, and donates two hydrogen bonds to the P2 and P1′ carbonyl oxygens of peptidomimetics (notation of Schechter and Berger[117]). This key water molecule has no counterpart in the related mammalian aspartic proteinases. Early on, it was realized that incorporation into an inhibitor of a structural mimic for this water molecule would be entropically favourable and should also result in improved selectivity.[56,118] However, the successful design of molecules fulfilling this requirement was achieved only very recently. In a landmark structure-based drug design study by Lam and co-workers, nonpeptide cyclic ureas were discovered which combine high potency with high oral bioavailability and high selectivity.[44]

The design strategy was based on previous structure–activity studies on linear C_2-symmetric diols.[119] These inhibitors, albeit very potent, could not be developed into useful drugs owing to their poor oral bioavailability.[119] The goal of Lam *et al.* was to find novel, small-molecular-weight HIV-PR inhibitors that would not retain any peptide character.[44] They hypothesized that a conformationally restricted, cyclic structure which would incorporate a diol as the transition-state mimic as well as a mimic for the structural water could meet these requirements. The design strategy involved the following steps[44] (Fig. 24.21). (i) A model of a C_2-symmetric diol bound to the HIV-PR was built using the crystal structure of a HIV-PR complex with a hydroxyethylamine inhibitor.[118] (ii) A pharmacophore model was generated, which featured two symmetry-related hydrophobic groups and a hydrogen-bond donor/acceptor group. (iii) A 3D database search was carried out using the pharmacophore model. (iv) The hit from the 3D search suggested that a cyclohexanone ring could represent a promising new substructure. (v) Since diol-containing C_2-symmetric peptidomimetics were known to be superior inhibitors of the HIV-PR in comparison to the mono-ol derivatives,[119] the cyclohexanone was modified to a cycloheptanone to incorporate the diol functionality. (vi) The target structure was further modified to a cyclic urea, in order to strengthen the hydrogen-bonded interactions with the flaps. (vii) The optimal stereochemistry and conformation for these cyclic ureas was correctly inferred from molecular modelling analyses. This is a remarkable result, since there are four chiral centres in these molecules and also because the preferred configuration for the P1/P1′ substituents counterintuitively corresponds to the non-natural D-phenylalanine. (viii) Several substituted cyclic urea derivatives were synthesized and tested. One of them, DMP323 (Fig. 24.21), was found to combine good potency against both the HIV-PR and the HIV virus *in vitro*, with significant oral bioavailability (27% in the rat, 37% in the dog).[44] This compound has been selected for further development and has entered phase I clinical studies.[44]

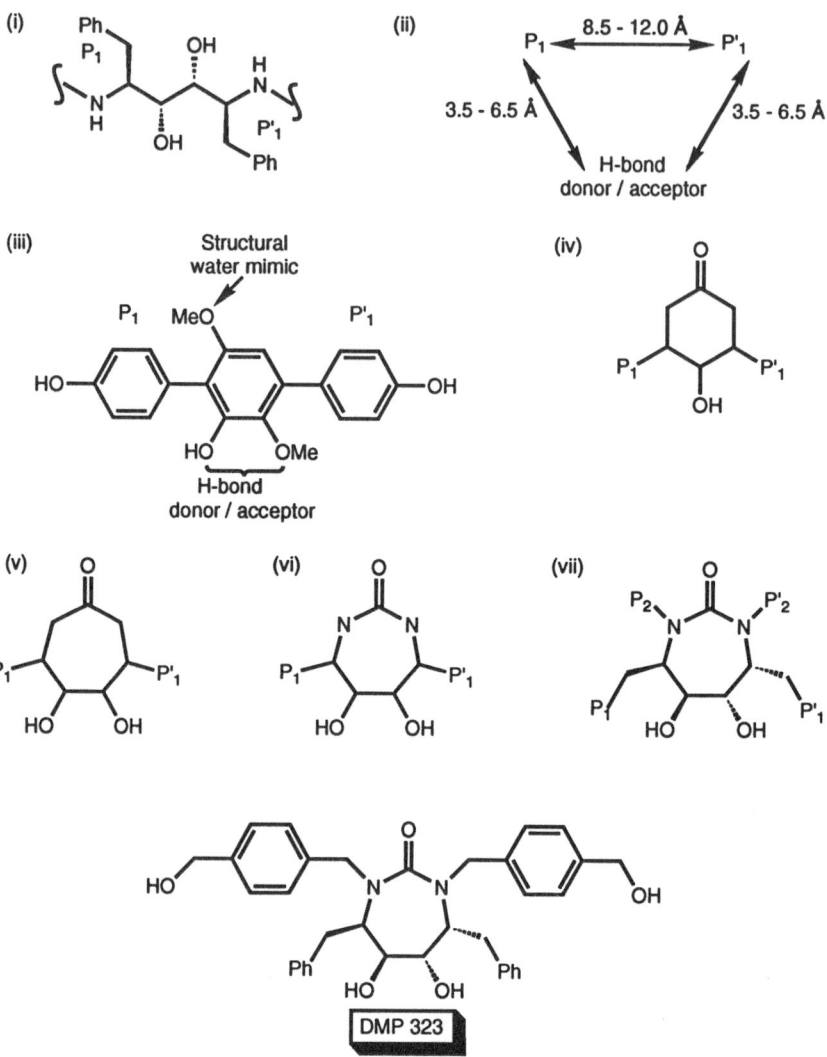

Fig. 24.21 Structure-based design of nonpeptide inhibitors of the aspartic proteinase from the human immunodeficiency virus. For explanation, see text. (Adapted, with permission, from Lam, P. Y. S. *et al.* (1994) *Science,* **263**: 380–384. Copyright © 1994 by the AAAS.)

VI.   FUTURE PROSPECTS

In view of the recent introduction of protein crystallography in the pharmaceutical industry and of the time required before a newly discovered lead is launched on the market, it is not too surprising if, among all marketed drugs today, only a handful of them benefited from structure-based drug design at the time they were discovered. Given the current blossoming of crystallographic studies in drug companies and recent success stories of structure-based drug design, there is no doubt that protein crystallography will have a major impact on drug discovery in the forthcoming years. Recent advances in technology and methodology have made X-ray structure determination routine and highly automated work, provided a good starting model is available for molecular replacement calculations. X-ray analysis of a protein of unknown fold is still time-consuming. However, the database of protein structures is expanding exponentially and we will probably have a reference fold for most protein sequences in the near future. Nevertheless, crystallization of membrane proteins remains a major hurdle, which, if not overcome, will hamper access to a whole range of important pharmaceutical targets.

The full potential of protein crystallography in drug discovery has clearly not yet been realized, mainly because of the current limitations of molecular modelling methods.[9,61] When better ways are devised to predict and evaluate more correctly ligand–protein interactions and free energies of binding,[120] structure–based drug design will certainly have an even stronger influence on future drug discovery programmes than it has today.

FURTHER READING

Green, N. M. (1994) Stereoimages. A practical approach. *Structure* 2: 85–87.
Ducruix, A. and Giege, R. (eds) (1992) *Crystallization of Nucleic Acids and Proteins: A Practical Approach.* Oxford University Press, Oxford.
McRee, D. E. (1993) *Practical Protein Crystallography.* Academic Press, San Diego.
Perutz, M. (1992) *Protein Structure. New Approaches to Disease and Therapy.* W.H. Freeman, New York.

REFERENCES

1. Shakespeare, W. (1977) *Macbeth.* Editions Aubier Montaigne, Paris.
2. Appelt, K., Bacquet, R. J., Bartlett, C. A. *et al.* (1991) Design of enzyme inhibitors using iterative protein crystallographic analysis. *J. Med. Chem.* **34**: 1925–1934.
3. Navia, M. A. and Murcko, M. A. (1992) Use of structural information in drug design. *Curr. Opin. Struct. Biol.* **2**: 202–210.
4. Kuntz, I. D. (1992) Structure-based strategies for drug design and discovery. *Science* **257**: 1078–1082.
5. Erickson, J. W. and Fesik, S. W. (1992) Macromolecular X-ray crystallography and NMR as tools for structure-based drug design. *Annu. Rep. Med. Chem.* **27**: 271–289.
6. Navia, M. A. and Peattie, D. A. (1993) Structure-based drug design: applications in immunopharmacology and immunosuppression. *Trends Pharmacol. Sci.* **14**: 189–195.
7. Reich, S. H. and Webber, S. E. (1993) Structure-based drug design (SBDD): every structure tells a story. *Perspect. Drug Dis. Des.* **1**: 371–390.
8. Bugg, C. E., Carson, W. M. and Montgomery, J. A. (1993) Drugs by design. *Sci. Am.* **269**: 60–66.
9. Greer, J., Erickson, J. W., Baldwin, J. J. and Varney, M. D. (1994) Application of the three-dimensional structures of protein target molecules in structure-based drug design. *J. Med. Chem.* **37**: 1035–1054.
10. Walkinshaw, M. D. (1992) Protein targets for structure-based drug design. *Med. Res. Rev.* **12**: 317–372.
11. Lolis, E. and Petsko, G. A. (1990) Transition-state analogues in protein crystallography: probes of the structural source of enzyme catalysis. *Annu. Rev. Biochem.* **59**: 597–630.
12. Verschueren, K. H. G., Seljée, F., Rozeboom, H. J., Kalk, K. H. and Dijkstra, B. W. (1993) Crystallographic analysis of the catalytic mechanism of haloalkane dehalogenase. *Nature* **363**: 693–698.

13. Strynadka, N. C. J., Adachi, H., Jensen, S. E., Johns, K., Sielecki, A., Betzel, C., Sutoh, K. and James, M. N. G. (1992) Molecular structure of the acyl-enzyme intermediate in β-lactam hydrolysis at 1.7 Å resolution. *Nature* **359**: 700–705.

14. Walsh, C. T. (1984) Suicide substrates, mechanism-based enzyme inactivators: recent developments. *Annu. Rev. Biochem.* **53**: 493–535.

15. Broom, A. D. (1989) Rational design of enzyme inhibitors: multisubstrate analogue inhibitors. *J. Med. Chem.* **32**: 2–7.

16. Wolfenden, R. and Radzicka, A. (1991) Transition-state analogues. *Curr. Opin. Struct. Biol.* **1**, 780–787.

17. Cohen, N. C., Blaney, J. M., Humblet, C., Gund, P. and Barry, D. C. (1990). Molecular modelling software and methods for medicinal chemistry. *J. Med. Chem.* **33**: 883–894.

18. Smith, T. J., Kremer, M. J., Luo, M., Vriend, G., Arnold, E., Kamer, G., Rossman, M. G., McKinlay, M. A., Diana, G. D. and Otto, M. J. (1986) The site of attachment in human rhinovirus 14 for antiviral agents that inhibit uncoating. *Science* **233**: 1286–1293.

19. Weber, C., Wider, G., von Freyberg, B., Traber, R., Braun, W., Widmer, H. and Wüthrich, K. (1991) The NMR structure of cyclosporin A bound to cyclophilin in aqueous solution. *Biochemistry* **30**: 6563–6574.

20. Fesik, S. W., Gampe, R. T., Jr., Eaton, H. L. *et al.* (1991) NMR studies of [U-13C]cyclosporin A bound to cyclophilin: bound conformation and portions of cyclosporin involved in binding. *Biochemistry* **30**: 6574–6583.

21. Altschuh, D., Vix, O., Rees, B. and Thierry, J.-C. (1992) A conformation of cyclosporin A in aqueous environment revealed by the X-ray structure of a cyclosporin–Fab complex. *Science* **256**: 92–94.

22. Thériault, Y., Logan, T. M., Meadows, R., Yu, L., Olejniczak, E. T., Holzman, T. F., Simmer, R. L. and Fesik, S. W. (1993) Solution structure of the cyclosporin A/cyclophilin complex by NMR. *Nature* **361**: 88–91.

23. Pflügl, G., Kallen, J., Schirmer, T., Jansonius, J.N., Zurini, M. G. M. and Walkinshaw, M. D. (1993) X-ray structure of a decameric cyclophilin–cyclosporin crystal complex. *Nature* **361**: 91–94.

24. Ke, H., Zhao, Y., Luo, F., Weissman, I. and Friedman, J. (1993) Crystal structure of murine cyclophilin C complexed with immunosuppressive drug cyclosporin A. *Proc. Natl. Acad. Sci. USA* **90**: 11850–11854.

25. Ke, H., Mayrose, D., Belshaw, P. J. Alberg, D. G., Schreiber, S. L., Chang, Z. Y., Etzkorn, F. A., Ho, S. and Walsh, C. T. (1994) Crystal structures of cyclophilin A complexed with cyclosporin A and N-methyl-4-[(E)-2-butenyl]-4,4-dimethylthreonine cyclosporin A. *Structure* **2**: 33–44.

26. Van Duyne, G. D., Standaert, R. F., Karplus, P. A., Schreiber, S. L. and Clardy, J. (1991) Atomic structure of FKBP-FK506, an immunophilin–immunosuppressant complex. *Science* **252**: 839–842.

27. Badger, J., Minor, I., Kremer, M. J. *et al.* (1988) Structural analysis of a series of antiviral agents complexed with human rhinovirus 14. *Proc. Natl. Acad. Sci. USA* **85**: 3304–3308.

28. Rich, D. H., Sun, C.-Q., Vara Prasad, J. V. N., Pathiasseril, A., Toth, M. V., Marshall, G. R., Clare, M., Mueller, R. A. and Houseman, K. (1991) Effect of hydroxyl group configuration in hydroxyethylamine dipeptide isosteres on HIV protease inhibition. Evidence for multiple binding modes. *J. Med. Chem.* **34**: 1222–1225.

29. Krohn, A., Redshaw, S., Ritchie, J. C., Graves, B. J. and Hatada, M. H. (1991) Novel binding mode of highly potent HIV-proteinase inhibitors incorporating the (R)-hydroxyethylamine isostere. *J. Med. Chem.* **34**: 3340–3342.

30. Lalezari, I., Lalezari, P., Poyart, C., Marden, M., Kister, J., Bohn, B., Fermi, G. and Perutz, M. F. (1990) New effectors of human hemoglobin: structure and function. *Biochemistry* **29**: 1515–1523.

31. Banner, D. W. and Hadváry, P. (1991) Crystallographic analysis at 3.0 Å resolution of the binding to human thrombin of four active site-directed inhibitors. *J. Biol. Chem.* **266**: 20085–20093.

32. Stubbs, M. T. and Bode, W. (1993) Crystal structures of thrombin and thrombin complexes as a framework for antithrombotic drug design. *Perspect. Drug Dis. Des.* **1**: 431–452.

33. Powers, J. C., Oleksyszyn, J., Narasimhan, S. L., Kam, C.-M, Radhakrishnan, R. and Meyer, E. F. Jr. (1990) Reaction of porcine pancreatic elastase with 7-substituted 3-alkoxy-4-chloroisocoumarins: design of potent inhibitors using the crystal structure of the complex formed with 4-chloro-3-ethoxy-7-guanidinoisocoumarin. *Biochemistry* **29**: 3108–3118.

34. Ealick, S. E., Babu, Y. S., Bugg, C. E., Erion, M. D, Guida, W. C., Montgomery, J. A. and Secrist,

J. A. III (1991) Application of crystallographic and modelling methods in the design of purine nucleoside phosphorylase inhibitors. *Proc. Natl. Acad. Sci. USA* **88**: 11540–11544.

35. Thompson, W. J., Fitzgerald, P. M. D., Holloway, M. K. *et al.* (1992) Synthesis and antiviral activity of a series of HIV-1 protease inhibitors with functionality tethered to the P_1 or P_1' phenyl substituents: X-ray crystal structure assisted design. *J. Med. Chem.* **35**: 1685–1701.

36. Clare, M. (1993) HIV protease: structure-based design. *Perspect. Drug Dis. Des.* **1**: 49–68.

37. Montgomery, J. A., Niwas, S., Rose, J. D., Secrist, J. A., III, Babu, Y. S., Bugg, C. E., Erion, M. D., Guida, W. C. and Ealick, S. E. (1993) Structure-based design of inhibitors of purine nucleoside phosphorylase. 1. 9-(Arylmethyl) derivatives of 9-deazaguanine. *J. Med. Chem.* **36**: 55–69.

38. Secrist, J. A., III, Niwas, S., Rose, J. D., Babu, Y. S., Bugg, C. E., Erion, M. D., Guida, W. C., Ealick, S. E. and Montgomery, J. A. (1993) Structure-based design of inhibitors of purine nucleoside phosphorylase. 2. 9-Alicyclic and 9-heteroalicyclic derivatives of 9-deazaguanine. *J. Med. Chem.* **36**: 1847–1854.

39. Erion, M. D., Niwas, S., Rose, J. D. *et al.* (1993) Structure-based design of inhibitors of purine nucleoside phosphorylase. 3. 9-Arylmethyl derivatives of 9-deazaguanine substituted on the methylene group. *J. Med. Chem.* **36**: 3771–3783.

40. Guida, W. C., Elliott, R. D., Thomas, H. J., Secrist, J. A., III, Babu, Y. S., Bugg, C. E., Erion, M. D., Ealick, S. E. and Montgomery, J. A. (1994) Structure-based design of inhibitors of purine nucleoside phosphorylase. 4. A study of phosphate mimics. *J. Med. Chem.* **37**: 1109–1114.

41. Baldwin, J. J., Ponticello, G. S., Anderson, P. S. *et al.* Thienothiopyran-2-sulfonamides: novel topically active carbonic anhydrase inhibitors for the treatment of glaucoma. *J. Med. Chem.* **32**: 2510–2513.

42. Appelt, K. (1993) Crystal structures of HIV-1 protease–inhibitor complexes. *Perspect. Drug Dis. Des.* **1**: 23–48.

43. Vacca, J. P., Fitzgerald, P. M. D., Holloway, M. K., Hungate, R. W., Starbuck, K. E., Chen, L. J., Darke, P. L., Anderson, P. S. and Huff, J. R. (1994) Conformationally constrained HIV-1 protease inhibitors. *Bioorg. Med. Chem. Lett.* **4**: 499–504.

44. Lam, P. Y. S., Jadhav, P. K., Eyermann, C. J. *et al.* (1994) Rational design of potent, bioavailable, nonpeptide cyclic ureas as HIV protease inhibitors. *Science* **263**: 380–384.

45. Morgan, B. P., Holland, D. R. Matthews, B. W. and Bartlett, P. A. (1994) Structure-based design of an inhibitor of the zinc peptidase thermolysin. *J. Am. Chem. Soc.* **116**: 3251–3260.

46. Thaisrivongs, S., Blinn, J. R., Pals, D. T. and Turner, S. R. (1991) Conformationally constrained renin inhibitory peptides: cyclic (3-1)-1-(carboxymethyl)-L-prolyl-L-phenylalanyl-L-histidinamide as a conformational restriction at the P_2–P_4 tripeptide portion of the angiotensinogen template. *J. Med. Chem.* **34**: 1276–1282.

47. Weber, A. E., Halgren, T. A., Doyle, J. J., Lynch, R. J., Siegl, P. K. S., Parsons, W. H., Greenlee, W. J. and Patchett, A. A. (1991) Design and synthesis of P2-P1'-linked macrocyclic human renin inhibitors. *J. Med. Chem.* **34**: 2692–2701.

48. Alberg, D. G. and Schreiber, S. L. (1993) Structure-based design of a cyclophilin–calcineurin bridging ligand. *Science* **262**: 248–250.

49. Selassie, C. D., Fang, Z.-X., Li, R.-L., Hansch, C., Debnath, G., Klein, T. E., Langridge, R. and Kaufman, B. T. (1989) On the structure selectivity problem in drug design. A comparative study of benzylpyrimidine inhibition of vertebrate and bacterial dihydrofolate reductase via molecular graphics and quantitative structure–activity relationships. *J. Med. Chem.* **32**: 1895–1905.

50. Roth, B. (1986) Design of dihydrofolate reductase inhibitors from X-ray crystal structures. *Fed. Proc. Fed. Am. Soc. Exp. Biol.* **45**: 2765–2772.

51. Dhanaraj, V., Dealwis, C. G., Frazao, C. *et al.* (1992) X-ray analyses of peptide–inhibitor complexes define the structural basis of specificity for human and mouse renins. *Nature* **357**: 466–471.

52. MacPherson, L. J., Bayburt, E. K., Capparelli, M. P., Bohacek, R. S., Clarke, F. H., Ghai, R. D., Sakane, Y., Berry, C. J., Peppard, J. V. and Trapani, A. J. (1993) Design and synthesis of an orally active macrocyclic neutral endopeptidase 24.11 inhibitor. *J. Med. Chem.* **36**: 3821–3828.

53. Brown, F. J., Andisik, D. W., Bernstein, P. R. *et al.* (1994) Design of orally active, non-peptidic inhibitors of human leukocyte elastase. *J. Med. Chem.* **37**: 1259–1261.

54. Varney, M. D., Marzoni, G. P., Palmer, C. L. *et al.* (1992) Crystal-structure-based design and synthesis of benz[cd]indole-containing inhibitors of thymidylate synthase. *J. Med. Chem.* **35**: 663–676.

55. Reich, S. H., Fuhry, M. A. M., Nguyen, D. *et al.* (1992) Design and synthesis of novel 6,7-imidazotetrahydroquinoline inhibitors of thymidylate synthase using iterative protein crystal structure analysis. *J. Med. Chem.* **35**: 847–858.

56. Erickson, J., Neidhart, D. J., VanDrie, J. *et al.* (1990) Design, activity, and 2.8 Å crystal structure of a C_2 symmetric inhibitor complexed to HIV-1 protease. *Science* **249**: 527–533.

57. Erickson, J. W. (1993) Design and structure of symmetry-based inhibitors of HIV-1 protease. *Perspect. Drug Dis. Des.* **1**: 109–128.

58. Hosur, M. V., Bhat, T. N., Kempf, D. J., Baldwin, E. T., Liu, B., Gulnik, S., Wideburg, N. E., Norbeck, D. W., Appelt, K. and Erickson, J. W. (1994) Influence of stereochemistry on activity and binding modes for C_2 symmetry-based diol inhibitors of HIV-1 protease. *J. Am. Chem. Soc.* **116**: 847–855.

59. Kuntz, I. D., Meng, E. C. and Shoichet, B. K. (1994) Structure-based molecular design. *Acc. Chem. Res.* **27**: 117–123.

60. Martin, Y. C. (1992) Database searching in drug design. *J. Med. Chem.* **35**: 2145–2154.

61. Blaney, J. M. and Dixon, J. S. (1993) A good ligand is hard to find: automated docking methods. *Perspect. Drug Dis. Des.* **1**: 301–319.

62. Desjarlais, R. L., Seibel, G. L., Kuntz, I. D., Furth, P. S., Alvarez, J. C., Ortiz de Montellano, P. R., DeCamp, D. L., Babe, L. M. and Craik, C. S. (1990) Structure-based design of nonpeptide inhibitors specific for the human immunodeficiency virus 1 protease. *Proc. Natl. Acad. Sci. USA* **87**: 6644–6648.

63. Bures, M. G., Hutchins, C. W., Maus, M., Kohlbrenner, W., Kadam, S. and Erickson, J. W. (1990) *Tetrahedron Comp. Methodol.* **3**: 673–680.

64. Shoichet, B. K., Stroud, R. M., Santi, D. V., Kuntz, I. D and Perry, K. M. (1993) Structure-based discovery of inhibitors of thymidylate synthase. *Science* **259**: 1445–1450.

65. Ring, C. S., Sun, E., McKerrow, J. H., Lee, G. K., Rosenthal, P. J., Kuntz, I. D. and Cohen, F. E. (1993) Structure-based inhibitor design by using protein models for the development of antiparasitic agents. *Proc. Natl. Acad. Sci. USA* **90**: 3583–3587.

66. McPherson, A., Jr. (1982) *Preparation and Analysis of Protein Crystals.* Wiley, New York.

67. Ducruix, A. and Giege, R. (eds) (1992) *Crystallization of Nucleic Acids and Proteins: A Practical Approach.* Oxford University Press, Oxford.

68. Blundell, T. L. and Johnson, L. N. (1976) *Protein Crystallography.* Academic Press, San Diego.

69. Wyckoff, H. (ed.) (1985) *Diffraction Methods for Biological Macromolecules. Methods in Enzymology,* vols. 114 and 115. Academic Press, San Diego.

70. McRee, D. E. (1993) *Practical Protein Crystallography.* Academic Press, San Diego.

71. Drenth, J. (1994) *Principles of Protein X-ray Crystallography.* Springer-Verlag, New York.

72. Viterbo, D. (1992) Solution and refinement of crystal structures. In Giacovazzo, C. (ed.) *Fundamentals of Crystallography,* pp. 319–401. Oxford University Press, Oxford.

73. Bernstein, F. C., Koetzle, T. F., Williams, G. J., Meyer, E. J., Brice, M. D., Rodgers, J. R., Kennard, O., Shimanouchi, T. and Tasumi, M. (1978) The protein data bank: a computer-based archival file for macromolecular structures. *Arch. Biochem. Biophys.* **185**: 584–591.

74. Bränden, C. -I. and Jones, T. A. (1990) Between objectivity and subjectivity. *Nature* **343**: 687–689.

75. Janin, J. (1990) Errors in three dimensions. *Biochimie* **72**: 705–709.

76. DeVos, A. M., Tong, L., Milburn, M. V., Matias, P. M., Jankarik, J., Noguchi, S., Nishimura, S., Miura, K. and Kim, S.-H. (1988) Three-dimensional structure of an oncogene protein: catalytic domain of human c-H-ras p21. *Science* **239**: 888–893.

77. Pai, E. F., Kabsch, W., Krengel, U., Holmes, K. C., John, J. and Wittinghofer, A. (1989) Structure of the guanine-nucleotide-binding domain of the Ha-ras oncogene product p21 in the triphosphate conformation. *Nature* **341**: 209–214.

78. Navia, M. A., Fitzgerald, P. M. D., McKeever, B. M., Leu, C.-T., Heimbach, J. C., Herber, W. K., Sigal, I. S., Drake, P. L. and Springer, J. P. (1989) Three-dimensional structure of aspartyl protease from human immunodeficiency virus HIV-1. *Nature* **337**: 615–620.

79. Wlodawer, A., Miller, M., Jaskolski, M., Sathyanarayana, B. K., Baldwin, E., Weber, I. T., Selk, L. M., Clawson, L., Schneider, J. and Kent, S. B. H. (1989) Conserved folding in retroviral proteases: crystal structure of a synthetic HIV-1 protease. *Science* **245**: 616–621.

80. Lapatto, R., Blundell, T., Hemmings, A. *et al.* (1989) X-ray analysis of HIV-1 proteinase at 2.7 Å resolution confirms structural homology among retroviral enzymes. *Nature* **342**: 299–302.

81. Howard, J. B. and Rees D. C. (1991) Perspectives on non-heme iron protein chemistry. *Adv. Protein Chem.* **42**: 199–280.
82. Brünger, A. T. (1992) Free R value: a novel statistical quantity for assessing the accuracy of crystal structures. *Nature* **355**: 472–475.
83. Jia, Z., Vandonselaar, M., Quail, J. W. and Delbaere L. T. J. (1993) Active-centre torsion-angle strain revealed in 1.6 Å-resolution structure of histidine-containing phosphocarrier protein. *Nature* **361**: 94–97.
84. Chevrier, B., Schalk, C., D'Orchymont, H., Rondeau, J.-M., Moras, D. and Tarnus, C. (1994) Crystal structure of *Aeromonas proteolytica* aminopeptidase: a prototypical member of the co-catalytic zinc enzyme family. *Structure* **2**: 283–291.
85. Perutz, M. (1992) *Protein Structure. New Approaches to Disease and Therapy.* W. H. Freeman, New York.
86. Brange, J., Ribel, U., Hansen, J. F. *et al.* (1988) Monomeric insulins obtained by protein engineering and their medical implications. *Nature* **333**: 679–682.
87. Cushman, D. W., Cheung, H. S., Sabo, E. F. and Ondetti, M. A. (1977) Design of potent competitive inhibitors of angiotensin-converting enzyme. Carboxyalkanoyl and mercaptalkanoyl amino acids. *Biochemistry* **16**: 5484–5491.
88. Hassall, C. H., Kröhn, A., Moody, C. H. and Thomas, W. A. (1982) The design of a new group of angiotensin-converting enzyme inhibitors. *FEBS Lett.* **147**: 175–179.
89. Attwood, M. R., Hassall, C. H., Kröhn, A., Lawton, G. and Redshaw, S. (1986) The design and synthesis of the angiotensin-converting enzyme inhibitor cilazapril and related bicyclic compounds. *J. Chem. Soc., Perkins Trans. 1* 1011–1019.
90. Blundell, T. L., Cooper, J., Foundling, S. I., Jones, D. M., Atrash, B. and Szelke, M. (1987) On the rational design of renin inhibitors: X-ray studies of aspartic proteinases complexed with transition-state analogues. *Biochemistry* **26**: 5585–5590.
91. Greenlee, W. J. (1990) Renin inhibitors. *Med. Res. Rev.* **10**: 173–236.
92. Lunney, E. A., Hamilton, H. W., Hodges, J. C. *et al.* (1993) Analyses of ligand binding in five endothiapepsin crystal complexes and their use in the design and evaluation of novel renin inhibitors. *J. Med. Chem.* **36**: 3809–3820.
93. Iizuka, K., Kamijo, T., Harada, H., Akahane, K., Kubota, T., Umeyama, H., Ishida, T. and Kiso, Y. (1990) Orally potent human renin inhibitors derived from angiotensinogen transition state: design, synthesis, and mode of interaction. *J. Med. Chem.* **33**: 2707–2714.
94. Bode, W., Meyer, E., Jr. and Powers, J. C. (1989) Human leukocyte and porcine pancreatic elastase: X-ray crystal structures, mechanism, substrate specificity, and mechanism-based inhibitors. *Biochemistry* **28**: 1951–1963.
95. Wlodawer, A. and Erickson, J. W. Structure-based inhibitors of HIV-1 protease. *Annu. Rev. Biochem.* **62**: 543–585.
96. von Itzstein, M., Wu, W.-Y., Kok, G. B. *et al.* (1993) Rational design of potent sialidase-based inhibitors of influenza virus replication. *Nature* **363**: 418–423.
97. Andrus, M. B. and Schreiber, S. L. (1993) Structure-based design of an acyclic ligand that bridges FKBP12 and calcineurin. *J. Am. Chem. Soc.* **115**: 10420–10421.
98. Holt, D. A., Luengo, J. I., Yamashita, D. S. *et al.* (1993) Design, synthesis, and kinetic evaluation of high-affinity FKBP ligands and the X-ray crystal structures of their complexes with FKBP12. *J. Am. Chem. Soc.* **115**: 9925–9938.
99. Fuh, G., Cunningham, B. C., Fukunaga, R., Nagata, S., Goeddel, D. B. and Wells, J. A. (1992) Rational design of potent antagonists to the human growth hormone receptor. *Science* **256**: 1677–1680.
100. Smythe, M. L. and von Itzstein, M. (1994) Design and synthesis of a biologically active antibody mimic based on an antibody–antigen crystal structure. *J. Am. Chem. Soc.* **116**: 2725–2733.
101. Ealick, S. E., Rule, S. A., Carter, D. C. *et al.* (1990) Three-dimensional structure of human erythrocyte purine nucleoside phosphorylase at 3.2 Å resolution. *J. Biol. Chem.* **265**: 1812–1820.
102. Burley, S. K. and Petsko, G. A. (1985) Aromatic–aromatic interaction: a mechanism of protein structure stabilization. *Science* **229**: 23–28.
103. Roques, B. P. and Beaumont, A. (1990) Neutral endopeptidase-24.11 inhibitors: from analgesics to antihypertensives? *TIPS* **11**: 245–249.

104. Brenner, B.M., Ballerman, B. J., Gunning, M. E. and Zeidel, M. L. (1990) Diverse biological actions of atrial natriuretic peptide. *Physiol. Rev.* **70**: 665–700.

105. Holden, H. M., Tronrud, D. E., Monzingo, A. F., Weaver, L. H. and Matthews, B. W. (1987) Slow- and fast-binding inhibitors of thermolysin display different modes of binding: crystallographic analysis of extended phosphonamidate transition-state analogues. *Biochemistry* **26**: 8542–8553.

106. Stein, R. L., Trainor, D. A. and Wildorger, R. A. (1985) Neutrophil elastase. *Annu. Rep. Med. Chem.* **20**: 237–246.

107. Takahashi, L. H., Radhakrishnan, R., Rosenfield, R. E., Jr., Meyer, E. F., Jr., Trainor, D. A. and Stein, M. (1988) X-ray diffraction analysis of the inhibition of porcine pancreatic elastase by a peptidyl trifluoromethylketone. *J. Mol. Biol.* **201**: 423–428.

108. Matthews, D. A., Appelt, K., Oatley, S. J. and Xuong, Ng. H. (1990) Crystal structure of *Escherichia coli* thymidylate synthase containing bound 5-fluoro-2′-deoxyuridylate and 10-propargyl-5,8-dideazafolate. *J. Mol. Biol.* **214**: 923–936.

109. Mohana Rao, J. K., Erickson, J. W. and Wlodawer, A. (1991) Structural and evolutionary relationships between retroviral and eucaryotic aspartic proteinases. *Biochemistry* **30**: 4663–4671.

110. Kohl, N. E., Emini, E. A., Schleif, W. A., Davis, L. J., Heimbach, J. C., Dixon, R. A. F., Scolnick, E. M. and Sigal, I. S. (1988) Active human immunodeficiency virus protease is required for viral infectivity. *Proc. Natl. Acad. Sci. USA* **85**: 4686–4690.

111. Spinelli, S., Liu, Q. Z., Alzari, P. M., Hirel, P. H. and Poljak, R. J. (1991) The three-dimensional structure of the aspartyl protease from the HIV-1 isolate BRU. *Biochimie* **73**: 1391–1396.

112. Mulichak, A. M., Hui, J. O., Tomasselli, A. G., Heinrikson, R. L., Curry, K. A., Tomich, C. -S., Thaisrivongs, S., Sawyer, T. K. and Watenpaugh, K. D. (1993) The crystallographic structure of the protease from human immunodeficiency virus type 2 with two synthetic peptidic transition state analog inhibitors. *J. Biol. Chem.* **268**: 13103–13109.

113. Poorman, R. A., Tomasselli, A. G., Heinrikson, R. L. and Kezdy, F. J. (1991) A cumulative specificity model for proteases from human immunodeficiency virus types 1 and 2, inferred from statistical analysis of an extended substrate data base. *J. Biol. Chem.* **266**: 14554–14561.

114. Babine, R. E., Zhang, N., Jurgens, A. R., Schow, S. R., Desai, P. R., James, J. C. and Semmelhack, M. F. (1992) The use of HIV-1 protease structure in inhibitor design. *Bioorg. Med. Chem. Lett.* **2**: 541–546.

115. Caflisch, A., Miranker, A. and Karplus, M. (1993) Multiple copy simultaneous search and construction of ligands in binding sites: application to inhibitors of HIV-1 aspartic proteinase. *J. Med. Chem.* **36**: 2142–2167.

116. Waller, C. L., Oprea, T. I., Giolitti, A. and Marshall, G. R. (1993) Three-dimensional QSAR of human immunodeficiency virus (I) protease inhibitors. 1. A CoMFA study employing experimentally-determined alignment rules. *J. Med. Chem.* **36**: 4152–4160.

117. Schechter, I. and Berger, A. (1967) On the size of the active site in proteases. 1. Papain. *Biochem. Biophys. Res. Commun.* **27**: 157–162.

118. Swain, A. L., Miller, M. M., Green, J., Rich, D. H., Schneider, J., Kent, S. B. H. and Wlodawer, A. (1990) X-ray crystallographic structure of a complex between a synthetic protease of human immunodeficiency virus 1 and a substrate-based hydroxyethylamine inhibitor. *Proc. Natl. Acad. Sci. USA* **87**: 8805–8809.

119. Kempf, D. J., Codacovi, L., Wang, X. C. *et al.* (1993) Symmetry-based inhibitors of HIV protease. Structure–activity studies of acylated 2,4-diamino-1,5-diphenyl-3-hydroxypentane and 2,5-diamino-1,6-diphenylhexane-3,4-diol. *J. Med. Chem.* **36**: 320–330.

120. Kollman, P. A. (1994) Theory of macromolecule–ligand interactions. *Curr. Opin. Struct. Biol.* **4**: 240–245.

121. Green, N. M. (1994) Stereoimages. A practical approach. *Structure* **2**: 85–87.

122. Knight, S., Andersson, I. and Brändén, C. -I. (1989) Reexamination of the three-dimensional structure of the small subunit of RuBisCO from higher plants. *Science* **244**: 702–705.

123. Curmi, P. M. G., Cascio, D., Sweet, R. M., Eisenberg, D. and Schreuder, H. (1992) Crystal structure of the unactivated form of ribulose-1,5-bisphosphate carboxylase/oxygenase from tobacco refined at 2.0 Å resolution. *J. Biol. Chem.* **267**: 16980–16989.

124. Stuart, D. I. and Phillips, D. C. (1985) On the deviation of dynamic information from diffraction data. *Methods Enzymol.* **115**: 117–142.

25

Protein Homology Modelling and Drug Discovery

MARCEL F. HIBERT

On croit savoir parce qu'on a vu, mais on ne verrait rien si on ne croyait pas.
Régis Debray, *L'Oeil Naïf* (1994)

THE PRACTICE OF MEDICINAL CHEMISTRY
ISBN 0-12-744640-0

I.   INTRODUCTION

One of the key steps in designing and optimizing products of therapeutic interest consists in trying to understand the molecular recognition process between ligands and a target host molecule. In most cases, the chemical structure of the ligands is available. In contrast, until very recently, very little was known about the structure of the target macromolecule (protein, glycoprotein, nucleic acid). In practice, the medicinal chemist has to face three possible situations to which correspond three different strategies (Fig. 25.1).

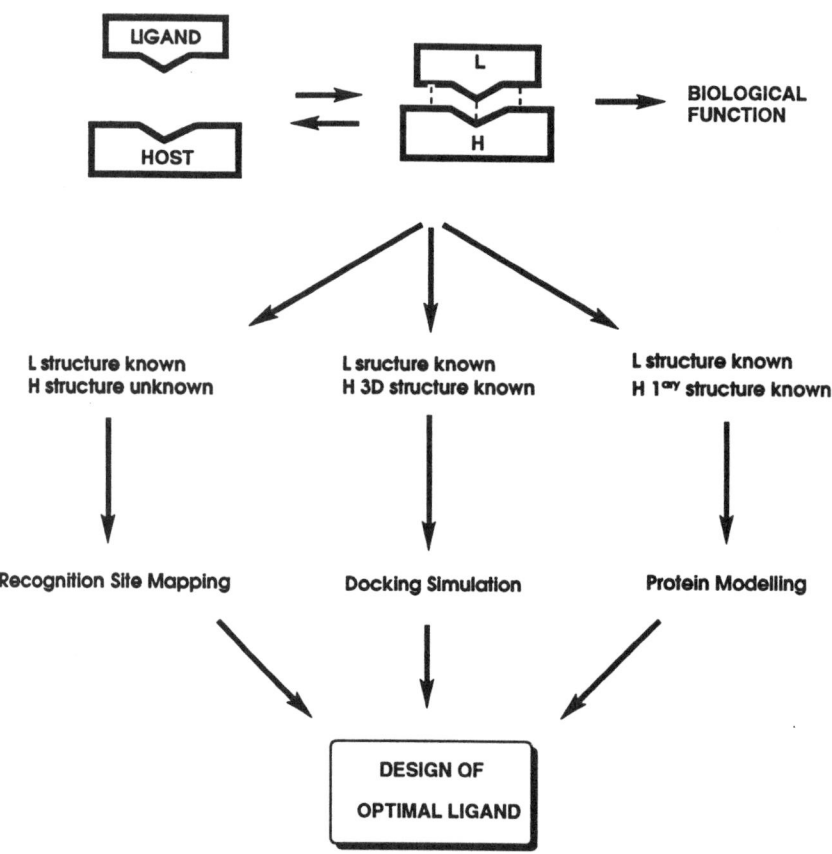

Fig. 25.1   Drug design strategies.

(1)   *The structure of the host molecule is unknown.* It has perhaps been characterized biochemically, pharmacologically and has been given a name; however, nothing is known about its chemical structure. In this case, the strategy that has been developed to study the ligand–host molecular recognition is called 'recognition site mapping' (or 'receptor mapping')[1] and is described in Chapter 22.

(2)   *The three-dimensional structure of the host molecules is known.* Using different techniques such as crystallography, electron microscopy, NMR, etc., the relative atomic coordinates of the host molecule have been characterized. In most cases, the structures of a number

of ligand–host complexes have also been resolved. Simple to sophisticated molecular modelling techniques can then be used to simulate ligand docking and receptor function, and ultimately to design the optimal ligand. This case is discussed in detail in Chapter 24 (see also Kollman[2]).

(3) *The primary structure of the host molecule is known.* The amino acid sequence (proteins) or the nucleotide sequence (nucleic acids) has been identified. Taking into account experimental data, molecular modelling strategies have been developed to generate a theoretical three-dimensional structure of the target, host, molecule. In this chapter, we will restrict ourselves to *protein modelling.* Nucleic acid modelling examples can be found elsewhere.[3,4]

II. PROTEIN STRUCTURE

The knowledge of a protein's 3D structure is a prerequisite for the proper understanding of its function, which is usually controlled by residues that are not sequential and whose role can be identified only from 3D structure analysis. Medicinal chemists are encouraged to refer to books fully dedicated to protein 3D structure description.[5] We give here some definitions and a brief outline of the main protein structural features (Fig. 25.2).

A. The primary structure

The identification of the sequence of amino acids along the protein polypeptide chain is the first important step towards the full structural characterization of a protein. This identification used to be achieved by protein purification, degradation and sequencing. Nowadays, molecular biology techniques represent a new and abundant source of protein primary sequences (see Chapter 10). These sequences are readily available from data banks.[6]

B. The secondary structure

The amino-acid sequence and the environment determine the formation of local structural features, the most important of which are α-helices and β-sheets (Fig. 25.3).

α-Helical secondary structure is found in proteins when a stretch of consecutive residues have their φ, ψ angle pair around −60° and −50°, respectively. Hydrogen bonds are formed between the carbonyl of the peptide bond of residue *n* and the N—H of the peptide bond of residue *n* + 4 (Fig. 25.3). This leads to a right-handed α-helical backbone having 3.6 residues per turn. Length varies from 4 to over 40 residues. Some amino acids are found preferably in α-helices (Ala, Leu, Met, Glu), while other are rarely found (Pro, Gly). The α-helix displays a strong dipole moment along its axis arising from the alignment in the same direction of peptide bonds.

A β-sheet is made of several β-strands. Each strand contains usually from 5 to 10 residues and its backbone is fully extended. β-strands are aligned adjacent to each other and connected by a network of hydrogen bonds between CO groups of one β-strand and NH groups on an adjacent β-strand (Fig. 25.3). β-sheets are 'pleated' and side-chains point alternately below and above the average plane.

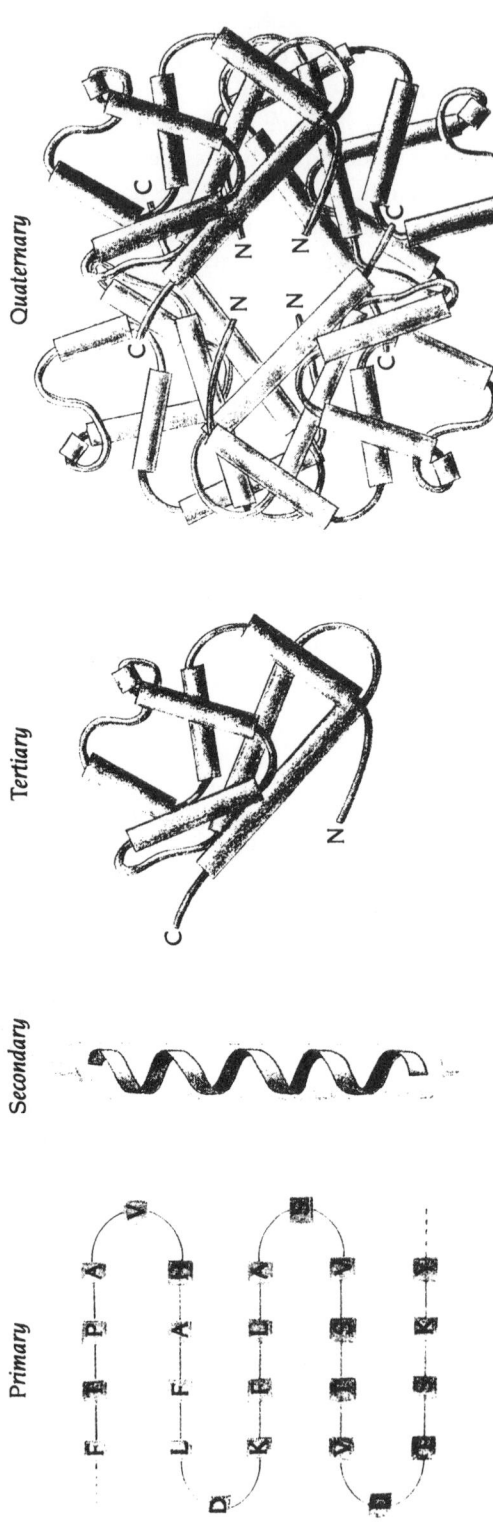

Fig. 25.2 Primary, secondary, tertiary and quaternary structures of a protein: schematic representation. (Reproduced from ref. 5, with permission of the authors and publisher.)

β-Sheets can be parallel or antiparallel according to the relative direction of neighbour peptide chains. In a few cases, a combination of parallel and antiparallel strands are found in the same sheet.

C. The tertiary structure

Connection of secondary structural features, α-helix and β-strands, with loops of various length leads to the protein three-dimensional (tertiary) structure. A number of structural motifs are often encountered (α-structures, β-structures, α/β structures) and combined to form domains. Domains have usually independent stable tertiary structures of their own. Large proteins can fold into several domains, usually associated with different structural or biological functions.

D. The quaternary structure

A number of biological host 'molecules' are in fact made up of highly associated identical or different polypeptide chains. The resulting homo- or heteromeric complex is characterized by its quaternary structure, that is the 3D structure of the complex. The quaternary structure most often determines the biological function. The challenge for medicinal chemists trying to rationalize drug design is to access the tertiary or quaternary structure of the target protein, in the absence of an experimental 3D structure. Molecular modelling represents the only available approach.

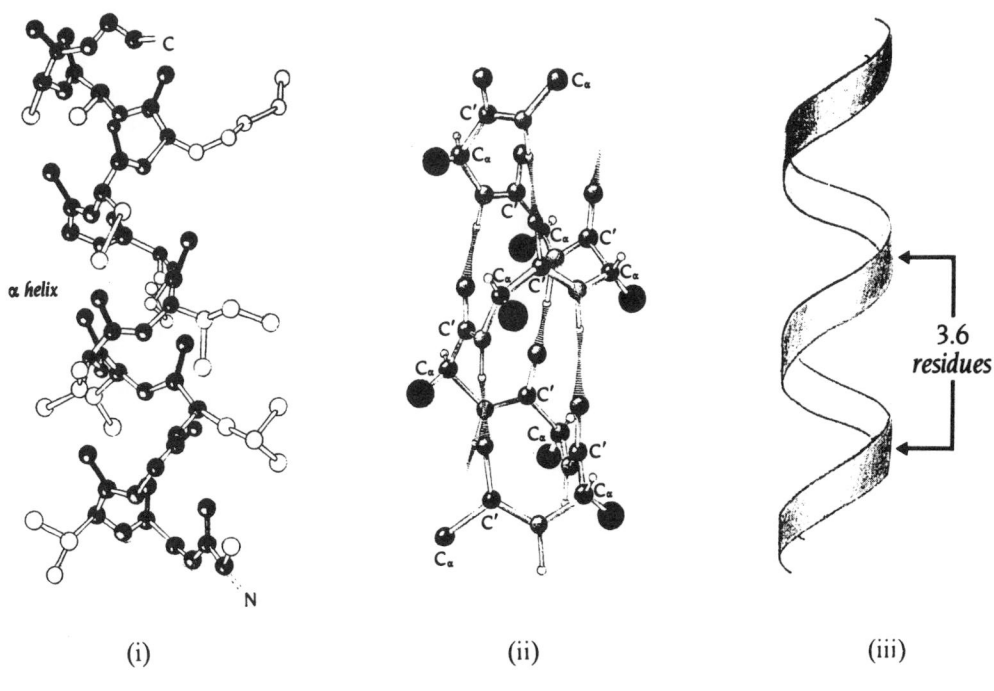

(i)   (ii)   (iii)

Fig. 25.3a

Continued overleaf

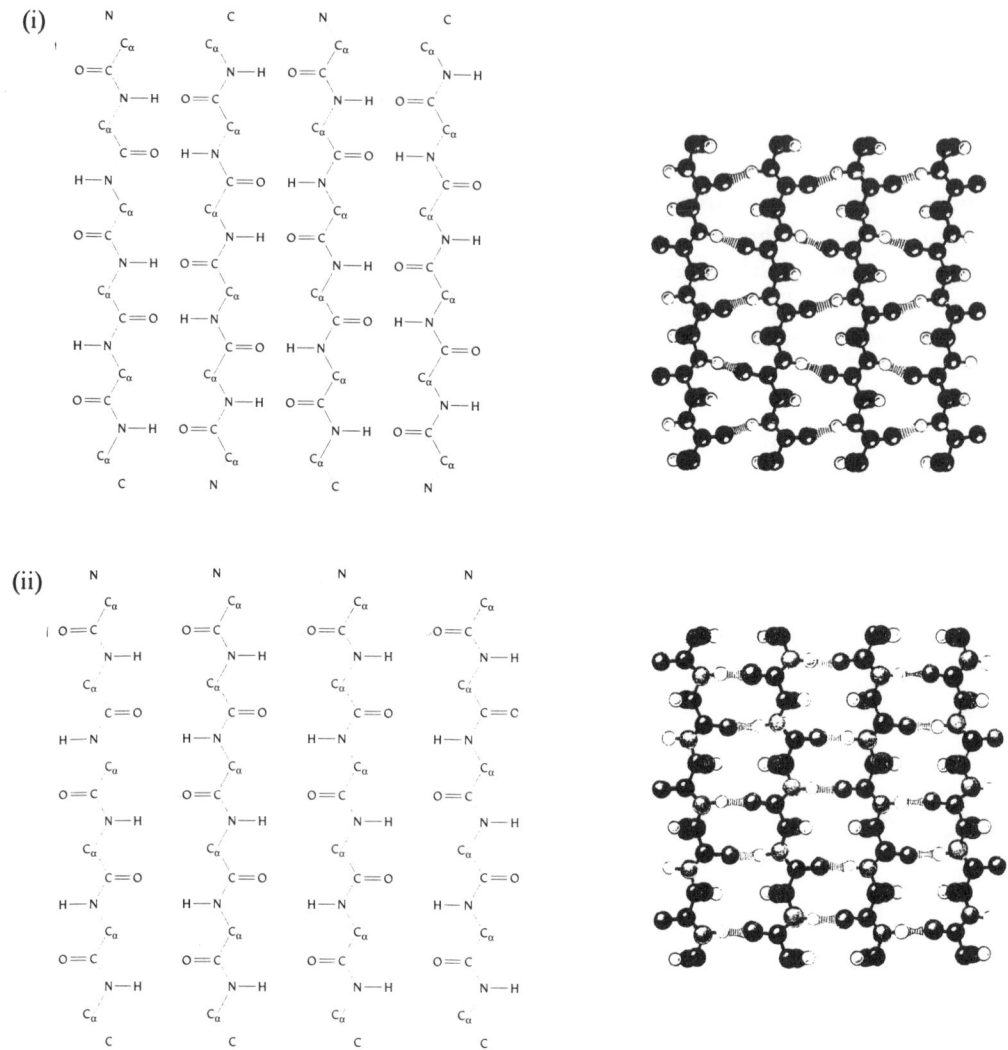

Fig. 25.3 (a) An α-helix: (i) the backbone atoms are in black, the side-chain atoms are displayed as open circles; (ii) only main chain- and Cα-atoms are displayed with the network of hydrogen bonds. (iii) 'ribbon' representation of the α-helix backbone. (b) β-Strands and β-sheets: (i) antiparallel pattern; (ii) parallel pattern. (Reproduced from ref. 5, with permission of the authors and publisher.)

III.   MODELLING STRATEGY

Attempts to predict protein folding *ab initio* from the primary sequence are still being made.[7] However, the likelihood of success remains very limited for several reasons: proteins are large molecules with a large number of possible conformations that are impossible to generate with current computing facilities; in addition, the difference in energy between most of these conformations, including the fully unfolded and the actual 3D structure, is usually small and does not permit the identification of the natural folding; furthermore, there is not necessarily a direct relationship between a sequence and its folding. For instance, local structural or environmental constraints might oblige the same sequence of amino acids to fold as an α-helix, a β-sheet or a loop. These observations appear rather discouraging. However, extensive structural analysis of existing 3D protein structures indicates that (i) there is a limited number of topologically different domain types; (ii) proteins with similar amino acid sequences usually have similar 3D structures; (iii) proteins might have similar 3D structures in spite of a lack of sequence homology; (iv) proteins belonging to the same structural class have similar core regions containing homologous secondary structural elements with similar relative positioning; (v) loop and backbone folding is not random and obeys certain rules.

In addition, experimental data can be extremely useful in guiding the prediction of protein folding. Hence, the only approach that has already proved to be of practical interest proceeds by analogy. Now it clearly appears to be possible, using information from related proteins, to model a protein from its sequence. The approach is usually termed 'modelling by homology'. The method relies on primary sequence homology only or may be extended to take into account structural information in a more systematic and automated way.[8-10]

The general strategy can be outlined as follows (Fig. 25.4).

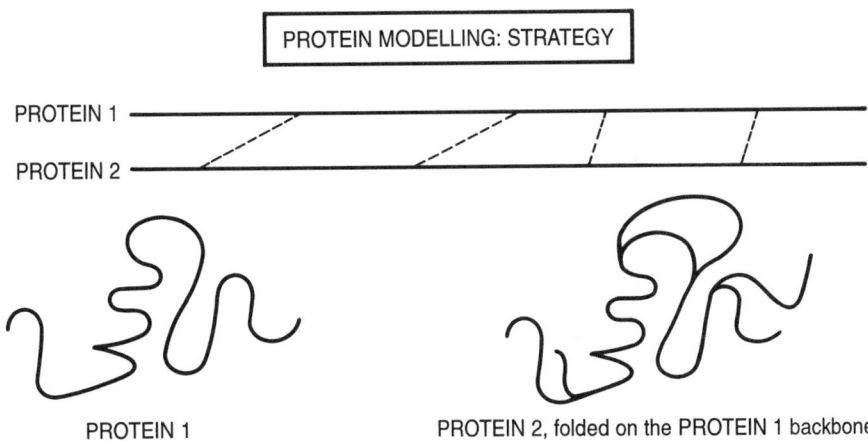

PROTEIN MODELLING: STRATEGY

PROTEIN 1

PROTEIN 2

PROTEIN 1   PROTEIN 2, folded on the PROTEIN 1 backbone

Fig. 25.4   Protein modelling by homology: strategy. There is some primary sequence homology between protein 1 and protein 2. An experimental 3D structure is available for protein 1. Protein 1 is used as a template to fold protein 2 by superimposition of homologous domains. Other methods (e.g. loop searching) are used to complete protein 2. The protein 2 model is optimized by energy minimization. The model is validated by experimental data.

(1) Search sequence databases[9-12] to find proteins related to the protein to be built (protein 2, Fig. 25.4).
(2) Analyse homologous primary sequences in order to characterize similar features (conserved amino acids, hydropathicity, secondary structure).
(3) Select among homologous proteins the reference protein (protein 1, Fig. 25.4) whose atomic coordinates are available.
(4) Set the conformation of protein 2 to be the same as that of protein 1 in each homologous region.

(5) Connect these regions with appropriate protein fragments in conformations derived from structural database searching[11] or loop generation.[12]

(6) Add side-chains in energetically permissible conformations.[13]

(7) Refine the model by energy minimization and molecular dynamics in the presence and absence of ligand.

(8) Validate the model experimentally.

The last point is unfortunately very often neglected, whereas it is the most crucial step in the whole process.

We will examine some of these steps in more detail and present three successful examples of such protein modelling studies.

A.   Sequence comparison and analysis (points (1) to (3))

More than 40 000 protein sequences are currently available in several databases.[9-12] This number will increase very rapidly with the appearance of new molecular biology techniques (such as the polymerase chain reaction, PCR) and recent progress towards the characterization of the human genome.

Software packages allowing a rapid analysis of primary sequence homology are available. One of the most popular can be obtained from the Wisconsin University Genetics Compter Group (GCG) and runs on personal computers.[14]

1.   Sequence alignment and amino acid homology

Several methods are used to investigate primary sequence homology. The prototype is the method developed by Needleman and Wunsch.[15] They consider the mutation rate of amino acid residues to derive optimal comparison scores and corresponding alignments. The method has been extended to take into account physicochemical parameters.[10,11] Aligned sequences are generated and percentages of identity or similarity can be calculated and displayed as matrices or as evolutionary trees (e.g. Table 25.1). Linear alignment methods are generally unreliable when the homology is lower than 20–25% .

2.   Conservation analysis

It is important to identify residues highly conserved in the class of proteins considered and those that are specific to subclasses or to a given protein. The first category of residues are likely to play a key role in the structure or the function that is common to all the members of the family, while the second are likely to play a specific role in a particular member of the protein family (e.g. recognition of a corresponding selective ligand). 'Visual' analysis of aligned sequences remains the best way to study the conservation pattern.

3.   Hydropathicity and secondary structure homology

In addition to primary sequence homology, it is important to seek structural features that are likely to be conserved in the 3D structures of homologous proteins. In this respect the hydropathicity profile and the putative secondary structure of proteins can be investigated and

Table 25.1 Percentage of identity (above diagonal) and similarity (below) between the transmembrane regions of 42 different GPCRs. Entry numbers correspond to receptors identified by their PDB code number, as listed below the table.

	1	2	3	4	5	6	7	8	9	10	11	12	13	14	15	16	17	18	19	20	21	22	23	24	25	26	27	28	29	30	31	32	33	34	35	36	37	38	39	40	41	42
1	//	35	53	35	42	43	44	43	41	46	48	41	45	41	43	36	36	35	35	35	31	32	36	23	24	27	26	27	23	25	28	16	19	20	19	21	26	24	14	9	11	8
2	63	//	39	76	39	35	42	39	36	38	39	39	41	41	39	30	29	33	29	33	23	31	30	25	21	21	23	22	20	21	22	25	13	16	19	15	20	15	20	12	11	14
3	75	64	//	39	39	42	45	43	36	41	46	42	43	38	38	33	32	35	33	35	35	33	25	27	22	21	22	25	23	23	23	25	17	21	17	17	18	21	21	11	13	15
4	61	92	65	//	39	37	42	37	35	38	40	41	41	37	38	29	29	34	29	35	21	28	26	21	20	23	23	18	21	20	26	12	17	20	16	19	17	19	14	13	14	9
5	69	71	66	71	//	41	43	39	40	42	47	39	42	39	43	33	33	33	34	34	39	24	26	27	25	27	25	27	25	25	23	27	16	23	18	21	20	19	11	12	11	9
6	68	67	63	67	69	//	45	41	37	83	43	43	44	41	39	29	31	31	31	30	25	31	33	27	29	28	29	23	22	24	23	29	17	16	24	17	20	19	11	11	12	9
7	67	73	65	72	69	65	//	76	53	47	49	49	43	41	43	32	32	33	34	33	29	35	36	28	27	29	23	25	27	24	16	21	19	17	22	20	25	10	11	15	7
8	65	67	65	66	63	63	85	//	55	45	46	45	43	39	43	31	31	29	30	30	25	31	33	27	29	27	22	24	23	29	16	27	26	14	17	20	25	27	8	14	17	9
9	60	66	59	65	63	60	73	74	//	41	41	45	43	36	41	34	35	32	30	32	25	31	31	25	25	23	23	24	24	24	18	19	18	15	21	22	27	11	11	11	10
10	69	69	63	69	71	93	67	64	61	//	43	47	47	42	42	33	31	33	32	33	28	27	29	25	23	25	27	19	21	21	23	15	17	23	20	23	21	12	12	14	12
11	72	65	69	64	71	67	68	66	61	70	//	43	48	42	47	30	31	29	33	32	28	29	34	28	31	29	30	24	26	27	26	15	21	20	19	21	22	21	9	14	13	11
12	69	67	67	67	65	67	74	67	66	70	73	//	47	44	70	37	37	36	36	39	27	31	32	24	23	25	21	18	23	23	14	21	21	21	18	25	23	11	7	11	7
13	65	71	67	68	71	67	69	64	63	70	75	71	//	70	70	33	29	33	30	33	27	34	34	26	26	26	22	25	21	28	17	18	23	19	20	23	22	9	11	13	10
14	69	65	72	63	70	69	67	64	61	69	72	70	85	//	62	33	29	34	33	31	22	29	31	26	28	29	29	21	26	19	24	15	18	23	23	24	22	11	15	12	9
15	67	66	65	67	66	68	65	64	67	66	69	70	66	81	77	//	77	33	31	25	33	25	33	32	33	30	27	27	21	26	17	16	20	18	24	20	23	11	7	11	9
16	62	63	61	62	61	58	57	57	57	59	61	63	59	61	63	//	71	76	75	80	28	26	25	19	24	23	24	26	21	23	14	15	18	20	22	19	18	12	11	10	12
17	64	61	63	60	61	57	57	56	59	59	61	64	59	57	53	86	//	77	86	71	27	24	24	21	23	25	25	25	23	21	27	15	19	17	19	21	17	20	9	9	11	14
18	63	64	64	63	62	60	58	55	55	57	62	64	63	63	57	92	88	//	75	79	31	25	27	20	21	22	25	24	23	23	27	13	18	18	19	21	19	19	9	10	11	14
19	63	61	61	62	59	57	59	55	57	59	60	63	59	57	54	87	95	89	//	74	27	26	24	23	25	23	26	25	21	27	14	16	16	20	21	18	18	10	10	10	13
20	64	61	61	62	62	58	57	56	57	61	64	65	63	60	57	91	88	93	89	//	29	24	27	22	22	22	23	25	24	25	24	13	17	17	19	21	18	18	10	13	10	14
21	56	55	55	54	51	49	50	48	51	54	51	53	53	50	53	56	55	56	56	//	22	24	21	22	21	19	21	22	18	20	23	18	17	17	16	23	21	8	7	10	16
22	58	59	51	59	55	53	60	55	57	54	59	63	59	54	57	49	51	51	52	49	53	//	60	22	24	25	23	25	20	27	17	17	17	19	20	22	19	7	12	14	8
23	57	54	52	53	53	51	61	53	55	53	60	60	55	51	55	47	50	50	49	51	56	79	//	25	25	25	28	25	27	23	31	15	25	22	22	23	21	21	9	15	16	8
24	48	50	49	50	49	47	51	50	49	51	48	51	52	51	48	46	49	49	49	47	50	40	41	//	65	47	23	25	21	20	24	26	10	4	9	10
25	53	51	49	49	49	49	52	45	46	53	49	49	51	48	45	49	49	51	44	46	45	47	43	51	51	79	//	67	27	26	27	21	15	21	21	23	24	11	12	13	7
26	50	50	47	51	51	46	49	49	45	48	52	49	51	49	50	49	49	47	43	51	47	47	43	51	47	85	84	//	27	27	27	25	21	17	21	21	22	21	24	23	8	7	11	7
27	57	52	52	51	56	55	53	49	45	56	57	49	57	58	55	51	54	51	54	47	51	52	58	57	56	//	39	45	29	26	19	24	21	21	22	19	23	9	9	9	11
28	58	52	53	51	50	49	52	50	46	49	55	49	50	49	49	55	49	50	49	47	48	53	53	52	55	56	66	//	73	27	21	18	19	19	17	22	21	21	10	7	8	12
29	55	51	51	51	50	51	51	49	48	51	56	47	50	49	49	47	51	51	50	51	50	53	53	53	55	69	91	//	25	20	18	24	19	20	20	21	25	13	9	11	9
30	53	55	51	53	53	50	55	56	47	51	50	50	52	47	50	51	52	47	50	51	51	54	49	49	55	55	57	57	//	20	18	29	15	16	19	23	11	11	11	10
31	50	53	47	50	53	44	47	54	48	52	47	56	53	52	49	50	53	48	53	50	53	52	48	46	49	52	49	51	//	15	21	21	16	22	21	24	8	12	13	13
32	47	48	47	47	46	41	43	42	38	45	47	45	49	44	46	37	43	42	41	40	47	45	45	42	42	45	45	43	47	47	//	17	15	18	17	16	19	11	9	7	13
33	48	49	46	47	48	47	49	50	44	46	52	47	45	46	45	46	44	45	43	45	50	45	45	49	50	45	51	45	45	58	45	39	//	20	25	19	18	25	11	13	10	9
34	49	49	41	51	47	45	45	39	40	45	52	44	49	50	47	45	45	46	47	45	44	45	47	43	50	51	46	46	49	50	43	48	45	//	71	71	21	23	6	9	6	8
35	49	49	44	51	47	45	45	40	43	45	52	48	51	52	49	47	48	47	48	49	44	49	49	47	50	49	49	43	44	44	46	40	47	89	//	67	23	22	7	10	9	7
36	51	52	45	51	49	45	47	41	44	47	52	47	53	52	52	47	45	45	47	45	51	52	47	45	51	44	50	41	45	43	46	30	50	66	67	//	23	21	7	9	5	7
37	53	49	47	45	49	49	48	49	49	49	45	46	48	45	48	45	41	45	52	48	48	53	52	45	42	45	43	47	36	40	46	44	47	47	//	39	9	7	9	10
38	51	47	47	48	47	45	51	50	49	45	48	45	42	45	47	46	47	49	45	47	44	46	48	51	53	52	51	46	44	49	49	44	47	47	46	51	61	//	13	10	9	11
39	35	40	31	43	35	33	41	35	39	35	36	39	35	35	33	33	37	35	37	35	32	35	39	35	37	32	31	33	32	35	35	31	30	27	27	28	32	38	//	38	35	7
40	35	38	33	39	31	31	36	31	40	37	37	35	37	35	34	34	33	33	35	37	40	28	35	31	35	35	31	35	28	30	30	28	31	65	//	69	11
41	37	39	37	39	35	37	41	37	39	38	41	42	39	37	37	34	37	37	36	38	40	39	31	39	35	39	37	37	38	37	34	31	27	29	28	32	34	59	86	//	11
42	29	37	30	33	27	34	31	33	29	37	36	30	35	33	28	29	35	32	33	33	37	31	32	27	26	27	31	33	33	31	30	33	29	29	29	27	28	29	30	37	35	//

(1) 5ht1a$Huma;(2) 5ht1c$Rat;(3) 5ht1d$Can;(4) 5ht2$$Rat;(5) His2$Cani;(6) D1dr$Huma;(7) D2dr$Huma;(8) D3dr$Ratt;
(9) D4dr$Huma;(10) D5dr$Huma;(11) A1ar$$Rat;(12) A2ar$Huma;(13) B1ar$Huma;(14) B2ar$Huma;(15) B3ar$Huma;(16) Acm1$Huma;
(17) Acm2$Huma;(18) Acm3$$Pig;(19) Acm4$Huma;(20) Acm5$Huma;(21) Cannabino;(22) Aden1$Can;(23) Aden2$Can;(24) Nk1r$$Rat;
(25) Nk2r$bovi;(26) Nk3r$$Rat;(27) Bombesinr;(28) Endo1rece;(29) Endo2rece;(30) Rdc1$Cani;(31) Trh$Mouse;(32) Txr$Human;
(33) Paf$Quine;(34) Lshr$Huma;(35) Tshr$Huma;(36) Fshr$Huma;(37) Opsr$Huma;(38) Oped$Huma;(39) Bac$Halba;(40) Bachh$alo;
(41) Bachn$att;(42) Mglutarec;

compared. There is always a very good compatibility between the hydrophobicity of a protein domain and its local environment. Thus, the 3D folding of a protein is such that hydrophobic residues are protected from the aqueous environment in the case of water-soluble proteins. In contrast, they are found at the surface of the protein domain embedded in the hydrophobic phospholipid bilayer in the case of membrane proteins. Hence the hydropathicity profile of a protein provides information on its folding and must be similar in proteins with similar 3D structures.[16–18]

The most usual approaches to predicting the hydropathicity profile of a given protein derive from the method developed by Kyte and Doolittle.[19] From database analysis they defined the

Table 25.2   Indices of hydrophobicity of the 20 amino acids. (From Kyte and Doolittle.[19])

Amino acid	Hydropathicity index	Amino acid	Hydropathicity index
Arginine	−4.5	Serine	−0.8
Lysine	−3.9	Threonine	−0.7
Asparagine	−3.5	Glycine	−0.4
Aspartic acid	−3.5	Alanine	1.8
Glutamine	−3.5	Methionine	1.9
Glutamic acid	−3.5	Cysteine	2.5
Histidine	−3.2	Phenylalanine	2.8
Proline	−1.6	Leucine	3.8
Tyrosine	−1.3	Valine	4.2
Tryptophan	−0.9	Isoleucine	4.5

hydropathicity index for each of the 20 amino acids (Table 25.2). They then scored the hydropathicity on a window of 9 to 11 amino acids, moving all along the protein sequence. This leads to diagrams such as those displayed in Fig. 25.5. The hydrophobic regions appear as positive peaks while the hydrophilic ones appear as negative peaks. The hydropathicity profiles of aligned sequences can be calculated and compared. For example, all receptors belonging to the seven-transmembrane-domain receptor family show in their hydropathicity profile at least seven positive peaks corresponding to the seven hydrophobic transmembrane regions. The potential and limits of these methods have been reviewed.[20]

The prediction of secondary structures is a key step in the modelling attempt. Several methods have been developed. They correspond to two different strategies: an extrapolation from a statistical analysis of known protein primary, secondary and tertiary structures, or a direct prediction based on physicochemical parameters.[21,22]

The most extensively used methods belong to the first class. The prototype is the Chou and Fassman method,[23] which takes into account the observed frequency of a given amino acid's occurrence in an α-helix, a β-strand or a turn, and the identity of the amino acids found in its immediate neighbourhood. The protein sequence is analysed linearly and average probability values for each residue of belonging to an α-helix, a β-strand and a turn are generated. Putative structural domains are identified this way.

A number of modified methods have been developed and their predictive power has been compared.[24-28] Their success rate reaches at best 65%. These methods are based on statistical parameters derived from existing X-ray crystallography structures. With very few exceptions, proteins that are available in the Brookhaven Protein Databank are water-soluble proteins. Accordingly, the reliability of secondary structure prediction methods for membrane proteins has been questioned.[24] It seems to vary significantly from one method to another but it will undoubtely be improved in the near future with extension of the experimental data set.

4.   Experimental data

Before undertaking the 3D modelling procedure, it is very important to collect as exhaustively as possible relevant experimental data which might be of significance helping to position the different protein domains. In addition, any available experimental data on one member of the protein family might be relevant to all the other members, including the protein of interest.

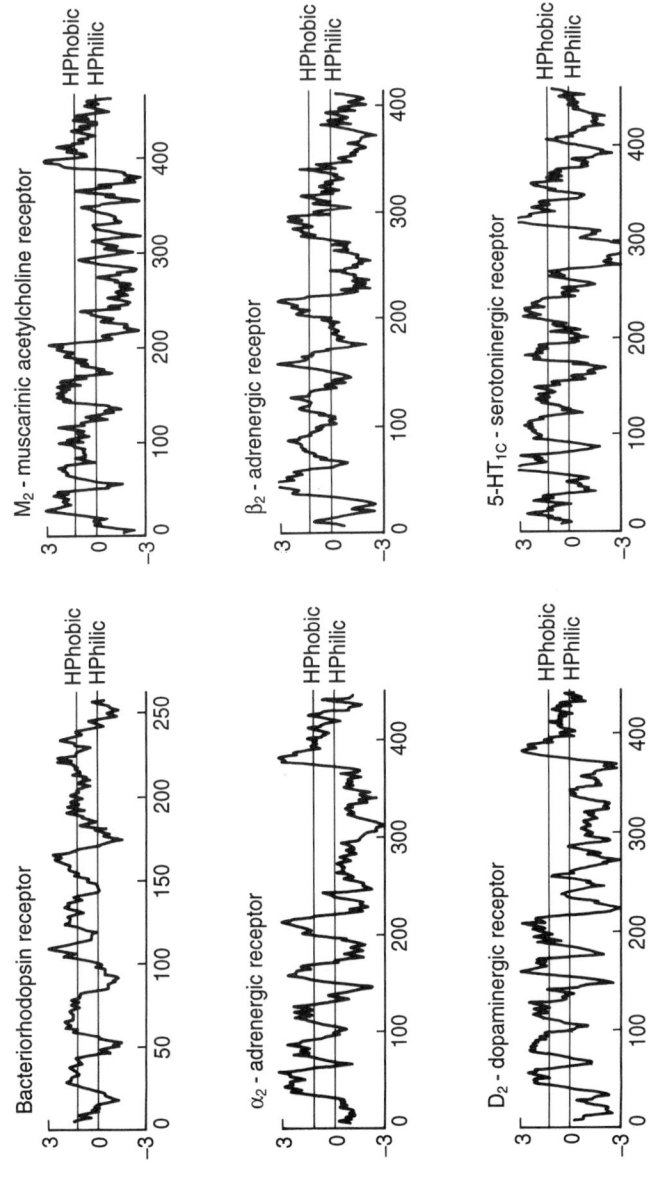

Fig. 25.5 Hydropathicity plots of some G-protein-coupled receptors: *x*-axis = hydrophobicity score; *y*-axis = residue number in the sequence. Positive peaks correspond to putative hydrophobic domains. (Reproduced with permission from Trumpp-Kallmeyer *et al.* (1992) *J. Med. Chem.* **35**: 3448–3462. Copyright (1992) American Chemical Society.)

Hence, a global knowledege of the structure–function relationship among the homologous proteins is most useful. For example, data such as circular dichroism, catalytic mechanism, ligand structure–activity relationships, accessibility to antibodies or enzymes, chemical labelling, site-directed mutagenesis, and so on should be taken into account during the folding process.

B.   The 3D modelling process

Once the homology between the primary and secondary structures of the reference protein and the protein of interest has been established, the next step consists in folding the backbone of the model protein in each homologous region. This can be achieved with commercially available molecular modelling packages,[29–32] allowing the generation of classical structural patterns (α-helix, β-strands) or fitting of a flexible molecule on a given rigid reference scaffold.

The next, more delicate, step is to connect these domains with loops or sequence fragments which show no homology with the reference 3D structure. If these loops are not too long (up to 12 amino acids), their structure is not random. Their backbone conformations usually cluster in sets of similar structures. Preliminary models of the loops can be extracted from the Brookhaven Protein Databank knowing the number of amino acids in the loop, the type of structural elements they connect and the distance and orientation of the N- and C-terminal peptidic connections. Typically, several clusters of conformers are found. Conformers representative of the different clusters are selected and incorporated into the model. Their relevance is probed by energy calculation.

Finally, side-chains are connected to the protein backbone. Their initial conformation is set according to energetic or statistical considerations. 'Manual' refinement of the initial positioning is usually necessary to optimize 'obvious' side-chain interactions (ion pairs, hydrogen bonds, aromatic–aromatic interactions, etc.).

The model is then refined through energy minimization and molecular dynamics to relieve the strain caused by unfavourable side-chain interactions or inappropriate loop topologies.

'Classical' protein energy minimization and molecular dynamics algorithms are readily available in commercial software. However, they should not be used without a clear under-standing of their potential and limits, which cannot be reviewed in this chapter.

The medicinal chemist now has in hand a 3D *model* of the target protein. One should keep in mind Magritte's painting 'The Perfidy of Images' showing a realistic depiction manner a smoker's pipe together with this warning *'Ceci n'est pas une pipe'* (This is not a pipe). The image that has been generated is not the protein. At best, it is a model which accounts to some extent for experimental facts. It is very important to bear in mind the assumptions that have been made all along the modelling process, as well as the inherent limits of the tools and methodologies that have been used. Additional theoretical calculations never *validate* a model; only appropriate experiments will do so.

C.   Experimental validation

As discussed above, experimental validation is one of the most critical steps in the modelling process. A proposed protein three-dimensional model must account for existing experimental data and should represent a source of novel hypotheses which can and should be tested and validated experimentally. As mentioned already, a battery of complementary experimental techniques is necessary to probe a model; for example, accessibility to antibodies, chemical labelling, site-directed mutagenesis, and biophysical techniques (CD, NMR, X-ray, etc.). Ultimately, the model should have a predictive value for ligand design or protein engineering. Considering the prerequisites (homology with a crystallized protein) and the numerous putative pitfalls of the modelling process, one might wonder whether the tertiary fold of a protein can indeed be successfully predicted and will be of any use. The answer to these questions is definitely yes, as illustrated by many studies. The first significant achievement is the work of Kirschner and co-workers, who were able to define a 3D model for the α-subunit of tryptophan synthase.[33] The X-ray structure of this protein has subsequently been determined and is in very good agreement with the proposed model. We will illustrate the protein homology strategy with two more recent examples of great therapeutic interest: the modelling of an enzyme, the HIV-protease, and the modelling of a class of membrane receptors, the G-protein-coupled receptors (GPCR).

IV. EXAMPLES

We will briefly illustrate the modelling process following the general strategic scheme detailed above: (i) choice of the target; (ii) sequence analysis; (iii) 3D modelling; (iv) experimental validation. Readers are refered to the original publications for more details.

A. HIV-protease

1. The target

The human immunodeficiency virus (HIV) requires a specific protease for the maturation of its components. Inhibiton of this protease might represent one of the therapeutic approaches to AIDS. The protease has been cloned and sequenced.[34] It contains 99 amino acids.

2. Sequence analysis

On the basis of a variety of experimental results, the HIV-protease has been shown to belong to the class of aspartic proteases. Pearl and Taylor[35] have found sequence homology between HIV-protease and one of the two symetrical domains of several cellular aspartic proteases. In the alignment, 30 residues out of 99 are identical and 11 additional ones correspond to conservative substitutions. The residues of the catalytic triad are conserved and could be aligned. Secondary structure analysis showed that the topology is conserved so that deletions are positioned in surface loops (Table 25.3).

3. 3D modelling

Pearl and Taylor used as the template for HIV-protease folding one of the two symetrical domains of endothiapepsin.[35] Loops were rebuilt to correspond to the lengths in HIV-protease. Analysis of the model led to the suggestion that retroviral proteases may be dimeric aspartic proteases. A dimer of the 3D model has been generated (Fig. 25.6). It shows a high structural

Table 25.3 Alignment of HIV-1 protease sequence stretches with aspartic proteases. Each line corresponds to a different protein sequence. (Reproduced with permission from Pearl, L. H. and Taylor, W. (1987) *Nature* **329**: 351–354. Copyright (1987) Macmillan Magazines Limited.)

```
Dr TE      --TGRKFSAISLGKPNYIIIKYKK------------EHHLKCILD TG STVNNTSKNIFDLPI---   -QHTSTFIHTSHQ-PLIVNKSIII--   -PSKILFPT   YQH LGRLLAEAKATISV
IAP-MIB    HLKKDCGAPERETRESRLCYRCGK------------GYHRASECGIT DSG DKSIISLHNWPKSWPT-   -UVSBHELQGLQSS-P-AISASAL--   -THRDAEGK   PQSL HGRDALGHHGHTLTH
RSU        PPAVSLAHTHEHKDRPLVRVILTHTGSHPVKORSVYITAL DSG ADITIISEEDWPTDWPVH   EAAHPQ-IHQIGGGIPHRKBRHIE   -LGUIHRDQ   RGSTL GHDCLGQLGLRLTH
BLU        --LS-IPLARS-RPSVAVVLSGI-PHLGPSONQAL HLD TG AEHIVLPQHNLVRDYP-   -RIPAA-VLGAGQUSRHVHRLGGP   -LTLALKPE   RGEL GFDULSRLGASIGI
SRU-I      GSSDIYHVGPIICQRPSLTLWLDD----KHFTQL D TG ADUIIKLEDWPPHWP-   ITDTLTHLRGIGGS--HHPKOSEK-   -YLTHRDKE   PUH HGRDLLSGHKIHHCS
STLU       ----LPIIPLDPARRPLIKAEUHI----QTSHPHIIIAL D IC ADNIVLPHALFSDIP-   -LKHTS-VLGAGGQTODHFKLTBLP   UL1RLPFRT   HHAT IGRDALGGCGGUVYL
HTLU-I     ----LPUIPLDPARRPUIKAQUDI----QISHPKIIIAL D IC ADNIVLPIALFSSNIP-   -LKHTS-VLGAGGQTOBHFKLTBLP   UL1RLPFRT   HHAT IGRDALGGCGQULYL
HTLU-II    DISILPLIPLROGQGPILGURISV----HGQTPQPIAAL D C DLIUFQTLVPGPVK-   -LHDIL-ILGHGGTHTQFKLLHP   LHIFLPFAR   KHTI IGRDAL QGCGGULYL
H?BEU      EDSICGCOCSGAPPCPRIILSVGG----HPITFLUD TC AOHSUA TGN---GPLS-   -SRTSH-UGGATG-BKHRHHTTD-   RTUHLGGGH   PYF LGRDLLTKLGAQIHF
FLU        -HIRVGRAATPPPFEPRIILKVGG----QPUTFLUD TC AOHSUA TGN--PGPLS-   -DRTAL-UGGATG-BKHYRHITD-   RVUQLATGK   PYF LGRDLLTKLKAGINF
Mo-HULU    ILDDOGGGGQDPPPFEPRIILTVGG----QPUTFLUD TG AOHSUA TQN--POPLS-   -BRSAH-UGGATG-BKHYRHITD-   RKVHLATGK   PYF LGRDLLTKLHUPDC
ANU-HULU   ILDOGGGOGOLPPPFEPRIILTVGG----QPUTFLUD TG AOHSUA TQN--POPLS-   -BRSAH-UGGATG-BKHYRHITD-   RKVHLATGK   PYF LGRDLLTKLKAGINF
Eqiau      QPGOFVGUYHLEKRPTIVLIHD------TPLHVLD TG ADTVLI TAHYHRLK-   -YRGRK-YGGTGI-IGUGGHHET?-   -STPVTIKK   PUTIL GRDILGDLGAHLVL
Viina      TCGAVRAPVVUTCAPPKIEIKUOT----RUKKLLUD TC ADKTIVISHOMSGIP-   -KGRILGOIGG-ICGEKHEG---   -UHLGYKD   PUDQL GRNHRRELGIGLIH
ANU-2      GTUSFNFPQITLHQRPLVTIRIGG----QLKEALD TG ADDIVLCCHHLPGHH-   -XPKH-IGGIGG--FIKVRGVD--   -QIPVEICQ   PUH IGRNLLTGIGCTLHF
HIU-1      GTUSFNFPQITLHQRPLVTIKIGG----QLKEALD TG ADDIVLEEHSLPGHW---   -KPKH-IGGIGG--FIKVRGVD--   -QILEICQ   PUH IGHLLTGIGCTLHF
```

(a) 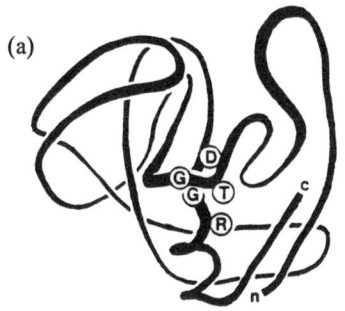 (b)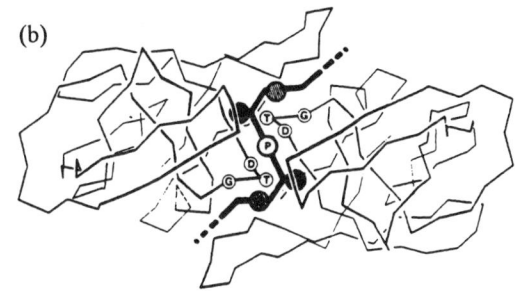

Fig. 25.6 Predicted tertiary structures of HIV-1 protease: (a) monomer folding and catalytic site residues; (b) proposed dimeric quaternary structure and schematic representation of the substrate in the binding site. (Reproduced with permission from Pearl, L. H. and Taylor, W. (1987) *Nature* **329**: 351–354. Copyright (1987) Macmillan Magazines Limited.)

homology with monomeric proteases with similar binding cleft and catalytic site. Subsequently, Wlodawer and co-workers solved the crystallographic structure of a retroviral aspartic protease, the Rous sarcoma virus (RSV) protease. As predicted for the HIV-protease, the RSV protease acts as a dimer with an active site very similar to monomeric cellular proteases. The 3D structure of RSV protease was used to define a refined model of HIV-protease[36] (Fig. 25.7). As in the model of Pearl and Taylor, the active site could be described in detail. The putative binding mode of substrates and inhibitors was derived from X-ray structures of protease—inhibitor complexes. A significant conformational change of two 'flap' regions has also been predicted. These two models provided sufficient insight into the structure and function of HIV-protease to be immediately useful for the rational design of potential inhibitors of this enzyme.

4. *Experimental validation*

The models proposed are consistent with results of site-directed mutagenesis. Moreover, the crystal structure of HIV-protease has been solved.[37] Comparison with previously proposed models shows remarkably good agreement. The location of the active site and substrate binding residues were very accurately predicted.[37] This story demonstrates that modelling of unknown structures based on the structures of related proteins can give accurate results and might have very important implications for drug design, as will be illustrated in Chapter 10.

B. **G-protein-coupled receptors**

1. *The target*

G-protein-coupled receptors (GPCRs) represent a very important structural and functional class of membrane-embedded receptors. They play a critical role in a large number of physiological processes and represent crucial targets for drug design. The general mechanism of action of GPCRs is illustrated in Fig. 25.8. An extracellular ligand binds to the receptor, which in turn couples to an intracellular heterotrimeric protein which dissociates and triggers an intracellular biological response.

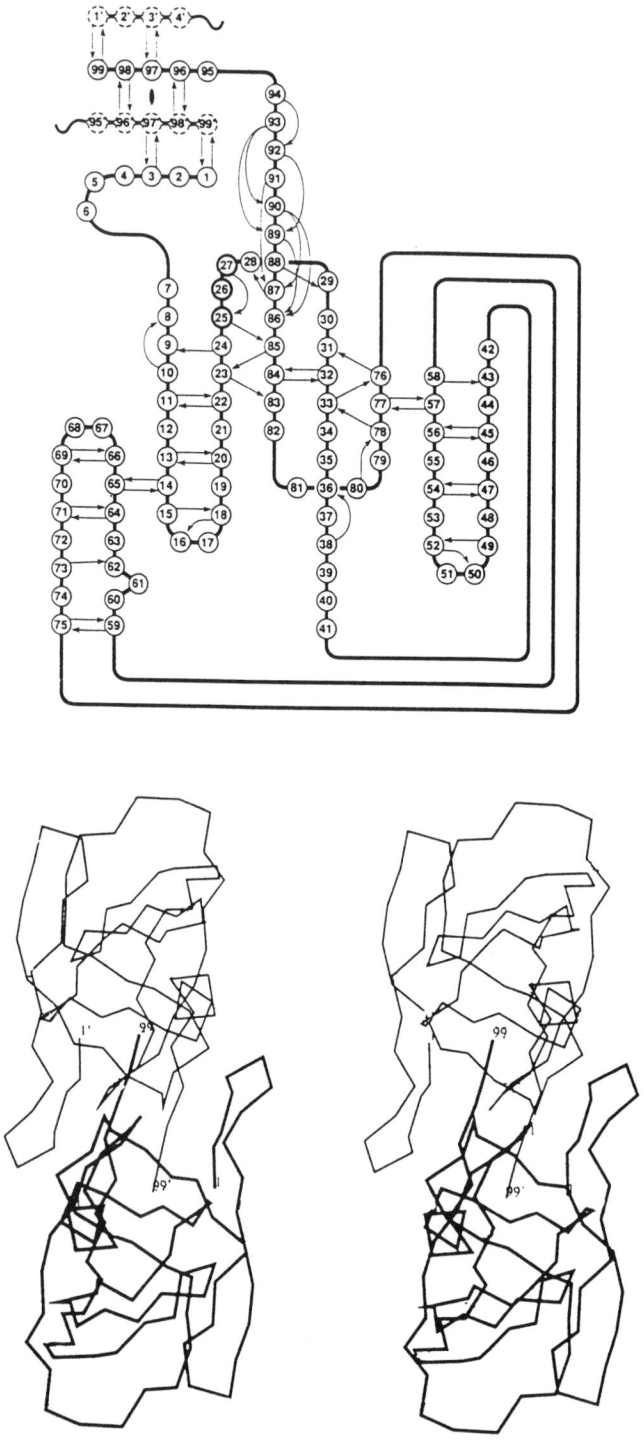

Fig. 25.7 Secondary (monomer, top) and 3D experimental (dimer, bottom) structures of HIV-1 protease. (Reprinted with permission from Weber, I. T. *et al.* (1989) Molecular modelling of the HIV-1 protease and its substrate binding site. *Science* **243**: 928–931. Copyright (1989) American Association for the Advancement of Science.)

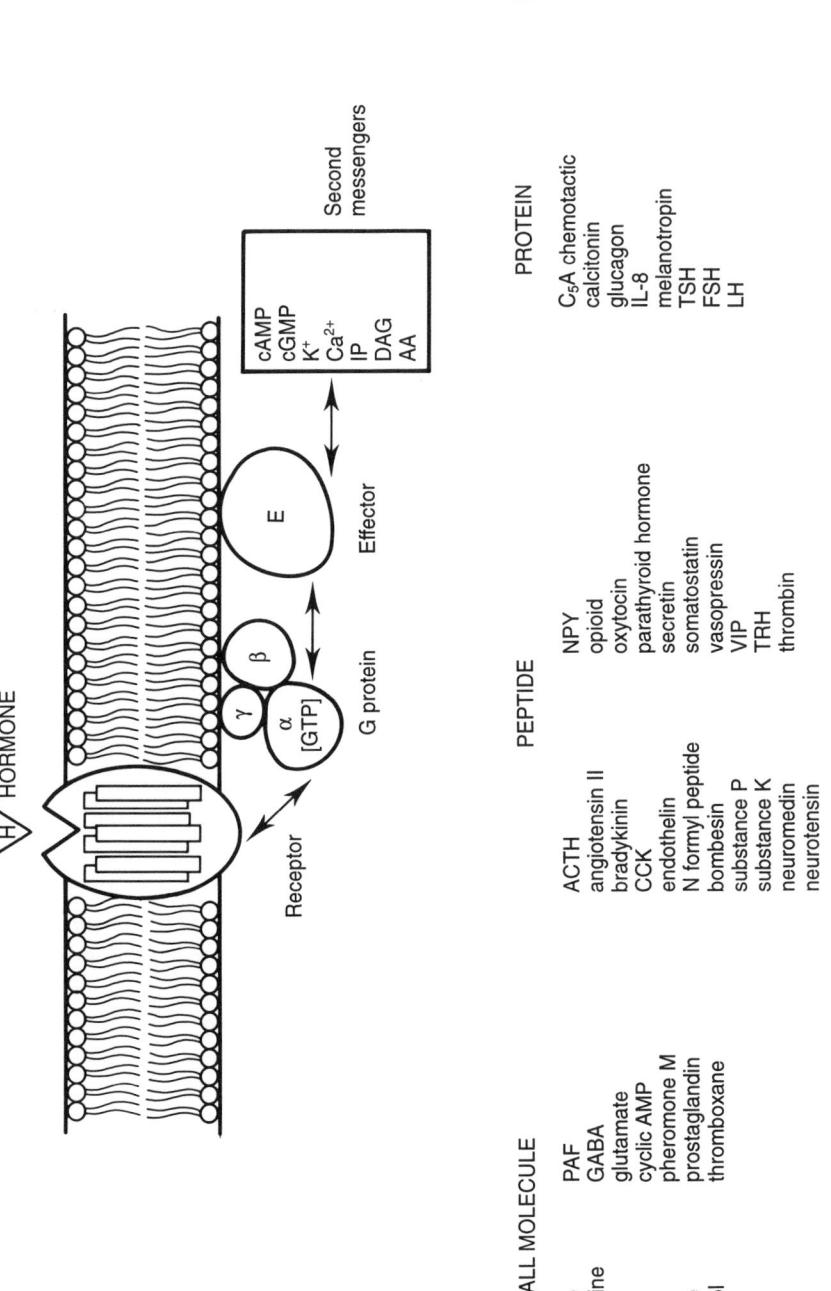

Fig. 25.8 Schematic representation of G-protein-coupled receptors and list of some of their endogeneous ligands.

It is of prime importance to understand the receptor–ligand recognition process in order to better understand the whole biological process and to rationalize drug design. Since the mid 1980s, a large number of GPCRs have been cloned and sequenced, offering the possibility of attempting 3D modelling. This study is briefly and schematically outlined below. Readers should refer to original articles for more details.[38–40]

2.   Homology analysis

Primary sequences of GPCRs are available from original articles or from databanks (e.g. EMBL). The GCG software[14] is one of the most convenient packages for extracting, aligning and analysing primary sequences and was used in this study. Sequence alignments were performed using the method of Needleman and Wunsch[15] (Table 25.4).

The degree of identity and similarity between the different GPCRs has been evaluated (Table 25.1). It is generally good (20–90%), as expected for family members. Seven domains containing 18–26 amino acids are clearly well conserved in all GPCRs.

The hydropathicity profiles were generated using the Kyte and Doolittle method[19] (Fig. 25.5). Positive peaks correspond to hydrophobic streches in the primary sequence. Seven of them are usually identified in GPCRs. They correspond to the most conserved domains and are likely to represent transmembrane regions of the proteins.

The secondary structure prediction tools are not fully validated for membrane proteins.[24] However, the amino acid sequences of the putative seven transmembrane regions and the lengths of these regions suggest α-helical structures.

In conclusion, sequence analysis suggests that GPCRs have in common seven α-helical transmembrane regions which could be identified.

3.   3D Modelling

It is of prime importance to consider all available experimental data derived from studies such as the accessibility of the receptors to enzymes or antibodies, chemical labelling, mutagenesis, structure–activity relationships, fluorescence, circular dichroism, and so on. For instance, such studies led to the definiton of a two-dimensional model of GPCRs and to the approximate localization of the ligand binding site (transmembrane region) and of the main G-protein-coupling domain (third intracellular loop).[41,42] The next step consisted in proposing a more detailed 3D model. This was achieved as follows.[38–40]

The reference protein chosen is bacteriorhodopsin. This protein shows no sequence or functional homology with GPCRs. However, it presents an activation system very similar to that of mammalian opsins (which are GPCR members) and contains seven transmembrane α-helical domains as postulated for GPCR.[43] A low-resolution (10 Å) crystallographic structure of bacteriorhodopsin[43] has been used as a scaffold to position the seven α-helical domains of GPCR relative to each other.

For a given receptor, each of the seven hydrophobic stretches of amino acids was built as an α-helix with the SYBYL program and energy-minimized with AMBER[44] and TRIPOS[29] force fields.

The seven helices were then assembled using bacteriorhodopsin as a template. The relative orientation of the helices meets three independent criteria: the hydrophobic face points to the outside, towards the hydrophobic membrane environment; the most conserved residues are found in the core of the protein; and the ligand binding residues converge to the inside of the protein.

Table 25.4 Sequence alignment of the seven putative transmembrane domains (TM) of 42 different G-protein-coupled receptors. (Reproduced with permission from Trumpp-Kallmeyer *et al.* (1992) *J. Med. Chem.* **35**: 3448–3462. Copyright (1992) American Chemical Society.)

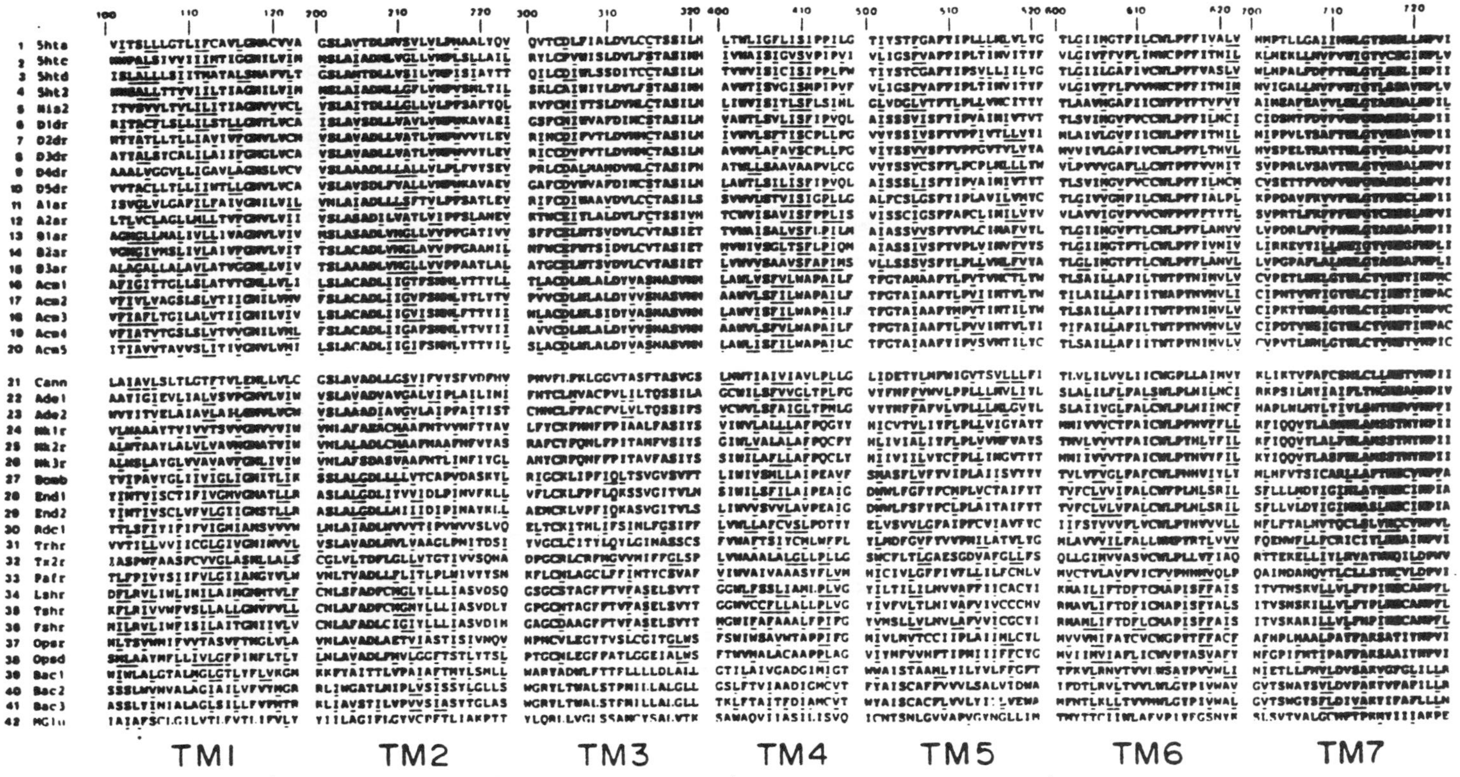

Loops were built with the loop search program in SYBYL. The whole structure was then extensively energy-minimized without or with ligands.

These models led to the proposal of a number novel hypotheses:

- The activation site of GPCRs is not close to the hydrophilic extracellular aqueous surface. It appears to be buried about 15 Å inside the structure.
- The putative binding sites of several important neurotransmitters have been described (Figs 25.9 and 25.10).[38–40] For instance, residues likely to interact directly with dopamine, adrenaline, serotonin, histamine, acetylcholine, adenosine, substance P, TSH, etc., have been identified.[38–40]
- A number of hypotheses regarding the receptor activation mechanisms and its dynamics have been proposed.[38–40]

The proposed model is in good qualitative agreement with the existing experimental results. However the next crucial step was to further validate these models experimentally and to examine their predictive value.

4. Experimental validation

Such models can be directly or indirectly tested by a number of experimental approaches, as discussed above. We mention here briefly some data providing support to the model.

- The predicted backbone architecture is in very good agreement with the first crystallography data on a GPCR (bovine opsin) published recently.[45] GPCRs do indeed have seven α-helical transmembrane domains, bundled very similarly to bacteriorhodopsin's domains.
- The depth of the binding site of small ligands is at least 11 Å as predicted and as demonstrated by fluorescence quenching experiments.[46]
- The binding site of a number of neurotransmitters has been probed by site directed mutagenesis. More than 100 mutants have been studied.[47] The observed shifts in ligand affinity are in most cases in good qualitative agreement with the models. The acetylcholine muscarinic M_1 receptor and the vasopressin receptor binding sites have been explored in a systematic way.[48,49]

These results show again the excellent predictive value of the models. They also highlight their limits. The complexity of the biological system and the subtlety of the dynamic receptor–ligand recogniton process do not allow any quantitative prediction at this stage. However, models have proved to be extremely valuable in leading to original working hypotheses which could be experimentally explored and usually validated. The next obvious step is the use of these models for drug design.

V.   GENERAL CONCLUSION

Access to a 3D representation of a target protein is crucial for the understanding of its function and the design of selective ligands. X-ray crystallography structure elucidation remains difficult and aleatory, more particularly in the case of membrane proteins. As illustrated previously, homology protein modelling represents a very valuable alternative way of generating a theoretical

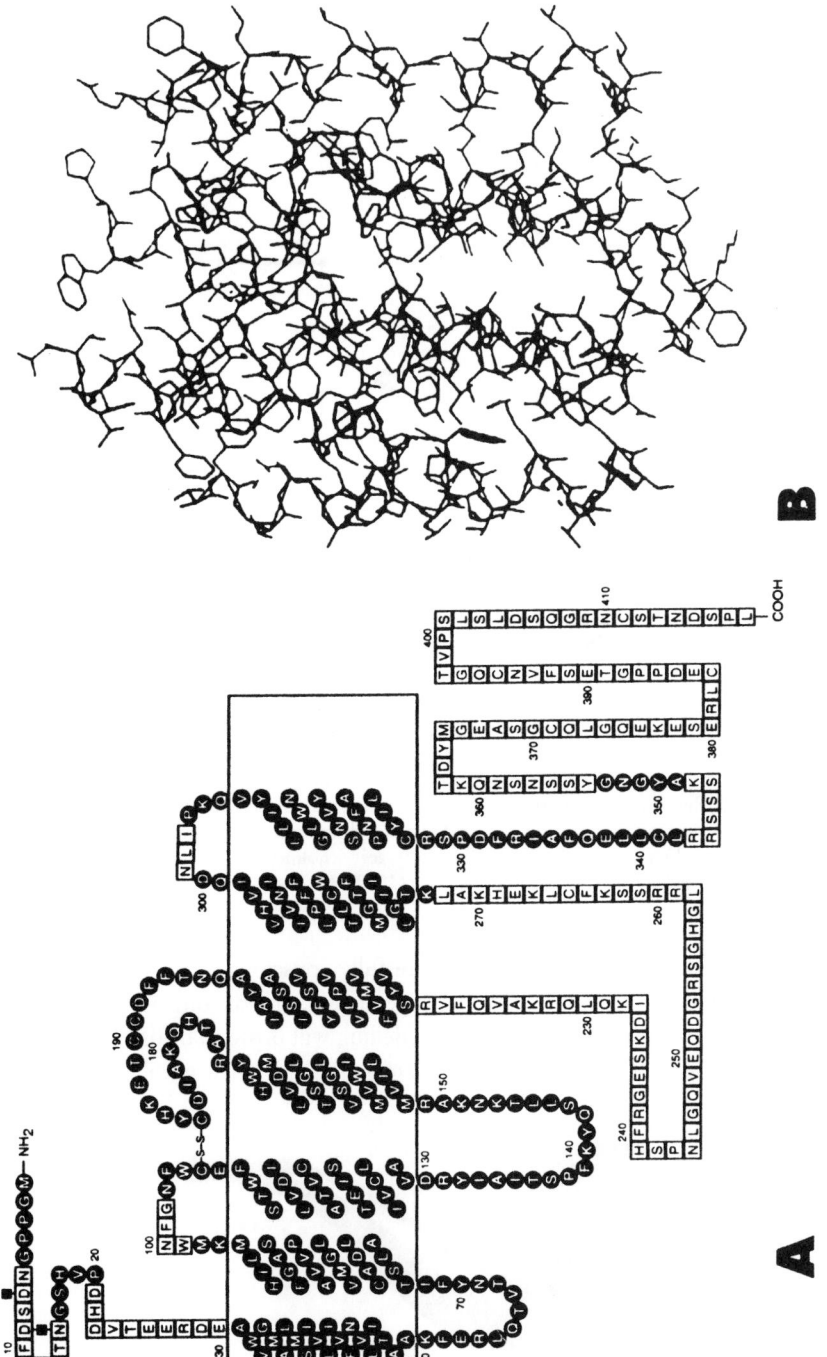

Fig. 25.9 Two dimensional (A) and three-dimensional (B) models of a GPCR.

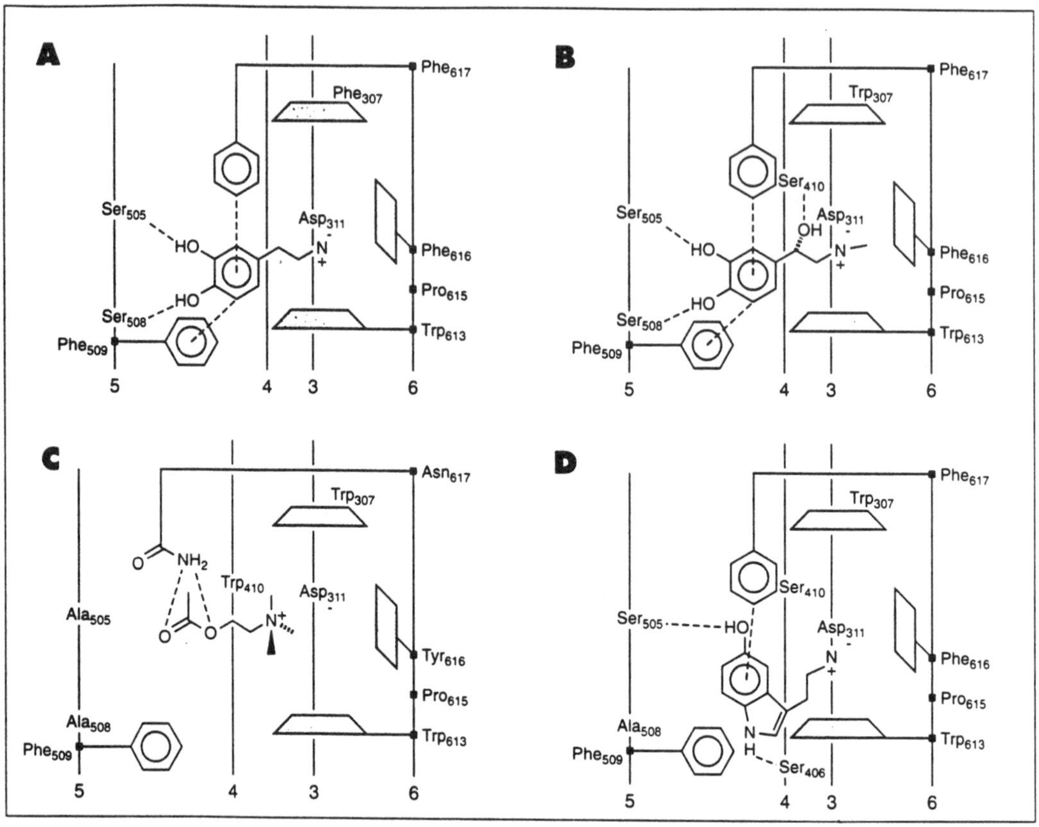

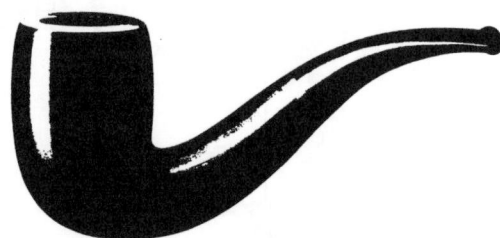

A Phe617, Phe307, Ser505, Asp311, Phe616, Pro615, Ser508, Trp613, Phe509 — 5 4 3 6

B Phe617, Trp307, Ser410, Ser505, Asp311, OH, Phe616, Pro615, Ser508, Trp613, Phe509 — 5 4 3 6

C Asn617, Trp307, NH2, Trp410, Asp311, Ala505, O, Tyr616, Pro615, Ala508, Trp613, Phe509 — 5 4 3 6

D Phe617, Trp307, Ser410, Ser505, Asp311, Phe616, Pro615, Ala508, Trp613, Phe509, Ser406 — 5 4 3 6

Fig. 25.10 Schematic representation of predicted neurotransmitter binding sites. Helix axes are represented as vertical lines and numbered 1 to 7. Residues surrounding the neurotransmitter are displayed schematically and numbered in a coded maner: the first digit indicates the transmembrane domain and the next two digits correspond to the rank of the residue un this domain. (A) Dopamine; (B) adrenaline; (C) acetylcholine; (D) serotonin. (Reproduced with the permission of the authors and publisher from *Médecine/Sciences* (1993) **9**: 31–40).

three-dimensional structure. As long as scientists are fully conscious of the limits of the methods and tools being used and of the models they have generated, and as long as they give priority to experimental validation of these models, protein modelling will prove to be of extraordinary value.

As a final warning, I would recommend readers to post above their graphics computer a copy of Magritte's painting, just in case!

Ceci n'est pas une pipe.

Fig. 25.11 'La Trahison des Images' (The Perfidy of Images) — Magritte.

REFERENCES

1. Humblet, C. and Marshall, G. (1980) Pharmacophore identification and receptor mapping. *Annu. Rep. Med. Chem.* **15**: 267–276.
2. Kollman, P. A. (1994) Theory of macromolecule–ligand interactions. *Curr. Op. Struct. Biol.* **4**: 240–245.
3. Beveridge, D. L. and Ravishanker, G. (1994) Molecular dynamics studies of DNA. *Curr. Op. Struct. Biol.* **4**: 246–255.
4. Michel, F. and Westhof, E. (1994) Slippery substrates. *Nature Struct. Biol.* **1**: 5–7.
5. Branden, C. and Tooze, J. (1991) *Introduction to Protein Structure*. Garland, New York.
6. (a) NBRF/PI, National Biomedical Research Foundation, 3900 Reservoir Road, NW. Washington, DC 20007, USA. (b) EMBL database, European Molecular Biology Laboratory, Postfach 10.22009, 6900 Heidelberg, Germany. (c) GenBank database, IntelliGenetics, Inc., 700 El Camino Real East, Mountain View, CA 94040, USA
7. Kolinski, A. and Skolnick, J. (1994) Simulations of protein folding. I. Lattice model and interaction scheme. *Proteins: Struct., Funct. Gen.* **18**: 338–352.
8. Greer, J. (1981) Comparative model building of the mammalian serine proteases. *J. Mol. Biol.* **153**: 1027–1042.
9. Sali, A., Overington, J. P., Johnson, M. S. and Blundell, T. (1990) From comparisons of protein sequences and structures to protein modelling and design. *Trends Biol. Sci.* **15**: 235–240.
10. Matthews, B. and Rossmann, M. G. (1985) Comparison of protein structures. *Methods Enzymol.* **115**: 397–420.
11. Jones, T. A. and Thirup, S. (1986) Using known substructures in protein model building and crystallography. *EMBO J.* **5**: 819–822.
12. Shenkin, P. S., Yarmush, D. L., Fine, R. M., Wang, H. J. and Levinthal, C. (1987) Predicting antibody hypervariable loop conformation. *Biopolymers* **26**: 2053, 2085.
13. Dunbrack, R. L. and Karplus, M. (1994) Conformational analysis of the backbone-dependent rotamer preferences of protein side-chains. *Nature Struct. Biol.* **1**: 334–339.
14. Genetics Computer Group: Sequence analysis software package, University of Wisconsin, Biotechnology Center, 1710 University Avenue, Madison, Wisconsin 53705, USA.
15. Needleman, S. B. and Wunsch, C. D. (1970) A general method applicable to the search of similarities in the aminoacid sequence of two proteins. *J. Mol. Biol.* **48**: 443–453.
16. Chotia, C. and Lesk, A. M. (1986) The relation between the divergence of sequence and structure in proteins. *EMBO J.* **5**: 823–826.
17. Hubbard, T. J. and Blundell, T. L. (1987) Comparison of solvent inaccessible cores of homologous proteins: definitions useful for protein modelling. *Protein Eng.* **1**, 159–181.
18. Taylor W. R. (1988) Pattern matching methods in protein sequence comparison and structure prediction. *Protein Eng.* **2**: 77–86.
19. Kyte, J. and Doolittle R. F. (1982) A simple method for displaying the hydropathic character of a protein. *J. Mol. Biol.* **157**: 105–132.
20. Jähning, F. (1990) Structure predictions of membrane proteins are not that bad, *Trends in Biol. Sci.* **15**: 93–95.
21. Lim, V. J. (1974) Algorithms for prediction of α-helical and β-structural regions in globular proteins. *J. Mol. Biol.* **88**: 973–994.
22. Sali, A. and Blundell, T. L. (1990) Definition of general topical equivalence in protein structures. *J. Mol. Biol.* **212**: 403–428.
23. Chou, P. Y. and Fassman, G. D. (1974) Prediction of protein conformation. *Biochemistry.* **13**: 222–245.
24. Fasman, G. D. and Gilbert W. A. (1990) The prediction of transmembrane protein sequences and their conformation: an evaluation. *Trends Biol. Sci.* **15**: 89–92.
25. Garnier, J., Osguthorpe, D. J. and Robson, B. (1978) Analysis of the accuracy and implications of simple methods for predicting the secondary structure of globular proteins. *J. Mol. Biol.* **120**: 97–120.
26. Eisenberg, D., Weiss, R. M. and Terwilliger, T. C. (1984) The hydrophobic moment detects periodicity in protein hydrophobicity. *Proc. Natl Acad. Sci. USA* **81**: 140–144.

27. Holley, L. H. and Karplus, M. (1989) Protein secondary structure prediction with a neural network. *Proc. Natl Acad. Sci. USA.* **86**: 152–156.

28. Lemesle-Varloot, L., Henrissat, B., Gaboriaud, C., Bissery, V., Morgat, A. and Mornon, J. P. (1990) Hydrophobic cluster analysis: procedure to derive structural and functional information from 2D-representation of protein sequences. *Biochimie* 72: 555–574.

29. SYBYL molecular modelling software, Tripos Associates Inc., St Louis MO 62117, USA.

30. Insight/Discover, Biosym, Inc., 9605 Scranton Rd, suite 101, San Diego, CA 92121, USA.

31. CHARMm/QUANTA, Molecular Simulations, MSI AG, Margarethenstrasse 47, CH-4053 Basel, Switzerland.

32. MAD/TSAR, Oxford Molecular Ltd, Magdalen Centre, Oxford Science Park, Stanford-on-Thames, Oxford OX4 4GA, England.

33. Luger, K., Szadkowski, H. and Kirschner K. (1990) An 8-fold βα-barrel protein with redundant folding possibilities. *Protein Eng.* **3**: 249–258.

34. Ratner, L., Haseltine, W, Patarea, R. *et al.* (1985) Complete nucleotide sequence of the AIDS virus, HTLV-III. *Nature* **313**: 277–286.

35. Pearl, L. H. and Taylor, W. (1987) A structural model for the retroviral proteases. *Nature* **329**: 351–354.

36. Weber, I. T., Miller, M., Jaskolski, M., Leis, J., Skalka, A. M. and Wlodawer, A. (1989) Molecular modeling of the HIV-1 protease and its substrate binding site. *Science* 243: 928–931.

37. Wlodawer, A., Miller, M., Jaskolski, M., Sathyanarayana, B., Baldwin, E., Weber, I., Selk, L., Clawson, L., Schneider, J. and Kent, S. (1989) Conserved folding in retroviral proteases: crystal structure of a synthetic HIV-1 protease. *Science* **245**: 616–621.

38. Hibert, M., Trumpp-Kallmeyer, S., Bruinvels, A. and Hoflack, J. (1991) Three-dimensional models of neurotransmitter G protein-coupled receptors. *Mol. Pharmacol.* **40**: 8–15.

39. Trumpp-Kallmeyer, S., Hoflack J., Bruinvels A. and Hibert M. (1992) Modelling of G protein-coupled receptors: application to dopamine, adrenaline, serotonin, acetylcholine and mammalian opsin receptors. *J. Med. Chem.* **35**: 3448–3462.

40. Hoflack, J., Trumpp-Kallmeyer, S. and Hibert M. (1993) Molecular modelling of G-protein-coupled receptors. In Kubinyi, H. (ed.) *3D QSAR in Drug Design: Theory, Method and Applications.* Escom, Leiden.

41. Lefkowitz, E. J. and Caron, M. G. (1988) Adrenergic receptor model for the study of receptor coupled to guanide nucleotides regulatory proteins. *J. Biol. Chem.* **263**: 4993–4996.

42. Dixon, R. A. F. and Strader, C. D. (1988) Structure and function of G protein-coupled receptors. *Annu. Rep. Med. Chem.* **23**: 221–223.

43. Henderson, R. J., Baldwin, J., Ceska, T. H., Zemlin, F., Beckman, L. and Downing, K. (1990) Model for the structure of bacteriorhodopsin based on high resolution cryomicroscopy. *J. Mol. Biol.* **213**: 899–929.

44. Weiner, S. J. and Kollman, P. A. (1986) An all atom force field for simulations of proteins and nucleic acids. *J. Comput. Chem.* 7: 230–252.

45. Schertler, G., Villa, C. and Henderson, R. (1993) Projection structure of rhodopsin. *Nature* 362: 770–772.

46. Tota, M., Candelore, M., Dixon, R. A. F. and Strader, C. (1991) Biophysical and genetic analysis of the ligand binding site of beta-adrenoceptor. *Trends Pharmacol. Sci.* **12**: 4–6.

47. Savarese, T. and Fraser C. (1992) In vitro mutagenesis in the search for structure–function relationship among G protein-coupled receptors. *Biochem. J.* **283**: 1–19.

48. Hibert, M., Hoflack, J., Trumpp-Kallmeyer, S., Paquet, J. L., Leppik, R., Barberis, C., Mouillac, B., Chini, B. and Jard, S. (1995) 3D models of hormone receptors: experimental validation. *Eur. J. Med. Chem.* **30:** 189–199.

49. Mouillac, B., Chini, B., Jard, S., Balestre, M. N., Elands, J., Trumpp-Kallmeyer, S., Hoflack, J., Hibert, M., Jard, S. and Barberis, C. (1995) The binding site of neuropeptide vasopressin V1a receptor. *J. Biol. Chem.* **27:** 1–7.

26

The Transition from Agonist to Antagonist Activity: Symmetry and Other Considerations

DAVID J. TRIGGLE

One side will make you grow taller, and the other side will make you grow shorter.
One side of what?, the other side of what?, thought Alice.
Lewis Carroll (1832–1898), *Alice's Adventures in Wonderland*

I. INTRODUCTION

Receptors are chiral entities and the interactions of many drugs and ligands at specific sites exhibit chirality of interaction.[1–3] Indeed, so common is this chirality of interaction that its occurrence is frequently used as a major index of discrete drug–receptor interactions in quantitative receptor analyses including, for example, receptor expression and radioligand binding assays. Chirality of drug–receptor interaction is the rule rather than the exception.[4]

The recognition that enantiomeric and diastereomeric drugs may differ both quantitatively and qualitatively in their therapeutic and toxic effects has generated considerable interest at the

THE PRACTICE OF MEDICINAL CHEMISTRY
ISBN 0-12-744640-0

regulatory level. Surveys of the chiral nature of natural/semisynthetic and totally synthetic drugs reveal that, as anticipated, the majority of the former are chiral and available as single enantiomers or isomers. For synthetic chiral drugs the majority are still available as racemates; however, the extent of availability of chiral drugs is increasing.[5] With new regulatory demands it is likely that there will be an increasing introduction of single-isomer species both as existing and as new chemical entities.[3,6–8] Accordingly, issues of the stereochemistry of drug–receptor interactions *and* of quantitative and qualitative differences between drug isomers will continue to assume increasing scientific and clinical importance.

The concept of specificity in drug–receptor interactions was certainly quite explicit in early considerations of these interactions. Thus, Crum-Brown and Fraser in their pioneering structure–activity studies on alkaloidal agents implicitly defined stereoselectivity as a component of the relationship between chemical constitution and biological activity.[9] Similarly, Paul Ehrlich and John Newton Langley in their pioneering work defining receptors recognized the importance of specific receptor-mediated interactions[10] mediated through 'a law for which both their (drugs') relative mass and chemical affinity for the substance (receptor) are factors',[11] and the significance of the receptor as a transducer which 'receives the stimulus and, by transmitting it, causes contraction (response)'.[12]

Specificity, stereoselectivity and the factoring of ligands and drugs as agonists and antagonists with quantitative and qualitative differences in activities have thus long been recognized as fundamental properties of drug–receptor interactions. Increasingly, it is recognized that ligands need to be regarded as a continuum of agonist–partial agonist–antagonist. Furthermore, a

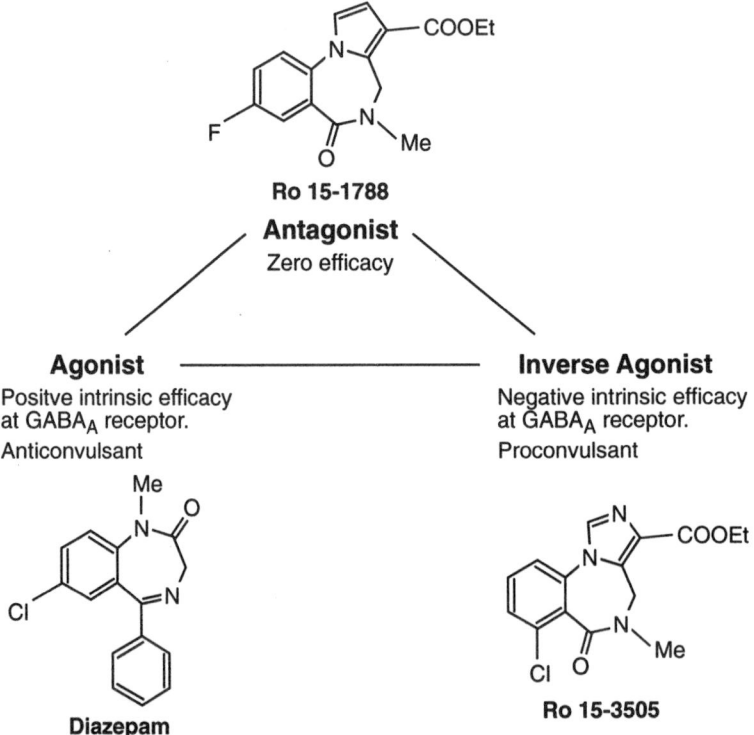

Figure 26.1 Agonist, antagonist and inverse agonist structures at the benzodiazepine receptor

symmetry is imposed on ligand–receptor interactions with the existence of agonists, antagonists and neutral antagonists. This concept is well illustrated with the benzodiazepine receptor, where agonists, antagonists and 'inverse agonists' serve as anticonvulsant, neutral and proconvulsant species, respectively (Fig. 26.1).[13]

II.   RECEPTORS AS CHIRAL ENTITIES

The inherent asymmetry of drug–receptor interactions derives from the chirality of the molecular building blocks of receptors — the L(S)-amino acids — although the origin of this fundamental chirality remains to be resolved.[14–16] Given that the underlying chirality of drug–receptor interactions derives from the chirality of the protein substrate, it may be expected that proteins derived from the enantiomeric D(R)-amino acids will have the same fundamental folding properties but will exhibit the opposite chirality from their naturally occurring counterparts.[15] Exactly this is achieved with HIV-1 protease (Fig. 26.2) where the D and L forms

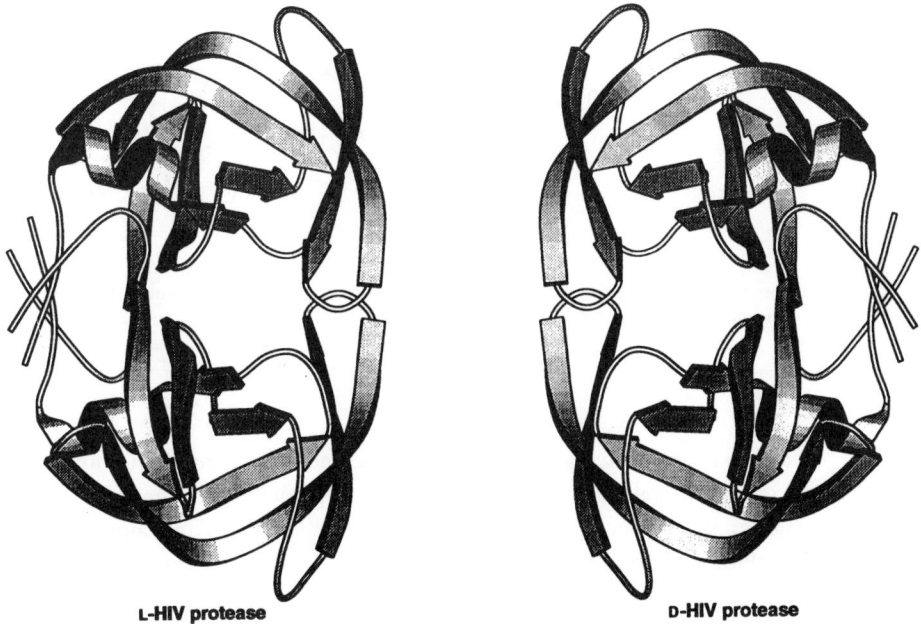

L-HIV protease   D-HIV protease

Figure 26.2   Ribbon representatives of the polypeptide backbone of the homodimeric HIV-protease. (Reproduced with permission from ref. 17.)

of the enzyme exhibit reciprocal chiral specificity with their substrates.[17] Such considerations are doubtless important to the drug regulatory agencies of alternate mirror worlds,[18] but there are also very important potential therapeutic considerations for the generation of peptide drugs with desirable biological properties. The Ca^{2+} binding protein calmodulin binds amphiphilic peptides as antagonists: the binding surface is remarkably sterically tolerant and similarly amphiphilic D-amino acid residue peptides also bind with high affinity to the native mellitin.[19] Experimental allergic encephalomyelitis is a major animal model of multiple sclerosis and the pathogenesis affecting the CD4⁺ helper T cell subset. Anti-CD4 antibodies are experimentally potentially effective therapeutic agents. A synthetic closed loop L-amino acid analogue of the CD4 surface in the complementarity-determining region (CDR3), a hairpin loop, was effective *in vitro* only, but the reverse engineered D-peptide was effective *in vivo* and was devoid of immunogenic activity (Fig. 26.3).[20]

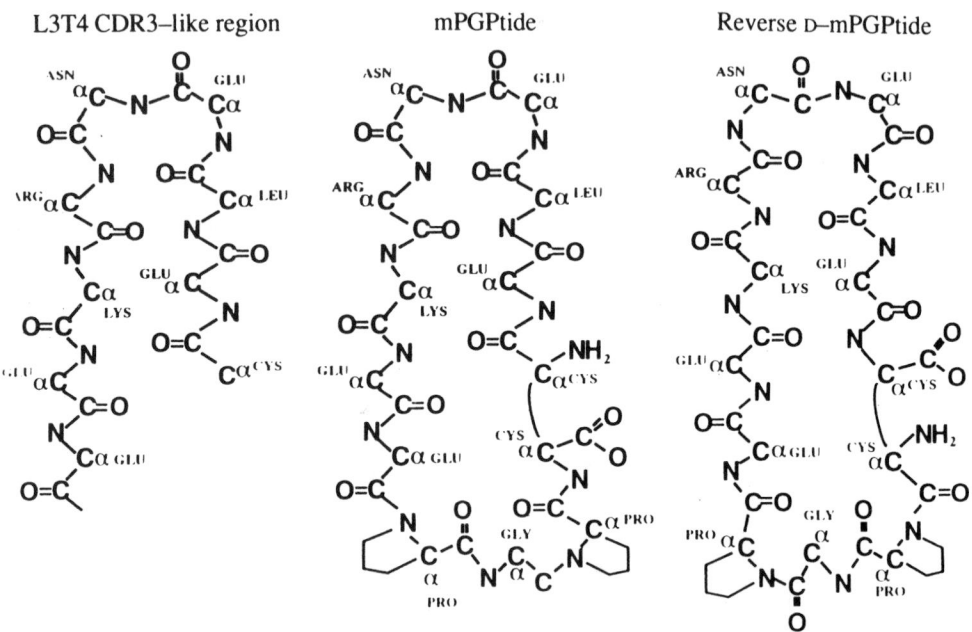

Figure 26.3 Structures of L-amino acid murine PGP (proline-glycine-proline) peptide analogue (mPGPtide) compared with the reverse D-amino acid structuree of the L3T4 CDR3 region of mouse CD4. (Reproduced with permission from ref. 20.)

Peptides containing D-amino acids are found in nature and it has long been known that they form part of bacterial cell walls and antibiotics including penicillin and gramicidin. Peptides containing D residues are, however, also found in vertebrate species. Thus, amphibians secrete opiod peptides including dermorphin (Tyr-D-Ala-Phe-Gly-Tyr-Pro-Ser-amide) from the skin secretions of *Phyllomedusa sauvagei*; dermorphin is some 1000 times more potent than morphine as an analgesic.[21,22] This and related peptides are apparently biosynthesized by post-translational processing of the precursor L-peptides.

There is ample documentation of the general chirality of drug interactions at many different receptor types and subtypes[1,23] In principle, isomers may differ in biological activities in several ways:

(1) Both (all) isomers are equally active and there is no observed stereochemistry of interaction.
(2) The isomers differ quantitatively in their activities: in the extreme situation one isomer may not exhibit detectable biological activity.
(3) The isomers differ qualitatively in their activities and the isomers exhibit distinct biological properties.

Examples of all of these situations are known. Of particular interest are those instances where isomers may exhibit agonist, partial agonist or antagonist properties. This can be seen with isoproterenol where the (−)- and (+)-enantiomers are agonist and antagonist, respectively, at α-adrenoceptors.[1] In this same series of catecholamines derived from norepinephrine with increasing *N*-alkyl substitution, there is both a progressive loss of α-stimulant activity and an increase in α-blocking activity with an inversion in stereoselectivity (Table 26.1). A further example is provided by the cardiovascular α,β-blocker labetalol, with two asymmetric centres and with different stereochemical demands on these adrenoceptors (Table 26.2). At the 5-HT$_{1A}$ receptor there are several examples of opposing enantiomeric activities (Fig. 26.4).[2] Both enantiomers of 11-hydroxy-10-methylaporphine bind strongly to these receptors, but the (*S*)- and (*R*)-enantiomers are antagonist and agonist respectively.[24,25] Of particular interest is UH-301, inactive as a racemate, but with enantiomers of opposing agonist and antagonist activity.[26] A number of similar examples are known with drugs that affect ion channels.[27,28]

Table 26.1   Stereoselectivity indices of catecholamines at α- and β-adrenoceptors.

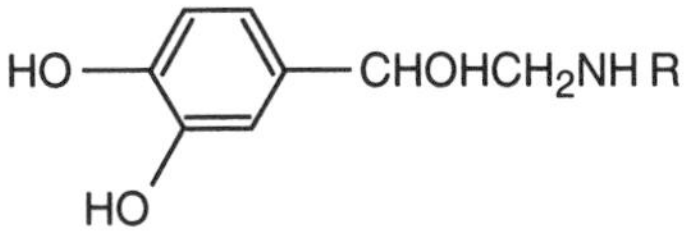

R	α	Ratio (−):(+)	β
H	4		20
Me	8		50
Pr^i		(−)agonist : (+)antagonist	> 500
—CHMeCH$_2$—⬡—OH	0.1		>1000

Data from Ariens.[1]

Table 26.2   Stereoselectivity of labetalol stereoisomers at adrenoceptors.

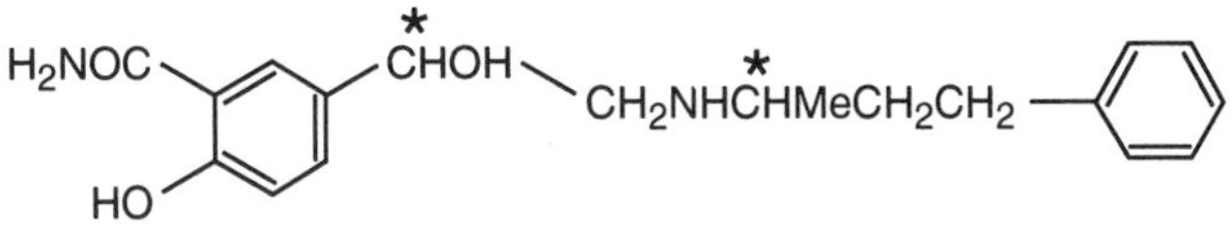

Stereoisomer (*,*)	α$_1$ (rabbit aorta) pA_2	β$_1$ (guinea pig atrium) pA_2	β$_2$ (guinea pig trachea) pA_2
RR	5.87	**8.26**	**8.52**
SS	5.98	6.43	<6.0
RS	5.5	6.97	6.33
SR	**7.18**	6.37	<6.0

Data from Ariëns.[1]

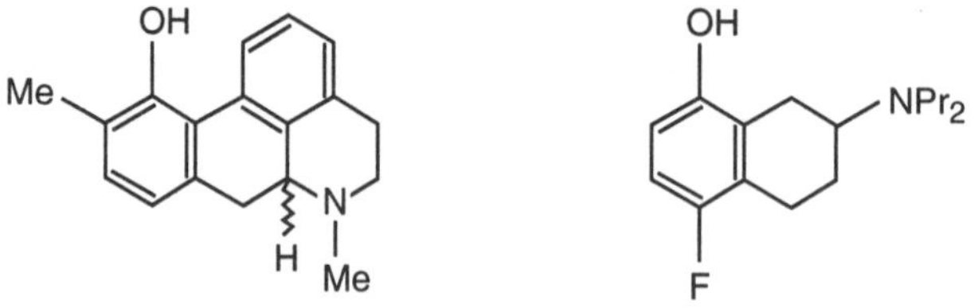

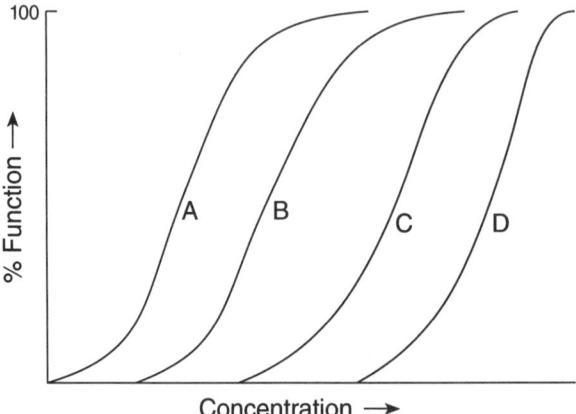

11-Hydroxy-10-Methylaporphine　　　　　　　**UH-301**

Figure 26.4　Ligands active at the 5-HT$_{1A}$ receptor.

III.　PROBLEMS OF DEFINITION

The linkage of biological response to the initial drug–receptor interaction and the definition of quantitative relationships presents a number of major problems. Response is the end stage of a multistep pathway:

$$A + \text{Receptor} \longrightarrow [A\text{–Receptor}] \xrightarrow{\text{intermediate steps}} \text{Response}$$

Accordingly, there may well be several possible dose-response curves defining the relationships between drug concentration and response (Fig. 26.5). Many specific examples have been provided and analysed.[29]

Figure 26.5　Dose–response curves for agonist–receptor interaction depicting binding, serveral intermediate steps and final response. A represents a tissue response, B and C biochemical events, and D binding of the agonist.

The dose–response curves may depend upon the cellular concentration of receptor or coupling protein: a drug which appears as an agonist in one cell or tissue may appear as an antagonist in another preparation. This is well illustrated with receptors coupled to G-proteins where the definition of agonists, partial agonists and antagonists can vary between systems according to the nature and stoichiometries of the component coupled entities.[30] Figure 26.6 depicts muscarinic receptor-mediated increases in phosphatidylinositol metabolism and inhibition of adenylate cyclase before and after reduction of receptor number by alkylation with

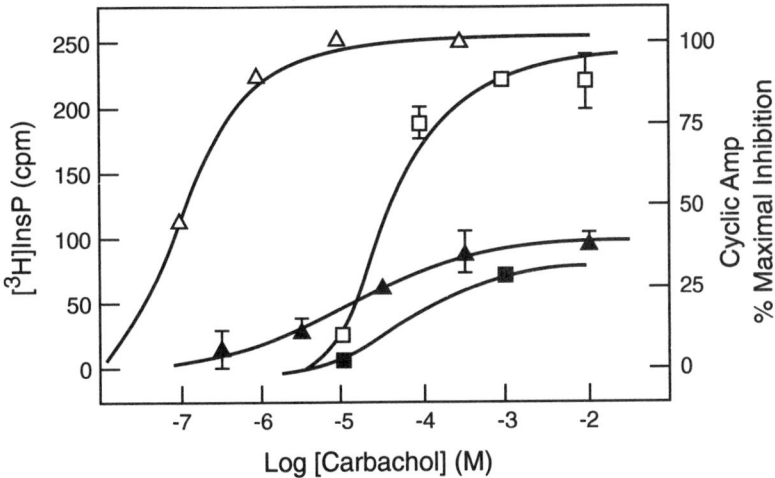

Figure 26.6 Dose–response curves for carbachol-mediated inhibition of cAMP formation (△,▲) and stimulation of phosphatidylinositol (InsP) hydrolosis (□,■) before (open symbols) and after (closed symbols) receptor inactivitation in chick heart cells. (Reproduced with permission from ref. 31.)

an irreversible receptor antagonist.[31] Carbachol, a full agonist, has been converted to a partial agonist by this process. Similarly, in a cell line expressing only the cloned m2 muscarinic receptor, quite separate dose–response curves occur for carbachol-mediated inhibition of adenylate cyclase and stimulation of phosphatidylinositol turnover (Fig. 26.7).[32] This reflects the different efficiencies of coupling of a single receptor subtype to different G-protein effectors.

In the immune system a T cell lymphokine, interleukin-2 (IL-2) stimulates both the differentiation of antigen-stimulated B cells into antigen-secreting species and their progression through the cell cycle. The IL-2 receptor consists of two components, 75 kDa and 55 kDa, that interact cooperatively to form the high-affinity binding site. The 75 kDa component transduces the signal for proliferation and J-chain (antibody) gene activation and the 55 kDa component

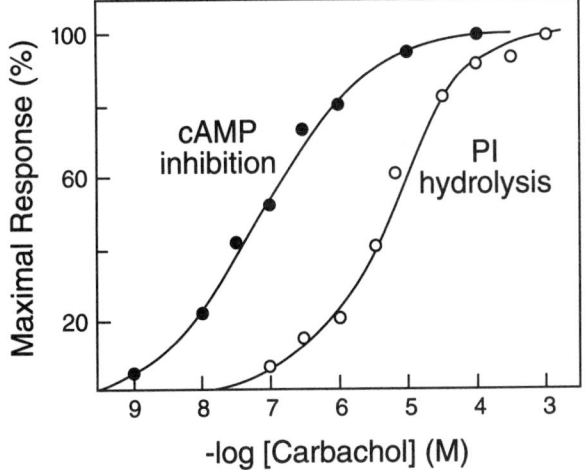

Figure 26.7 Dose-response curves for carbachol-mediated inhibition of cAMP formation and stimulation of phosphtidylinostil (PI) hydrolysis in clonal m₂-muscarinic receptors. (Reproduced with permission from ref. 32.)

amplifies the binding affinity of IL-2. Both events are thus mediated through a single receptor and transduction pathway and a common tyrosine kinase mediates different translations of a single message.[33]

That competitive agonists and antagonists share common binding sites has long been accepted and validated in a number of receptor systems, notably the G protein-coupled receptors for the small neurotransmitters including norepinephrine and acetylcholine.[34]

Occupancy of a common site is not, however, an obligatory prerequisite for agonist/antagonist interactions. For the substance P receptor (neurokinin-1), mutants have been constructed that bind the nonpeptide antagonist CP 96345, but not substance P itself (Fig. 26.8).[35] Similarly, the binding of the benzodiazepine antagonists L 365260 and L 364718 to the brain cholecystokinin B/gastrin receptors in humans and rodents differs according to the residue at equivalent positions 319 (human) and 355 (rodent) — valine and leucine, respectively. However, agonist binding is unaffected.[36]

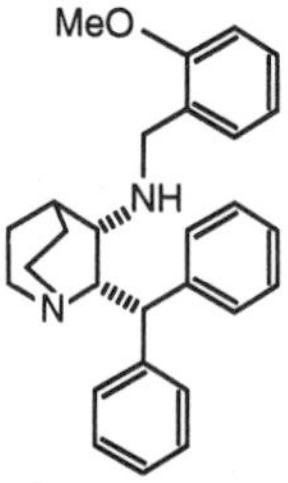

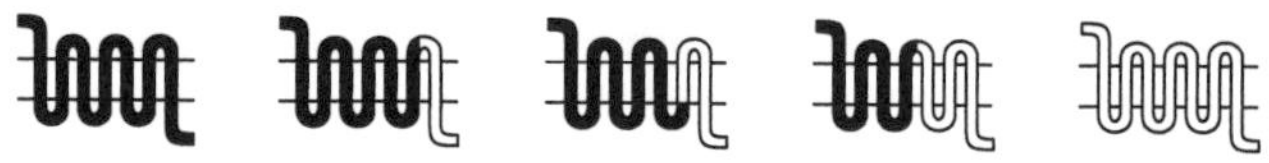

	Wild type NK-1	CR NK1 (NK3-TM7)	CR NK1 (NK3-TM6-7)	CR NK1 (NK3-TM5-7)	Wild type NK-3
Substance P	0.14±0.03	0.49±0.04	1.1±0.2	0.9±0.1	300±80
Eledoisin	16±5	4.6±1.3	12±3.5	4.5±0.6	4.7±1.1
(CP 96345)	14±6	5.4±0.9	330±60	>>10,000	>>10,000

Figure 26.8 Substance P and CP 96345 interaction (K_0, nM) at chimeric NK-1/NK-3 receptors. (Data from Getler et al.[35])

Other factors that determine the potency and the quality of a drug–receptor interaction include receptor clustering whereby ligand–induced association of receptors initiates response,[37] membrane potential where agonist–antagonist transitions occur according to the polarized or depolarized state of the cell,[27,28] and mutations in receptors whereby receptors may become constitutively active in the absence of activator.[38]

IV. QUANTITATIVE APPROACHES TO AGONISM AND ANTAGONISM

To measure agonism and antagonism it is necessary to define both the affinity of the ligand for its receptor site *and* the ability of the ligand to initiate biological response. These parameters are not simple to measure without ambiguity, but quantitative determinations are necessary to facilitate drug discovery and evaluation.[29,39] The roles of both agonist and antagonist drugs in

Table 26.3   Roles of agonists and antagonists in receptor discrimination studies

Binding	Function
1. Radioactive ligand selective affinity	Agonist selective affinity intrinsic efficacy
2. Antagonist selective affinity	Antagonist selective affinity
3. Receptors relative density	Receptors relative density coupling to effectors
4. –	Effector transduction coupling efficiency

From Kenakin and Bond.[40]

the drug discovery process through binding and functional studies illustrate the discriminant role that agonists may play (Table 26.3).[40,41]

In the original formalism of Clark it was assumed that the dose–response relationship represented an occupancy curve and that biological response was directly proportional to receptor occupancy:[42]

$$\frac{R_A}{R_{max}} = \frac{[R.A]}{[R_{tot}]} \tag{1}$$

Clearly, this simple relationship does not accommodate the frequently observed phenomenon in homologous series of partial agonists and a transition from agonism to antagonism (Fig. 26.9).

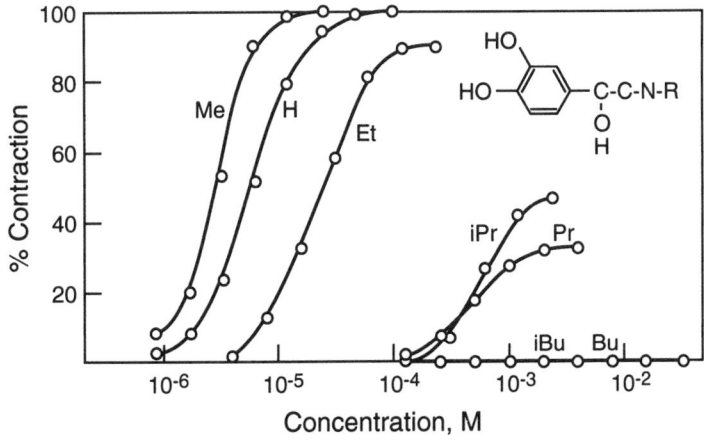

Figure 26.9   Dose–response curves for a homologous series of catecholamines depicting the gradual transistion in agonist properties with increasing molecular substitution. Quite frequently the molecules without detectable agonist activity function as competitive antagonists, indicating that they have not lost receptor recognition capacity.

The term 'intrinsic activity' (i.a.) introduced by Ariens[43] provides a phenomenological descriptor for the relative ability of a drug to produce a response relative to some standard where i.a. = 1:

$$\frac{R_A}{R_{max}} = i.a. \frac{[R.A]}{[R_{tot}]} \tag{2}$$

The experimental observations indicating that a 'receptor reserve' exists whereby only fractional occupancy of receptors might be necessary to produce maximum biological response was accommodated by Stephenson[44] in his parameter stimulus [S] defined as

$$S = e\frac{[R.A]}{[R_{tot}]} \tag{3}$$

where e is a dimensionless parameter (efficacy), that denotes the ability of a drug to produce response, whereby

$$\frac{R_A}{R_{max}} = f[S] = fe\frac{[A]}{[A] + K_A} \tag{4}$$

By dissociating receptor stimulus and tissue response as directly proportional quantities, Stephenson accommodated the existence of a receptor reserve. An immediate corollary of this treatment is that response can be generated from drugs with low efficacy and high receptor occupancy or with high efficacy and low receptor occupancy. With the introduction of the term intrinsic efficacy, ϵ, by Furchgott,[45]

$$\epsilon = \frac{e}{[R_{tot}]} \tag{5}$$

where (R_{tot}) is the total tissue concentration of receptors,

$$\text{Response} = f\epsilon\ \frac{[R_{tot}]}{1} + \frac{K_A}{[A]} \tag{6}$$

A further modification of this approach may be seen in the operational model of Black and Leff.[46] In this model the initiation of response may be viewed as two successive saturable hyperbolic functions. First, the binding of drug to receptor and, second, the interaction of the drug–receptor complex ('operational binding') with one or more response elements or coupling functions (adenylyl cyclase, ion channel, etc.) from which the biological response is initiated. Accordingly,

$$\frac{R_A}{R_{max}} = [A]\ \epsilon/K_A + (\epsilon + 1\ )\ [A] \tag{7}$$

where ϵ is equal to R_{max}/K_E and K_E is the value of [A.R] which generates 50% response.

The interactions of drugs with receptors is not, however, independent of changes in protein conformation and/or selective affinity of drugs for one or other interconvertible protein conformation. Accordingly, in a receptor existing in the R and T states, with an equilibrium constant L, the microscopic affinities of drugs will be given by K_{AR} and K_{AT} (Fig. 26.10). If R and T represent active and inactive conformations, respectively, of the receptor, then selective

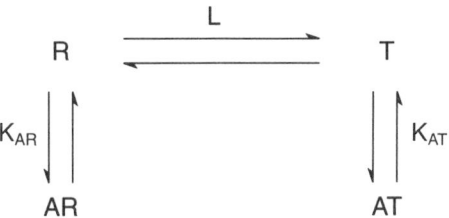

Figure 26.10   The allosteric model of drug–receptor interaction where the receptor exists (minimally) in two slots R and T. K_{AR} and K_{AT} are the equilibrium constants for drug (A) binding to slots R and T. L is the equilibrium constant of the R-to-T transition.

and nonselective interactions of drug with these states will be associated with varying degrees of agonism and antagonism and

$$\epsilon = \frac{K_{AR}}{K_{AT}} - 1 \tag{8}$$

V.   OPERATIONAL DEFINITIONS AND EXAMPLES

A.   G-protein-coupled receptors

The G-proteins are a major family of heterotrimers made up of α-, β- and γ-subunits which cycle between GDP- and GTP-ligated states and which have intrinsic GTPase activity.[47–49] This enzyme activity is critical to the cascade initiated by receptor activation and to the termination of the events, and is mediated by a specific domain of the G_a subunit that is regulated by interaction with an activated receptor.[50,51] This interaction initiates a cycle in which GDP is replaced by GTP to produce an active GTP-α subunit and a β,γ subunit which interact with discrete effectors (Fig. 26.11). These systems provide additional definitions of both efficacy and of agonist–antagonist transitions. For β-adrenergic and opiate receptors coupled through $G_{a(s)}$ and $G_{a(i)}$ to stimulate or inhibit adenylyl cyclase, intrinsic activity at the level of cyclase correlates well with intrinsic activity at the level of GTPase (Fig. 26.12).[52,53]

The function of the agonist in these G-protein-coupled receptors is to promote coupling of the receptor to G_a in a ternary complex of ligand, receptor and G-protein. This coupling is achieved dominantly through the third cytoplasmic loop of the seven-helical transmembrane receptor. The activated coupling conformation of the receptor is achievable in the absence of agonists in constitutively active mutants of α- and β-adrenoceptors.[38,54,55] Thus, in the α_2 receptor a single mutation in this loop of threonine[38] produces constitutively active receptors that mediate agonist-independent inhibition of adenylate cyclase. Constitutively active β_2-adrenoceptors have been expressed *in vivo* where they increase myocardial baseline function including adenylyl cyclase and contractile activity; this enhanced baseline activity is independent of endogenous catecholamines and is insensitive to neutral antagonists such as propranolol.[56] It will be important to determine whether such constitutively active receptors may contribute, by virtue of their 'spontaneous activity', to disease states. Receptors active without ligands pose an interesting challenge to the definition of agonism and antagonism.

The ternary complex model of drug–receptor interactions also permits a symmetry-based view of agonists and antagonists in which agonists promote receptor–effector coupling, neutral

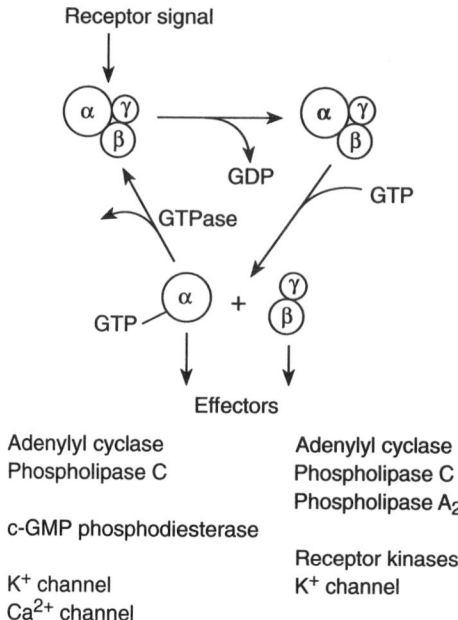

Figure 26.11 The receptor–G-protein sequence. An activated receptor interacts with the trimeric GDP-ligated receptor to produce an interchange of GDP and GTP and dissociation into the activated $G_\alpha GTP$ and $G_{\beta\gamma}$ subunits: these then interact with a variety of effectors. The activated receptor acts as a switch for the G-protein complex.

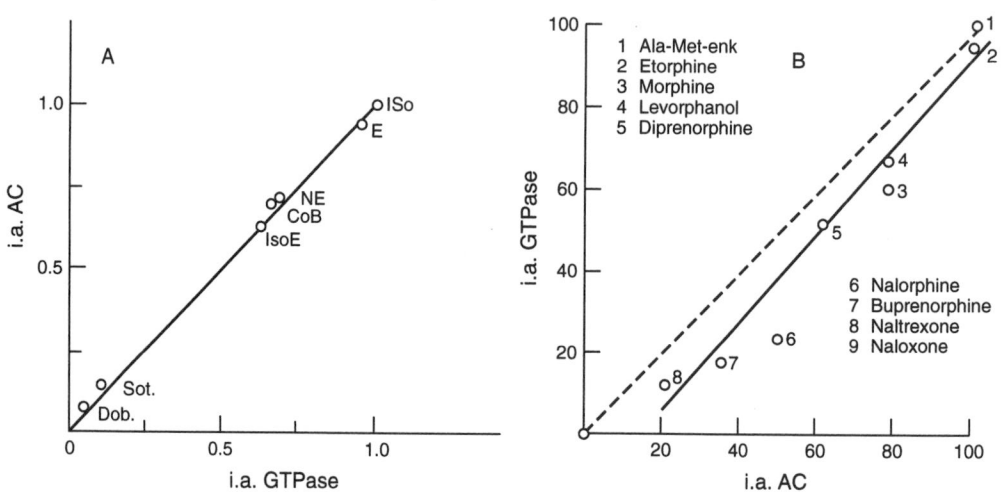

Figure 26.12 Correlations of intrinsic activities for agonists mediated via stimulation of adenylyl cyclase by catecholamine (A) or inhibition by opiates (B) with GTPase activity. (Reproduced from refs 52 and 53 with permission of the American Society of Biological Chemists.)

antagonists do not affect receptor–effector coupling but prevent the effect of agonists, and negative antagonists reduce spontaneous receptor–effector coupling.[57–59] In a constitutively active β_2-adrenoceptor mutant, some β-blockers, including betaxolol and ICI 118551, are negative antagonists that depress basal (spontaneous) adenylyl cyclase activity, a process that is competitively blocked by the neutral antagonist propranolol (Fig. 26.13).[60] Similarly, negative competitive antagonists have also been found for the G-coupled delta-opiate receptor.[61]

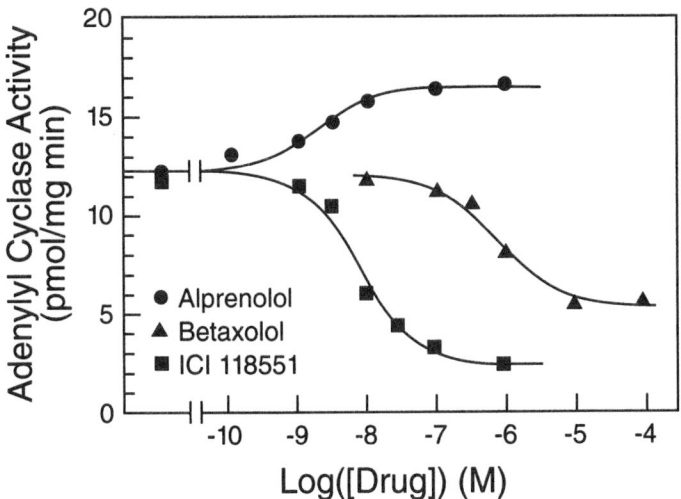

Figure 26.13 The actions of β-adrenoceptor antagonists on the activity of adenyl cyclase in constitutively active β_2-receptors expressed in CHO cells. (Reproduced with permission from ref. 60.)

B. Mono- and bivalent interactions

For a number of receptor systems, notably those for polypeptide hormones, receptor dimerization and aggregation appear to be critical components of the activation and transduction pathways.[37] For such systems, agonist-independent receptor activation and agonist–antagonist interconversion according to ligand geometry may both occur.

Gonadotropin-releasing hormone (GnRH; Fig. 26.14) stimulates pituitary luteinizing

pyroGlu-His-Trp-Ser-Tyr-Gly-Leu-Arg-Pro-Gly-CONH$_2$

GnRH : agonist

pyroGlu-His-Trp-Ser-Tyr-Lys

GnRH : antagonist

pyroGlu His-Trp-Ser-Tyr-Lys(12-15Å)Lys-Tyr-Ser-Trp-His-Glupyro

GnRH dimer : antagonist

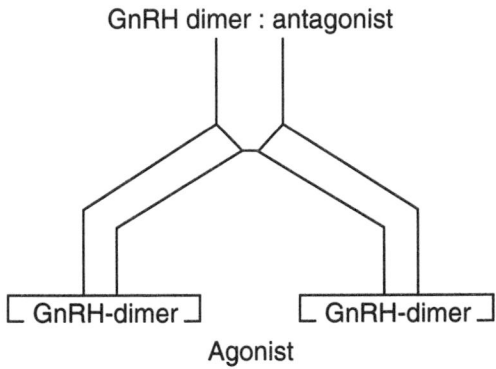

Figure 26.14 Studies of GnRH and a GnRH peptide antagonist. A dimer of the GnRH antagonist also serves as an antagonist, but when expressed as a divalent antibody it functions as an agonist. (Based on work by Conn and co-workers.[64])

hormone release by a process that involves receptor microassociation.[62,63] The hexapeptide D-pyroGlu-D-His-D-Trp-D-Ser-D-Tyr-D-Lys is an antagonist of GnRH with no detectable agonist-like properties. The dimeric hexapeptide (Fig. 26.14) is also an antagonist: however, the product of this dimeric antagonist and antibody to GnRH yields a species (Fig. 26.14) that functions as an agonist to release LH from pituitary cells.[64,65] An antagonist–agonist transition has thus been achieved through a symmetrical arrangement of monovalent antagonist species at a peptide receptor. Consistent with the hypothesis that the geometry of binding site occupancy is a critical determinant of agonist activity at GnRH receptors, dimeric analogues of the hormone separated by some 24 Å show increased activity relative to the parent monomer.[66]

C.   Receptor–ligand entities

Thrombin is a potent physiological activator of platelet aggregation, a signal critical to both haemostasis and thrombosis.[67,68] Additionally, thrombin plays a multiplicity of roles in inflammatory and repair responses.[69] These events are mediated through interactions at the thrombin receptor. This receptor is a member of the G-protein-coupled seven-transmembrane domain family which includes the receptors for many neurotransmitters and polypeptide hormones.[70,71]

The thrombin receptor activation process is quite remarkable. The large *N*-terminal region of the receptor contains within it both a proteolytic site 41 residues from the terminal *and* a masked endogenous activator. Cleavage at this site reveals a new *N* terminus which serves as a 'tethered' ligand to activate the receptor (Fig. 26.15).[72,73] Thus, the thrombin-activated receptor is actually a self-contained receptor–ligand (agonist) entity. The structure–function requirements for agonist activity of the proteolytically unmasked *N*-terminal peptide have been established:[70-73] the pentapeptide Ser-Phe-Leu-Leu-Arg-NH$_2$ is an agonist and the 14-residue Ser-Phe-Leu-Leu-Arg-Asn-Pro-Asn-Asp-Lys-Tyr-Glu-Pro-Phe-NH$_2$ is a full agonist. The critical domains responsible for peptide binding appear to be extracellular and associated with the extracellular loop linking transmembrane domains 4 and 5.[74]

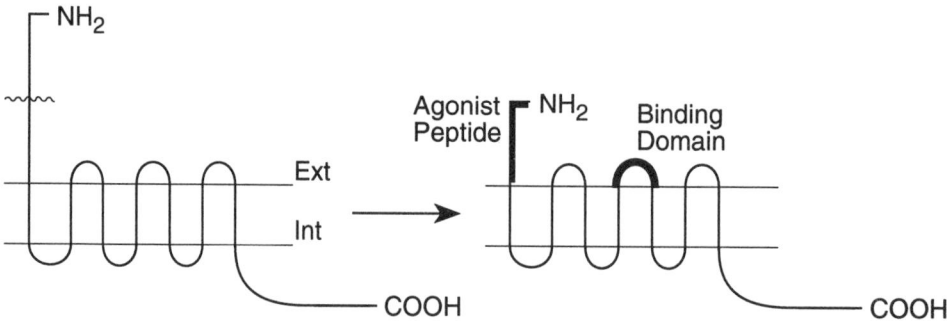

Figure 26.15 The thrombin receptor, subsequent to proleolytic cleavage, expresses an endogenous *N*-terminal sequence that functions as a tethered ligand.

The existence of a receptor which contains a permanently tethered agonist ligand and is activated by a necessarily all-or-none proteolytic process raises questions of fundamental significance to the issues of graded responses and termination of the responses initiated. How does a cell distinguish between low and high thrombin concentrations, since all receptors will ultimately be cleaved to generate the agonist peptide? A correlation has been observed between receptor cleavage and the accumulation of the messenger IP_3, indicating that each 'quantum' of phosphatidylinositol hydrolysis is followed by receptor turn-off despite the permanent presence of the built-in ligand.[75] Thus, the cells generate dose–response curves through different rates of receptor cleavage according to thrombin concentration, rather than through conventional fractional receptor occupancy. The presence of permanently tethered agonist ligands at this receptor raises the issue of how antagonists might be generated. The development of competitive antagonists would appear to be problematic.[75]

Analogous tethered ligands also exist for voltage-gated ion channels. Early work by Armstrong and Bezanilla[76] on the inactivation of K^+ channels led to a physical 'ball and chain model' whereby this cytoplasmic component would physically occlude the channel pore. This model has been confirmed by demonstrations that the *N*-terminal sequence of K^+ channel expressed by the Shaker gene of *Drosophila* carries the properties of voltage-dependent channel inactivation.[77,78] The *N*-terminal residues 1–19 are characterized by 11 consecutive hydrophobic or uncharged residues and a subsequent 8 hydrophilic and charged residues. This sequence could mimic the charged quaternary ammonium ions, including tetraethylammonium, known to produce open-channel block. Indeed, an *N*-terminal peptide alone can restore inactivation to K^+ channels mutated to a noninactivating state (Fig. 26.16). Since K^+ channels are believed to be tetrameric in the functional state, each heteromeric complex possesses, in principle, four

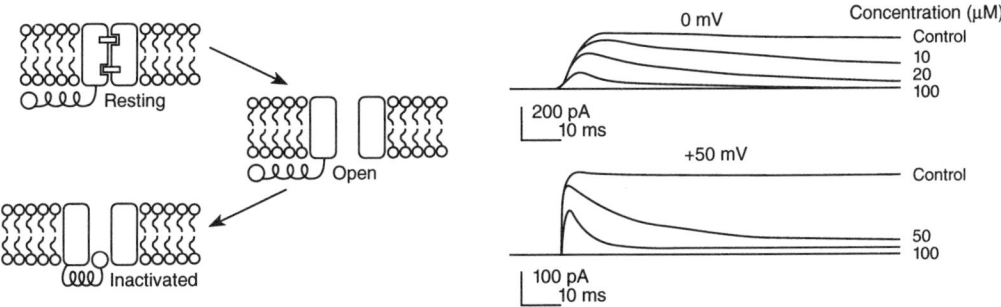

Figure 26.16 (a) Schematic representation of the 'ball and chain' model of the K^+ channel inactivation process depicting the *N*-terminal sequence as constituting the inactivation particle. (b) The effects of a peptide (administered intracellularly) representing the first 20 residues of the *N*-terminal region of the ShB K^+ channel (from *Drosophila*) on the mutant ShB K^+ channel (Δ6-46) expressed in *Xenopus*. (Reproduced with permission from ref. 78.)

tethered antagonist ligands: however, only one ligand is required to produce inactivation.[79] A similar tethered antagonist ligand also exists in Na^+ channels where the cytoplasmic loop linking domains III and IV of the channel protein is critical to the inactivation process. A peptide containing a hydrophobic sequence expressed in this region is capable of conferring inactivation properties on mutant noninactivating Na^+ channels.[80]

D. The immune receptor

Immune protection in mammalian species is afforded by the T and B lymphocytes. Antigen receptors on these lymphocytes are capable of recognizing virtually any molecule; the necessary diversity of receptors is generated during lymphocyte development by a selection sequence. The T cell recognition process is unique since it involves recognition of processed or degraded antigen by the T cell receptor (TCR) in association with molecules encoded by the major histocompatibilty complex (MHC) and further accessory species, including notably CD3. The MHC molecules are extremely polymorphic and serve as an effective guidance system for the T cells.[81] Given the diversity of both T cell receptors and MHC, it is critical that control processes be in place to avoid autoimmune responses.

The T cell recognition process has been considered to be a binary, or all-or-none, event. Either the processed and presented antigen is recognized and the immune responses are initiated, or it is not recognized and there is no corresponding initiation of response. The responses include Ca^{2+} mobilization, phosphatidylinositol turnover, protein kinase C translocation and cytokine secretion. However, the T cell system is analogous to the previously discussed pharmacological receptors since there exists a continuum of presented ligands with agonist, partial agonist and antagonist functions.[82] Analogues of immunogenic peptides in which the TCR contact residues have been altered show this spectrum of properties from full activation to full antagonism, a process depicted in Fig. 26.17.[82–84]

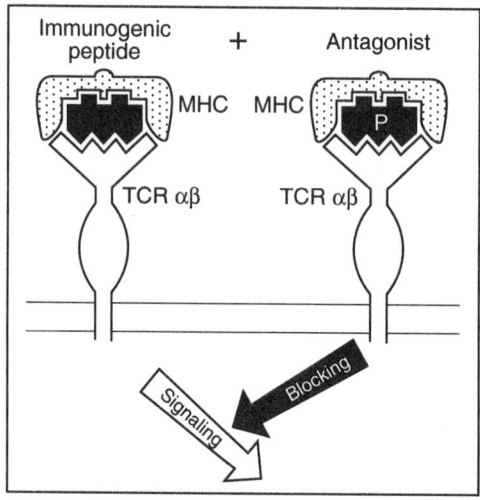

Figure 26.17   Representation of T cell agonism and antagonism. (Reproduced with permission from ref. 82.)

There are important therapeutic consequences of the concept of an agonist–antagonist continuum of analogue peptides at the T cell receptor. Antagonist species may be useful in the control of autoimmune diseases including experimental autoimmune encephalomyelitis and adjuvant arthritis.[85,86] Additionally, both the affinity of peptides and their agonist/antagonist quality may be important to the process of positive selection of T cells whereby precursor T cells mature, or do not mature (negative selection), according to the interaction with MHC self-alleles and peptide in the thymus. Accordingly, peptide ligands with low efficacy may mediate positive selection whereas high-efficacy ligands mediate negative selection and cell apoptosis.[87,88]

E.   Ion channels

Ion channels are pharmacological receptors. They exist as homologous protein families; they possess specific drug binding sites for both activator and antagonist ligands; some ion channels are directly linked to guanine nucleotide binding proteins; and they are regulated by both homologous and heterologous influences and during disease states.[27,28,89] In fact, ion channels are best regarded as multiple pharmacological receptors with a plethora of functional drug binding sites, as illustrated for the voltage-gated Ca^{2+} channel (Fig. 26.18). Since channels exist in a number of states or families of states — resting, open and inactivated — according to membrane potential and state of ligation,[90] the interpretation of structure–activity relationships may be complex. According to the modulated receptor treatment of drug–receptor interactions at ion channels, drugs may bind to or access preferentially one or other channel state, with the following consequences.[91–93]

(1)   Different channel states have different affinities for drugs
(2)   Drugs may exhibit structure–activity relationships, including stereochemistry, that exhibit qualitative and quantitative differences according to channel state.

These factors have been reviewed previously.[27,28,94] Two examples are illustrative. The local anaesthetic RAC 109 shows a stereoselectivity of blockade of voltage-gated Na^+ channels that differs according to stimulus mode (Table 26.4).[95] This may be interpreted as an absence of stereoselectivity when RAC 109 interacts with the resting channel state and an enhanced stereoselectivity upon interaction with the inactivated channel state. The 1,4-dihydropyridines constitute a potent series of activators and antagonists at the L-type of voltage-gated Ca^{2+} channel.[96,97] Of particular interest to this structure are observations that very small structural changes distinguish potent antagonists and activators *and* that in some series the enantiomeric forms have opposing biological activities (Fig. 26.19).[98–100] Of even greater interest, the property of channel activation/antagonism may be state-dependent and vary according to membrane

Table 26.4   Stereoselectivity of local anaesthetic action.

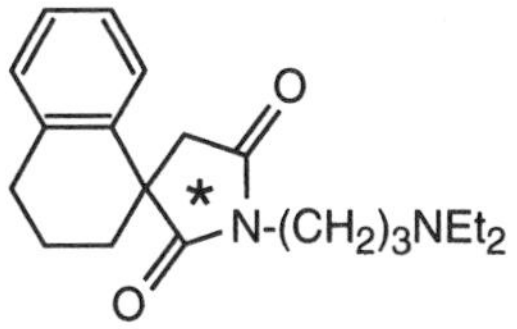

RAC 109 enantiomer	RAC 421 EC$_{50}$, (mmol^{-1})		
	Block at rest	Conditioned block $E_c = 0$ mV	$E_c = +80$ mV
RAC-109 (−)	0.85	0.14	0.034
RAC-109 (+)	1.30	0.79	0.49
RAC-421 (−)	1.48	0.10	0.042
RAC-421 (+)	2.09	0.98	0.42

Data from Yeh.[95]

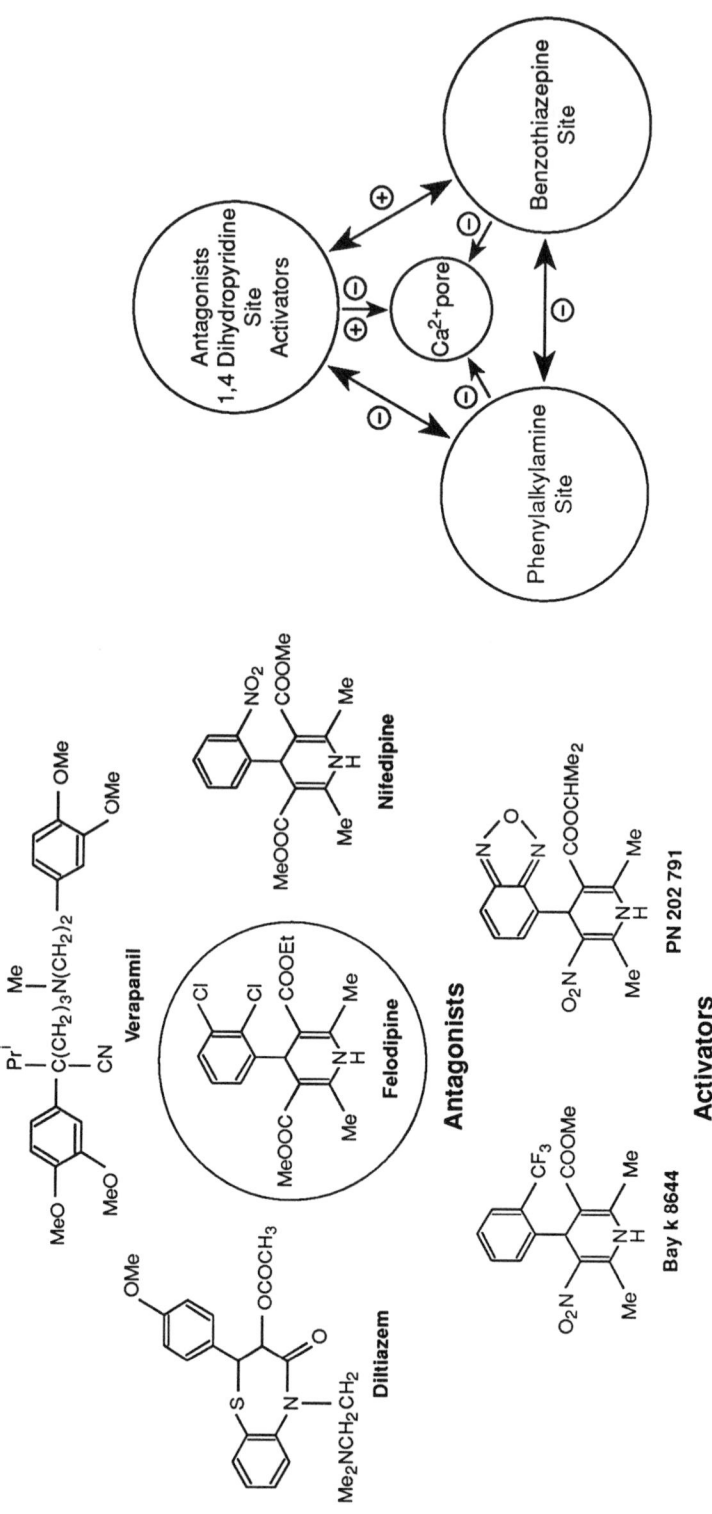

Figure 26.18 Multiple drug binding sites on the L-type voltage-gated Ca^{2+} channel

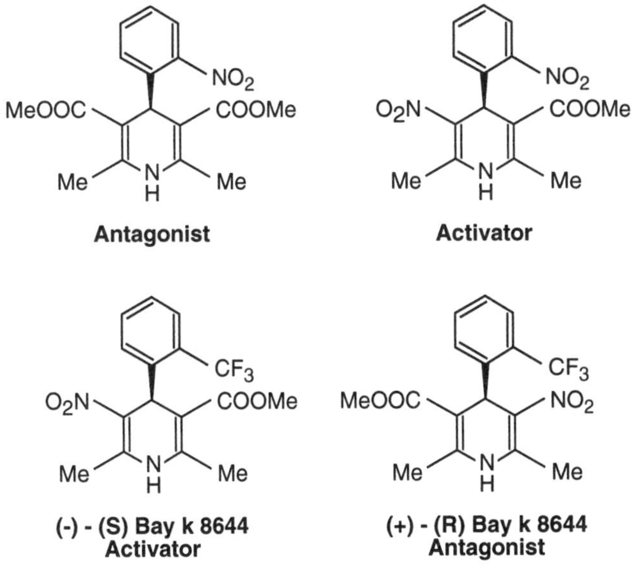

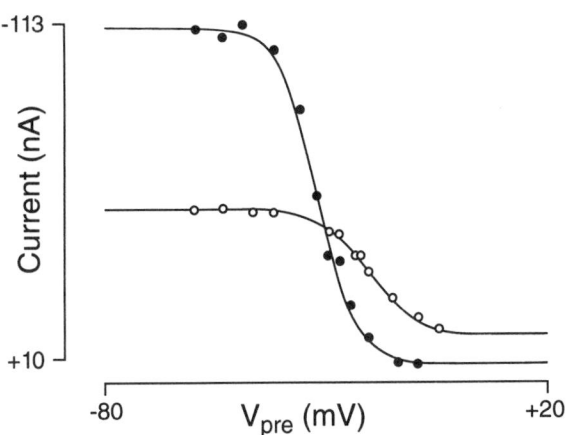

Figure 26.19   Activator/antagonist pairs of enantiomeric 1,4-dihdropyridines.

Figure 26.20   The availability of Ca^{2+} current in calf Purkinje fibres as modified by the 1,4-dihydropydrine Bay K 8644. Channel availability was determined by measuring currents in response to test pulses to 0 mV after 500 ms steps to conditioning voltages. (Reproduced with permission from ref. 102.)

potential, switching between activation and antagonism with decreasing membrane potential (Fig. 26.20).[101,102] Thus, the 1,4-dihydropyridines may be molecular chameleons of the Ca^{2+} channel, changing properties according to channel state.

VI.   SUMMARY AND CONCLUSIONS

The issue of agonist-to-antagonist transitions and their definition are central themes in medicinal chemistry and are linked to factors that determine the symmetry of drug–receptor interactions. It is clear that agonist/antagonist properties are not simple properties of the ligand alone, but rather are also properties of the receptor and its associated coupled effectors. The nature and stoichiometry of the receptor–effector components are critical determinants of the characteristics of the response. Additionally, receptors may initiate responses in the absence of a physiological ligand because they are constitutively active, and receptors may also contain ligands as an integral component of the receptor structure itself. Receptors and ligands enjoy a complementarity and symmetry of interaction that befits their mutual dependence. This mutual dependence raises issues of the coevolution of receptor–ligand systems and of the relative origin of ligands and receptors.[103]

REFERENCES

1. Ariëns, E. J., Soudijn, W. and Timmermans, P. B. M. W. M. (eds) (1983) *Stereochemistry and Biological Activity of Drugs*. Blackwell Scientific, Oxford.
2. Crossley, R. (1993) The relevance of chirality to the study of biological activity. *Tetrahedron*. **48**: 8155–8178.
3. Stinson, S. C. (1993) Chiral drugs. *Chem. Eng. News*, Sept. 27: 38–65.
4. Cushny, A. R. (1926) *Biological Relations of Optically Isomeric Substances*. Williams and Wilkins, Baltimore.
5. Millership, J. S. and Fitzpatrick, A. (1993) Commonly used chiral drugs: a survey. *Chirality* **5**: 573–576.
6. Ariens, E. J. (1953) Nonchiral, homochiral and composite chiral drugs. *Trends Pharmacol. Sci.* **14**: 68–75.
7. Gross, M., Cartwright, A., Campbell, B., Bolton, R., Holmes, K., Kirkland, K., Salmonson, T. and Robert, J.-L. (1993) Regulatory requirements for chiral drugs. *Drug Inf. J.* **27**: 453–457.
8. Editorial: FDA's policy statement for the development of new stereoisomeric drugs. *Chirality* (1992) **4**: 338–340.
9. Crum-Brown, A. and Fraser, T. R. (1865) *On the Connection Between Chemical Constitution and Biological Activities*. Neill and Company, Edinburgh.
10. Ehrlich, P. (1901) Croonian Lecture. On immunity with special reference to cell life. *Proc. R. Soc., London, Ser B.* **66**: 424–448.
11. Langley, J. N. (1878) On the physiology of the salivary secretion. *J. Physiol.* **1**: 339–367.
12. Langley, J. N. (1906) Croonian Lecture: On nerve endings and on special excitable substances in cells. *Proc. R. Soc. London, Series B* **78**: 170–194.
13. Fryer, R. I. (1990) Ligand interactions at the benzodiazepine receptor. In Emmett, J. C. (ed.) *Comprehensive Medicinal Chemistry*, vol. 3, *Membranes and Receptors*, pp. 539–566. Pergamon Press, Oxford.
14. Mason, S. F. (1988) Biomolecular handedness. Origins and significance. *Biochem. Pharmacol.* **37**: 1–7.
15. Petsko, G. A. (1992) On the other hand. . . . *Science* **256**: 1403–1404.
16. Eliel, E. L. and Wilen, S. H. (1994) *Stereochemistry of Organic Compounds*, pp. 209–214. Wiley-Interscience, New York.
17. de L Milton, R. C., Milton, S. C. F. and Kent, S. B. H. (1992) Total chemical synthesis of a D-enzyme: the enantiomers of HIV-1 protease show demonstration of reciprocal chiral substrate specificity. *Science* **256**: 1445–1448.
18. Triggle, D. J. (1993) The future of medicinal chemistry: through a glass darkly. *Annu. Rep. Med. Chem.* **28**: 343–350.
19. Fisher, P. J., Prendergast, F. G., Ehrhardt, M. R., Urbauer, J. L., Ward, A. J., Sedarous, S. S., McCormick, D. J. and Buckley, P. J. (1994) Calmodulin interacts with amphiphilic peptides composed of all D-amino acids. *Nature*, **368**: 651-653.
20. Jameson, B. A., McDonnell, J. M., Marini, J. C. and Korngold, R. (1994) A rationally designed CD4 analogue inhibits experimental allergic encephalomyelitis. *Nature* **368**: 744–746.

21. Montecucchi, P. C., deCastiglione, R., Piani, S., Gozzini, L. and Erspamer, V. (1981) Amino acid composition and sequence of dermorphin, a novel opiate-like peptide from the skin of *Phyllomedusa sauvagei. Int. J. Peptide Protein Res.* **17**: 275–283.
22. Kreil, G. (1994) Peptides containing a D-amino acid from frogs and molluscs. *J. Biol. Chem.* **269**: 10967–10970.
23. Wainer, I. W. and Drayer, D. E. (eds) (1993) *Drug Stereochemistry, Analytical Methods and Pharmacology,* 2nd edn. Marcel Dekker, New York.
24. Cannon, J. G., Mohan, P., Bojarski, J., Long, J. P., Bhatnagar, R. K., Leonard, P. A. Flynn, J. R. and Chatterjee, T. K. (1988) (*R*)-(−)-10-Methyl-11-hydroxyaporphine: a highly selective serotonergic agonist. *J. Med. Chem.* **31**: 313–318.
25. Cannon, J. G., Moe, S. T. and Long, J. P. (1991) Enantiomers of 11- hydroxy-10-methyl-aporphine having opposing pharmacological effects at 5HTl$_A$ receptors. *Chirality* **3**: 19–23.
26. Hillver, S.-E., Bjork, L., Li, Y.-L., Svensson, B., Ross, S., Anden, N.-E. and Hacksel, U. (1990) (*S*)-5-Fluoro-8-hydroxy-2-(dipropylamino)tetralin: a putative 5-HTl$_A$-receptor antagonist. *J. Med. Chem.* **33**: 1541–1544.
27. Kwon, Y.-W. and Triggle, D. J. (1991) Chiral aspects of drug action at ion channels. A commentary on the stereoselectivity of drug actions at voltage-gated ion channels with particular reference to verapamil actions at the Ca^{2+} channel. *Chirality* **3**: 393–404.
28. Triggle, D. J. (1994) On the other hand: the stereoselectivity of drug action at ion channels. *Chirality* **6**: 58–62.
29. Kenakin, T. (1993) *Pharmacological Analysis of Drug–Receptor Interactions,* 2nd edn. Raven Press, New York.
30. Hoyer, D. and Boddeke, H. W. G. M. (1993) Partial agonists, full agonists, antagonists: dilemmas of definition. *Trends Pharmacol. Sci.* **14**: 270–275.
31. Brown, J. H. and Goldstein, D. (1986) Differences in muscarinic receptor reserve for inhibition of adenylate cyclase and stimulation of phosphoinositide hydrolysis in heart cells. *Mol. Pharmacol.* **30**: 566–570.
32. Ashkenazi, A., Winslow, J. W., Peralta, E. G., Peterson, G. L., Schimerlik, M. I., Capon, D. J. and Ramachandran, J. (1987) An M2 muscarinic receptor subtype coupled to both adenylyl cyclase and phosphoinositide turnover. *Science,* **238**: 672–674.
33. Tigges, M. A., Casey, L. S. and Koshland, M. E. (1989) Mechanisms of interleukin-2 signaling: mediation of different outcomes by a single receptor and transduction pathway. *Science* **243**: 781–786.
34. Strader, C. D., Sigal, I. S., Candelore, M. R., Rands, E., Hill, W. S. and Dixon, R. A. F. (1988) Conserved aspartic acid residues 79 and 113 of the β-adrenergic receptor have different roles in receptor function. *J. Biol. Chem.* **263**: 10267–10271.
35. Getler, V., Johansen, T. E., Snider, R. M., Lowe III, J. A., Nakanishi, S. and Schwartz, T. W. (1993) Different binding epitopes on the NKl receptor for substance P and a nonpeptide antagonist. *Nature* **362**: 345–348.
36. Beinhorn, M., Lee, Y.-M., McBride, E. W., Quinn, S. M. and Kopin, A. S. (1993) A single amino acid of the cholecystokinin-B1 gastrin receptor determines specificity for non-peptide antagonists. *Nature* **362**: 348–350.
37. Lauffenburger, D. A. and Linderman, J. J. (1993) *Models for Binding, Trafficking and Signaling.* Oxford University Press, Oxford.
38. Ren, Q., Kurose, H., Lefkowitz, R. J. and Cotecchia, S. (1993) Constitutively active mutants of the β-adrenergic receptor. *J. Biol. Chem.* **268**: 16483–16487.
39. Kenakin, T. (1990) Drugs and receptors. An overview of the current state of knowledge. *Drugs* **40**: 666–687.
40. Kenakin, T. R. and Bond, R. A. (1992) Theoretical and practical advantages and limitations of techniques used in functional pharmacological classification of drug receptors. In Angeli, P., Giulini, U. and Quagley, W. (eds) *Trends in Receptor Research,* pp. 31–42. Elsevier, Amsterdam.
41. Leff, P. and Dougall, I. G. (1992) Is pharmacological analysis of agonist action useful in medicinal chemistry?. In Angeli, P., Giulini, U. and Quagley, W. (eds) *Trends in Receptor Research,* pp. 43–60. Elsevier, Amsterdam.
42. Clark, A. J. (1937) General pharmacology. In *Heffners Handbook der Experimental. Pharmakologie,* vol. 4. Springer, Berlin.

43. Ariens, E. J. (1954) Affinity and intrinsic activity in the theory of competitive antagonism. *Arch. Int. Pharmacodyn.* **99**: 32–49.

44. Stephenson, R. P. (1956) A modification of receptor theory. *Br. J. Pharmacol.* **11**: 379–393.

45. Furchgott, R. (1966) The use of 2-haloalkylamines in the differentiation of dissociation constants of receptor agonist complexes. *Adv. Drug Res.* **3**: 21–55.

46. Black, J. W. and Leff, P. (1983) Operational models of pharmacological agonism. *Proc. R. Soc. London, Ser. B.* **220**: 141–162.

47. Bourne, H. R., Sanders, D. A. and McCormick, F. (1990) The GTPase superfamily: a conserved switch for diverse cell function. *Nature* **348**: 125–132.

48. Kazino, Y., Itoh, H., Kozasa, T., Nafafuki, M. and Stoh, T. (1991) Structure and function of signal-transducing GTP- binding proteins. *Annu. Rev. Biochem.* **60**: 349–400.

49. Neer, E. I. (1994) G proteins: critical control points of transmembrane signals. *Protein Sci.* **3**: 3–14.

50. Noel, J. P., Hamm, H. and Sigler, P. B. (1993) The 2.2 Å crystal structure of transducin-α complexed with GTP γS. *Nature* **336**: 654–663.

51. Bourne, H. R. (1993) A turn-on and or surprise. *Nature* **366**: 628–629.

52. Pike, L. J. and Lefkowitz, R. J. (1981) Correlation of beta-adrenergic receptor-stimulated (^{3}H)GDP release and adenylate cyclase activation. *J. Biol. Chem.* **256**: 2207–2212.

53. Koski, G., Streaty, R. A. and Klee, W. A. (1982) Modulation of sodium-sensitive GTPase by partial opiate agonists. *J. Biol. Chem.* **257**: 14035–14040.

54. Cottecchia, S., Exum S., Caron, M. G. and Lefkowitz, R. J. (1990) Regions of the α_1-adrenergic receptor involved in coupling to phosphatidylinositol hydrolysis and enhanced sensitivity of biological function. *Proc. Natl. Acad. Sci. USA* **87**: 2896–2900.

55. Samama, P., Cotecchia, S., Costa, T. and Lefkowitz, R. J. (1993) A mutation-induced activated state of the β_2-adrenergic receptor. *J. Biol. Chem.* **268**: 4625–4636.

56. Milano, C. A., Allen, L. F., Rockman, H. A., Dolber, P. C., Chien, K. R., Johnson, T. D., Bond, R. A. and Lefkowitz, R. J. (1994) Enhanced myocardial function in transgenic mice overexpressing the β_2-adrenergic receptor. *Science* **264**: 582–586.

57. Karlin, A. (1967) On the application of a 'plausible' model of allosteric proteins to the receptor for acetylcholine. *J. Theor. Biol.* **16**: 306–320.

58. Costa, T., Ogino, Y., Munson, P. J., Onaran, H. O. and Rodbard, D. (1992) Drug efficacy of guanine nucleotide-binding regulatory protein-linked receptors; thermodynamic interpretation of negative antagonism and of receptor activity in the absence of ligand. *Mol. Pharmacol.* **41**: 549–560.

59. Schutz, W. and Freissmuth, M. (1992) Reverse intrinsic activity of antagonists on G protein-coupled receptors. *Trends Pharmacol. Sci.* **13**: 376–380.

60. Samama, P., Pei, G., Costa, T., Cotecchia, S. and Lefkowitz, R. J. (1994) Negative antagonists promote an inactive conformation of the β_2-adrenergic receptor. *Mol. Pharmacol.* **451**: 390–394.

61. Costa, T. and Herz, A. (1989) Antagonists with negative intrinsic activity at opiod receptor coupled to GTP binding proteins. *Proc. Nat. Acad. Sci. USA* **86**: 7321–7325.

62. Hopkins, C. R., Semoff, S. and Gregory, H. (1981) Regulation of gonadotropin secretion in the anterior pituitary. *Phil. Trans. R. Soc. London, Ser B.* **296**: 73–81.

63. Gregory, H., Taylor, C. L. and Hopkins, C. R. (1982) Luteinizing hormone release from dissociated pituitary by dimerization of occupied LHR H receptors. *Nature* **300**: 269–271.

64. Conn, P. M., Rogers, D. C., Stewart, J. M., Niedel, J. and Sheffield, T. (1982) Conversion of a gonadotropin-releasing hormone antagonist to an agonist. *Nature* **296**: 653–655.

65. Blum, J. J. and Conn, P. M. (1982) Gonadotropin-releasing hormone stimulation of luteinizing hormone release: a ligand–receptor–effector model. *Proc. Natl. Acad. Sci. USA* **79**: 7307–7311.

66. Kitajima, Y., Catt, K. J. and Chen, H.-C. (1989) Enhanced biological activity of dimeric gondadotropin releasing hormone. *Biochem. Biophys. Res. Commun.* **159**: 893–898.

67. Walz, D. A., Fenton, J. W. and Shuman, M. A. (eds) (1986) Regulatory functions of thrombin. *Ann. NY Acad. Sci.* **485.**

68. Eidt, J. F., Allison, P., Nobel, S., Ashton, J., Golino, P., McNatt, J., Buja, L. M. and Willerson, J. T. (1989) Thrombin is an important mediator of platelet aggregation in stressed canine coronory arteries with endothelial injury. *J. Clin. Invest.* **84**: 18–27.

69. Shuman, M. A. (1986) Thrombin-cellular interactions. *Ann. New York Acad. Sci.* **485**: 349–368.

70. Vu, T.-K. H., Hung, D. T., Wheaton, V. I. and Coughlin, S. R. (1991) Molecular cloning of a functional thrombin receptor reveals a novel proteolytic mechanism of receptor activation. *Cell* **64**: 1057–1068.

71. Watson, S. and Arkinstall, S. (1994) *The G-Protein Linked Receptor Facts Book.* Academic Press, London and San Diego.

72. Vu, T.-K. H., Wheaton, V. I., Hung, D. T., Charo, I. and Coughlin, S. R. (1991) Domains specifying thrombin–receptor interaction. *Nature* **353:** 674–677.

73. Scarborough, R. M., Naughton, M. A., Teng, W., Hing, D. T., Rose, J., Vu, T.-K. H., Wheaton, V. I., Turck, C. W. and Coughlin, S. R. (1992) Tethered ligand agonist peptides. *J. Biol. Chem.* **267:** 13146–13149.

74. Gerszten, R. E., Chen, J., Ishii, M., Ishii, K., Wang, L., Nanevicz, T., Turck, C. W., Vu, T.-K. H. and Coughlin, S. R. (1994) Specificity of the thrombin receptor for agonist peptide is defined by its extra cellular surface. *Nature* **368:** 648–651.

75. Ishii, K., Hein, L., Kobilka, B. and Coughlin, S. R. (1993) Kinetics of thrombin receptor cleavage on intact cells. Relation to signaling. *J. Biol. Chem.* **268:** 9780–9786.

76. Armstrong, C.M. and Bezanilla, F. (1977) Inactivation of the sodium channel. II. Gating current experiments. *J. Gen. Physiol.* **70:** 567–590

77. Hoshi, T., Zagotta, W. N. and Aldrich, R. W. (1990) Biophysical and molecular mechanisms of shaker potassium channel inactivation. *Science* **250:** 533–538.

78. Zagotta, W. N., Hoshi, T. and Aldrich, R. W. (1990) Restoration of inactivation in mutants of Shaker potassium channels by a peptide derived from ShB. *Science* **250:** 568–571.

79. MacKinnon, R., Aldrich, R. W. and Lee, A. W. (1993) Functional stoichiometry of Shaker potassium channel inactivation. *Science* **262:** 757–759.

80. Eaholtz, G., Scheuer, T. and Catterall, W. A. (1994) Restoration of inactivation and block of open sodium channels by an inactivation gate peptide. *Neuron* **12:** 1041–1048.

81. Owen, M. J. and Lamb, J. R. (1988) *Immune Recognition.* IRL Press, Oxford.

82. Evavold, B. D., Sloan-Lancaster, J. and Allen P. M. (1993) Tickling the TCR: selective T-cell functions stimulated by altered peptide ligands. *Immunol. Today* **14:** 602–609.

83. Evavold, B. D. and Allen, P. M. (1992) Separation of IL-4 production for T cell proliferation by an altered T cell receptor ligand. *Science* **252:** 1308–1310.

84. DeMagistris, M. T., Alexander, J., Coggeshall, M., Altman, A., Gaeta, F. C. A., Grey, H. M. and Sette, A. (1992) Antigen analog-major histocompatibility complexes act as antagonists of the T cell receptor. *Cell* **68:** 625–634.

85. Smilek, D. E., Wraith, D. C. and Hodgkinson, S. (1991) *Proc. Natl. Acad. Sci. USA* **88:** 9633–9677.

86. Wauben, M. H. M., Boog, C. J. P. and van der Zee, R. (1992) Disease inhibition by major histocompatability complex binding peptide analogues of disease-associated epitopes: more than blocking alone. *J. Exp. Med.* **176:** 667–677.

87. Hogquist, K. A., Jameson, S. C., Heath, W. R., Howard, J. L., Bevan, M. J. and Carbone, F. R. (1994) T cell receptor antagonist peptides induce positive selection. *Cell* **76:** 17–27.

88. Marrack, P. and Parker, D. C. (1994) A little of what you fancy. *Nature* **368:** 397–398.

89. Rampe, D. and Triggle, D. J. (eds) (1994) Ion channels as targets for drug design. *Drug Dev. Res.* **33.**

90. Hille, B. (1993) *Ion Channels,* 2nd edn. Sinauer Press, Sunderland, MA.

91. Hille, B. (1977) Local anesthetics: hydrophilic and hydrophobic pathways for the drug–receptor reaction. *J. Gen. Physiol.* **69:** 497–515.

92. Hondeghem, L. M. and Katzung, B. G. (1977) Time- and voltage dependent interactions of antiarrhythmic drugs with sodium channels. *Biochim. Biophys. Acta* **472:** 373–398.

93. Hondeghem, L. M. and Katzung, B. G. (1984) Antiarrhythmic agents: the modulated receptor mechanism of action of sodium and calcium channel-blocking drugs. *Annu. Rev. Pharmacol.* **24:** 387–423.

94. Triggle, D. J. (1989) Structure-function correlations of 1,4-dihyropyridine calcium channel antagonists and activators. In Hondeghem, L. M. (ed.) *Molecular and Cellular Mechanisms of Antiarrhythmic Agents,* pp. 269–292. Futura Publishing, Mt. Kisco, NY.

95. Yeh, J. Z. (1980) Blockade of sodium channels by stereoisomers of local anesthetics. In Fink, B. R. (ed.) *Molecular Mechanisms of Anesthesia,* pp. 35–44. Raven Press, New York.

96. Triggle, D. J., Langs, D. A. and Janis, R. A. (1989) Ca^{2+} channel ligands. Structure–function relationships of the 1,4-dihydropyridines. *Med. Res. Rev.* **9:** 123–180.

97. Goldmann, S. and Stoltefuss, J. (1991) 1,4-Dihydropyridines: effects of chirality and conformation on the calcium antagonist and calcium agonist activities. *Angew. Chem. Int. Ed. Engl.* **30:** 1559–1578.

98. Hof, R. P., Ruegg, U.-T., Hof, A. and Vogel, A. (1985) Stereoselectivity at the calcium channel: opposite actions of the enantiomers of a 1,4-dihydropyridine. *J. Cardiovasc. Pharmacol.* **7**: 689–693.

99. Franckowiak, G., Bechem, M., Schramm, M. and Thomas, G. (1985) The optical isomers of the 1,4-dihydropyridine Bay K 8644 show opposite effects on Ca channels. *Eur. J. Pharmacol.* **114**: 223–226.

100. Wei, X.-Y., Luchowski, E. M., Rutledge, A., Su, C. M. and Triggle, D. J. (1986) Pharmacologic and radioligand binding analysis of the actions of 1,4-dihydropyridine activator–antagonist pairs in smooth muscle. *J. Pharmacol. Exp. Ther.* **239**: 144–153.

101. Kass, R. (1987) Voltage-dependent modulation of cardiac calcium channel current by optical isomers of Bay K 8644: implications for channel gating. *Circ. Res.* **61** (supplement 1): 1–5.

102. Sanguinetti, M. C., Krafte, D. S. and Kass, R. S. (1986) Voltage dependent modulation of Ca channel current in heart cells by Bay K 8644. *J. Gen. Physiol.* **88**: 369–392.

103. Moyle, W. R., Campbell, R. K., Myers, R. V., Bernard, M. P., Han, Y. and Wang, X. (1994) Co-evolution of ligand–receptor pairs. *Nature* **368**: 251–255.

27

Design of Peptidomimetics

HIROSHI NAKANISHI and MICHAEL KAHN

It's not just what we inherit from our mothers and fathers that haunts us. It's all kinds of old defunct theories, all sorts of old defunct beliefs, and things like that.
Henrik Ibsen, *Ghosts* (1881)

I. INTRODUCTION

Peptides and proteins control all biological processes at some level (transcriptional, translational or post-translational). Yet, at the molecular level, our understanding of the relationship between structure and function remains rudimentary. The problems involved in clarifying these issues are somewhat different for peptides and proteins. The dissection of multidomain proteins into small synthetic conformationally restricted components is an important step in the design of low-molecular-weight nonpeptides that mimic the activity of

THE PRACTICE OF MEDICINAL CHEMISTRY
ISBN 0-12-744640-0

the native protein. Mimetics of critical functional domains might possess beneficial properties in comparison to the intact proteinaceous species with regard to specificity and therapeutic potential, and are valuable probes for the study of molecular recognition events.[1] On the other hand, peptides are characteristically highly flexible molecules whose structure is strongly influenced by their environment.[2] Their random conformations in solution complicate their use in determining their receptor-bound or bioactive structures.[3,4] Conformational constraints can significantly aid this determination.[5] Peptide mimetics are powerful tools for the study of molecular recognition and are providing a unique opportunity to dissect and investigate structure–function relationships in peptides and complex proteins.

II.   NONPEPTIDE MIMETICS

The isolation and identification in 1975 of the endogenous opioid pentapeptides methionine and leucine enkephalin[6] represents the intellectual groundbreaking in the field of peptidomimetics. The work described demonstrated that, despite their highly disparate structures, these linear pentapeptides and the condensed heterocyclic species morphine elicit their biological response, analgesia, by binding to the opiate receptor. However, despite intensive efforts to understand this relationship, it is fair to say that some 20 years later it remains far from clear.

III.   SCREENING

To date, unquestionably the greatest success in developing nonpeptide leads for peptide ligands has come from a screening approach. A wide array of ligands, often bearing little, if any, structural resemblance to the endogenous peptide ligand which they mimic, have been uncovered through receptor-based screening programmes.[7] What lessons can be learned from these screening leads? Importantly, they have validated many of the critical concepts which underlie the rational design of peptidomimetics, in that they prove that compounds lacking amide bonds, obvious pharmacophore similarity and flexibility can be potent and selective ligands for peptide receptors. However, a very sobering note is that these relationships provide us with very limited information with regard to developing generic solutions for rationally traversing the pathway from peptides to mimetics.

IV.   DESIGN OF NONPEPTIDE MIMETICS

There has been an increasing effort to rationally design and synthesize highly active analogues of biologically significant peptides and proteins. It is anticipated that these drugs of the future will possess greater selectivity, and fewer side-effects than their present-day counterparts.[8] The complex problems associated with the rational design of mimetics are constantly being reduced, owing to advances in molecular biology, spectroscopy and computational chemistry. The determination of the receptor-bound conformation of a peptide or protein ligand is invaluable for the rational design of mimetics. However, with few exceptions this information is not readily available.[9,10] Conformational constraints constitute one of the most promising avenues for the solution of this problem, particularly if the constraint is such that only one conformation of the ligand is significantly populated. Rigid analogues pay a lower entropy cost upon binding to their receptor and therefore should bind more avidly, assuming appositive placement of pharmacophoric residues.[11] Proteolytic enzymes generally prefer conformationally adaptable substrates; therefore, constrained analogues are generally endowed with increased proteolytic stability. Additionally, selectivity can be enhanced by the preclusion of conformers that produce undesired bioactivity.[12]

V. THE SECONDARY STRUCTURE APPROACH

One approach to the design of peptidomimetics has been guided by the simple elegance which nature has employed in the molecular architecture of proteinaceous species.[13] Three basic building blocks (α-helices, β-sheets and reverse turns) are utilized for the construction of all proteins. The design and synthesis of peptidomimetic prosthetic units to replace these three architectural motifs is affording an opportunity to dissect and investigate complex structure–function relationships in proteins through the use of small synthetic conformationally restricted components. This is a critical step towards the rational design of low-molecular-weight nonpeptide pharmaceutical agents that are devoid of the shortcomings of conventional peptides. A recent symposium in print is devoted to this topic.[14]

VI. REVERSE TURN (β-TURNS AND γ-TURNS)

The surface localization of turns in proteins, and the predominance of residues containing potentially critical pharmacophoric information, has led to the hypothesis that turns play critical roles in a myriad of recognition events.[15] Reverse turns are classified into γ-turns consisting of three residues (sometimes referred to as a C7 conformation) and the more common β-turns (C10 conformation) formed by a tetrapeptide. An excellent review by Ball and Alewood in 1990[16] summarized the progress to that point in reverse turn mimetics. More recently, Baca *et al.*[17] made use of Nagai's thiazolidine lactam type II′ β-turn mimetic[18] to replace the type I′ β-turn between Gly16 and Gly17 in HIV-1 protease. The β-turn mimetic-containing enzyme dimerized similarly to the native enzyme. It was fully active, possessed the same substrate specificity as the native enzyme, and showed enhanced thermal stability. Nicolaou *et al.*[19] utilized 3-deoxy-β-D-glucose (Fig. 27.1) as a scaffold to synthesize the first nonpeptidic analogue of the receptor-recognizing β-turn (Phe7, Trp8, Lys9, Thr10) of somatostatin (Fig. 27.2). This mimetic binds to the pituitary gland somatostatin receptor with an IC_{50} value of 1.3 µM. Interestingly, in a functional assay this mimetic displayed agonist activity at 3 µM (less frequently observed with peptidomimetics).

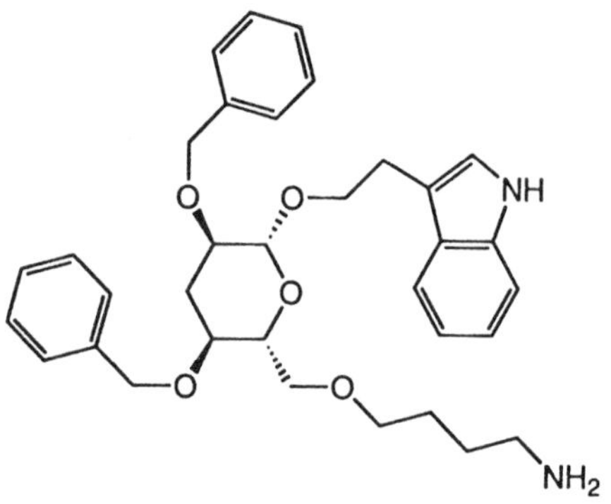

Fig. 27.1

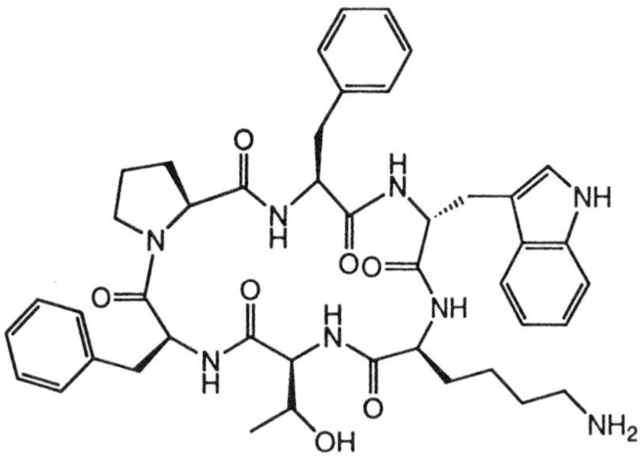

Fig. 27.2

An interesting recent application involved the design of a benzodiazepine peptidomimetic to inhibit the enzyme *Ras* farnesyl transferase (Fig. 27.3). The benzodiazepine system is intended to mimic the proposed β-turn in the CAAX sequence of the enzyme substrate[20] and has an IC_{50} < 1 nM. Interestingly, the structurally related lipophilic conformationally restricted mimic of the tripeptide (*Z*)-PheHisLeu is a potent inhibitor of angiotensin converting enzyme (ACE) (Fig. 27.4).[21] Presumably in this instance, by analogy with other metalloprotease substrate interactions,[22] the enzyme-bound substrate adopts an extended structure.

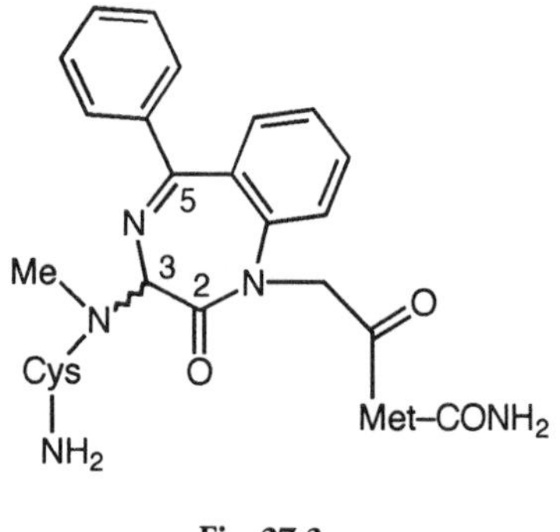

Fig. 27.3

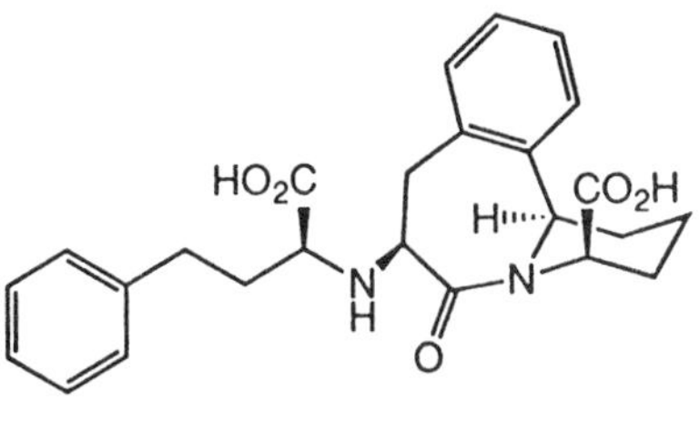

Fig. 27.4

VII. RECENT ADVANCES

In the design of reverse turn mimetic systems, there are a number of concerns and criteria which need to be addressed. β-Turns comprise a rather diverse group of structures. β-Turns are classified according to the φ and ψ angles, of the $i+1$ and $i+2$ residues. In addition to a number of turn types (I, I′, II, II′, III, III′, IV, V, Va, VIa, VIb, VII and VIII) the C_i^α to C_{i+3}^α distance varies from 4 to 7 Å.[23] From this cursory discussion, it should be readily apparent that no one structure can accurately mimic this diversity of turns. The interaction of the amino acid side-chains with their complementary receptor groups is the critical determinant of biological specificity. A successful peptidomimetic must correctly position the appropriate functional groups on a relatively rigid framework. Therefore, an idealized mimetic design should incorporate the ability to accurately display critical pharmacophoric information in the same manner in which it is presented in native reverse turns. This is a far from trivial synthetic problem, in that it requires the stereo- and enantiocontrolled introduction of a minimum of four noncontiguous asymmetric centres. Furthermore, the nonpeptidic character of these molecules best promises to overcome the inherent problems of peptides. Synthetic expediency is a major concern that should not be lightly regarded, particularly at an early stage when the delineation of structure–activity relationships is critical and requires the synthesis and evaluation of a series of related structures.

The major breakthrough in peptide synthesis was the development of a solid-phase format by Merrifield, for which he was awarded the Nobel Prize in 1985.[24] Therefore we desired to capture the modular component nature and automated facility of SPPS (solid-phase peptide synthesis) in our approach to peptidomimetics. This is additionally allowing us to develop libraries of conformationally constrained peptidomimetics.[25] With this mandate, it became relatively facile to propose a retrosynthetic strategy to accomplish this goal (Fig. 27.5). The synthesis of the reverse turn mimetic can be performed in solution; however, it is designed to be and is fully compatible with SPPS protocols. In essence, it involves the coupling of the first modular component piece (**1**) to the amino terminus of a growing peptide chain (**2**). Coupling of the second component (**3**), removal of the protecting group P′, and subsequent coupling of the third modular component (**4**) provides the nascent β-turn (**5**). The critical step in this sequence involves the use of an azetidinone as an activated ester to effect the macrocyclization reaction.[26] Upon nucleophilic opening of the azetidinone by the X moiety, a new amino terminus is generated for continuation of the synthesis. An important feature of this scheme is the ability to alter the X-group linker, in regard to both length and degree of rigidity/flexibility.

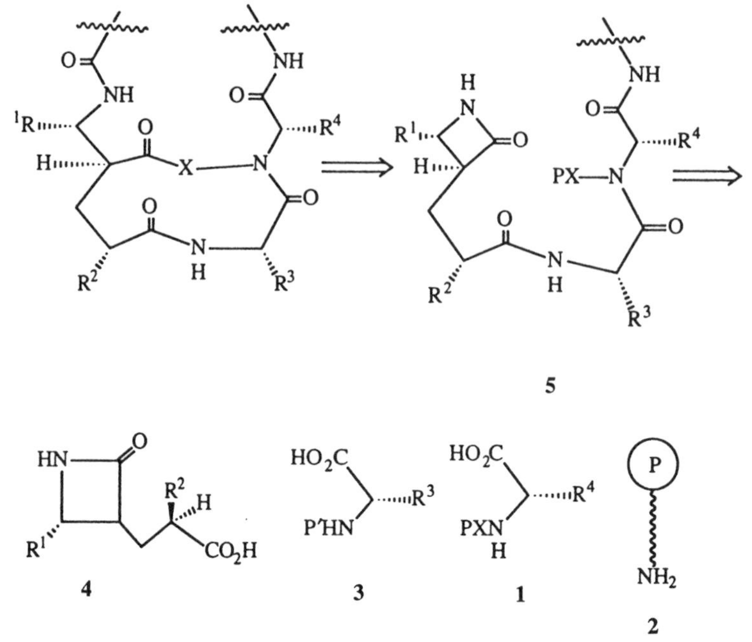

Fig. 27.5

The requisite stereogenic centres are readily derived, principally from the 'chiral pool'. The synthesis allows for the introduction of natural or non-natural amino acid side-chain functionality in either L or D configuration. Additionally, deletion of the second modular component (3) provides access to γ-turn mimetics[27] (Fig. 27.6).

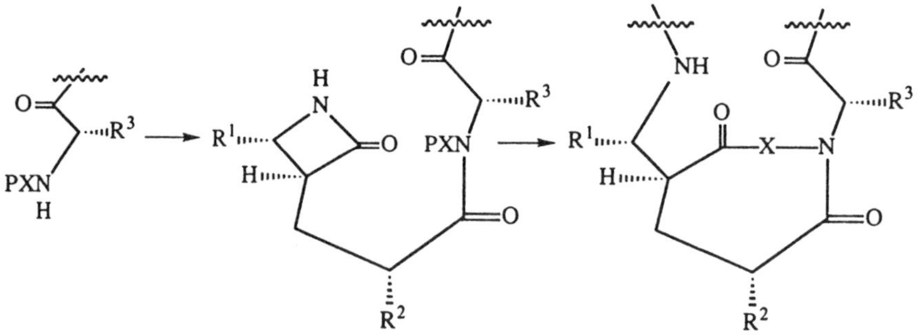

Fig. 27.6

We have used this mimetic system to explore structure–function relationships among molecules of the immunoglobulin gene superfamily. Immunoglobulins are constructed from a series of antiparallel β-pleated sheets connected by loops.[28,29] The specificity of these molecules is determined by the sequence and size of the canonical hypervariable complementarity-determining regions (CDRs).[30,31]

Reo 323 I V S Y S G S G L N 332

mAb 87.92.6 46 L L I Y S G S T L Q 55

● identical

○ conservative substitution

Fig. 27.7

The monoclonal antibody 87.92.6 (mAb 87.92.6) is an anti-idiotype antibody which binds to the cellular receptor of the type 3 reovirus. Sequence analysis revealed an intriguing homology between the two proteinaceous ligands which bind the receptor (Fig. 27.7).[32] In particular, a region within the CDR2 of the light chain of mAb 87.92.6 and the haemagglutinin of the type 3 reovirus exhibited strong primary sequence homology. The V_L CDR 2 canonically exists in a reverse turn conformation.[33] On the basis of this analysis, we designed and synthesized a reverse turn mimetic (Fig. 27.8), which incorporated the sequence Y, S, G, S, S. Importantly, it displayed similar binding properties to the cellular reovirus receptor and to mAb 9BG5, and had the same inhibitory effect on cell proliferation as did the native antibody 87.92.6.

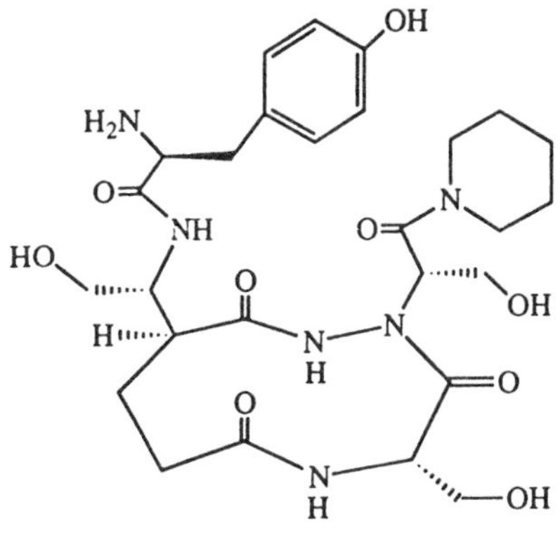

Fig. 27.8

We have also designed a mimetic of the CDR2-like region of human CD4. CD4 is a 55-kDa glycoprotein, primarily found on the cell surface of the helper class of T cells. It binds the human immunodeficiency virus glycoprotein (HIV gp120) with high affinity ($K_d \approx 1$–4 nM), and is an important route of cellular entry for the virus. Extensive mutagenesis[35,36] and peptide mapping[37] experiments have shown that the region of amino acids 40–55 within the CDR2-like domain of CD4 is critical for gp120 binding. X-ray crystallographic analysis showed that residues Gln40 through Phe43 reside on a highly surface-exposed β-turn connecting the C′ and C″ β-strands. A first-generation mimetic of this region (Fig. 27.9) was designed and synthesized.

NMR and molecular modelling analysis confirmed that the 10-membered ring system (Fig. 27.9) closely mimicked the conformation of this loop. Importantly, this small-molecule mimic (molecular weight 810 as its trifluoroacetate salt) abrogates the binding of HIV-1 (IIIB) gp120 to CD4$^+$ cells at low micromolar levels and reduces syncytium formation 50% at 250 µg ml^{-1} (ref. 1).

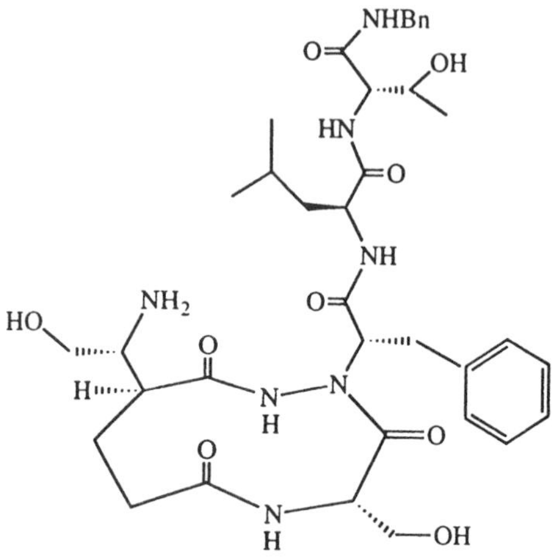

Fig. 27.9

Recently, we have been addressing a problem previously described concerning the relationship between morphine and enkephalin. The inherent mobility of the enkephalin framework, its rapid degradation *in vivo*[38] and the existence of multiple receptor subtypes[39,40] have hampered the assessment of its bioactive conformations. Conformationally constrained peptides or peptidomimetics[41–44] should facilitate this task. Several turn conformations have been proposed based upon computational models,[45–48] X-ray crystallography[49,50] and spectroscopic studies.[51–53]

In 1976, Bradbury *et al.* proposed a β-bend model stabilized by an intramolecular hydrogen bond between the N—H of Phe4 and the C=O of Tyr1, which produces a spatial disposition between the Phe4 aromatic ring and the tyramine segment of Tyr1, analogous to that existing between the corresponding moieties in the potent morphine analogue PEO.[54,55] Further support for the relevance of this conformation was provided by energy calculations on the potent [D-Ala2, Met5] enkephalin analogue, the lowest-energy conformer[56–58] of which contained a folded structure with a turn centred on residues 2 and 3. However, evidence contrary to the biological significance of a 4→1 β-turn has been presented by Freidinger,[59] and additionally by Schiller in the analysis of the conformations of 13- and 14-membered rigid cyclic analogues.[60]

To examine further this hypothetical bioactive confirmation, we have synthesized a family of 4→1 β-turn mimetics (Fig. 27.10, (1)–(4)). The lowest-energy conformer of the 10-membered ring system is an excellent mimic of an idealized type I' β-turn (6 atom r.m.s. deviation, 0.22 Å) and displays excellent overlap with the critical Phe^4 aromatic ring and tyramine moieties of PET (Fig. 27.11), yet it is essentially devoid of biological activity. Only the 14-membered ring analogue (Fig. 27.10), (1), which has a rather expanded loop structure, demonstrates any, albeit minimal, binding activity at the µ receptor. The results of this investigation can be interpreted

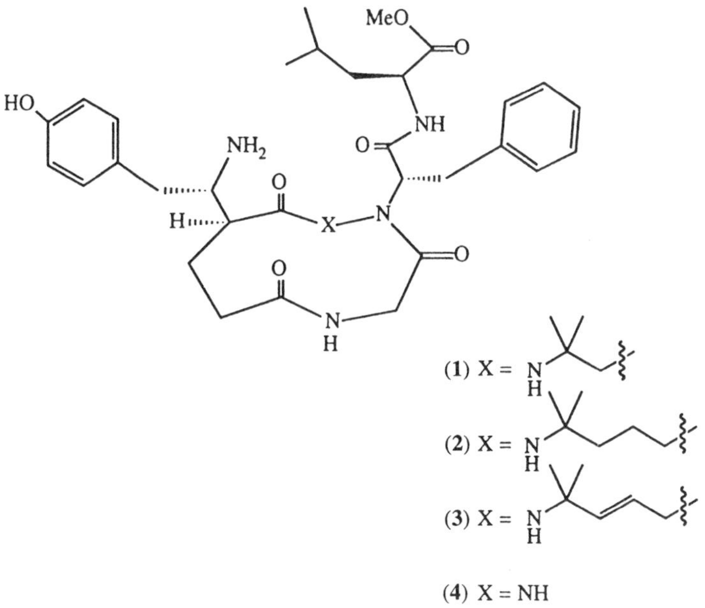

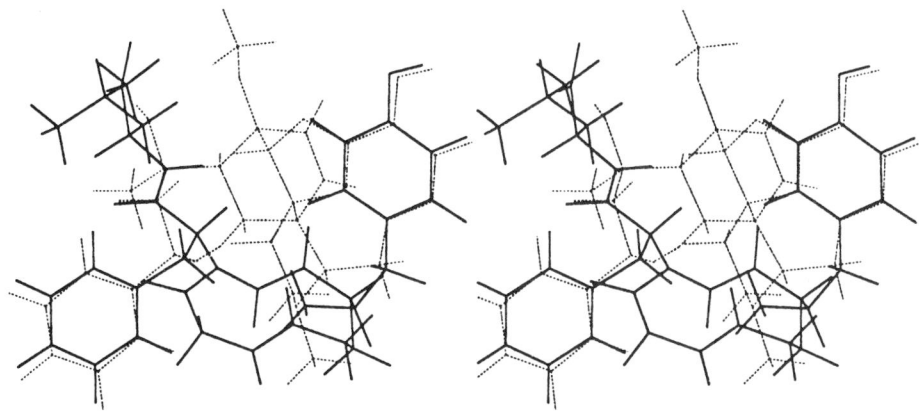

Fig. 27.10

Fig. 27.11 The tyramide and phenyl ring moieties of enkaphalin mimetic (solid line) can be perfectly aligned with those of the morphine analogue PET, 7-[1-phenyl-3-hydroxybutyl-3-]endoethenotetrahydrothebaine (dashed line) by a flexible fitting procedure without any steric conflict.

as casting significant doubt on the biological relevance of a 4→1 β-turn conformation for enkephalin.

A similar series of experiments involving conformationally constrained analogues of 5→2 enkephalin β-turn mimetics is underway.[61] It is hoped that this type of a systematic approach to the synthesis of constrained reverse turn analogues in conjunction with multiple peptide synthetic strategies will clarify the situation regarding the biological significance of these and other proposed receptor-bound reverse turn conformations.

VIII.   α-HELIX

Helices are the most common secondary structural element found in globular proteins, accounting for just over one-third of all residues.[62] Extensive effort has been directed towards an understanding of helix formation, its stability and amino acid propensities.[63–69] Yet, as noted by Kemp and Curran,[70] little attention has been given to the design of helical templates. This is due in large part to the inherently more difficult task of mimicking the approximately 12 amino acids (i.e. three turns of an α-helix) required to form a stabilized, isolated helical peptide. The formation of an α-helix involves two steps: initiation and propagation. To date, most of the effort in the design and synthesis of α-helix mimetics has centred around N-terminal initiation motifs.

Arrhenius and Satterthwait used a hydrazone-ethylene bridge to replace the 5→1 backbone hydrogen bond in one turn of an α-helix to afford the cyclic peptide shown in Fig. 27.12.[71,72] Conformational analysis of both the methyl ester and amide were performed in CDCl$_3$ and DMSO-d$_6$ by NMR spectroscopy. Based upon 1D nuclear Overhauser effect (nOe) measurements, both compounds seem to prefer the cis-N-methyl peptide bond conformation in DMSO and an equilibrium mixture in CDCl$_3$. Based on this analysis, the formation of an α-helix inducing conformation in these macrocyclic compounds is inconclusive. A pentapeptide Ala-(Glu-γ-ethylester)$_4$-ethyl ester was subsequently added to the carboxy terminus of the macrocyclic template (Fig. 27.12). The conformations of the pentapeptide with and without the macrocyclic template were monitored by NMR utilizing 3J coupling constants, sequential nOe and H/D exchange rates of the amide protons in deuterated trifluoroethanol. The observed 3.8 Hz 3J coupling constant[73] observed for the alanine residue, together with the smaller exchange rates, tends to indicate the formation of an α-helical conformation.

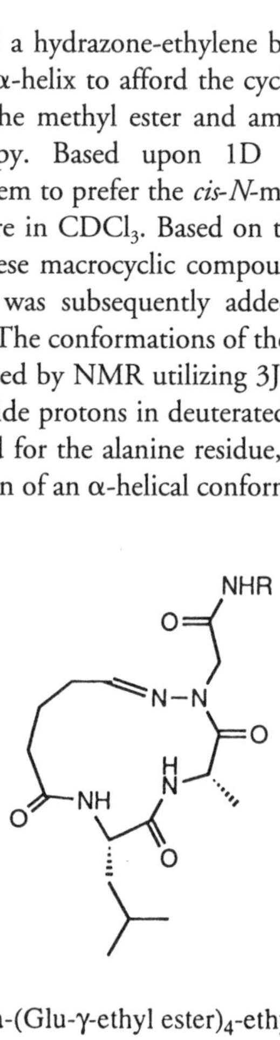

R=Ala-(Glu-γ-ethyl ester)$_4$-ethyl ester

Fig. 27.12

The proper alignment of two or more hydrogen-bond acceptors is crucial for the design of a successful helix nucleation template. Kemp et al., by restraining two proline rings with a thiamethylene bridge, thereby forming a tricyclic template (Fig. 27.13),[70] intended to orient the three amide carbonyls at the proper pitch and spacing for a right-handed α-helix. Observation of an nOe from the acetyl methyl to the following proline αH in CDCl$_3$[74] leads one to believe that the carbonyl oxygen of the acetyl group at the N-terminus is improperly positioned

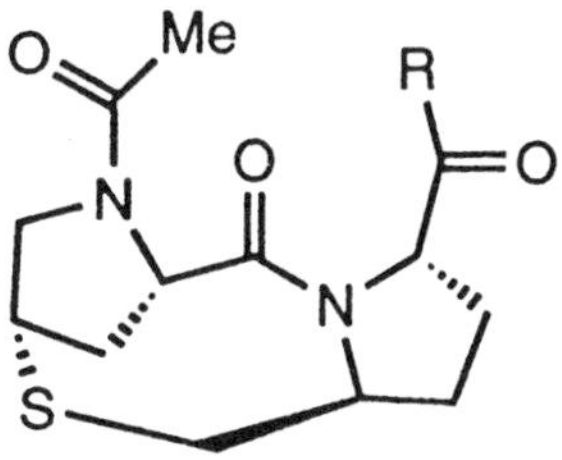

R=OMe or (Ala)$_n$
where n=1-6

Fig. 27.13

(i.e. oriented *cis*), presumably to avoid the dipole–dipole repulsion of the aligned carbonyls. However, NMR investigation of (poly-alanine) ($n=1–6$) conjugated to this template in CDCl$_3$ indicated the existence of a conformational equilibrium between an intramolecularly hydrogen-bonded structure with a *trans* N-terminal acetamide bond, and a non-hydrogen bonded structure derived from the *cis* conformer.[75] The *trans*-to-*cis* ratio (which correlates with the observed helix-to-random coil ratio) is found to be length and solvent dependent for the poly(alanine) oligomers.[76]

In a subsequent design, the number of hydrogen-bond donor sites was increased to four by using a cyclic triproline helix template (Fig. 27.14).[77] X-ray and NMR studies determined that the template exists largely in a non-helical conformation. This finding was in agreement with molecular mechanics calculations which suggested that a helical conformation is approximately 4 kcal mol^{-1} less stable. Appending a poly(alanine) ($n=1–3$) sequence to the template generated a peptide that adopted largely a 3$_{10}$ helical conformation.

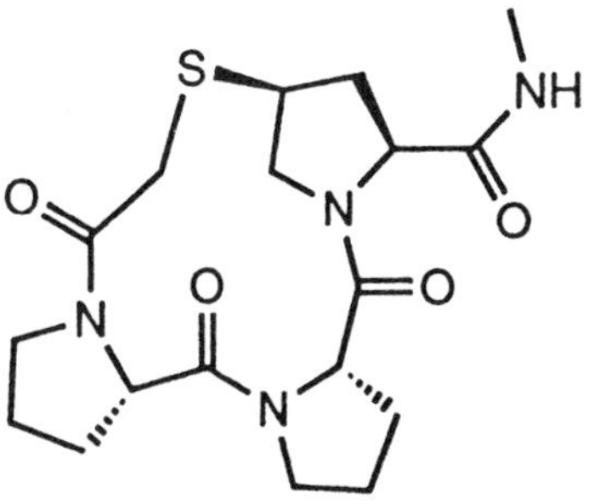

Fig. 27.14

A template which affords rigid alignment of three carbonyl oxygens was devised by Müller *et al.*[78] They utilized the cage compound (Fig. 27.15) which is readily accessible via a series of electrocyclic addition reactions. A nonapeptide (mixture of Ala and Aib) coupled to this cage compound showed significantly increased α-helicity compared with the linear nonapeptide in 1:1 water–TFE solution as judged by CD spectra. On the other hand, the same nonapeptide coupled to the enantiomeric template (Fig. 27.16), where the three carbonyl groups are aligned

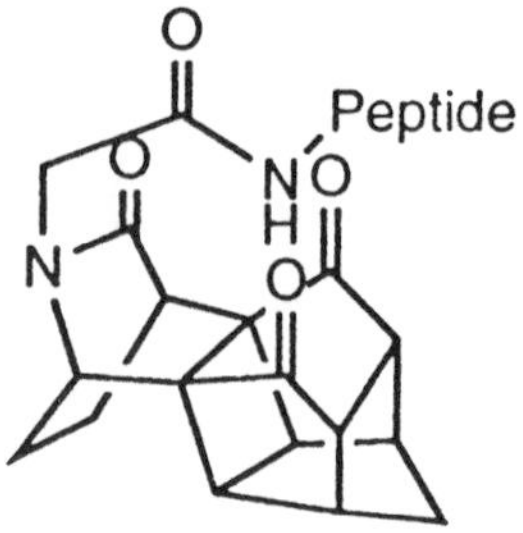

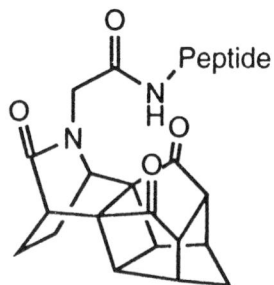

Fig. 27.15

as in a left-handed helix, exhibited decreased helicity under the same conditions. Estimated α-helicity based on the CD-ellipticities at 222 nm are 40%, 70% and 25% for the N-Boc protected linear, right-handed conjugate (Fig. 27.15) and left-handed conjugates (Fig. 27.16) respectively.[78]

Fig. 27.16

IX. β-SHEET

Despite a wide array of potential applications for β-sheet mimetics (e.g. enzyme inhibitors,[79] antigen presentation,[80] disruption of dimerization[81] and second messenger signalling[82]), limited effort in this area has been reported to date. The difficulty in forming a well-defined β-sheet in unaggregated form has hindered understanding of β-sheet properties. In proteins, β-sheets form as the result of an extensive hydrogen-bond network and side-chain–side-chain interactions. Providing hydrogen-bond donors, acceptors and side-chain functional groups in the proper arrangement is a significant synthetic challenge.[83]

Kemp *et al.* described the first β-sheet mimetic which utilizes a diacylaminoepindolidione template. This template was linked to a dipeptide Pro-D-Ala, which is presumed to adopt a β-turn conformation. Subsequent coupling of a urea, which perforce inverts the directionality of the peptide chain, permits the formation of an antiparallel sheet structure (Fig. 27.17).[83–85] Removal of the urea allows for the formation of a parallel β-sheet (Fig. 27.18).[83] The existence of a β-sheet conformation was confirmed by the observation of nOe's between the α-hydrogens of glycine and the H-1 of the epindolidione, and between the hydrogens of the

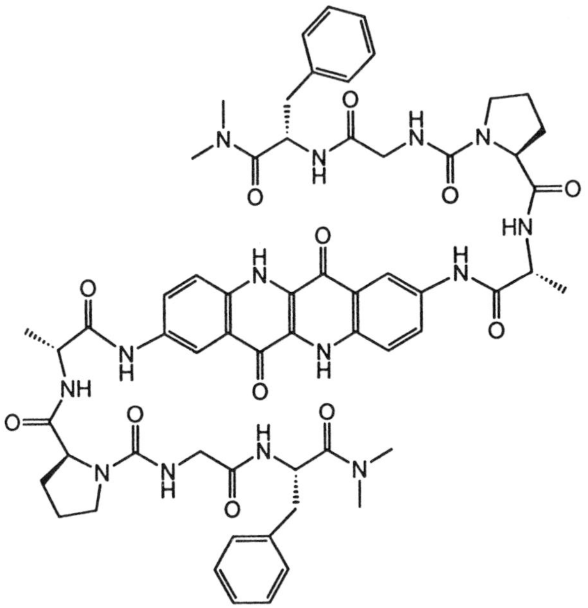

Fig. 27.17

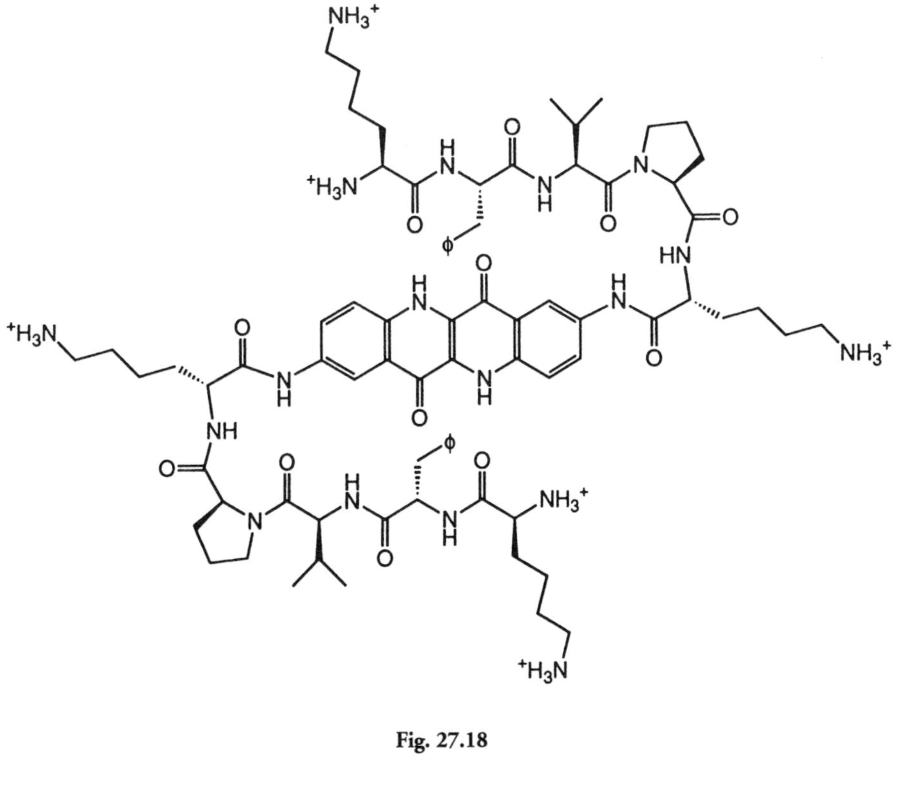

Fig. 27.18

N-methyls and H-10 of the epindolidione in DMSO. Additional supporting evidence was provided by the temperature dependence of amide proton chemical shifts, and geminal coupling constants. The β-turn-forming sequence Pro-D-Ala was replaced by Sar-Gly (Sar = *N*-methylglycine) to examine the effect of the β-turn on the formation of the antiparallel β-sheet. The CD spectrum for this substance, in solvents ranging in polarity from THF to DMSO, exhibited no bands in the range 300–500 nm, indicating no significant interaction between the two amino acid asymmetric centres and the epindolidione, consistent with there being no significant secondary structure.[86] Although the epindolidiones may provide valuable information on the nucleation and stability of parallel and antiparallel β-sheets, a significant shortcoming is the difficulty of incorporating side-chain functionality into this template, which would be required for many biological applications. The use of 3,5-linked pyrrolin-4-ones[87,88] overcomes this problem at the expense of a displaced NH group (Fig. 27.19). Initial modelling indicated that a β-strand would be the favoured conformation. The X-ray crystal structure of this compound confirmed that it exists in a β-strand conformation and that the side-chain orientations closely mimic a natural β-strand in angiotensin. It was also determined from examination of the unit cell that the mimetic dimer adopts an antiparallel β-pleated sheet. Aspartic proteinase inhibitor analogues (for renin and HIV-1) were constructed using the pyrrolinone template based upon previously reported inhibitors. The limited examples disclosed displayed encouraging binding affinities, selectivities, and improved transport properties.[89]

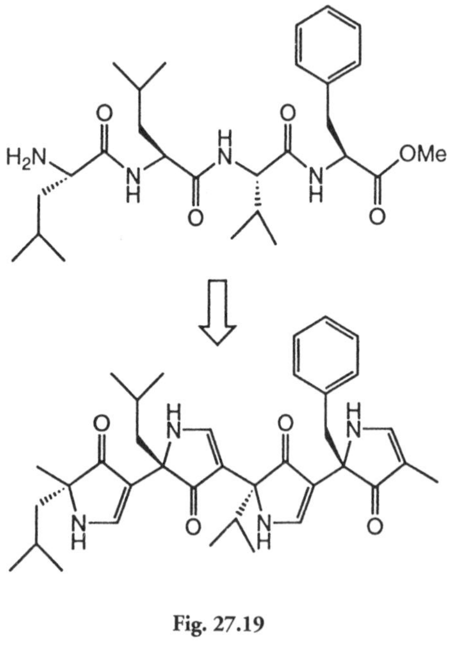

Fig. 27.19

In an attempt to lock the peptide backbone in a β-sheet conformation, Martin *et al.*[90] have used a trisubstituted cyclopropane in a renin inhibitor. Vinylogous polypeptides have also been used to constrain the peptide backbone conformation.[91] They were found to adopt either antiparallel or parallel β-sheets as crystals depending on the side-chain substituents. Elongated vinylogous polypeptides seem to adopt a helical conformation. Flexibility and lack of hydrogen-bond donor/acceptor capacity may hinder their generic application for enzyme inhibition, although cyclotheonamide B, a naturally occurring vinylogous polypeptide, is a relatively potent inhibitor of thrombin.[92]

Using a dibenzofuran as a β-turn template (Fig. 27.20)[93,94] Kelly *et al.* were able to nucleate and stabilize a β-sheet conformation. Similarly, a tricyclic xanthene template was used to mimic the β-loop structure of the snake toxin flavoridin (Fig. 27.21). This analogue displayed approximately 50-fold higher affinity to the fibrinogen receptor gp-IIb/IIIa than the corresponding linear peptide.[78] It is interesting to note that in both cases, in addition to orienting the proper hydrogen-bonding networks, hydrophobic clustering at the turn template seems to stabilize and nucleate the β-sheet.[94]

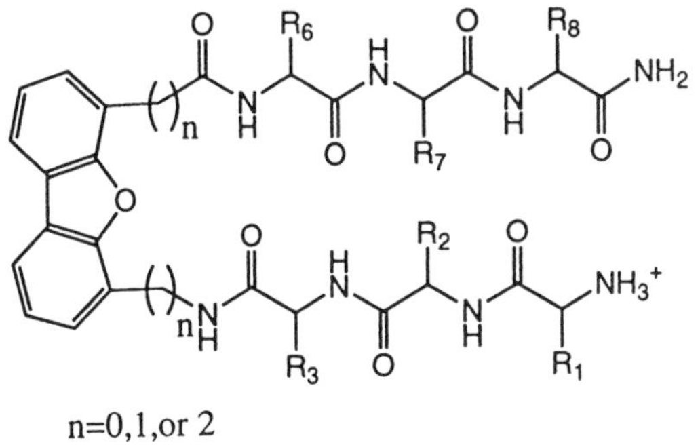

n=0,1,or 2

Fig. 27.20

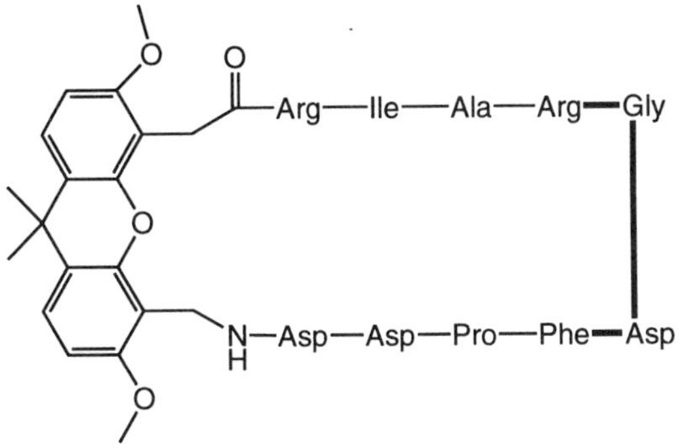

Fig. 27.21

X.   CONCLUSION

The advent of molecular biology (in particular cDNA cloning and monoclonal antibodies) has provided enormous opportunities for structural as well as functional analysis of a wide array of proteinaceous species. The critical roles that proteins play at all levels of biological regulation have opened virtually limitless potential for therapeutic intervention with recombinant proteins. However, with some notable exceptions (EPO, tPA, etc.), the therapeutic applications of proteinaceous species have been severely restricted. Proteins are subject to poor bioavailability, and rapid proteolytic degradation and clearance, and are potentially antigenic. One approach to overcome these liabilities is to develop small molecule mimics.

Recently, there has been an increasing effort to rationally design and synthesize biologically active nonpeptide analogues of peptides and proteins. It is anticipated that these drugs of tomorrow will possess greater selectivity, and hence fewer side-effects, than their present-day counterparts. A number of approaches to this task have been outlined in this chapter. Perhaps the most fascinating feature to emerge in the field of peptidomimetics is the enormous structural diversity and creativity that is being utilized to mimic the ingenious simplicity of nature.

REFERENCES

1. Chen, S., Chrusciel, R. A., Nakanishi, H. *et al.* (1992) Design and synthesis of a CD-4 β-turn mimetic that inhibits human immunodeficiency virus envelope glycoprotein gp120 binding and infection of human lymphocytes. *Proc. Natl. Acad. Sci. USA.* **89**: 5872–5876.
2. Marshall, G. R., Gorin, F. A. and Moore M. L. (1978) *Annu. Rev. Med. Chem.* **13**: 227–238.
3. Fauchère, J. L. (1987) In Hadzi, D. and Jerman-Blazic, B. (eds) *QSAR in Drug Design and Toxicology.* Elsevier, Amsterdam, pp. 22.
4. Hruby, V. J. (1987) Implications of the X-ray structure of deamino-oxytocin to agonist/antagonist–receptor interactions. *Trends Pharmacol. Sci.* **8**: 336.
5. Hruby, V. J., Al-Oeidi, F. and Kazmierski, W. (1990) Emerging approaches in the molecular design of receptor-selective peptide ligands: conformational, topographical and dynamic considerations. *Biochem. J.* **268**: 249–262.
6. Hughes, J., Smith, T. W., Kostelitz, H. W., Fothergill, L. A., Morgan, B. A. and Morris, H. R. (1975) Identification of two related pentapeptides from the brain with potent opiate agonist activity. *Nature.* **258**: 577–579.
7. For example, see Hagan, R.M. and McClem, S. (1993) Vineyard peptide conference bears fruit. *Trends Pharmacol. Sci.* **14**: 315–318.
8. Fauchère, J. L. (1986) Elements for the rational design of peptide drugs. *Adv. Drug Res.* **15**: 29–69.
9. Milner-White, J. (1989) Predicting the biologically active conformations of short polypeptides. *Trends Pharmacol. Sci.* **10**: 70–74.
10. de Vos, A. M., Ultsch, M. and Kossiakoff, A. A. (1992) Human growth hormone and extracellular domain of its receptor: crystal structure of the complex. *Science,* **255**: 306–312.
11. Miklavc, A., Kocjan, D., Avbelj, F. and Hadzi, D. (1987) In Hadzi, D. and Jerman-Blazic, B. (eds) *QSAR in Drug Design and Toxicology,* pp. 185. Elsevier, Amsterdam.
12. Veber, D. F., Holly, F. W., Paleveda, W. J., Nutt, R. F., Bergstrand, S. J., Torchiana, M., Glitzer, M. S. and Saperstein, R. (1979) Highly active cyclic and bicyclic somatostatin analogues of reduced ring size. *Nature* **280**: 512–514.
13. Kaiser, E. T. and Kezdy, F. J. (1983) Secondary structures of proteins and peptides in amphilic environments (a review). *Proc. Natl. Acad. Sci. USA* **80**: 1137–1143.
14. Kahn, M. (1993) (ed.) In *Peptide Secondary Structure Mimetics.* Tetrahedron Symposia-in-Print Number 50. Pergamon Press, Oxford.
15. Rose, G. D., Gierash, L. M. and Smith, J. A. (1985) Turns in peptides and proteins. *Adv. Protein Chem.* **37**: 1–109.
16. Ball, J. B. and Alewood, P. F. (1990) Conformational constraints: non-peptide β-turn mimics. *J. Mol. Recog.* **3**: 55–64.
17. Baca, M., Alewood, P. F., Kent and S. B. H. (1993) Structural engineering of the HIV-1 protease molecule with a β-turn mimic of fixed geometry. *Protein Sci.* **2**: 1085–1091.
18. Nagai, U. and Sato, K. (1985) Synthesis of a bicyclic dipeptide with the shape of β-turn central part. *Tetrahedron Lett.* **26**: 647–650.
19. Nicolaou, K. C., Salvino, J. M., Raynor, K., Pietranico, S., Reisine, T., Freidinger, R. M. and Hirschmann, R. (1990) Design and synthesis of a pentidomimetic employing β-D glucose for scaffolding. *Peptide Chem. Struct. Biol. Proc. 11th Am. Peptide Symp,* pp. 881–884.

20. James, G. L., Goldstein, J. L., Brown, M. S. *et al.* (1993) Benzodiazepine peptidomimetics: potent inhibitors of *Ras* farnesylation in animal cells. *Science* **260:** 1937–1942.

21. Flynn, G. A., Giroux, E. L. and Dage, R. C. (1987) An acyl-iminium ion cyclization route to a novel conformationally restricted dipeptide mimic: applications to angiotensin converting enzyme inhibition. *J. Am. Chem. Soc.* **109:** 7914–5.

22. Borkakoti, N., Winkler, F. K., Williams, D. H., D'Arcy, A., Broadhurst, M. J., Brown, P. A., Johnson, W. H. and Murray, E. J. (1994) Structure of the catalytic domain of human fibroblast collagenase complexed with an inhibitor. *Struct. Biol.* **1:** 106–110.

23. Wilmot, C. M. and Thornton, J. M. (1988) Analysis and prediction of the different types of β-turn in proteins. *J. Mol. Biol.* **197:** 221–232.

24. Merrifield, R. B. (1985) Solid phase synthesis (Nobel Lecture). *Angew. Chem. Int. Ed. Engl.* **24:** 799–810.

25. Kahn *et al.*, unpublished results.

26. Wasserman, H. H. (1982) Transamidation reactions using β-lactams. The synthesis of homaline. *Tetrahedron Lett.* **23:** 465–468.

27. Sato, M., Lee, J. Y. H., Nakanishi, H., Johnson, M. E., Chrusciel, R. A. and Kahn, M. (1992) Design, synthesis and conformational analysis of γ-turn peptide mimetics of bradykinin. *Biochem. Biophys. Res. Commun.* **187:** 999–1006.

28. Kabat, E. A. (1978) *Adv. Protein Chem.* **32:** 1–75.

29. Amzel, L. M. and Poljak, R. J. (1979) *Annu. Rev. Biochem.* **48:** 961–997.

30. Martin, A. C. R., Cheetham, J. C. and Rees, A. R. (1989) Modelling antibody hypervariable loops: a combined algorithm. *Proc. Natl. Acad. Sci. USA* **86:** 9268–9272.

31. Chothia, C., Lesk, A. M., Tramontano, A. *et al.* (1989) Conformations of immunoglobulin hypervariable regions. *Nature* **342:** 877–883.

32. Bruck, C., Co, M. S., Slaoui, M., Gaulton, G. N., Smith T., Fields, B N., Mullins, J. I. and Greene, M. I. (1986) Nucleic acid sequence of an internal image-bearing monoclonal anti-idiotype and its comparison to the sequence of the external antigens. *Proc. Natl. Acad. Sci. USA* **83:** 6578–6582.

33. Chothia, C. and Lesk, A. M. (1987) Canonical structures for the hypervariable regions of immunoglobulins. *J. Mol. Biol.* **196:** 901–917.

34. Saragovi, H. U., Fitzpatrick, D., Raktabutr, A., Nakanishi, H., Kahn, M. and Greene, M. I. (1991) Design and synthesis of a mimetic from an antibody complementarity-determining region. *Science* **253:** 792–797.

35. Landau, N. R., Warton, M. and Littman, D. R. (1988) The envelope glycoprotein of the human immunodeficiency virus binds to the immunoglobulin-like domain of CD4. *Nature* **334:** 159–162.

36. Ashkenazi, A., Presta, L. G., Marsters, S. A., Camerato, T. R., Rosenthal, K. A., Fendly, B. M. and Capon, D. J. (1990) Mapping the CD4 binding site for human immunodeficiency virus by alanine-scanning mutagenesis. *Proc. Natl. Acad. Sci. USA* **87:** 7150–7154.

37. Jameson, B. A., Rao, P. E., Kong. L. I., Hahn, B. H., Shaw, G. M., Hood, L. E. and Kent, S. B. H. (1988) Location and chemical synthesis of a binding site for HIV-1 on the CD4 protein. *Science.* **240:** 1335–1339.

38. Roques, B. P., Garbary-Jaureguiberry, C., Oberlin, R., Anteunis, M. and Lala, A. K. (1976) Enkephalin degrading enzyme inhibitors: a physiological way to new analgesics and psychoactive Agents. *Nature* **262:** 778.

39. Mansour, A., Khachturian, H., Lewis, M. E., Akil, H. and Watson, S. J. (1988) Anatomy of CNS opioid receptors. *Trends Neurosci.* **11:** 308–314.

40. Rapaka, R. S., Barnett, G. and Hawks, R. L. (1986) (eds) *Opioid Peptides: Medicinal Chemistry.* NIDA Research Monograph 69. Rockville, MD.

41. Su., T., Nakanishi, H., Xue, L., Chen, B., Tuladhar, S., Johnson, M. E. and Kahn, M. (1993) Nonpeptide β-turn mimetics of enkephalin. *Bioorg. Med. Chem. Lett.* **5:** 835–840.

42. Hansen, P. E., Morgan, B. A. (1990) Structure–activity relationships in enkephalin peptides. In Udenfried, S. and Meienhofer, J. (eds) *The Peptides: Analysis, Synthesis, Biology,* 6th edn., pp. 269–321. Academic Press, Orlando.

43. Schiller, P. W. (1990) Conformation analysis of enkephalin and conformation–activity relationships. In Udenfried, S. and Meienhofer, J. (eds) *The Peptides: Analysis, Synthesis, Biology,* 6th edn., pp. 219–268. Academic Press, Orlando.

44. Bélanger, P. C., Dufresne, C., Scheigetz, J., Young, R. N., Springer, J. P. and Dmitrienko, G. I. (1982) Design and synthesis of nonpeptide compounds as mimics of a conformation of methionine enkephalin. *Can. J. Chem.* **60**: 1019–1029.

45. Hassan, M. and Goodman, M. (1986) Computer simulations of cyclic enkephalin analogues. *Biochemistry* **25**: 7596–7606 and references therein.

46. Chew, C., Villar, H. O. and Loew, G. H. (1991) Theoretical study of the flexibility and solution conformation of the cyclic opioid peptide [D-Pen², D-Pen⁵] enkephalin and [D-Pen, L-Pen⁵] enkephalin. *Mol. Pharmacol.* **39**: 502–510.

47. Pettitt, B. M., Matsunaga, T., Al-Obeidi, F., Gehrig, C., Hruby, V. J., Karplus, M., Ohlmeyer, M. H., Swanson, R. M., Dillard, L. W. and Reader, J. C. (1991) *Biophys. J.* **60**: 1540.

48. Smith, P. E., Dana, L. X. and Pettitt, B. M. (1991) Simulation of the structure and dynamics of the bis(penicillamine) enkephalin zwitterion. *J. Am. Chem. Soc.* **113**: 67.

49. Aubry, A., Birlirakis, N., Sakarellos-Daitsiotis, M., Sakarellos, C. and Marroud, M. A (1989) Crystal molecular conformation of leucine-enkephalin related to the morphine molecule. *Biopolymers* **28**: 27–40.

50. Griffin, J. F. and Smith, G. D. (1988) X-ray diffraction studies of enkephalins and opiates. In Rapaka, R. S. and Dhawan, B. N. (eds) *Opioid Peptides: An Update*, pp. 41–59. NIDA Research Monograph 87. Washington, DC.

51. Hruby, V. J., Kao, L. F., Pettitt, B. M. and Karplus, M. (1988) The conformational properties of the delta opioid peptide [D-Pen², D-Pen⁵] enkephalin in aqueous solution determined by NMR and energy minimization calculations. *J. Am. Chem. Soc.* **110**: 3351–3359.

52. Picone, D., D'Ursi, A., Motta, A., Tacredi, T. and Temussi, P. A. (1990) Conformational preferences of [Leu⁵] enkephalin in biomimetic media. *Eur. J. Biochem.* **192**: 433–439.

53. Mosberg, H. I., Sobczyk-Kojiro, K., Subramanian, P., Crippen, G. M., Ramalingam, K. and Woodard, R. W. (1990) Combined use of stereospecific deuteration, NMR, distance geometry, and energy minimization for the conformational analysis of the highly δ opioid receptor selective peptide [D-Pen²,D-Pen⁵] enkephalin. *J. Am. Chem. Soc.* **112**: 822–829.

54. Bradbury, A. F., Smyth, D. G. and Snell, C. R. (1976) Biosynthetic origin and receptor conformation of methionine enkephalin. *Nature* **260**: 165–166.

55. Loew, G. H. and Burt, S. K. (1978) Energy confirmation study of met-enkephalin and its D-Ala² analogue and their resemblance to rigid opiates. *Proc. Natl. Acad. Sci. USA* **75**: 7–11.

56. Humblet, C. and DeCoen, J. L. (1977) In Goodrum, M. and Meienhofer, J. (eds) *Peptides: Proceedings of the Fifth American Peptide Symposium*, pp. 88–91. Wiley, New York.

57. Balodis, Y. Y., Nikiforovich, G. V., Grinsteine, I. V., Vegner, R. E. and Chipens, G. I. (1978) *FEBS Lett.* **86**: 239–242.

58. Manavalan, P. and Momany, F. A. (1980) Conformational energy studies on N-methylated analogues of thyrotropin releasing hormone enkephalin and luteinizing hormone-releasing hormones. *Biopolymers* **19**: 1943–1973.

59. Freidinger, R. M. (1981) In Rich, D. H. and Gross, E. (eds) *Peptides, Synthesis, Structure, Function*, pp. 673–683. Pierce Chemical Co., Rockford

60. DiMaio, J. and Schiller, P. W. (1980) A cyclic enkephalin analog with high in vitro opiate activity. *Proc. Natl. Acad. Sci. USA* **77**: 7162–7166.

61. Gardner, B., Nakanishi, H. and Kahn, M. (1993) Conformationally constrained nonpeptide β-turn mimetics of enkephalin. *Tetrahedron* **49**: 3433–3448.

62. Barlow, D. J. and Thornton, J. M. (1988) Helix geometry in proteins. *J. Mol. Biol.* **201**: 601–619.

63. Padmanabhan, S., Marqusee, S., Ridgeway, T., Laue, T. M. and Baldwin, R. L. (1990) Relative helix-forming tendencies of non-polar amino acids. *Nature* **344**: 268–270.

64. Chakrabartty, A., Schellman, J. A. and Baldwin, R. L. (1991) Large differences in the helix propensities of alanine and glycine. *Nature* **351**: 586–588.

65. Padmanabhan, S. and Baldwin, R. L. (1991) Straight-chain non-polar amino acids are good helix formers in water. *J. Mol. Biol.* **219**: 135–137.

66. Chakrabartty, A., Kortemme, T., Padamanabhan, S. and Baldwin, R. L. (1993) Aromatic side-chain contribution to far-ultraviolet circular dichroism of helical peptides and its effect en measurement of helix propensities. *Biochemistry* **32**: 5560–5565.

67. Blaber, M., Zhang, X-J and Matthews, B. W. (1993) Structural basis of amino acid α-helix propensity. *Science* **260**: 1637–1640.

68. Hermans, J., Anderson, A. G. and Yun, R. H. (1992) Differential helix propensity of small apolar side chains studied by molecular dynamics simulations. *Biochemistry* **31**: 5646–5653.

69. Komeiji, Y., Uebayashi, M., Someya, J-I. and Yamato, I. (1993) A molecular dynamics study of solvent behavior around a protein. *Proteins* **16**: 268–277.

70. Kemp, D. S. and Curran, T. P. (1988) (2*S*, 5*S*, 8*S*, 11*S*)-1-Acetyl-1,4-diaza-3-keto-5-carboxy-10-thia-tricyclo-[2.8.0^{4,8}]-tridecane. 1. Synthesis of prolyl-proline-derived, peptide-functionalized templates for α-helix formation. *Tetrahedron Lett.* **29**: 4931–4934.

71. Arrhenius, T., Lerner, R. A. and Satterthwait, A. C. (1987) The chemical synthesis of structured peptides using covalent hydrogen bond mimics. In Oxender, D. (ed.) *Protein Structure, Folding and Design*, pp. 453–465. Alan R. Liss, New York.

72. Arrhenius, T. and Satterthwait, A. C. (1989) The substitution of an amide-amide backbone hydrogen bond in an α-helical peptide with a covalent hydrogen bond mimic. In Rivier, J. E. and Marshall, G. R. (eds) *The 11th American Peptide Symposium* pp. 870–872. Escom, Leiden.

73. Pardi, A., Billeter, M. and Wuthrich, K. (1984) Calibration of the angular dependence of the amide proton-Cα proton coupling constants, $^3J_{HN\alpha}$, in a globular protein. *J. Mol. Biol.* **180**: 741–751.

74. Kemp, D. S. and Curran, T. P. (1988) The preferred conformation of 1 (1 = αTemp-OH) and its peptide conjugates αTemp-L-(Ala)n-OR (n=1 to 4) and αTemp-L-Ala-L-Phe-L-Lys (ε Boc)-L-Lys (εBOC)-NHMe. *Tetrahedron Lett.* **29**: 4935–4938.

75. Kemp, D. S., Allen, T. J. and Oslick, S. L. (1991) Development of a 3-state equilibrium model for the helix-nucleation template Ac-Hel$_1$-OH. In Smith, J. A. and Rivier, J. E. (eds) *Peptides Chemistry and Biology: Proceedings of the 12th American Peptide Symposium*, pp. 352–355. Escom, Leiden.

76. Kemp, D. S., Curran, T. P., Boyd, J. G. and Allen, T. J. (1991) Studies of *N*-terminal templates for α-helix formation. Synthesis and conformational analysis of (2*S*, 5*S*, 8*S*, 11*S*)-1-acetyl-1,4-diaza-3-keto-5-carboxy-10-thiatricyclo [2.8.1.0^{4,8}]-tridecane (Ac-Hel$_1$-OH). *J. Org. Chem.* **56**: 6672–6682.

77. Kemp, D. S. and Rothman, J. H. (1992) 3$_{10}$ helix nucleation with a macrocyclic triproline template. In Smith, J. A. and Rivier, J. E. (eds) *Peptides: Chemistry and Biology, Proceedings of the 12th American Peptide Symposium*, pp. 350–351. Escom, Leiden.

78. Müller, K., Obrecht, D., Knierzinger, A. *et al.* (1993) Building blocks for the induction or fixation of peptide conformations. In Testa, B., Kyburz, E., Fuhrer, W. and Giger, R. (eds) *Perspectives in Medicinal Chemistry*, pp. 513–531. Verlag Helvetica Chimica Acta, Basel.

79. Borkakoti, N., Winkler, F. K., Williams, D. H., D'Arcy, A., Broadhurst, M. J., Brown, P. A., Johnson, W. H. and Murray, E. J. (1994) Structure of the catalytic domain of human fibroblast collagenase complexed with an inhibitor. *Struct. Biol.* **1**: 106–110.

80. Bjorkman, P. J., Saper, M. A., Samraoui, B., Bennett, W. S., Strominger, J. L. and Wiley, D. C. (1987) The foreign antigen binding site and T-cell recognition regions. *Nature* **329**: 512–518.

81. Schramm, H. J., Nakashima, H., Schramm, W., Wakayama, H. and Yamamoto, N. (1991) HIV-1 reproduction is inhibited by peptide derived from the N- and C-termini of HIV-1. *Biochem. Biophys. Res. Commun.* **179**(2), 847–851.

82. Waksman, G., Kominos, D., Robertson, S. C. *et al.* (1992) Crystal structure of the phosphotyrosine recognition domain SH2 of v-Src complexed with tyrosine-phosphorylated peptides. *Nature.* **358**: 646–653.

83. Kemp, D. S., Blanchard, D. E. and Muendel, C. C. (1991) Studies on the nucleation in DMSO and water of β-sheet structures with peptide epinolodione conjugates. In Smith, J. A. and Rivier, J. E. (eds) *Peptides; Chemistry and Biology, Proceedings of the 12th American Peptide Symposium*, pp. 319–322. Escom, Leiden.

84. Kemp, D. S. and Bowen, B. R. (1988) Synthesis of peptide-functionalized diacyl-aminoependolidiones as templates for β-sheet formation. *Tetrahedron Lett.* **29**: 5077–5080.

85. Kemp, D. S. and Bowen, B. R. (1988) Conformational analysis of peptide-functionalized diacyl-aminoepindolidiones: ^{1}H NMR evidence for β-sheet formation. *Tetrahedron Lett.* **29**: 5081–5082.

86. Kemp, D. S. and Bowen, B. R. (1990) Diacyclaminepindolidiones as templates for β-sheets. In Gierasch, L. M. and King, J. (eds) *Protein Folding: Deciphering the Second Half of the Genetic Code*, pp 293–303. AAAS, Washington, DC.

87. Smith, A. B., III, Keenan, T. P., Holcomb, R. C., Sprengler, P. A., Guzman, M. C., Wood, J. L., Carroll, P. J. and Hirschmann, R. (1992) Design, synthesis, and crystal structure of a pyrrolinone-based peptidomimetic possessing the conformation of a β-strand: potential application to the design of novel inhibitors of proteolytic enzymes. *J. Am. Chem. Soc.* **114**: 10672–10674.

88. Smith, A. B. III, Holcomb, R. C., Guzman, M. C., Keenan, T. P., Sprengler, P. A. and Hirschmann, R. (1993) An effective synthesis of scalemic 3,5,5-trisubstituted pyrrolin-4-ones. *Tetrahedron Letts.* **34:** 63–66.

89. Smith, A. B. III, Hirschmann, R., Pasternak, A. *et al.* (1994) Design and synthesis of peptidomimetics inhibitors of HIV-1 protease and renin. Evidence for improved transport. *J. Med. Chem.* **37**(2): 215–218.

90. Martin, S. F., Austin, R. E., Oalmann, C. J. et al. (1992) 1,2,3-Trisubstituted cyclopropanes as conformationally restricted peptide isosteres: application to the degree and synthesis of novel renin inhibitors. *J. Med. Chem.* **35:** 1710–1721.

91. Hagihara, M., Anthony, N. J., Stout, T. J., Clardy, J. and Schrieber, S. L. (1992) Vinylogous polypeptides: an alternative backbone. *J. Am. Chem. Soc.* **114:** 6568–6570.

92. Fusetani, N., Matsunaga, S., Matsumoto, H. and Takebayashi, Y. (1990) Cyclotheonamides, potent thrombin inhibitors from a marine sponge *Theonella SP. J. Am. Chem. Soc.* **112:** 7053–7054.

93. Diaz, H., Tsang, K. Y., Choo, D., Espina, J. R. and Kelly, J. W. (1993) Design, synthesis and partial characterization of water-soluble β-sheets stabilized by a dibenzofuran-based amino acid. *J. Am. Chem. Soc.* **115:** 3790–3791.

94. Tsang, K. Y., Diaz, H., Graciani, N. and Kelly, J. W. (1994) Hydrophobic cluster formation is necessary for dibenzofuran-based amino acids to function as β-nucleators. *J. Am. Chem. Soc.* **116:** 3988–4005.

PART VI

Chemical Modifications Influencing the Pharmacokinetic Properties

28

The Fate of Xenobiotics in Living Organisms

FRANS M. BELPAIRE AND MARC G. BOGAERT

To explain all nature is too difficult a task for any one man or even for any one age. 'T is much better to do a little with certainty, and leave the rest for others that come after you, than to explain all things.
Isaac Newton

Most drugs exert their effect through reversible binding to receptors. Onset, duration and intensity of the effect will depend on the concentration of the drug in the fluid surrounding the receptors, i.e. the biophase. Only exceptionally are drugs applied *in situ*; in most cases drugs are

THE PRACTICE OF MEDICINAL CHEMISTRY
ISBN 0-12-744640-0

transferred from the site of administration to the biophase via the plasma. Indeed, after absorption, the drug is distributed via the circulation to the different parts of the organism, including the organ(s) in which the biophase for the drug is localized. The drug is also distributed to organs such as the kidneys and the liver, which excrete it unchanged into the urine or the bile, and to organs, mainly the liver, which metabolize it. The metabolites formed are either further metabolized or excreted unchanged. As a consequence of elimination (excretion and biotransformation), the concentration of the drug in the organism, i.e. in the biophase, decreases, usually resulting in a decrease of the effect. The processes involved in drug disposition (absorption, distribution and elimination) are shown schematically in Fig. 28.1. The concentrations of a drug in the biophase and elsewhere in the organism depend upon the dose administered, and upon the rate and extent of absorption, distribution and elimination. Pharmacokinetics is the study of the drug concentration as a function of time in the different parts of the organism.

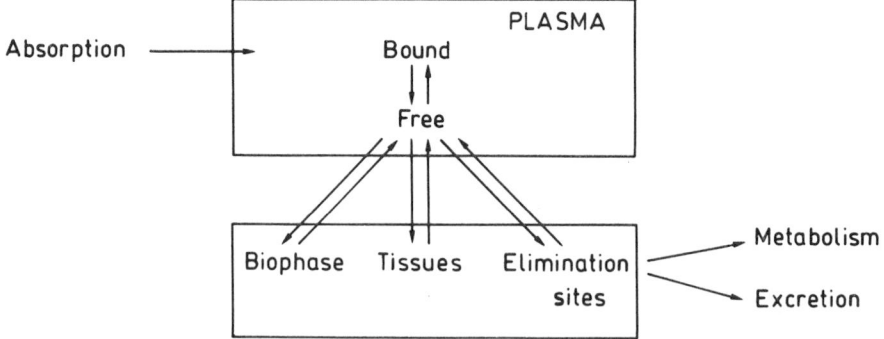

Fig. 28.1   Schematic representation of drug absorption, distribution and elimination.

Drug disposition involves passage through biological membranes. In this overview, first the mechanisms of the passage of drugs through membranes will be discussed, and then the different processes of drug disposition will be described.

I.   PASSAGE OF DRUGS THROUGH MEMBRANES

After administration, a drug often encounters several cell membranes before it reaches the biophase and other parts of the organism, e.g. the elimination sites. Cellular membranes are composed of a lipoidal matrix covered on both sides by proteins. Cell membranes contain small pores, and narrow, water-filled channels exist between cells. Drugs cross membranes by passive or, in some cases, carrier-mediated mechanisms.

A.   Passive processes

1.   Filtration

If hydrostatic pressure is applied or if an osmotic gradient is imposed across a cell membrane, water, together with small solutes, will pass through the cell membrane pores. There is a considerable variation in the estimated pore size of various membranes and, correspondingly, in the size of the molecules that can pass through these pores. In most cell membranes the pores have a diameter of about 7 Å; substances with a molecular weight below 100 daltons, such as water and urea can pass through them, but most drugs have molecular weights above 100 daltons.

The channels between cells are usually rather narrow, but between capillary endothelial cells the intercellular channels measure about 40 Å. These allow passage of molecules with molecular weight below 60 kDa. Most drugs have molecular weight lower than 1 kDa. Most proteins have molecular weight larger than 60 kDa and cannot pass through these channels, and this is also true for proteins to which drugs are bound. Albumin (68 kDa) passes to a limited extent from the plasma to the extracellular fluid. The capillaries of the glomeruli of the kidney are composed of a particularly thin endothelium, which is very rich in intercellular pores, so that this membrane is far more permeable to solutes than are the capillaries elsewhere. The endothelial cells of the brain capillaries are surrounded by a layer of glial cells, which have tight intercellular junctions. To move from blood to brain and vice versa, materials must pass through the cells rather than between them. Filtration is not possible, and this constitues the so called 'blood–brain barrier'.

2.   Passive diffusion

Passive diffusion is the most important mechanism for passage of drugs through membranes. Lipid-soluble drugs penetrate lipid membranes with ease. Polar molecules, and all ionized compounds, partition poorly into lipids and are not able to pass through membranes, or do so at a much lower rate than do lipophilic molecules. Transmembrane diffusion is driven by the transmembranar concentration gradient of the drug. The rate of diffusion depends, apart from the lipid/water partition coefficient of the drug (P) and the concentration gradient ($C_{out} - C_{in}$), on membrane properties such as the membrane area (A), the thickness of the membrane (h), and the diffusion coefficient (D) of the drug in the membrane, according to Fick's law:

$$\text{Rate of diffusion} = -\frac{D \cdot A \cdot P \cdot (C_{out} - C_{in})}{h}$$

Many drugs are acidic or basic compounds which in aqueous medium are ionized to a certain degree, depending on their dissociation constant (pK_a) and the pH of the solution, according to the Henderson–Hasselbalch equation.

For acidic drugs

$$pH = pK_a + \log\frac{\text{Ionized concentration}}{\text{Unionized concentration}}$$

For basic drugs

$$pH = pK_a + \log\frac{\text{Unionized concentration}}{\text{Ionized concentration}}$$

Very weak acids with pK_a values higher than 7.5 are essentially unionized at the pH values encountered in the organism. For these drugs, transport is rapid and independent of pH, provided the unionized form is lipid-soluble. For acidic drugs with a pK_a value between 3.0 and 7.5, the fraction of unionized drug changes importantly with the changes in pH encountered in the organism, and for these drugs a change in the rate of transport with pH is expected. For acidic drugs with a pK_a lower than 2.5, the fraction of unionized drug is low so that diffusion across membranes is very slow. A similar analysis can be done for bases.

At equilibrium the concentrations of unionized molecules on each side of the membrane are equal. If the pH on each side of the membrane is equal, the concentration of ionized molecules, and thus the total concentration of the molecules, will be the same on each side of the membrane. If there is a difference in pH, as for example between plasma (pH 7.4) and the stomach contents (pH 1–3), at equilibrium the concentration of the ionized molecules and therefore the total concentration will be much higher on one side of the membrane than on the other. This phenomenon is called ion-trapping.

B. Carrier-mediated processes

For some substances, including those which are lipid-insoluble or ionized, the transfer through some membranes can be facilitated by specialized processes, e.g. passive facilitated diffusion and active transport. Facilitated transport is carrier-mediated and operates along a concentration gradient, without expenditure of energy. At equilibrium the solute will attain the same concentrations on each side of the membrane; at high concentrations of the drug, the rate of transport reaches a maximum. The process is rather specific, and substances can inhibit each other's passage. Passive facilitated diffusion seems to play a minor role in drug transport. An example is the transport of vitamin B_{12} across the gastrointestinal wall.

Active transport also has the characteristics of a carrier-mediated transport outlined above but, in addition, the molecules move against a concentration gradient, and energy is required. Active transport can explain renal and biliary excretion of many drugs, e.g. the renal tubular secretion of penicillins.

II. ABSORPTION

Absorption can be defined as the passage of a drug from its site of administration into the circulation. If a drug is administered directly into the vascular system, e.g. by intravenous administration, absorption is not needed. Drugs can be administered by enteral and parenteral routes. Enteral administration occurs through contact of the drug with the buccal mucosa (sublingual), through swallowing (oral) or by rectal administration. With parenteral administration, the gastrointestinal tract is bypassed; examples are the intravenous and intramuscular routes. Drugs can also be absorbed through the skin or through the mucosa of various organs (bronchial, nasal, vaginal, ...). In some cases a drug is applied for its local effect, and no absorption is intended.

To express the extent to which and at which rate a drug reaches the systemic circulation, the term *bioavailability* is used. Bioavailability of a drug is (1) the fraction of the administered dose which reaches the systemic circulation, and (2) the rate at which this occurs. After intravenous administration, bioavailability is by definition 100%; for all other routes of administration, the bioavailability can vary between 0 and 100%.

Bioavailability is influenced by several factors, such as drug characteristics (solubility, particle size, crystalline form, pK_a, lipid/water partition coefficient), formulation (pharmaceutical dosage

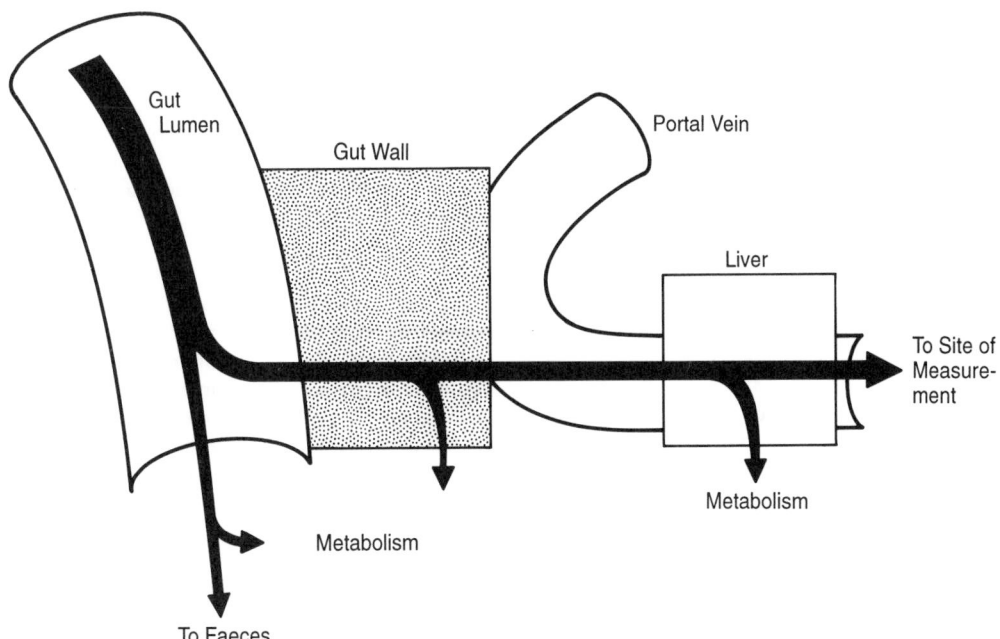

Fig. 28.2   After oral administration, a drug must pass from the gut lumen, through the gut wall and then through the liver before reaching the systemic circulation. Biotransformation may occur in the lumen before absorption, in the gut wall during absorption, and/or in the liver after absorption but before reaching the systemic circulation. (From Rowland and Tozer (1989) *Clinical Pharmacokinetics*, Lea & Febiger, Philadelphia. Reproduced with permission.)

form), changes at the site of administration (pH, blood flow), the presence of other drugs or food, and the route of administration. The last is very important; after absorption from the gastrointestinal tract, a drug has to pass the liver before gaining access to the systemic circulation (Fig. 28.2). Both the gastrointestinal tract wall and the liver are capable of metabolizing drugs. This presystemic metabolism, termed the 'first pass effect', can result in an appreciable fraction of the dose not reaching the systemic circulation. This first pass phenomenon also exists after intraperitoneal and, partially, after rectal administration. It does not exist for other routes of administration. Drugs that undergo extensive first pass metabolism often have low and variable bioavailability.

In this chapter we will describe in detail drug administration by the oral route. Some characteristics of other common routes of drug administration are listed in Table 28.1. For more details on these various routes, the reader is referred to the literature.

The rate and extent of absorption after oral administration are determined first by disintegration and dissolution. Before a drug is absorbed from the gastrointestinal tract it has to dissolve in the aqueous medium of the stomach and the intestine. Dissolution of the drug will depend on the water solubility, particle size, chemical form and crystalline characteristics of the drug, and the pH of the surrounding medium. Many drugs are taken as tablets or capsules and these have to disintegrate before dissolution and liquid dosage forms are, in general, more rapidly absorbed than solid forms. Disintegration can be controlled and in recent years various modified drug products have been developed to alter the timing of the release of the active drug from the the drug product. The term 'controlled release' has been used to describe various types

Table 28.1 Common routes of drug administration.

Route	Bioavailability	Advantages	Disadvantages
Parenteral routes			
Intravenous bolus (i.v.)	Complete (100 %) systemic drug absorption. Rate of bioavailability considered instantaneous.	Drug is given for immediate effect.	Increased chance for adverse reaction. Possible anaphylaxis.
Intravenous infusion (i.v. inf)	Complete (100 %) systemic drug absorption. Rate of drug absorption controlled by infusion pump.	Plasma drug levels more precisely controlled. May inject large fluid volumes. May use drugs with poor lipid solubility and/or irritating drugs.	Requires skill in insertion of infusion set. Tissue damage at site of injection (infiltration, necrosis, or sterile abscess).
Intramuscular injection (i.m.)	Rapid absorption from aqueous solution. Slow absorption from nonaqueous (oil) solutions.	Easier to inject than by intravenous injection. Larger volumes may be used compared to subcutaneous solutions.	Irritating drugs may be very painful. Different rates or absorption depending upon muscle group injected and blood flow.
Subcutaneous injection (s.c.)	Prompt from aqueous solution. Slow absorption from repository formulations.	Generally, used for insulin injection.	Rate of drug absorption depends upon blood flow and injection volume.
Enteral routes			
Buccal or sublingual (s.l.)	Rapid absorption from lipid-soluble drugs.	No 'first-pass' effects.	Some drug may be swallowed. Not for most drugs or drugs with high doses.
Oral (p.o.)	Absorption may vary. Generally, slower absorption rate compared to i.v. bolus or i.m. injection.	Safest and easiest route of drug administration. May use immediate-release and modified-release drug products.	Some drugs may have erratic absorption, be unstable in the gastrointestinal tract, or be metabolized by liver prior to systemic absorption.
Rectal (p.r.)	Absorption may vary from suppository. More reliable absorption from enema (solution).	Useful when patient cannot swallow medication. Used for local and systemic effects.	Absorption may be erratic. Suppository may migrate to different position. Some patient discomfort.

(Continued)

Table 28.1 *Continued*

Route	Bioavailability	Advantages	Disadvantages
Other routes			
Transdermal	Slow absorption, rate may vary. Increased absorption with occlusive dressing.	Transdermal delivery system (patch) is easy to use. Used for lipid-soluble drugs with low dose and low MW.	Some irritation by patch or drug. Permeability of skin variable with condition, anatomic site, age, and gender. Type of cream or ointment base affects drug release and absorption.
Inhalation	Rapid absorption. Total dose absorbed is variable.	May be used for local or systemic effects.	Particle size of drug determines anatomic placement in respiratory tract. May stimulate cough reflex. Some drug may be swallowed.

Reproduced with permission from Shargel,L. and Yu, A. B. C. (1993) *Applied Biopharmaceutics and Pharmacokinetics* (third edition). Prentice-Hall International Editions p. 120.

of oral extended release rate dosage forms (such as sustained release, prolonged release) and delayed release dosage forms (e.g. enteric coated). One of the newer systems for controlled release is the osmotic pump: drug delivery is driven by an osmotically controlled device that pumps a constant amount of water through the system, dissolving and releasing a constant amount of drug per unit time.

Once the drug is dissolved, it can be absorbed, mostly by passive diffusion, and pass into the capillaries of the gastrointestinal wall and then into the portal venous system. For some drugs with high lipid solubility, absorption via the lymphatic system is possible. As drug molecules move through the gastrointestinal tract, they encounter environments which vary in pH, enzyme content, and fluidity of contents as well as in the area available for absorption. For acids and bases only the nonionized molecules can be absorbed. At all physiological pH values weak acids and bases exist mostly in the unionized form and can be absorbed as well from the stomach as from the intestine. Strong bases such as the quaternary ammonium compounds are to a large extent ionized at all physiological pH values, and are hardly absorbed at all.

Absorption is also influenced by the gastric emptying time. The residence time of drugs in the stomach varies from a few minutes to several hours and is dependent on the volume, viscosity and composition of the stomach content. A drug taken with food will stay longer in the stomach. Under normal conditions, gastric emptying is rapid and the stomach's role in drug absorption is modest. The small intestine is then the most important site for drug absorption in the gastrointestinal tract. The intestinal mucosa is covered by numerous villi and microvili, providing a surface area of approximately $250 \, m^2$ available for passive diffusion. In theory, weakly acidic drugs are better substrates for passive diffusion at the pH of the stomach than at that of the intestine. However, the limited residence time of the drug in the stomach and the relatively small surface area of the stomach more than balance the influence of pH in determining the optimal site of absorption. Factors that promote gastric emptying will increase the absorption rate of most drugs, but not necessarily the total amount of drug eventually absorbed. The motility of the intestine can also influence the absorption: when peristalsis increases, disintegration and dissolution of the drug are often accelerated.

After absorption from the gastrointestinal tract the drug reaches the systemic circulation via the portal system and the liver. Some drugs are largely metabolized during this first hepatic passage. For this reason, some drugs which are well absorbed through the gastrointestinal membrane still have a low bioavailability.

III. DRUG DISTRIBUTION

After absorption, the drug is distributed from plasma to the various organs. The rate and extent of distribution depend on blood flow to each organ, tissue size, binding of drugs to plasma proteins and tissue components, and permeability of tissue membranes. The latter factor depends on the physicochemical properties of the drug. Blood flow is different from tissue to tissue. For lipid-soluble drugs, rapid equilibration occurs between blood on one hand and lungs, kidney, liver, heart and brain — organs with a high blood flow — on the other hand; less rapid equilibration is found in skeletal muscle, bone and adipose tissue, which receive a considerably smaller volume of blood per unit mass. For most lipophilic drugs the tissue membranes effectively present no barrier, and distribution depends essentially on the perfusion rate of the tissue. This is termed 'perfusion rate-limited distribution'. Tissue uptake of a drug continues until equilibrium is reached between the diffusible form of the drug in the tissue and the blood perfusing it, i.e. until the free concentrations in plasma water and tissue water are equal. Drugs can be present in tissues in higher concentrations than in plasma as a consequence of pH gradients (ion trapping), but mainly as a consequence of binding to tissue constituents or of dissolution in fat.

A. Volume of distribution

The apparent volume of distribution is a proportionality constant relating the total amount of drug present in the organism to its plasma concentration at the same time. It is in fact the volume in which the drug apparently distributes in a concentration equal to its concentration in plasma. This calculated value does not necessarily correspond to an anatomical or physiological part of the organism and can be much larger than the volume of total body water. It is therefore called the 'apparent' volume of distribution. Drugs can have apparent volumes of distribution from $0.04 \, l \, kg^{-1}$ to $20 \, l \, kg^{-1}$, i.e. 2.8–1400 litres for a 70-kg person.

Total body water (42 litres in a normal 70-kg man) consist of plasma (3 litres), interstitial fluid (11 litres) and intracellular fluid (28 litres). If a drug is not bound in plasma or tissues and distributes over total body water, the apparent volume of distribution will be 42 litres per 70 kg; this is the case, for example, for antipyrine. If a drug is likewise not bound in plasma and tissues but does not penetrate cells, the distribution will be limited to the extracellular space, equalling 14 litres. The apparent volumes of such drugs approximate their true volume of distribution. However, most substances bind to plasma and tissue proteins. For a drug which is preferentially bound to plasma proteins, for equal free concentrations the total concentrations will be higher in plasma than in the intracellular space. In this case the apparent volume of distribution will be smaller than 42 litres. If, on the other hand, a drug binds preferentially to tissue proteins, the total concentration of drug will be lower in plasma than in tissues and the apparent volume of distribution will be larger than 42 litres. A typical example is digoxin, with an apparent volume of distribution of 600 litres.

The following equation describes the relationship between apparent volume of distribution, drug binding and anatomical volumes:

$$V_d = V_B + V_T \frac{f_B}{f_T}$$

where V_d is the apparent volume of distribution, V_B is the blood volume, V_T is the extravascular volume and f_B and f_T are the free fractions of drug in blood and extravascular space, respectively. From this equation it is apparent that the apparent volume of distribution increases with increases in anatomical volumes or tissue binding, and decreases with increases in plasma or blood binding.

Many acidic drugs, e.g. salicylates, sulfonamides, penicillins and anticoagulants, are highly bound to plasma proteins or are not lipophilic enough to distribute intracellularly, and therefore have small volumes of distribution (<20 litres). Basic drugs, on the other hand, are often highly distributed in tissues: their concentration in plasma is low and their apparent volume of distribution is large. Table 28.2 shows the apparent volume of distribution for some drugs.

Table 28.2 Apparent volume of distribution of some drugs in $l\ kg^{-1}$.

Drug	V_d	Drug	V_d
Warfarin	0.11	Cimetidine	2.1
Ibuprofen	0.14	Propranolol	3.9
Salicylic acid	0.17	Digoxin	8.0
Gentamicin	0.25	Imipramine	30.0
Digitoxin	0.51	Chloroquine	235
Atenolol	0.70		

B.   Binding to plasma proteins

Many drugs are bound to some extent to plasma proteins. The plasma protein binding is expressed as the ratio of bound concentration over total (bound plus free) concentration, i.e. fraction bound, or, if the value is multiplied by 100, percentage bound. Free fraction equals one minus bound fraction.

Many acidic drugs bind to albumin. Basic drugs also bind to α_1-acid glycoprotein and to lipoproteins. α_1-Acid glycoprotein is an acute-phase reactant and its concentration in plasma rises in inflammation. For most drugs the binding to plasma proteins is a reversible process with extremely rapid rates of association and dissociation, and can be described by the law of mass action. The degree of binding is determined by affinity (expressed as the association constant), capacity (the number of binding sites per molecule protein), protein concentration and drug concentration. The number of binding sites is limited. At therapeutic drug concentrations usually only a small fraction of the available binding sites is occupied; for a given protein concentration the free fraction is then relatively constant and independent of drug concentration. In some instances the drug concentrations are so high that most binding sites are occupied and the free fraction becomes concentration-dependent. Concentration-dependent changes in drug binding are most likely to occur with drugs which have a high affinity for the proteins and which are given in large doses, e.g. acetylsalicylic acid, phenylbutazone, some penicillins and cephalosporins.

The plasma binding of drugs is altered in some physiological and pathological conditions. This often results from a change in plasma protein concentration. In various disease states (such as renal failure, liver disease, inflammation), in pregnancy and in the neonatal period, hypoalbuminaemia is observed; α_1-acid glycoprotein concentrations rise in inflammatory diseases, stress and malignancy, and fall in liver disease. A change in affinity can also lead to a change in binding. This can occur through competition between endogenous compounds and drug molecules for common binding sites. Free fatty acids, for example, bind strongly to albumin; when their concentration in plasma increases due to fasting, exercise or infection, the drug can be displaced from its binding sites. Accumulation of endogenous compounds also occurs in disease states such as renal failure or liver disease; hyperbilirubinaemia, for example, can decrease the binding of other drugs. Binding can also be changed by competition between drugs. Such an interaction is to be expected when the molar concentration of the 'displacer' is about the same as that of the protein binding sites, resulting in a decrease of the available binding sites for the 'displaced' drug. How do changes in binding, i.e. in free fraction, influence the free drug concentration in plasma? The changes of free concentration (calculated as total concentration times free fraction) will always be less than the changes of free fraction because of redistribution of the displaced drug to the tissues, and, often, because of its more rapid elimination. The change of free drug concentration as a consequence of a change in plasma binding will be largest for drugs with smaller initial distribution volumes. Drug interactions due to competition for protein binding sites are more likely to be clinically significant when the displaced drug is highly plasma bound (> 90%) and has a relatively small volume of distribution and a narrow toxic-therapeutic index. These conditions are not often met, however. Examples are the displacement of coumarin anticoagulant drugs by phenylbutazone or other nonsteroidal antiinflammatory drugs.

IV. DRUG ELIMINATION

Elimination covers both excretion (i.e. elimination of unchanged drug from the body) and biotransformation (metabolism). Some drugs are excreted in the bile and may be eliminated with the faeces, others are excreted in saliva. General anaesthestics are often excreted by the lungs. However, renal excretion and hepatic biotransformation are the major routes of drug elimination and these phenomena will be discussed, together with biliary excretion.

A. Excretion

1. Renal excretion

The renal excretion of drugs involves one or more of the processes of glomerular filtration, tubular reabsorption and active tubular secretion (Fig. 28.3).

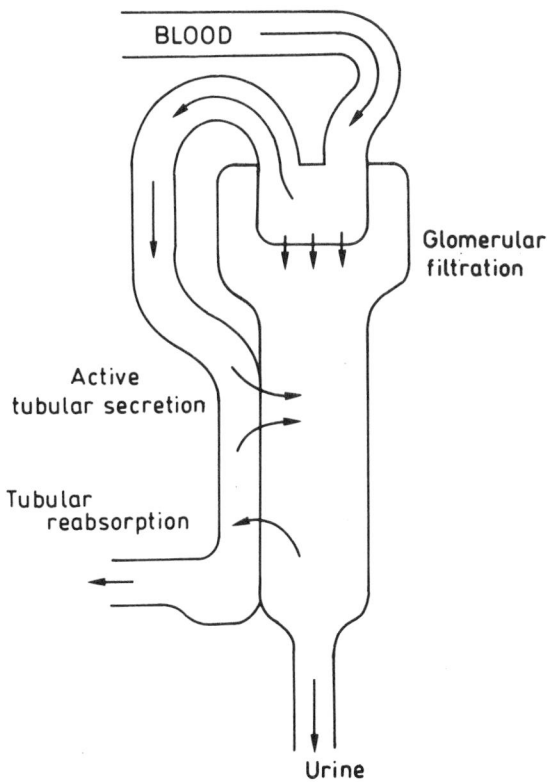

Fig. 28.3   Schematic representation of renal excretion of drugs.

(a) Glomerular filtration.   Blood flow to the kidneys is about $1.2–1.5 \, l \, min^{-1}$. About 10% of this volume is filtered through the glomeruli, which amounts to a filtrate of about 125 ml min^{-1} or 180 litres per 24 h. The pores of the glomerular capillaries are sufficiently large to permit passage of most drug molecules, but do not allow passage of blood cells and of large molecules (> 60 kDa) such as plasma proteins. Drugs bound to plasma proteins are thus not filtered.

(b) Tubular reabsorption.   More than 99% of the original 180 litres of protein-free filtrate is reabsorbed via the tubular cells; only about 1.5 litres is excreted as urine. Solutes and drugs dissolved in this filtrate can also be reabsorbed. For different drugs, tubular reabsorption varies from almost absent to almost complete. For most drugs, reabsorption is a passive process (passive diffusion). The drugs diffuse from tubular fluid to plasma in accordance with their concentration gradient, lipid/water partition coefficient, degree of ionization and molecular weight. The pH of the urine varies between 4.5 and 7.0, and pH changes can influence passive reabsorption and thus the excretion of the drug (see the Henderson–Hasselbalch equation in the introduction). Acidifying the urine favours the reabsorption of weak acids such as salicylates and retards their excretion, whereas the reverse is true for weak bases. Alkalinization of the urine increases the excretion of weak acids. On the other hand, the urinary excretion of weak bases is low in alkaline urine. It is possible, for example, to shorten the half-life of

phenobarbital, a weak acid, by administration of sodium bicarbonate, say to a patient in the case of overdose.

Increased urinary volume (diuresis) also increases the renal excretion of drugs that are extensively reabsorbed; the concentration gradient between tubular fluid and plasma is decreased by the increased tubular water load.

(c) Active tubular secretion.

By this process drug is transported against a concentration gradient from the blood capillaries across the tubular membranes to the tubular fluid. In the proximal renal tubuli, two systems are primarily responsible for the active tubular secretion of drugs, one for organic anions and one for organic cations. The anionic system transports organic acids such as penicillins, indomethacin and glucuronides. The cationic system transports organic bases such as morphine, procaine and quaternary ammonium compounds. These transport systems are saturable at high drug concentrations and competition is possible between drugs which are transported by the same transport mechanism. This characteristic has been used to decrease the urinary excretion of penicillin by probenicid, a weak organic acid, thereby prolonging penicillin's effect.

Plasma protein binding does not affect the rate of tubular secretion as the affinity of drugs for this transport system is much higher than for the plasma proteins.

(d) Renal clearance.

A fraction of the drug presented to the kidneys along with the renal arterial blood is removed by the above-mentioned processes. The efficiency of the renal excretion of a drug can be expressed as 'renal clearance'. The renal clearance of a drug is the volume of plasma which is cleared of that drug per unit time. Substances such as inulin and creatinine are eliminated by glomerular filtration and are not subject to either tubular secretion or reabsorption, and are not bound to plasma proteins. Their renal clearance in adults with normal renal function will be around 125 ml min^{-1}, corresponding to the volume of plasma filtered. The clearance for inulin or creatinine can therefore be used as an index of the glomerular filtration rate. For substances which are filtered but also actively secreted, renal clearance is higher than 125 ml min^{-1} and can be as high as 650 ml min^{-1}, which is the total plasma flow through the kidneys. Such values are found for p-aminohippuric acid and penicillins, for example. For a drug which is filtered but reabsorbed, or if a drug is bound in plasma, clearance values lower than 120 ml min^{-1}. are found. The renal clearance of a drug relative to the glomerular filtration rate therefore provides information on the mechanisms of renal excretion.

The renal clearance of a drug can be calculated by dividing the amount of drug excreted in the urine over a given time interval by the concentration of the drug in blood or plasma at the time corresponding to the midpoint of the urine collection interval.

2. Biliary excretion

Some drugs are actively secreted into the bile and pass as such into the intestine. In the rat, only compounds with a molecular weight greater than 350 daltons are extensively secreted in the bile. In humans, the molecular weight threshold for appreciable biliary excretion is in the order of 400–500 daltons.

A drug (and/or its metabolites) entering the intestine from the bile may be excreted in the faeces. However, substances secreted with the bile can be reabsorbed from the intestine and thus undergo 'enterohepatic cycling', as shown in Fig. 28.4. Drug conjugates, e.g. glucuronides, can be hydrolysed in the gut, by bacteria, for example, with liberation and reabsorption of the parent drug. This has be found for chloramphenicol and steroids.

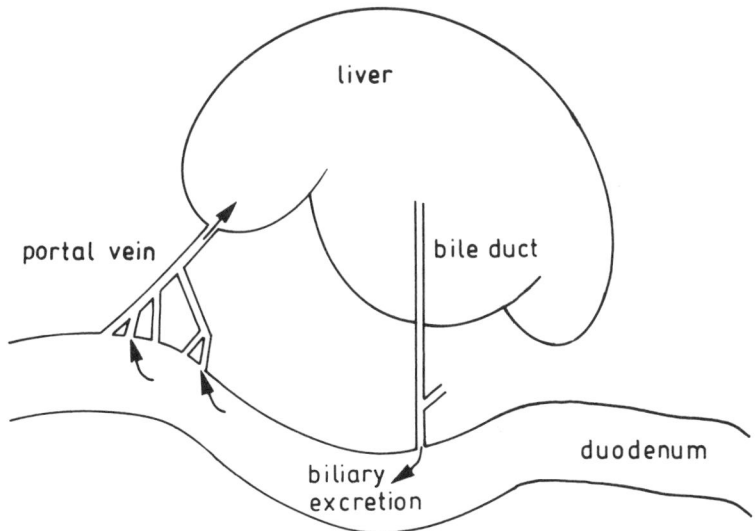

Fig. 28.4   Schematic representation of enterohepatic cycling of drugs.

B.   Biotransformation

Many drugs are lipophilic and are only partially ionized at the pH values encountered in the organism. After glomerular filtration these compounds are largely reabsorbed from the renal tubules. The metabolites formed by metabolization are generally more hydrophilic, therefore allowing their excretion by the kidneys. Biotransformation usually inactivates a drug, but in some cases active metabolites are formed. For some drugs, the activity may reside wholly in one or more metabolites: drugs that only become active after biotransformation are termed 'prodrugs'. Prodrugs are sometimes developed to improve absorption. They are often more lipid-soluble than the parent compound and after absorption are rapidly converted to the parent compound in the gut wall or in the liver. An example is pivampicillin, an ester of ampicillin, which is rapidly and completely hydrolysed to ampicillin during absorption.

The main drug biotransformation site is the liver, but biotransformation can also take place in intestinal mucosa, lung, kidneys, skin, placenta and plasma. Most of biotransforming enzymes are found in the microsomes, a cellular fraction derived from the endoplasmic reticulum. Liver or other organs are homogenized, and the homogenate is centrifuged at $9000g$ to $12\,000g$ for 30 min. The supernatant is centrifuged at $105\,000g$ for 1 h. The sediment collected is the microsomal fraction and the supernatant contains the cytosol.

Two phases can be distinguished in the various pathways of biotransformation. Phase I involves addition of functionally reactive groups by oxidation, reduction or hydrolysis. Phase II consists of conjugation of reactive groups, present either in the parent molecule or after phase I transformation. Phenacetin, for example, is first dealkylated to expose a reactive hydroxyl group, which then conjugates with glucuronic acid. The various phase I and phase II reactions are summarized in Tables 28.3 and 28.5.

Table 28.3   Phase I reactions.

Oxidation via microsomal P450 system
  Aliphatic hydroxylation (pentobarbital)
  Aromatic hydroxylation (propranolol)
  Deamination (amphetamine)
  N-Dealkylation (imipramine)
  O-Dealkylation (phenacetin)
  S-Dealkylation (thiopental)
  Dehalogenation (halothane)
  Desulfuration (parathion)
  Epoxidation (carbamazepine)
  N-Hydroxylation (trimethylamine)
  Sulfoxidation (chlorpromazine)

Oxidation via non-microsomal mechanisms
  Alcohol dehydrogenase (ethanol)
  Monoamine oxidase (tyramine)
  Purine oxidase (theophylline)

Reduction
  Azoreduction (sulfasalazine)
  Nitroreduction (chloramphenicol)

Hydrolysis
  Ester hydrolysis (procaine)
  Amide hydrolysis (procainamide)

---

1. Phase I reactions

(a) Oxidation.   Most oxidative processes take place in liver microsomes and are catalysed by monooxygenase enzymes known as mixed-function oxidases. These processes require reduced nicotinamide–adenine dinucleotide phosphate, molecular oxygen and a complex of enzymes in the endoplasmic reticulum. The terminal oxidizing enzyme is cytochrome P450, a haemoprotein. The notation 'P450' refers to the ability of the reduced (ferrous) form of the haemoprotein to react with carbon monoxide, yielding a complex with an absorption peak at 450 nm. For each molecule of substrate oxidized, one molecule of oxygen is consumed; one oxygen-atom is introduced into the substrate, and the other is reduced to form water. The P450s represent a superfamily of enzymes. Initially it was believed that there were only two forms, termed P450 and P448. Nowadays more than 20 different P450s have been identified in humans. To unify the nomenclature, P450s are grouped in families within which the amino acid sequence homology is higher than 40%. The majority of P450s involved in drug metabolism belong to three distinct families, CYP1 (formerly known as P450I), CYP2 (P450II) and CYP3 (P450III). Each P450 family is further divided into subfamilies, designated by capital letters, which in mammals contain proteins that share more than 55% amino acid sequence homology. In each subfamily, specific enzymes are denoted by an arabic number. Each isoenzyme has more or less distinct substrate specificity requirements. Only a few of these 20 isoforms play a role in clinically important oxidative drug metabolism. CYP3A4, CYP2D6 and CYP2C9 are the most important cytochrome families in regard to

Table 28.4 Substrates for, and inducers of some human liver cytochrome P450 enzymes.

Enzyme	Substrate	Inducer
CYP1A2	Caffeine, paracetamol, phenacetine, theophylline	Cigarette smoke, omeprazole
CYP2C	Diazepam, imipramine, S-mephenytoin, omeprazole, propranolol, tolbutamide	
CYP2D6	Debrisoquine, dextromethorphan, encainide, fluoxetine, imipramine, metoprolol, sparteine	
CYP2E1	Chlorzoxazone, ethanol, paracetamol	Ethanol, isoniazid
CYP3A	Cyclosporin A, diltiazem, erythromycin, lidocaine, midazolam, nifedipine, quinidine, verapamil	Carbamazepine, phenobarbital, rifampicin, phenytoin, glucocorticoids

drug metabolism. Cytochromes CYP1A2 and CYP1A1 are involved essentially in the metabolism of environmental chemicals and of a much smaller number of drugs (see Table 28.4). Sometimes a single substrate is metabolized by a single P450 enzyme, while other substrates can be oxidized to varying degrees by multiple P450 enzymes.

In addition to cytochrome P450s, hepatic microsomes contain another class of monooxygenases, the flavin-containing monooxygenases (FMO). These enzymes catalyse oxidation at nucleophilic nitrogen, sulfur and phosphorus atoms rather than direct oxidation at carbon atoms, for phenothiazines, ephedrine, norcocaine and the monoether and carbamate-containing pesticides.

Some oxidations are mediated by hepatic enzymes localized outside the microsomal system. Alcohol dehydrogenase and aldehyde dehydrogenase, which catalyse a variety of alcohols and aldehydes such as ethanol and acetaldehyde, are found in the soluble fraction of the liver. Xanthine oxidase, mainly found in the liver and small intestine but also present in kidneys, spleen and heart, oxidizes mercaptopurine to 6-thiouric acid. Monoamine oxidase, a mitochondrial enzyme found in liver, kidney, intestine and nervous tissue, oxidatively deaminates several naturally occurring amines (catecholamines, serotonin) as well as a number of drugs.

(b) Reduction. Reduction, for example azo- and nitro-reduction, is a less common pathway of drug metabolism. Reductase activity has been found in the microsomal fraction and the cytosol of the hepatocyte. Anaerobic intestinal bacteria in the lower gastrointestinal tract are also rich in these reductive enzymes. A historical example is that of Prontosil®, a sulfonamide prodrug. It is metabolized by azo-reduction to form the active metabolite, sulfanilamide. Sulfasalazine is also cleaved via azo-reduction by intestinal bacteria to form aminosalicylate, the active component, and sulfapyridine. Chloramphenicol is metabolized by nitro-reduction to an amine in bacteria and some tissues.

(c) Hydrolysis. Hydrolysis of esters and amides is a common pathway of drug metabolism. The liver microsomes contain nonspecific esterases, as do other tissues and plasma. Hydrolysis

of an ester results in the formation of an alcohol and an acid; hydrolysis of an amide results in the formation of an amine and an acid. The ester procaine, a local anaesthetic, is rapidly hydrolysed by plasma cholinesterases and to a lesser extent by hepatic microsomal esterase. An example of a hydrolysed amide is the antiarrhythmic drug procainamide. Enalapril, a prodrug, is hydrolysed by esterases to the active metabolite enalaprilate, which inhibits the angiotensin converting enzyme.

2. Phase II reactions

Compounds having polar constituents such as —OH, —NH$_2$ or —COOH, or acquiring them by a phase I reaction, may undergo a phase II, or conjugation reaction. The major conjugation reactions are listed in Table 28.5.

Table 28.5   Phase II, or conjugation reactions.

Conjugation	Localization	Conjugating agent	Functional groups
Glucuronidation	Microsomes	UDPGA[a]	—OH,—COOH, —NH$_2$, —SH
Sulfation	Cytosol	PAPS[b]	—OH, —NH$_2$
Acetylation	Cytosol	Acetyl-CoA	—COOH
Glutathion	Cytosol	Glutathion	Epoxides, arene oxides
Methylation	Cytosol	SAM[c]	—OH, —NH$_2$
Amino acid	Cytosol	Glycine	—COOH

[a]UDPGA: uridine diphosphoglucuronic acid. [b]PAPS: 3′-phosphoadenosine-5′-phosphosulfate. [c]SAM: S-adenosylmethionine.

The reactive group interacts with endogenous compounds such as glucuronic acid, sulfate, glycine, acetate or glutathione. Glucuronide formation is the most common conjugation process. Conjugation reactions may involve an active, high-energy form of the conjugating agent, such as uridine diphosphoglucuronic acid (UDPGA) and acetyl-CoA, which in the presence of the appropriate transferase enzyme combines with the drug to form the conjugate. For other conjugating reactions, the drug is activated to a high-energy compound that then reacts with the conjugating agent in the presence of a transferase enzyme. Glutathione, for example, reacts via the enzyme glutathione S-transferase with reactive electrophilic oxygen intermediates of certain drugs, such as paracetamol.

Conjugates are usually pharmacologically inactive; they are more hydrophilic than the parent compounds and are easily excreted by the kidneys or the bile. Certain conjugates such as morphine-6-glucuronide and acetyl procainamide are pharmacologically active.

3. Stereoselective metabolism

Synthesis of a drug with an asymmetrical or chiral centre usually results in two enantiomers, mirror images that cannot be superimposed. Such a 50:50 mixture is called a racemate. The enantiomers of a racemic drug often differ in pharmacodynamic and/or pharmacokinetic properties as a consequence of stereoselective interaction with optically active biological macromolecules. Stereoselective metabolism of chiral xenobiotics is a well recognized. Both phase I and phase II metabolic reactions are capable of discriminating between enantiomers.

Stereoselective metabolism of chiral drugs implies the preferential enzymatic removal of one enantiomeric form over the other.

Stereoselective drug metabolism may be divided into three groups: substrate, product, and substrate–product stereoselectivity.

Substrate stereoselectivity is characterized by the preferential enzymatic metabolism of one enantiomer; metabolism can occur with retention or with loss of stereoisomerism. Most examples of stereoselective metabolism belong to this group. Several chiral nonsteroidal anti-inflammatory agents of the 2-arylpropionic acid group undergo an unusual metabolic reaction whereby (*R*)-enantiomers are inverted to the active (*S*)-antipodes. The extent of inversion varies considerably depending on the drug, but is also species-dependent.

Product stereoselectivity is observed when a prochiral drug is preferentially metabolized to one or more chiral products. There are only few examples of this type of stereoselectivity, e.g. the 5-hydroxylation of phenytoin and the 4-hydroxylation of debrisoquine, both with preferential formation of the (*S*)-enantiomer of the hydroxylated product.

Substrate–product stereoselectivity. The enantiomers of a drug which possess both asymmetrical and prochiral characterstics can undergo stereoselective metabolism whereby a second chiral centre is introduced. Examples are the hydroxylation of perhexiline and the keto-reduction of warfarin.

Stereoselective metabolism is the most important process responsible for the stereoselectivity observed in pharmacokinetics. Verapamil has received considerable attention as a classical example of substrate stereoselective pharmacokinetics in humans. After oral administration, the drug undergoes an important stereoselective first pass metabolism, so that (−)-verapamil, the active enantiomer, has a 2–3 times lower bioavailability than its antipode. The (−)/(+) plasma concentration ratio is therefore higher after intravenous than after oral administration.

4.   Factors influencing biotransformation

Many factors can influence the metabolism of drugs, leading to large intra- and interindividual differences in the elimination of drugs. Some factors are genetically determined, others environmentally.

(a) Species differences.

There are large differences in drug metabolism between species. Rates of metabolism may differ; in general, smaller animals metabolize faster than larger animal species. Different species may also show differences in individual metabolic pathways. In the rat, for example, amphetamine is mainly hydroxylated, whereas in humans and dogs it is mainly deaminated. A specific pathway may be absent in a particular species; for example, the cat is unable to form glucuronic acid conjugates of some drugs; dogs are unable to *N*-acetylate aromatic amino groups and hydrazides.

The problems posed by species differences for the development and screening of new drugs are considerable. Knowledge of the mechanism of biotransformation of a new chemical agent in animals is, however, fundamental to its safety evaluation.

(b) Genetic factors.

It has been established by twin studies and other means that interindividual differences in drug metabolism are largely under genetic control. For drugs such as phenylbutazone, antipyrine and dicoumarol, fraternal twins show wide variations in metabolic rate, as generally seen in human populations, whereas each pair of identical twins shows similar metabolic rates.

Family studies have suggested that metabolism is under *polygenetic* control. Frequency distribution plots of metabolic parameters usually yield continuous, unimodal curves similar to the normal distribution curve.

The metabolism of some drugs, however, is under *monogenetic* control and shows a bimodal distribution with genetic polymorphism in the population. Genetic polymorphism was first described for the *N*-acetylation of isoniazid and other drugs (e.g. procainamide, hydralazine, dapsone, sulfadimidine). Two phenotypes are found in the population, fast and slow acetylators. Genetic polymorphism was later also recognized for drug oxidations. The best-known example is the deficiency of 4-hydroxylation of the antihypertensive agent debrisoquine by the CYP2D6 isoform. Two distinct modes in the frequency distribution of debrisoquine metabolic ratios are observed, which represent two distinct phenotypes, poor and extensive metabolizers (Fig. 28.5). The prevalence of poor metabolizers of debrisoquine in Caucasian populations varies between 5% and 10%; in other ethnic groups the frequencies range from 0 (among Japanese) to 30% (in a small population of Chinese living in Canada). Studies with subjects phenotyped for debrisoquine have shown that the metabolism of more than 30 other drugs co-segregates with debrisoquine hydroxylation. These drugs include sparteine, β-adrenergic blockers such as metoprolol and propranolol, the antitussive opioid dextromethorphan, tricyclic antidepressants and the antiarrhythmic agents encainide and propafenone.

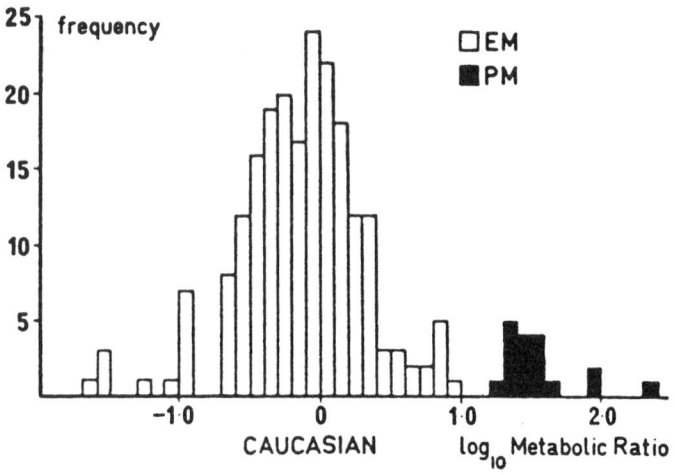

Fig. 28.5 Semilog frequency–distribution histogram of debrisoquine 4-hydroxylation (i.e. metabolic ratio) in 229 British Caucasians. Excretion as percentage of dose of debrisoquine and 4-hydroxydebrisoquine in measured after oral administration of 12.4 mg debrisoquine sulfate. The metabolic ratio was calculated by dividing the percentage excretion of debrisoquine by the percentage excretion of 4-hydroxydebrisoquine in urine collected during an 8 hour period after administration of debrisoquine sulfate. (From Woodhouse, N. M. *et. al.* (1979) Debrisoquine hydroxylation polymorphism among Ghanaians and Caucasians. *Clin. Pharmacol. Ther.* **26**: 584–591. Reproduced with permission.)

Another intensively studied genetic polymorphism of drug oxidation concerns the antiepileptic drug mephenytoin. This deficiency, resulting from an inherited defect in the CYP2C19 enzyme, affects only the (*S*)-enantiomer of mephenytoin. (*S*)-Mephenytoin undergoes rapid and complete oxidation to a *p*-hydroxylated product, while the (*R*)-antipode is subject to a much slower *N*-demethylation pathway. The poor metabolizer phenotype occurs with a frequency of 2–5% in Caucasians, but with a frequency above 20% in Japanese. The metabolism of drugs such as phenytoin, propranolol, diazepam, omeprazole and hexobarbital co-segregates with that of mephenytoin.

Two cytochrome P450 isoenzymes, CYP2D6 and CYP2C19, are involved in the metabolism of propranolol. The 4-hydroxylation of propranolol co-segregates with the debrisoquine polymorphism, but the side-chain oxidation to naphthoxylactic acid is catalysed in part by the mephenytoin isoenzyme.

The clinical consequences of polymorphism depend on the characteristics of the drug in extensive metabolizers (e.g. presence or absence of hepatic first pass), on the quantitative importance of the defective pathway(s) in the overall elimination of the drug, but also on the concentration–response relationship and the therapeutic index of the drug. The presence of the slow hydroxylator phenotype can result in accumulation of the parent drug, with stronger or prolonged effects and/or adverse reactions, or may lead to a decreased effect if the effect is related to an active metabolite.

(c) Gender.   Important sex-related differences in metabolism have been found in rats. Male rats metabolize certain drugs faster than females, and these differences also occur for oxidative pathways and for glucuronide and glutathione conjugations of certain substrates. Studies in the rat have shown not only quantitative differences in the amount of cytochrome P450 isoenzymes between sexes, but also qualitative differences; there are male-specific and female-specific P450 isoenzymes. Sex hormones, especially androgens, play an important role in defining the differences in cytochrome P450 composition of male and female rats.

In humans, too, sex differences in metabolism exist, but the differences are small and usually not clinically important. The clearance of benzodiazepines eliminated by metabolic conjugation (temazepam, oxazepam, lorazepam) is significantly less in women than in men. These differences parallel those found in rats, but are much smaller. It was recently shown that gastric alcohol dehydrogenase activity is much lower in women than in men, explaining in part the higher ethanol blood levels found in women for the same dose.

(d) Age.   In most rodents the fetus is essentially devoid of hepatic cytochrome P450-linked drug-metabolizing enzymes. After birth, however, the system develops very rapidly and attains adult levels within a few days or weeks. Unlike the fetuses of common laboratory animals, the human fetus is able to oxidize drugs, although not all drugs and not at the rates achieved in adults. These activities begin to develop during the first trimester, reach a plateau until parturition, and then rise gradually for several weeks until the adult level is reached. Sulfate conjugation seems to be as efficient in newborns as in adults, but most other conjugation pathways are poorly developed in the fetus. Conjugation with glucuronic acid reaches adult levels only at 3 years of age. This is responsible for the serious adverse reactions observed in newborns after administration of chloramphenicol, a drug that is ordinarily conjugated with glucuronic acid, leading to the 'grey syndrome'.

Certain drugs (e.g. antipyrine, diazoxide, carbamazepine, theophylline) are metabolized faster in older infants and children than in adults.

In male rats oxidative metabolism of some drugs declines with ageing. In female rats, as in mice and monkeys, the oxidative activities are well preserved during ageing. The decrease in enzyme activity in the male rat liver is due to the loss of the male-specific cytochrome P450 isoenzyme and the appearance of the female-specific cytochrome P450 form. In humans, cytochrome P450-mediated enzyme activities do not decrease with ageing. In many *in vivo* studies, however, a decreased hepatic biotransformation was described in the elderly, which can probably be explained by a reduction in liver size and hepatic blood flow.

(e) Drug interactions. Numerous drugs or environmental chemicals can potentiate or inhibit the pharmacological and toxicological effects of other drugs by altering the activity of drug metabolizing enzymes.

Enzyme induction. Chronic administration of a substance can stimulate its own biotransformation (autoinduction) or the biotransformation of other substances (heteroinduction). Examples of inducers include drugs, steroids, industrial chemicals, pesticides, herbicides, polycyclic hydrocarbons and diet constituents. Phenobarbital and some polycyclic hydrocarbons such as 3-methylcholanthrene, benzpyrene, and constituents of cigarette smoke have been extensively studied as inducers. Enzyme systems inducible by xenobiotics are cytochrome P450s, glutathione S-transferase, glucuronyl transferase and epoxide hydrolase. The stimulation of the activity of enzymes involves new protein synthesis and, in most cases, an increase in the rate of gene transcription; it is true enzyme induction and not activation of latent enzyme. Inducing agents have no effect *in vitro*; animals have to be pretreated and a period of time has to elapse, corresponding to known rates of protein synthesis. In the case of cytochrome P450, the effect of the inducer is to increase its microsomal concentration. Not all P450 isoenzymes are inducible. Each inducer specifically increases the synthesis of certain P450 isoenzymes, as shown in Table 28.4. The former concept of 'phenobarbital-type inducers' or 'polycyclic hydrocarbon inducers' is no longer valid. At least three other distinct major inducer categories are now recognized. P450 induction by phenobarbital in the liver is accompanied by a substantial increase in the content of smooth endoplasmic reticulum within the liver cells and by an increase in liver weight. Such morphological changes are, however, far less prominent with inducers from most other categories and during induction in nonhepatic tissues.

Clinically important enzyme inducers are carbamazepin, phenobarbital, phenytoin and rifampicin. A potent enzyme inducer such as rifampicin can markedly alter enzyme activity within 48 hours after its administration, while for other inducers several days are necessary. Enzyme induction is dose-dependent.

Enzyme inhibition. The metabolism of drugs can be inhibited by exogenous and endogenous compounds. Several mechanisms are involved. Some potent inhibitors of P450 form inactive complexes with the haemoprotein; many of these inhibitors are nitrogenous compounds, such as cimetidine. The most common mechanism, however, is competitive inhibition. In theory, any two drugs that are metabolized by the same P450 isoenzyme have a potential for competitive interaction. Using an *in vitro* preparation of human hepatic microsomes or a recombinant preparation of the specific enzyme, it is possible to predict such interactions. The clinical significance of such a competitive interaction will depend on the drugs' affinities for binding to the P450 isoenzyme, the concentrations of the drugs in the endoplasmic reticulum, the dependence on the P450 isoenzyme for elimination, and the therapeutic index of the inhibited drug. Some drugs act as competitive inhibitors of a P450 isoenzyme although they are not metabolized by that P450 isoenzyme. In humans quinidine, for example, selectively inhibits CYP2D6 but is not metabolized by that isoenzyme.

Inhibitors for nonmicrosomal enzymes are also known: disulfiram, for example, inhibits alcohol and aldehyde dehydrogenase, laevodopa inhibits dopa decarboxylase, allopurinol inhibits xanthine oxidase, and phenelzine inhibits monoamine oxidase.

5. Hepatic clearance

Hepatic clearance (Cl_H) of a drug may be defined as the volume of blood perfusing the liver that is cleared of the drug per unit of time. The pharmacokinetic concept of hepatic clearance takes into consideration the anatomical and physiological facts that drug is transported to the liver by the portal vein and the hepatic artery and leaves the organ by the hepatic vein. It diffuses from plasma water to reach the metabolic enzymes. There are therefore at least three major parameters to consider in quantifying drug elimination by the liver: blood flow through the organ (Q), which reflects transport to the liver; free fraction of drug in blood (f_u) which affects access of drug to the enzymes; and intrinsic ability of the hepatic enzymes to metabolize the drug, expressed as intrinsic clearance (Cl'_{int}). Intrinsic clearance is the ability of the liver to remove drug in the absence of flow limitations and blood binding. Taking in account these three parameters, the hepatic clearance can be expressed by

$$Cl_H = Q \frac{f_u \cdot Cl'_{int}}{Q + f_u \cdot Cl'_{int}}$$

It is obvious that the hepatic clearance cannot be larger than the total volume of blood reaching the liver per unit time, i.e. the liver blood flow Q. The ratio of the hepatic clearance of a drug to the hepatic blood flow is called the extraction ratio of the drug (E). The value of the extraction ratio can vary between 0 and 1. It is 0 when $f_u \cdot Cl'_{int}$ is zero, i.e. when the drug is not metabolized in the liver. It is 1 when the hepatic clearance equals the hepatic blood flow (about $1.5\,l\,min^{-1}$ in humans).

When $f_u \cdot Cl'_{int}$ is very small in comparison to hepatic blood flow ($f_u \cdot Cl'_{int} < Q$), the equation reduces to

$$Cl_H = f_u \cdot Cl'_{int}$$

In that case, clearance is not blood-flow-dependent but depends on enzymatic activity and blood binding. Binding to blood will limit the elimination. This is called 'restrictive elimination'. Drugs with restrictive elimination have a low extraction ratio (<0.3). Examples are antipyrine, phenytoin and warfarin. When $f_u \cdot Cl'_{int}$ is very large in comparison to hepatic blood flow ($f_u \cdot Cl'_{int} > Q$), the equation reduces to

$$Cl_H = Q$$

In this case, clearance is dependent on hepatic blood flow and independent of Cl'_{int} and f_u. This is termed 'blood-flow-dependent' or 'nonrestrictive' elimination. Drugs with such an elimination have a high extraction ratio (>0.7). Bound and free molecules are eliminated, as the affinity for the hepatic enzymes is larger than for the binding proteins in blood. The decrease in hepatic blood flow which occurs in hepatic disease and cardiac failure and after administration of β-blockers leads to decreased clearance. Examples of drugs with a high extraction ratio are nitroglycerine, propranolol and lidocaine. When a drug with a high extraction ratio is given orally, an important first pass elimination occurs. This is called 'presystemic elimination'. The higher the extraction ratio of a drug, the lower its bioavailability. For a drug which is completely absorbed from the gastrointestinal tract and metabolized in the liver, bioavailability equals $1 - E$.

REFERENCES

1. Brosen, K. (1990) Recent developments in hepatic drug oxidation. Implications for clinical pharmacokinetics. *Clin. Pharmacokinet.* **18**: 220–239.
2. Gibaldi, M. (1991) *Biopharmaceutics and Clinical Pharmacokinetics.* Lea and Febiger, Philadelphia.
3. Gonzalez, F. J. G. and Idle, J. R. (1994) Pharmacogenetic phenotyping and genotyping. Present status and future potential. *Clin. Pharmacokinet.* **26**: 59–70.
4. Murray, M. (1992) P450 enzymes. Inhibition, mechanisms, genetic regulation and effects of liver disease. *Clin. Pharmacokinet.* **23**: 132–146.
5. Pratt, W. B. and Taylor, P. (1990) *Principles of Drug Action.* Churchill Livingstone, New York.
6. Rowland, M. and Tozer, T. N. (1989) Clinical pharmacokinetics: concepts and application. Lea and Febiger, Philadelphia.
7. Shargel, L. and Yu, A. B. C. (1993) *Applied biopharmaceutics and Pharmacokinetics.* Prentice-Hall, Englewood Cliffs, NJ.
8. Watkins, P. B. (1992) Drug metabolism by cytochromes P450 in the liver and small bowel. *Gastrointest. Pharmacol.* **21**: 511–526.

29

Biotransformation Reactions

CAMILLE G. WERMUTH AND BERNARD TESTA

Plus ils sont solubles, moins ils sont toxiques.
The more soluble they are, the less toxic they are.
M. C. Richet[1]

THE PRACTICE OF MEDICINAL CHEMISTRY
ISBN 0-12-744640-0

I. INTRODUCTION

The objective of this chapter is to make medicinal chemists aware of the chemical processes involved in the biotransformation of drugs and to encourage them to further study[2–9] so as to be able to use the acquired knowledge in the design of new drug entities. The apparent function of drug metabolism is the transformation of foreign compounds into water-soluble derivatives which can easily be eliminated via the renal route. Indeed, *lipophilic* molecules are poorly eliminated in the urine but undergo recycling by glomerular reabsorption or by an enterohepatic cycle. The vast majority of drugs are substrates for biotransformation reactions, as are most other xenobiotics (i.e. compounds foreign to the body such as pesticides, food additives, industrial and technical chemicals, pollutants, and leisure substances).

As a rule, the metabolism of xenobiotics takes place in two steps, known as phase I and phase II reactions. During phase I, a *functionalization reaction* of the xenobiotic is achieved. New polar groups such as CO_2H, OH or NH_2 are introduced or unveiled from pre-existing functions through oxidative, reductive or hydrolytic reactions. The polar group created or released then serves as an anchor point for the second metabolic step (Fig. 29.1). The phase II reactions, known as *conjugation reactions*, link an endogenous solubilizing moiety either to the original drug (if polar functions are already present) or to the phase I metabolite. Common solubilizing groups are glucuronic acid, various amino acids, or even sulfuric acid. The conjugate molecule, being more polar and water-soluble, is usually excreted via the renal route.

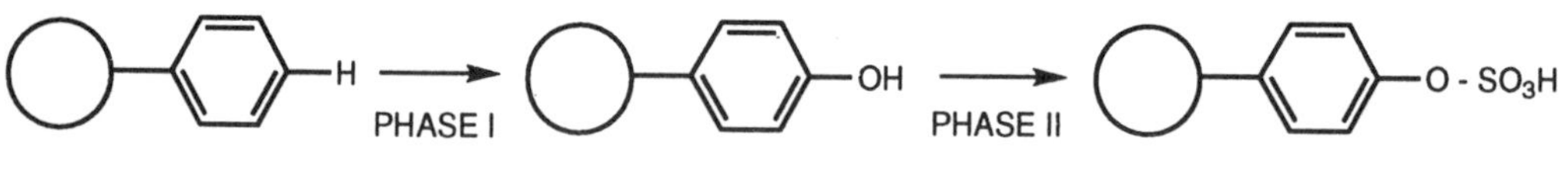

Fig. 29.1   A phenyl ring in a xenobiotic first undergoes a functionalization reaction (phase I) and is then conjugated (phase II).

Phase I metabolites are sometimes excreted prior to conjugation. Conversely, reactions of functionalization (mainly hydrolyses and oxidations) can occur *after* conjugation reactions. Some small molecules generated by metabolic cleavage (e.g. carbon dioxide, methylamine, some thiols and thioethers) are gaseous and can be eliminated via the lungs. Finally, two categories of xenobiotics are not or are barely subject to metabolic transformations, namely highly hydrophilic compounds (e.g. saccharine, strong acids or bases), and highly lipophilic, polyhalogenated xenobiotics such as some insecticides. The former cannot penetrate intracellular compartments and enter in contact with the enzymes, while the latter are sterically shielded from metabolic attack.

The global result of phase I and II transformations should normally be the inactivation and detoxication of the xenobiotic. However, innumerable examples exist of metabolic reactions *not* leading to inactivation or detoxication. For example, it happens rather frequently that a phase I metabolite will possess its own activity which will be similar to or different from that of the parent drug. Metabolic precursors can even be intentionally prepared which release the active species only *in vivo*. Such compounds are called *prodrugs* (see Chapters 31 and 32). Other metabolites may be highly reactive entities able to bind covalently to soluble or membrane proteins, to enzymes (mechanism-based, irreversible inactivators), or to DNA (mutagenic and carcinogenic compounds). Metabolism-induced toxicity is discussed in Chapter 30. In this context, it becomes obvious that for long-term treatment of chronic diseases a thorough study of the drug metabolism is indispensable, including an assessment of the activities and side-effects of each identified metabolite.

Because most drug candidates giving rise to a toxic metabolite are not developed beyond the preclinical or clinical stages, reactions of toxication are rather uncommon in drug metabolism. The situation is different for many nontherapeutic xenobiotics, e.g. pollutants and industrial chemicals. Thus, 4-fluorobutyric acid is metabolized to fluoroacetic acid, which enters the tricarboxylic acid cycle in place of acetic acid to yield fluorocitric acid, a specific inhibitor of the enzyme aconitase.[10] This effectively blocks the tricarboxylic acid cycle, an essential supplier of energy to the cell (Fig. 29.2).

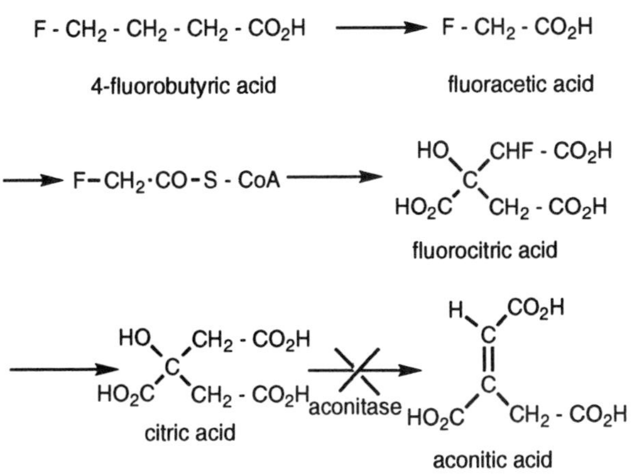

$$F - CH_2 - CH_2 - CH_2 - CO_2H \longrightarrow F - CH_2 - CO_2H$$

4-fluorobutyric acid — fluoracetic acid

$$\longrightarrow F-CH_2 \cdot CO-S-CoA \longrightarrow$$

fluorocitric acid

citric acid — aconitase — aconitic acid

Fig. 29.2 The incorporation of fluoroacetic acid, the final metabolite of the even-numbered ω-fluorocarboxylic acids, in the Krebs cycle achieves a lethal synthesis in blocking the enzyme aconitase.[10]

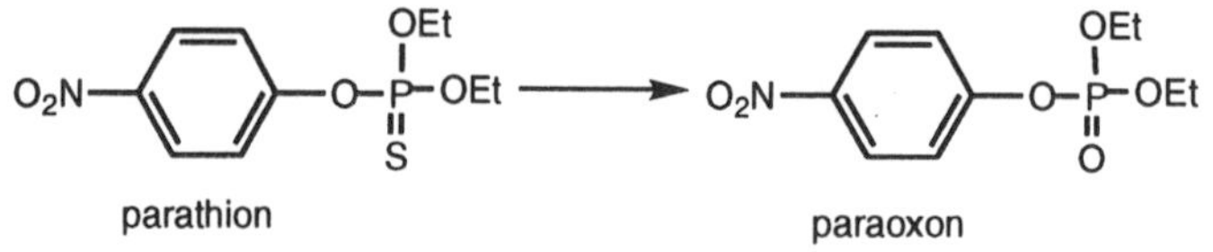

Fig. 29.3 Metabolic conversion of the nontoxic insecticide parathion to paraoxon, a potent acetylcholinesterase inhibitor.

Such a mechanism of toxication is known as *lethal synthesis*. A classic example of lethal synthesis is provided by the metabolic conversion of the nontoxic insecticide parathion into its oxygenated isostere paraoxon, a potent acetylcholinesterase inhibitor (Fig. 29.3).

II.   REACTIONS OF FUNCTIONALIZATION (PHASE I)

Phase I reactions, which often create anchor points in the xenobiotic molecule for subsequent conjugation, comprise oxidations (electron removal, dehydrogenation and hydroxylation), reductions (electron donation, hydrogenation and removal of oxygen), and hydrolytic reactions. Many metabolic reactions take place in the endoplasmic reticulum of the liver cells, but other organs, particularly kidneys and lungs, also participate in drug metabolism. In addition, a variety of other tissues have the capacity to metabolize xenobiotics.

A.   Oxidations catalysed by monooxygenases

1.   The endoplasmic reticulum and cytochrome P450

The endoplasmic reticulum forms a network containing two structures called the smooth and the rough reticulum. The rough form contains small and dense organelles, the ribosomes, which play an essential role in the synthesis of proteins. The smooth form is bereft of ribosomes but contains oxidative enzymes. When the hepatic tissue is homogenized, the endoplasmic reticulum is broken down to form small vesicles called microsomes. In the laboratory, microsomal preparations are obtained by centrifuging the homogenate at $10\,000\,g$ for 10 min in order to sediment nuclei, mitochondria and cellular debris, and then by centrifuging again at $100\,000\,g$ for 1 h. The deposit obtained in this manner consists of microsomes that are separated from the supernatant fraction (the cytosol).

The major redox system present in the endoplasmic reticulum catalyses the reductive cleavage of molecular oxygen, transferring one atom of oxygen to the substrate and forming one molecule of H_2O with the other atom:

$$R{-}H + O_2 + NADPH + H^+ \rightarrow R{-}OH + NADP^+ + H_2O$$

This reaction is known as a monooxygenation, the major microsomal monooxygenase being cytochrome P450. The two electrons necessary for the reaction are transferred by NADPH-

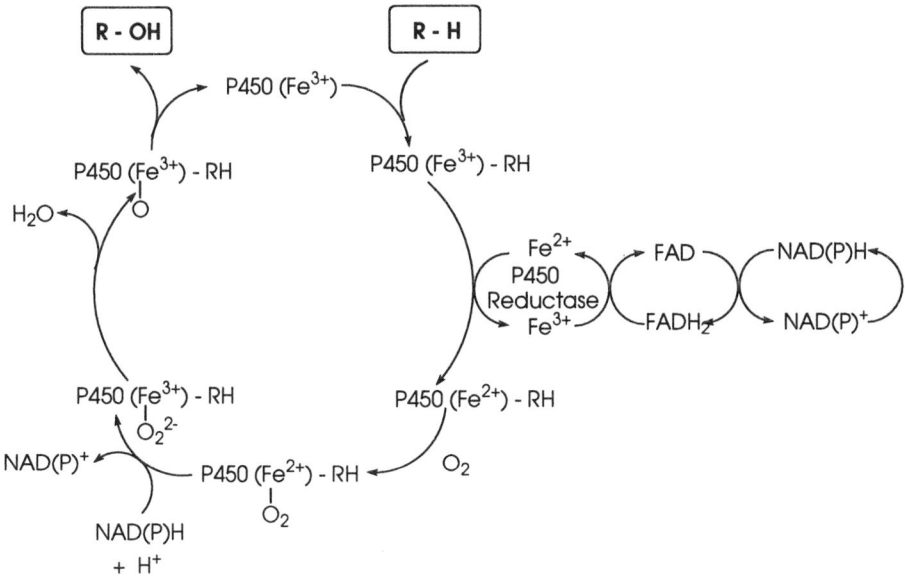

Fig. 29.4   The simplified cytochrome P450 redox cycle.

cytochrome P450 reductase; the second electron in some cases comes from NADH-cytochrome b_5 reductase and cytochrome b_5. The mechanism of the cytochrome P450 redox system is represented in Fig. 29.4.

Cytochromes P450 (CYP) are by far the most important xenobiotic- and endobiotic-metabolizing monooxygenases. They are made of a molecule of haem, protoporphyrin IX, and a variable protein of MW ~50 kDa. Cytochromes P450 form a very large group of haemoproteins encoded by the *CYP* gene superfamily and classified into families and subfamilies. The major xenobiotic-metabolizing cytochromes P450 in humans are found in family 1 (CYP1A1 and CYP 1A2), family 2 (CYP2B6, CYP2C8, CYP2C9, CYP2C18, CYP2D6 and CYP2E1), family 3 (CYP3A), and family 4 (CYP4A9, CYP4A11 and CYP4B1).

In the resting state, the central iron atom of protoporphyrin IX is in a hexacoordinated, ferric form. The substrate R—H binds reversibly to the enzyme and the complex undergoes reduction to the ferrous state. This allows molecular oxygen to bind as a third partner. Following the second reduction step, molecular oxygen is ultimately reduced to a hydroperoxide, which is cleaved with liberation of H_2O and formation of a monooxygen known as oxene. The oxene, which is electrophilic and quite reactive, can act on the substrate in a manner which depends on the reactivity of the substrate itself. Thus, the oxene can (a) be transferred directly to the substrate (oxygen insertion or addition), (b) remove an electron, or more frequently (c) pull a hydrogen radical away from the substrate and transfer back a formal HO· radical (a reaction known as oxygen rebound). The latter is the mechanism by which RR'R''C—H is oxidized to RR'R''C—OH. After release of the product, the regenerated cytochrome P450 is ready for a new cycle. As illustrated below, the substrates to be oxidized are very diverse, the oxidation involving C, Si, N, P, S, Se and other atoms (Fig. 29.5).

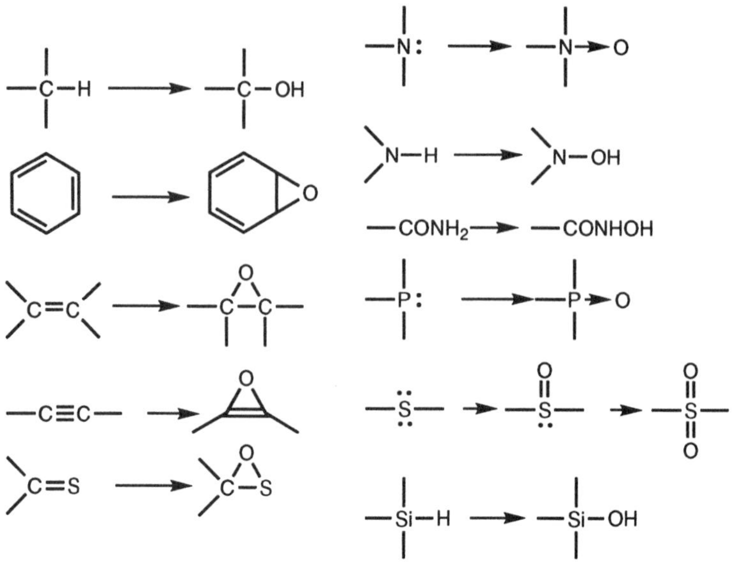

Fig. 29.5   Major reactions of oxygenation catalysed by cytochrome P450.

2.   Reactions of carbon oxidation

The reactions of C-oxidation represent the most common metabolic attacks on xenobiotics. From a mechanistic point of view it is convenient to distinguish between saturated (sp³) and unsaturated (sp² and sp) carbon atoms.

(a) Hydroxylation of saturated aliphatic carbon atoms.   The saturated aliphatic carbons hydroxylated by cytochrome P450 are found in complex molecules as well as in saturated hydrocarbons (alkanes and cycloalkanes). Steroids offer a telling example, as seen with progesterone, which is hydroxylated in positions 11β, 17α, and 21 to yield hydrocortisone. In

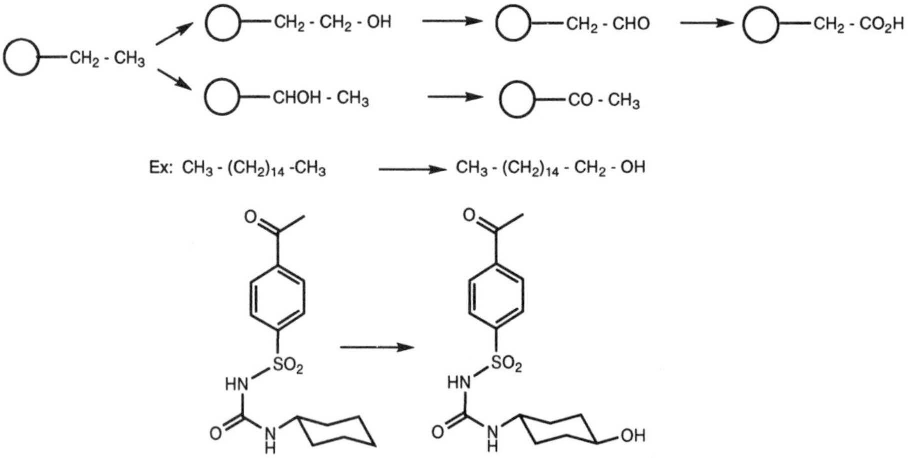

Fig. 29.6   Hydroxylations on saturated carbon atoms.

practice a nonactivated alkyl group undergoes mainly ω and ω − 1 oxidation. *n*-Hexadecane, for example, is ω-hydroxylated in the liver to yield hexadecanol, which is further oxidized to hexadecanoic acid. For shorter chains, both terminal and ω−1 oxidations are observed (Fig. 29.6). Cyclic aliphatic systems are usually hydroxylated on the least-hindered or most-activated carbon atoms.

(b) Hydroxylation at activated sp³ carbon atoms.

For activated sp³ carbon atoms in allylic, propynylic or benzylic positions, the ω and ω−1 rule no longer holds and the activated atoms are hydroxylated preferentially (Fig. 29.7).

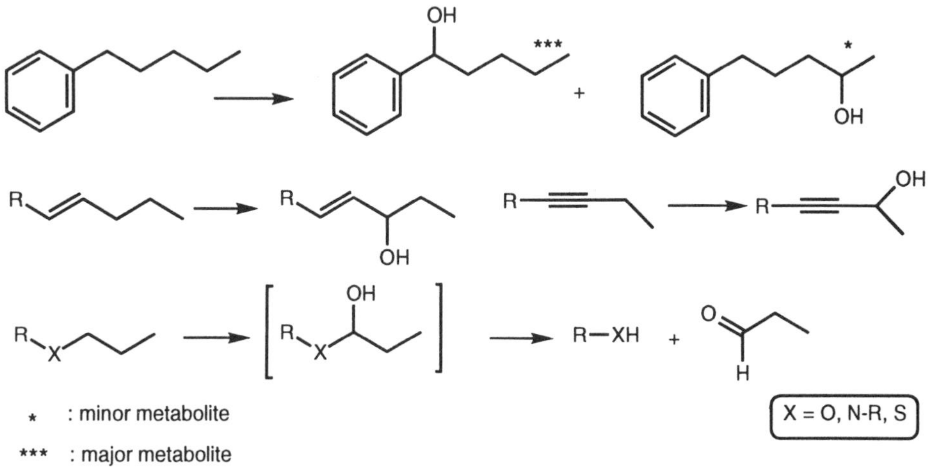

*   : minor metabolite

***   : major metabolite

X = O, N-R, S

Fig. 29.7   Regioselectivity of hydroxylation at activated sp³ carbon atoms.

The same is true for carbons in a position α to a heteroatom such as N, O or S (Fig. 29.8). With amines, hydroxylation leads to a hydroxy-aminal which is immediately hydrolysed. The final result is *dealkylation* when a secondary or a tertiary amine loses an alkyl substituent, and *deamination* when the substrate loses an amino group. But here again, positions other than the α one can be hydroxylated, albeit to a lesser extent (Fig. 29.8).

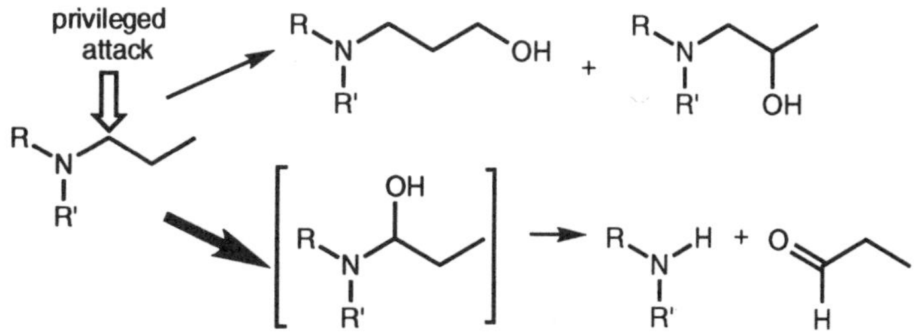

Fig. 29.8   For long-chain amines, α, ω and ω−1 attacks coexist, but α attacks are privileged.

Aromatic ethers undergo a similar a-hydroxylation, followed by hydrolysis of the hemiacetal to a phenol and an aldehyde (Fig. 29.9).

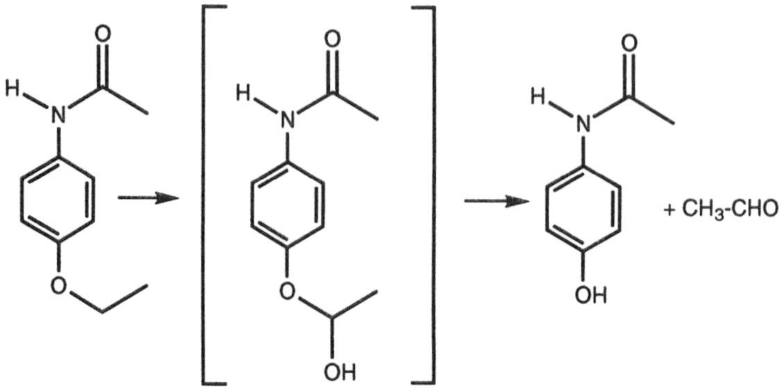

Fig. 29.9   The oxidative O-dealkylation of phenacetin yields paracetamol.

Note: Dealkylation reactions can also result from *direct* oxidation of the heteroatom (N, S) as opposed to that of the α-carbon (see below).

Chlorinated or brominated aliphatic derivatives can similarly be metabolized by successive hydroxylation and elimination of HCl or HBr. Dehalogenated carbonyl compounds are thus formed (Fig. 29.10).

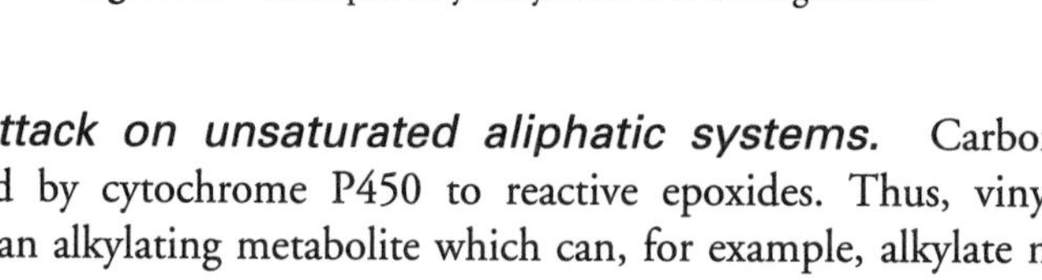

Fig. 29.10   Example of hydroxylation α to a halogen atom.

(c) Oxidative attack on unsaturated aliphatic systems.   Carbon–carbon double bonds are oxidized by cytochrome P450 to reactive epoxides. Thus, vinyl chloride yields epoxychlorethane, an alkylating metabolite which can, for example, alkylate nucleic acids (Fig. 29.11).

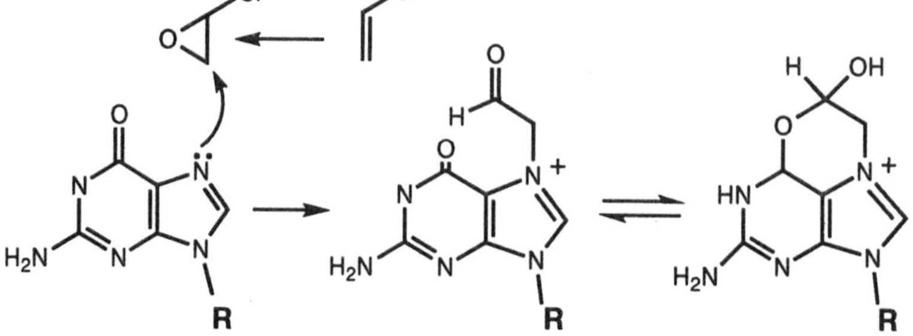

Fig. 29.11   Oxidative alkylation of a guanine rest by vinyl chloride.

The synthetic estrogen diethylstilbestrol undergoes a similar attack. Despite its relatively hindered character, the central double bond is converted to the corresponding epoxide, which was once believed to be the ultimate carcinogenic metabolite (Fig. 29.12).

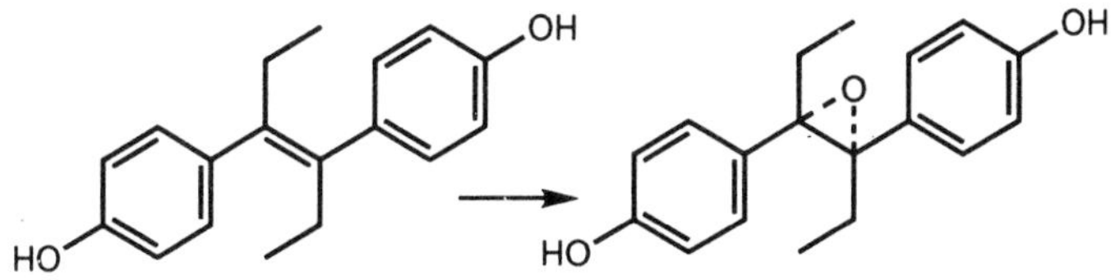

Fig. 29.12 Epoxidation of diethylstilbestrol.

With carbon–carbon triple bonds, oxygen insertion yields an oxirene which opens by heterolytic C—O bond cleavage to form a highly reactive intermediate which binds covalently to the enzyme. In the case of 17a-ethynyl steroids the reaction can also result in an extension of ring D (Fig. 29.13).

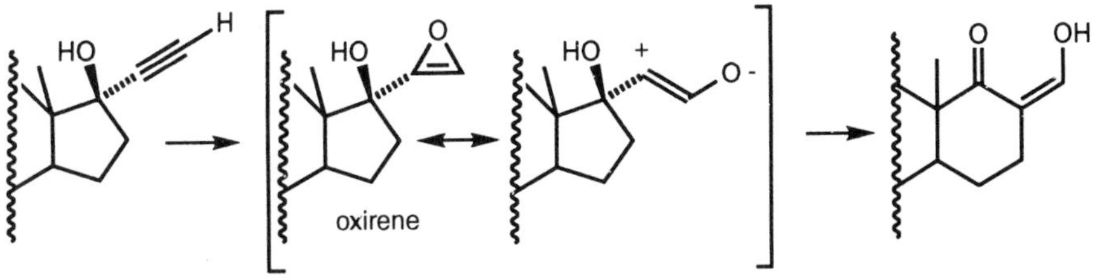

Fig. 29.13 The triple bond in a 17α-ethynyl steroid is first epoxidated to an oxirene, which then undergoes a rearrangement and an extension of ring D.

(d) Hydroxylation of aromatic rings. Aromatic rings are frequently oxidized to phenols, followed by conjugation and excretion. The mechanism of the reaction is discussed later, and we shall first consider an example of phenol formation. In the hydroxylation of chlorobenzene, all three isomers are produced, i.e. *ortho-*, *meta-* and *para*-chlorophenol, but in different amounts (Fig. 29.14). As a rule, hydroxylation occurs on the less-hindered site, usually the *para* position. Electronic factors are also operative. This is seen in the hydroxylation of many drugs, two of which are shown in Fig. 29.15.

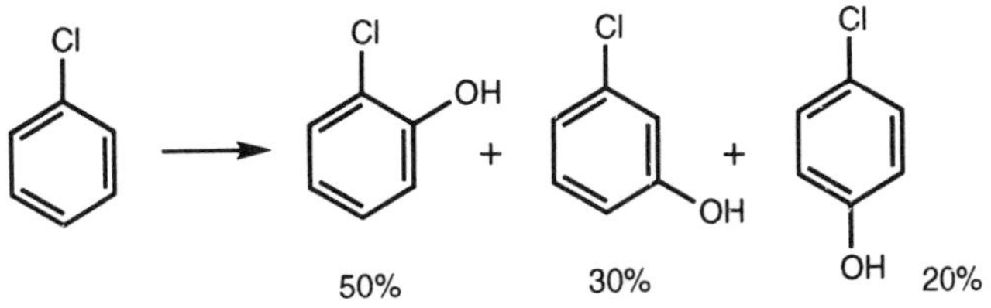

Fig. 29.14 Hydroxylation of chlorobenzene in the rat yields the three isomers, i.e. *o-*, *m-* and *p*-chlorophenol.

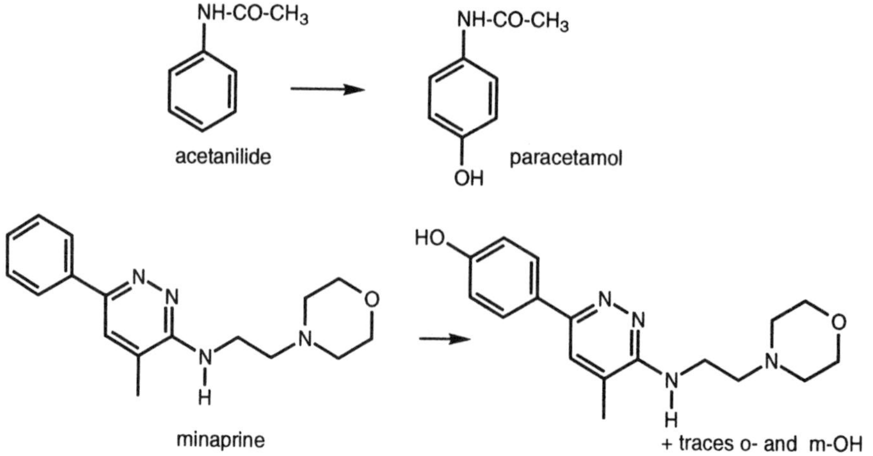

Fig. 29.15 Aromatic rings are predominantly hydroxylated in the *para* position.

The mechanism of the oxidative attack catalysed by cytochrome P450 involves the addition of an activated oxene species to the aromatic ring (Fig. 29.16). The resulting tetrahedral intermediate usually rearranges, forming an intermediate epoxide. Epoxides (also called arene oxides or oxiranes) are electrophiles which are detoxified by a number of routes, e.g. protonation and rearrangement to a phenol (often the most efficient pathway), hydration by epoxide hydrolase, and conjugation with glutathione. The toxicity of a number of aromatic compounds is due to the epoxide reacting with cellular constituents (cytotoxicity, mutagenesis), or to the further oxidation of phenols to diphenols and then to semiquinones and quinones.

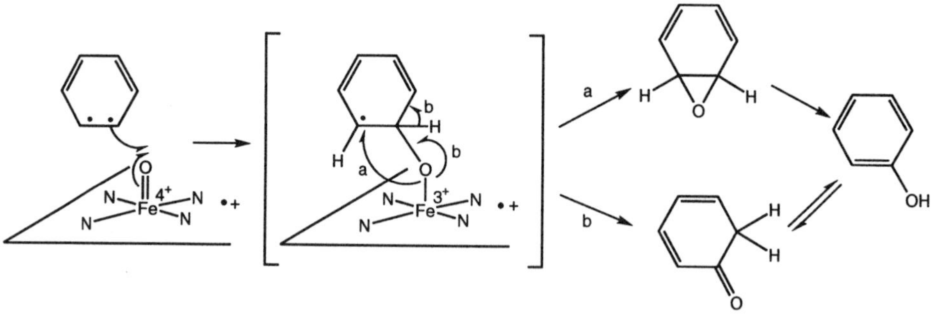

Fig. 29.16 Addition–rearrangement mechanism for arene oxide formation and proton-catalysed rearrangement of an arene oxide to a phenol. (After Silverman.[3])

(e) The NIH-shift. The *NIH-shift* is a particular intramolecular rearrangement occurring during the hydroxylation of aromatic rings and resulting in the migration of a hydrogen or a halogen atom. In the case of a hydrogen atom, the migration is not apparent but becomes observable with deuterium or tritium. This transposition was first observed in 1967 at the National Institutes of Health (Bethesda, MD, USA), when the enzymatic hydroxylation of

4-[³H]-phenylalanine unexpectedly yielded 3-[³H]-para-tyrosine with a retention of 90% of the radioactivity (Fig. 29.17).

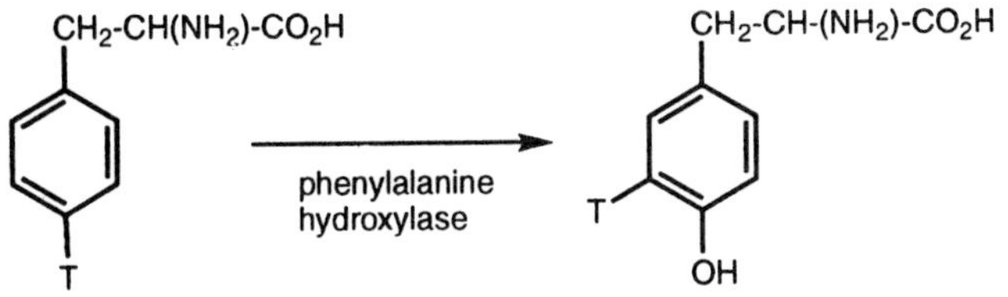

Fig. 29.17 NIH shift in the hydroxylation of tritiated phenylalanine to *p*-tyrosine.

The percentages of retention and migration depend on the nature of the label (hydrogen isotope or halogen atom) and of the substituent(s) carried by the aromatic ring. When the substituent R cannot provide a proton, good retention (40–60%) of the label is observed. This is the case for R = Cl, CN, OCH₃, NO₂, CONH₂ and C₆H₅, the predominant mechanism then being that shown in Fig. 29.18.

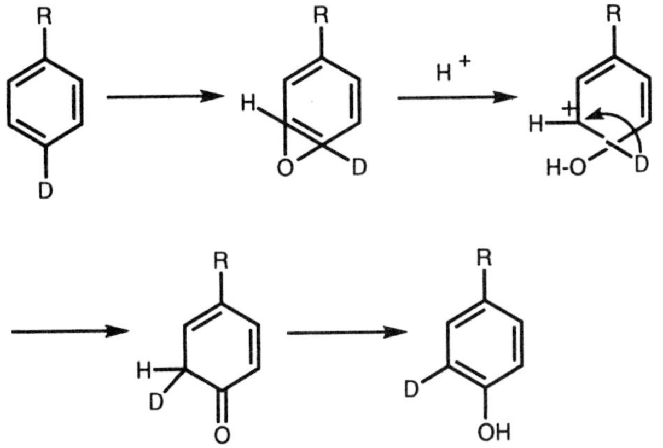

Fig. 29.18 Mechanism of the NIH shift when the substituent R is not a hydrogen donor.

When the R substituent is a proton donor (R = CO_2H, NH_2, SO_2NH_2, $NH-CO-R_1$, etc.), only little retention (0–30%) and migration is achieved. The mechanism shown in Fig. 29.19 accounts for the reaction. The acidic hydrogen competes with the deuterium atom, and two pathways are possible, namely elimination of H⁺ (pathway *a*) or elimination of D⁺ (pathway *b*).

(f) The NIH-shift and obstructive halogenation. In order to decrease the metabolism of an aromatic ring, one can block the *para* position with a halogen atom. However, owing to the NIH-shift, *para*-substituted rings can still be oxidized (Fig. 29.20). In drug design, obstructive halogenation is justified when the duration of action of an aromatic compound must be prolonged.

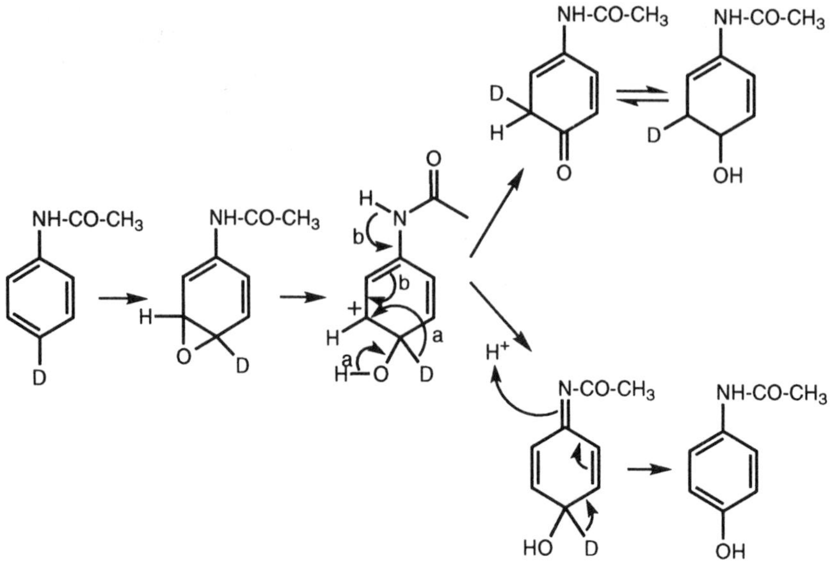

Fig. 29.19 Mechanism of the NIH shift when the substituent R is a proton donor.

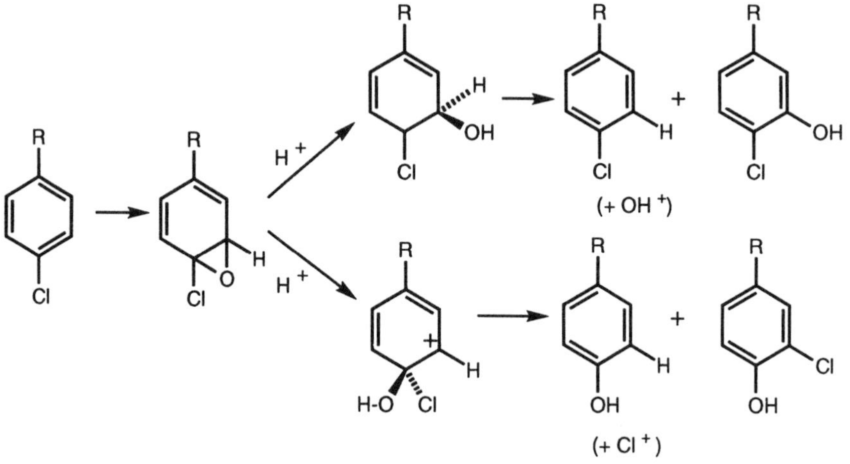

Fig. 29.20 Example of oxidation of a *para*-halogenated ring.

3. Reactions of N-oxygenation

Enzymatically, *N*-oxygenation can be catalysed by cytochrome P450 and/or by the FAD-containing monooxygenase, depending on substrate and conditions. From a chemical viewpoint, the oxidation of nitrogen atoms in organic compounds can be summarized as follows.

Tertiary aliphatic amines are usually oxidized to the corresponding N-oxides, but the reaction is strongly affected by steric hindrance. Usual substrates are *N,N*-dimethylamino aliphatic and aromatic tertiary amines (e.g., *N,N*-dimethylaniline) (Fig. 29.21A), saturated *N*-methylaza heterocycles (e.g. *N*-methylpiperidines), and aromatic aza heterocycles (e.g. pyridine).

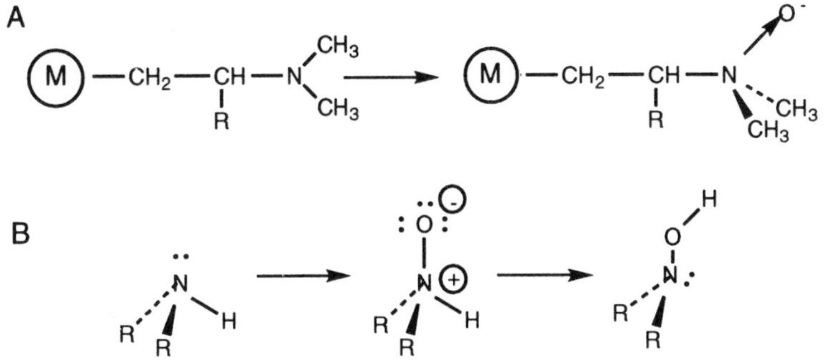

Fig. 29.21   *N*-Oxygenation of tertiary aliphatic amines (A) and secondary amines (B).

Secondary and primary amines are *N*-oxygenated to hydroxylamines as shown in Fig. 29.21B. The intermediate is believed to be an *N*-oxide.

Note that a drug very seldom undergoes a single metabolic reaction but is substrate of several competitive pathways. *N*-Benzylamphetamine offers an example in the present context (Fig. 29.22).[4]

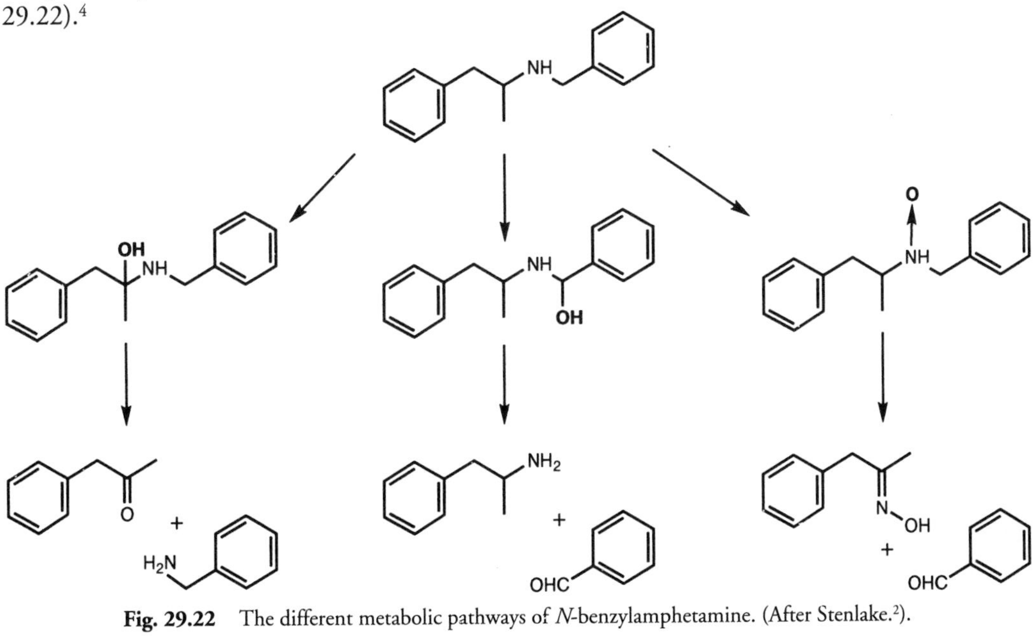

Fig. 29.22   The different metabolic pathways of *N*-benzylamphetamine. (After Stenlake.[2]).

Amides can be *N*-oxygenated to hydroxylamides. This is true for primary and secondary amides. For example, urethane and *N*-acetylfluorene are converted into a highly carcinogenic hydroxylamides (Fig. 29.23). The toxicity of phenacetin has similarly been attributed to an *N*-hydroxylated metabolite.

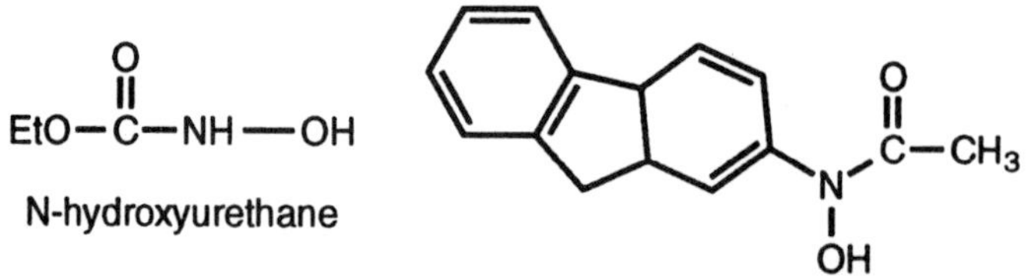

Fig. 29.23   Examples of hydroxylamides resulting from the *N*-oxygenation of amides.

4. Reactions of S-oxidation

Thiol compounds can be oxidized to disulfides, or to sulfenic, sulfinic and finally to sulfonic acids. Similarly sulfides are easily converted by monooxygenases to sulfoxides and then to sulfones.

Thiocarbonyl derivatives are also substrates of monooxygenases, forming *S*-monooxides (sulfines) and then *S*-dioxides (sulfenes). The latter are highly reactive metabolites, especially towards nucleophilic sites in biological macromolecules, and are believed to account for the carcinogenicity of a number of thioamides. *S*-Monooxides can also rearrange to the corresponding carbonyl by expelling a sulfur atom (oxidative desulfuration of thioamides, thioureas and thiobarbiturates).

B. Oxidations Catalysed by other Oxidoreductases

1. Enzymes

Besides the monooxygenases discussed above, a number of other oxidoreductases can oxidize xenobiotics. These enzymes are mostly but not exclusively nonmicrosomal, being present in the cytosol or mitochondria of the liver and extrahepatic tissues. The list includes alcohol dehydrogenases, aldehyde dehydrogenases, dihydrodiol dehydrogenases, haemoglobin, monoamine oxidases, xanthine oxidase and aldehyde oxidase. Some of these enzyme systems are discussed below.

2. Reactions of oxidation

Alcohol dehydrogenases catalyse the oxidation of primary and secondary alcohols to aldehydes and ketones, respectively. Typical primary alcohols acting as substrates are ethanol, benzylic alcohol, phenylethanol, geraniol and retinol. Methanol is a poor substrate and is oxidized only slowly at high concentrations. Secondary alcohols are more difficult to oxidize, while tertiary alcohols are resistant towards dehydrogenation. This explains in part the greater potency of tertiary alcohols as hypnotics (e.g. methylpentynol, amylene hydrate).

Alcohol dehydrogenases are zinc enzymes that use NAD$^+$ as coenzyme according to the reaction.

$$CH_3-CH_2-OH + NAD \rightarrow CH_3-CHO + NADH + H^+$$

The reaction involves the transfer of a hydride ion to the nicotinamide part of NAD$^+$ and is stereospecific.

Aldehyde dehydrogenases transform aldehydes into carboxylic acids (e.g. succinaldehyde dehydrogenase). As with alcohol dehydrogenases, the key step of the reaction is the cleavage of the α-C$=$H bond, with a hydride transfer to NAD$^+$.

Monoamine oxidases (MAO) are mitochondrial enzymes existing in two forms, MAO-A and MAO-B. Their physiological function is to deaminate endogenous amines, in particular catecholamines, but their involvement in the oxidation of xenobiotics is exemplified by the toxication of MPTP (1-methyl-1,2,3,6–tetrahydropyridine) and analogues to the corresponding pyridinium ions.

C. Reductions

A number of reactions of reduction have been demonstrated in the metabolism of xenobiotics. From a quantitative viewpoint, they are less important than oxidations since the human organism is mostly an aerobic one. From a qualitative viewpoint, however, reactions of reduction may be of great pharmacological or toxicological significance when they generate active metabolites or toxic metabolic intermediates.

1.   Reductions at carbon atoms

The major reactions of reduction at carbon atoms can be found in Fig. 29.24. Thus, aldehydes and ketones are readily reduced to primary and secondary alcohols, respectively. Quinones can be reduced to dihydrodiols either by a two-electron mechanism (carbonyl reductase and quinone reductase) or by two single-electron steps (cytochrome P450 and some flavoproteins). Reduction of olefinic groups, i.e. the reverse of desaturation, is documented for a few drugs bearing an α,β-ketoalkene function. Dehalogenation reactions can also proceed reductively. Reductive dehalogenations involve replacement of a halogen by a hydrogen, or *vic*-bisdehalogenation. Some radical species formed as intermediates may have toxicological significance.

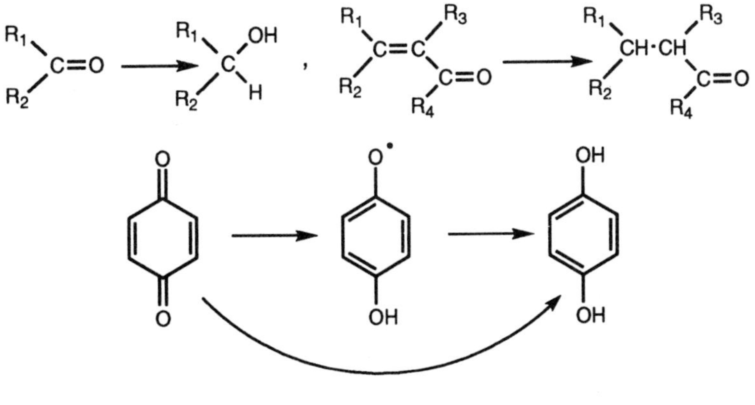

Fig. 29.24   Some reactions of reduction at carbon atoms.

2.　Reductions at other atoms

Various reactions of *N*-oxidation are reversible, cytochrome P450 and other reductases being able to deoxygenate *N*-oxides back to the amine (see Fig. 29.25). The same is true for aromatic nitro compounds, aromatic nitroso compounds and hydroxylamines, and imines and oximes, which can ultimately be reduced to primary amines. Azo and azoxy compounds can be reduced to hydrazines. An important pathway of hydrazines is their reductive cleavage to primary amines. A toxicologically significant pathway thus exists for the reduction of some aromatic azo compounds to potentially toxic primary aromatic amines.

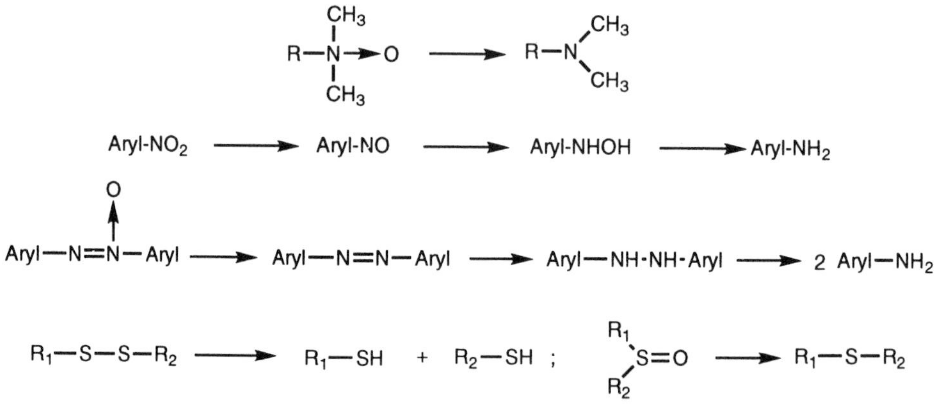

Fig. 29.25　Some reactions of reduction at nitrogen and sulfur atoms.

Other reductions involve sulfur (Fig. 29.25) and a few other atoms. Thus, disulfides are reduced to thiols, and there are numerous examples of the reduction of sulfoxides. In contrast, the reduction of sulfones has never been found to occur.

D.　Hydrolytic reactions

1.　Hydrolases

Hydrolases constitute a very complex ensemble of enzymes, many of which are known or suspected to be involved in xenobiotic metabolism. Relevant enzymes among the serine hydrolases include carboxylesterases, arylesterases, cholinesterase, and a number of serine endopeptidases. Other hydrolases worth mentioning are arylsulfatases, aryldialkylphosphatases, β-glucuronidases, epoxide hydrolases, cysteine endopeptidases, aspartic endopeptidases and metalloendopeptidases.

2.　Reactions of hydration and hydrolysis

Hydrolases catalyse the addition of a molecule of water to a variety of functional groups. Thus, epoxide hydrolase hydrates epoxides to yield *trans*-dihydrodiols. This reaction is documented for many arene oxides, in particular metabolites of aromatic compounds, and epoxides of olefins.

Here, a molecule of water is added to the substrate without loss of a molecular fragment; hence the use of the term 'hydration' sometimes found in the literature. The main reactions of hydrolytic cleavage (hydrolysis) are shown in Figure 29.26. They are frequent for organic esters, inorganic esters such as nitrates, and amides. These reactions are catalysed by esterases, peptidases or other enzymes, but nonenzymatic hydrolysis is also known to occur for sufficiently labile compounds under biological conditions of pH and temperature. Such reactions are of particular significance in the activation of ester prodrugs. Another reaction of interest is the hydrolysis of carbamate esters. Hydrolysis, which is often found to proceed readily, liberates the carbamic acid. The latter is unstable and breaks down to the amine and carbon dioxide.

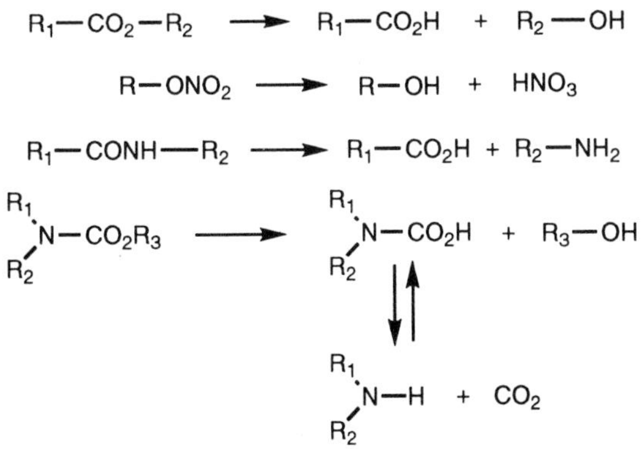

$$R_1\text{—}CO_2\text{—}R_2 \longrightarrow R_1\text{—}CO_2H + R_2\text{—}OH$$

$$R\text{—}ONO_2 \longrightarrow R\text{—}OH + HNO_3$$

$$R_1\text{—}CONH\text{—}R_2 \longrightarrow R_1\text{—}CO_2H + R_2\text{—}NH_2$$

$$\begin{matrix} R_1 \\ \quad N\text{—}CO_2R_3 \\ R_2 \end{matrix} \longrightarrow \begin{matrix} R_1 \\ \quad N\text{—}CO_2H + R_3\text{—}OH \\ R_2 \end{matrix}$$

$$\begin{matrix} R_1 \\ \quad N\text{—}H + CO_2 \\ R_2 \end{matrix}$$

Fig. 29.26   Some reaction of hydrolysis.

III.   REACTIONS OF CONJUGATION (PHASE II)

A.   Introduction

As already defined above, conjugation reactions link an endogenous moiety (an endocon) either to the original drug (if polar functions are already present) or to the phase I metabolite. Conjugates are usually devoid of pharmacological activities, but there are notable exceptions. In addition, they are often more polar and water-soluble than the parent drug, and readily excreted via the renal route. However, certain conjugation reactions do *not* result in decreased lipophilicity, e.g. acetylations and some reactions of methylation.

Reactions of conjugation are characterized by the following criteria, none of which is a *sine qua non.*

(1)   They are catalysed by enzymes known as *transferases.*
(2)   They involve a *cofactor* which binds to the enzyme in the close proximity of the substrate and carries the endogenous molecule or moiety to be transferred.
(3)   Except for methylations and acetylations, this endocon is highly polar and its size is comparable to that of the substrate.

B.   Methylation

1.   Biochemistry

Methylation is a important reaction in the biosynthesis of endogenous compounds such as adrenaline and melatonin, in the inactivation of biogenic amines such as the catecholamines, serotonin and histamine, and in modulating the activities of macromolecules such as proteins and nucleic acids. The number of xenobiotics that are methylated is comparatively modest, yet this reaction is seldom devoid of pharmacodynamic consequences (toxication or detoxication). Reactions of methylation imply the transfer of a methyl group from the onium-type cofactor S-adenosylmethionine (SAM) to the substrate by means of a methyltransferase. The activated methyl group from SAM is transferred to the acceptor molecules $R-XH$ or RX, as shown in Fig. 29.27.

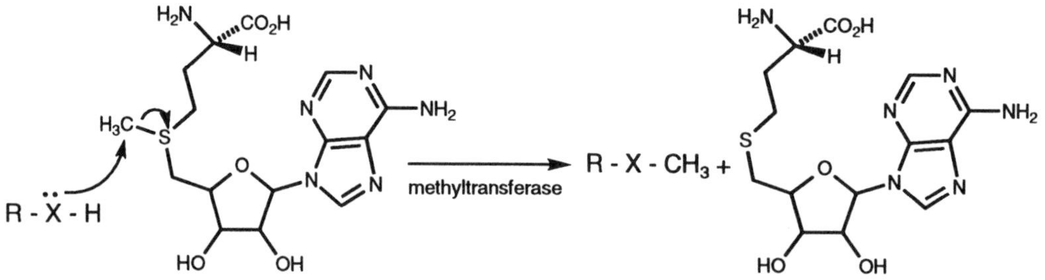

Fig. 29.27   Mechanism of methylation.

A number of methyltransferases are able to methylate small molecules on a phenolic, an amino or a thiol group. The major enzyme responsible for O-methylations is catechol O-methyltransferase (COMT), a cytosolic enzyme that also exists in membrane-bound form. N-Methylations are catalysed by several enzymes such as nicotinamide N-methyltransferase, histamine methyltransferase, phenylethanolamine N-methyltransferase (noradrenaline N-methyl-transferase) and a nonspecific amine N-methyltransferase (arylamine N-methyltransferase, tryptamine N-methyltransferase). S-Methylations are catalysed by the membrane-bound thiol methyltransferase and the cytosolic thiopurine methyltransferase.

2.   Methylation reactions

O-Methylation of xenobiotic catechols occurs preferentially at the *meta* position, L-dopa and isoproterenol being classical examples. Frequently *O*-methylation is a late event in the metabolism of aryl groups, after they have been oxidized to catechols. Thus the anti-inflammatory drug diclofenac yields in humans 3'-hydroxy-4'-methoxydiclofenac as the major metabolite with a very long plasmatic half-life. Noncatechol diphenols are not subject to methylation, e.g. terbutaline. A few monophenols can also undergo methylation to a limited extent.

The *N-methylation* of xenobiotics occurs with primary and secondary amines (e.g. amphetamine and tetrahydroisoquinolines, respectively), with pyrrol-type nitrogen atoms (as exemplified by imidazole, histamine and thiabendazole), and with pyridine-type nitrogen atoms.

The latter reaction of *N*-methylation is an effective route of detoxication. It leads to quaternary ammoniums which are stable to *N*-demethylation and more polar (having a permanent positive charge) than the parent compound. Known substrates are nicotinamide, pyridine, and a number of related heterocyclic compounds.

S-Methylation is known for aromatic sulfhydryl groups such as thiophenols, 6-mercaptopurine and propylthiouracil, as well as for aliphatic thiols like captopril. Once formed, such methylthio metabolites can be further processed to sulfoxides and sulfones before being excreted.

C. Acetylation and acylation

All cases discussed in this section involve the reaction between an amine and an acyl group to yield an amide. The high-energy cofactor required is in most cases an acyl-coenzyme A derivative (acyl-S-CoA) where the acyl moiety is bound by a thioester linkage.

1. Acetylation reactions

The most common reactions of acylation are in fact acetylations of xenobiotics containing a primary amino group. The cofactor of acetylation is acetyl-coenzyme A (acetyl-S-CoA), the reaction being catalysed by a variety of *N*-acetyltransferases. Arylamine *N*-acetyltransferase (NAT) is the most important enzyme, but aromatic-hydroxylamine *O*-acetyltransferase and *N*-hydroxyarylamine *O*-acetyltransferase are also involved in the acetylation of some aromatic amines and hydroxylamines.

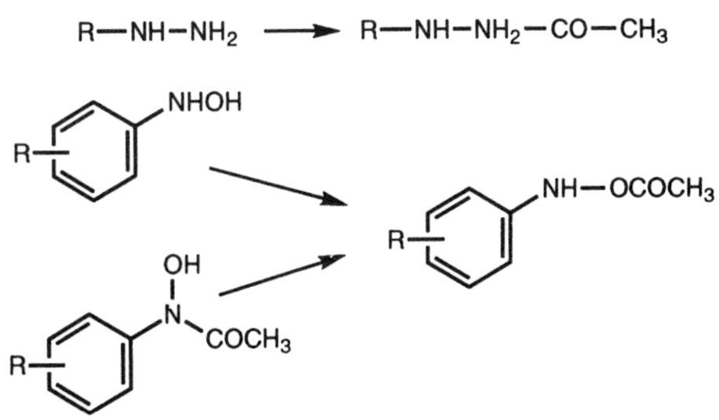

Fig. 29.28 Major reactions of *N*-acetylation.

The major reactions of *N*-acetylation are listed in Fig. 29.28. A large variety of primary aromatic amines are *N*-acetylated, often to a large extent; they include several drugs such as sulfonamides and *p*-aminosalicylic acid, not to mention various carcinogenic amines such as benzidine. Other substrates include a few aliphatic amines, cysteine conjugates, and mainly hydrazines and hydrazides. Medicinal examples of the latter include isoniazid and hydralazine. The metabolites resulting from *N*-acetylation are uncharged amides; when the parent xenobiotic is an amine of high basicity, acetylation may result in decreased water solubility. Genetic differences exist in some animal species and in humans, where one distinguishes between slow and fast acetylators. Examples of drugs exhibiting acetylation polymorphism are the antibacterial drug sulfamethazine, the antituberculosis drug isoniazid, and the antileprosy agent dapsone.

2.   Other reactions of acylation

Cholesteryl ester synthase and fatty acid synthase, and also sterol *O*-acyltransferase, perform conjugations of various xenobiotic alcohols (e.g. ethanol, tetrahydrocannabinol and codeine) with fatty acids such as palmitic, oleic, linoleic and linolenic acids. A limited number of *N*-formylation reactions of aromatic amines are catalysed by arylformamidase in the presence of *N*-formyl-L-kynurenine.

D.   Acyl-coenzyme A thioesters as metabolic intermediates

1.   Biochemistry

The reactions described in this section all have in common the fact that they involve xenobiotic carboxylic acids (R—COOH) coupling with coenzyme A (CoA-SH) to form an acyl-CoA metabolic intermediate (R—CO-S-CoA). The reaction requires ATP and is catalysed by various acyl-CoA ligases of overlapping substrate specificity, e.g. acetate-CoA ligase, butyrate-CoA ligase, long-chain fatty acid-CoA ligase, benzoate-CoA ligase and phenylacetate-CoA ligase.

The acyl-CoA conjugates thus formed are seldom excreted, but undergo further transformation by a considerable variety of pathways.

- Hydrolysis (by thiolester hydrolases)
- Formation of amino acid conjugates
- Formation of hybrid triglycerides and phospholipids
- Formation of cholesteryl esters and bile acid esters
- Formation of acylcarnitines
- Protein acylation
- Unidirectional chiral inversion of arylpropionic acids
- Dehydrogenation and β-oxidation
- 2-Carbon chain elongation.

2.   Amino acid conjugation

This is a major route for many xenobiotic acids, involving the formation of an amide bond between the xenobiotic acyl-CoA and the amino acid. Glycine is the amino acid most frequently used for conjugation, forming conjugates with the general structure R—CO—NHCH$_2$COOH. A few glutamine conjugates have also been characterized in humans. The enzymes catalysing these transfer reactions are various *N*-acyltransferases, for example glycine *N*-acyltransferase, glutamine *N*-phenylacetyltransferase, glutamine *N*-acyltransferase and glycine *N*-benzoyltransferase. The xenobiotic acids undergoing amino acid conjugation are mainly benzoic acids such as benzoic acid itself and salicylic acid, which form hippuric acid and salicyluric acid, respectively. Phenylacetic acid derivatives can yield glycine and glutamine conjugates. In addition, other amino acids can be used for conjugation in various animal species, e.g. alanine and taurine, as well as some dipeptides.

3.   Other reactions

Incorporation of xenobiotic acids into lipids is of rather recent characterization and forms highly lipophilic metabolites that may burden the body as long-retained residues. In the majority of cases, triacylglycerol analogues or cholesterol esters are formed. In some cases, acyl-CoA conjugates formed from xenobiotic acids can also enter the physiological pathways of fatty acids catabolism or anabolism. Thus, intermediate metabolites of β-oxidation may be observed, as exemplified by valproic acid. The enzymes catalysing this pathway are clearly those involved in the metabolism of fatty acids. In addition, a few examples are known of xenobiotic alkanoic and arylalkanoic acids undergoing two-carbon chain elongation, or chain shortening by two carbons or even four or six carbons.

E.   Glucuronidation

1.   Biochemistry

In glucuronidation (i.e. glucuronic acid conjugation), one molecule of glucuronic acid is transferred to the substrate from uridine-5′-diphospho-α-D-glucuronic acid (UDPGA), a cofactor that is synthesized from glucose-1-phosphate via uridine triphosphate (Fig. 29.29). The

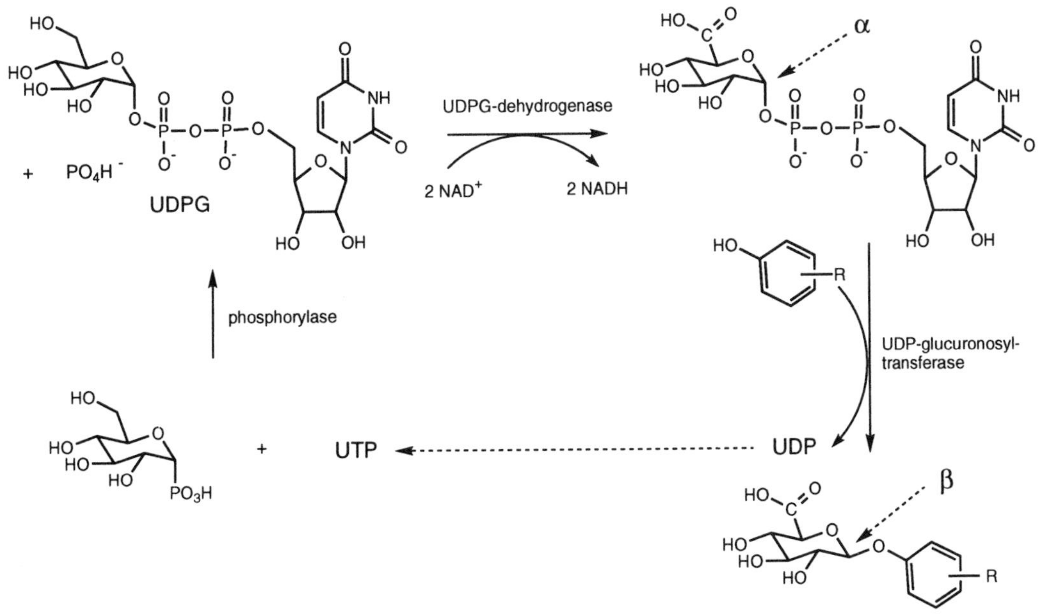

Fig. 29.29   Synthesis of uridine-5′-diphospho-α-D-glucuronic acid (UDPGA) and glucuronyltransferase-catalysed glucuronidation of a phenol.

reaction is catalysed by glucuronyltransferase (UDPGT), an enzyme which consists in a number of products of the *UGT* gene superfamily. According to a recent nomenclature, the human UDPGT isozymes are the products of two gene families, *UGT1* and *UGT2*, whose products are the phenol/bilirubin UGTs and steroid UGTs, respectively. Individual enzymes include UGT1*1 and UGT1*4, UGT1*6, UGT2B4, UGT2B7, UGT2B8, UGT2B9 and UGT2B10.

2. Reactions of glucuronidation

The mechanism of glucuronidation is one of nucleophilic substitution with inversion of configuration, α-D-glucuronic acid in UDPGA forming β-D-glucuronides. The functional groups able to undergo glucuronidation are shown in Fig. 29.30. A common characteristic of these groups, despite their great chemical variety, is their nucleophilic character. As a consequence of this diversity, the products of glucuronidation are classified as *O-*, *N-*, *S-* and *C-*glucuronides.

The *O-glucuronidation* of phenolic xenobiotics or metabolites is often in competition with *O-*sulfation, with the latter reaction predominating at low doses and the former at high doses. Another major group of substrates are alcohols, be they primary, secondary or tertiary. An interesting example is that of morphine, which is conjugated on its phenolic and secondary alcohol groups to form the 3-*O*-glucuronide (a weak opiate antagonist) and the 6-*O*-glucuronide (a strong opiate agonist), respectively.

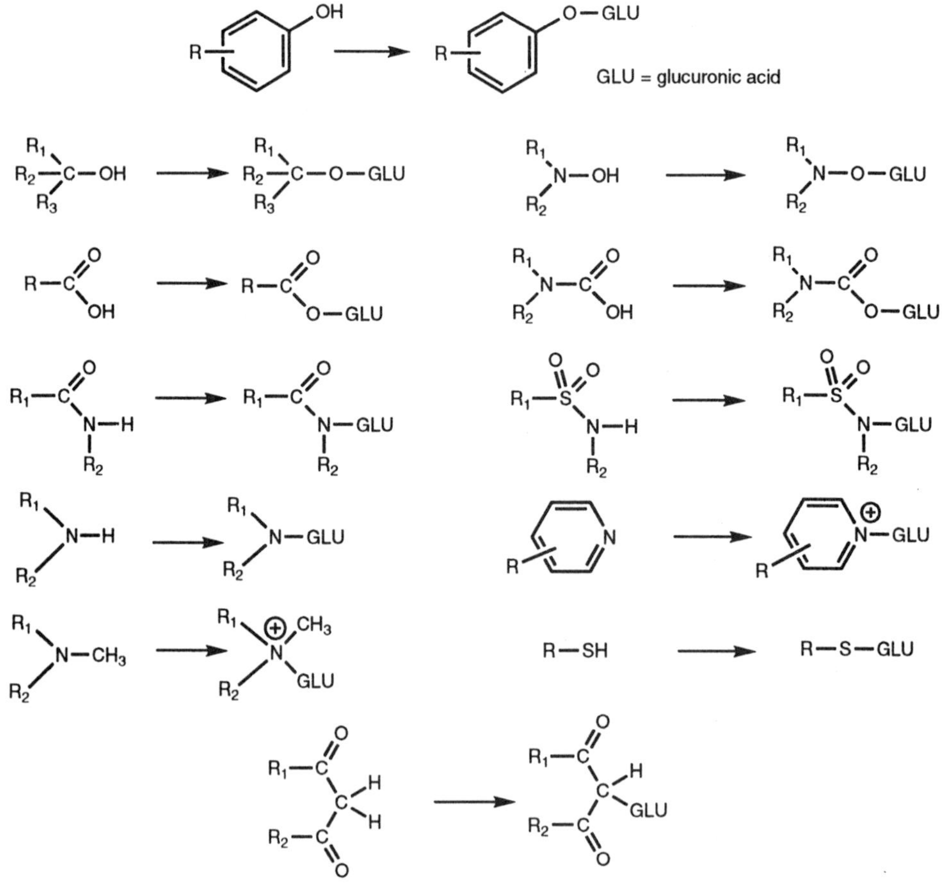

Fig. 29.30 Reactions of glucuronidation in xenobiotic metabolism.

Another important pathway of *O*-glucuronidation is the formation of acylglucuronides. Good substrates are arylacetic acids and aliphatic acids. These metabolites are relatively reactive, rearranging to positional isomers and binding covalently to plasmatic and seemingly also tissular proteins. Thus, acylglucuronide formation cannot be viewed solely as a reaction of inactivation and detoxication. A special class of acyl glucuronides is that formed by carbamic acids which themselves are not stable enough to be characterized. An increasing number of primary and secondary amines are found to yield this type of glucuronide, whose chemical and biochemical reactivity remains to be better elucidated. Hydroxylamines and hydroxylamides may also form *O*-glucuronides. Thus, a few drugs and a number of aromatic amines are known to be *N*-hydroxylated and then *O*-glucuronidated. The reactivity of *N-O*-glucuronides to undergo heterolytic cleavage and form nitrenium ions does not appear to be well characterized.

Second in importance to *O*-glucuronides are the *N-glucuronides* formed from carboxamides, sulfonamides, and various amines. The reaction has special significance for antibacterial sulfanilamides, producing highly water-soluble metabolites which do not crystallize in the kidneys. *N*-Glucuronidation of aromatic and aliphatic amines and pyridine-type nitrogens has been observed in only a few cases. A reaction of greater significance in human drug metabolism is the *N*-glucuronidation of lipophilic, basic tertiary amines containing one or two methyl groups.

Some *S-glucuronides* are formed from aliphatic thiols, aromatic thiols and dithiocarboxylic acids. *C-Glucuronidation* is seen in humans for 1,3-dicarbonyl drugs such as sulfinpyrazone.

F. Sulfate conjugation

In reactions of sulfoconjugation, a sulfate molecule is transferred from the cofactor (3'-phosphoadenosine 5'-phosphosulfate, PAPS) to the substrate by cytosolic enzymes known as sulfotransferases (Fig. 29.31). These include aryl sulfotransferase, alcohol sulfotransferase, amine sulfotransferase, estrone sulfotransferase, tyrosine-ester sulfotransferase, steroid sulfotransferase, and cortisol sulfotransferase. The former three enzymes are of particular significance in the metabolism of xenobiotics.

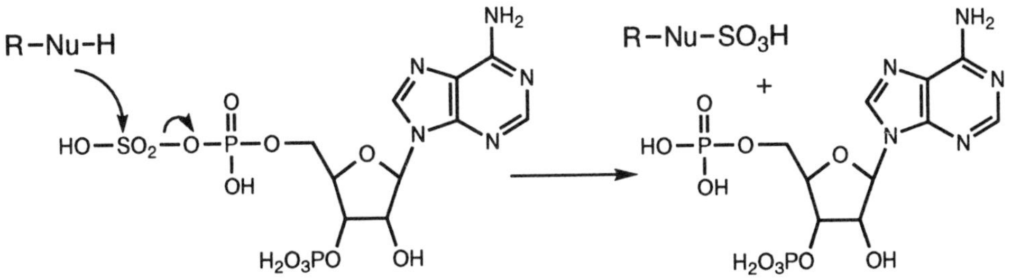

Fig. 29.31 The structure of 3'-phosphoadenosine 5'-phosphosulfate (PAPS).

The sulfate moiety in PAPS will bind to an electrophilic $-OH$ or $-NH-$ site in the substrate, forming an ester sulfate $(R-O-SO_3^-)$ or a sulfamate $(RR'NSO_3^-)$. Sulfoconjugation of alcohols leads to metabolites of different stabilities. Endogenous hydroxysteroids (i.e. cyclic secondary alcohols) form relatively stable sulfates, while some secondary alcohol metabolites of xenobiotics (e.g. safrole and oestragole) form genotoxic carbocations. Primary alcohols, e.g. methanol and ethanol, can also form low amounts of sulfates whose alkylating capacity is well known. In contrast to some alcohols, phenols form stable sulfate esters. The reaction is usually of high affinity, but the limited availability of PAPS restricts the amounts of conjugate being produced.

Aromatic hydroxylamines and hydroxylamides are good substrates for some sulfotransferases and yield unstable sulfate esters ($RR'N-OSO_3^-$). Indeed, heterolytic $N-O$ cleavage produces highly electrophilic nitrenium ions believed to account for part or all of the cytotoxicity of arylamines and arylamides. In contrast, significantly more stable products are obtained upon formation of sulfamates from amines such as primary and secondary alkyl- and arylamines.

G.   Conjugation with glutathione

1.   Biochemistry

Glutathione (GSH, γ-glutamylcysteinylglycine) is a thiol-containing tripeptide of capital significance in the detoxication and toxication of drugs and other xenobiotics. Glutathione reacts with endogenous and exogenous compounds in a variety of manners. First, the nucleophilic properties of the thiol group make it an effective conjugating agent. Second, glutathione can act as a reducing or oxidizing agent depending on its redox state (i.e. GSH or GSSG). Furthermore, the reactions of glutathione can be enzymatic (e.g. conjugations catalysed by glutathione S-transferases, and peroxide reductions catalysed by glutathione peroxidase) or nonenzymatic (e.g. some conjugations and various redox reactions).

The glutathione transferase (GST) comprises multifunctional proteins coded by a multigene family. These enzymes are mainly localized in the cytosol as homodimers and heterodimers, and exist as four classes in mammals. The human enzymes comprise the dimers: A1-1, A1-2, A2-2, A3-3 (alpha class), M1a-1a, M1a-1b, M1b-1b, M1a-2, M2-2, M3-3 (mu class), P1-1 (pi class), T1-1 (theta class), and a microsomal enzyme (MIC). The GST A1-1 and A1-2 are also known as ligandin when they act as binding or carrier proteins, a property also displayed by M1a-1a and M1b-1b. The nucleophilic character of glutathione is due to its thiol or rather thiolate group. As a result, GSTs transfer glutathione to a very large variety of electrophilic groups (see below) in nucleophilic reactions categorized as either substitutions or additions. With compounds of sufficient reactivity, these reactions can also occur nonenzymatically. Once formed, glutathione conjugates (GS-R) are seldom excreted as such but usually undergo further biotransformation. Cleavage of the glutamyl moiety by glutamyl transpeptidase and of the cysteinyl moiety by cysteinylglycine dipeptidase or aminopeptidase M leaves a cysteine conjugate (Cys-S-R) which is further N-acetylated by cysteine-S-conjugate N-acetyltransferase to yield an N-acetylcysteine conjugate (CysAc-S-R). The latter type of conjugates are known as mercapturic acids. These may be either excreted or further transformed, since cysteine conjugates can be substrates of cysteine-S-conjugate β-lyase to yield thiols ($R-SH$). These in turn can rearrange or be S-methylated and then S-oxygenated to yield thiomethyl conjugates ($R-S-Me$), sulfoxides ($R-SO-Me$) and sulfones ($R-SO_2-Me$).

2. Reactions of conjugation

The major reactions of glutathione are shown in Fig. 29.32. Nucleophilic addition to epoxides yields nonaromatic conjugates which may undergo further transformation as described above. This reaction is well documented for the arene oxide metabolites of numerous drugs and xenobiotics containing a aromatic moiety. The same reaction can also occur readily for epoxides of olefins. An important pathway of substitution exists for $-CH_2X$ moieties. Various electron-withdrawing leaving groups X may be involved, for example the chorine atom at the NCH_2CH_2Cl group of anticancer alkylating agents.

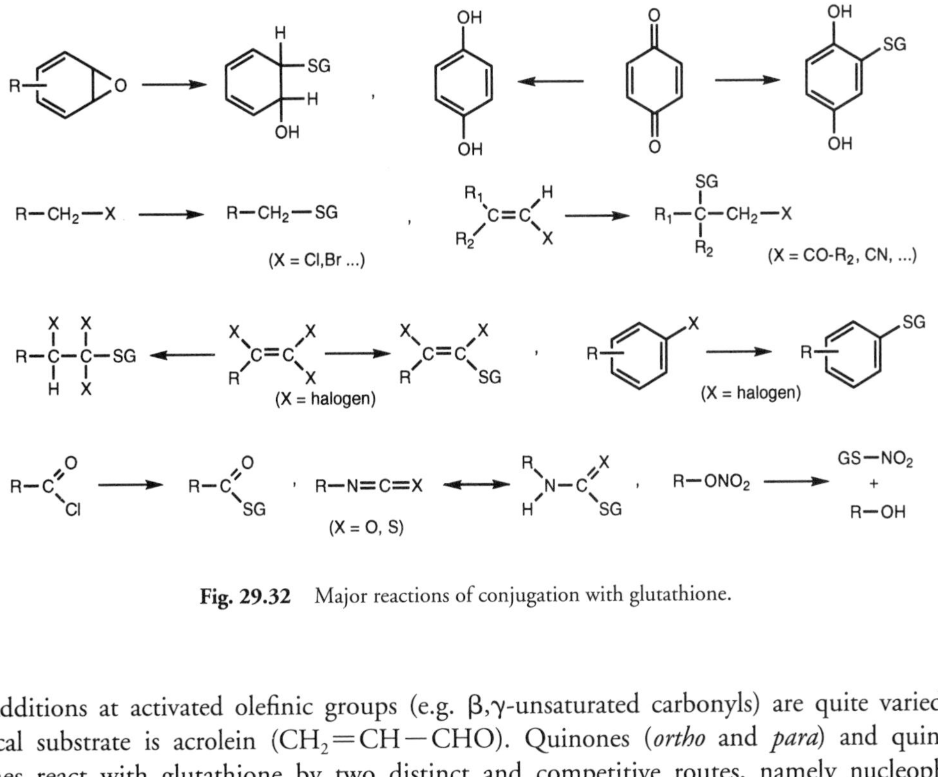

Fig. 29.32 Major reactions of conjugation with glutathione.

Additions at activated olefinic groups (e.g. β,γ-unsaturated carbonyls) are quite varied. A typical substrate is acrolein ($CH_2=CH-CHO$). Quinones (*ortho* and *para*) and quinone imines react with glutathione by two distinct and competitive routes, namely nucleophilic addition to form a conjugate, and reduction to the hydroquinone or the aminophenol. The conjugates produced by addition may undergo reoxidation to S-glutathionylquinones or S-glutathionylquinone imines of considerable reactivity.

Haloalkenes may react with GSH either by substitution or by addition. Formation of mercapturic acids occurs as for other glutathione conjugates, but in this case $S-C$ cleavage of the S-cysteinyl conjugates by the renal β-lyase yields thiols of significant toxicity since they rearrange to form highly reactive thioketenes ($XRC=C=S$) and/or thioacyl halides. With a good leaving group and adequate substituents, nucleophilic aromatic substitution reactions also occur at aromatic rings. A good example of the detoxication of acyl halides with glutathione is provided by phosgene ($O=CCl_2$), an extremely toxic metabolite of chloroform which is inactivated to the diglutathionyl conjugate $O=C(SG)_2$. The addition of glutathione to isocyanates and isothiocyanates is of significance owing to its reversible character. Substrates of the reaction are xenobiotics such as the well-known toxin methyl isocyanate, whose glutathione conjugate behaves as a transport form able to carbamoylate various macromolecules, enzymes and membranes structures.

Organic nitrate esters such as nitroglycerine are vasodilators whose action results from their reduction to nitric oxide (NO). Glutathione and other thiols play an important role in this activation, a thionitrate being formed in the first step. N-Reduction may then proceed by various routes having nitrite (NO_2^-) or S-nitrosoglutathione (GS-NO) as an intermediate.

H. Other reactions of conjugation

A number of other routes of xenobiotic conjugation have been reported, but their importance is restricted to a few exogenous substrates. While phosphorylation is of great significance in the processing of endogenous compounds and macromolecules, relatively few xenobiotics form phosphate esters. The enzymes involved are various phosphotransferases. Thus, a number of antiviral nucleoside analogues yield the mono-, di- and triphosphates *in vitro* and *in vivo*, e.g. zidovudine (AZT).

The reaction of hydrazines with endogenous carbonyls occurs nonenzymatically and involves a variety of carbonyl compounds, namely aldehydes (mainly acetaldehyde) and ketones (e.g. acetone, pyruvic acid, and α-ketoglutaric acid). The products thus formed are hydrazones which may be excreted as such or undergo further transformation.

IV. CONCLUSION

The knowledge of the pathways for drug biotransformation is an essential tool for the drug designer. It allows the prediction, at least in a qualitative manner, of the probable metabolites of a drug candidate. Thus it represents a valuable selection criterion when the decision has to be taken to develop one drug candidate rather than another. Of particular importance is the capacity to forecast the probability of appearance of toxic metabolites, as discussed in Chapter 30. The basic laws of drug metabolism can also be used in a prospective manner for the design of drugs with improved pharmacokinetic and biopharmaceutical properties. Such improved derivatives of a given active compound are called prodrugs and will be treated in Chapters 31 and 32.

REFERENCES

1. Richet, M.C. (1893) Note sur le rapport entre la toxicité et les propriétés physiques des corps. *Compt. Rend. Soc. Biol. (Paris)* **45**: 775–776.
2. Stenlake, J. B. (1979) *Foundations of Molecular Pharmacology.* vol. 2, *The Chemical Basis of Drug Action.* The Athlone Press-University of London, London.
3. Silverman, R. B. (1992) *The Organic Chemistry of Drug Design and Drug Action.* Academic Press, San Diego.
4. Testa, B. and Jenner, P. (1976) *Drug Metabolism. Chemical and Biochemical Aspects.* Marcel Dekker, New York.

5. Jenner, P. and Testa, B. (eds) (1980 and 1981). *Concepts in Drug Metabolism*. Parts A and B. Marcel Dekker, New York.
6. Testa, B. Drug metabolism. In Wolff, M. (ed) *Burger's Medicinal Chemistry*, 5th edn, vol. 1. Wiley, New York, in press.
7. Testa, B. (1995) *The Metabolism of Drugs and Other Xenobiotics – Biochemistry of Redox Reactions*. Academic Press, London.
8. Mulder, G. J. (ed.) (1990) *Conjugation Reactions in Drug Metabolism*. Taylor & Francis, London.
9. International Union of Biochemistry and Molecular Biology (1992) *Enzyme Nomenclature 1992*. Academic Press, San Diego.
10. Peters, R. A., Wakelin, R. W., Rivett, D. E. A. and Thomas, L. C. (1953) Fluoroacetate poisoning: comparison of synthetic fluorocitric acid with the enzymatically synthesized fluorotricarboxylic acid. *Nature* **171**: 1111–1112.

Chemical Aspects of Biotransformations Leading to Toxic Metabolites

ANDRÉ PICOT and ANNE-CHRISTINE MACHEREY

'La matière demeure et la forme se perd'
'The matter remains and the form is lost'
Ronsard

THE PRACTICE OF MEDICINAL CHEMISTRY
ISBN 0-12-744640-0

I. INTRODUCTION

Toxicity is the result of the more or less harmful action of chemicals on a living organism. Toxicology, the study of toxicity, is situated at the border of chemistry, biology and, in some cases, physics. Molecular toxicology tries to elucidate the mechanisms by which chemicals exert their toxic effects. Because many foreign chemicals enter the body in inert but unexcretable forms, biotransformations are an important aspect of the fate of xenobiotics.[1,2] In the case of drugs, metabolic conversions may be required for therapeutic effect ('prodrugs'). In other cases, metabolism results in a loss of the biological activity. Sometimes, biotransformations produce toxic metabolites. The last process is called toxication or bioactivation. It should be emphasized that the general principles of pharmacology embrace the occurrence of toxic events: although biotransformation processes are often referred to as detoxication, the metabolic products are, in a number of cases, more toxic than the parent compounds. For drugs, whether biotransformations lead to the formation of toxic metabolites or to variations in therapeutic effects depends on intrinsic factors (such as the genetic polymorphism of some metabolic pathways) and extrinsic factors (such as the dose, the route or the duration). The biochemical conversions are usually of an enzymatic nature and yield reactive intermediates which may be implicated in the toxicity as far as the final metabolites. The primary events which constitute the beginning of the toxic effect may result, after metabolism, from an inhibition of a specific (and in most cases enzymatic) cellular function, an alkylating attack or an oxidative stress.

With regard to the toxicity arising from metabolites ('indirect toxicity'), three cases may be distinguished[3,4] (Fig 30.1).

A. Biotransformation begins with the transient formation of a reactive intermediate, whose lifetime is long enough to allow an attack on cellular components. This occurs when a reactive intermediate (such as a radical or a carbenium ion) is formed and reacts rapidly

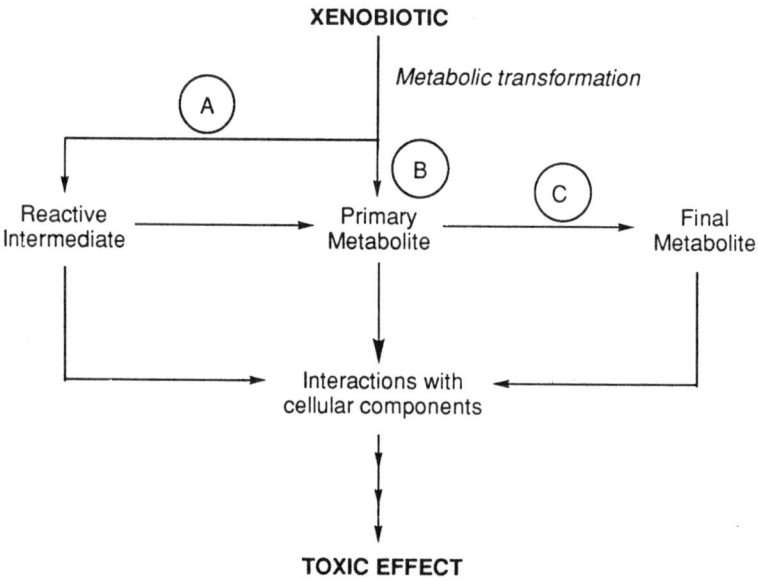

Fig. 30.1   Indirect toxicity.

with nucleophilic functions in cellular macromolecules (such as unsaturated lipids, proteins, nucleic acids), thus leading to their degradation and finally to cellular necrosis.

B.   The first step of the metabolic process yields a primary metabolite which can, in some cases, accumulate in the cell and reacts with cellular components before being transformed.

C.   The final metabolites, when in excess, may accumulate and react with cellular macromolecules.

Usually, metabolic conversions are divided into two major types of reactions. Phase I reactions, or functionalization reactions, involve the introduction of a polar functionality such as a hydroxyl group into the xenobiotic structure. During phase II reactions, this group is subsequently coupled (or conjugated) with an endogenous cofactor which contains a functional group that is usually ionized at physiological pH. This ionic functional group facilitates active excretion into the urinary and/or hepatobiliary system.

Because bioactivation is mainly an activation of xenobiotics to electrophilic forms which are entities capable of reacting irreversibly with tissue nucleophiles, biotransformations leading to toxic metabolites are in most cases phase I reactions. But phase II reactions may also give rise to toxic phenomena, e.g. when conjugation produces a toxic metabolite or when it is responsible for a specific target organ toxicity by acting as a delivery form to particular sites in the body where it is hydrolysed and exerts a localized effect. Also, the final toxic metabolite may be formed by combinations of several phase I and phase II reactions.

II.   REACTIONS INVOLVED IN THE BIOACTIVATION PROCESS

During the biotransformations affecting xenobiotics, four major kinds of chemical reactions may occur: oxidations (by far the most important), reductions, substitutions and eliminations. As phase I and II reactions are parts of this classification, these four classes of reactions can give rise to toxic metabolites.

A.   Oxidation

Several enzymatic systems are involved during the oxidative transformations of xenobiotics. Whether substances are acted upon by one enzyme rather than another depends not only on its specific function but also on the electromolecular environment. The most important is the microsomal drug metabolizing system known as cytochrome P450 monooxygenase, which is localized mainly in the liver and which is involved in virtually all biological oxidations of xenobiotics. Those include *C*-, *N*- and *S*-oxidations, *N*-, *O*- and *S*-dealkylation, deaminations and certain dehalogenations. Under anaerobic conditions it can also catalyse reductive reactions. The cytochrome P450 monooxygenase system is a multienzymatic complex constituted by the cytochrome P450 haemoprotein, the flavoprotein enzyme NADPH cytochrome P450 reductase, and the unsaturated phospholipid phosphatidylcholine. The catalytic mechanism of cytochrome P450 involves a formal $(FeO)^{3+}$ complex formed by the elimination of H_2O from the iron site after two electrons have been added (Fig. 30.2).

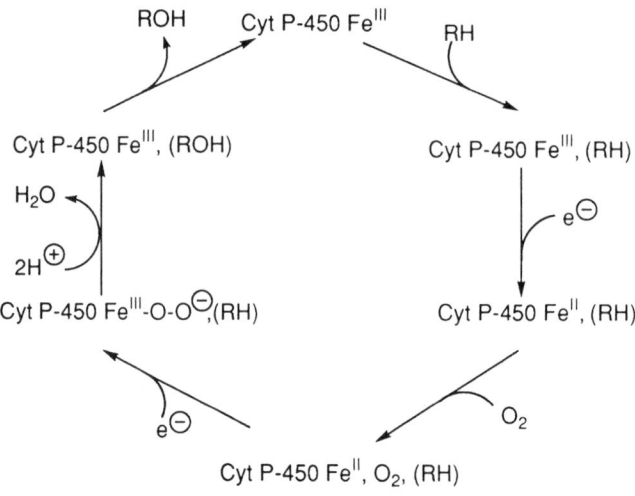

Fig. 30.2   Catalytic cycle of cytochrome P450 monooxygenase.

Another oxidative enzyme is the FAD-containing monooxygenase, which is capable of oxidizing nucleophilic nitrogen, sulfur and organophosphorus compounds. The flavoprotein binds NADPH, oxygen and then the substrate. The oxidized metabolite is released, followed by NADPH. Alcohol dehydrogenase and aldehyde dehydrogenase catalyse the oxidation of a variety of alcohols and aldehydes into aldehydes and acids in the liver. Xanthine oxidase oxidizes several purine derivatives such as theophylline. The monoamine oxidase (MAO) and diamine oxidase convert amines into alkyl or aryl aldehydes by means of the abstraction of two hydrogen atoms, one from the nitrogen and the other from the α carbon, and a subsequent hydrolysis. Peroxidases are oxidative enzymes which couple the reduction of hydrogen peroxide and lipid hydroperoxides to the oxidation of other substrates. This co-oxidation is responsible for the production of reactive electrophiles from aromatic amines (e.g. the highly carcinogenic benzidine), phenols, hydroquinone and polycyclic aromatic hydrocarbons.

The oxidation reactions can be described in terms of a rather common chemistry that involves the abstraction of either a hydrogen atom or a nonbonded (or π) electron by the iron-oxo porphyrin complex (Fig. 30.3). This one-electron oxidation yields transient radicals (Fig. 30.4) which are transformed into more stable forms. They can incorporate an oxygen atom by a radical recombination with dioxygen. This yields an oxidized derivative that may be sometimes more toxic than the parent compound or susceptible to further metabolic conversions. Free

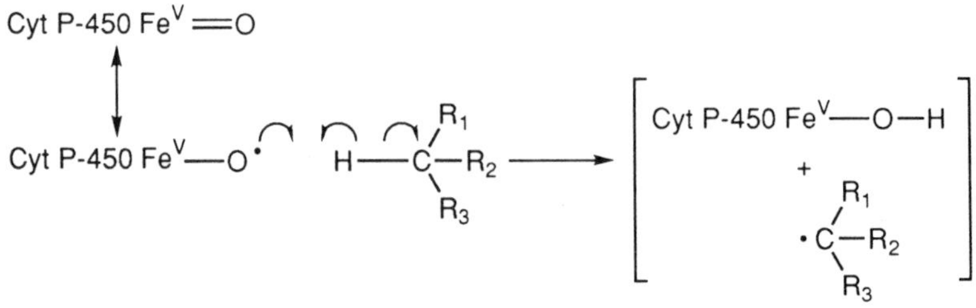

Fig. 30.3   Cytochrome P450 oxidation process.

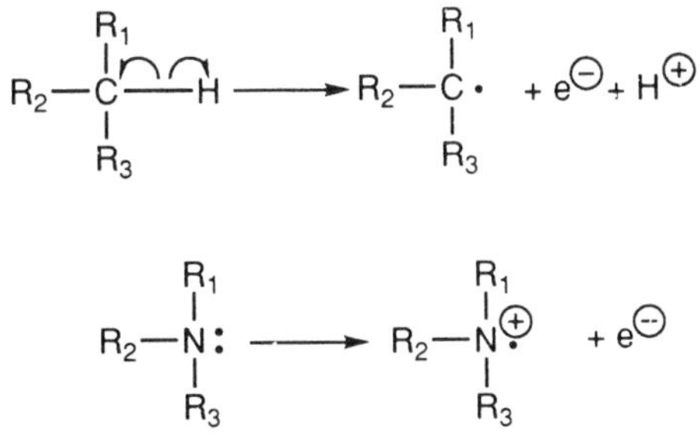

$$R_2-\overset{\overset{\displaystyle R_1}{|}}{\underset{\underset{\displaystyle R_3}{|}}{C}}-H \longrightarrow R_2-\overset{\overset{\displaystyle R_1}{|}}{\underset{\underset{\displaystyle R_3}{|}}{C}}\cdot \quad + e^{\ominus} + H^{\oplus}$$

$$R_2-\overset{\overset{\displaystyle R_1}{|}}{\underset{\underset{\displaystyle R_3}{|}}{N}}: \longrightarrow R_2-\overset{\overset{\displaystyle R_1}{|}}{\underset{\underset{\displaystyle R_3}{|}}{N}}^{\oplus}\cdot \quad + e^{\ominus}$$

Fig. 30.4 One-electron oxidation.

radicals may also bind to the site of their formation, thus leading to inhibition or inactivation of the enzyme. When the radical is not efficiently controlled by the iron, it may leave the active site. The subsequent 'free' radical is able to produce damage to unsaturated fatty acids, thus leading to lipid peroxidation and destruction of the cellular structure. Another mode of radical stabilization is a second one-electron oxidation, which consists of the loss of another electron. The fate of free radicals is now extensively studied because of their great capacities for forming covalent bonds with cellular macromolecules.[5-7]

1. C−H bond oxidations

These oxidations, which are usually catalysed by cytochrome P450 monooxygenases, produce hydroxylated derivatives.[8] When the C−H bond is located in the α position to a heteroatom (such as O, S, N, halogen), the α-hydroxylated derivative obtained is often unstable and may be further oxidized or cleaved (Fig. 30.5).

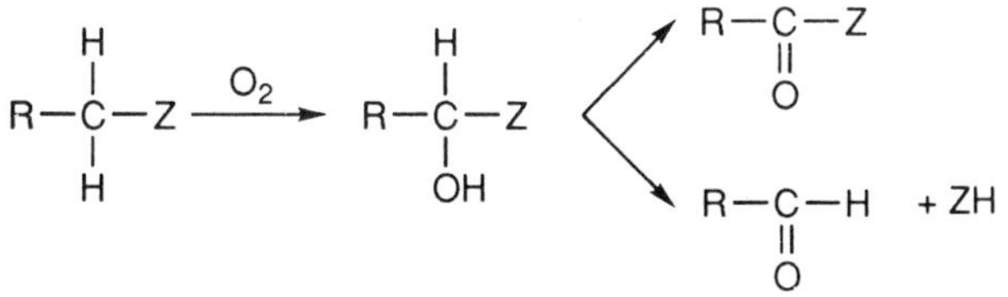

$$R-\overset{\overset{\displaystyle H}{|}}{\underset{\underset{\displaystyle H}{|}}{C}}-Z \xrightarrow{O_2} R-\overset{\overset{\displaystyle H}{|}}{\underset{\underset{\displaystyle OH}{|}}{C}}-Z \left\langle \begin{array}{l} R-\overset{\overset{\displaystyle}{C}}{\underset{\underset{\displaystyle O}{\parallel}}{}}-Z \\[2em] R-\overset{\overset{\displaystyle}{C}}{\underset{\underset{\displaystyle O}{\parallel}}{}}-H \quad + ZH \end{array} \right.$$

Fig. 30.5 C−H bond oxidation in the α-position to a heteroatom.

The antibiotic chloramphenicol is oxidized by cytochrome P450 monooxygenase to chloramphenicol oxamyl chloride formed by the oxidative dechlorination of the dichloromethyl moiety of chloramphenicol.[9] The reactive metabolite binds to the ε-amino group of a lysine residue in the cytochrome P450 (Fig. 30.6). This yields an adduct that blocks the electron transport from NADPH cytochrome P450 reductase.[10] This type of mechanism is termed a suicide-substrate mechanism.

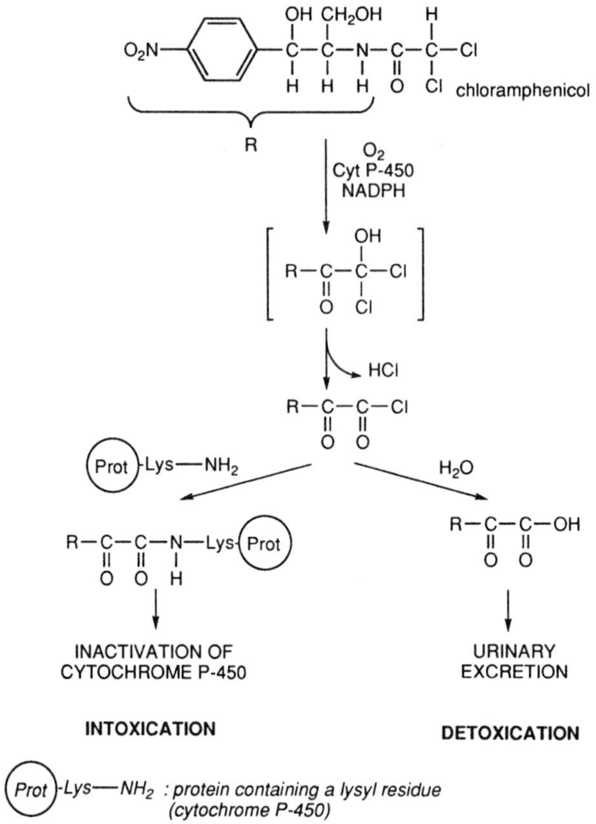

Fig. 30.6   Metabolic activation of chloramphenicol.

In the case of chloroform, the unstable trichloromethanol loses hydrochloric acid and forms phosgene, which is very reactive (Fig. 30.7).

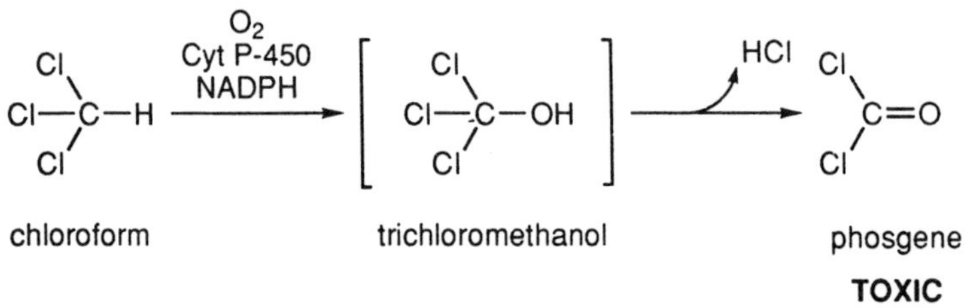

Fig. 30.7   Oxidation of chloroform.

Tertiary amines containing at least one hydrogen on the α carbon may either be *N*-oxidized (leading to an *N*-oxide in the case of tertiary amines), or *C*-oxidized, thus leading to a carbinolamine. The latter, often being unstable, usually splits into a secondary amine and a aldehyde moiety (Fig. 30.8).

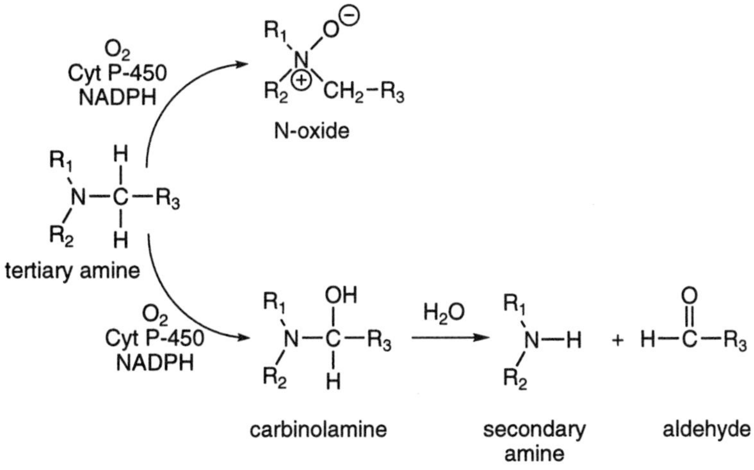

Fig. 30.8 Oxidation of a tertiary amine.

During the oxidation of nitrosamines, the hydroxylated derivative formed cleaves spontaneously into highly reactive metabolites capable of alkylating nucleophilic sites in the cellular components.

2. Unsaturated bond oxidations

Double bonds are oxidized by cytochrome P450 monooxygenases into epoxides, which are generally very reactive. Epoxides are considered responsible for the toxicity of the unsaturated compounds.

The hepatocarcinogenicity of aflatoxin B_1 (AFB$_1$) is known to be due to the epoxide (AFB$_1$-oxide) formed, which binds directly with the N-7 atom of a guanine molecule in DNA (Fig. 30.9).

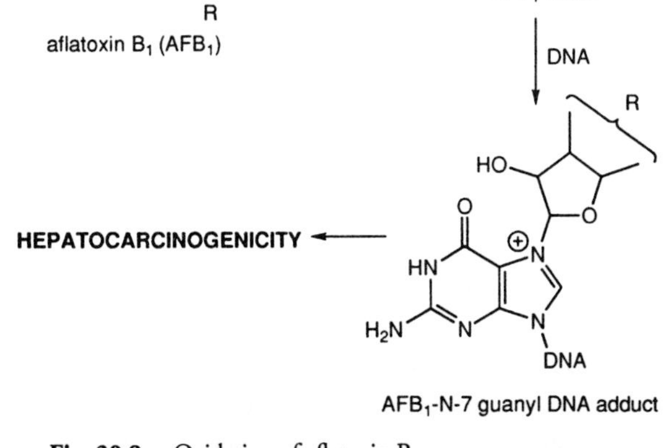

Fig. 30.9 Oxidation of aflatoxin B_1.

Aromatic chemicals are metabolized into unstable arene-oxides, which, as epoxides, are comparable to potentially equivalent electrophilic carbocations. These metabolites react easily with thiol groups derived from proteins, leading, for example, to hepatotoxicity. Bromobenzene (Fig. 30.10) is oxidized into a 3-4 epoxide, which does not exhibit mutagenic or carcinogenic activity but reacts nonenzymatically with liver proteins and produces hepatic necrosis.

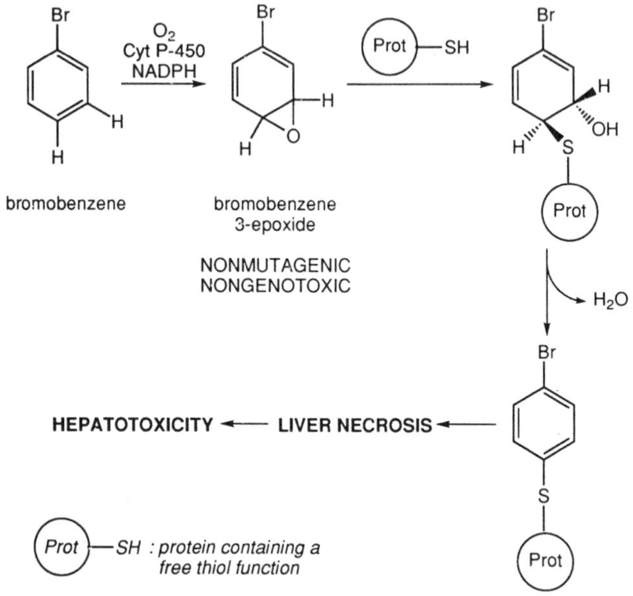

Fig. 30.10 Metabolism of bromobenzene.

3. N-oxidations

Tertiary amines are transformed into N-oxides (generally less toxic), but primary and secondary amines are oxidized into hydroxylated derivatives (hydroxylamines). This oxidation is responsible for the hepatotoxicity of 2-acetylaminofluorene (Fig. 30.11).

Nitrenium ions may occur during bioactivation of aromatic amines and amides, which are usually N-oxidized into N-hydroxylated derivatives. By direct elimination or esterification followed by elimination, the latter may be transformed into highly reactive nitrenium ions. Nitrenium ions are of great importance because of the equilibrium with their mesomeric carbocationic forms and the subsequent reactivity with cellular nucleophilic macromolecules (nucleic acids, etc.).

4. Heteroatom oxidations

Heteroatoms such as nitrogen or sulfur are oxidized on their free peripheral electrons (Fig. 30.12) as described for thiophene.[11] Halogenated aromatic compounds may also be oxidized by cytochrome P450 monooxygenases, yielding hypervalent halogenated compounds.

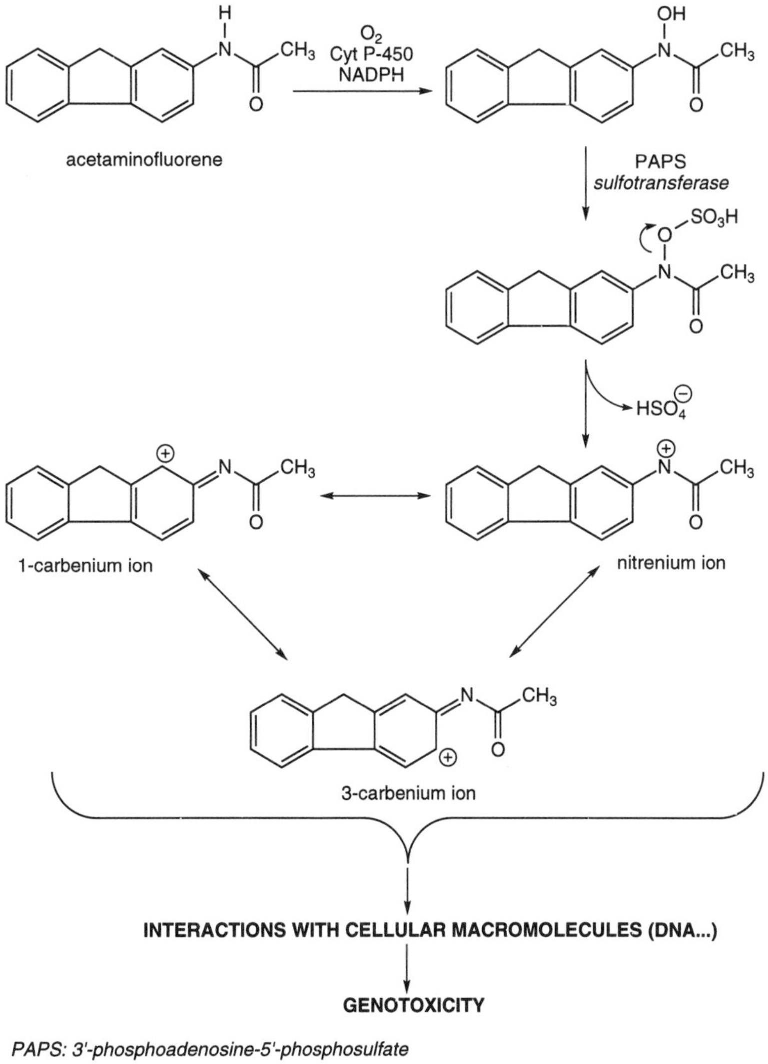

Fig. 30-11 *N*-oxidation of acetylaminofluorene.

B. Oxidative stress

Oxidative stress has been defined as a disturbance in the pro-oxidant–antioxidant balance in favour of pro-oxidant state resulting from alterations in the redox state of the cell. The stepwise reduction of oxygen into superoxide anion, hydrogen peroxide, hydroxyl radical and finally water, which accounts for about 5% of the normal oxygen reduction (versus 95% by means of the mitochondrial electron-transport chain), may be increased by the redox cycling of some xenobiotics such as quinones or nitro-aromatic derivatives. These compounds are susceptible to one-electron reduction which yields radical structures which may be back-oxidized to the parent compound. During this reoxidation, oxygen is reduced into superoxide anion. The oxygen reduction products are highly reactive entities that attack all the cellular components, especially

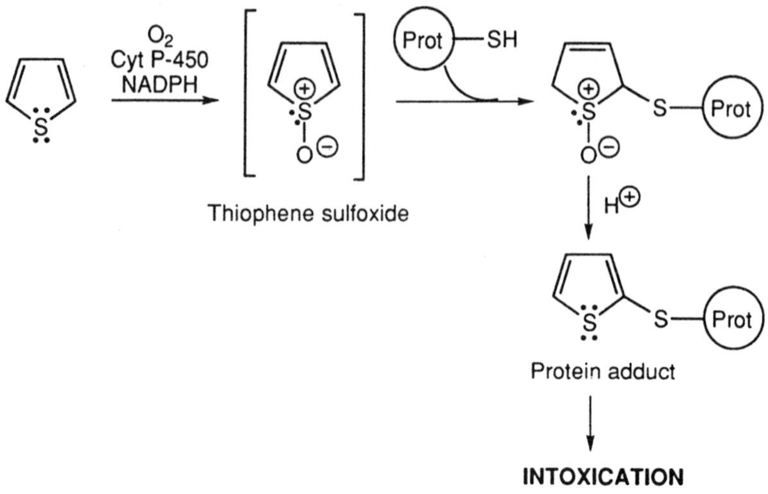

Fig. 30.12   Oxidation of thiophene.

when their normal degradation systems (superoxide dismutase, glutathione peroxidase, catalase) are overburdened. The polyunsaturated lipids are especially sensitive to these attacks because they are susceptible to a membrane-degrading peroxidation.

C.   Reduction

Reductive biotransformations of several compounds such as polyhalogenated, keto, nitro and azo derivatives are catalysed by a variety of enzymes which differ according to the substrates and the species. The liver cytochrome P450-dependent drug-metabolizing system is capable of reducing N-oxide, nitro and azo bonds, whereas the cytosolic nitrobenzene reductase activity is mainly due to cytochrome P450 reductase, which transforms nitrobenzene into its hydroxylamino derivative. NADPH cytochrome c reductase is also able to catalyse the reduction of nitro compounds. These metabolic conversions may also be brought about by gastrointestinal anaerobic bacteria.

Reductive processes that occur during the metabolism of xenobiotics involve either one-electron reduction or a two-electron transfer. Ionic reduction using a hydride occurs *in vivo* during the reduction catalysed by NADH or NADPH enzyme, whereas one-electron reduction releases a radical structure which may contribute to the toxic effect. Figure 30.13 illustrates the biotransformations affecting the anthracycline antitumour drug daunomycin.[12]

1.   Polyhalogenated compound reduction

Some polyhalogenated compounds such as CCl_4, $BrCCl_3$, halothane ($CF_3-CHBrCl$), when in the presence of the reduced form of cytochrome P450, may undergo a reductolysis[13] (Fig. 30.14) which leads to a radical that may be transformed by different pathways. The radical formed may add directly on the unsaturated lipid bonds, or initiate an unsaturated lipid

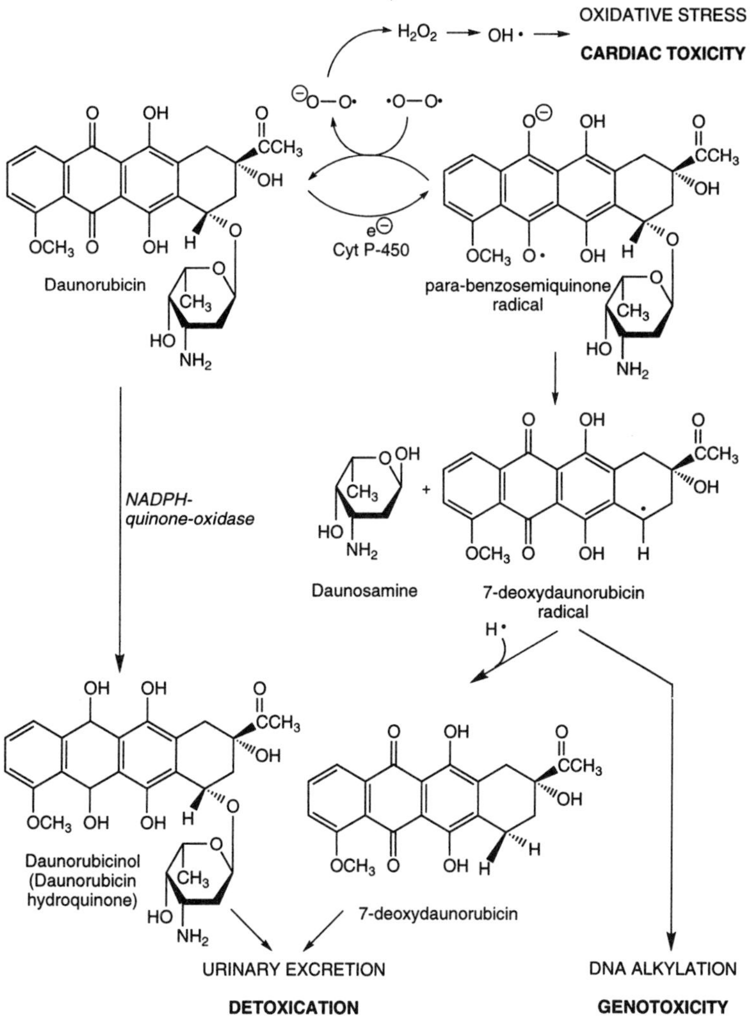

Fig. 30.13   Biotransformations of daunorubicin.

peroxidation, or undergo another one-electron reduction. The last reaction yields a carbene that can form a carbenic complex with the iron of the reductive form of cytochrome P450. Polyhalogenated compound reductions give rise to several reactive intermediates: radicals, carbenes and peroxides, whose participation in the toxic effect varies greatly.

2.   Nitro compound reduction

The different steps of the biotransformations that produce a primary amine from an aromatic nitro compound involve the nitro radical-anion, the nitroso derivative, the nitroxyl radical, the hydroxylamine and then the primary amine (Fig. 30.15). Each of these different intermediates may contribute to the toxicity. Hydroxylamines are often responsible for methaemoglobinaemia, whereas mutagenic and carcinogenic activity may be due to the combination of nitro radical-anion, nitroso derivatives or esterified hydroxylamines (such as sulfate derivatives) with cellular macromolecules.

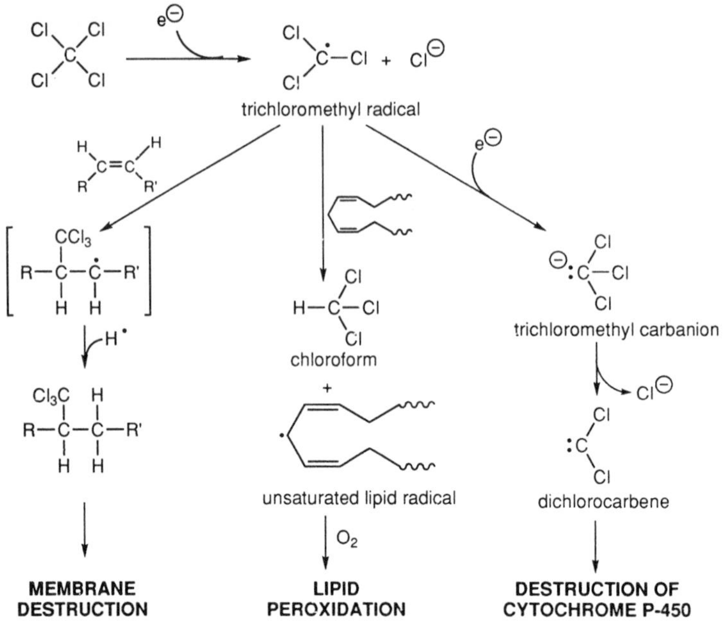

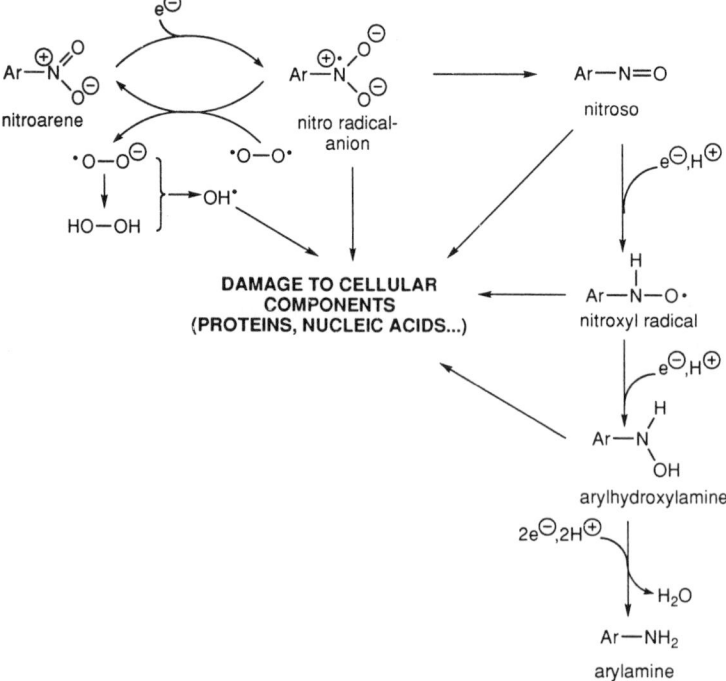

Fig. 30.14   Reduction of polyhalogenated compounds.

Fig. 30.15   Reductive biotransformation of nitro arene compounds.

Carcinogenicity may also be the result of the oxidative stress subsequent to the formation of oxygen-reduction products (superoxide anion, hydrogen peroxide, hydroxyl radical) during the redox cycling of the nitro radical-anion, which restores the parent nitro compound.

3.   Azo compound reduction

Azo compounds are susceptible to reduction, first to hydrazo intermediates which are reductively cleaved into the appropriate amines. It has been proposed that the first step, as with nitro compounds, is the formation of an azo-anion radical.

D.   Substitutions: hydrolysis and conjugation

Among substitution reactions, ester and amide hydrolyses are of common occurrence, and often operate during detoxication processes. In addition to specific enzymes, the stomach and the kidney are areas where acid-catalysed hydrolyses may occur, whereas base-catalysed reactions may be assisted by the alkaline pH of the intestine.

Phase II, or conjugation reactions are also substitution reactions, which proceed by means of an endogenous and generally activated nucleophile. In mammals, six major conjugation reactions of xenobiotics exist and are mediated by transferase enzymes. The specificity for the endogenous agent is high, but the specificity for the xenobiotic is broader. To a great extent, conjugation produces excretable and nontoxic metabolites and thus is referred to as detoxication, but exceptions exist in each class of conjugation reaction.

1.   Glucuronic acid conjugation

This substitution involves the transfer of a glucuronic acid from uridine diphosphate glucuronic acid (UDPGA) to a functional group in the xenobiotic substrate. The group may be a hydroxyl, carboxylic acid, amino or sulfur function. Glucuronides are never directly implicated in toxicity but are sometimes responsible for target-organ toxicity. Aromatic amines may be converted in the liver into N-glucuronides, which are excreted in the urine and broken down in the bladder (because of the acidic pH) to liberate the proximate hydroxylamine carcinogen.

2.   Sulfation

Sulfate conjugation gives a polar and ionized conjugate by means of the esterification of a hydroxyl group with sulfate ion (in the form of 3'-phosphoadenosine-5'-phosphosulfate or PAPS). The reaction is catalysed by a hydrosoluble sulfotransferase. Sulfation sometimes gives rise to reactive intermediates that may undergo further reactions to yield electrophilic metabolites. In the case of 2-acetylaminofluorene, the O—sulfate moiety is a facile leaving group, and this cleavage produces nitrenium ions which act as alkylating agents for DNA (Fig. 30.11).

3.   Acetylation

Acetylation is a very common metabolic reaction which occurs with amino, hydroxyl or sulfhydryl groups. The acetyl group is transferred from acetyl-coenzyme A and the reaction is catalysed by acetyltransferases. An important aspect of this kind of substitution is the genetic polymorphism of one acetyltransferase in humans, who are divided into fast and slow acetylators. In a few cases, the conjugates are further metabolized to toxic compounds, as is seen with isoniazid. Some evidence exists that acetylation of the antitubercular isoniazid leads to enhanced hepatotoxicity of the drug.[14] Acetylation followed by hydrolysis and cytochrome P450-dependent oxidation yields free acetyl radicals[15] or acylium cations which may acetylate the nucleophilic macromolecule functions (Fig. 30.16).

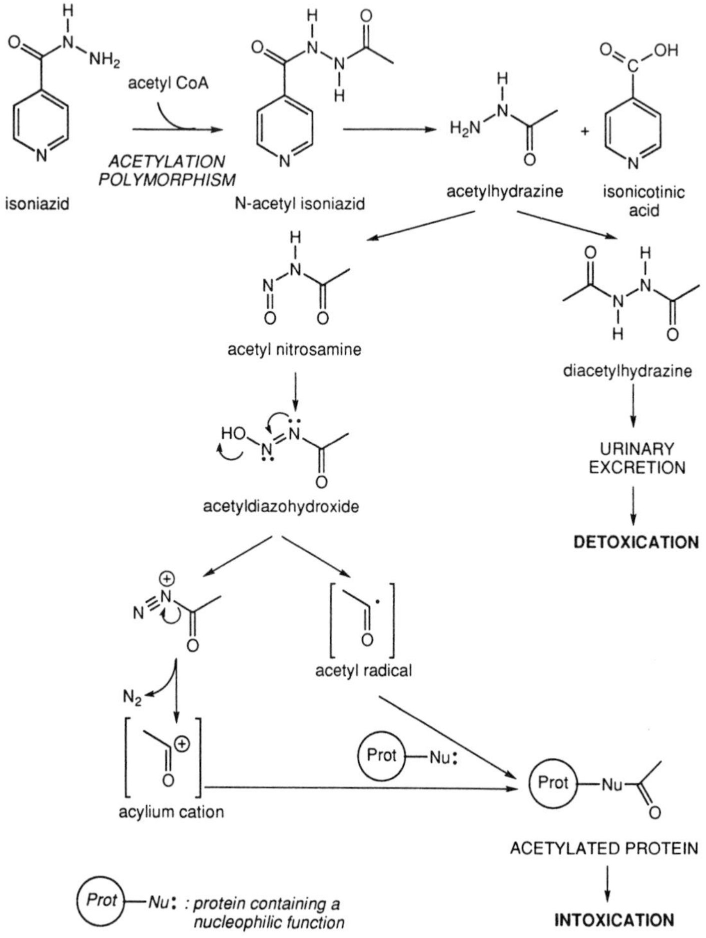

Fig. 30.16 Bioactivation of isoniazid.

4.   Glutathione conjugation

Substitution reactions of xenobiotics with glutathione are the most important and contribute efficiently to detoxication. Nevertheless, in some cases such as vicinal dihalogenated compounds, glutathione conjugation produces monosubstituted derivatives which may cycle into a highly electrophilic sulfonium ion (Fig. 30.17).

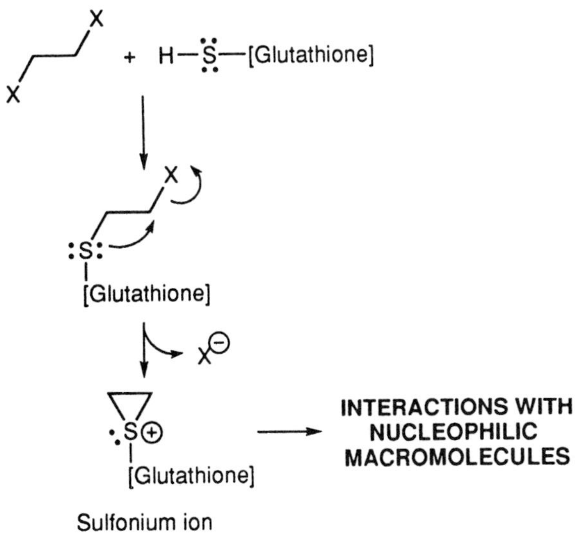

Fig. 30.17   Bioactivation to sulfonium ion.

5.   Methylation

Methylation is rarely of quantitative importance in the metabolization of xenobiotics. The methyl group is transferred from the nucleotide S-adenosyl-L-methionine (SAM) by means of a methyl transferase. The functional groups include primary, secondary and tertiary amines, pyridines, phenols, catechols, thiophenols, etc. The azaheterocycle pyridine is metabolized to the N-methylpyridinium ion, which is more toxic than pyridine itself[16] (Fig. 30.18). The binding properties of the ionized metabolite are disturbed by the loss of its hydrophobic feature, resulting from the polarity inversion.

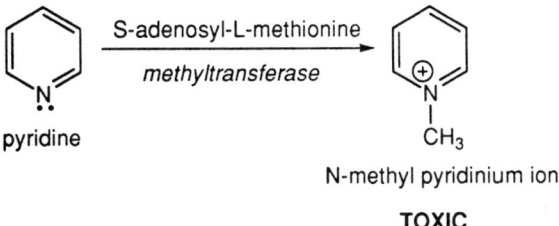

pyridine

N-methyl pyridinium ion

TOXIC

Fig. 30.18   Bioactivation of pyridine.

E.   Eliminations

Eliminations of hydrohalide or halogen occur sometimes during the metabolism of halogenated xenobiotics and lead to an alkene. The double bond may be oxidized into an epoxide by means of oxidative enzyme systems as discussed earlier. Dehydrogenation, dehydrochloration and dechloration are (with oxidation) the different metabolic pathways of the γ-isomer of the insecticide hexachlorocyclohexane (lindane).

F.   Further biotransformations leading to the ultimate toxicant

Other reactions must be mentioned besides the major reactions described above. These reactions may be responsible for the transformation of a toxic metabolite into the ultimate toxicant.[17] Rearrangements and cyclizations are examples of reactions involved in these processes. In the case of the solvent hexane (Fig. 30.19), the toxic metabolite 2,5-hexanedione is formed by four successive oxidations of the molecule.[3,18] The condensation of the γ-diketone with the lysyl amino group of a neurofilament protein is followed by cyclization according to a Paal–Knorr-type reaction. This is the initial process that explains hexane-induced neurotoxicity.[3,19] A further auto-oxidation of the N-pyrrolyl derivatives leads to the cross-linking of the axonal intermediate filament proteins and the subsequent occurrence of peripheral neurotoxicity.

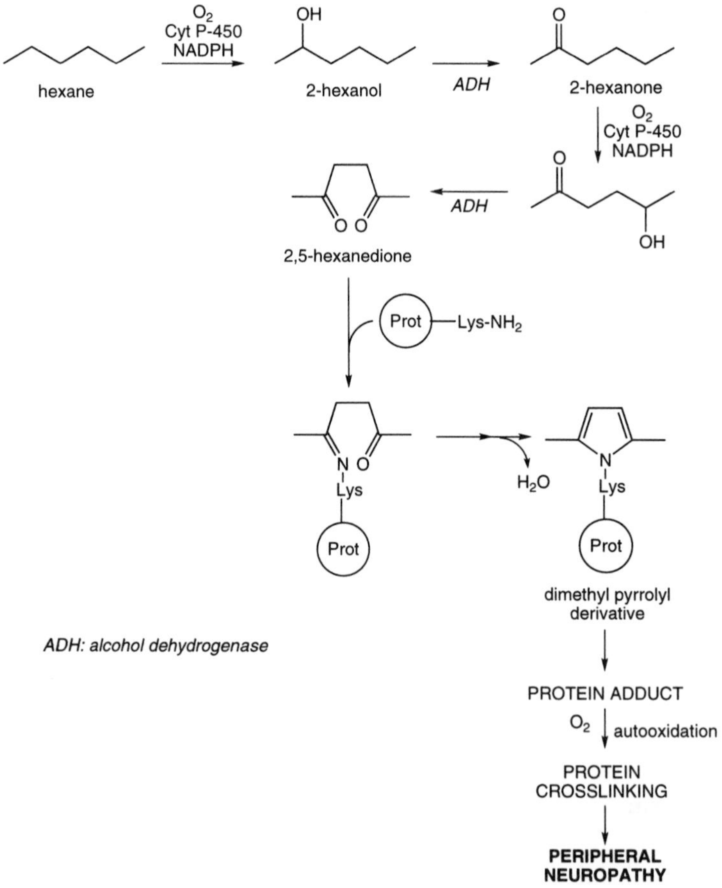

Fig. 30.19   Bioactivation of hexane.

III. EXAMPLES OF METABOLIC CONVERSIONS LEADING TO TOXIC METABOLITES

The formation of toxic metabolites and/or intermediates during the metabolization of drugs may occur by a considerable variety of pathways which are mediated by several enzyme systems. The following five examples do not represent an exhaustive list of the bioactivation processes, but are samples of original, significant and/or well-known drugs whose biotransformations lead to toxic compounds by the four main types of reactions discussed above. Two of them (acetaminophen, tienilic acid) are cytochrome P450 mediated oxidations. Halothane acts through both oxidative and reductive biotransformations. Valproic acid is toxic through its elimination product, and the toxicity (which, in the case of antitumour drugs, is also the expected effect) of mechlorethamine results from intramolecular substitution.

A. Acetaminophen

The analgesic acetaminophen (4-hydroxyacetanilide, paracetamol) exhibits hepatotoxicity when administered in very high doses (approximately 250 mg kg^{-1}).[20] The metabolite responsible is

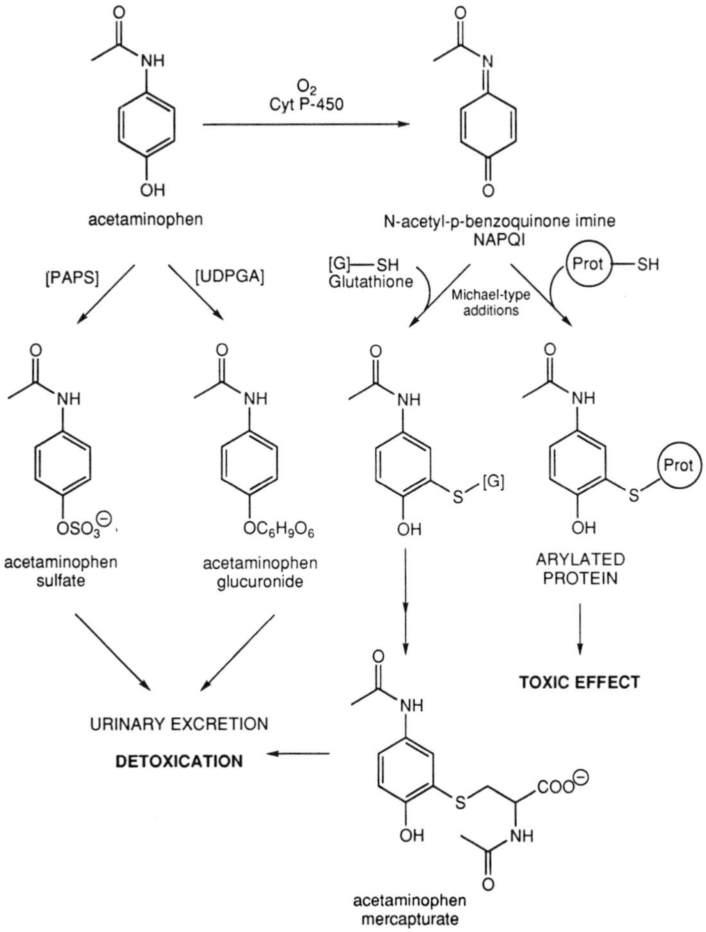

Fig. 30.20 Biotransformation pathway of acetaminophen.

known to be the *N*-acetyl-*p*-benzoquinone imine (NAPQI) (Fig. 30.20). The formation of NAPQI may proceed via the cytochrome P450 monooxygenase, but also via peroxidases such as prostaglandin hydroperoxidase.

The most commonly described mechanism proposes that metabolic activation occurs through *N*-oxidation of acetaminophen to *N*-hydroxyacetaminophen, followed by dehydratation to NAPQI (Fig. 30.21).[21]

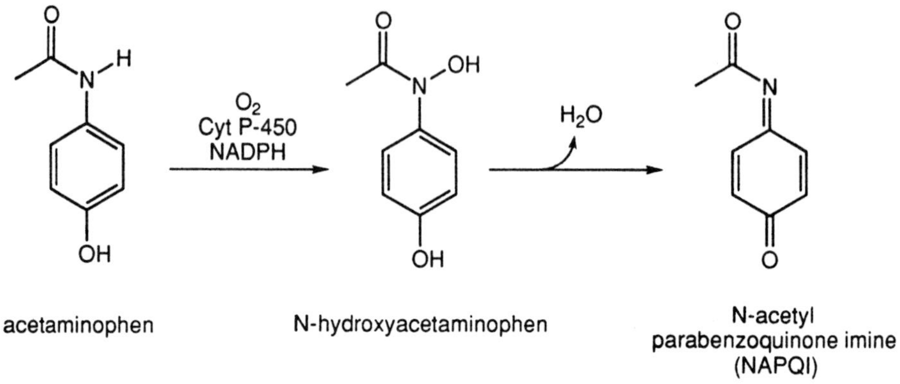

acetaminophen   N-hydroxyacetaminophen   N-acetyl
                                                                          parabenzoquinone imine
                                                                          (NAPQI)

Fig. 30.21   Oxidation of acetaminophen according to the '*N*-hydroxyacetaminophen pathway'.

However, it seems that *N*-hydroxyacetaminophen is not a major intermediate in the oxidation of acetaminophen. The formation of *N*-acetyl-*p*-benzoquinone imine probably proceeds by two successive one-electron oxidations[22] (Fig. 30.22). During the first step, a one-electron oxidation yields a phenoxy radical (Ar-O·).[23] The presence of the radical was supported by fast flow ESR spectroscopy in the presence of horseradish peroxidase. In the second one-electron oxidation, the phenoxy radical is oxidized to NAPQI. As described in Fig. 30.20, the highly electrophilic NAPQI may easily react with glutathione or protein thiol groups according to a Michael-type addition. The attack on liver protein thiol groups and the subsequent adduct formation is frequently mentioned in the mechanism of acetaminophen hepatotoxicity.

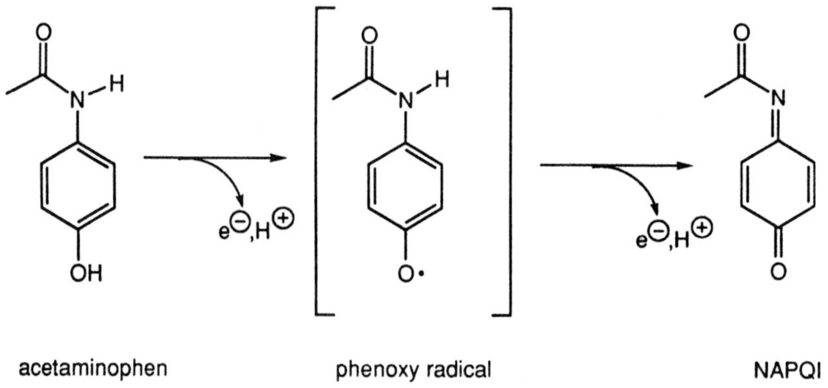

acetaminophen   phenoxy radical   NAPQI

Fig. 30.22   Oxidation of acetaminophen by means of the phenoxy radical.

Another hypothesis for the mechanism of toxicity is supported by the oxidative potency of NAPQI, but still suffers from lack of evidence.[24] NAPQI is a good oxidant for thiol functions of cellular components and pyridine nucleotides. Moreover, it may undergo a redox cycling with formation of superoxide anion by means of an oxygen one-electron reduction (Fig. 30.23). The stepwise reduction of oxygen produces hydrogen peroxide and finally a hydroxyl radical, which is a strong oxidant implicated in cellular oxidative stress. This oxidative stress causes a glutathione depletion, a disruption of the cellular calcium regulation, and modifications of cellular proteins, thus leading to cell death.

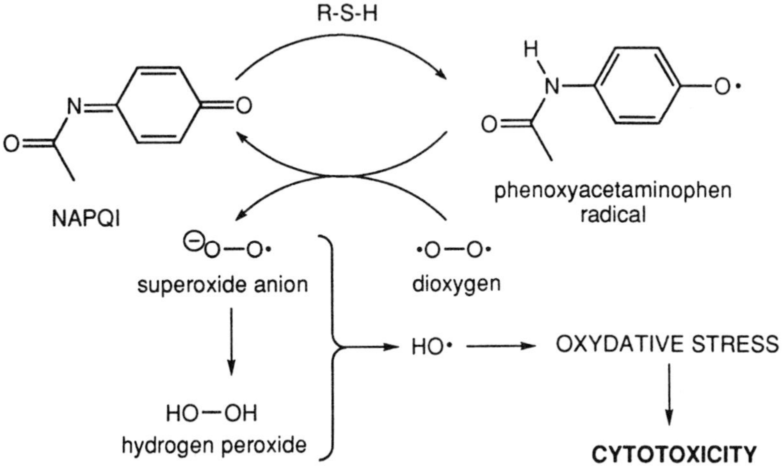

Fig. 30.23   Redox cycling of *N*-acetylparabenzoquinone imine.

It therefore, appears that both covalent (e.g. alkylation) and noncovalent (e.g. oxidative stress) interactions play major roles in the pathogenesis of acute lethal cell injury caused by NAPQI.[25] At present, it is not possible to identify which of these two interactions is the critical event in initiating acetaminophen hepatotoxicity.

B.   Tienilic acid

Tienilic acid is a uricosuric diuretic drug that may cause immunoallergic hepatitis in 1 in 10 000 patients, a side-effect that resulted in its withdrawal from circulation. The immunoallergic hepatitis was associated with the appearance of circulating anti-reticulum antibodies called anti-LKM$_2$ antibodies which are directed towards a liver endoplasmic reticulum protein.[26] From these observations, the mechanism of the immunotoxicity associated with the prolonged use of tienilic acid was elucidated by the Mansuy team.[27,28]

Tienilic acid is oxidized in the liver by the cytochrome P450 monooxygenase to 5-hydroxytienilic acid, which is the major urinary metabolite (about 50% in humans). This oxidation occurs through an electrophilic intermediate capable of alkylating the cytochrome P450. This suicide-substrate inactivation is also observed with many xenobiotics such as alkenes with terminal unsaturation, alkynes, strained cycloalkylamines, 4-alkyldihydropyridines, benzodioxoles and some tertiary amines. The irreversible binding of the compound with cytochrome P450 leads to the appearance of antibodies against the modified protein and the subsequent destruction of hepatocytes.

In humans, the bioactivation of tienilic acid as its reactive intermediate depends on cytochrome P450 2C9. This isoform is one of the major forms of cytochrome P450 in the human liver. It has been recently demonstrated that in the presence of cytochrome P450 thiophene is oxidized *in vivo* to yield thiophene sulfoxide (Fig. 30.12). This unusual function is a very electrophilic species capable of reacting with thiol group nucleophiles such as glutathione (detoxication) or proteins. This interaction with free proteins that contain thiol groups may give rise to an adduct and the potential associated toxicity.

In the case of tienilic acid, a sulfoxide is probably formed,[29] and this electrophile would be especially strong because of the mesomeric effect caused by the keto function. Addition of water to the sulfoxide, according to the Michael reaction, may occur at the activated position on the thiophene ring, thus yielding a 5-hydroxydihydrothiophene sulfoxide, which, after dehydration, should give 5-hydroxytienilic acid. Similarly, an amino acid nucleophilic function of the active site of cytochrome P450 monooxygenase apoprotein may react with the same electrophilic centre, thus giving rise to an adduct between the activated tienilic acid and cytochrome P450 2C9.

The inactivation of cytochrome P450 2C9 by covalent binding with the active metabolite of tienilic acid seems correlated with the appearance of anti-LKM$_2$ antibodies in patients showing an immunoallergic hepatitis (Fig. 30.24).

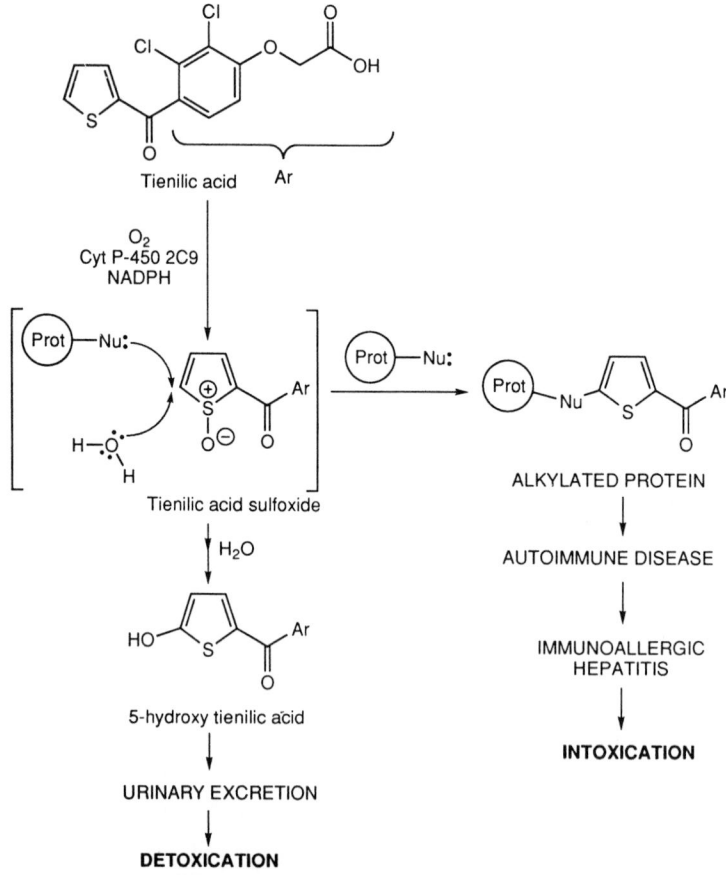

Fig. 30.24   Tienilic acid biotransformation to tienilic acid sulfoxide.

C. Halothane

Halothane is a widely used anaesthetic that occasionaly results in severe hepatitis. About 60–80% of the dose is eliminated in unmetabolized form during the 24 hours following administration to patients; 15% is metabolized in the presence of cytochrome P450 monooxygenase according to the two main pathways[8] depicted in Fig. 30.25.

The major biotransformation pathway involves an oxidative step with introduction of an oxygen atom and the subsequent formation of a halohydrin. The unstable halohydrin loses hydrobromic acid to yield trifluoroacetyl chloride, which in turn is hydrolysed to trifluoroacetic acid. This final metabolite is found in the urine.[30]

In conditions of low levels of oxygen, a reductive pathway (10%) is enhanced and yields a free-radical intermediate characterized as the 1-chloro-2,2,2-trifluoroethyl radical. Another one-electron reduction produces the 1-chloro-2,2,2-trifluoroethyl carbanion, which may undergo

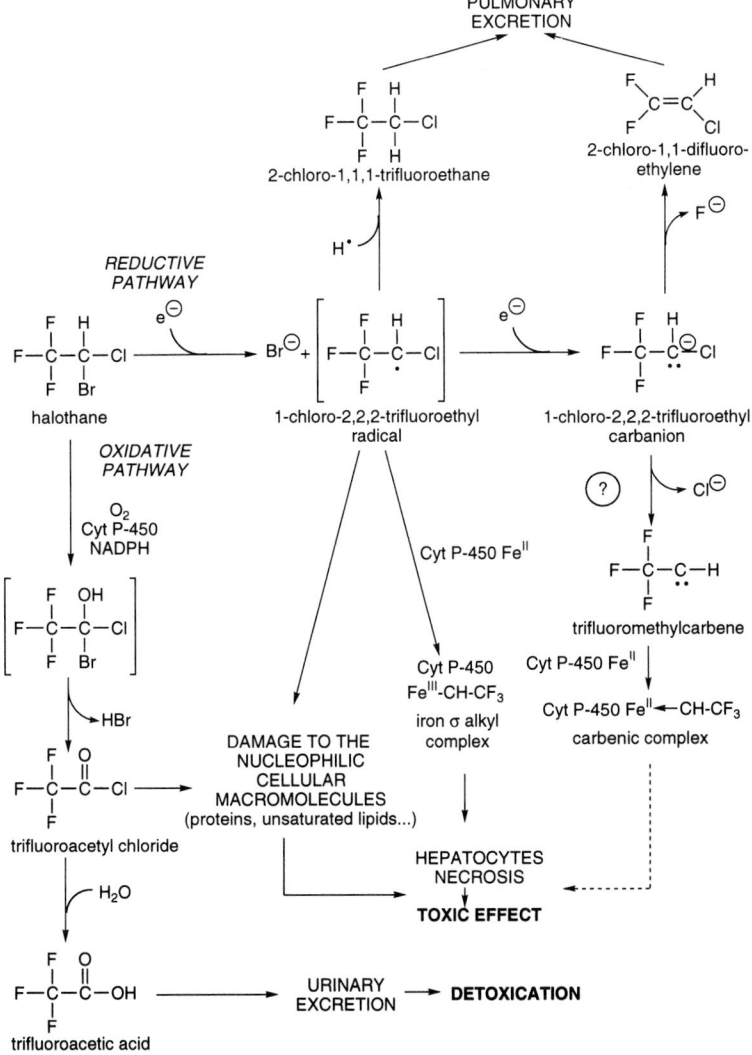

Fig. 30.25 The major metabolic pathways of halothane.

two possible kinds of elimination. One is the abstraction of a fluoride ion according to a E1Bc elimination, which yields 2-chloro-1,1-difluoroethylene. This metabolite is eliminated by exhalation. Early studies suggested that a second elimination process might be a α-elimination of a chloride ion, which produces trifluoromethylcarbene,[31] but this was later reconsidered.[32] It was hypothesized that a carbenic complex with the Fe[II] in the active site might lead to inactivation of the cytochrome P450, but this inactivation is now thought to be due to the formation of an iron-σ-alkyl complex derived from the 1-chloro-2,2,2-trifluoroethyl radical.

The initially formed 1-chloro-2,2,2-trifluoroethyl radical may also cause a radical attack on polyunsaturated lipids which produces 2-chloro-1,1,1-trifluoroethane. This mechanism is identical to the pathway described with the trichloromethyl radical formed during the one-electron reduction of carbon tetrachloride (Fig. 30.14). The trichloromethyl radical may initiate peroxidation of the unsaturated lipids from the membrane and the subsequent liberation of chloroform.

Several studies have demonstrated that halothane hepatotoxicity is mainly due to an immune reaction towards modified proteins of the liver. In fact, these proteins are trifluoroacetylated on their ε-NH$_2$-lysyl residue by the trifluoroacetyl chloride formed during the oxidative metabolisation of halothane.[33,34] The product of the reaction can act as a foreign epitope and the drug–protein conjugate, called neoantigen, elicits an immune response toward the liver[35] (Fig. 30.26).

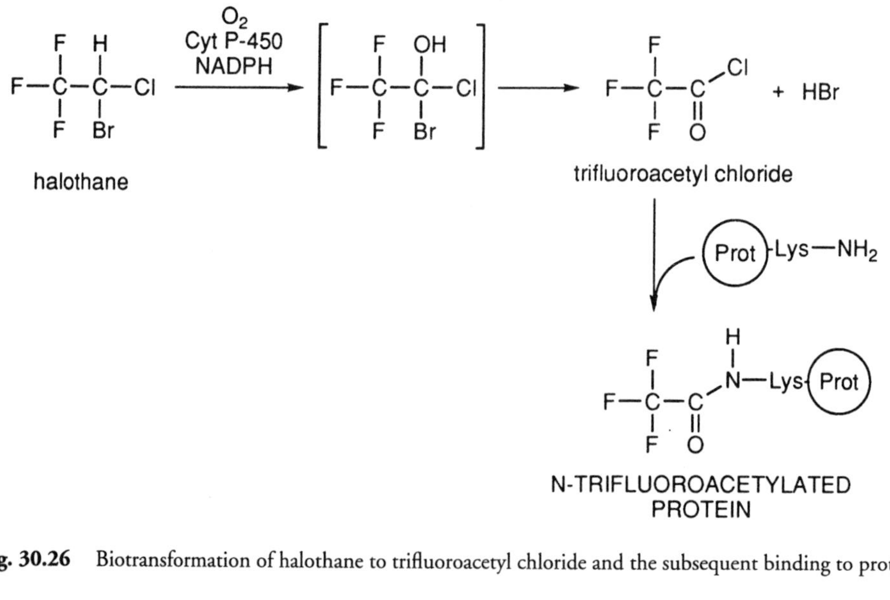

Fig. 30.26   Biotransformation of halothane to trifluoroacetyl chloride and the subsequent binding to protein.

D.   Valproic acid

Valproic acid is an anticonvulsant agent used in the therapy of epilepsy which occasionally results in hepatotoxicity in young children. The toxicity is characterized by mitochondrial damage, impairment of fatty acid β-oxidation and lipid accumulation.

It has been proposed that hepatotoxicity is a consequence of the further biotransformation of the valproic acid metabolite 2-propyl-4-pentenoic acid (also called Δ^4-VPA).[36] As depicted in Fig. 30.27, Δ^4-VPA is not formed by dehydration of 4- or 5-hydroxyvalproic acids, which are,

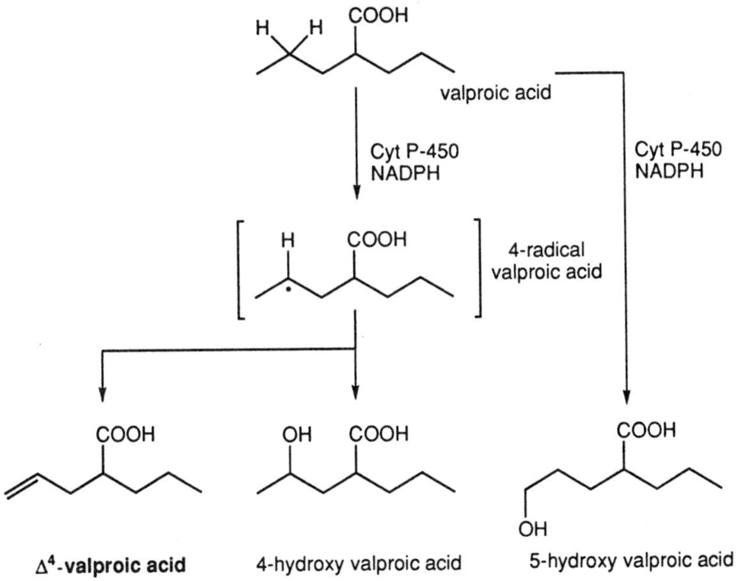

Fig. 30.27 Bioactivation of valproic acid to Δ⁴-VPA.

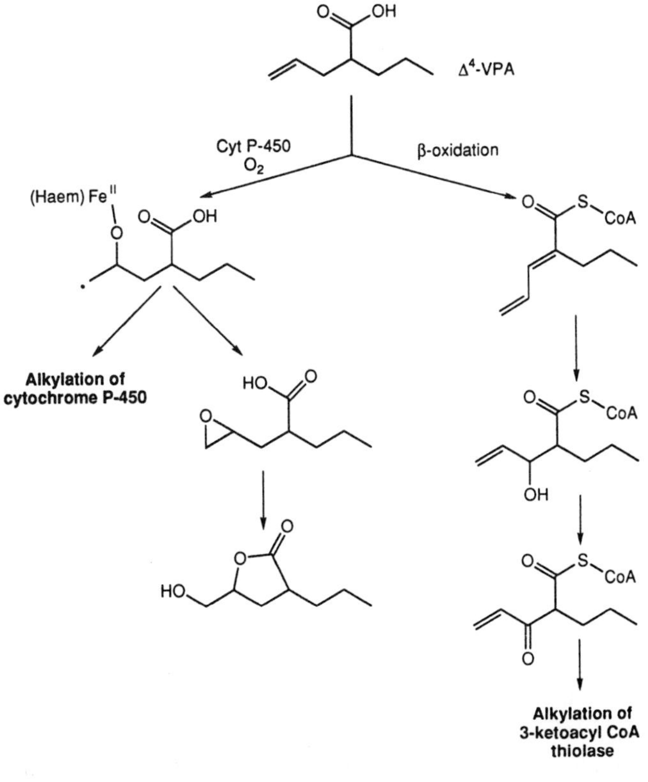

Fig. 30.28 Bioactivation of Δ⁴-VPA.

with the glucuronide conjugate, the major metabolites of valproic acid.[37] The mechanism is proposed to involve an initial hydrogen abstraction to generate a transient free radical intermediate. It has been demonstrated that the carbon-centred radical is localized at the C-4 position. The radical undergoes both recombination (which yields 4-hydroxyvalproic acid) and elimination (which produces the unsaturated derivative Δ^4-VPA). The formation of these metabolites is catalysed by the cytochrome P450 mixed-function oxidase.

Further biotransformations of Δ^4-VPA involve both the liver microsomal cytochrome P450 enzymes and the fatty acid β-oxidation pathway (Fig. 30.28). The mixed-function oxidase system metabolizes the unsaturated metabolite to a γ-butyrolactone[38] derivative through a chemically reactive entity that is a suicide-substrate inhibitor of cytochrome P450. The alkylation of the prosthetic haem by means of the radical occurs prior to the formation of the epoxide.[39] Thus the epoxide is not involved in the cytochrome P450 inhibition.

The β-oxidation cycle activates Δ^4-VPA to its coenzyme A derivative and, through sequential steps of β-oxidation, yields 3-oxo 2-propyl-4-pentenoic acid.[40] This final metabolite is believed to be a reactive electrophilic species that alkylates 3-ketoacyi-CoA thiolase (the terminal enzyme of β-oxidation) by means of a Michael-type addition through nucleophilic attack at the olefinic terminus.[41] In addition to its direct toxicity, Δ^4-VPA is a strong teratogenic compound in animal models.

E.   Mechlorethamine

The antineoplastic drug 2-chloro-N-(2-chloroethyl)-N-methylethanamine (mechlorethamine) is a direct alkylating agent. It is very unstable in aqueous solution and reacts almost completely in the body within a few minutes. The mechanism by which this nitrogen mustard becomes covalently bonded to the N-7 atoms of two guanine residues in DNA is based on intramolecular substitutions yielding cyclic carbocations[42] (Fig. 30.29).

In the first step, the tertiary amine mechlorethamine is converted to a quaternary ammonium compound. The 2-chloroethyl side-chain undergoes a first-order intramolecular substitution (SNi) which produces an ethyl eniminium intermediate. This strong electrophilic entity may react with the N-7 atom of a guanine through the formation of a carbenium ion (or transition complex intermediate) by reaction which resembles an SN2 substitution. This reaction gives rise to a covalent linkage. The unshared electrons of the 7-nitrogen atom in guanine are sterically available and thus are the key target for alkylating mutagens. The adduct formed may undergo another identical metabolic transformation on the second arm to yield cross-linked guanines. The adduct is intermolecular if it occurs in the complementary strand, and the cross-linking may prevent strand separation during the DNA replication.

IV.   CONCLUSION

In the foregoing it has been emphasized that almost all metabolic reactions are capable of producing reactive metabolites. This bioactivation yields toxic compounds which may act directly or indirectly[3,25] (Fig. 30.30). The emergence of toxicity may be the outcome of the interactions of metabolites or reactive intermediates with biological targets such as cellular macromolecules. Often, covalent bonds are formed during a phenomenon which may be

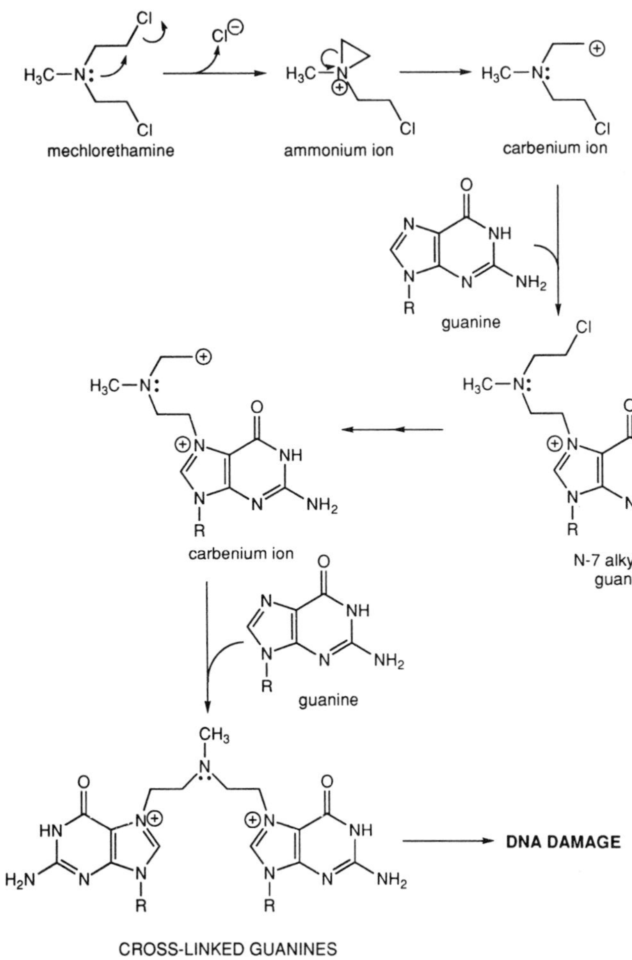

Fig. 30.29 Biotransformation of mechlorethamine.

referred to as alkylating stress. The specific inhibition of an enzyme by its own substrate (suicide-substrate) is a peculiar feature of alkylating stress. Other compounds exhibit their toxicity by inducing the generation of reactive oxygen species, thus producing alterations in the redox state of the cell.

Generally, the formation of toxic metabolites is not the only pathway of biotransformation, and the overall metabolism comprises detoxication and bioactivation processes. The toxic metabolites are themselves often further detoxified. The duality between a beneficial detoxication phenomenon (metabolism, drug resistance) and the occurrence of a toxic effect represents the cost of a rapid adaptation to the transformation of any xenobiotic.[3]

ACKNOWLEDGEMENTS

The authors gratefully aknowledge D. Mansuy, P. Dansette, M. Delaforge and D. Cornish-Bowden for their scientific help and valuable assistance in reviewing the manuscript.

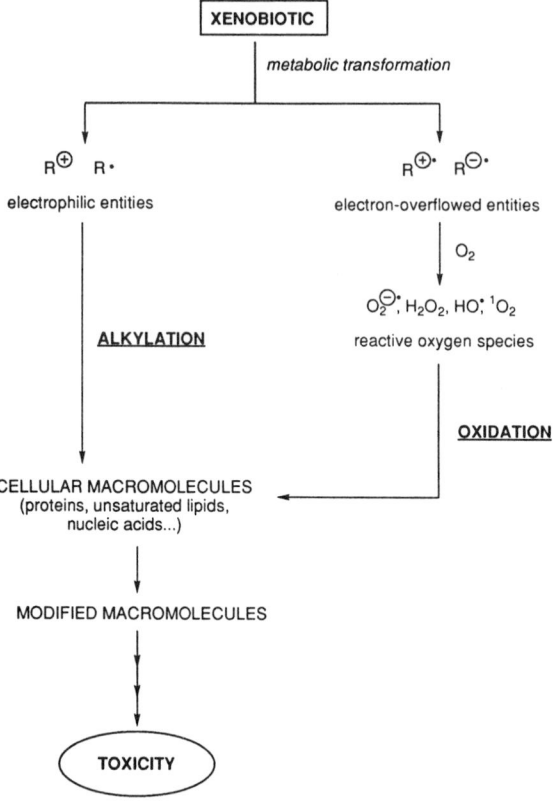

Fig. 30.30   Alkylating and oxidative stresses.

REFERENCES

1. Sipes, G., and Gandolfi, A. J. (1991) Biotransformation of toxicants. In Amdur, M. O., Doull J. and Klaassen, C. D. (eds) *Casarett and Doull's Toxicology: The Basic Science of Poisons,* 4th edn. Pergamon Press, New York.
2. Alvares, A. P. and Pratt, W. B. (1990) Pathways of drug metabolism. In Pratt, W. B. and Taylor, P. (eds) *Principles of Drug Action: The Basis of Pharmacology,* 3rd edn. Churchill Livingstone, New York.
3. Picot, A. (1979) *Aspects biochimiques de la toxicité de diverses substances chimiques (solvants, produits mutagènes, cancérogènes . . .).* CNRS. Gif-sur-Yvette.
4. Picot, A. and Louis, J.-M. (1995) Toxicologie moléculaire. *Notions de biologie et de chimie appliquées.* Tec. Doc. Lavoisier, Paris.
5. Mason, R. P. and Chignell, C. F. (1982) Free radicals in pharmacology and toxicology: selected topics. *Pharmacol. Rev.* **33**: 189–211.
6. Aust, S. D., Chignell, C. F., Bray, T. M., Kalyanaraman, B. and Mason, R. P. (1993) Free radicals in toxicology. *Toxicol. Appl. Pharmacol.* **120**: 168–178.
7. Singal, P. K., Petkau, A., Gerrard, J. M., Hrushovetz, S. and Foerster, J. (1988) Free radicals in health and disease. *Mol. Cell. Biochem.* **84**: 121–122.
8. Anders, M. W. and Pohl, L. R. (1985) Halogenated alkanes. In Anders, M. W. (ed.) *Bioactivation of Foreign Compounds.* Academic Press: Orlando.
9. Pohl, L. R., Nelson, S. D. and Krishna, G. (1978) Investigation of the mechanism of metabolic activation of chloramphenicol by rat liver microsomes: identification of a new metabolite. *Biochem. Pharmacol.* **27**: 491–496.

10. Halpert, J. R., Miller, N. E. and Gorsky, L. D. (1985) On the mechanism of the inactivation of the major phenobarbital-inducible isozyme of rat liver cytochrome P-450 by chloramphenicol. *J. Biol. Chem.* **260**: 8397–8403.

11. Dansette, P. M., Do Cao Thang, El Amri, H. and Mansuy, D. (1992) Evidence for thiophene-*S*-oxide as a primary reactive metabolite of thiophene *in vivo*: formation of a dihydrothiophene sulfoxide mercapturic acid. *Biochem. Biophys. Res. Commun.* **186**: 1624.

12. Gaudiano, G. and Koch, T. H. (1991) Redox chemistry of anthracycline antitumor drugs: a use of captodative radicals as tools for its elucidation and control. *Chem. Res. Toxicol.* **4**: 2–16.

13. Butler, T. S. (1961) Reduction of carbon tetrachloride *in vivo* and reduction of carbon tetrachloride and chloroform *in vitro* by tissues and tissue constituents. *J. Pharmacol. Exp. Ther.* **134**: 311–319.

14. Timbrell, J. A., Mitchell, J. R., Snodgrass, W. R. and Nelson, S. D. (1980) Isoniazid hepatotoxicity: the relationship between covalent binding and metabolism *in vivo*. *J. Pharmacol. Exp. Ther.* **213**: 364–369.

15. Sinha, B. K. (1987) Activation of hydrazine derivatives to free radicals in the perfused rat liver: a spin-trapping study. *Biochim. Biophys. Acta* **924**: 261–269.

16. D'Souza, J., Caldwell, J. and Smith, R. L. (1980) Species variations in the *N*-methylation and quaternization of [^{14}C]pyridine. *Xenobiotica* **10**: 151–157.

17. Miller, E. C. and Miller, J. A. (1981) Mechanisms of chemical carcinogenesis. *Cancer.* **47**: 1055–1064.

18. Picot, A., Archieri, M.-J. and Guery, J. (1995) *Monographies de Toxicochimie: Hydrocarbures saturés.* CNRS: Gif-sur-Yvette.

19. De Caprio, A. P., Strominger, L. N. and Weber, P. (1983) Neurotoxicity and protein binding of 2,5-hexanedione in the hen. *Toxicol. Appl. Pharmacol.* **68**: 297–307.

20. Thomas, S. H. L. (1993) Paracetamol (acetaminophen) poisoning. *Pharmacol. Ther.* **60**: 91–120.

21. Mitchell, J. R., Jollow, D. J., Gillette, J. R. and Brodie, B. B. (1973) Drug metabolism as a cause of drug toxicity. *Drug Metab. Dispos.* **1**: 418–423.

22. Rao, D. N. R., Fischer, V. and Mason, R. P. (1990) Glutathione and ascorbate reduction of the acetaminophen radical formed by peroxidase. Detection of the glutathione disulfide radical formed by the ascorbyl radical. *J. Biol. Chem.* **265**: 844–847.

23. Fischer, V., West, P. R., Harman, L. S and Mason, R. P. (1985) Free-radical metabolites of acetaminophen and a dimethylated derivative. *Environ. Health Perspect.* **64**: 127–137.

24. Rosen, G. M., Singletary, W. V. Jr., Rauckman, E. J. and Killenberg, P. G. (1983) Acetaminophen hepatotoxicity. An alternative mechanism. *Biochem. Pharmacol.* **32**: 2053–2059.

25. Nelson, S. D. and Pearson, P. G. (1990) Covalent and noncovalent interactions in acute lethal cell injury caused by chemicals. *Annu. Rev. Pharmacol. Toxicol.* **30**: 169–195.

26. Homberg, J. C., André, C. and Abuaf, N. (1984) A new anti-liver-kidney microsome antibody (anti-LKM$_2$) in tienilic acid-induced hepatitis. *Clin. Exp. Immunol.* **55**: 561–570.

27. Lopez-Garcia, M. P., Dansette, P. and Mansuy, D. (1994) Thiophene derivatives as new mechanism-based inhibitors of cytochromes P450: inactivation of yeast-expressed human liver cytochrome P450 2C9 by tienilic acid. *Biochemistry* **33**: 166–175.

28. Lecoeur, S., Bonierbale, E., Challine, D., Gautier, J.-C., Valadon, P., Dansette, P. M., Catinot, R., Ballet, F., Mansuy, D. and Beaune, P. H. (1994) Specificity of *in vitro* binding of tienilic acid metabolites to human liver microsomes in relationship to the type of hepatotoxicity: comparison with two directly hepatotoxic drugs. *Chem. Res. Toxicol.* **7**: 434–442.

29. Lopez-Garcia, P. M., Dansette, P., Valadon, P., Amar, C., Beaune, P. H., Guengerich, F. P. and Mansuy, D. (1993) Human liver P-450 expressed in yeast as tools for reactive-metabolite formation studies. Oxidative activation of tienilic acid by P450 2C9 and P450 2C10. *Eur. J. Biochem.* **213**: 232–232.

30. Harris, J. W., Pohl, L. R., Martin, J. L. and Anders, M. W. (1991) Tissue acylation by the chlorofluorocarbon substitute 2,2-dichloro-1,1,1-trifluoroethane. *Proc. Natl. Acad. Sci. USA* **88**: 1407–1410.

31. Mansuy, D., Nastainczyk, W. and Ullrich, V. (1974) The mechanism of halothane binding to microsomal cytochrome P450. *Naunyn-Schmiedeberg's Arch. Pharmacol.* **285**: 315–324

32. Ahr, H. J., King, L. J., Nastainczyk, W. and Ullrich, V. (1982) The mechanism of reductive dehalogenation of halothane by liver cytochrome P-450. *Biochem. Pharmacol.* **31**: 383–390

33. Pohl, L. R. (1993) An immunochemical approach of identifying and characterizing protein targets of toxic reactive metabolites. *Chem. Res. Toxicol.* **6**: 786–793.

34. Kenna, J. G., Neuberger, J. and Williams, R. (1988) Evidence for expression in human liver of halothane-induced neoantigens recognized by antibodies in sera from patients with halothane hepatitis. *Hepatology* **8**: 1635–1641.

35. Pohl, L. R., Kenna, J. G., Satoh, H. and Christ, D. (1989) Neoantigens associated with halothane hepatitis. *Drug Metab. Rev.* **20**: 203–217.

36. Baillie, T. A. (1988) Metabolic activation of valproic acid and drug-mediated hepatotoxicity. Role of the terminal olefin 2-*n*-propyl-4-pentenoic acid. *Chem. Res. Toxicol.* **1**: 195–199.

37. Rettie, A. E., Rettenmeier, A. W., Howald, W. N. and Baillie, T. A. (1987) Cytochrome P450-catalyzed formation of Δ^4-VPA, a toxic metabolite of valproic acid. *Science* **235**: 890–893.

38. Prickett, K. S. and Baillie, T. A. (1986) Metabolism of unsaturated derivative of valproic acid in rat liver microsomes and destruction of cytochrome P-450. *Drug Metab. Dispos.* **14**: 221–229.

39. Ortiz de Montellano, P. R., Yost, G. S., Mico, B. A., Dinizo, S. E., Correia, M. A. and Kambara, H. (1979) Destruction of cytochrome P450 by isopropyl-4-pentenamide and methyl-2-isopropyl-4-pentenoate: mass spectrometric characterization of prosthetic heme adducts and nonparticipation of epoxide metabolites. *Arch. Biochem. Biophys.* **197**: 524–533.

40. Rettenmeier, A. W., Gordon, W. P., Prickett, K. S., Levy, R. H. and Baillie, T. A. (1986) Biotransformation and pharmacokinetics in the rhesus monkey of 2-*n*-propyl-4-pentenoic acid, a toxic metabolite of valproic acid. *Drug Metab. Dispos.* **14**: 454–464.

41. Rettenmeier, A. W., Prickett, K. S., Gordon, W. P., Bjorge, S. M., Chang, S.-L., Levy, R. H. and Baillie, T. A. (1985) Studies on the biotransformation in the perfused rat liver of 2-*n*-propyl-4-pentenoic acid, a metabolite of the antiepileptic drug valproic acid. Evidence for the formation of chemically reactive intermediates. *Drug Metab. Dispos.* **13**: 81–96.

42. Calabresi, B. A. and Chabner, B. A. (1990) Antineoplastic agents. In Goodman Gilman, A., Rall, T. W., Nies, A. S. and Taylor, P. (eds) *Goodman and Gilman's The Pharmacological Basis of Therapeutics* 8th edn. Pergamon Press, New York.

31

Designing Prodrugs and Bioprecursors I: Carrier Prodrugs

CAMILLE G. WERMUTH, JEAN-CYR GAIGNAULT AND
CHRISTIAN MARCHANDEAU

La façon de donner vaut mieux que ce que l'on donne.
The manner of giving counts more that what one gives
Piere Corneille, *Le Menteur*, Act 1, Scene 1.

THE PRACTICE OF MEDICINAL CHEMISTRY
ISBN 0-12-744640-0

I.   GENERAL INTRODUCTION

Therapeutic approaches based on molecular pharmacology mostly use *in vitro* models (membrane or enzyme preparations, cell or microorganism cultures, isolated organs, etc.). In the last decade they have led to the discovery of numerous potent and quite selective agents. As examples we can mention the GABAergic agonist muscimol,[1] the H_2 histamine antagonists burimamide and cimetidine,[2] the $GABA_A$ receptor antagonist gabazine,[3,4] the hydroxymethylglutaryl-CoA reductase inhibitor mevastatin,[5,6] the cholecystokinin antagonist asperlicin,[7] the anticancer drugs taxol[8,9] and neocarzinostatin[10] and the neurotensin antagonist SR 48692.[11]

However, the bioavailability of molecules exclusively screened through *in vitro* assays can be low. Because of the polarity of the functional groups present in the molecule, they may be poorly absorbed or incorrectly distributed. They may also, as a result of their vulnerability, be the subject of early metabolic destruction such as by first-pass effects or any other kind of degradation leading to a short biological half-life. For such molecules the *in vivo* administration is limited to the parenteral route and their clinical usefulness is thus restricted. Sometimes an adequate pharmaceutical formulation (microencapsulation, sustained-release or enterosoluble preparations) can overcome these drawbacks, but often the galenic formulation is inoperant and a chemical modification of the active molecule is necessary to correct its pharmacokinetic insufficiencies. This *chemical formulation* process, whose objective is to convert an interesting active molecule into a clinically acceptable drug, often involves design of a so-called 'prodrug'.

Initially the term prodrug was introduced by Albert to describe 'any compound that undergoes biotransformation prior to exhibiting its pharmacological effects'.[12] Such a broad definition includes accidental historical prodrugs (aspirin and salicylic acid), active metabolites (imipramine and desmethylimipramine) and compounds intentionally prepared to improve the pharmacokinetic profile of an active molecule. From this point of view the term 'drug latentiation' proposed by Harper[13] is more appropriate for prodrug design as it indicates that there is intention. Drug latentiation is defined as 'the chemical modification of a biologically active compound to form a new compound that, upon *in vivo* enzymatic attack, will liberate the parent compound'. Even this definition is too broad and a survey of the specialized literature led us to divide prodrugs into two classes: the carrier-prodrugs, and the bioprecursors.[14,15]

The *carrier-prodrugs* result from a temporary linkage of the active molecule with a transport moiety that is frequently of lipophilic nature. A simple hydrolytic reaction cleaves this transport moiety at the correct moment (e.g. bacampicillin, progabide). Such prodrugs are *per se* less active than the parent compounds, or even inactive. The transport moiety (carrier group) will be chosen for its nontoxicity and its ability to ensure the release of the active principle with efficient kinetics.

The *bioprecursors* do not involve a temporary linkage between the active principle and a carrier group but result from a molecular modification of the active principle itself. This modification generates a new compound, able to be a substrate for the metabolizing enzymes, the metabolite being the expected active principle. This approach exemplifies the active metabolite concept in the prospective application (e.g., sulindac, fenbufen).

II.   THE CARRIER-PRODRUG PRINCIPLE

The carrier-prodrug principle (Fig. 31.1) consists of 'the attachment of a carrier group to the active drug to alter its physicochemical properties and then the subsequent enzyme attack to release the active drug moiety'.[13] 'Prodrugs can thus be viewed as drugs containing specialized nontoxic protective groups used in a transient manner to alter or eliminate undesirable properties in the parent molecule'.[16]

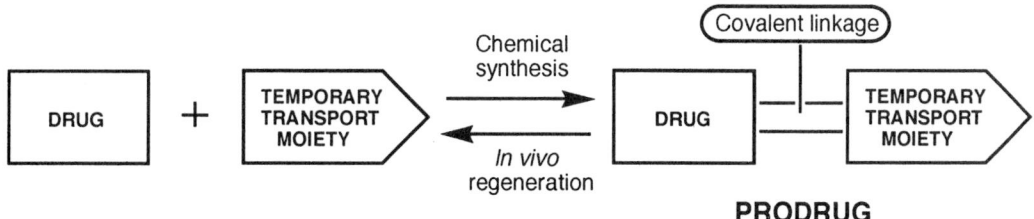

Fig. 31.1   The carrier-prodrug principle.[19]

A well-designed carrier-prodrug satisfies the following criteria.[17,18]

(1) The linkage between the drug substance and the transport moiety is usually a covalent bond.
(2) As a rule the prodrug is inactive or less active than the parent compound.
(3) The linkage between the parent compound and the transport moiety must be broken *in vivo*.
(4) The prodrug, as well as the transport moiety released *in vivo*, must be nontoxic.
(5) The generation of the active form must take place with rapid kinetics to ensure effective drug levels at the site of action and to minimize either direct prodrug metabolization or gradual drug inactivation.

An example of prodrug design taking into account these criteria is found in orally active ampicillin derivatives.[20–22] Ampicillin is one of the main β-lactam antibiotics. It is widely used as a broad-spectrum antibiotic but it suffers from poor absorption when administered orally: only about 40% of the drug is absorbed. In other words, to achieve the same clinical efficiency and the same blood level one must give two to three times more ampicillin by mouth than by intramuscular injection. The clinical tolerance of orally given ampicillin may be affected, the nonabsorbed part of the drug destroying the intestinal flora. Accordingly, numerous attempts have been made to improve these poor absorption properties.

Figure 31.2 represents two prodrugs of ampicillin: pivampicillin and bacampicillin. They both result from the esterification of the polar carboxylic group with a lipophilic, enzymatically labile ester. The main properties of these prodrugs can be summarized as follows.

(1) The absorption of these compounds is nearly quantitative (98–99%).
(2) The generation of free ampicillin in the bloodstream is rapid (less than 15 min).
(3) The released carrier molecules are formaldehyde and pivalic acid (trimethylacetic acid) for pivampicillin, and acetaldehyde, ethanol and carbon dioxide in the case of bacampicillin. These latter three compounds are natural metabolites in the human body. This may explain the better tolerance of bacampicillin compared to pivampicillin.

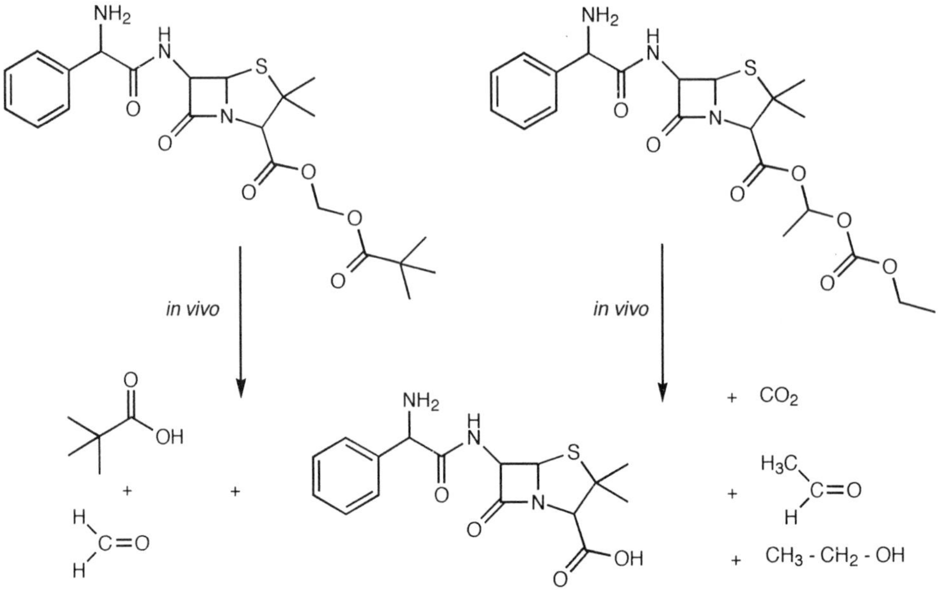

Fig. 31.2   Prodrugs derived from ampicillin.[20–22]

(4) The serum levels attained following oral administration of bacampicillin are similar to those obtained after intramuscular injection of an equimolecular amount of free ampicillin.

(5) Clinical trials confirm the efficiency and the safety of the prodrugs. Owing to their good absorption, the drugs are given at lower dosage than ampicillin: 0.8–1.0 g daily is sufficient in common infections as compared to 2.0 g daily for ampicillin.

(6) It has been shown, and this seems to be a rule for prodrugs, that pivampicillin and bacampicillin are inactive *per se*, the antibiotic potency appearing only *in vivo* after the release of free ampicillin.

III.   PRACTICAL APPLICATIONS OF CARRIER-PRODRUG DESIGN

The domain of application of the prodrug approach is illustrated in Fig. 31.3. In practice, carrier prodrugs usually achieve one of the five following goals: increased lipophilicity, increased duration of pharmacological effects, increased site-specificity, decreased toxicity and adverse reactions, improvement in drug formulation (stability, water solubility, suppression of an undesirable organoleptic or physicochemical property). The present chapter concentrates on problems related to the *pharmacokinetic phase,* such as improving the biomembrane passage, achieving site-specific delivery and obtaining sustained release. Prodrug problems related to the *pharmaceutical phase* (chemical solutions to formulation problems) will be treated in Chapters 34 and 35 (water solubility) and 38 (increasing chemical stability, dealing with mesomorphic crystalline forms, transforming liquids into solids, alleviating gastrointestinal irritation and painful injections, suppressing undesirable organoleptic properties, etc.). For applications in the field of insecticides, see Drabek and Neumann.[23]

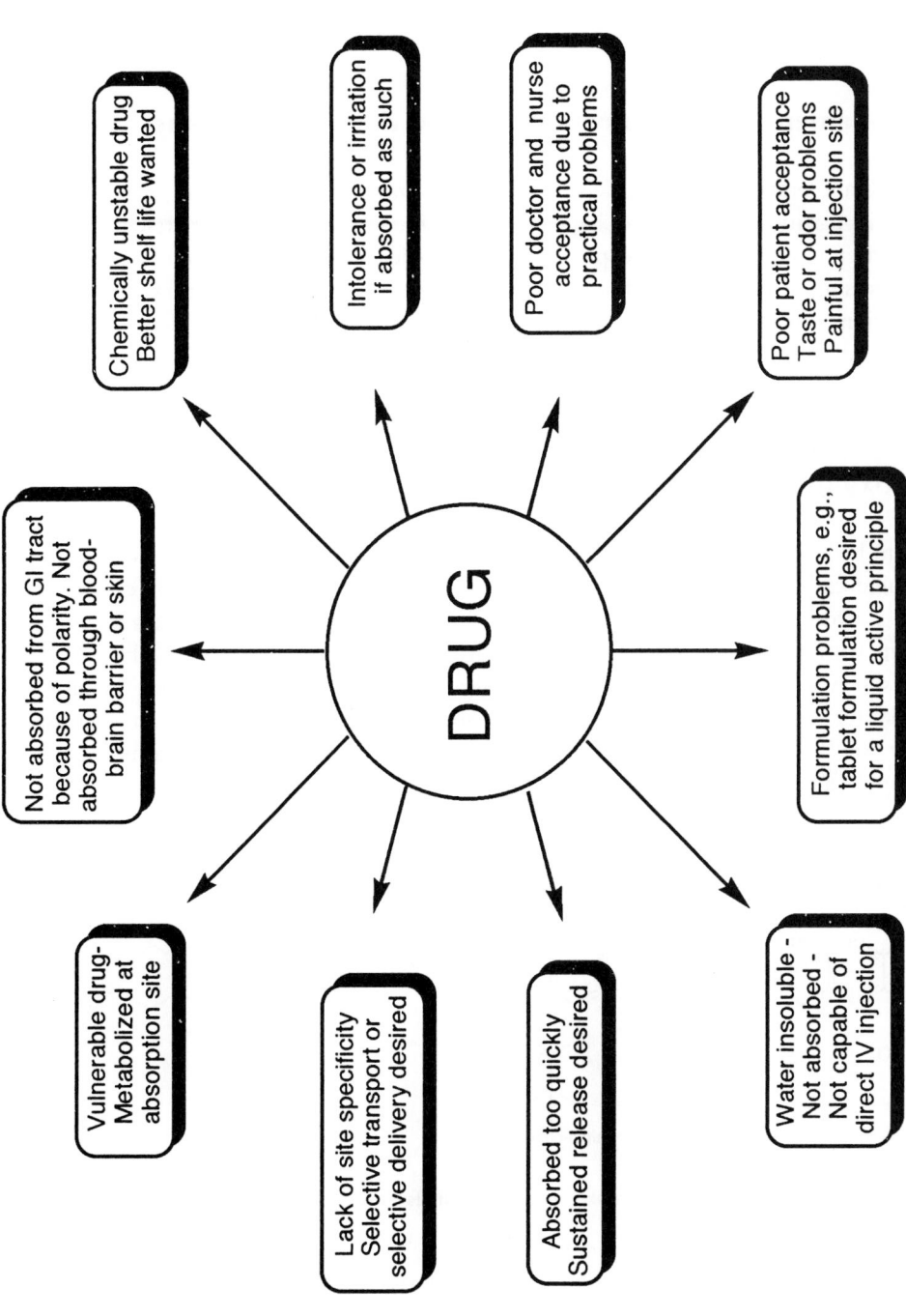

Fig. 31.3 Shortcomings that may be overcome through chemical formulation.[17,19,24]

Bioactive compounds and drugs usually bear a limited number of polar functional groups suitable for prodrug synthesis. Among these, the most frequent are the alcoholic and the phenolic hydroxyls, the amino group, and the carboxylic function. The aim of the next sections is to illustrate how such groups can be used to prepare prodrugs with improved pharmacokinetic properties.

A.   Improvement of the bioavailability and the biomembrane passage

The biomembrane passage of a drug depends primarily on its physicochemical properties and especially on its partition coefficient (Chapters 19 and 28). Thus, the transient attachment of a lipophilic carrier group to an active principle can provide better bioavailability, mostly by facilitating crossing of the cell membrane by passive diffusion. As well as peroral absorption, rectal absorption, ocular drug delivery and dermal drug delivery are also dependent on passive diffusion. Finally, lipophilic carriers can sometimes be useful in reducing first-pass metabolism.[25]

1.   Derivatization of drugs containing alcoholic or phenolic hydroxy groups

Starting from hydroxylic derivatives, high lipophilicity can be obtained simply by esterification with lipophilic carboxylic acids. Dipivaloylepinephrine, for example (Fig. 31.4) crosses the cornea and is used in the treatment of glaucoma.[26] The β-blocker timolol contains a secondary amino group with a pK_a of 9.2 and, since this group is highly protonated at pH 7.4, the compound shows a low lipophilicity at physiological pH ($\log P = -0.04$), which in turn is unfavourable for corneal penetration. The corresponding butyryl ester has an increased lipophilicity ($\log P = 2.08$) and causes a 4- to 6-fold increase in the corneal absorption of timolol following topical administration to rabbits.[25]

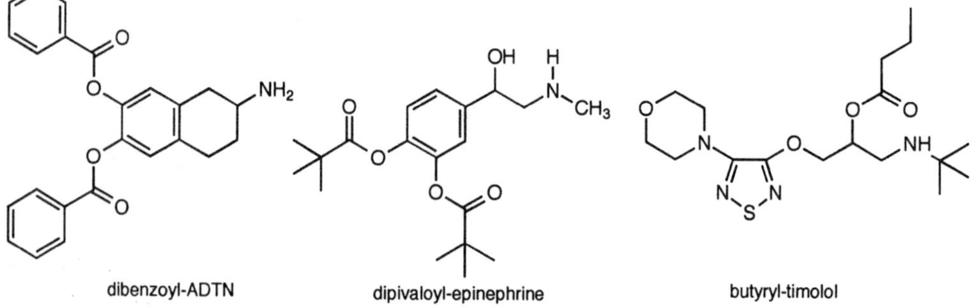

| dibenzoyl-ADTN | dipivaloyl-epinephrine | butyryl-timolol |

Fig. 31.4   Lipophilic prodrugs of hydroxy compounds with facilitated membrane penetration.[25–28]

In a similar manner, dibenzoyl-2-amino-6,7-dihydroxytetrahydronaphthalene (DB-ADTN) reaches the central nervous system, whereas the parent dopamine agonist ADTN does not.[27,28] For dipivaloylepinephrine and dibenzoyl-ADTN, the selective acylation of the phenolic hydroxyl groups was achieved in a strong acidic medium, the amino function being protected by protonation.[27,29] Acylated thymidine analogues such as 3'-O-hexyl-5'-amino-2'-

deoxythymidine are prodrugs for topical application against herpes simplex type 1 viruses (HSV-1).[30] Diacetyl and dipropionyl guanine derivatives, given orally to mice, provided concentrations of the parent drug that were more than 15-fold higher than those observed after dosing with the nonacylated parent drug.[31] In augmenting the lipophilicity and simultaneously destroying the crystal lattice energy, the 2′,3′-diacetate of the antiviral agent 6-methoxypurine arabinoside allowed a 5-fold increase in bioavailability and a 3-fold increase in water solubility in comparison to the nonacetylated drug.[32] As a consequence, an intravenous formulation could be developed.

2. Derivatization of drugs containing a carbonyl function: aldehydes and ketones

The ethylene ketal derivative of prostaglandin E_2 (dinoprostone) possesses much improved solid-state stability (see Chapter 38). Functionalized spirothiazolidines of hydrocortisone and hydrocortisone 21-acetate (Fig. 31.5), prepared with cysteine esters or related β-aminothiols, have improved topical anti-inflammatory activity. It is speculated that the Schiff base intermediate formed upon ring-opening may accumulate in the skin by binding (through its SH function) to thiol groups in the skin.[33]

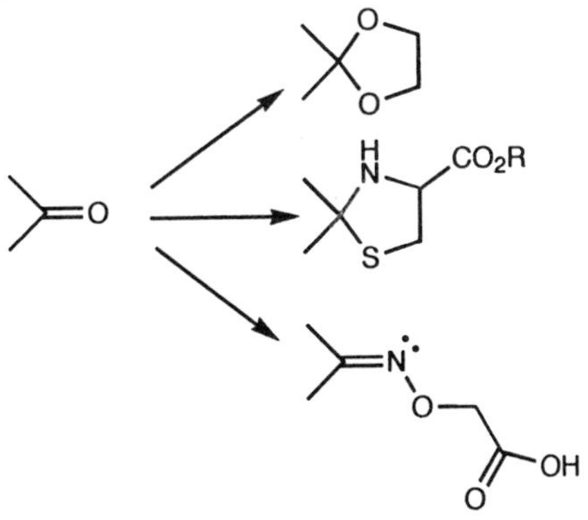

Fig. 31.5 Prodrug possibilities starting from aldehydes or ketones.

Simple and substituted oximes are biostable unless intramolecular assistance is provided. This is the case for the oximes derived from oxyamino acetic acid, which are possible water-soluble prodrugs of ketones and aldehydes (see Chapter 35).

3. Derivatization of drugs containing a carboxylic acid function

Lipophilic prodrugs can also be derived from a carboxylic function, the most commonly used derivatives being carboxylic esters. Simple esters of aliphatic alcohols are attractive as they are cheap to prepare, chemically stable, and yield harmless hydrolysis products.[34] Typical representatives of such prodrugs are tyrosine methyl ester,[35] nipecotic acid ethyl ester,[36] enalaprilat ethyl ester,[37,38] trandolapril,[39] γ-aminobutyric acid cetyl ester,[40,41] and methotrexate cetyl ester.[42]

Lipoidal prodrugs, in which the carboxyl function esterifies the free alcoholic hydroxyl of

1,2- or 1,3-diglycerides, are well absorbed and show high lymphotropism. Applied to the anti-inflammatory agent naproxen, this approach yielded the 2-ester of 1,3-dipalmitoylglycerol (Fig. 36.6), which produces less gastric irritation and higher plasma levels than the parent compound.[43]

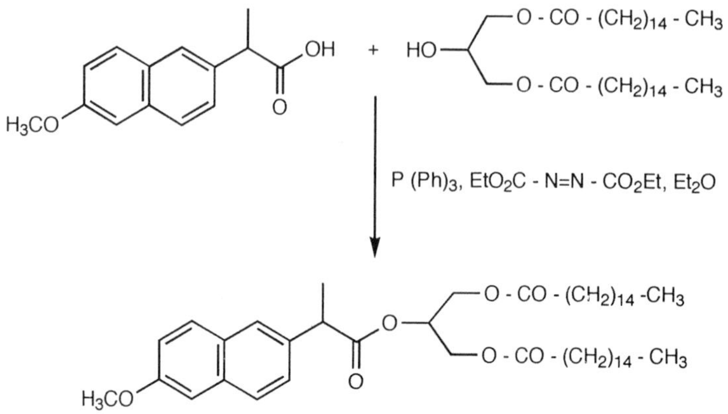

Fig. 31.6   Synthesis of the naproxen-2-glyceride.[43]

The rationale for the design of lipoidal prodrugs is based on well-established principles concerning the intestinal absorption of natural triglycerides.[43,44] As described by Jones[43] (see Fig. 31.7):

> Orally ingested fat enters in the intestinal tract and, as a result of the churning action of stomach musculature, forms an oil-in-water emulsion which passes down the duodenum where it comes into contact with pancreatic lipase. This enzyme acts at the interface of the emulsion particles and specifically cleaves the triglycerides, releasing the fatty acids derived from the 1 and 3 positions, giving 2-monoglycerides as the predominant product. The 2-monoglycerides, free fatty acids and bile salts form negatively charged polymolecular aggregates termed micelles. Only small quantities of diglycerides and triglycerides are present in these micellar particles, but these quantities can apparently be absorbed intact. During the conversion of fats from an emulsion phase (diameter 5000 Å) to a micellar phase (diameter 40–50 Å), the particle size has been greatly decreased. These micellar particles are now small enough to allow free access to the microcillous spaces and absorption into the mucosal cell, where resynthesis occurs under the influence of intracellular enzymes. The triglycerides are finally released from the mucosal cells to the lymphatic circulation as chylomicron particles.

Glyceride prodrugs were also prepared starting from aspirin,[45,46] indomethacin,[47] chlorambucil,[48] and GABA.[49,50] An extension of the use of lipoidal transport groups was made to phospholipids.[51,52] Despite their interest, lipoidal prodrugs have low chances being developed, mostly because they do not crystallize well and can be obtained pure only with difficulty.

The widespread use of acyloxymethyl esters in antibiotic chemistry, as illustrated above for bacampicillin, was initiated by Jansen and Russel[53] at Wyeth Laboratories and successfully applied to pivampicillin,[20] talampicillin[22] and cephalosporins.[54] In each of these cases, the oral absorption of the antibiotic was improved by some 2–3-fold over that of the parent compound. The acyloxymethyl derivatization was also extended to amino acids such as α-methyldopa,[55] isoguvacine[56] and tranexamic acid,[57] anti-inflammatory drugs such as niflumic acid[58] or indomethacin,[59] and quinolone antibacterials such as norfloxacin.[60]

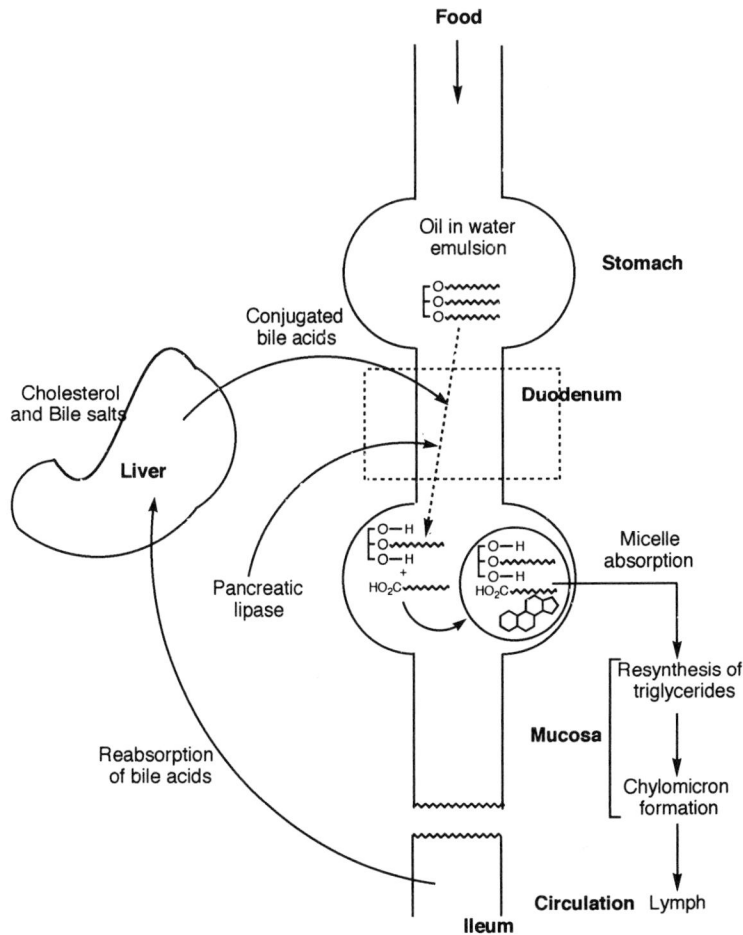

Fig. 31.7 Absorption of fats in the gastrointestinal tract.[43]

Primary amides of carboxylic acids are easily converted in humans to the corresponding acid (e.g. depamide, progabide) and can thus be used in prodrug design. Amides of ketoprofen-derived arylacetic acids possess a therapeutic index one order of magnitude greater than that of indomethacin.[61]

4. Derivatization of amines

Owing to the slow *in vivo* cleavage rate of the *N*-substituted amides, acylation of amines is generally not recommended. Better possibilities are offered by activated amides, peptides, imines and soft quaternary ammonium salts. However, the use of simple *N*-acyl derivatives must not be systematically discarded. The *N*-benzoyl or *N*-pivaloyl derivatives of the inhibitory neurotransmitter GABA are examples of compounds able to penetrate the blood–barrier and to abolish pentetrazole- and bicuculline-induced convulsions. It was also demonstrated in rats that, following subcutaneous injection, rat-brain homogenates liberate free GABA from these amides.[62] There is even some biochemical and pharmacological evidence suggesting that *N*-pivaloyltaurine crosses the blood–brain barrier.[63]

Imines[64] and enamines,[65,66] stabilized through hydrogen bonds, can also be effective prodrugs of primary amines (Fig. 31.8).

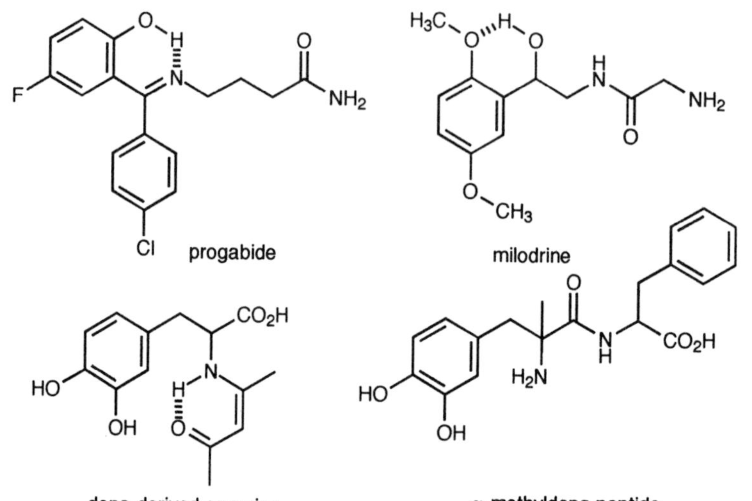

progabide

milodrine

dopa-derived enamine

α-methyldopa peptide

Fig. 31.8 Imine, enamine and peptide prodrugs derived from amino functions.

Small peptides constitute an alternative way of derivatizing amines. The hypotensive drug milodrine, for example (Fig. 31.8), is the well-absorbed transport from which 2-(2,5-dimethoxyphenyl)-2-hydroxyethylamine (ST-1059) is liberated by enzymic cleavage of the glycine residue.[67] Given orally to fasted Wistar rats, the *N*-(*Z*-alanyl)amide of the hypoglycaemic sulfonylurea carbutamide demonstrated a 4–6 times higher potency than the parent sulfonamide. The compound is well tolerated and is metabolized to the parent drug, the amino acid moiety just modifying the bioavailability.[68] Among the numerous variations made around the α-methyldopa molecule, acylation with a glycyl-glycyl residue was claimed to improve the oral bioavailability.[69] For a series of anticandidal di- and tripeptides containing *m*-fluorophenylalanine (m-FPhe), competitive antagonism studies supported peptide transport-mediated entry of the warhead m-FPhe inside the cell.[70] Dipeptides derived from α-methyldopa (Fig. 31.8) show a 10–20-fold better penetration of the intestinal wall than α-methyldopa itself.[71]

5. Prodrugs for compounds with acidic NH functions

Prodrugs obtained by *N*-alkoxycarbonyloxymethylation of 5-fluorouracil show improved delivery properties. Both 1- and 3-alkoxycarbonyloxymethyl derivatives are hydrolysed quantitatively to 5-fluorouracil but the 3-substituted derivatives show greater promise as prodrugs since they combine adequate stability in aqueous solution with a high susceptibility to hydrolysis in plasma.[72] Sulfonamides, but also carboxamides, carbamates and other NH-acidic compounds (Fig. 31.9) can be acylated with various groups[73] or converted into phthalidyl derivatives.[74]

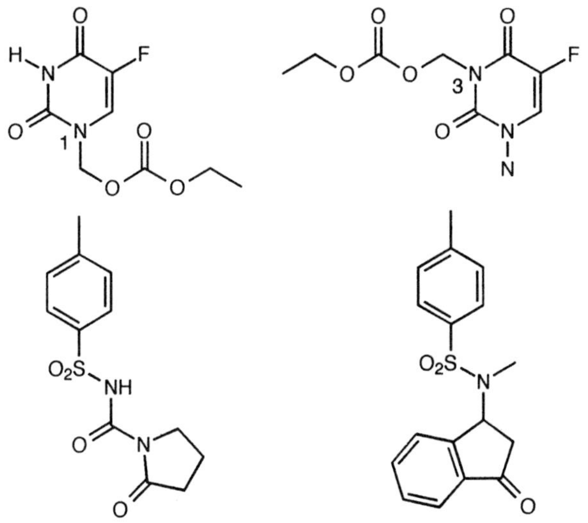

Fig. 31.9 Prodrugs of acidic NH functions.

Hetacillin[75,76] and droxicam[77] are examples of simultaneous cyclic protections of an acidic NH function and an amino or a hydroxylic groups located in the vicinity (Fig. 31.10).

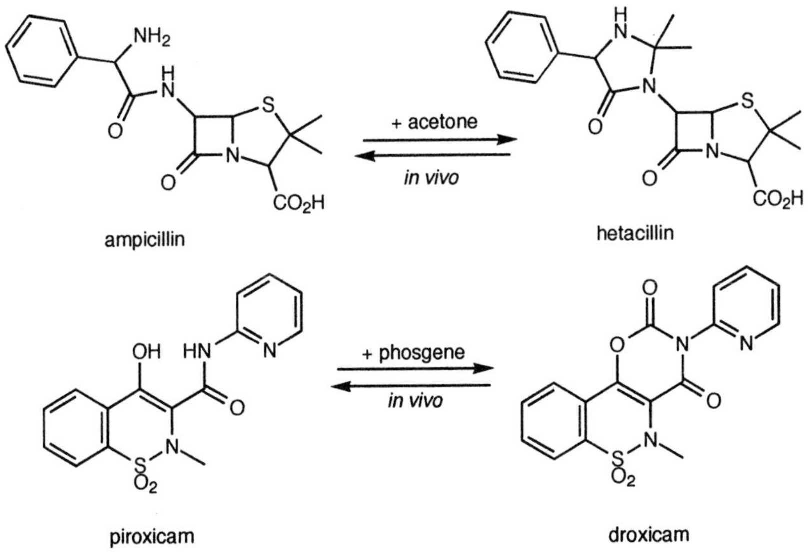

Fig. 31.10 Cyclic protections of two neighbouring functions.

B. Site-specific delivery

Many hopes were put in the prodrug approach as a means to achieving the targeting of drugs for specific sites in the body. Actually only a few convincing examples are found in the literature and we are becoming somewhat disillusioned about the real possibilities of the approach. In principle two targeting possibilities can be considered:[25] first, one can design a prodrug that affords an increased or selective transport of the parent drug to the site of action (*site-directed drug delivery*); second, one can design a derivative that goes everywhere but undergoes bioactivation only inside the target organ (*site-specific* drug release).

1. Site-directed drug delivery

Most of the successes in achieving site-directed drug delivery through prodrugs have been through localized delivery of lipophilic prodrugs (eyes, skin) with increased permeability characteristics. Systemic site-directed delivery, that is delivery to a specific internal site or organ through selective transport, is very difficult to achieve. Nevertheless, some possibilities of local enrichment or of privileged entry into the central nervous system are found in the literature. Thus the L-glutamic analogue of iproniazid presents preferential monoamine oxidase inhibition in the brain,[78] whereas the palmitoyl isopropylhydrazide demonstrates clear cardiac selectivity (Table 31.1).

Table 31.1   Effect of the acyl group in isopropyl hydrazide on selective transport.[78]

Isopropyl hydrazide	% Monoamine increase		Ratios
	Cardiac catecholamines	Cerebral 5-HTP	
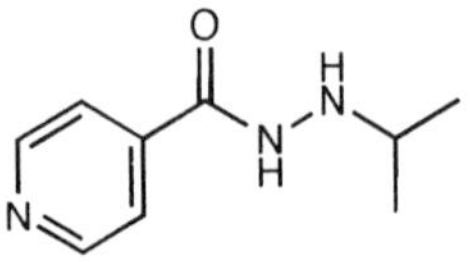	100	100	1.0
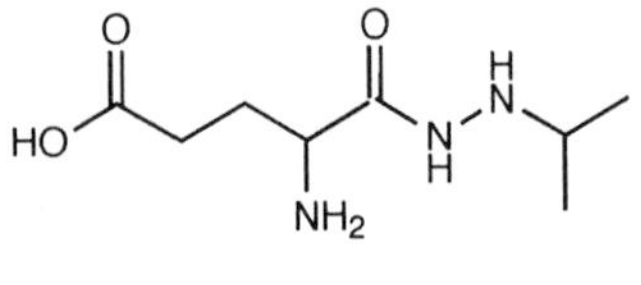	75	250	3.3
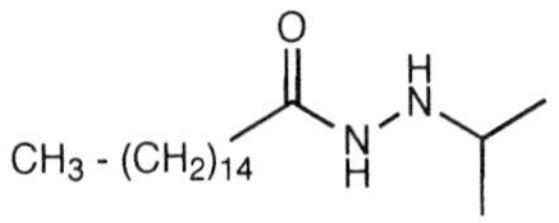	145	60	0.4

The propensity of fatty chains to concentrate in cardiac tissue is also illustrated by findings in the field of myocardial imaging agents. An iodine- and tellurium-containing fatty acid (Fig. 31.11) has a high heart uptake, and heart/blood ratios remained high for several hours: $13:1$ after 1 hour and $9:1$ after 4 hours.[79]

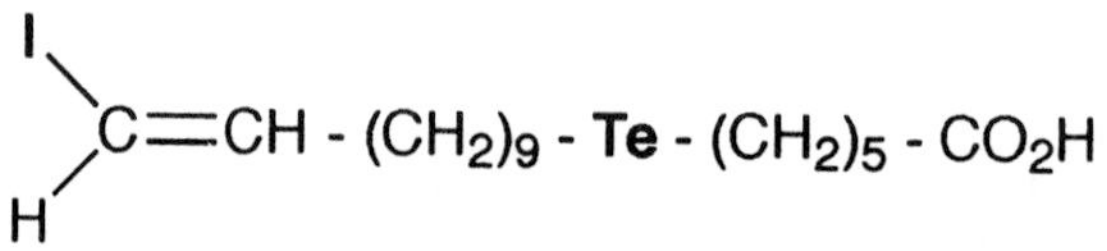

$$I \diagdown C=CH - (CH_2)_9 - Te - (CH_2)_5 - CO_2H$$
$$H \diagup$$

Fig. 31.11   Myocardial imaging agent.

Coupling of drugs to modified bile acids was recently proposed for liver-specific targeting.[80] The rationale is based on the recognition of bile acid-linked drugs by the endogenous bile acid transport system. Chlorambucil, an alkylating cytostatic agent, HR-780, an inhibitor of HMG-CoA reductase, and an oxaproline peptide, an inhibitor of prolyl-4-hydroxylase, were chosen for conjugation to bile acids (Fig. 31.12).

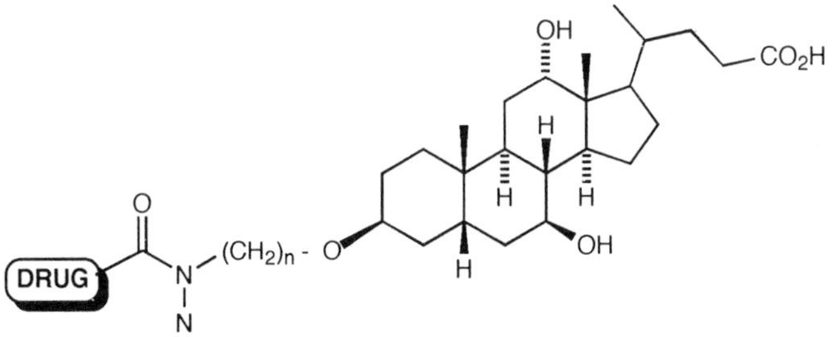

Fig. 31.12 Bile acids for liver specific targeting.[80]

The 2,3-dichlorophenoxyacetic moiety of ethacrynic acid was claimed to have a high affinity for the renal tissue,[81] and 2-thiouracil and 6-propylthiouracil exhibit marked affinities for melatonin-producing tissues.[82,83] They were therefore (unsuccessfully) tested for the treatment of malignant melanoma.[84] Many other examples of selective conducting moieties are found in X-ray contrast media and radioisotope imaging agents.[85] Similar efforts were made to find selective cancer chemotherapeutics, and a variety of drugs that are known to accumulate selectively in particular tissues have also been tried. Mustard derivatives of amino acids, steroid hormones, tetracyclines, quinacrine and uracil are examples.[86] Site-directed cancer chemotherapy can involve drugs bound to specific antibodies. Daunomycin, conjugated via an oxidized dextran bridge with anti-B-cell lymphoma 38C-13 cell-surface IgM antibodies, given to 38C-tumour-bearing mice gave increased life span and even complete cure.[87] Descriptions of some other attempts to achieve delivery to the central nervous system will be found in Chapters 37 and 38.

2. Site-specific drug release

The whole strategy of site-specific release of a given drug lies in the discovery of an enzyme present in high concentrations in the target organ and effectively absent elsewhere. An appropriate prodrug can then be designed using the selective cleavage possibility offered by the enzyme.

A selective renal vasodilatation, for example, is produced by administration of γ-glutamyldopa. It is well known that L-dopa is a precursor of the neurotransmitter dopamine, which plays an important role in the central nervous system and in the kidneys. The association of L-dopa with a peripheral dopa-decarboxylase inhibitor allows preferential dopamine production in the brain and can be considered at present the best therapeutic possibility for Parkinson's disease.

On the renal side, a prodrug of L-dopa, γ-glutamyl-L-3,4-dihydroxyphenylalanine (γ-glutamyldopa), produces a specific vasodilatation of the renal tissue. Indeed, the γ-glutamyl derivatives of amino acids and peptides accumulate in the kidneys, where they undergo a selective metabolic process (for a review see Magnan *et al.*[88]). The successive actions of two enzymes present in high concentration in the kidney, γ-glutamyl transpeptidase and L-aromatic amino acid decarboxylase, release dopamine locally from γ-glutamyldopa (Fig. 31.13).

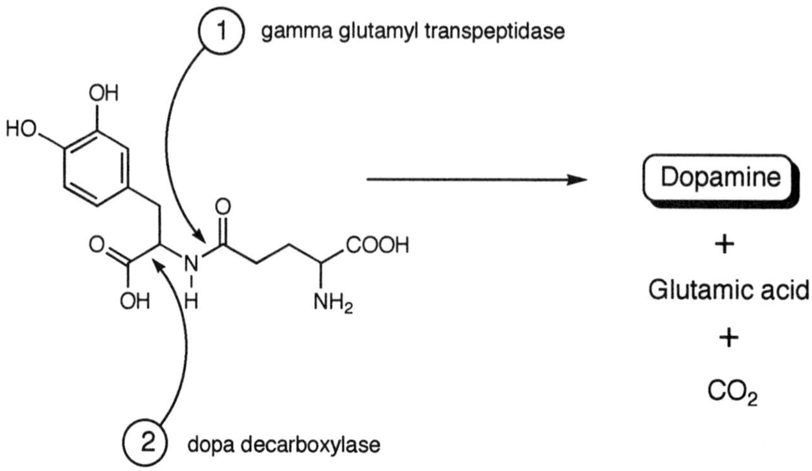

Fig. 31.13   Selective renal vasodilatation with γ-glutamyl-dopa.[89]

In mice, the renal levels of dopamine, after γ-glutamyldopa, are five times higher than after an equimolar administration of L-dopa. A perfusion of 10 μM g^{-1} per 30 min of γ-glutamyldopa in rats produces a 60% increase of the renal plasmatic flux.[89] The same dose of L-dopa induces no vasodilatation. Massive administration of γ-glutamyldopa (20 times the preceding dose) produces only a weak pressor effect, demonstrating that the systemic effects of the prodrug are low. The same principle was used for the synthesis of γ-glutamyl derivatives of dopamine itself and diacyldopamines.[90,91]

Similarly, it is possible to obtain a kidney-selective accumulation of sulfamethoxazole by administering the drug in the form of *N*-acetyl-γ-glutamate.[92] The regeneration of the free sulfamide requires the initial deacylation of the glutamic moiety thanks to an *N*-acylamino acid deacylase which is also present in the kidney in high concentrations (Fig. 31.14). The γ-glutamyl strategy for confining drug action to the kidney and the urinary tract implies that the prodrug under consideration can function as a substrate for γ-glutamyl transpeptidase and, eventually, for *N*-acylamino acid deacylase.

The unique glucosidase activity of the colonic microflora has been utilized to deliver selectively steroid prodrugs useful in treating inflammatory bowel disease.[93] Dexamethasone 21-β-D-glucoside appeared to be a good candidate as nearly 60% of an oral dose of the prodrug reached the caecum in the form of free steroid. Given orally, the parent dexamethasone was absorbed almost exclusively from the small intestine and less than 1% reached the caecum.[94] In various tumour tissues the activity of the enzyme uridine phosphorylase is markedly higher than in the surrounding normal tissues. This observation prompted the synthesis of 5-fluorouracil prodrugs. Among them, 5'-deoxy-5-fluorouracil shows high antitumour activity and less host toxicity compared to fluorouracil. This favourable therapeutic index is attributed to a preferential bioactivation by uridine phosphorylase in the tumour cells.[95,96]

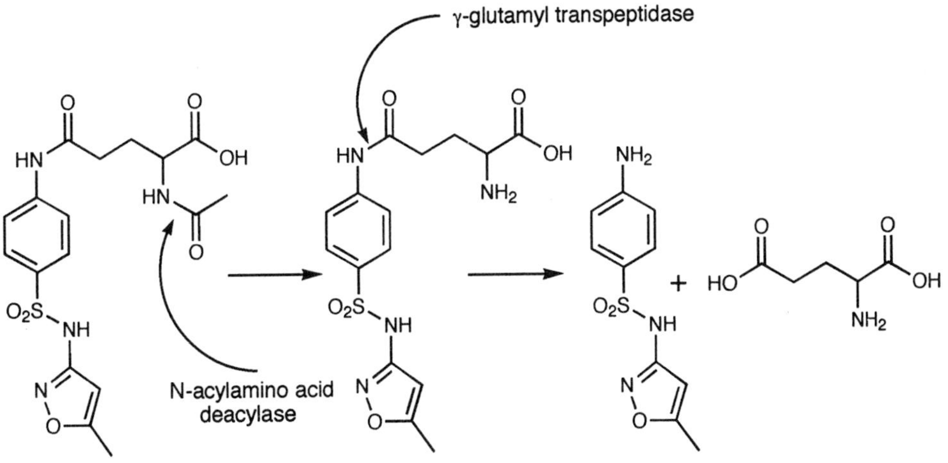

Fig. 31.14 Kidney-selective release of sulfamethoxazole.[92]

C. Prolonged duration of action

Unless they are accumulated in the fatty tissues, orally administered drugs are not expected to act much longer than their transit period in the gastrointestinal tract (12–48 h). For drugs rapidly cleared from the body, the duration of activity is even shorter, and a frequent dosing within the 24-h period is required to maintain adequate plasma concentrations. This frequent dosing of short-half-life drugs results in sharp peak–valley plasma concentration–time profiles, and consequently patient compliance is often poor.[97] However, for therapeutic, epidemiological, sociological or political reasons, durations of action prolonged over weeks or months are desired. The easiest administration route is then represented by intramuscular injection of depot preparations. The most successful applications are found in the domains of hormonal steroids, of antipsychotic drugs and, to a lesser extent, of antibiotics. The general strategy consists in preparing lipophilic prodrugs, dissolved or suspended in oily vehicles, and administering them by deep intramuscular injection.

1. Contraceptive steroids

Progestogens such as norethysterone enanthate and medroxyprogesterone acetate (MPA) have long durations of activity (3 months) owing primarily to slow release from the injection site and storage in the fatty tissues.[98] Progestogen–estrogen combinations such as dihydroxyprogesterone acetophenide–estradiol enanthate or MPA–estradiol cypionate (=cyclopentylpropionate) are administered on a monthly basis.

2. Treatment of menopause

The symptomatic treatment of menopause (sweating, hot flushes, depression) has been successfullly accomplished by the use of 200 mg of dehydroepiandrosterereone-3-heptanoate and 4 mg of estradiol 17-β-valerate in a suspension of a castor oil–benzyl benzoate vehicle.[99]

In the estradiol prodrug estradiol 3-benzoate 17-β-cyclooctenyl ether (EBCO), the phenolic hydroxyl group is masked as a benzoyl ester and the alcoholic 17-γ-hydroxyl as an enol ether derived from cyclooctanone (Fig. 31.15). Given to rats orally as a suspension in sesame oil, this derivative was active for 1 to 2 weeks because it was stored in body fat.[100]

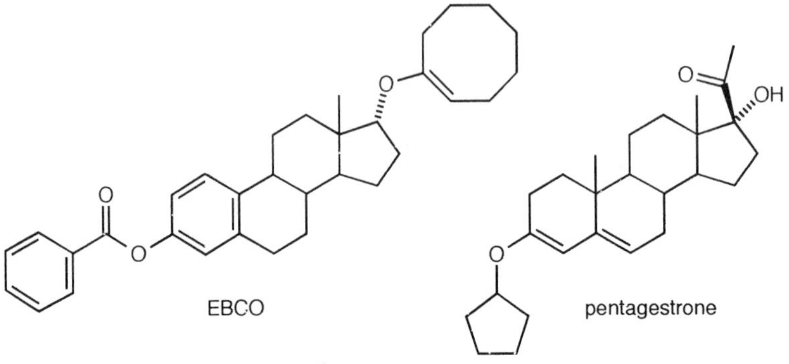

Fig. 31.15   Enol ethers as long-lasting steroid prodrugs .[100,101]

Enol ethers were also used for the synthesis of other long-lasting steroidal drugs such as penmestrol or pentagestrone.[101]

3.   Antipsychotics

Clinically, depot neuroleptics possess several advantages over the short-acting oral forms. Among these, the main advantages are (a) ease of administration, (b) reliable therapeutic effect with no increase in tolerance, (c) enhanced patient compliance, (d) reduced relapse and rehospitalization rate, and (f) enhanced rate and incidence of 'normal life' reintegration and resocialization.[98]

IV.   THE USE OF CASCADE PRODRUGS

Classical carrier-linked prodrugs may sometimes be ineffective because the prodrug linkage is too stable (amides, nonactivated esters). In such cases a β-assistance provided by a nuclophile easily generated *in vivo* can represent an interesting solution. The release of the active molecule from the prodrug proceeds through a two-step trigger mechanism for which the name 'cascade latentiation' was coined by Cain in 1975.[102,103]

The concept, also called distal hydrolysis[34] or the double prodrug concept,[25,106] is illustrated by the use of 2-acyloxymethylbenzoic acids as amine protective functions providing amides with the lability of esters (Fig. 31.16A) and by the use of substituted vinyl esters [= (2-oxo-1,3-dioxol-yl)methyl esters] as lipophilic cascade carriers for carboxylic acid-containing drugs such as ampicillin[104] or α-methyldopa[105] or various cephalosporins[12,21,30,107] (Fig. 31.16B).

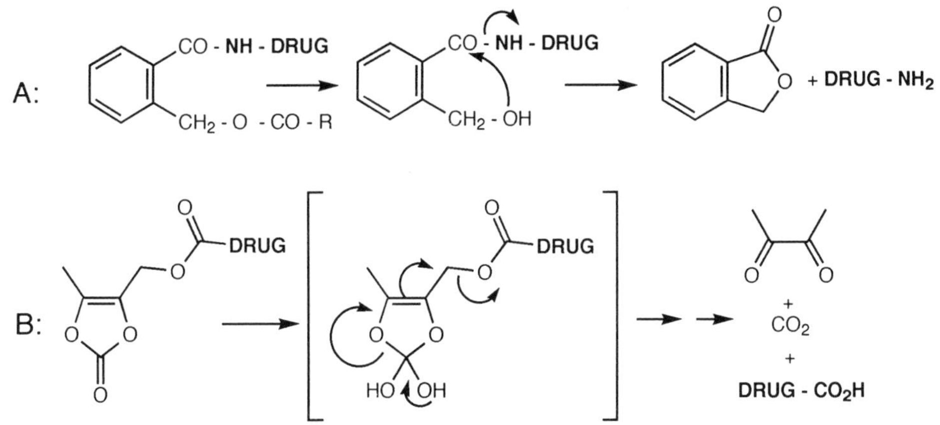

A:

B:

Fig. 31.16 (A) 2-Acyloxymethylbenzoic acids provides amides with the lability of esters.[102,103] (B) Substituted vinyl esters as lipophilic cascade carriers for carboxylic acid containing drugs.[104,105]

A. Water-soluble taxol prodrugs

Taxol is a potent microtubule-stabilizing agent that has been approved for cancer treatment. Despite taxol's therapeutic promise, its aqueous insolubility ($<0.004\,\mathrm{mg\,ml^{-1}}$) hampers its clinical application. Nicolaou *et al.*[108] report the design, synthesis and biological activity of prodrugs designed to improve water solubility and which can also be considered as cascade prodrugs (Fig. 31.17).

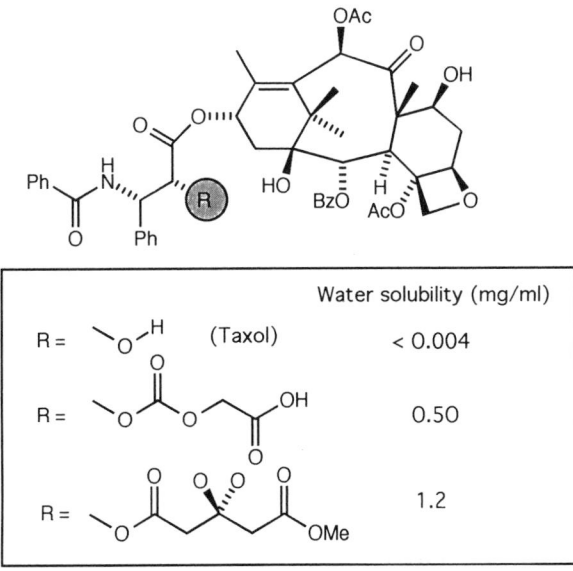

Fig. 31.17 Water-soluble protaxols.[108]

The mechanistic rationale of the design of these protaxols lies in the spontaneous decomposition of the carbonate ester after the abstraction of one of the activated protons or of an acidic proton (Fig. 31.18).

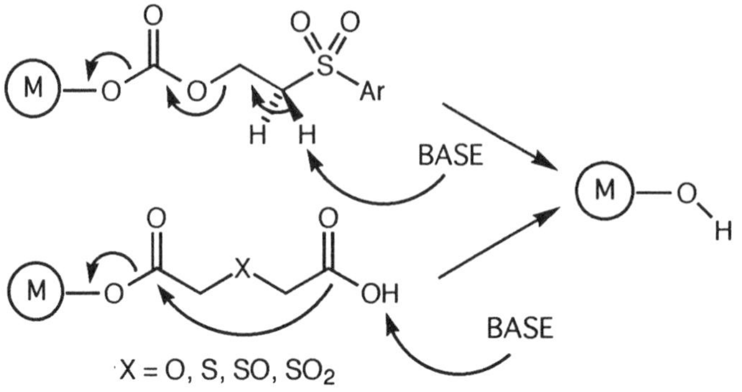

Fig. 31.18   Taxol release mechanisms from protaxols.[108]

B.   Bioactivation of an antibacterial prodrug

Although the amino acid (**1**) in Fig. 31.19 is a potent inhibitor of CMP-KDO synthetase, a key enzyme in the biosynthesis of the lipopolysaccharide of Gram-negative bacteria, it is unable to reach its cytoplasmic target and is therefore inactive as an antibacterial agent. Simple lipophilic esters are not useful for enhancing the delivery of the amino acid (**1**) since they are not cleaved by the bacteria. The double prodrug (**3**) on the other hand, has recently been found to solve the problem.[109] Upon entry into bacterial cells, the disulfide bond in compound (**3**) is reduced by sulfydryl compounds present in the intracellular milieu, resulting in the formation of the thiol (**2**). This is highly unstable and the active amino acid (**1**) is formed by a rapid intramolecular displacement.

C.   Double prodrugs derived from pilocarpine

Monoesters of pilocarpic acid are potentially useful prodrug forms for ocular administration and enable an efficient penetration through the corneal membrane. Unfortunately, they suffer from poor solution stability as in aqueous solution they cyclize spontaneously to pilocarpine.[110] However, double esters derived from pilocarpic acid (Fig. 31.20) possess high stability in aqueous solution (shelf-lives of more than 5 years at 20°C were estimated). At the same time, they are readily converted to pilocarpine under conditions simulating those occurring *in vivo* through a sequential process involving enzymatic hydrolysis of the *O*-acyl bond followed by spontaneous lactonization of the intermediate pilocarpic monoester.[111]

D.   Double prodrugs for peptides

Amsbery and Borchard[112,113] have applied Cain's cascade concept to prepare lipophilic

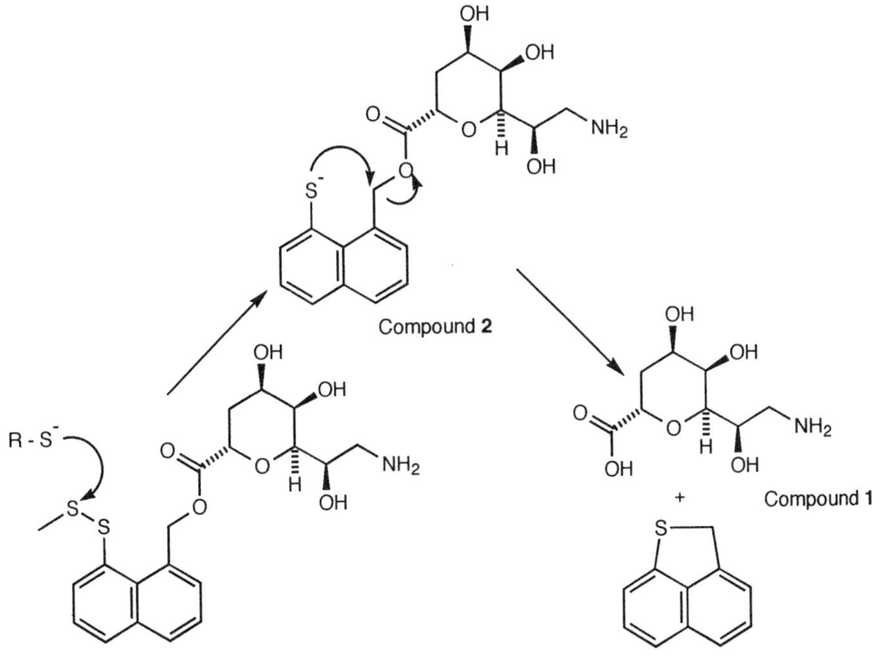

Fig. 31.19 Bioactivation of the antibacterial prodrug of an impermeant inhibitor of 3-deoxy-D-manno-2-octulosonate cytidylyltransferase.[109]

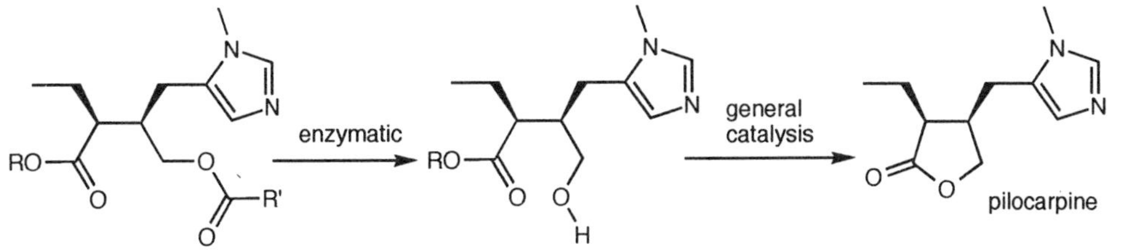

Fig. 31.20 Double esters derived from pilocarpic acid are readily converted to pilocarpine under conditions simulating those occurring *in vivo*.[111]

polypeptide prodrugs. The amine functionality of the polypeptide is coupled to 2'-acylated derivatives of 3-(2',5'-dihydroxy-4',6'-dimethylphenyl)-3,3-dimethylpropionic acid (Fig. 31.21). Under simulated physiological conditions the parent amine is regenerated in a two-step process: enzymatic hydrolysis of the phenolic ester, followed by a nonenzymatic intramolecular cyclization leading to the release of the free amine (polypeptide) and a lactone. The lactoniztion step is highly favoured because of the steric pressure created by the three methyl groups ('trimethyl lock' concept). An alternative to the hydrolytic first step involves a bioreductive generation of the intermediate phenolic amide (Fig. 31.21).

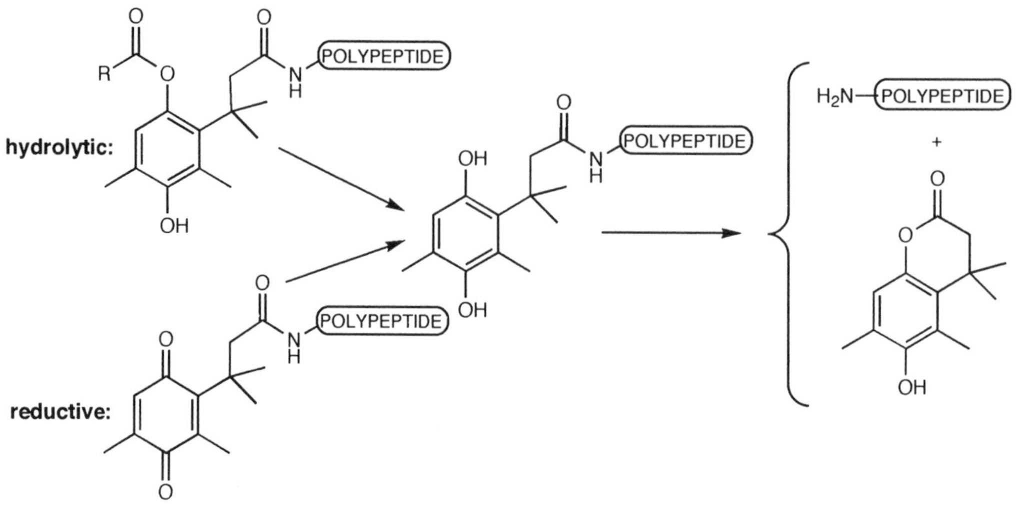

Fig. 31.21   Proposed conversion of esterase-sensitive and redox-sensitive double prodrugs of peptides.[112,113]

V. SOFT DRUGS

The 'soft' quaternary ammonium salts developed by Bodor[114–117] are vulnerable derivatives of their 'hard' analogues. In general, they show the same type of activity but with a much shorter half-life, as is the case for the soft analogue of cetylpyridinium chloride (Fig. 31.22). Both compounds have the same hydrophobic chain length, and thus similar surface-active and antimicrobial properties. However, the soft analogue is about 40 times less toxic than its hard analogue in terms of LD_{50}.[115] This is because the soft analogue undergoes a fast and easy hydrolytic deactivation resulting in the simultaneous destruction of the positive quaternary head and the surface-active properties.

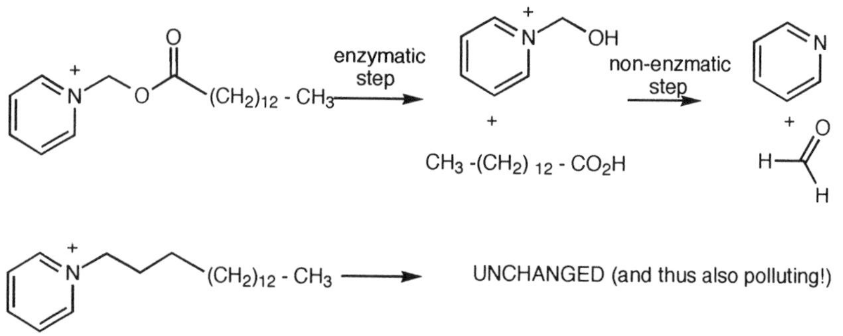

Fig. 31.22   The soft analogue of cetylpyridinium chloride.[115]

In a similar way, the tetradecyloxymethyl quaternary salt of pilocarpine allows enhanced penetration through the cornea followed by a facile hydrolytic cleavage to pilocarpine (Fig. 31.23). The corresponding hard analogue (*N*-cetylpilocarpine) is unable to regenerate the parent drug and lacks any activity.[118]

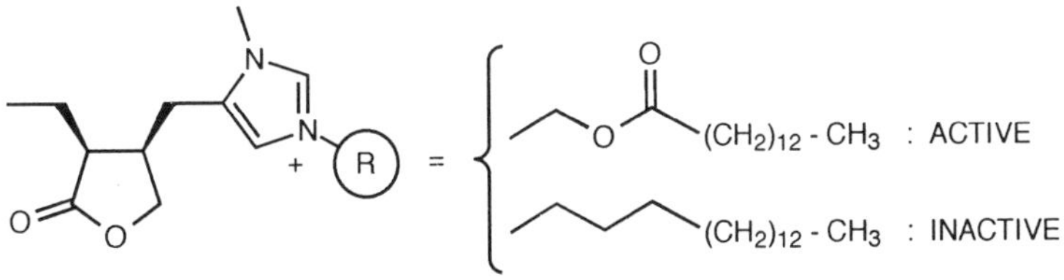

Fig. 31.23   The soft quaternary derivative of pilocarpine allows an enhanced penetration through the cornea.[118]

VI. CONCLUSION

The carrier-prodrug approach is particularly successful in the antibiotics field and in the improvement of some pharmacokinetic parameters. Other prodrug examples are less convincing; they have nevertheless been included in this chapter to illustrate the 'state of the art'.[119] Probably most of them have never been tested in man or laboratory. The design of carrier-prodrugs represents in medicinal chemistry the counterpart of the design of protective groups in organic chemistry. The approaches have much in common; in both of them imagination has no limits and reigns as master. However, among the enormous number of candidates, only very few attain real success and celebrity.

REFERENCES

1. Johnston, G. A. R., Curtis, D. R., DeGroat, W. C. and Duggan, A. W. (1968) Central actions of ibotenic acid and muscimol. *Biochem. Pharmacol.* **17:** 2488–2489.
2. Ganellin, C. R. (1993) Discovery of cimetidine, ranitidine and other H2-receptor histamine antagonists. In Ganellin, C. R. and Roberts, S. M. (eds) *Medicinal Chemistry. The Role of Organic Chemistry in Drug Research*, pp. 228–255. Academic Press, London.
3. Wermuth, C. G. and Bizière, K. (1986) Pyridazinyl-GABA derivatives: a new class of synthetic GABA_A antagonists. *Trends Pharmacol. Sci.* **7:** 421–424.
4. Rognan, D., Boulanger, T., Hoffmann, R., Vercauteren, D., André, J. -M., Durant, F. and Wermuth, C. G. (1992) Structure and molecular modeling of GABA_A receptor antagonists. *J. Med. Chem.* **35:** 1969–1977.
5. Endo, A. (1985) Compactin (ML-236B) and related compounds as potential cholesterol-lowering agents that inhibit HMG-CoA reductase. *J. Med. Chem.* **28:** 401–405.
6. Lee, T. J. (1987) Synthesis, SARs and therapeutic potential of HMG-CoA reductase inhibitors. *Trends Pharmacol. Sci.* **8:** 442–446.
7. Chang, R. S. L. and Lotti, V. Y. (1986) Biochemical and pharmacological characterization of an extremely potent and selective nonpeptide CCK antagonist. *Proc. Natl. Acad. Sci. USA* **83:** 4923–4926.
8. Wani, M. C., Taylor, H. L., Wall, M. E., Coogan, P. C. and McPail, A. J. (1971) Plant antitumor

agents. IV. The isolation and structure of taxol, a novel antileukemic and antitumor agent from *Taxus brevifolia. J. Am. Chem. Soc.* **93:** 2325–2327.

9. Schiff, P. B., Fant, J. and Horwitz, S. B. (1979) Promotion of microtubule assembly *in vitro* by Taxol. *Nature* **277:** 665–669.

10. Silverman, R. B. (1992) *The Organic Chemistry of Drug Design and Drug Action,* pp. 266–270. Academic Press, San Diego.

11. Gully, D., Canton, M., Boigegrain, R. *et al.* (1993) Biochemical and pharmacological profile of a potent and selective nonpeptide antagonist of the neurotensin receptor. *Proc. Natl. Acad. Sci. USA* **90:** 65–69.

12. Albert, A. (1958) Chemical aspects of selective toxicity. *Nature (London)* **182:** 421–423.

13. Harper, N. J. (1959) Drug latentiation. *J. Med. Pharm. Chem.* **1:** 467–500.

14. Wermuth, C. G. (1983) Bioprécurseurs contre prodrogues. In Briot, M., Cautreds, W. and Roncucci, R. (eds) *Drug Metabolism and Drug Design: Quo Vadis?* pp. 253–271. Sanofi-Clin-Midy, Montpellier.

15. Wermuth, C. G. (1984) Designing prodrugs and biprecursors. In Jolles, G. and Wooldrige, K. R. M. (eds) *Drug Design: Fact or Fantasy?* pp. 47–72. Academic Press, London.

16. Sinkula, A. A. (1977) Prodrugs, protective groups and the medicinal chemist. In Mathieu, J. (ed.) *Medicinal Chemistry.* pp. 125–133. Elsevier, Amsterdam.

17. Stella, V. (1975) Pro-drugs: an overview and definition. In Higuchi, T. and Stella, V. (eds) *Pro-drugs as Novel Drug Delivery Systems,* pp. 1–115. American Chemical Society, Washington DC.

18. Wermuth, C. G. (1980) Les prodrogues, des médicaments plus sûrs et plus maniables. *Bull. Soc. Pharm. Bordeaux* **119:** 107–129.

19. Wermuth, C. G. (1981) Modulation of natural substances in order to improve their pharmacokinetic properties. In Beal, J. L. and Reinhard, E. (eds) *Natural Products as Medicinal Agents.* pp. 185–216. Hippokrates Verlag, Stuttgart.

20. Daehne, W. V., Frederiksen, E., Gundersen, E., Lund, F., March, P., Petersen, H. J., Roholt, K., Tybring, L. and Godtfredsen, W. O. (1970) Acyloxymethyl esters of ampicillin. *J. Med. Chem.* **13:** 607–612.

21. Bodin, N. O., Ekström, B., Forsgren, U., Jalar, L. P., Magni, L., Ramsey, C. H. and Sjöberg, B. (1975) Bacampicilline: a new orally well-absorbed derivative of ampicillin. *Antimicrob. Agents Chemother.* **8:** 518–525.

22. Clayton, J. P., Cole, M., Elson, S. W., Ferres, H., Hanson, J. C., Mizen, L. W. and Sutherland, R. (1976) Preparation, hydrolysis, and oral absorption of lactonyl esters of penicillin. *J. Med. Chem.* **19:** 1385–1391.

23. Drabek, J. and Neumann, R. (1985) Proinsecticides. In Hutson, D. H. and Roberts, T. R. (eds) *Progress in Pesticide Biochemistry and Toxicology,* pp. 35–86. Wiley, Chichester.

24. Higuchi, T. and Stella, V. (1975) *Pro-drugs as Novel Drug Delivery Systems.* ACS Symposium Series, A.C. vol. 14. American Chemical Society. Washington DC.

25. Bundgaard, H. (1991) Design and application of prodrugs. In Krogsgaard-Larsen, P. and Bundgaard, H. (eds) *A Textbook of Drug Design and Development,* pp. 113–191. Harwood Academic Publishers, Chur.

26. McClure, D. (1975) The effect of a pro-drug of epinephrine (dipivaloyl-epinephrine) in glaucoma – general pharmacology, toxicology and clinical experience. In Higuchi, T. and Stella, V. (eds) *Pro-Drugs as Novel Drug Delivery Systems,* pp. 224–235. American Chemical Society, Washington DC.

27. Horn, A. S. (1980) Pro-drugs of domaminergic agonists. *Chem. Ind.* 441–444.

28. Westerink, B. H. C., Dijkstra, D., Feenstra, M. G. P., Grol, C. J., Horn, A. S., Rollema, H. and Wirix, E. (1980) Dopaminergic prodrugs: brain concentration and neurochemical effects of 5,6- and 6,7-ADTN after administration as dibenzoyl esters. *Eur. J. Pharmacol.* **61:** 7–15.

29. Tullar, B. F., Minatoya, H. and Lorenz, R. R. (1976) Esters of *N*-tert-butylarterenol. Long-acting new bronchodilators with reduced cardiac effects. *J. Med. Chem.* **19:** 834–838.

30. Lin, T. S. (1984) Synthesis and in vitro antiviral activity of 3′-*O*-acyl derivatives of 5′-amino-2′-deoxy thymidine: potential prodrugs for topical application. *J. Pharm. Sci.* **73:** 1568–1571.

31. Harnden, M. R., Jarvest, R. L., Boyd, M. R., Sutton, D. and Vere hodge, R. A. (1989) Prodrugs of the selective antiherpesvirus agent 9-[4-hydroxy-3-(hydroxymethyl)but-1-yl]guanine (BRL 39123) with improved gastrointestinal absorption properties. *J. Med. Chem.* **32:** 1738–1743.

32. Jones, L. A., Moorman, A. R., Chamberlain, S. D., Miranda, P. D., Reynolds, D. J., Burns, C. L.

and Krenitzky, T. A. (1992) Di- and triester prodrugs of the varicella-zoster antiviral agent 6-methoxypurine arabinoside. *J. Med. Chem.* **35:** 56–63.

33. Bodor, N., Sloan, K. B., Little, R. J., Selk, S. H. and Caldwell, L. (1982) Soft drugs 4. 3-Spirothiazolidines of hydrocortisone and its derivatives. *Int. J. Pharm.* **10:** 307–321.

34. Collis, A. J. (1993) Drugs access and prodrugs. In Gannellin C. R. and Roberts, S. M. (eds) *Medicinal Chemistry – The Role of Organic Chemistry in Drug Research*, pp. 61–82. Academic Press, London.

35. Anden, N. E., Corrodi, H., Dahlström, A., Fuxe K. and Högfelt, T. (1966) Effects of tyrosine hydroxylase inhibition on the amine levels of central monoamine neurons. *Life Sci.* **5:** 561–568.

36. Frey, H. H., Popp, C. and Löscher, W. (1979) Influence of inhibitors of the high affinity GABA uptake on seizure threshold in mice. *Neuropharmacology.* **18:** 581–590.

37. Ulm, E. H., Hichens, M., Gomez, H. J., Till, A. E., Hand, E., Vassil, T. C., Biollaz, J., Brunner, H. R. and Schelling, J. L. (1982) Enalapril maleate and a lysine analogue (MK-521): Disposition in man. *Br. J. Pharmacol.* **14:** 357–362.

38. Swanson, B. L., Vlasses, P. H., Ferguson, R. K., Berquist, P. A., Till, A. E., Irvin, J. D. and Harris, K. (1984) Influence of food on the bioavailability of enalapril. *J. Pharm. Sci.* **73:** 1655–1657.

39. Zannad, F. (1993) Trandolapril, how does it differ from other angiotensin converting enzyme inhibitors? *Drugs* **46:** 172–183.

40. Tsybina, N. M., Ostrovskaya, R. U., Protopova, T. V., Parin, V. V., Selezneva, N. I. and Skolainov, A. P. (1974) Synthesis and pharmacological activity of gamma-aminobutyric acid derivatives. *Khim. Pharm. Zh.* **17:** 10–13.

41. Ostrovskaya, R. U., Parin, V. V. and Tsybina, N. M. (1972) The comparative neurotropic potency of gamma-aminobutyric acid and its cetyl esters. *Byul. Eksp. Biol. Med.* **73:** 51–55.

42. Beardsley, G. P. and Rosowsky, A. (1980) Effect of methotrexate γ-monohexadecyl ester (γ-MHxMTX) on nucleoside uptake by human leukemic cells. *Proc. Am. Assoc. Cancer Res.* **21** (71st Meeting).

43. Jones, G. (1980) Lipoidal pro-drug analogues of various anti-inflammatory agents. *Chem. Ind. (London)* 452–456.

44. Akesson, B., Gronowitz, S., Herslof, B. and Ohlson, R. (1978) Absorption of synthetic, stereochemically defined acylglycerols in the rat. *Lipids* (1978) **13:** 338–343.

45. Paris, G. Y., Garmaise, D. L., Cimon, D. G., Swett, L., Carter, G. W. and Young, P. (1979) Glycerides as prodrugs. 1. Synthesis and antiinflammatory activity of 1,3-bis(alkanoyl)-2-(O-acetylsalicyloyl) glycerides (aspirin triglycerides). *J. Med. Chem.* **22:** 683–687.

46. Paris, G. Y., Garmaise, D. L., Cimon, D. G., Swett, L., Carter, G. W. and Young, P. (1980) Glycerides as prodrugs. 2. 1,3-Dialkanoyl-2-(2-methyl-4-oxo-1,3-benzodioxan-2-yl) glycerides (cyclic aspirin triglycerides) as antiinflammatory agents. *J. Med. Chem.* **23:** 79–82.

47. Paris, G. Y., Garmaise, D. L., Cimon, D. G., Swett, L., Carter, G. W. and Young, P. (1980) Glycerides as prodrugs. 3. Synthesis and antiinflammatory activity of [1-(p-chlorobenzoyl)-5-methoxy-2-methylindole-3-acetyl] glycerides (indomethacin glycerides). *J. Med. Chem.* **23:** 9–12.

48. Garzon Aburpeh, A., Poupaert, J. H., Claesen, M., Dumont, P. and Atassi, G. (1983) 1,3-Dipalmitoylglycerol ester of chlorambucil as a lymphotropic orally administrable antineoplastic agent. *J. Med. Chem.* **26:** 1200–1203.

49. Jacob, J. N., Hesse, G. W. and Shashoua, V. E. (1987) Gamma-aminobutyric acid esters. 3. Synthesis, brain uptake, and pharmacological properties of C-18 glyceryl lipid esters of GABA with varying degrees of unsaturation. *J. Med. Chem.* **30:** 1573–1576.

50. Deverre, J. R., Loiseau, P., Couvreur, P., Letourneux, Y., Gayral, P. and Benoit, J. P. (1989) In-vitro evaluation of filaricidal activity of GABA and 1,3-dipalmitoyl-2-(4-aminobutyryl) glycerol HCl; a diglyceride prodrug. *J. Pharm. Pharmacol.* **41:** 191–193.

51. Hong, C. I., An, S.-H., Schliselfeld, L., Buchheit, D. G., Nechaev, A., Kiritsis, A. J. and West, C. R. (1988) Nucleoside conjugates. 10. Synthesis and antitumor activity of 1-β-D-arabinofuranosylcytosine 5'-diphosphate-1,2-dipalmitins. *J. Med. Chem.* **31:** 1793–1798.

52. Namane, A., Gouyette, C., Fillion, M. -P., Fillion, G. and Huynh-Dinh, T. (1992) Improved brain delivery of AZT using a gycosyl phosphotriester prodrug. *J. Med. Chem.* **35:** 3039–3044.

53. Jansen, A. B. A. and Russel, T. J. (1965) Some novel penicillin derivatives. *J. Chem. Soc.* 2127–2132.

54. Binderup, E., Godtfredsen, W. O. and Roholt, K. (1971) Orally active cephaloglycin esters. *J. Antibiot.* **24:** 767–773.

55. Saari, W. S., Freedman, M. B. and Hartman, R. D. (1978) Synthesis and antihypertensive activity of some ester progenitors of methyldopa. *J. Med. Chem.* (1978) **21:** 746–753.

56. Falch, E., Krogsgaard-Larsen, P. and Christensen, A. V. (1981) Esters of isoguvacine as potential prodrugs. *J. Med. Chem.* **24:** 285–289.

57. Svahn, C. M., Merenyi, F., Karlson, L., Widlund, L. and Grälls, M. (1986) Tranexamic acid derivatives with enhanced absorption. *J. Med. Chem.* **29:** 448–453.

58. Torriani, H. (1979) Talniflumate. *Drugs Future* **4:** 448–450.

59. Torriani, H. (1982) Talmetacin. *Drugs Future* **7:** 823–824.

60. Alexander, J., Fromtling, R. A., Bland, J. A., Pelak, B. A. and Gilfillan, E. C. (1991) (Acyloxy)alkyl carbamate prodrugs of norfloxacin. *J. Med. Chem.* **34:** 78–81.

61. Walsh, D. A., Moran, H. W., Shamblee, D. A., Welstead, Jr, W. J., Nolan, J. C., Sancilio, L. F. and Graff, G. (1990) Antiinflammatory agents. 4. Synthesis and biological evaluation of potential prodrugs of 2-amino-3-benzoylbenzeneacetic acid and 2-amino-3-(4-chlorobenzoyl)benzeneacetic acid. *J. Med. Chem.* **33:** 2296–2304.

62. Galzinga, L., Garbin, L., Bianchi, M. and Marzotto, A. (1978) Properties of two derivatives of γ-aminobutyric acid (GABA) capable of abolishing cardiazol- and bicuculline-induced convulsions in the rat. *Arch. Int. Pharmacodyn.* **235:** 73–85.

63. Ahtee, L., Halmekoski, J., Heinonen, H. and Koskimies, A. (1979) Comparison of the central nervous system actions of taurine and *N*-pivaloyltaurine. *Br. J. Pharmacol.* **66:** 480P.

64. Kaplan, J. P., Raizon, B., Desarmenien, M., Feltz, P., Headley, P. M., Worms, P., Lloyd, K. G. and Bartholini, G. (1980) New anticonvulsants: Schiff bases of γ-aminobutyric acid and γ-aminobutyramide. *J. Med. Chem.* **23:** 702–704.

65. Jensen, N. P., Friedman, J. J., Kropp, H. and Kahan, F. M. (1980) Use of acetylacetone to prepare a prodrug of cycloserine. *J. Med. Chem.* **23:** 6–8.

66. Bodor, N. S., Sloan, K. B. and Hussain, A. A. Novel transient pro-drug forms of L-DOPA. U.S. Patent 3 891 696 (24 June 1975; Inter'X Res. Corp.).

67. Koch, H. (1981) ST-1059. *Drugs Future* **6:** 244–246.

68. Vicentini, C. B., Guarneri, M. and Sarto, G. (1983) Hypoglycemic compounds. Sulfonylurea derivatives containing amino acids and dipeptides. *Farmaco, Ed Sci.* **38:** 595–608.

69. Boehringer. Dérivés de la L-(3,4-dixhydroxy-phényl)-2-méthyl alanine et leur préparation. Belgian Patent 839 362 (9 March 1976; Boehringer Mannheim GmbH).

70. Kinsbury, W. D., Boehm, J. C., Mehta, R. J. and Grappel, S. F. (1983) Transport of antimicrobial agents using peptide carrier systems: anticandidal activity of *m*-fluorophenylalanine peptide conjugates. *J. Med. Chem.* **26:** 1725–1729.

71. Hu, M., Subramanian, P., Mosberg, H. I. and Amidon, G. L. (1989) Use of the peptide carrier system to improve the intestinal absorption of L-α-methyldopa: carrier kinetics, intestinal permeabilities, and *in vitro* hydrolysis of dipeptidyl derivatives of L-α-methyldopa. *Pharm. Res.* **6:** 66–70.

72. Buur, A., Bundgaard, H. and Falch, E. (1986) Prodrugs of 5-fluorouracil. VII. Hydrolysis kinetics and physiocochemical properties of *N*-ethoxy- and *N*-phenoxycarbonylmethyl derivatives of 5-fluorouracil. *Acta Pharm. Suec.* **23:** 205–216.

73. Larsen, J. D. and Bundgaard, H. (1987) Prodrug forms for the sulfonamide group. I. Evaluation of *N*-acyl derivatives, *N*-sulfonylamidines, *N*-sulfonyl-sulfinimines and sulfonylureas as possible prodrug derivatives. *Int. J. Pharm.* **37:** 87–95.

74. Bundgaard, H., Buur, A., Hansen, K. T., Larsen, J. D., Moss, J. and Olsen, L. (1988) Prodrugs as drug delivery systems. 77. Phthalidyl derivatives as prodrug forms for amides, sulfonamides, carbamates and other NH-acidic compounds. *Int. J. Pharm.* **45:** 47–57.

75. Hardcastle, G. A., Johnson, D. A., Panetta, C. A., Scott, A. I. and Sutherland, S. A. (1966) The preparation and structure of hetacillin. *J. Org. Chem.* **31:** 897–899.

76. Bundgaard, H. (1985) Design of prodrugs: bioreversible derivatives for various functional groups and chemical entities. In Bundgaard, H. (ed.) *Design of Prodrugs*, pp. 1–92. Elsevier, Amsterdam.

77. Anonymous (1986) Droxicam. *Drugs Future* **11:** 835–836.

78. Zeller, P., Pletscher, A., Gey, K. F., Gutmann, H., Hegedus, B. and Staub, O. (1959) Amino acid and fatty acid hydrazides: chemistry and action on monoamine oxides. *Ann. N.Y. Acad. Sci.* **80:** 555–567.

79. Knapp, F. F. J., Goodman, M. M., Callahan, A. P., Ferren, L. A., Kabalka, G. W. and Sastry,

K. A. R. (1983) New myocardial imaging agents: stabilization of radioiodine as a terminal vinyl iodide moiety on tellurium fatty acids. *J. Med. Chem.* **26:** 1293–1300.

80. Wess, G., Kramer, W., Schubert, G., Bickel, M., Hoffman, A. and Baringhaus, K. H. (1993) Coupling of drugs to modified bile acids for liver specific targeting. *Abst. Pap. 205th Meet. Am. Chem. Soc.* Pt. 1, MEDI 152.

81. Biel, J. H. and Martin, Y. C. (1971) Organic synthesis as a source of new drugs. In American Chemical Society (ed.) *Drug Discovery – Science and Development in a Changing Society.* pp. 81–111. American Chemical Society, Washington DC.

82. Whittaker, J. R. (1971) Biosynthesis of a thiouracil pheomelanin in embryonic pigment cells exposed to thiouracil. *J. Biol. Chem.* **246:** 6217–6226.

83. Dencker, L., Larsson, B., Olander, K., Ullberg, S. and Yokota, M. (1979) False precursors of melanin as selective melanoma seekers. *Br. J. Cancer* **39:** 449–452.

84. Wätjen, F., Buchardt, O. and Langvad, E. (1982) Affinity therapeutics. 1. Selective incorporation of 2-thiouracil derivatives in murine melanomas. Cytostatic activity of 2-thiouracil arotinoids, 2-thiouracil retinoids, arotinoids and retinoids. *J. Med. Chem.* **25:** 956–960.

85. Ariëns, E. J. (1971) Modulation of pharmacokinetics by molecular manipulation. In Ariëns, E. J. (ed.) *Drug Design.* pp. 1–127. Academic Press, New York.

86. Ariëns, E. J. (1975) Pharmacological basis of cancer therapy. In *Twenty-Seventh Annual Symposium on Fundamental Cancer Research, 1974.* The University of Texas M.D. Anderson Hospital and Tumor Institute at Houston: The Williams and Wilkins Company, Baltimore.

87. Hurwitx, E., Kashi, R., Burowsky, D., Arnon, R. and Haimovitch, J. (1983) Site-directed chemotherapy with a drug bound to anti-idiotypic antibody to a lymphoma cell-surface IgM. *Int. J. Cancer* **31:** 745–748.

88. Magnan, S. D. J., Shirota, F. N. and Nagasawa, H. T. (1982) Drug latentiation by γ-glutamyl transpeptidase. *J. Med. Chem.* **25:** 1018–1021.

89. Wilk, S., Mizoguchi, H. and Orlowski, M. (1978) Gamma-gutamyl-DOPA: a kidney specific dopamine precursor. *J. Pharmacol. Exp. Ther.* **206:** 227–232.

90. Kynel, J. J., Minard, F. N. and Jones, P. H. (1979) Peripheral dopamine receptors. In Imbs, J. L. and Schwartz, J. (eds) *Symposium on Peripheral Dopaminergic Receptors – Strasbourg, July 1978,* pp. 369–380. Pergamon Press, Oxford.

91. Jones, P. H., Kyncl, J., Ours, C. W. and Somani, P. (1977) Esters of γ-glutamyl amide of dopamine. US Patent 4 017 636 (12 April 1977; to Abott Laboratories).

92. Orlowski, M., Mizoguchi, H. and Wilks, S. (1979) *N*-Acyl-γ-glutamyl derivatives of sulfamethoxazole as models of kidney-selective prodrugs. *J. Pharmacol. Exp. Ther.* **212:** 167–172.

93. Friend, D. R. and Chang, G. W. (1985) Drug glycosides: potential prodrugs for colon-specific drug delivery. *J. Med. Chem.* **28:** 51–57.

94. Friend, D. R. and Chang, G. W. (1984) A colon-specific drug-delivery system based on drug glycosides and the glycosidases of colonic bacteria. *J. Med. Chem.* **27:** 261–266.

95. Cook, A. F., Holman, M. J., Kramer, M. J. and Trown, P. W. (1979) Florinated pyrimidine nucleoside. 3. Synthesis and antitumor activity of a series of 5′-deoxy-5-fluoropyrimidine nucleosides. *J. Med. Chem.* **22:** 1330–1335.

96. Au, J. L. -S., Walker, J. S. and Rustman, Y. (1983) Pharmacokinetic studies of 5-fluorouracil and 5′-deoxy-5-fluorouridine in rats. *J. Pharmacol. Exp. Ther.* **227:** 174–180.

97. Stella, V. J., Charman, W. N. A. and Naringrekar, V. H. (1985) Prodrugs: do they have advantages in clinical practice? *Drugs,* **29:** 455–473.

98. Sinkula, A. A. (1985) Sustained drug action accomplished by the prodrugs approach. In Bundgaard, H. (ed.) *Design of Prodrugs,* pp. 157–176. Elsevier, Amsterdam.

99. Dusterberg, B. and Wendt, H. (1983) Plasma levels of dehydroepiandrosterone and 17β-estradiol after intramuscular administration of Gynodian-Depot® in 3 women. *Hormone Res.* **17:** 84–89.

100. Falconi, G., Galetti, F., Celasco, G. and Gardi, R. (1972) Oral long-lasting estrogenic activity of estradiol 3-benzoate 17-cyclooctenyl ether. *Steroids* **20:** 627–632.

101. Ercoli, A. and Gardi, R. (1960) Δ^4-3-Keto steroidal ethers. Paradoxical dependency on their effectiveness on the administration route. *J. Am. Chem. Soc.* **82:** 746–748.

102. Cain, B. F. (1975) The role of structure–activity studies in the design of antitumor agents. *Cancer Chemother. Rep.* **59:** 679–683.

103. Cain, B. F. (1976) 2-Acyloxymethylbenzoic acids. Novel amine protective functions providing

amides with the lability of esters. *J. Org. Chem.* **41:** 2029–2031.

104. Sakamoto, F., Ikeda, S. and Tsukamoto, G. (1984) Studies on prodrugs. II. Preparation and characterization of (5-substituted 2-oxo-1,3-dioxolen-4-yl)methyl esters of ampicillin. *Chem. Pharm. Bull.* **32:** 2241–2248.

105. Saari, W. S., Halczenko, W., Cochran, D. W., Dobrinska, M. R., Vincek, W. C., Titus, D. C., Gaul, S. L. and Sweet, C. S. (1984) 3-Hydroxy-α-methyltryrosine progenitors: synthesis and evaluation of some (2-oxo-1,3-dioxol-4-yl)methyl esters. *J. Med. Chem.* **27:** 713–717.

106. Bundgaard, H. (1991) Novel chemical approaches in prodrug design. *Drugs Future* **16:** 443–458.

107. Borgman, R. J., Smith, R. V. and Keiser, J. E. (1975) The acetylation of apomorphine. An improved method for the selective preparation of diacetylapomorphine utilizing trifuoroacetic acid/acetyl bromide. *Synthesis* 249–250.

108. Nicolaou, K. C., Riemer, C., Kerr, M. A., Rideout, D. and Wrasidlo, W. (1993) Design, synthesis and biological activity of protaxols. *Nature (London)* **364:** 464–466.

109. Norbeck, D. W., Rosenbrook, W., Kramer, J. B., Grampovnik, D. J. and Lartey, P. A. (1989) A novel prodrug of an impermeant inhibitor of 3-deoxy-D-manno-2-octulosonate cytidylyl-transferase has antibacterial activity. *J. Med. Chem.* **32:** 625–629.

110. Bundgaard, H., Falch, E., Larsen, C. and Mikkelson, T. J. (1986) Pilocarpine prodrugs I. Synthesis, stability, bioconversion, and physiocochemical properties of sequentially labile pilocarpine acid diesters. *J. Pharm. Sci.* **75:** 36–44.

111. Bundgaard, H., Falch, E., Larsen, C., Mosher, G. L. and Mikkelson, T. J. (1986) Pilocarpine prodrugs II. Synthesis, stability, bioconversion and physiocochemical properties of sequentially labile pilocarpine acid diesters. *J. Pharm. Sci.* **75:** 775–783.

112. Amsberry, K. L. and Borchardt, R. T. (1991) Amine prodrugs which utilize hydroxy-amide lactonization. I. A potential redox-sensitive amide prodrug. *Pharm. Res.* **8:** 323–330.

113. Amsberry, K. L. Gerstenberger, A. E. and Borchardt, R. T. (1991) Amine prodrugs which utilize hydroxy-amide lactonization. II. A potential esterase-sensitive prodrug. *Pharm. Res.* **8:** 455–461.

114. Bodor, N. S. (1977) Novel approaches for the design of membrane transport properties of drugs. In Roche, E. B. (ed.) *Design of Biopharmaceutical Properties through Prodrugs and Analogs,* pp. 98–135. American Pharmaceutical Association, Washington DC.

115. Bodor, N. S., Kaminski, J. J. and Selk, S. (1980) Soft drugs. 1. Labile quaternary ammonium salts as soft antimicrobials. *J. Med. Chem.* **23:** 469–474.

116. Bodor, N. S. and Kaminski, J. J. (1980) Soft drugs. 2. Soft alkylating compounds as potential antitumor agents. *J. Med. Chem.* **232:** 566–569.

117. Bodor, N. S., Woods, R., Raper, C., Kearney, P. and Kaminski, J. J. (1980) Soft drugs. 3. A new class of anticholinergic agents. *J. Med. Chem.* **23:** 474–480.

118. Bodor, N. (1985) Prodrugs versus soft drugs. In Bundgaard, H. (ed.) *Design of Prodrugs.* pp. 333–354. Elsevier, Amsterdam.

119. Pitman, I. H. (1981) Pro-drugs of amides, imides and amines. In *Medicinal Research Reviews.* pp. 189–214. Wiley, New York.

Designing Prodrugs and Bioprecursors II: Bioprecursor Prodrugs

CAMILLE G. WERMUTH

Although a detailed knowledge of permeability and enzymes can assist a designer in finding pro-agents...
(they) will have in mind an organism's normal reaction to a foreign substance is to burn it up as food
Adrien Albert[1]

THE PRACTICE OF MEDICINAL CHEMISTRY
ISBN 0-12-744640-0

I. THE ACTIVE METABOLITE CONCEPT AND ITS PROSPECTIVE APPLICATION

The pioneering experiments of the collaborators of Fourneau[2] demonstrated that Prontosil rubrum is inactive *in vitro* and is converted *in vivo* into sulfanilamide, the true active principle. Since then the possibility of metabolic bioactivation has been clearly recognized and largely developed, especially by Brodie.[3] Table 32.1 summarizes some early recognized active metabolites.

Table 32.1   Early recognized active metabolites.

Drug	Active metabolite
Acetanilide	Paracetamol
Proguanil	Cycloguanil
Imipramine	Desmethylimipramine
Chloral hydrate	Trichloroethanol
Phenylbutazone	Oxyphenylbutazone
L-Dopa	Dopamine

Further metabolic studies made the distinction between phase I reactions that involve the transformation of specific groupings in a substrate molecule and the creation of new functional groups, and phase II reactions that are conjugations of the functions thus created with convenient, mostly solubilizing, moieties.[4]

A survey of a great number of examples of active metabolites shows that they belong exclusively to the phase I products and result from one of the reactions mentioned in Table 32.2. As such reactions follow some general rules, they can often be predicted. Taking into account the common metabolic pathways, one can imagine the design of a given molecule so that it will be converted *in vivo* into the desired compound by one or more of the phase I reactions. In other

Table 32.2   Phase I reactions.[4]

Oxiditative reactions
Oxidation of alcohol, carbonyl, and acid functions, hydroxylation of aliphatic carbon atoms, hydroxylation of alicyclic carbon atoms, oxidation of aromatic carbon atoms, oxidation of carbon–carbon double bonds, oxidation of nitrogen-containing functional groups, oxidation of silicon, phosphorus, arsenic and sulfur, oxidative *N*-dealkylation, oxidative *O*- and *S*-dealkylation, oxidative deamination, other oxidative reactions

Reductive reactions
Reduction of carbonyl groups, reduction of alcoholic groups and carbon–carbon double bonds, reduction of nitrogen-containing functional groups, other reductive reactions

Reactions without change in the state of oxidation
Hydrolysis of esters and ethers, hydrolytic cleavage of carbon–nitrogen single bonds, hydrolytic cleavage of nonaromatic heterocycles, hydration and dehydration at multiple bonds, new atomic linkages resulting from dehydration reactions, hydrolytic dehalogenation: removal of hydrogen halide molecules, various reactions

words, the active metabolite concept can be used in a forward-looking way ('metabolic synthesis'). By analogy with the retrosynthetic reasoning usual in organic chemistry, we can envisage retrometabolic reasoning in prodrug design. Such reasoning can lead to a particular group of prodrugs for which we have proposed the term *bioprecursors* or *bioprecursor prodrugs*.[5,6]

The following examples illustrate the approach, although the intentional use of bioprecursor design is relatively recent and in some cases there are some doubts about the prospective or retrospective character of the design. The first examples relate to oxidative bioactivations; they are followed by examples of reductive bioactivations, and finally by nonredox reactions. Often, however, the active species results from a cascade of metabolic reactions involving oxidative as well as reductive processes, complicated by hydrolytic reactions or hydration–dehydration sequences.

II. OXIDATIVE BIOACTIVATIONS

A. Dexpanthenol and 3-pyridine-methanol as provitamins

A simple example of bioprecursor prodrugs is found in dexpanthenol and 3-pyridine-methanol (Fig. 32.1). These primary alcohols are the reduced forms of the vitaminic factors pantothenic acid and nicotinic acid, respectively. Dexpanthenol has the advantage over the parent drug of being more stable, especially towards racemization.

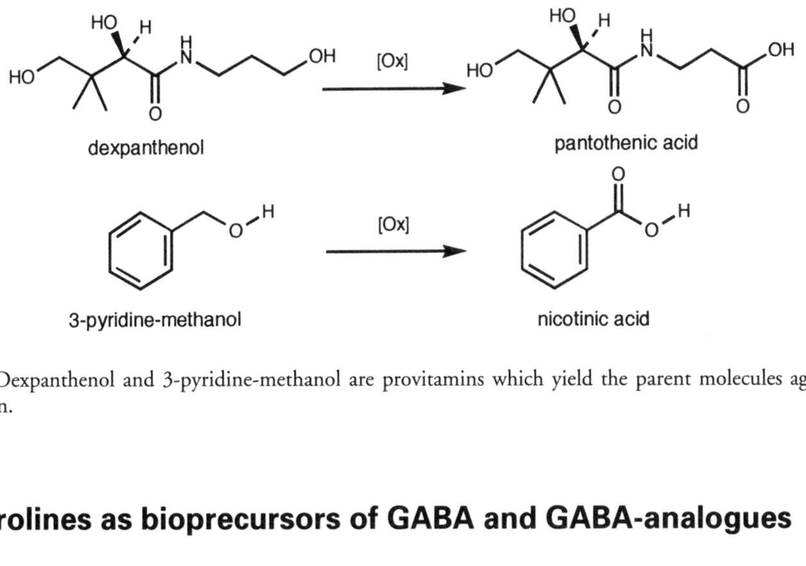

dexpanthenol   [Ox]   pantothenic acid

3-pyridine-methanol   [Ox]   nicotinic acid

Fig. 32.1 Dexpanthenol and 3-pyridine-methanol are provitamins which yield the parent molecules again after *in vivo* oxidation.

B. Pyrrolines as bioprecursors of GABA and GABA-analogues

A major obstacle to the design of potential therapeutic agents acting through the GABA system is the poor brain-penetrating properties of active compounds. The approach taken by Callery *et al.*,[7] for the design of brain-penetrating compounds active on the GABA system, centres on the hypothesis that Δ^1-pyrroline and its analogues are bioprecursors of GABA and GABA-analogues (Fig. 32.2). This hypothesis is inspired by the fact that putrescine was reported to be a precursor of GABA in mammalian systems,[8] and that the proposed pathway (Fig. 32.3) involves the conversion of Δ^1-pyrroline to GABA.

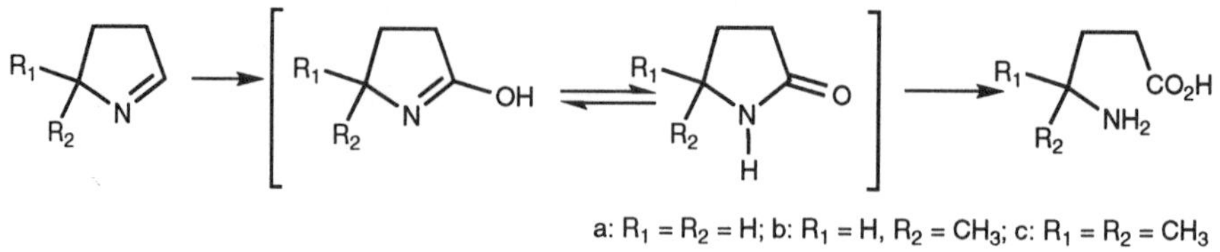

a: $R_1 = R_2 = H$; b: $R_1 = H$, $R_2 = CH_3$; c: $R_1 = R_2 = CH_3$

Fig. 32.2   Pyrrolines as bioprecursors of GABA and GABA-analogues.[7]

The capacity of brain tissue to carry out this conversion was demonstrated by *in vivo* brain studies. After an intraperitoneal injection of 200 mg kg^{-1} of 5-methyl-Δ^{-1}-pyrroline to mice, the brain concentrations of 4-methyl-GABA were 170 and 270 μM, 0.5 and 5 hours, respectively, after administration. These levels far exceeded the IC$_{50}$ value of 3.5 μM reported for inhibition of GABA-binding *in vivo* by 4-methyl-GABA.[9] On the other hand, 4-methyl-GABA did not penetrate the central nervous system in measurable quantities following intraperitoneal administration to mice in high doses (400 mg kg^{-1}).

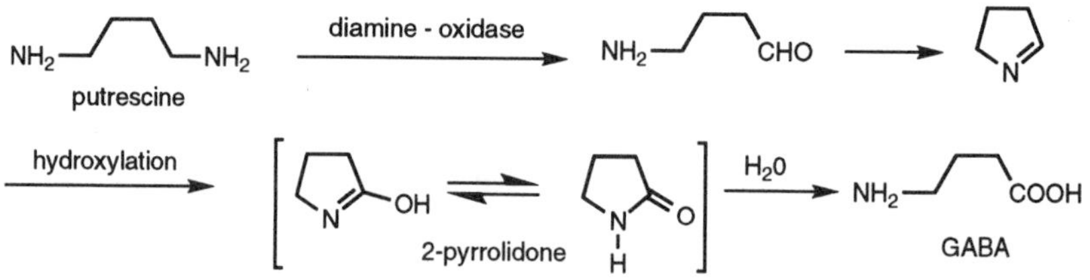

Fig. 32.3   Putrescine is a precursor of GABA in mammalian systems.[8]

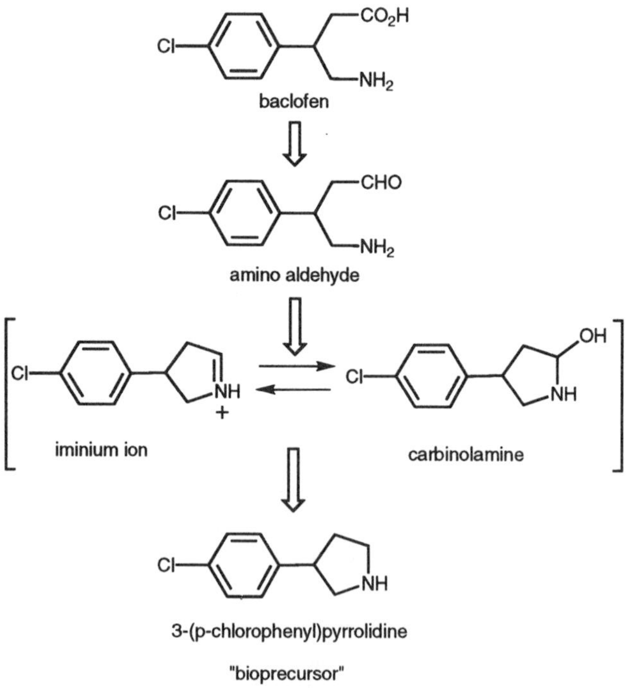

Fig. 32.4   3-(*p*-Chlorophenyl)pyrrolidine acts as a prodrug for baclofen.[10]

In a similar way, 3-(*p*-chlorophenyl) pyrrolidine acts as a prodrug for baclofen (Fig. 32.4) Its administration by the parenteral route achieves detectable brain levels of baclofen and demonstrates some activity of the prodrug in the isoniazid-induced (GABA-inhibited) convulsion model.[10]

It is noteworthy that the lactam of baclofen is active on various models of anticonvulsant activity (maximal electroshock seizure test, pentylenetetrazol seizure threshold test, bicuculline seizure test) with ED_{50} values ranging from 68 to 143 mg kg^{-1} i.p. in rats. Baclofen itself is practically inactive in these tests.

C. Cyclophosphamide[11]

Cyclophosphamide is a cytotoxic (cytostatic), cell cycle-nonspecific, antiproliferative agent which is used in such diverse medical problems as neoplasia, tissue transplantation, and inflammatory diseases.[12] Chemically it is an inert bioprecursor for a potent nitrogen mustard alkylation agent (Fig. 32.5).

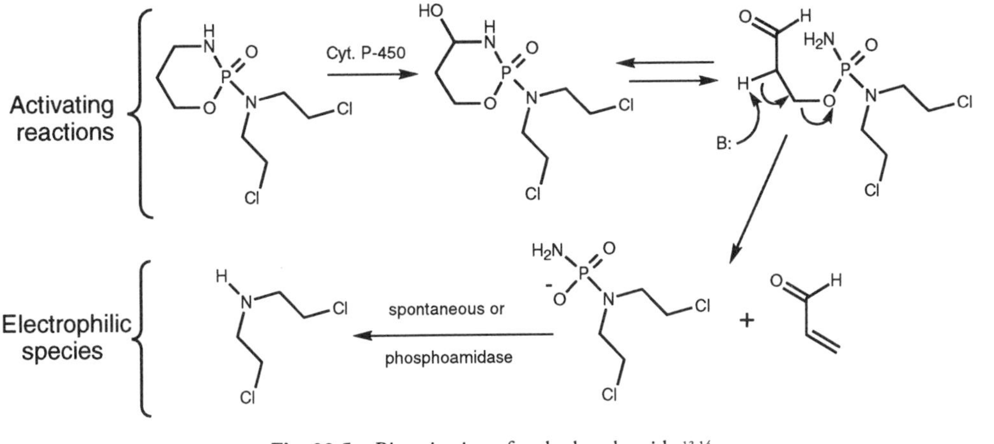

Fig. 32.5 Bioactivation of cyclophosphamide.[13,14]

Cyclophosphamide was synthesized by Arnold and co-workers[15–17] in the hope that it would be inert until activated by enzymes present in the body, especially in the tumour. The activation mechanism is believed to require an initial oxidative dealkylation, similar to that described above for pyrroline, followed by a spontaneous or phosphoramidase-catalysed hydrolysis to the parent nitrogen mustard.[13,14]

D. 6-Deoxyacyclovir as a bioprecursor of acyclovir

The antiherpetic agent acyclovir suffers from poor oral bioavailability, only 10–20% of an oral dose being absorbed in humans. This can essentially be ascribed to a low water solubility owing to strong interaction forces in the crystal lattice. The corresponding deoxo derivative (6-deoxyacyclovir) was shown by Krenitsky[18] to be 18 times more water-soluble and to be rapidly oxidized to the parent drug by xanthine oxidase *in vivo* (Fig. 32.6). Studies in rats and in human volunteers showed that orally administered 6-deoxyacyclovir has a 5–6 times greater bioavailability than has acyclovir.[18,19]

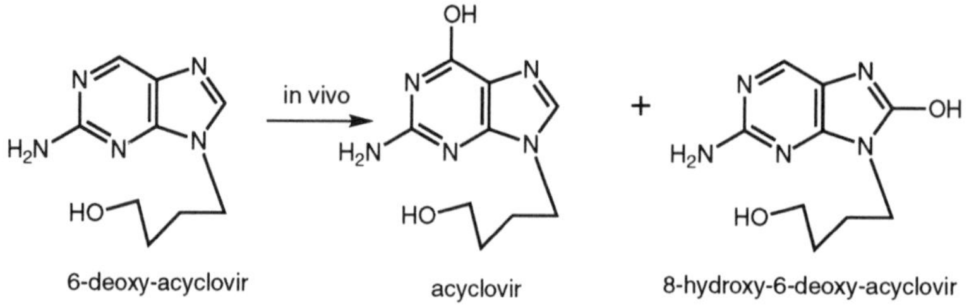

Fig. 32.6   6-Deoxyacyclovir as a bioprecursor of acyclovir.[18,19]

E.   L-2-Oxothiazolidine-4-carboxylate: a cysteine delivery system

The enzyme 5-oxo-L-prolinase which catalyses the conversion of 5-oxo-L-proline to L-glutamate coupled to the consumption of ATP (Fig. 32.7), was shown by Williamson and Meister[20] to act also on a synthetic substrate, L-2-oxothiazolidine-4-carboxylate, which is an analogue of 5-oxoproline with the 4-methylene group replaced by sulfur.

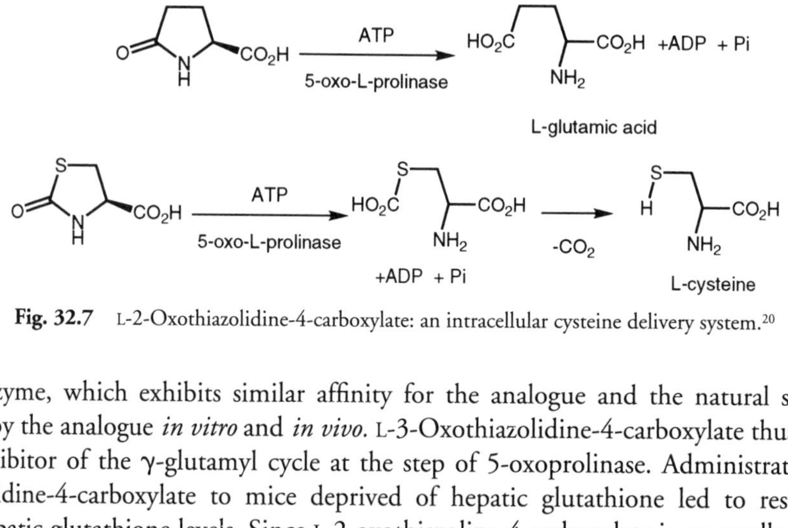

Fig. 32.7   L-2-Oxothiazolidine-4-carboxylate: an intracellular cysteine delivery system.[20]

The enzyme, which exhibits similar affinity for the analogue and the natural substrate, is inhibited by the analogue *in vitro* and *in vivo*. L-3-Oxothiazolidine-4-carboxylate thus serves as a potent inhibitor of the γ-glutamyl cycle at the step of 5-oxoprolinase. Administration of L-2-oxothiazolidine-4-carboxylate to mice deprived of hepatic glutathione led to restoration of normal hepatic glutathione levels. Since L-2-oxothiazoline-4-carboxylate is an excellent substrate of the enzyme, it may serve as an intracellular delivery system for cysteine and thus have potential as a therapeutic agent for conditions in which there is depletion of hepatic glutathione.

F.   Site-specific delivery of the acetylcholinesterase reactivator 2-PAM to the brain

N-Methylpyridinium-2-carbaldoxime (2-PAM, (**a**); in Fig. 32.8, constitutes the most potent reactivator of acetylcholinesterase poisoned through organophosphorus acylation. However, owing to its quaternary nitrogen, 2-PAM penetrates the biological membranes poorly and does not appreciably cross the blood–brain barrier. For this compound, Bodor and colleagues[21] designed an ingenious dihydropyridine-pyridinium salt type of redox delivery system. The active drug is administered as its 5,6-dihydropyridine derivative (Pro-2-PAM, (**b**)), which exists as a stable immonium salt (**c**). The lipoidal (**b**) (pK_a = 6.32) easily penetrates the blood–brain barrier where it is oxidized to the active (**a**).

A dramatic increase in the brain delivery of 2-PAM by the use of Pro-2-PAM is thus achieved, resulting in a reactivation of phosphorylated brain acetylcholinesterase *in vivo*.[22,23]

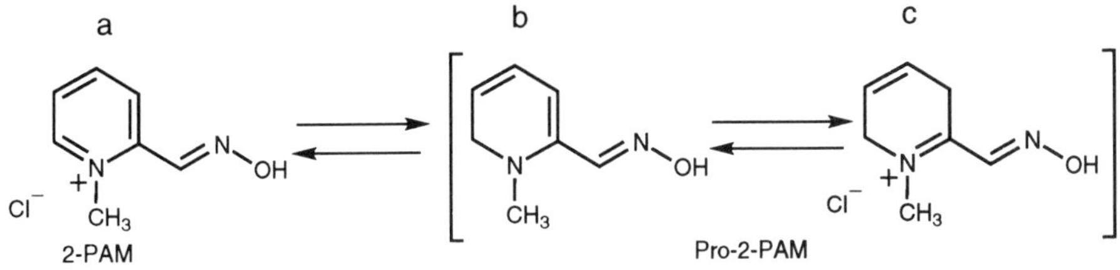

Fig. 32.8 Dihydro derivatives of 2-PAM.[21]

G. Methylenedioxy derivatives as bioprecursors of catechols

Various substituted and unsubstituted methylenedioxy derivatives of apomorphine and *N-n*-propylnorapomorphine have been studied by Baldessarini,[24] and one of these (10,11-methylenedioxy-*N-n*-propylnorapomorphine) was found to be both a long-acting and an orally efficient prodrug (Fig. 32.9). The oral activity of the compound can be ascribed to the protection of the catechol system from the first pass effect by the methylenedioxy group. The conversion to the free catechol is possible thanks to the hepatic microsomal enzymes (see Chapters 28 and 29 on drug metabolism).

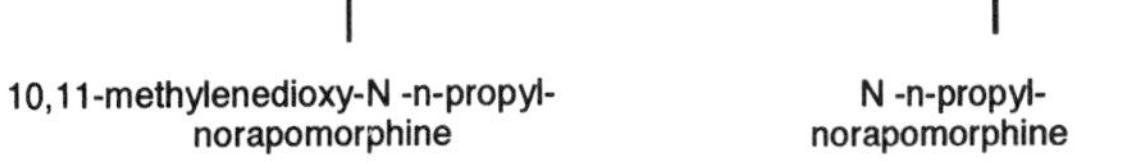

10,11-methylenedioxy-N -n-propyl-
norapomorphine

N -n-propyl-
norapomorphine

Fig. 32.9 Methylenedioxy derivatives as bioprecursors of catechols.[24]

H. Conversion of *N*-alkylaminobenzophenones to benzodiazepines *in vivo*

N-Dealkylation of tertiary amines is a frequently encountered metabolic process[4] and may be successfully used in bioprecursor design. A practical example is found in the case of *N*-alkylaminobenzophenones, which are open-ring analogues of the corresponding

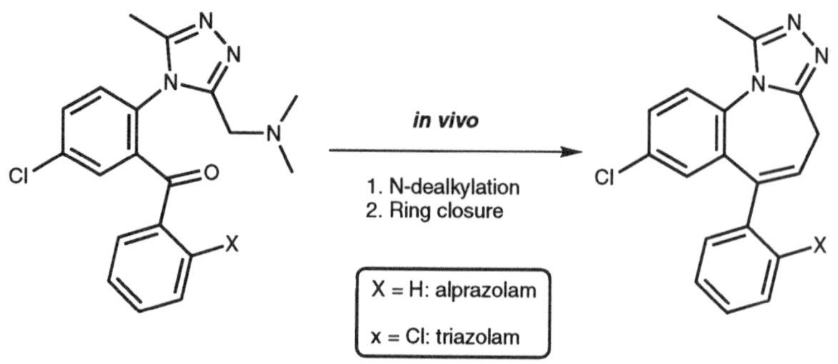

Fig. 32.10 Conversion of *N*-alkylaminobenzophenones to benzodiazepines *in vivo*.[26]

benzodiazepines.[25] These compounds possess potent sedative and muscle-relaxing activities and, in addition, antagonize pentylenetetrazole-induced clonic convulsions. It was demonstrated[26] that, *in vivo*, they undergo *N*-dealkylation and ring closure to form the corresponding benzodiazepine (Fig. 32.10). The *in vivo* conversion was found to occur in mice, rats and monkeys. These findings suggest that their observed pharmacological activity may be due to the formation of the corresponding benzodiazepine. The conversion was confirmed by a comparison of retention times in gas chromatography as well as through the use of GC-mass spectrometry. However, the conversion seems to be slow and/or incomplete and the open analogue is only about one-fifth as active as alprazolam itself (Table 32.3).

Table 32.3 Comparison of the anticonvulsant activity and bioavailability of alprazolam and its open analogue.[26]

Measured parameter	Open analogue	Alprazolam
DE_{50} antimetrazole (mg kg^{-1}, mice)	1.1	0.2
Cerebral level of alprazolam, $\frac{1}{2}$ h after administration of 20 mg kg^{-1} alprazolam or open analogue (mice)	224	1060

III. REDUCTIVE BIOACTIVATIONS

A. Reductive bioactivation of sulindac

Sulindac, *cis*-5-fluoro-2-methyl-1-[*p*-(methylsulphinyl)benzylidene]indene-3 acetic acid,[27] is a nonsteroidal anti-inflammatory agent having a broad spectrum of activity in animal models and in man. The two quantitatively significant biotransformations undergone by sulindac in laboratory species[28] and in man[29,30] involve only changes in the oxidation state of the sulphinyl substituent, viz., irreversible oxidation of the parent (sulindac) to sulfone and reversible reduction to sulfide (Fig. 32.11), the latter being the active species.[31] In two *in vitro* models of inflammation — prostaglandin synthetase inhibition and inhibition of platelet aggregation — the sulfide has activities comparable to those of indomethacin, whereas sulindac itself is devoid

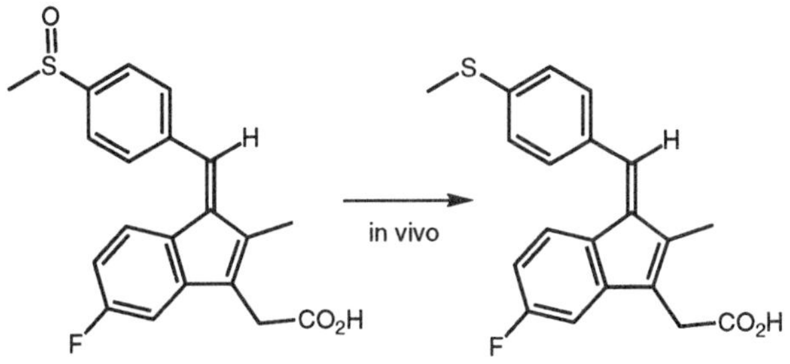

Fig. 32.11   Reductive bioactivation of sulindac.[31]

of activity. Nevertheless, sulindac is the preferred compound for clinical applications: an oral dosage of this inactive bioprecursor will circumvent initial exposure of gastric and intestinal mucosa to the active drug, and might thus provide a therapeutic advantage in comparison with the sulfide dosing.

B.   Reductive bioactivation of nitrogen mustards

Many conventional anticancer drugs display relatively poor selectivity for neoplastic cells, and solid tumours are particularly resistant both to radiation and chemotherapy. However, in solid tumours there are some unique and important microenvironmental properties such as localized hypoxia, nutrient deprivation and low pH.[32] On the other hand, as shown above for sulindac, sulfoxides can undergo two major biotransformations: reversible reduction to the sulfide and irreversible oxidation to the sulfone. The oxidation to the sulfone is the dominant process under normal physiological conditions, but the reduction to the sulfide becomes significant under anaerobic conditions.[33] Taking advantage of these findings, Kwon *et al.*[34] devised a hypoxia-selective alkylating bioprecursor prodrug (Fig. 32.12).

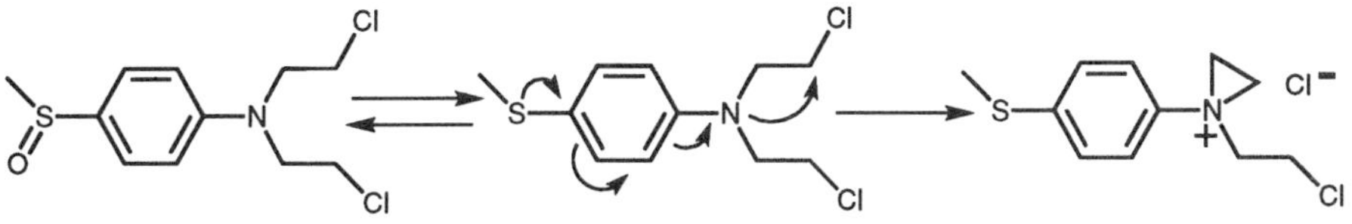

Fig. 32.12   Hypoxia-selective nitrogen mustard.[34]

The initial sulfoxide is relatively stable because of the electron-withdrawing effect exerted by the sulfoxide function in the *para* position; hence the nitrogen lone pair is not available to readily form the aziridinium species. However, after reduction in the hypoxic tumour cells, the electron-donating sulfide is generated, which promotes the cyclization into the alkylating aziridinium ion.

A similar bioreductive activation mechanism hads already been proposed by Connors[35] some years before for agents specifically designed for the treatment of primary hepatocytic cancers of the liver. It consists in oral administration of an azobenzene-derived nitrogen

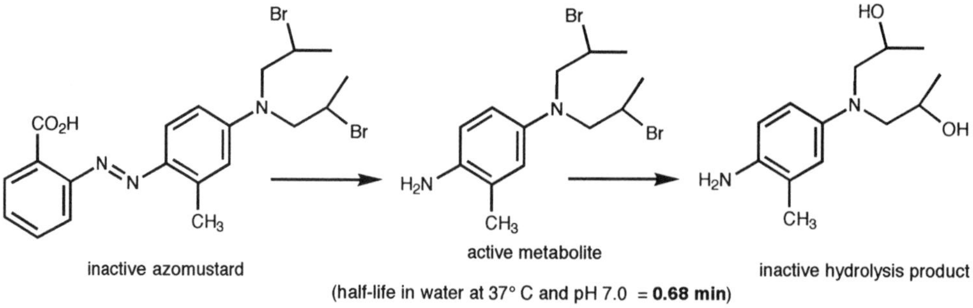

Fig. 32.13 Bioreductive activation of azomustards.[35]

mustard (Fig. 32.13). Such a compound is inactive *per se* but is completely activated on its first passage through the liver.

The alkylating *N-p*-aminophenyl mustard generated by the hepatic azoreductases has an extremely short half-life, thus confining cytotoxic alkylations to the liver cells. Little damage is caused to the liver, presumably because of its low mitotic index.

C. Reductive bioactivation of omeprazole

Omeprazole effectively inhibits gastric secrection by inhibiting the gastric H^+, K^+-ATPase.[36] This enzyme is responsible for gastric acid production, and is located in the secretory membranes of parietal cells. Thus omeprazole is proposed as an antiulcerative drug, specially in the treatment of Zollinger–Ellison syndrome.[37]

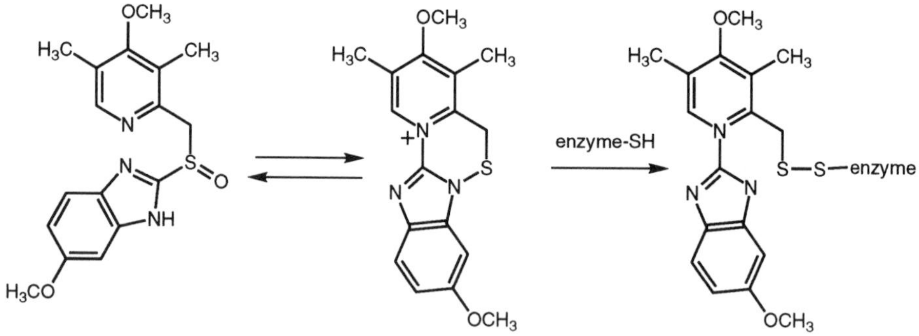

Fig. 32.14 Reductive bioactivation of omeprazole.

In vivo, omeprazole is transformed into the active inhibitor, a cyclic sulfenamide (Fig. 32.14), which forms disulfide bridges with the thiol groups of the enzyme and thus inactivates it.[38,39] The high specificity in the action of omeprazole (pK_a = 4.0) is due to its preferential concentration in the rather acidic parietal cells where it is activated. In neutral regions of the body, omeprazole is rather stable and only partially converted to the active species.

D. The bioreductive alkylation concept

This concept of bioreductive alkylation was put forward by Lin, Cosby, Shansky and Sartorelli.[40] Here again the challenge is to design biologically inactive forms of the compounds that become potent alkylating agents after *in vivo* reduction. One of the models proposed by Sartorelli, Lin and co-workers[40–43] is that of simple quinone methides (Fig. 32.15). Certain simple quinones substituted by one or more —CH$_2$—X groups present marked antineoplastic activity. These compounds may function as alkylating agents after reduction to the corresponding hydroquinones, which in turn yield quinone methides, the key alkylating agents *in vivo*.

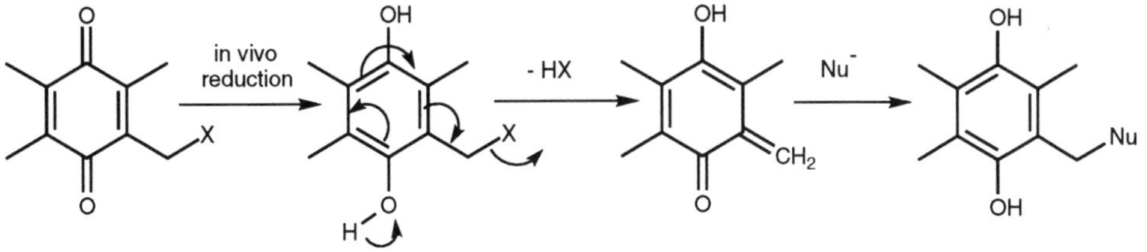

Fig. 32.15 The bioreductive alkylation concept.[44]

In a review article, Moore[44] discussed the concept of bioreductive alkylation as the mechanism of action of many naturally occurring and synthetic antitumour agents and antibiotics. Four models are presented: activated enamines, vinylogous quinone methides, simple quinone methides and α-methylene lactones or lactams. These may account for the activity of a large number of well-known agents such as mitomycin, doxorubicin, daunorubicin and camptothecin.

IV. MIXED ACTIVATION MECHANISMS

A. Arylacetic acids from aroylpropionic precursors

The metabolic pathways involved in the biotransformation of nicotine and haloperidol involve the initial formation of aroylpropionic acids (3-nicotinoylpropionic and 3-(*p*-fluorobenzoyl) propionic acid, respectively). These aroylpropionic acids subsequently undergo a progressive degradation of the oxobutyric side-chain and yield finally arylacetic acids[4] (Fig. 32.16).

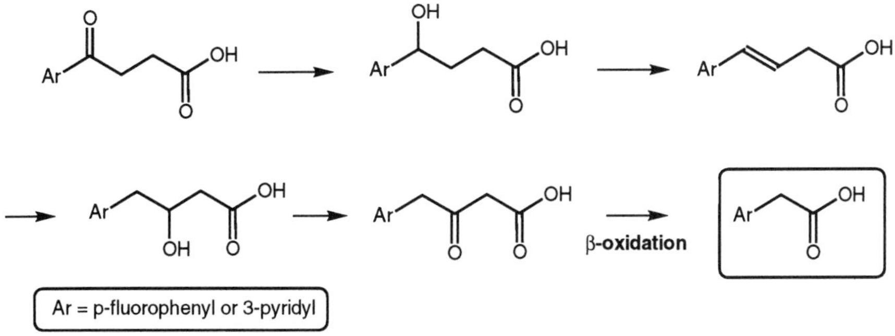

Ar = p-fluorophenyl or 3-pyridyl

Fig. 32.16 Progressive metabolic degradation of β-aroylpropionic acids into arylacetic acids.[4]

This information was used to design bucloxic acid,[45,46] fenbufene[47,48] and furobufene,[49] all of which are three bioprecursor forms of anti-inflammatory arylacetic acids (Fig. 32.17). For all these compounds the bioactivation takes place through a multistep process implying reductive, oxidative and hydration–dehydration sequences.

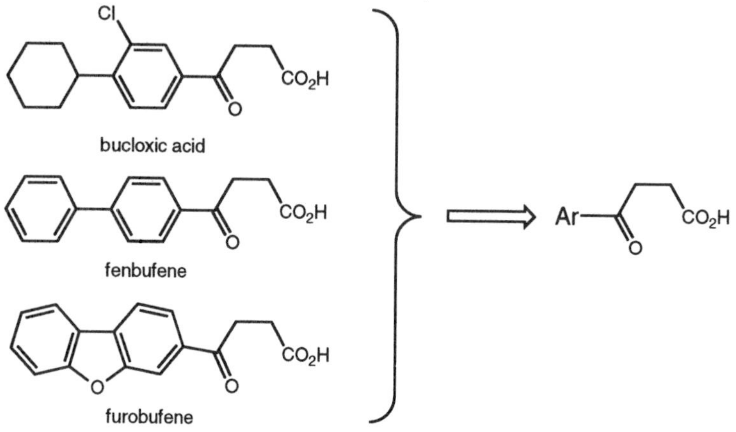

Fig. 32.17 Anti-inflammatory agents presenting the aroylpropionic structure.[45,47,49]

More recently, arylhexenoic acids were shown to undergo a similar metabolic degradation to arylacetic acids.[50] The hexenoic analogue of indomethacin (Fig. 32.18) acts as prodrug of indomethacin and provides sustained analgesia at oral doses of $30\,mg\,kg^{-1}$ to mice (phenylquinone writhing test) or to rats (yeast-induced hyperalgesia test).

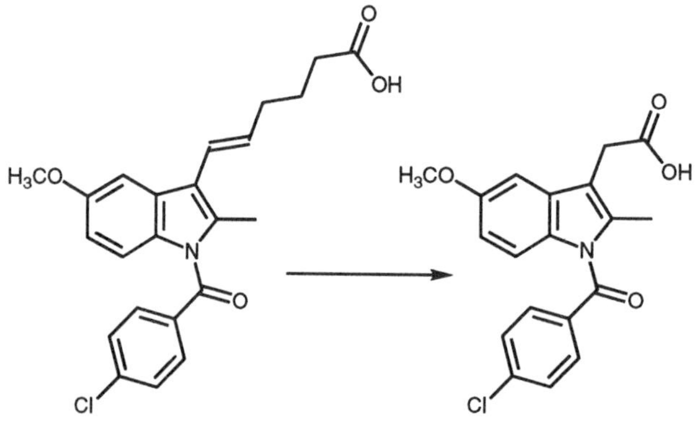

Fig. 32.18 The hexenoic analogue of indomethacin as prodrug of indomethacin.

B. Intracellular delivery of phenylglyoxylic acids

In the context of ischaemic heart disease, particularly following myocardial infarction, the stimulation of the multienzyme complex pyruvate dehydrogenase (PDH) offers a means of 'switching over' myocardial metabolism from fatty acid utilization to glucose, which is more economical in terms of oxygen consumption.[51] Among the agents able to promote carbohydrate oxidation by increasing PDH levels in the heart, α-keto acids and especially phenylglyoxylic acids proved to be valuable candidates.[52] Attempts to increase the *in vivo* activity of *p*-hydroxyphenyl-glyoxylic acid and to prolong the duration of its action by delivering it into cells as a prodrug suggested the use of L-(+)-2-(4-hydroxyphenyl)glycine, or oxfenicin (Fig. 32.19).[52] Amino acids are known to be transported across lipid membranes by an active transport process. In addition, it is known that L-(+)-α-amino acids are converted to α-keto acids by transaminase enzymes.

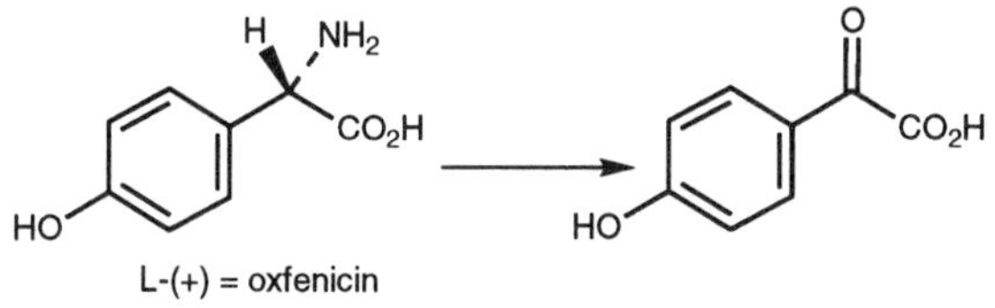

L-(+) = oxfenicin

Fig. 32.19 Intracellular delivery of phenylglyoxylic acids.[52]

Oxfenicin was effective for over 3 hours in stimulating rat heart PDH activity whether given by oral, intravenous or subcutaneous routes of administration.[53,54] Moreover, pharmacokinetic studies in rats, dogs and man have shown that *p*-hydroxyphenylglyoxylic acid appears in the blood soon after administration of oxfenicin. Oxfenicin is undergoing clinical trials for ischaemic heart disease.

V. DISCUSSION

A. Bioprecursors versus carrier-prodrugs

A comparative balance-sheet established for the two prodrug approaches leads to the following conclusions (Table 32.4).

- The *bioavailability* of carrier-prodrugs is modulated using a transient transport moiety; such a linkage is not implied for bioprecursors which result from a molecular modification of the active principle itself.
- The *lipophilicity* is generally the subject of a profound alteration of the parent molecule in the case of carrier-prodrugs, whereas it remains practically unchanged for bioprecursors.
- The *bioactivation* process is exclusively hydrolytic for carrier-prodrugs; it involves mostly redox systems for bioprecursors.
- The *catalysis* leading to the active principle is hydrolytic (either through general catalysis or through extrahepatic enzymes) for carrier-prodrugs. For bioprecursors, it seems largely restricted to phase I metabolizing enzymes.

Table 32.4 Bioprecursors versus carrier prodrugs.

	Prodrugs	
	Carrier prodrugs	Bioprecursors
Constitution	Active principle + carrier group	No carrier group
Lipophilicity	Strongly modified	Slightly modified
Bioactivation	Hydrolytic	Oxidative or reductive
Catalysis	Chemical or enzymic	Only enzymic

B. Existence of mixed-type prodrugs

In some cases the design of mixed-type prodrugs can be advantageous, as illustrated in the following examples.

1. Disulfide thiamin prodrugs

The thiamin (vitamin B$_1$) molecule contains a quaternary ammonium functionality and is thus badly absorbed. In healthy patients the necessary amounts of thiamine are absorbed thanks to an active transport mechanism coupled with ATP consumption. However, these mechanisms are rapidly saturable and easily inhibited, specially by chronic alcoholic consumption. As a consequence of the insufficient absorption of thiamin, alcoholism often entails Wernicke's encephalopathy (neurological disorders such as nystagmus, ocular motor nerve paralysis, memory losses, disorientation). The design of lipophilic prodrugs able to reach the CNS by passive diffusion was then undertaken: compounds like (**a**) and (**b**) in Fig. 32.20 result from lipophilic disulfide derivation of the open-ring thiolate anion corresponding to thiamin.

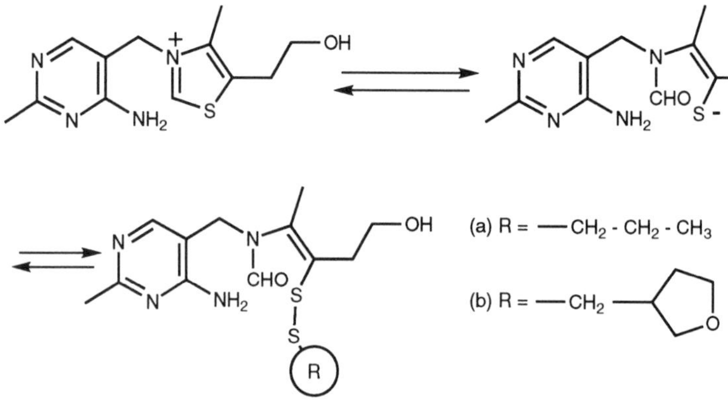

Fig. 32.20 Disulfide thiamin prodrugs as examples of mixed-type prodrugs.[55]

Such compounds can also be considered as carrier-prodrugs, in so far as the thiolate is linked to an *n*-propylthio (**a**) or a tetrahydrofuranylmethylenethio (**b**) transport moiety, or as bioprecursors, in so far as a bioreductive cleavage in the thiolate anion is needed to generate the active thiamin; the thiolate anion then functions as a less polar (no quaternary ammonium function) precursor form of thiamin. After oral administration, higher thiamin blood levels were observed, in both healthy volunteers and cirrhotic patients with the prodrug, than with thiamin hydrochloride.[56]

2. Trigonelline esters and amines

Generalizing the dihydropyridine ⟷ pyridinium salt redox delivery system, successfully applied to 2-PAM, Bodor and co-workers proposed an astute sustained-release methodology for brain delivery based on the mixed-type prodrugs.[57] The biologically active compound is linked to a lipoidal dihydropyridine carrier that easily penetrates the blood–brain barrier (Fig. 32.21). Enzymatic oxidation *in vivo* of the carrier part to the ionic pyridinium salt by the NAD ⟷ NADH system prevents its elimination from the brain, while elimination from the general

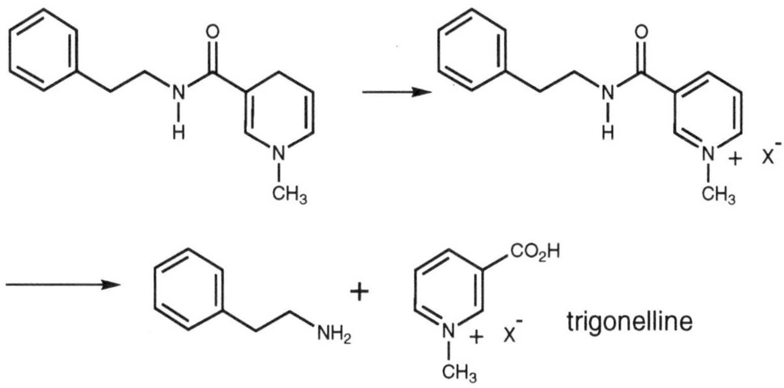

Fig. 32.21   Trigonelline amides (or esters) as examples of mixed-type prodrugs.[57]

circulation is accelerated. Subsequent cleavage of the quaternary carrier-drug species results in sustained delivery of the drug in the brain and a facile elimination of the nontoxic carrier part (trigonelline or its *N*-benzyl analogue).

C.   DIFFICULTIES AND LIMITATIONS

The introduction of prodrugs in human therapy gave successful results in overcoming undesirable properties such as poor absorption, too fast biodegradation, or formulation problems. It can be expected that an increasing number of medicinal chemists will be tempted by this approach. However, they must keep in mind that prodrug design can also give rise to a large number of new difficulties, especially in the assessment of pharmacological, pharmacokinetic, toxicological and clinical properties.

At the *pharmacological level*, for example, because bioactivation is necessary to create the active species, these compounds cannot be submitted to preliminary *in vitro* screening tests, namely binding studies, neurotransmitter re-uptake, and measurements of enzymatic inhibition and activity on isolated organs.

The measurements of *pharmacokinetic parameters* can lead to numerous misinterpretations. Thus, pivampicillin has a half-life of 103 min in a buffered aqueous solution at 37°C, but this falls to less than 1 min after addition of only 1% of mouse or rat serum. In the presence of human serum (10%), however, it is 50 min, whereas in whole human blood it is only 5 min. These results exemplify the care required to avoid incorrect conclusions. In addition, when a prodrug and the parent molecule are compared, one must take into account the differences in their respective time-courses of action. The maximum activity can appear later for the prodrug than for the parent compound, and often comparison of the area under the curve would constitute a better criterion.

At the *toxicological level*, even when prodrugs derive from well-known active principles, they have to be regarded as new entities. Undesirable side-effects can appear which are directly related to the prodrug (allergy to bucloxic acid) or derived from the bioactivation process (formation of unwanted or unexpected metabolites) or which can be attributed to the temporary transport moiety (digestive intolerance to pivampicillin, antivitamin-PP activity of nicafenine). This latter case is particularly illustrative: apparently innocent carrier groups such as *N*-hydroxyethylnicotinamide appeared as promising candidates for improving the absorption of acidic anti-inflammatory drugs or clofibric acid.[58-60] However, during the clinical studies, side-effects similar to vitamin PP deficiency appeared, suggesting that *N*-hydroxyethylnicotinamide could function as a nicotinamide antimetabolite. The compounds then had to be withdrawn (H. Cousse, Pierre Fabre & Co, personal communication).

In a review of potential hazards of the prodrug approach, Gorrod[61] cites four toxicity mechanisms:

(1) Formation of a toxic metabolite of the total prodrug, which is not produced by the parent drug.
(2) Consumption of a vital constituent (for example, glutathione) during the prodrug activation process. As L-cysteine is needed for the biosynthesis of glutathione, a supply from L-cysteine prodrugs can eventually confer some protection of the hepatic cells.[62]
(3) Generation of a toxic derivative from a transport moiety supposed to be 'inert'.
(4) Release of a pharmacokinetic modifier (causing enzymatic induction, displacing protein-bound molecules, altering drug excretion, etc.).

At the eventual *clinical stage*, the predictive value of animal experiments is also questionable. Thus, for two prodrugs derived from α-methyldopa, the active doses in the rat were identical; none the less, they turned out to be very different during clinical investigations. One compound was just as active as α-methyldopa, whereas the other was 3–4 times more active.[63,64]

An application file for a new prodrug should take into account all these aspects and can in no way be regarded simply as a complement to the main file.

VI. CONCLUSION

In the future it would be preferable to distinguish the carrier-prodrug and the bioprecursor approaches. The first, consisting in the attachment of a temporary carrier group to an active principle, has largely proved its utility in the design of orally active antibiotics and more generally wherever high bioavailability in plasma or peripheral organs is required. The CNS delivery of drugs using carrier-prodrugs, is less convincing in so far as usually high dosages are needed to ascertain clinical efficiency (1–2 g progabide per day, for example).

The design of bioprecursors, which represents a prospective creative application of the active metabolite concept, seems *a priori* better suited for CNS delivery, but it still has to prove its clinical usefulness.

Mixed-type approaches gave good results for thiamin and appear to be an interesting alternative when each approach fails individually.

REFERENCES

1. Albert, A. (1965) *Selective Toxicity*, 3rd edn. Wiley, New York.
2. Tréfouël, J., Tréfouël, T., Nitti, F. and Bovet, D. (1935) Activité du p-aminophénylsulfamide sur les infections streptococciques expérimentales de la souris et du lapin. *CR Séances Soc. Biol.*, **120**: 756–758.
3. Brodie, B. B. (1964) Difficultés de transposer à l'homme les résultats expérimentaux obtenus sur l'animal. In Hazard, R. and Cheymol, J. (eds) *Actualités Pharmacologiques*, pp. 1–40. Masson, Paris.

4. Testa, B. and Jenner, P. (1976) *Drug Metabolism, Chemical and Biochemical Aspects.* Marcel Dekker, New York.

5. Wermuth, C. G. (1983) Bioprécurseurs contre prodrogues. In Briot, M., Cautreels, W. and Ronucci, R. (eds) *Drug Metabolism and Drug Design: Quo Vadis?*, pp. 253–271. Sanofi-Clin-Midy, Montpellier.

6. Wermuth, C. G. (1984) Designing prodrugs and bioprecursors. In Jollès, G. and Wooldridge, K.R.H. (eds) *Drug Design: Fact or Fantasy?*, pp.47–72. Academic Press, London.

7. Callery, P. S., Geelhaar, L. A., Balachandran Nayar, M. S., Stogniev, M. and Gurudath Rao, K. (1982) Pyrrolines as prodrugs of γ-aminobutyric acid analogues. *J. Neurochem.* **38**: 1063–1067.

8. Tabor, H. and Tabor, C. W. (1964) Spermidine, spermine and related amines. *Pharmacol. Rev.* **16**: 245–300.

9. Iversen, L. L., Bird, E., Spokes, E., Nicholson, S.H. and Suckling, C. J. (1978) Agonist specificity of GABA binding sites in human brain and GABA in Huntington's disease and schizophrenia. In Krogsgaard-Larsen, P., Schel-Krüger, J. and Kofod, H. (eds) *GABA Neurotransmitters*, pp. 179–190. Academic Press, New York.

10. Wall, G. M. and Baker, J. K. (1989) Metabolism of 3-(*p*-chlorophenyl)pyrrolidine. Structural effects in conversion of a prototype γ-aminobutyric acid prodrug to lactam and γ-aminobutyric acid type metabolites. *J. Med. Chem.* **32**: 1340–1348.

11. Maxwell, R. A. and Eckhardt, S. B. (1990) *Drug Discovery. A Casebook and Analysis*, pp. 265–280. Humana Press, Clifton.

12. Gershwin, M. E., Goetzl, E. J. and Steinberg, A. D. (1974) Cyclophosphamide: use in practice. *An. Intern. Med.* **80**: 531–540.

13. Silverman, R. B. (1992) *The Organic Chemistry of Drug Design and Drug Action*, p. 380. Academic Press, San Diego.

14. Zon, G. (1982) Cyclophosphamide analogues. In Ellis, G. P. and West, G. B. (eds) *Medicinal Chemistry*, pp. 205–246. Elsevier, Amsterdam.

15. Arnold, H., Bourseaux, F. and Brock, N. (1958) NeuartigeKrebs-Chemotherapeutika aus der Gruppe der zyklischen *N*-Lost-phosphamidester. *Naturwissenschaften* **45**: 64–66.

16. Arnold, H., Bourseaux, F. and Brock, N. (1958) Chemotherapeutic action of a cyclic nitrogen mustard phosphamide ester (B518-ASTA) in experimental tumors of the rat. *Nature* **181**: 931.

17. Arnold, H. (1967) Ueber die Chemie neuer zytostatisch wirksamer N-Chloroethyl-phosphorsäureesterdiamide. In Spitzy, K. and Haschek, H. (eds) *Proceedings of the Fifth International Congress on Chemotherapy*, pp.751–754. Verlag der Wiener Medizinischen Akademie, Wien.

18. Krenitsky, T. A., Hall, W. W., de Miranda, P., Beauchamp, L. M., Schaeffer, H. J. and Whiteman, P. D. (1984) Deoxyacyclovir: a xanthine oxidase-activated prodrug of acyclovir. *Proc. Natl. Acad. Sci. USA* **31**: 3209–3213.

19. Whiteman, P. D., Bye, A., Fowle, A. S. E., Jeal, S., Land, G. and Posner, J. (1984) Tolerance and pharmacokinetics of A515U, an acyclovir analogue in healthy volunteers. *Eur. J. Clin. Pharmacol.* **27**: 471–475.

20. Williamson, J. M. and Meister, A. (1981) Stimulation of hepatic glutathione formation by administration of L-2-oxothiazolidine-4-carboxylate, a 5-oxo-1-prolinase substrate. *Proc. Natl. Acad. Sci. USA* **78**: 936–939.

21. Bodor, N., Shek, E. and Higuchi, T. (1976) Improved delivery through biological membranes. 1. Synthesis and properties of 1-methyl-1,6-dihydropyridine-2-carbaldoxime, a pro-drug of *N*-methylpyridinium-2-carbaldoxime chloride. *J. Med. Chem.* **19**: 102–107.

22. Shek, E., Higuchi, T. and Bodor, N. (1976) Improved delivery through biological membranes. 2. Distribution, excretion, and metabolism of *N*-methyl-1,6-dihydropyridine-2-carbaldoxime hydrochloride, a pro-drug of *N*-methylpyridinium-2-carbaldoxime chloride. *J. Med. Chem.* **19** 108–112.

23. Shek, E. and Higuchi, T. (1976) Improved delivery through biological membranes. 3. Delivery of *N*-methylpyridinium-2-carbaldoxime chloride through the blood–brain barrier in its dihydropyridine pro-drug form. *J. Med. Chem.* **19**: 113–117.

24. Baldessarini, R. J., Neumeyer, J. L., Campbell, A., Sperk, G., Ram. V. J., Arana, G. W. and Kula, N. S. (1982) An orally effective, long-acting dopaminergic prodrug: (−)-10,11-methylenedioxy-*N*-propylnorapomorphine. *Eur. J. Pharmacol.* **77**: 87–88.

25. Gall, M., Hester Jr, J. B., Rudzik, A. D. and Lahti, R. A. (1976) Synthesis and pharmacology of novel anxiolytic agents derived from 2-[(dialkylamino)methyl-4*H*-triazol-4-yl] benzophenones and related heterocyclic benzophenones. *J. Med. Chem.* **19**: 1057–1064.

26. Lathi, R. A. and Gall, M. (1976) Conversion of *N*-alkylaminobenzophenones to benzodiazepines *in vivo. J. Med. Chem.* **19**: 1064–1067.

27. Shen, T. I., Witzel, B. E., Jones, H., Linn, B. O., McPherson, J., Greenwald, R., Fordice, M. and Jacobs, A. (1972) Synthesis of a new anti-inflammatory agent, *cis*-5-fluoro-2-methyl-1-[*p*-(methylsulfinyl)benzylidenyl]-indene-3-acetic acid. *Fed. Proc.* **31**: 577.

28. Hucker, H. B., Stauffer, S. C., White, S. D., Rhodes, R. A., Arrison, B. H., Umbenhauer, E. R., Bower, R. J. and McMahon, F. G. (1973) Physiological disposition and metabolic fate of a new anti-inflammatory agent, *cis*-5-fluoro-2-methyl-1-[*p*-(methylsulfinyl)benzylidenyl]-indene-3-acetic acid in the rat, dog, rhesus monkey, and man. *Drug Metab. Dispos.* **1**: 721–736.

29. Duggan, D. E., Hare, L. E., Ditzler, C. A., Lei, B. W. and Kwan, K. C. (1977) The disposition of sulindac. *Clin. Pharmacol. Ther.* **21**: 326–335.

30. Duggan, D. E., Hooke, K. F., Noll, R. M., Hucker, H. B. and Van Arman, C. G. (1978) Comparative biodisposition of solindac and metabolites in five species. *Biochem. Pharmacol.* **27**: 2311–2320.

31. Duggan, D. E., Hooke, K. F., Risley, E. A., Shen, T. Y. and Van Arman, C. G. (1977) Identification of the biologically active form of sulindac. *J. Pharmacol. Exp. Ther.* **201**: 8–13.

32. Kennedy, K. A., Teicher, B. A., Rockwell, S. and Sartorelli, A. C. (1980) The hypoxic tumor cell: a target for selective cancer chemotherapy. *Biochem. Pharmacol.* **29**: 1–8.

33. Davis, P. J. and Guenthner, L. E. (1985) Sulindac oxidation/reduction by microbial cultures; microbiol models for mammalian metabolism. *Xenobiotica* **15**: 845–857.

34. Kwon, C. -H., Blanco, D. R. and Baturay, N. (1992) *p*-(Methylsulfinyl)phenyl nitrogen mustard as a novel bioreductive prodrug selective against hypoxic tumors. *J. Med. Chem.* **35**: 2137–2139.

35. Connors, T. A. (1976) Bioactivation and cytotoxicity. In Bridges, J. W. and Chasseaud, L. F. (eds) *Progress in Drug Metabolism*, pp. 41–75. Wiley, London.

36. Wallmark, B., Brändström, A. and Larsson, H. (1984) Evidence for acid-induced transformation of omeprazole into an active inhibitor of $(H^+ + K^+)$-ATPase within the parietal cell. *Biochim. Biophys. Acta* **778**: 549–558.

37. Lamers, C. B. H. W., Lind, T., Moberg, S., Jansen, J. B. M. and Olbe, L. (1984) Omeprazole in Zollinger–Ellison syndrome. *N. Engl. J. Med.* **310**: 758–761.

38. Im, W. I., Shi, J. C., Blakeman, D. P. and McGrath, J. P. (1985) Omeprazole, a specific inhibitor of gastric $(H^+ - K^+)$-ATPase, is a H^+-activated oxidizing agent of sulfhydryl groups. *J. Biol. Chem.* **260**: 4591–4597.

39. Lindberg, P., Nordberg, P., Alminger, T. Brändström, A. and Wallmark, B. (1986) The mechanism of action of the gastric acid secretion inhibitor omeprazole. *J. Med. Chem.* **33**: 1685.

40. Lin, A. J., Cosby, L. A., Shansky, C. W. and Sartorelli, A. C. (1972) Potential bioreductive alkylating agents. 1. Benzoquinone derivatives. *J. Med. Chem.* **15**: 1247–1252.

41. Lin, A. J., Pardini, R. S., Cosby, L. A., Lillis, B. J., Shansky, C. W. and Sartorelli, A. C. (1973) Potential bioreductive alkylating agents. 2. Antitumor effect and biochemical studies of naphtoquinone derivatives. *J. Med. Chem.* **16**: 1268–1271.

42. Lin, A. J. and Sartorelli, A. C. (1973) 2,3-Dimethyl-5,6-bis(methylene)-1,4-benzoquinone. The active intermediate of bioreductive alkylating agents. *J. Org. Chem.* **38**, 813–815.

43. Lin, A. J., Lillis, B. J. and Sartorelli, A. C. (1975) Potential bioreductive alykylating agents. 5. Antineoplastic activity of quinoline-5,8-diones, naphthazarins, and naphtoquinones. *J. Med. Chem.* **18**: 917–921.

44. Moore, H. W. (1977) Bioactivation as a model for drug design bioreductive alkylation. *Science* **197**: 527–532.

45. Krausz, F., Demarne, H., Vaillant, J., Brunaud, M. and Navaro, J. (1974) Anti-inflammatoires non stéroidiques: dérivés de l'acide phényl-4-butyrique et phényl-4, oxo-4, butyrique. *Arzneimittel-Forsch. (Drug Res.)* **24**: 1360–1364.

46. Gros, P. M., Davi, H. H., Chasseaud, L. F. and Hawkins, D. R. (1974) Metabolic and pharmacokinetic study of bucloxic acid. *Arzneimittel-Forsch. (Drug Res.)* **24**: 1385–1390.

47. Kohler, C., Tolman, E., Wooding, W. and Ellenbogen, L. (1980) A review of the effects of fenbufen and a metabolite, biphenylacetic acid, on platelet biochemistry and function. *Arzneimittel Forsch. (Drug Res.)* **30**: 702–707.

48. Chicarelli, F. S., Eisner, H. J. and Van Lear, G. E. (1980) Disposition and metabolism of fenbufen in several laboratory animals. *Arzneimittel-Forsch. (Drug Res.)* **30**: 707–715.

49. Martel, R. R., Rochefort, J. G., Klicius, J. and Dobson, T. A. (1974) Anti-inflammatory properties of furobufen. *Can. J. Physiol. Pharmacol.* **52**: 669–673.

50. Gilard, J. W. and Belanger, P. (1987) Metabolic synthesis of arylacetic acid antiinflammatory drugs from arylhexenoic acids. 2. Indomathacin. *J. Med. Chem.* **30**: 2051–2058.

51. Neely, J. R. and Morgan, H. E. (1974) Relationship between carbohydrate and lipid metabolism and the energy balance of heart muscle. *Ann. Rev. Physiol.* **36**: 413–559.

52. Barnish, I. T., Cross, P. E., Danilevicz, J. C., Dickinson, R. P. and Stopher, D. A. (1981) Promotion of carbohydrate oxidation in the heart by some phenylglyoxylic acids. *J. Med. Chem.* **24**: 399–404.

53. Blackburn, K. J., Burges, R. A., Gardiner, D. G, Higgins, A. J., Morville, M. and Page, M. G. (1979) Protection against experimental myocardial ischaemia by L-4-hydroxyphenylglycine, a new agent which alters myocardial metabolic balance in favour of carbohydrate utilization. *Br. J. Pharmacol.* **66**: 443P–444P.

54. Higgins, A. J., Burges, R. A., Gardiner, D. G., Morville, M., Page, M. G. and Blackburn, K. J. (1980) Oxphenicine diverts rat muscle metabolism from fatty acid to carbohydrate oxidation and protects the ischaemic rat heart. *Life Sci.* **27**: 963–970.

55. Matsukawa, T., Yuruki, S. and Oka, Y. (1962) The synthesis of *S*-acylthiamine derivatives and their stability. *Ann. N.Y. Acad. Sci.* **98**: 430–444.

56. Thomson, A. D., Frank, O., Baker, H. and Leevy, C. M. (1971) Thiamine propyl disulphide: absorption and utilization. *Ann. Intern. Med.* **74**, 529–534.

57. Bodor, N., Farag, H. H. and Brewster III, M. E. (1981) Site-specific, sustained release of drugs to the brain. *Science* **214**: 1370–1372.

58. Cousse, H., Casadio, S. and Mouzin, G. (1978) L'hydroxy éthyl nicotinamide vecteur d'acides thérapeutiquement actifs. *Trav. Soc. Pharm. Montpellier* **38**: 71–76.

59. Casadio, S., Couse, H. and Mouzin, G. (1977) Nouvelles formes modulées de médicaments utilisant les *N*-hydroxy alcoyl pyridine carboxamides comme vecteur. French Patent 77.13478 (2 May 1977, to P. Fabre S. A.).

60. Vezin, J. C., Mouzin, G., Cousse, H. and Casadio, S. (1979) Nicafenine, a new analgesic. *Arzneimittel-Forsch.* **29**: 1659–1661.

61. Gorrod, J. W. (1980) Potential hazards of the pro-drug approach. *Chem. Ind.*: 457–461.

62. Roberts, J. C., Nagasawa, H. T., Zera, R. T., Fricke, R. F. and Goon, D. J. W. (1987) Prodrugs of 1-cysteine as protective agents against acetaminophen-induced hepatotoxicity. 2-(Polyhydroxyalkyl) and 2-(polyacetoxyalkyl)thiazolidine-4(*R*)-carboxylic acids. *J. Med. Chem.* **30**: 1891–1896.

63. Saari, W. S., Freedman, M. B., Hartman, R. D. *et al.* (1978) Synthesis and Antihypertensive activity of some ester progenitors of methyldopa. *J. Med. Chem.* **21**: 746–753.

64. Vickers, S., Duncan, C. A., White, S. D., Breault, G. O. Boyds, R. B., de Shepper, P. J. and Tempero, K. F. (1978) Evaluation of succinimidoethyl and pivaloyloxyethyl esters as progenitors of methyldopa in man, rhesus monkey, dog, and rat. *Drug. Metab. Dispos.* **6**: 640–646.

33

Macromolecular Carriers for Drug Targeting

ETIENNE H. SCHACHT, STEFAN VANSTEENKISTE
AND LEN SEYMOUR

*It is a capital mistake to theorize before one has data. Insensibly one
begins to twist facts to suit theories instead of theories to suit facts.*

Conan Doyle

I. INTRODUCTION

One of the major problems in chemotherapy is the limited selectivity of most common drugs. Following administration, the active agent is distributed all over the body. Only a certain fraction reaches the target cells. The undesired interaction with healthy cells can lead to severe side-effects. This is a major problem in cancer chemotherapy. Over the past three decades intensive efforts have been made to design novel systems able to deliver the drug more efficiently to the target site.

THE PRACTICE OF MEDICINAL CHEMISTRY
ISBN 0-12-744640-0

Most approaches are based on combinations of the drug with a polymer. The latter serves as a carrier system wherein the drug is dispersed or dissolved, or to which it is covalently linked. Cells, microspheres, nanospheres, liposomes, proteins, antibodies, hormones, natural and synthetic polymers, and others systems have been used as carriers. For a detailed discussion of these systems the readers is referred to some recent reviews and books.[1–8]

The objective of this chapter is to demonstrate the possibility of achieving drug targeting by linking drugs with soluble polymers. The aim is to discuss concepts and structure–property relationships and to illustrate applications with some selected examples. The term 'carrier' in this chapter will be restricted to water-soluble polymers to which a drug is covalently linked. Polymer–drug complexes will not be included.

II. CONCEPT

From the mid-1950s onwards, a large variety of drugs have been covalently attached to many natural or synthetic polymers. Initially, the only rationale was that converting the drug into a macromolecular prodrug might reduce renal excretion and hence increase the duration of activity. There was at that time little concern about the cellular uptake and processing of these conjugates. In 1975 Ringsdorf proposed a more rationalized model for macromolecular prodrugs[9] (Fig. 33.1). He upgraded enormously the potential of this concept by calling attention to the possibility of introducing onto the polymeric carrier not only the drug moiety but also groups that can influence the solubility properties as well as groups that can alter the body distribution and promote cell selectivity.

In this model the polymeric carrier can be either an inert or a biodegradable polymer. The drug can be fixed directly or via a spacer group onto the polymer backbone. If the polymeric conjugate is pharmacologically active as a whole, the product can be regarded as a polymer drug.

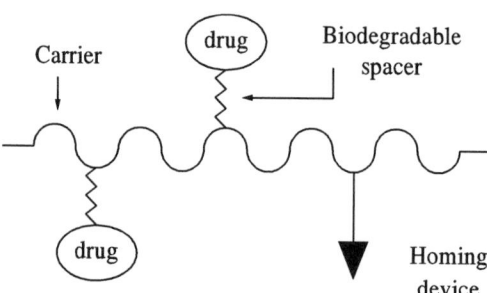

Fig. 33.1   Ringsdorf model.

Conjugates that are active after release of the parent drug are termed macromolecular prodrugs. The hydrophilic–lipophilic balance of the polymer conjugate can be varied by proper selection of the backbone and side-group constituents.The proper selection of this spacer opens the possibility of controlling the site and the rate of release of the active drug from the conjugate by hydrolytic or enzymatic cleavage. The most challenging aspect of this model is the possibility of altering the body distribution and cell uptake by attaching cell-specific or nonspecific uptake enhancers (homing devices). This model, although still oversimplified, has been an important mark in the history of polymeric prodrug design. It made clear that a more rational design was needed based on information arising from biological work. This remarkable paper has also catalysed the interest of biologists and pharmacists in synthetic polymers. As more information becomes available from cell biology and molecular biology, polymer chemists are trying to design tailor-made polymeric carriers that better fulfil the specified requirements.

III.   TYPE OF CARRIERS USED

The selection of polymers as candidate carriers is made on the basis of the following criteria:

- Chemical composition: availability of suitable functional groups for covalent coupling with drugs
- Biocompatibility: preferably nontoxic, nonimmunogenic
- Biodegradability
- Availability

A number of reviews cover what has been done over the past 20 years in the field of soluble polymers as potential drug carriers.[10–15] The polymers selected for preparing macromolecular prodrugs can be categorized according to (a) the chemical nature (vinylic or acrylic polymers, polysaccharides, poly(α-amino acids)); (b) the backbone stability (biodegradable polymers, stable polymers); (c) the origin (natural polymers, synthetic polymers); and (d) the molecular weight (oligomers, polymers). Examples of frequently used carriers are listed in Table 33.1.

Vinyl polymers can be easily prepared by radical polymerization of the corresponding vinyl monomer. Enormous variability in the polymer composition and properties can be achieved by copolymerization of selected monomers. This makes it possible to tailor-make the structure to meet the requirements of any system under consideration. For that reason, vinyl-type polymers are interesting drug carrier candidates. However, vinyl polymers are not biodegradable. Hence, in order to avoid undesirable storage, the molecular weight should at least be below the renal filtration limit (40–50 kDa) and for this reason the future of nondegradable polymeric carriers is questionable. The answer has to come from ongoing clinical evaluations of some polyvinylic-type macromolecular prodrugs. At present the most intensively studied vinyl polymers are copolymers of N-(2-hydroxypropyl)methacrylamide (PHPMA).[48–53] These polymers have been used as carriers for several drug molecules. A vast amount of information is available about biodistribution, immunogenicity and biological activity. PHPMA proved to be nontoxic and nonimmunogenic *in vivo* in animals. It was demonstrated that PHPMA-adriamycin conjugates are remarkably less toxic than the free drug. One conjugate carrying adriamycin (Fig. 33.2) has reached the stage of clinical evaluation.

Another polyvinylic prodrug that has reached clinical stage is a conjugate (SMANCS, Fig. 33.3) of a low-molecular-weight styrene maleic anhydride copolymer (SMA, 1.6 kDa) and neocarcinostatin (NCS).

Synthetic poly(α-amino acids) like poly(L-lysine), poly(L-glutamic acid) or poly[(N-hydroxyalkyl) glutamines] can be made by ring-opening polymerization of the N-carboxyanhydride monomers (Fig. 33.4). These polymers have functionalities in their side-groups (amine, hydroxyl, carboxyl) that allow covalent coupling with drug molecules. Generally, poly(L-amino acids) are biodegradable, whereas their D-enantiomers are not. The cationic nature of poly(L-lysine) in plasma causes it to interact easily with most cell membranes.

Table 33.1 Overview of macromolecular prodrug conjugates.

Drug carrier	Drug	Ref.
Vinyl polymers		
N(2-Hydroxypropyl)methacrylamide copolymers	Adriamycin	16–18
	Various others	
Poly(1-vinyl-2-pyrrolidone-co-maleic anhydride)	Quinidine	19
	6-Purinethiol	19
	5-Aminosalicylic acid	20
Poly(1-vinyl-2-pyrrolidone-co-vinylamine)	Chlorambucil	21
Poly(styrene-co-maleic anhydride)	Neocarcinorstatin	22
Poly(divinylether-co-maleic anhydride)	Cyclophosphamide	23
	Methotrexate	24
Polysaccharides		
Dextran	Procainamide	25,26
	Daunomycin	27
	interferon	28
	Mitomycin C	29,30
Inulin	Procainamide	26
	Antibiotics	31
Biozan R	Ampicilin	32
Carboxymethyldextran	Daunomycin	33
Chitosan	5-Fluorouracil	34
Synthetic poly(α-amino acids)		
Poly(L-lysine)	Methotrexate	35
Poly(L-aspartic acid)	Daunorubricin	36
Poly(2-hydroxyethyl)-D,L-aspartamide	Naproxen and others	37–39
Poly[(2-hydroxyethyl)-L-glutamine]	Mitomycin C	40
Proteins		
Human serum albumin	Primaquine	41
Bovine serum albumin	Methotrexate	42
Poly(ethylene glycol)		
	Enzymes/drugs	43,44
	Asparaginase	45
	Insulin	46
	Ibuprofen	47

Unfortunately the polymer is toxic.[54] Succinylation of the polymer converts it into a less toxic polyacid that still can be used as drug carrier[55] (Fig. 33.5).

Polysaccharides are another interesting class of drug carriers. Much attention has been directed to the use of dextran. Sezaki and his group prepared dextran-mitomycin conjugates by coupling mitomycin C with dextran modified with either aminocaproic acid or 6-bromohexanoic acid[29,30] (Fig. 33.6). The pharmacokinetics of these conjugates proved to be dependent on the molecular weight and the electrical charge of the polymer derivative.

The selection of dextran as drug carrier has mostly been based on its clinical use as a plasma expander and its claimed biodegradability. However, it was demonstrated by Vercauteren that

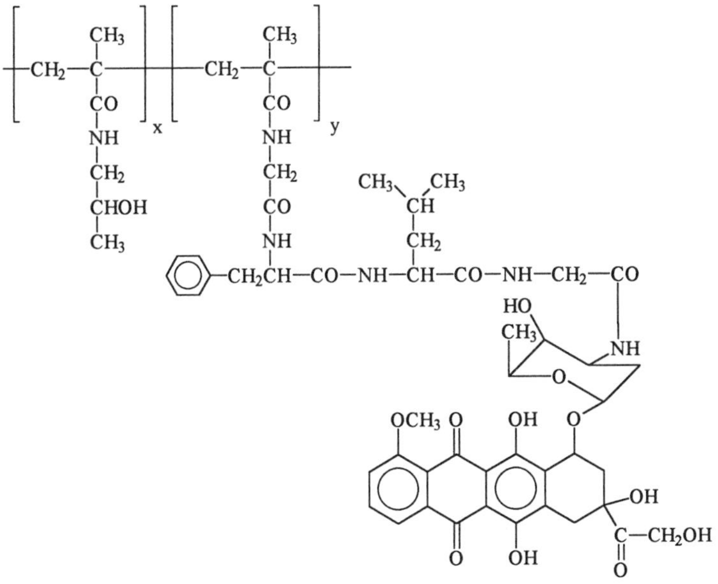

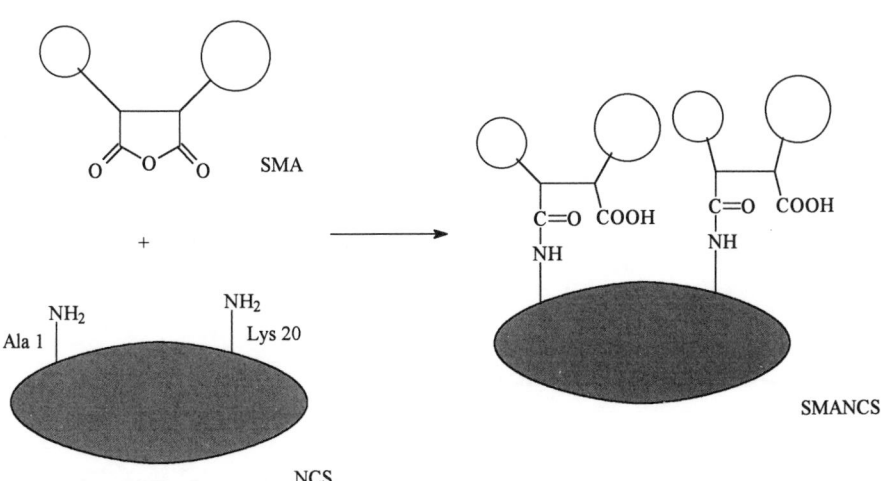

Fig. 33.2 Structure of HMPA copolymer containing adriamycin.

Fig. 33.3 Diagrammatic representation of the reaction between SMA and NCS to produce the conjugate SMANCS.

the *in vitro* degradation of dextrans in the presence of lysosomal glucosidases or endodextranases is rather slow. Moreover, it was shown that chemical modification of the dextran further reduces its biodegradability.[56]

Proteins such as serum albumin have also frequently been used for preparing polymeric prodrugs. An interesting example is the work of Meijer and co-workers, who used mannosylated

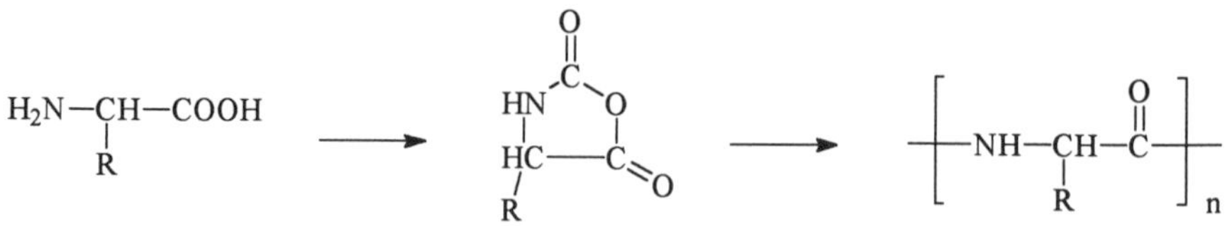

Fig. 33.4   Ring-opening polymerization of the N-carboxyanhydride monomers.

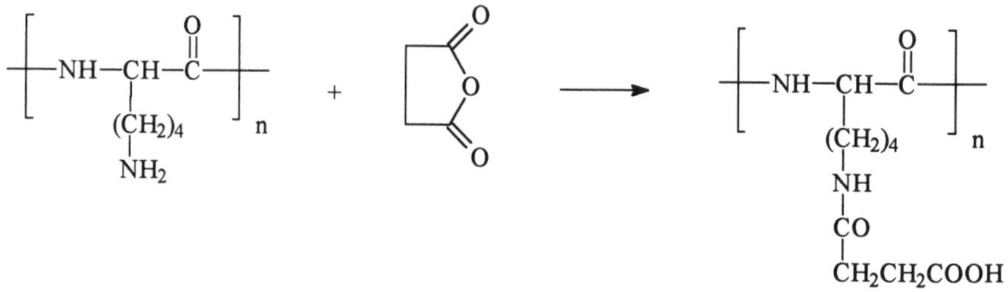

Fig. 33.5   Succinylation of poly(L-lysine).

serum albumin as carriers for antiviral drugs.[57,58] A disadvantage of proteins is their complexity in chemical composition, which complicates the identification of the final conjugates.

Poly(ethylene glycol) (PEG) has been used to modify a number of therapeutically interesting proteins. It has been clearly demonstrated by Abuchowski[44,45] that grafting of PEG onto proteins reduces their immunogenicity, improves their resistance to proteolytic degradation and improves their thermostability.

Micelle-forming block copolymers have been introduced by Yokoyama and colleagues.[59-61] Conjugates of adriamycin with poly(ethylene glycol)–poly(aspartamide) block copolymers tend to form micelles (Fig. 33.7). It was demonstrated that these systems have a very high *in vivo* antitumour activity.

IV.   METHODS OF DRUG RELEASE

Drug molecules are generally linked to the polymeric carrier via a spacer group. The drug can be released during plasma circulation or after cell uptake. Low-molecular-weight molecules can enter cells by diffusion. Macromolecules normally do not pass across plasma membranes and their capture by cells is restricted to passive or active endocytosis. The endocytic capture of macromolecules and its significance for drug delivery have been discussed in depth by Duncan.[62] In an endocytic process, polymers enter the cell in pinocytic vesicles which rapidly join the endosomal compartment before moving on to fuse with lysosomes containing a variety of enzymes, including peptidases. If the spacer is a good substrate for these lysosomal enzymes, lysosomotropic drug delivery is feasible. Lysosomotropic drug delivery depends on the choice of

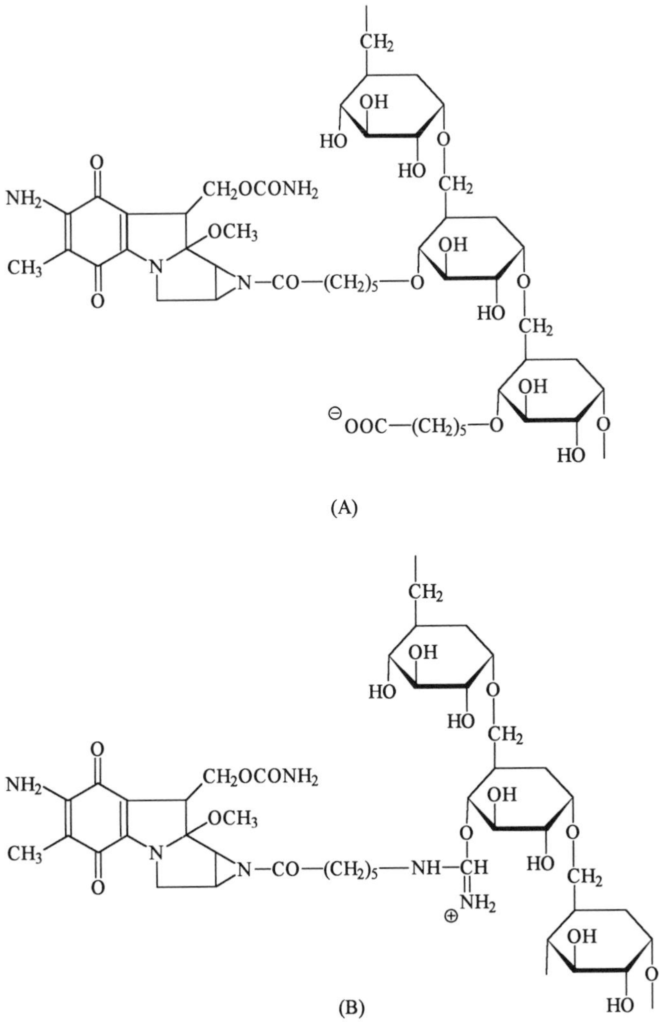

(A)

(B)

Fig. 33.6   Chemical structure of (A) anionic and (B) cationic mitomycin C-dextran conjugates.

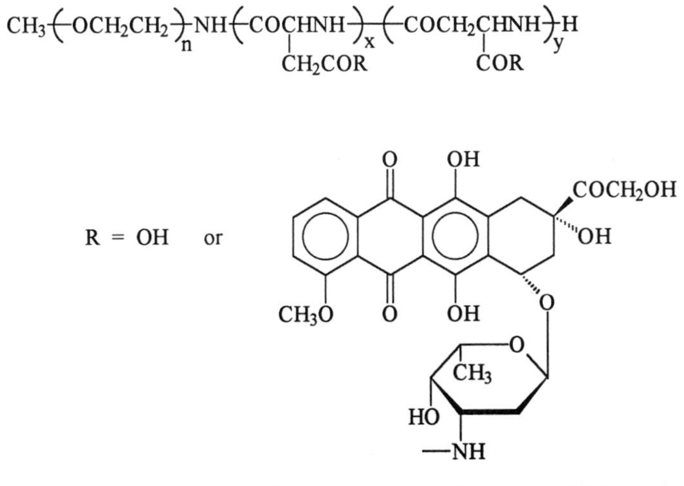

Fig. 33.7   Adriamycin-conjugated poly(ethylene glycol)–poly(aspartic acid) block copolymer.

drug, carrier and linkage between drug and carrier. The *in vivo* release can be due to passive hydrolysis or can be caused by a more specific mode of cleavage, such as enzymatic release or pH-controlled release.

(a) Passive hydrolysis. Esters, carbonates, amides and urethanes are susceptible to hydrolysis. Drugs linked with the spacer via such bonds will be released in aqueous media. The rate of release will decrease in the order ester > carbonate > urethane > amide. Cleavage may also occur at the level of the spacer–backbone bond so that spacer–drug moieties can be released as well.

(b) Enzyme-assisted hydrolysis. This is likely to occur for conjugates having oligopeptide spacers. The rate and site of the cleavage will depend on the composition of the peptide. Trouet and co-workers prepared albumin–adriamycin conjugates with oligopeptide spacers between the drug and the carrier.[63] As shown in Table 33.2 *in vitro* release of adriamycin increased with increasing length of the peptidic spacer. Only conjugates with tri- or tetrapeptide spacers expressed high *in vivo* anticancer activity observed by prolonged lifespan of the treated mice. Since the conjugates with tri- or tetrapeptide spacers released minor amounts of free drug in serum, the significant antitumour effect was attributed to lysosomal drug release. From these data it follows that site-specific drug release by proper molecular design of the conjugate is feasible. This is further substantiated by the excellent work of Kopececk and Duncan who evaluated a series of PHPMA–adriamycin conjugates with different oligopeptide spacers.[62,64] *In vitro* release studies in media containing lysosomal enzymes clearly demonstrated that drug release can be tailored by the length and composition of the peptide spacer (Table 33.2). *In vivo* experiments confirmed that the pharmacological activity of the polymer–drug conjugate depends on the nature of the spacer.

Table 33.2   Degradation of HPMA copolymers by rat liver lysosomal enzymes, effect of peptidyl side-chain.

Spacer	Percentage of doxorubicin released after 24 h
P-Gly-Phe-Gly-Dox	64
P-Gly-Leu-Gly-Dox	18.5
P-Gly-Phe-Leu-Gly-Dox	59.3
P-Gly-Leu-Phe-Gly-Dox	70.7

The importance of the spacer composition to the drug release was also demonstrated by De Marre for poly[(2-hydroxyethyl)-L-glutamine] PHEG peptide–mitomycin C conjugates.[40,65] Conjugates with a spacer having glycine as C-terminal amino acid were more susceptible to hydrolytic release in aqueous buffer or serum than those having a more hydrophobic terminal amino acid. Tetrapeptide spacers were more susceptible to cleavage by lysosomal enzymes than were tripeptides (Table 33.3).

Table 33.3 Release of mitomycin C (MMC) by hydrolysis of PHEG-tripeptide or tetrapeptide–MMC conjugates by tritosomes at pH 5.5 after 3 h.

Tripeptide spacers	Percentage MMC released	Tetrapeptide spacer	Percentage MMC released
Gly-Phe-Leu	2.4	Gly-Gly-Phe-Leu	3.1
Gly-Gly-Phe	2.5	Gly-Phe-Leu-Gly	57.7
Gly-Phe-Phe	2.7	Gly-Phe-Ala-Leu	74.6
Gly-Phe-Gly	7.1	Ala-Leu-Ala-Leu	81.0

(c) pH-controlled drug release. Polymers entering the endosomal or lysosomal compartment are exposed to an acidic medium (pH 4.5–5.5). Shen and Ryser developed a concept for pH-controlled intracellular drug release.[66] Daunorubicin was linked with aminoethyl polyacrylamide beads (Affi-gel 701) or poly(D-lysine) via an *N-cis*-aconityl spacer (Fig. 33.8). The *cis*-aconityl linkage between drug and carrier was readily hydrolysed at pH 4 but not appreciably at pH 6. Poly(D-lysine) conjugates caused 90% inhibition of growth of WEH 1-5 cells cultured *in vitro*. The conjugate was able to enter the cells by pinocytosis and, on reaching the lysosomal compartment, liberate daunorubicin. Drug release must be due to pH sensitivity of the *cis*-aconityl linkage, since the poly(D-lysine) is not biodegradable.

(d) Reduction-sensitive spacers. Shen and Ryser coupled methotrexate via a disulfide containing spacer with poly(D-lysine).[67] The conjugate was able to enter methotrexate-resistent cell lines cultured *in vitro*. There was evidence for a reductive cleavage of the spacer in the cytosol compartment. This example indicates another possibility for achieving intracellular release of drugs from polymeric conjugates by proper selection of the spacer.

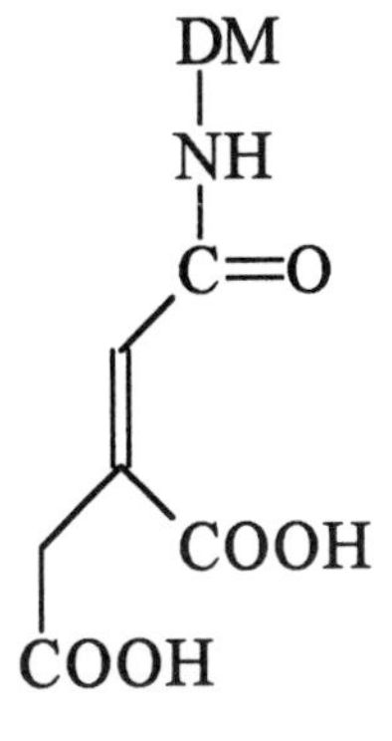

Fig. 33.8 *N-cis*-Aconityl daunorubicin.

V. MODIFICATION OF PHARMACOKINETICS AND IMMUNOGENICITY BY POLYMER CONJUGATION

The profile of plasma concentration of drugs is an important determinant of their quantitative access to peripheral targets. The plasma profile is usually measured as the area under the curve (AUC). In general, slow renal elimination and metabolic inactivation promote better access of drugs to remote targets, although this can also cause elevated toxicity. Many drugs in routine use are membrane permeable because their sites of action are intracellular, and such drugs typically exhibit high volumes of distribution and rapid plasma clearance. Conjugation to hydrophilic macromolecular carriers can prevent rapid renal excretion and restrict drug entry into cells to pinocytic mechanisms, markedly prolonging plasma circulation time.[68,69] It is important that polymers used for this type of pharmacokinetic modification are well tolerated, showing good biocompatibility with blood and tissues. To date the greatest success has been gained using neutral or slightly negatively charged polymers, since these materials have limited interaction with the negatively charged chondroitin sulphates and heparin sulphates of the endothelial wall and remain in circulation for a prolonged time.[70,71]

Molecular size is important in determining rates of glomerular filtration of large water-soluble molecules circulating in the plasma. For example, small proteins (<40 kDa) are rapidly excreted in the urine with half-lives of only a few minutes.[53,72] Conjugation of small peptides or proteins to hydrophilic soluble polymers can prevent rapid glomerular filtration and lead to much greater AUC. In most cases the resulting polymer–protein conjugate is thought to take the form of a colloid, with the protein core protected from interaction with other macromolecular plasma components by a hydrophilic polymeric shield. Hence, this procedure also decreases the immunogenicity of the protein component and permits repeated administration of foreign proteins.[44,73] One disadvantage of the approach is that the derivatized protein usually has decreased access to macromolecular substrates and cell surfaces. Hence, modification of murine antibodies for drug targeting has been largely unsuccessful.[51] However, the approach is particularly useful where the protein is an enzyme with a low-molecular-weight substrate found in plasma. For example, L-asparaginase is an enzyme which hydrolyses L-asparagine to yield L-aspartic acid and ammonia. The depletion of L-asparagine from blood plasma can be used to inhibit growth of certain tumours. In clinical trials, however, the enzyme displayed a very short plasma half-life ($T_{1/2} = 1.5$ h) and an anti-L-asparaginase antibody was soon produced in patients, which nullified the pharmacological activity. These problems were solved simultaneously by conjugating the enzyme with poly(ethylene glycol) (PEG). The immunogenic potential of the conjugated enzyme was decreased by 99% compared with the native form, and plasma circulation was greatly extended.[74] Polymer-tailored L-asparaginase is now being developed for clinical applications in the United States.

VI. ACTIVE TARGETING

A. Intra-arterial injection and embolization

An important physical means of achieving tumour-selective delivery of drugs is by direct injection into the artery feeding the tumour. Although it is usually impossible to gain access to arteries supplying exclusively tumour tissue, the regional selectivity of exposure to cytotoxic drugs that can be achieved in this way is much better than for intravenous injection. In addition, physiological differences between the vascular supply to tumour and normal tissues can sometimes be exploited to give additional selectivity of action; for example, the use of vasoconstricting agents to decrease the relative blood supply through normal vasculature, which is reported to be more responsive than tumour vasculature.[75-77] The artery most widely used for this type of clinical treatment is the hepatic artery, which supplies most of the blood to advanced hepatic metastases of colorectal carcinomas as well as primary liver tumours. Recently, great effort have been expended in developing techniques for injection into arteries supplying breast and renal tumours.

Apart from direct injection of drugs into tumour-feeding arteries, various attempts have been made to embolize the tumour capillary bed using microparticulate formulations of drugs. A range of drugs and delivery vehicles (simple aqueous solutions, oils or particulate formulations) have undergone evaluation.[78] One approach of particular note involving soluble macromolecular drug carriers is SMANCS. In the clinical formulation, neocarcinostatin (NCS) (molecular weight 10 700) is conjugated to two chains of a styrene–maleic anhydride copolymer (SMA) (molecular weight average 1500, polydispersity <1.2) through primary amino functions at NCS positions 1 (alanine) and 20 (lysine).[68,79] The SMA copolymer is itself derivatized with an alkyl group (usually butyl) which determines the overall hydrophobicity of the conjugate.[80] Although the resulting conjugate is sometimes applied intravenously, when it binds to albumin and shows prolonged circulation compared with parent NCS, the more successful use of SMANCS has followed its dissolution in lipiodol and hepatic arterial injection to treat primary hepatocellular carcinoma.

Primary hepatoma usually exhibits a leaky, sinusoidal, endothelial layer, permitting relatively easy interstitial access of oils administered intraarterially.[81] The lack of organized lymphatic drainage from the tumour (see later) results in long-term retention of oils that can be exploited for angiographic imaging of primary hepatic tumour masses. When SMANCS is dissolved in lipiodol, it remains selectively associated with the oily phase, diffusing out slowly into adjacent tumour tissues over a period of many weeks. One obvious strength of the SMANCS approach is that cytotoxicity of the conjugate depends on the rate of diffusion of SMANCS out of the lipidol; variations in alkyl derivatization of the polymeric SMA component can influence the oil–plasma partition coefficient of SMANCS, permitting development of drugs with precisely optimized release rates. This approach has been widely investigated in Japan for treatment of primary hepatoma, with remarkable response rates.[82,83] Phase I/II clinical trials are now being undertaken at the Queen Elizabeth Hospital, Birmingham, United Kingdom.

B. Antibody conjugates

Antibodies represent the most universally applicable active targeting agent, having exquisite selectivity for recognition of small antigenic epitopes. The antibody–antigen interaction can be so strong that antitumour effects of drug–antibody conjugates can be improved many times compared with the free drug.[84] Frequently, however, the quantity of drug that can be selectively targeted is limited by the number of antigens available. Hence in cancer therapy the targeted-drug approach has been most successful for extremely potent agents such as the plant toxins, which in conjugation with antibodies have been termed 'immunotoxins'.[85] Unfortunately, selectivity of immunotoxin delivery in human subjects, particularly where the target is a solid tumour, has been inadequate to mediate reproducible therapeutic responses.[86] One factor limiting this approach is the poor access of antibodies to tumour cells deep within the tumour interstitium, and recently greater attention has shifted to identifying antigens associated specifically with the vasculature serving the tumour.[87] Tumour-associated endothelial cells represent a target that is accessible, vulnerable and crucial to tumour survival; initial reports on selective destruction have been encouraging.[88]

One approach of particular note in cancer therapy has been the use of antibodies for tumour-targeted delivery of enzymes capable of activating innocuous prodrugs to highly cytotoxic species[89,90] (Fig. 33.9). This approach is known by the acronym ADEPT (antibody-directed-enzyme-prodrug therapy) and one major advantage over conventional antibody-targeting is the inherent amplification stage, meaning that for every successful enzyme-targeting event a very large number of prodrug molecules can be activated.[91,92] The novelty of this approach is such that it has attracted very great interest and certain versions have already received clinical appraisal. Initial results have been promising, though dogged with such problems as poor water-solubility of prodrugs, and the approach is currently being refined for further development.

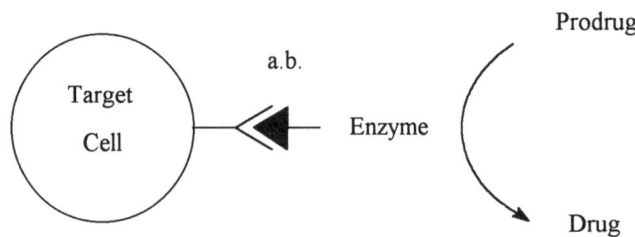

Fig. 33.9　Schematic representation of the ADEPT concept.

C.　Macromolecular glycoconjugates as carrier systems

Sugar-specific receptors are plasma membrane components (either glycoproteins or glycolipids, called lectins[93]) of many mammalian cells. The first membrane lectin was characterized on hepatocytes by the group of Ashwell and Morell.[94] Endogenous lectins, generally multivalent in their binding and recognition capacities, are found on numerous normal and malignant cells (Table 33.4). Biologically they are vital elements in a complex network of 'biosignalling', acting as sugar-specific receptors and/or mediating endocytosis of specific glycoconjugates.[95,96] Therefore, glycoconjugates may be used as carriers to specifically deliver biologically active agents such as metabolite inhibitors, toxic drugs, biological response modifiers or genetic material to intracellular compartments (e.g. lysosomatropic delivery[97]).

The possibility of using hepatic lectins recognizing galactose as targets for drug delivery is particularly attractive and has been investigated exhaustively. A well-known target is the asialoglycoprotein receptor (ASGP-R),[98] which is easily accessible to the vascular circulation, being situated predominantly on the sinusoidal surfaces of hepatocytes. Moreover, it is present in relatively large numbers, allowing the delivery of therapeutic doses of bioactive agents. In addition, the hepatocyte constitutes a valuable target for treatments of various diseases including

Table 33.4 Membrane lectins from various sources.[78,79]

Origin	Sugar specificity
Murine liver macrophages	D-Mannose, L-fucose, D-galactose and *N*-acetyl-D-glucosamine
Rat and human hepatocytes	D-Galactose
Mouse spleen	D-Galactose/*N*-acetyl-D-glucosamine
Human fibroblasts	D-Mannose-6-phosphate
Mouse L1210 leukaemia cells	L-Fucose

lysosomal storage diseases, metabolic deficiencies, hepatitis, parasitic infections (e.g. malaria) and cancer treatment (e.g. liver metastasis).

The feasibility of liver targeting is well documented. As an example, Vansteenkiste and colleagues[99] prepared a range of copolymers based on the carbohydrate dextran substituted with pendent side-chains terminated in 1-*O*-linked monosaccharides, including mannose and galactose (mono-gal) as well as clusters of three galactose molecules (tris-gal).[100] Following intravenous injection (50 µg) to rats, both galactosylated dextrans were cleared rapidly with plasma half-lives of <2 min, mainly into the liver. However, a significant difference in liver disposition was demonstrated between the tris-gal-substituted dextran (71% of the injected dose) and its mono-gal analogue (43%). Moreover, subcellular distribution experiments[101] indicated that mono-gal dextran is accumulated within the lysosomal compartment of liver hepatocytes. In contrast, the tris-gal-substituted polymer shows a greater affinity for the galactose-specific receptor *in vivo* and also shows a high level of association with the cell surface. This phenomenon offers the possibility of targeting prodrugs to the external surface of hepatocytes (a variation of the ADEPT concept).

Drug delivery to macrophages (e.g. Kupffer cells) offers a second potentially attractive goal in the development of targeted treatment of various malfunctions, notably parasitic disorders such as Leishmaniasis or enzyme deficiencies such as Gaucher's syndrome. Moreover, since macrophages are part of the immune system, they can be activated and rendered tumoricidal by immunostimulating agents (e.g. *N*-acetylmuramyldipeptide, MDP).

Mannosylated carriers can also fulfil an important role not only in active drug targeting but also in receptor blocking. It was demonstrated that mannosylated dextrans were useful as transient receptor blockers *in vivo* for a 791T/36-ricin toxin A immunotoxin.[100] The circulation half-life of the immunotoxin was prolonged by a factor 3–4 up to 40 min. following co-injection of an excess of mannosylated dextran. The liver disposition of the immunotoxin was markedly reduced from 43% to 18% of the recovered dose. The influence of the molecular size as well as the sugar loading of the competing polysaccharide was demonstrated to be small.

VII. PASSIVE TARGETING

Numerous studies over the past 40 years have reported an apparent passive targeting of soluble macromolecules to solid tumours. Various causes have been suggested, including rapid pinocytosis by tumour cells *in vivo*, although the most likely explanation was proposed by

Matsumura and Maeda (1986)[102] and results from the absence of organized lymphatic drainage of solid tumours. Slow or absent convection of fluid through solid tumour masses results in the formation of hypoxic regions and the elevation of interstitial hydrostatic pressure.[103] In response to poor nutritional supply, the tumours produce angiogenic and capillary-permeabilizing factors which result in nonspecific leakiness of the tumour vasculature and the extravasation and subsequent extravascular retention of macromolecules (and soluble drug conjugates) from the bloodstream. This effect, termed the 'enhanced permeability and retention effect' (EPR effect) is thought to be important for nutrition and for the laying down of new tumour stroma. Similar phenomena are observed in processes of wound healing.[104] Intensive studies are underway to elucidate factors controlling tumour vascular hyperpermeability, although the effect is already being examined clinically using anthracyclines conjugated to hydrophilic macromolecular carriers.

A number of macromolecular drug conjugates have taken advantage, sometimes inadvertently, of the EPR effect.[105–109] One of the best-characterized is the conjugate of doxorubicin (DOX) with copolymers based on N-(2-hydroxypropyl)methacrylamide (HPMA) which is now on phase I/II clinical trial in the United Kingdom.[110] The form under clinical evaluation has weight-average molecular weight of approximately 25 000 and the anthracycline is attached via a tetrapeptide side-chain designed as a substrate for lysosomal thiol-proteases. In preclinical studies the conjugate has shown a passive tumoritropism to subcutaneous tumours, together with sustained activation of the drug conjugate *in situ*. Following intravenous administration to mice bearing solid subcutaneous B16F10 melanomas, free DOX (5 mg DOX per kg body weight) produced tumour levels of only 0.55 µg DOX per g tumour, while the same dose of DOX administered as polymer conjugate achieved levels up to 7.5 µg per g tumour. The decreased peripheral toxicity of polymer-conjugated DOX permits the use of greater doses, and administration of doses of 18 mg DOX per kg results in tumour levels of drug up to 22 µg per g.[111] Hence the impressive anticancer activity observed is thought to result from a combination of passive tumoritropism and decreased peripheral toxicity.[110]

Some of the parameters influencing the tumoritropic behaviour of soluble macromolecules have now been elucidated,[68,112] permitting development of more sophisticated approaches using biodegradable carriers and linkages carefully designed for selective cleavage by tumour-associated enzymes.

VIII. ORAL DRUG DELIVERY

The preferred mode for drug administration is undoubtedly the oral route, but the efficiency of oral administration is often limited by premature uptake or degradation. For drugs that need to enter systemic circulation, the adsorption window is situated in the upper intestine. For treatment of inflammations in the lower part of the GI tract, uptake in the small intestine is to be avoided. A typical example is the treatment of ulcerative colitis and Crohn's disease with 5-aminosalicylic acid (5-ASA). The parent drug is not efficient because of premature uptake in the upper intestine. One possible solution is the use of polymeric conjugates of 5-ASA linked to a polymeric carrier via an azo bond. It is well known that the colon is a reductive medium that can split azo bonds with formation of the amino constituents. It is anticipated that a polymer–5-ASA conjugate will pass intact through the upper part of the GI tract and reach the colon, where 5-ASA will be released. We have prepared in our laboratory a series of azo-coupled polymer–5-ASA conjugates[113] (Fig. 33.10). *In vitro* experiments carried out in a bioreactor simulating the human intestinal microbial environment (SHIME) demonstrated that the parent drug is readily cleaved from the carrier in the colon-simulating part of the reactor.[114] Independently of our work, Kopececk and his group also prepared polymeric prodrugs of 5-ASA using PHPMA as carrier.[115]

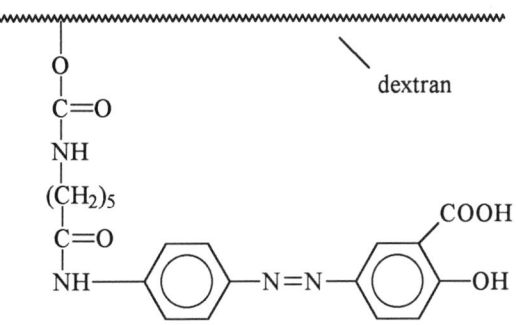

Fig. 33.10   Structure of azo-coupled dextran–5-ASA prodrug.

REFERENCES

1. Robinson, J. R. and Lee, H. L. (eds) (1987) *Controlled Drug Delivery: Fundamentals and Applications*, 2nd edn. Marcel Dekker, New York.
2. Duncan, R. and Seymour, L. W. (1989) *Controlled Release Technologies: A Survey of Research and Commercial Applications*. Elsevier Advanced Technology, Oxford.
3. Kim, S. W., Kopecek, J. and Knutsen, K. (1992) In Anderson, J. M. (ed.) *Advances in Drug Delivery Systems*, part 5. Elsevier, Amsterdam.
4. Kim, S. W., Kopecek, J. and Knutsen, K. (1994) In Anderson, J. M. (ed.) *Advances in Drug Delivery Systems*, part 6. Elsevier, Amsterdam.
5. Baker, R. (1987) *Controlled Release of Biologically Active Agents*. Wiley, New York.
6. Vert, M. (1986) Polyvalent polymeric drug carriers. *CRC Crit. Rev. Ther. Drug Carrier Syst.* **2**: 291–327.
7. Okano, T., Yui, N., Yokoyama, M. and Yoshida, R. (1994) *Advances in Polymeric Systems for Drug Delivery*. Gordon and Breach Science Publishers, Tokyo.
8. Barry, B. W. (1983) Drug delivery systems. *CHEMTECH* 38–44.
9. Ringsdorf, H. (1975) Structure and properties of pharmacologically active polymers. *J. Polym. Sci. Symp.* **51**: 135–153.
10. Donaruma, L. G. (1974) Synthetic biologically active polymers. *Prog. Polym. Sci.* **4**: 1–25.
11. Batz, H. G. (1977) Polymeric drugs. *Adv. Polym. Sci.* **23**: 25–53.
12. Ottenbrite, R. M. (1980) Introduction to biology and medicine. In Donaruma, L. G., Otenbrite, R. M. and Vogl, O. (eds) *Anionic Polymeric Drugs*. Wiley, New York.
13. Duncan, R. and Kopecek, J. (1984) Soluble synthetic polymers as potential drug carriers. *Adv. Polym. Sci.* **57**: 51–101.
14. Ferruti, P. and Tanzi, M. C. (1986) New polymeric and oligomeric matrices as drug carriers. *CRC Crit. Rev. Ther. Drug Carrier Syst.* **2**: 175–244.
15. Kim, S. W., Peterson, R. V. and Feijen, J. (1980) Polymeric drug delivery systems. In Arlens, E. (ed.) *Drug Design*, vol. X, pp. 193–250. Academic Press, New York.
16. Kopecek, J., Rejmanova, P., Duncan, R. and Lloyd, J. B. (1985) Controlled release of drug model from *N*-(2-hydroxypropyl)methacrylamide copolymers. *Ann. NY Acad. Sci.* **446**: 93–104.

17. Rihova, B., Ulbrich, K., Stohalm, J., Vetvicka, V., Bilej, M., Duncan, R. and Kopecek, J. (1989) Biocompatibility of N-(2-hydroxypropyl)methacrylamide copolymers containing adriamycin. Immunogenecity, effect on haematopoietic stem cells in bone marrow *in vivo* and effect on mouse splenocytes and human peripheral blood lymphocytes *in vitro*. *Biomaterials* **10**: 335–342.

18. Duncan, R. (1992) Drug-polymer conjugates: potential for improved chemotherapy. *Anticancer Drugs* **3**: 175–210.

19. Pato, J., Azori, M. and Tudos, F. (1987) Quinidine convently bound to a dextran carrier. *J. Bioact. Biocomp. Polymers* **2**: 142–147.

20. Mora, M., Pato, J. and Tudos, F. (1989) Polymeric prodrugs, 6. Synthesis and examination of 6-purinethiol bound to poly(1-vinyl-2-pyrrolidone-co-maleic acid). *Makromol. Chem.* **190**: 1967–1974.

21. Soutif, J. C., Mouity-Moussounda, F. and Brosse, J. C. (1983) Polymeric carriers of glycerol derivatives, 2. Chlorambucil derivatives. *Makromol. Chem. Rapid Commun.* **4**: 61–64.

22. Yasuhiro, M. and Maeda, H. (1986) A new concept for macromolecular therapeutics in cancer chemotherapy: mechanism of tumourotropic accumulation of proteins and the antitumour agent smancs. *Cancer Res.* **46**: 6387–6392.

23. Hirano, T., Ringsdorf, H. and Zaharko, D. Z. (1980) Antitumour activity of monomeric and polymeric cyclophosphamide derivatives compared with *in vitro* hydrolysis. *Cancer Res.* **40**: 2263–2267.

24. Przybylski, E., Fell, E., Ringsdorf, H. and Zaharko, D. Z. (1978) Pharmacologically active polymers, 17. Synthesis and characterization of polymeric derivatives of the antitumour agent methotrexate. *Makromol. Chem.* **179**: 1719–1733.

25. Remon, J. P., Duncan, R. and Schacht, E. (1984) Polymer–drug combinations: pinocytic uptake of modified polysaccharides containing procaimide moieties by rat visceral yolk sacs cultured *in vitro*. *J. Controlled Rel.* **1**: 47–56.

26. Schacht, E. (1985) Use of polysaccharides as drug carriers. *Ann. Natl. Acad. Sci. USA* **446**: 199–212.

27. Bernstein, A., Hurwitz, E., Maron, R., Arnon, R., Sela, M. and Wilchek, M. (1978) Higher antitumour efficacy of daunomycin when linked to dextran, *in vivo* and *in vitro* studies. *J. Natl. Cancer Inst.* **60**: 379–384.

28. Konieezny, M., Charytonowicz, D. and Inglot, A. D. (1982) Search for carriers for non-covalent binding of interferon among 1,3,5-triazine derivatives of dextran. *Arch. Immunol. Ther. Exp.* **30**: 1–10.

29. Sezaki, H. and Hashida, M. (1984) *CRC Crit. Rev. Therap. Drug Carrier Syst.* **1**: 1–38.

30. Matsumoto, S., Yamamoto, A., Takakura, Y., Hashida, M. and Sezaki, H. (1986) Cellular interaction and *in vitro* antitumour activity of mitomycin C–dextran conjugate. *Cancer Res.* **46**: 4463–4468.

31. Molteni, L. (1979) Dextrans as drug carriers. In Gregoriadis, G. (ed.) *Drug Carriers in Biology and Medicine*, pp. 107–125. Academic Press, London.

32. Simonescu, C. R., Popa, M. I. and Dimitriu, S. (1984) Bioactive polymers. XIV. Immobolization of ampicillin on biozan R. *Z. Naturforsch.* **39C**, 397–401.

33. Hurwitz, E., Wilchek, M. and Pitha, J. (1980) Soluble macromolecules as carriers of daunomycin. *J. Appl. Biochem.* **2**: 25–36.

34. Ouchi, Y., Banba, T., Matsumoto, T., Suzuki, S. and Suzuki, M. (1989) Antitumour activity of chitosan and chitin immobilized 5-fluorouracils through hexamethylene spacers via carbamoyl bonds. *J. Bioact. Biocomp. Pol.* **4**: 362–371.

35. Ryser, H. and Shen, W. C. (1978) Conjugation of methotrexate to poly(L-lysine) increases drug transport and overcomes drug resistance in cultured cells. *Proc. Natl. Acad. Sci. USA* **75**: 3867–3870.

36. Zunino, F., Giulliani, F., Savi, G., Dasdia, T. and Gambetta, R. (1982) Anti-tumour activity of daunorubicin linked to poly-L-aspartic acid. *J. Pharmacol. Exp. Ther.* **30**: 465–469.

37. Giammona, G., Puglisi, G., Carlisi, B., Pignatello, R., Spadaro, A. and Caruso, A. (1989) Polymeric prodrugs: α-β-poly(N-hydroxyethyl)-DL-aspartamide as macromolecular carrier for some non-steroidal anti-inflammatory agents. *Int. J. Pharm.* **57**: 55–62.

38. Friedmann, G., Aichaoui, H. and Brini, M. (1981) Polymères à propriétés pharmacologiques potentiels: greffage par liaison amide et (ou) ester d'un hypoglycémiant. *Makrol. Chem.* **182**: 337–347.

39. De Machado, M., Neuse, E. W. and Perlwitz, A. G. (1992) Water-soluble polyamides as potential drug carriers. V. Carboxy-functionalized polyaspartamides and copolyaspartamides. *Angew. Makromol. Chem.* **195**: 35–56.

40. De Marre, A., Soyez, H. and Schacht, E. (1994) Synthesis of macromolecular mitomycin C derivatives. *J. Controlled Rel.* **32**: 129–137.

41. Trouet, A., Baurain, R., Deprez-De Campaneere, D., Masquelier, M. and Pirson, P. (1982) Targeting of antitumoral antiprotozoal drugs by covalent linkage to protein carriers. In Gregoriadis, G., Senior, J. and Trouet, A. (eds) *Targeting of Drugs*, pp. 19–30. Plenum Press, New York.

42. Chu, B. C. F. and Whiteley, J. M. (1979) Control of solid tumour metastases with a high molecular weight derivative of methotrexate. *J. Natl. Cancer Inst.* **62**: 79–82.

43. Harris, J. M. (1992) Introduction to biotechnical and biomedical applications of poly(ethylene glycol). In Harris, J. M. (ed.) *Poly(ethylene glycol) Chemistry: Biotechnical and Biomedical Applications*, pp. 1–14. Plenum Press, New York.

44. Abuchowski, A., Van Es, T. and Palczuk, N. C. (1977) Alteration of immunological properties of bovine serum albumin by covalent attachment of polyethylene glycol. *J. Biol. Chem.* **252**: 3578–3581.

45. Abuchowski, A., Kazo, G. M., Verhoest, C. R. Jr., Van Es, T., Kafkewitz, D., Vian, A. T. and Davis, F. F. (1984) Cancer therapy with chemically modified enzymes. 1. A property of polyethylene glycol asparaginase conjugates. *Cancer Bio. Chem. Biophys.* **7**: 175–186.

46. Abuchowski, A. and Davis, F. F. (1981) In Hosenberg, J. and Roberts, J. (eds) *Enzymes as Drugs*. Wiley, New York.

47. Cecchi, R., Rusconi, L., Tanzi, M. C., Danusso, F. and Ferruti, P. (1981) Synthesis and pharmacological evaluation of 4-isobutylphenyl-2-propionic acid (ibuprofen). *J. Med. Chem.* **24**: 622–625.

48. Duncan, R., Kopecek, J. and Lloyd, J. B. (1983) Development of *N*-(2-hydroxypropyl)-methacrylamide copolymers as carriers of therapeutic agents. In Chiellini, E. and Guisti, P. (eds) *Polymers in Medicine: Biomedical and Pharmacological Applications*, pp. 97–14. Plenum Press, New York.

49. Lloyd, J. B., Duncan, R. and Pratten, M. K. (1983) Soluble synthetic polymers as targetable agents for intracellular drug release. *Br. Polym. J.* **15**: 158–159.

50. Duncan, R., Kopecek, J., Rejmanova, P. and Lloyd, J. B. (1983) Targeting of *N*-(2-hydroxypropyl)methacrylamide copolymers to liver by incorporation of galactose residues. *Biochem. Biophys. Acta* **755**: 518–521.

51. Seymour, L. W., Flanagan, P. A., Al-Shamkhani, A., Subr, V., Ulbrich, K., Cassidy, J. and Duncan, R. (1991) Synthetic polymers conjugated to monoclonal antibodies: vehicles for tumour-targeted drug delivery. *Select. Cancer Ther.* **7**: 59–73.

52. Flanagan, P. A., Kopeckova, P., Kopecek, J. and Duncan, R. (1989) Evaluation of antibody-*N*-(2-hydroxypropyl)methacrylamide copolymer conjugates as targetable drug-carriers. 1. Binding, pinocytic uptake and intracellular distribution of transferrin and anti-transferrin receptor antibody-conjugates. *Biochim. Biophys. Acta* **993**: 83–91.

53. Seymour, L. W., Duncan, R., Strohalm, J. and Kopecek, J. (1987) Effect of molecular weight (MW) of *N*-(2-hydroxypropyl)methacrylamide copolymers on body distribution and rate of excretion after subcutaneous, intraperitoneal and intravenous administration to rats. *J. Biomed. Mater. Res.* **21**: 1341–1358.

54. Sela, M. and Katchalski, E. (1959) Biological properties of poly-α-amino acids. *Adv. Protein Chem.* **14**: 391–478.

55. Monsigny, M., Roche, A. C., Midoux, P. and Mayer, R. (1994) Glycoconjugates as carriers for specific delivery of therapeutic drugs and genes. *Adv. Drug Del. Rev.* **14**: 1–24.

56. Vercauteren, R., Schacht, E. and Duncan, R. (1992) Effect of the chemical modification of dextran on the degradation by rat liver lysosomal enzymes. *J. Bioact. Biocomp. Polym.* **7**: 346–357.

57. Franssen, E. J.F., Moolenaar, F., De Zeeuw, D. and Meijer, D. K. F. (1994) Drug targeting to the kidney with low-molecular-weight proteins. *Adv. Drug Del. Rev.* **14**: 67–88.

58. Seymour, L. W. (1994) Soluble polymers for lectin-mediated drug targeting. *Adv. Drug Del. Rev.* **14**: 89–112.

59. Yokoyama, M., Miyauchi, M., Yamada, N., Okano, T., Sakurai, Y., Kataoka, K. and Inoue, S.

(1990) Characterization and anticancer activity of the micelle forming polymeric anti-cancer drug adriamycin-conjugated poly(ethylene glycol)–poly(aspartic acid) block copolymer. *Cancer Res.* **50**: 1693–1700.

60. Yokoyama, M., Okano, T., Sakurai, Y., Ekimoto, H., Shibazaki, C. and Kataoka, K. (1991) Toxicity and anti-tumour activity against solid tumours of micelle-forming polymeric anti-cancer drug and its extremely long circulation in blood. *Cancer Res.* **51**: 3229–3236.

61. Yokoyama, M. (1992) Block copolymers as drug carriers. *Crit. Rev. Ther. Drug Carrier Syst.* **9**: 213–248.

62. Duncan, R. (1987) Selective endocytosis of macromolecular drug carriers. In Robinson, J. R. and Lee, V. H. (eds) *Controlled Drug Delivery: Fundamentals and Applications*, 2nd edn, pp. 581–607. Marcel Dekker, New York.

63. Trouet, A., Masquelier, M., Baurain, R and Deprez-De Campeneere, D. (1982) A covalent linkage between daunorubicin and protein that is stable in serum and reversible by lysosomal hydrolases, as required for a lysosomotropic drug-carrier conjugate: *in vitro* and *in vivo* studies. *Proc. Natl. Acad. Sci. USA* **79**: 626–629.

64. Subr, V., Strohalm, J., Ulbrich, K., Duncan, R. and Hume, Z. (1992) Polymers containing enzymatically degradable bonds, XII. Effect of spacer structure on the rate of release of daunomycin and adriamycin from poly[N-(2-hydroxypropyl)-methacrylamide] copolymer drug carriers *in vitro* and antitumour activity measured *in vivo*. *J. Controlled Rel.* **18**: 123–132.

65. De Marre, A., Seymour, L. W. and Schacht, E. (1994) Evaluation of the hydrolytic and enzymatic stability of macromolecular mitomycin C derivatives. *J. Controlled Rel.* **31**: 89–97.

66. Shen, W. C. and Ryser, H. J. P. (1981) Cis-aconityl spacer between daunomycin and macromolecular carriers: a model of pH-sensitive linkage releasing drug from a lysosomotropic conjugate. *Biochem. Biophys. Res. Commun.* **102**: 1048–1054.

67. Shen, W. C., Ryser, H. J. P. and La Manna, L. (1985) Disulfide spacer between methotrexate and poly(D-lysine). *J. Biol. Chem.* **260**: 10905–10908.

68. Maeda, H., Seymour, L. W. and Miyamoto, Y. (1992) Conjugates of anticanter agents and polymers: advantages of macromolecular therapeutics *in vivo*. *Bioconj. Chem.* **3**: 351–362.

69. Seymour, L. W., Ulbrich, K., Strohalm, J. and Duncan, R. (1990) The pharmacokinetics of polymer-bound adriamycin. *Biochem. Pharmacol.* **39**: 1125–1131.

70. Takakura, Y., Kitajima, M., Matsumoto, S., Hashida, M. and Sezaki, H. (1987) Development of a novel polymeric prodrug of mitomycin C, mitomycin C–dextran conjugate with anionic charge. 1. Physicochemical characteristics and *in vitro* and *in vivo* antitumour activities. *Int. J. Pharm.* **37**: 135–143.

71. Sezaki, H. and Hashida, M. (1984) Macromolecule-drug conjugates in targeted cancer chemotherapy. *CRC Crit. Rev. Ther. Drug Carrier Syst.* **1**: 1–38.

72. Ogino, T., Inoue, M., Ando, Y., Arai, H. and Morino, Y. (1988) Chemical modification of superoxide dismutase. Extension of plasma half-life of the enzyme through its reversible binding to circulating albumin. *Int. J. Peptide Protein Res.* **32**: 153–159.

73. Abuchowski, A., McCoy, J. R., Palczuk, N. C., Es, T. V. and Davis, F. F. (1977) Effect of covalent attachment of polyethylene glycol on immunogenicity and circulating life of bovine liver catalase. *J. Biol. Chem.* **252**: 3582–3586.

74. Kamisaki, Y., Wada, H., Yagura, H., Matsushima, A. and Inada, Y. (1981) Reduction in immunogenicity and clearance rate of *Escherichia coli* L-asparaginase by modification with monomethoxypoly(ethylene glycol). *J. Pharmacol. Exp. Ther.* **216**: 410–414.

75. Li, C. J., Miyamoto, Y., Kojima, Y. and Maeda, H. (1993) Augmentation of tumour delivery of macromolecular drugs with reduced bone marow delivery by elevating blood pressure. *Br. J. Cancer* **67**: 975–980.

76. Suzuki, M., Hori, K., Abe, I., Saito, S. and Sato, H. (1981) A new approach to cancer chemotherapy: a selective enhancement of tumour blood flow with angiotensin II. *J. Natl. Cancer Inst.* **67**: 663–669.

77. Hori, K., Suzuki, M., Tanda, S., Saito, S., Shinozaki, S. and Zhang, Q. H. (1991) Fluctuation in tumour blood flow under normotension and the effect of angiotensin II induced hypertension. *Jpn. J. Cancer Res.* **82**: 1309–1316.

78. Willmott, N. (1987) Chemoembolisation in regional cancer chemotherapy: a rationale. *Cancer Treat. Rev.* **14**: 143–156.

79. Maeda, H. (1991) SMANCS and polymer-conjugated macromolecular drugs: advantages in cancer chemotherapy. *Drug Delivery Rev.* **6**: 181–202.

80. Hirayama, S., Sato, F., Oda, T. and Maeda, H. (1986) Stability of high molecular weight anticancer agent SMANCS and its transfer from oil-phase to water-phase. *Jpn. J. Antibiot.* **39**: 815–822.

81. Maeda, H. (1992) The tumour blood vessel as an ideal target for macromolecular anticancer agents. *J. Controlled Release* **19**: 315–324.

82. Konno, T., Maeda, H., Iwai, K., Tashiro, S., Maki, S., Morinaga, T., Mochinaga, M., Hiraoka, T. and Yokoyama, I. (1983) Effect of arterial administration of high-molecular-weight anticancer agent SMANCS with lipid lymphographic agent on hepatoma: a preliminary report. *Eur. J. Cancer Clin. Oncol.* **19**: 1053–1065.

83. Konno, T. and Maeda, H. (1987) Targeting chemotherapy of hepatocellular carcinoma: aterial administration of SMANCS/lipidol. In Okuda, K. and Ishak, K. G (eds) *Neoplasms of the Liver*, chap. 27, pp. 343–352. Springer-Verlag, New York.

84. Trail, P. A., Willner, D., Lasch, S. J., Henderson, A. J., Hofstead, S., Casazza, A. M., Firestone, R. A. and Hellstrom, K. E. (1993) Cure of xenografted human carcinomas by BR96-doxorubicin immunoconjugates. *Science* **261**: 212–215.

85. Wawrzynczak, E. J. and Derbyshire, E. J. (1992) Immunotoxins: the power and the glory. *Immunology Today* **13**: 381–383.

86. Vitetta, E. S., Stone, M., Amlot, P. *et al.* (1991) Phase I immunotoxin trial in patients with B-cell lymphoma. *Cancer Res.* **51**: 4052–4058.

87. Wang, J. M., Kumar, S., Pye, D., Van Agthoven, A. J. Krupinski, J. and Hunter, R. D. (1993) A monoclonal antibody detects heterogenicity in vascular endothelium of tumours and normal tissues. *Int. J. Cancer* **54**: 363–370.

88. Burrows, F. J. and Thorpe, P. E. (1993) Eradication of large solid tumours in mice with an immunotoxin directed against tumour vasculature. *Proc. Natl. Acad. Sci.* **90**: 8996–9000.

89. Bagshawe, K. D., Springer, C. J., Searle, F., Antoniw, P., Sharma, S. K., Melton, R. G. and Sherwood, R. F. (1988) A cytotoxic agent can be generated selectively at cancer sites. *Br. J. Cancer* **58**: 700–703.

90. Springer, C. J., Bagshawe, K. D., Sharma, S. K., Searle, F., Boden, J. A., Antoniw, P., Burke, P. J., Rogers, G. T., Sherwood, R. F. and Melton, R. G. (1991) Ablation of human choriocarcinoma xenografts in nude mice by antibody-directed enzyme prodrug therapy (ADEPT) with three novel compounds. *Eur. J. Cancer* **27**: 1361–1366.

91. Senter, P. D., Su, P. D. D., Katsuragi, T., Sakai, T., Cosand, W. L., Hellstrom, I., Hellstrom, K. E. (1991) Generation of 5-fluorouracil from 5-fluorocytosine by monoclonal antibody–cytosine deaminase conjugates. *Bioconjugate Chem.* **2**: 447–451.

92. Sharma, S. K., Bagshawe, K. D., Springer, C. J., Burge, P. J., Rogers, G. T., Boden, J. A., Antoniw, P., Melton, R. G. and Sherwood, R. F. (1991) Antibody directed enzyme prodrug therapy (ADEPT): a three phase system. *Disease Markers* **9**: 225–231.

93. Goldstein, I. J., Hughes, R. C., Monsigny, M., Osawa, T. and Sharon, N. (1980) What should be called a lectin? *Nature* **285**: 66.

94. Ashwell, G. and Harford, J. (1982) Carbohydrate-specific receptors of the liver. *Annu. Rev. Biochem.* **51**: 531–554.

95. Sharon, N. and Lis, H. (1989) Lectins as cell recognition molecules. *Science* **246**: 227–234.

96. Monsigny, M., Roche, A. C. and Midoux, P. (1988) Endogenous lectins and drug targeting. *Ann. NY Acad. Sci.* **551**: 399–414.

97. De Duve, C., De Barsy, T., Poole, B., Trouet, A., Tulkens, P. and Van Hoof, F. (1974) Lysosomoropic agents. *Biochem. Pharmacol.* **23**: 2495–2531.

98. Schwartz, A. L. (1984) The hepatic asialoglycoprotein receptor. *CRC Crit. Rev. Biochem.* **16**: 207–233.

99. Vansteenkiste, S., Schacht, E., Duncan, R., Seymour, L., Pawluczyk, I. and Baldwin, R. (1991) Fate of glycosylated dextrans after *in vivo* administration. *J. Controlled Rel.* **16**: 91–100.

100. Vansteenkiste, S., De Marre, A. and Schacht, E. (1992) Synthesis of glycosylated dextrans. *J. Bioact. Compat. Polymers* **7**: 4–14.

101. Anderson, D., Vansteenkiste, S., Schacht, E. H., Sen, S. V. and Seymour, L. W. (1994) Differential internalisation of some galactosylated dextrans by hepatocytes. *Eur. J. Pharm.*, in press.

102. Masumura, Y. and Maeda, H. (1986) A new concept for macromolecular therapeutics in cancer chemotherapy: mechanism of tumouritropic accumulation of proteins and antitumour agent SMANCS. *Cancer Res.* **46**: 6387–6392.

103. Jain, R. K. (1991) Vascular and interstitial barriers to the delivery of therapeutic agents in tumours. *Cancer Metast. Rev.* **9**: 253–266.

104. Senger, D. R., Van de Water, L., Brown, I. F., Nagy, J. A., Yeo, K. T., Berse, B., Jackman, R. W., Dvorak, A. M. and Dvorak, H. F. (1993) Vascular permeability factor in tumour biology. *Cancer Metastasis Reviews* **12**: 303–324.

105. Berstein, A., Hurwitz, E., Maron, R., Arnon, R., Sela, M. and Wilchek, M. (1978) Higher antitumour efficacy of daunomycin when linked to dextran: *in vivo* and *in vitro* studies. *J. Natl. Cancer Inst.* **60**: 379–384.

106. Zunino, F., Pratesi, G. and Pezzoni, G. (1987) Increased therapeutic efficacy and reduced toxicity of doxorubicin linked to pyran copolymer via the side chain of the drug. *Cancer Treat. Rep.* **71**: 367–373.

107. Trouet, A. and Jolles, G. (1984) Targeting of daunorubicin by association with DNA or proteins: a review. *Semin. Oncol.* **11**: 64–73.

108. Seymour, L. W. (1992) Passive tumour targeting of soluble macromolecules and drug conjugates. *Crit. Rev. Ther. Drug Carrier Syst.* **9**: 135–187.

109. Cassidy, J., Duncan, R., Morrison, G. J., Strohalm, J., Plocova, D., Kopecek, J. and Kaye, S. B. (1989) Activity of *N*-(2-hydroxypropyl)methacrylamide copolymers containing daunomycin against a rat tumour model. *Biochem. Pharmacol.* **38**: 875–880.

110. Duncan, R., Seymour, L. W., O'Hare, K. B. *et al.* (1992) Preclinical evaluation of polymer-bound doxorubicin. *J. Controlled Rel.* **18**: 123–132.

111. Seymour, L. W., Ulbrich, K., Steyger, P. S., Brereton, M., Subr, V., Strohalm, J. and Duncan, R. (1994) Tumourtropism and anticancer efficacy of polymer-based doxorubicin prodrugs in the treatment of subcutaneous murine B16F10 melanoma. *Br. J. Cancer* **70**(4): 636–641.

112. Seymour, L. W., Miyamoto, Y., Maeda, H., Brereton, M., Strohalm, J., Ulbrich, K. and Duncan, R. (1994) Influence of molecular weight on passive tumour accumulation of a soluble macromolecular drug carrier. *Eur. J. Cancer*, in press.

113. Callant, D. and Schacht, E. (1990) Macromolecular prodrugs of 5-aminosalicylic acid, 1. Azo-conjugates. *Makromol. Chem.* **191**: 529–536.

114. Molly, K., Legesse, W., Van de Woestyne, M., Verstraete, W., De Saeyer, N., De Roose, N. and Schacht, E. (1994) Evaluation of the release of 5-aminosalicylic acid from polymeric prodrugs. Simulator of the human instestinal microbial ecosystem. (SHIME-reactor). *J. Controlled Rel.*, in press.

115. Kopeckova, P. and Kopecek, J. (1990) Release of 5-aminosalicylic acid from bioadhesive *N*-(2-hydroxypropym)methacrylamide copolymers by azoreductases *in vitro*. *Makromol. Chem.* **191**: 2037–2045.

PART VII

Pharmaceutical and Chemical Formulation Problems

34

Preparation of Water-Soluble Compounds Through Salt Formation

BRADLEY D. ANDERSON AND KARL P. FLORA

There is nothing in the Universe but alkali and acid, from which Nature composes all things.
Otto Tachenius (1671)

I. THE CASE FOR WATER-SOLUBLE SALTS IN THE EARLY STAGES OF DRUG EVALUATION

Historically, little attention has been devoted to the selection of the optimal form (i.e. parent drug, prodrug, or salt) of a given compound during the early stages of the drug discovery/development process. Thus, the candidate evaluated in *in vitro* and *in vivo* screens for pharmacological activity will most likely have been the compound which proved to be easiest for the synthetic chemist to prepare and isolate in pure crystalline form. In the traditional development process, the formulation and drug metabolism scientists become intensively

THE PRACTICE OF MEDICINAL CHEMISTRY
ISBN 0-12-744640-0

involved only after a lead candidate has been identified. As these scientists will avow, this is often too late, for it is quite likely that they will determine that the lead compound does not exhibit optimal physicochemical properties such as high water solubility, oral bioavailability, low hygroscopicity, stability, and processability. When such physicochemical property-related difficulties arise, there is considerable reluctance to delay the lead candidate's development by initiating a programme of salt and/or prodrug evaluation because that would entail repeating the biological, toxicological, preformulation and formulation studies already completed. Therefore, the development team must often attempt to solve such problems using 'formulation approaches', which may result in delays in development, increased production costs, and a diminished competitive advantage in the marketplace.

While the importance of selecting the optimal salt form for a drug prior to dosage form design has long been recognized,[1-3] procedures that facilitate the rapid selection of the optimal salt or other chemical form of a potential drug candidate at the outset of the development programme are of increasing interest.[2,3] The focus of this chapter is confined to the problem of water-soluble salt selection and evaluation. A water-soluble form of a drug candidate is often the preferred form for a variety of reasons. In the preclinical evaluation of drug toxicity and bioavailability, a parenteral solution dosage form, often containing high concentrations of the active agent, is desirable so that maximum toxicity can be elicited and so that a reference intravenous pharmacokinetic profile can be established for bioavailability assessment. Water-soluble salts may be the optimal choice even for candidates ultimately intended for oral use, as the oral bioavailability may be governed by the drug dissolution rate, which in turn depends on aqueous solubility. This is not to say that the most water-soluble salt should necessarily be the candidate of choice, for there are many other criteria, discussed in this chapter, which must be considered in selecting the optimal form of a given candidate.

II. APPROVED PHARMACEUTICAL SALTS/COUNTERION PROPERTIES

Table 34.1 lists salts of commercially marketed prescription drugs which were approved on the basis of safety and efficacy by the US Food and Drug Administration at 31 January 1994.[4] Prior to 1938, drugs were approved on the basis of safety issues only. These drugs are not included in this review. The list does include several drugs (<1%) which were withdrawn from the market by the manufacturer. For purposes of this review, only salts of organic active ingredients have been included. Inorganic salts (e.g. aluminium, ammonium, magnesium, lithium, carbonate, etc.), salt forms of inactive ingredients (e.g. edetate, benzoate, etc.) and amino acids or other nutritional agents which may also be suitable as salt-forming agents (arginine, lysine, glutamate, etc.) are not listed in Table 34.1. unless salts of organic actives containing these agents have been approved.

III. MEASUREMENT OF AQUEOUS SOLUBILITY OF SALTS

A. pH–solubility profiles of weak acids, weak bases and their salts

The correct interpretation of an apparent solubility value for a given salt requires a quantitative (i.e. mathematical) understanding of the ionic equilibria governing the pH–solubility behaviour

Table 34.1 FDA -approved salts of prescription drugs in the United States.

	Percentage of total[a]		Percentage of total[a]
		ANIONS	
Acetate	2.7	Lactobionate	<1
Adipate	<1	Maleate	3.1
Besylate[b]	<1	Mesylate[i]	2.0
Bromide	2.9	Methylbromide	<1
Camsylate[c]	<1	Methylsulfate	<1
Chloride	2.3	Napsylate	<1
Citrate	1.8	Nitrate	1.6
Edisylate[d]	<1	Oleate	<1
Estolate[e]	<1	Pamoate[j]	<1
Fumarate	<1	Phosphate	2.0
Gluceptate[f]	<1	Polygalacturonate	<1
Gluconate	<1	Stearate	<1
Glucuronate	<1	Succinate	<1
Hippurate	<1	Sulfate	6.8
Hyclate[g]	<1	Sulfosalicylate	<1
Hydrobromide	<1	Tannate	<1
Hydrochloride	38.2	Tartrate	2.7
Iodide	<1	Terephthalate	<1
Isethionate[h]	<1	Tosylate[k]	<1
Lactate	<1	Triethiodide	<1
		CATIONS	
Benzathine[l]	<1	Potassium	1.2
Calcium	1.4	Procaine	<1
Diolamine[m]	<1	Sodium	17.8
Meglumine[n]	1.4	Tromethamine[p]	<1
Olamine[o]	<1	Zinc	<1

[a]Percentage of total is based on the total salts (anions and cations) of active ingredients approved for safety and efficacy at the time of the cited 1994 publication.
[b]Benzenesulfonate, [c](+)-7,7-dimethyl-2-oxobicyclo[2.2.1]heptane-1-methanesulfonic acid; [d]1,2-ethane-disulfonate; [e]dodecyl sulfate; [f]glucoheptonate; [g]hydrochloride hemiethanolate; [h]2-hydroxyethanesulfonate; [i]methanesulfonate; [j]4,4'-methylenebis[3-hydroxy-2-naphthalenecarboxylic acid]; [k]p-toluenesulfonate; [l]N,N'-bis(phenylmethyl)-1,2-ethanediamine; [m]2,2'-iminobis(ethanol); [n]1-deoxy-1-(methylamino)-D-glucitol; [o]2-aminoethanol; [p]2-amino-2-(hydroxymethyl)-1,3-propanediol.

of the neutral form of the drug and that of its salts. To illustrate, consider two compounds which exhibit classical pH-solubility behaviour — the weak carboxylic acid, flurbiprofen (**I**),[5] and the weakly basic amine, dexoxadrol (**II**)[6] (Fig. 34.1). The pH–solubility profile for flurbiprofen, pH-adjusted with NaOH, is shown in Fig. 34.2 (upper curve) and that for dexoxadrol pH-adjusted with HCl is shown in Fig. 34.3. Mathematical relationships describing the curves are developed below.

There are two key regions in the pH–solubility profiles depicted in Fig. 34.2, determined by the nature of the solid phase present in equilibrium with the drug in solution. These will be discussed separately. As shown in Fig. 34.2 (upper curve), at pH < 7.3 the solid phase present is

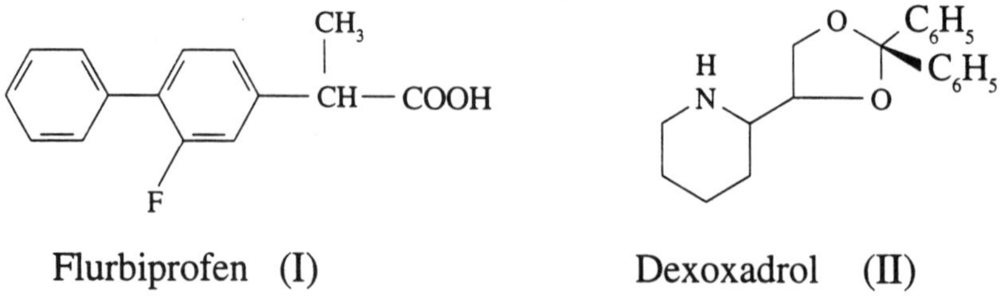

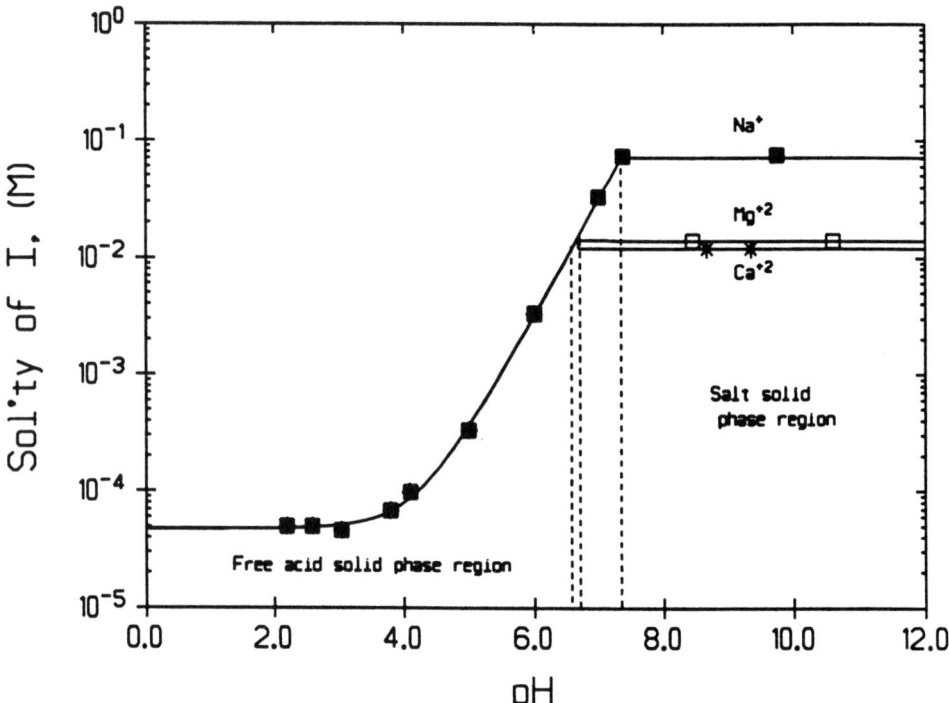

Fig. 34.1   Chemical structures of flurbiprofen (**I**) and dexoxadrol (**II**).

Fig. 34.2   Solubility of flurbiprofen free acid and its sodium, magnesium and calcium salts versus pH. Lines represent theoretical solubilities.

the free acid (neutral form, HA). As long as the free acid is present in solid form, the concentration [HA] of free acid in solution in equilibrium with the solid phase is fixed at a constant value, referred to as the intrinsic solubility, S_0. The overall solubility, S, under these conditions is

$$S = [HA] + [A^-] = S_0\left(1 + \frac{K_d}{[H^+]}\right) \tag{1}$$

where the concentration of anion, [A⁻], is obtained from the equilibrium expression for the ionization of a weak acid,

$$K_a = \frac{[H^+][A^-]}{[HA]} \tag{2}$$

It is evident from equation (2) that the logarithm of the solubility of a slightly soluble weak acid is a constant at $pH \ll pK_a$, while it increases linearly with pH at $pH \gg pK_a$. This simple linear relationship ends abruptly, however, at a certain pH – the pH at which the solid phase in equilibrium with the solution is no longer the free acid form but a salt. Then solubility is governed by the K_{sp}. For a sodium salt this relationship is

$$S = \left(1 + \frac{[H^+]}{K_a}\right)\sqrt{K_{sp}} \tag{3}$$

where

$$K_{sp} = [Na^+][A^-] \tag{4}$$

The pH–solubility profile for a weak base, as illustrated in Fig. 34.3 for dexoxadrol, appears to be nearly the mirror image of the curves shown in Fig. 34.2.

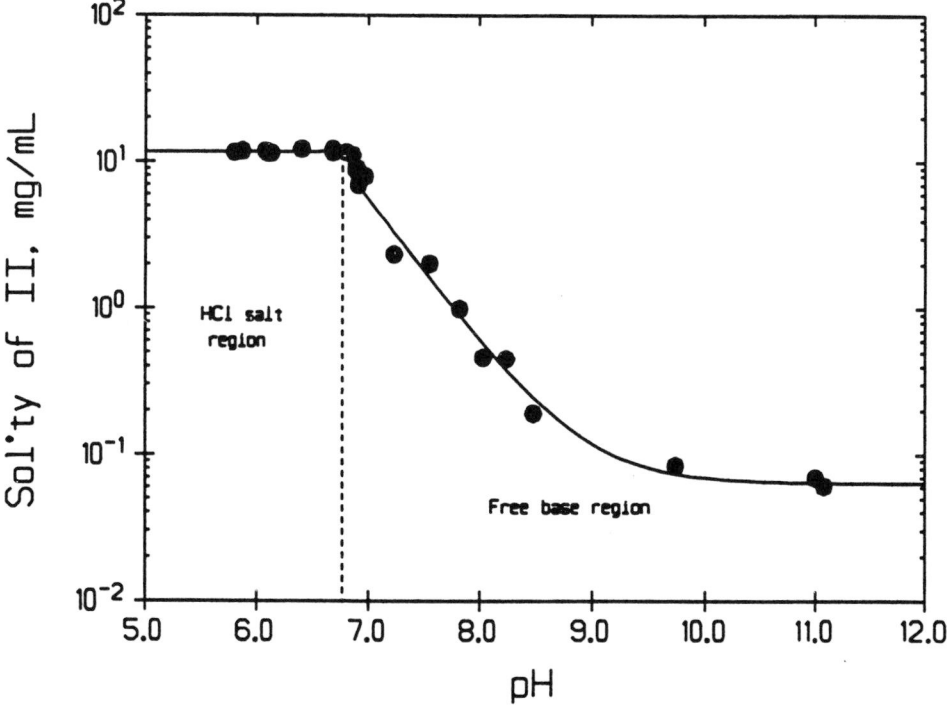

Fig. 34.3   Solubility of dexoxadrol and its HCl salt versus pH. Lines represent model calculated solubilities.

Again there are two key regions. At pH > 6.7 the solid phase present (actually an oil phase in the case illustrated) is the free base (neutral form, B). Therefore, the concentration of free base in solution, [B], is fixed at the intrinsic solubility, S_0. The overall solubility, S, under these conditions is

$$S = [BH^+] + [B] = S_0(1 + [H^+]/K_a) \tag{5}$$

where the concentration of the protonated conjugate acid species, [BH$^+$], is obtained from the pK$_a$ relationship

$$K_a = \frac{[H^+][B]}{[BH^+]} \tag{6}$$

It is evident from equation (5) that the logarithm of the solubility of dexoxadrol is a constant at pH $\gg$ pK$_a$, while it increases linearly with decreasing pH (slope = -1) at pH < pK$_a$. This simple linear relationship also ends abruptly, however, at the pH at which the HCl salt becomes the solid phase. At a pH below the apparent break point at pH $\sim$7, the solubility is governed by the K$_{sp}$ relationship

$$S = \left(1 + \frac{[K_a]}{[H^+]}\right)\sqrt{K_{sp}} \tag{7}$$

$$K_{sp} = [BH^+][Cl^-] \tag{8}$$

These profiles highlight an important point regarding the measurement of aqueous solubility of salts. The K$_{sp}$ or salt solubility is reflected only within a certain region of the pH–solubility profile. Shown in the lower curves in Fig. 34.2, for example, are the pH–solubility profiles for the magnesium and calcium salts of flurbiprofen. As observed previously for the sodium salt, the logarithm of solubility is constant below the pK$_a$ and increases linearly with pH until a break point occurs. This break point, which is at a different pH for each salt, represents the pH above which the solid phase at equilibrium is the salt rather than the free acid. Thus, salt solubility or K$_{sp}$ determinations should be conducted at pH values within these plateau regions.

B.   'Pitfalls' in the determination of salt solubilities

The most frequently encountered difficulty in determining the solubility of a given salt is that of complete or partial conversion (i.e. 'hydrolysis') of the salt to the free acid or free base form when the salt is initially added to water. For this reason, it is important to establish the identity of the solid phase *at equilibrium* in interpreting solubility data. This is illustrated in Fig. 34.4, which describes the apparent solubility of the tromethamine salt of flurbiprofen (curve I), which has an actual solubility of 0.069 M, versus the amount of 1 : 1 salt added to water.

Typically in experiments to measure salt solubilities, an amount of salt thought to represent an excess is added, and after an appropriate equilibration time the sample is observed for evidence of remaining suspended solid. If remaining solid is detected, equilibrium with respect to the salt solid phase is assumed. Figure 34.4 (curve II) shows, however, that excess solid may exist at equilibrium well below the point at which the system is saturated with respect to the 1 : 1 salt, but the solid phase is the free acid! This phenomenon can be understood by referring again to Fig. 34.2. When the 1 : 1 tromethamine salt of flurbiprofen is added to deionized water, some of it initially dissolves, resulting in a weakly buffered solution. The pH of this buffer, composed of equal concentrations of a weak acid and a weak base, is equal to $\frac{1}{2}$(pK$_{tromethamine}$ + pK$_{flurbiprofen}$) (= 6.15). From Fig. 34.2, the solubility of the free acid at pH 6.15 is only 4.3 $\times$ 10^{-3} M, well below the saturation solubility of the salt. The suspended solid remaining in the region where the amount of 1 : 1 salt initially added is between 4.3 $\times$ 10^{-3} M and $\sim$0.08 M contains only free acid, not 1 : 1 salt. The *apparent* solubility continually increases

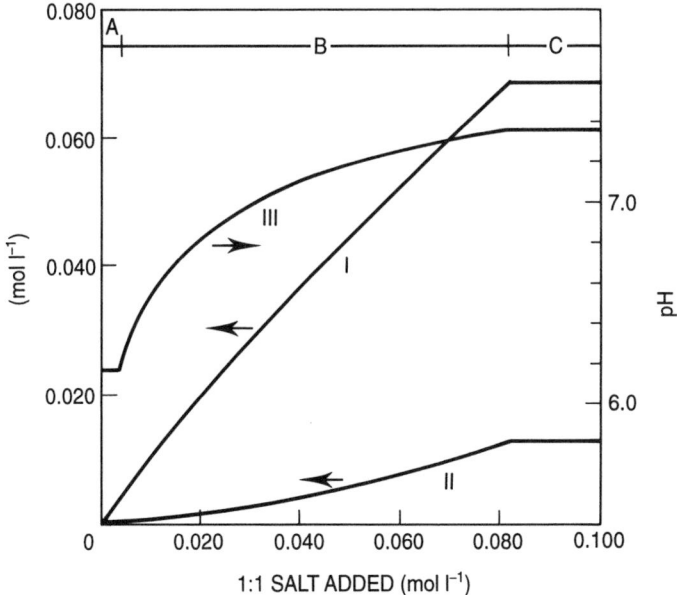

Fig. 34.4 Apparent equilibrium solubility (curve I), concentration of excess free acid solid phase (curve II) and pH (curve III) in aqueous solutions to which various quantities of the tromethamine salt of flurbiprofen have been added.

as more 1 : 1 salt is added, because more of the free acid precipitates, causing an increase in pH and an accompanying increase in solubility.

Owing to these difficulties, some salt solubilities reported in the literature may be in error. One method of evaluating the reliability of a solubility value generated for a given salt is to compare it with the solubility predicted at the same pH when the solid phase is the free acid or base. If the 'salt' solubility value is approximately the same as that predicted for the neutral solid phase at the same pH, partial or complete conversion to the free acid or base probably occurred. If this were so, the solubility value obtained may not be that for the salt.

A more subtle example of the importance of characterizing the solid phase is shown in the analysis of the pH–solubility profile for the anti-AIDS candidate (±)-3TC (Fig. 34.5).

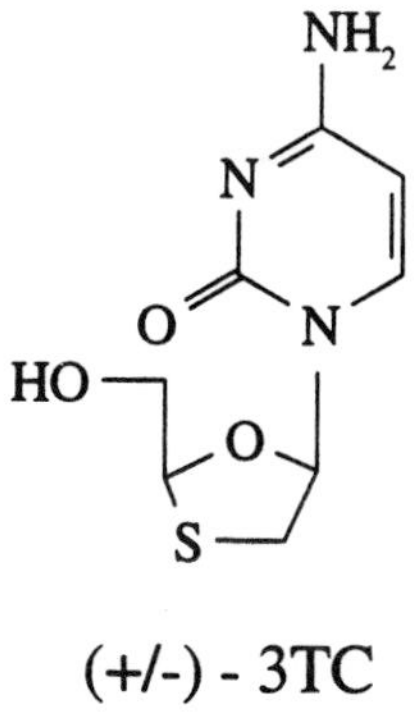

(+/-) - 3TC

Fig. 34.5 Chemical structure of the anti-AIDS drug candidate (±)-3TC.

When an excess of the free base, the conjugate acid of which has a pK_a of 4.2, is added to water and pH is adjusted downwards with HCl, the pH–solubility profile exhibits classical behaviour as described by equation (5) above pH ~4.5. Below this pH the logarithm of the solubility of (±)-3TC does not appear to increase linearly with decreasing pH with a slope of 1, as expected if the free base were the solid phase over the entire pH range, nor does the solubility remain constant below pH 4.5, as expected if the HCl salt were the solid phase. Analysis of the solid phase removed from these suspensions after equilibrium was established revealed that the solid phase below pH 3 was indeed the 1:1 HCl salt with K_{sp} = [BH$^+$][Cl$^-$] = 0.0436 M^2. Between pH 3 and ~4.5, the solid phase was a 2:1 hemisalt, consisting of one mole of free base [B] and one mole of the protonated species [BH$^+$] per mole of chloride with K_{sp} = [B][BH$^+$][Cl$^-$] = 5.3 × 10^{-4} M^3. The upper solid curve constructed in Fig. 34.6 is the theoretical curve in a solution containing no added KCl assuming the existence of these two HCl salt forms. The lower theoretical curve and data points reflect the solubility behaviour of (±)-3TC in 1 M KCl solution, assuming the same K_{sp} values. The presence of a common ion (Cl$^-$) dramatically lowers the solubility of both the 1:1 and 2:1 salts without affecting the free base solubility.

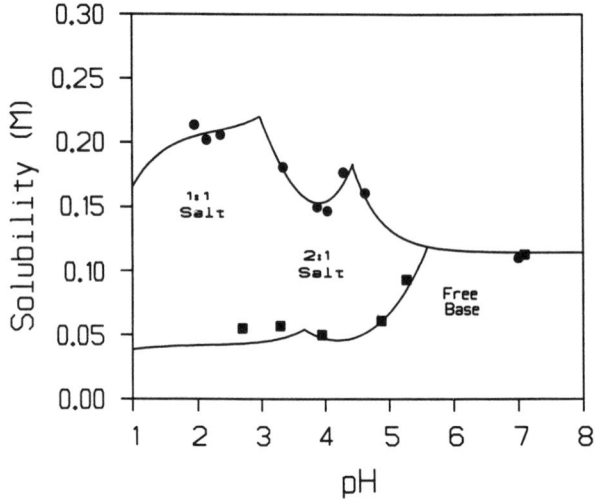

Fig. 34.6 Solubility of (±)-3TC, its 2:1 hemisalt and its HCl salt in aqueous solutions. Lines represent model calculated solubilities: (●) pH adjusted with HCl, no added KCl; (■) solubility in 1 M KCl.

IV.   COUNTERION STRUCTURE–SOLUBILITY RELATIONSHIPS

A.   Counterion pK_a

Successful salt formation generally requires that the pK_a of the conjugate acid be less than the pK_a of the conjugate base to ensure sufficient proton transfer from the acid to the basic species. Thus, strong mineral acids such as HBr (pK_a = −8.0), HCl (pK_a = −6.1) or H$_2$SO$_4$ (pK_a = −3.0) or one of the sulfonic acids (pK_a < 2.0) would be suitable acids for the preparation of salts of weakly basic amines having pK_a values < 4, whereas weaker acids (benzoate, acetate, etc.) would not be expected to form salts with such compounds.

Table 34.2 Theoretical equations for determining pH of salt solutions. (Salt concentration = $C \, \text{mol} \, l^{-1}$.)

Salt	Equation
Weak acid/strong base	$\text{pH} = \frac{1}{2}(pK_a + pK_w + \log C)$
Weak base/strong acid	$\text{pH} = \frac{1}{2}(pK_a - \log C)$
Weak acid/weak base	$\text{pH} = \frac{1}{2}[pK_a(\text{acid}) + pK_a(\text{base})]$

The equations listed in Table 34.2 describe the theoretical pH of aqueous solutions of various salts. Calculations of pH using the equations in Table 34.2 and consideration of the relationships governing the pH–solubility behaviour of weak acids and bases when the solid phase is the un-ionized form of the drug (discussed in the previous section) lead to the conclusion that it is advantageous in general to select conjugate acids (bases) having pK_a values well below (above) the pK_a of a weakly basic (acidic) drug as salt-forming counterions. As an example, consider the possible salts of chlordiazepoxide, a weakly basic drug having a pK_a of 4.8 and an intrinsic solubility of only 2 mg ml^{-1}. Whereas a 50 mg ml^{-1} solution of the HCl salt of chlordiazepoxide would have a calculated pH of ~2.8 and therefore be well below its predicted solubility (based on the free base solubility) of 200 mg ml^{-1} at this pH, a solution of the acetate (pK_a = 4.76) salt would form a buffer having a pH of ~4.78, allowing a water solubility (again governed by the free base intrinsic solubility) of only 4 mg ml^{-1}.

The above guideline favouring strong acid salts of weakly basic drugs and strong base salts with weakly acidic compounds is derived from the pH–solubility behaviour of the neutral solid form of a given drug. Other factors, particularly the K_{sp} of the salt, common-ion effects and hygroscopicity, may disfavour certain salts, such as hydrochloride salts or sodium salts in some cases, which might appear by the above criteria to be the first choice. Despite the fact that hydrochloride salts account for nearly half of the FDA-approved salts of weakly basic drugs listed in Table 34.1, there are numerous documented examples where hydrochloride salts exhibited lower solubilities than salts with other anions.[7-11] Solubility and, particularly, dissolution rates of hydrochloride salts administered orally in tablet form may be further suppressed by the common-ion effect, since chloride ion is present at high concentrations in gastric fluid.[12,13] Bogardus and Blackwood, for example, demonstrated that the compressed pellets of the free base form of doxycycline dissolved 6-fold faster in 0.1 M HCl than the more water-soluble hydrochloride salt owing to the influence of the common ion.[14]

Others have noted additional potential disadvantages of hydrochloride and sodium salts. The solution pH of hydrochloride salts may be excessively low, for example, which may lead to physiological compatibility or stability problems.[10,15,16] The pH of injectable formulations should ideally be 7.4, the pH of the blood. Above pH 9, tissue necrosis often occurs, while injections below pH 3 may cause extreme pain and phlebitis.[17] However, parenteral formulations are marketed having formulation pH as low as 2.0 (Tetracycline Injection[18]) and as high as 12 (Phenytoin Sodium Injection[18]) but extra precautions are necessary in their administration. Ideally, the optimal pH of a solution formulation should also be set at the minimum in the pH–degradation rate profile if other factors (e.g. solubility, physiological compatibility, etc.) allow. This pH may not coincide with the equilibrium pH obtained from a given salt. This is not to say that it is the selection of a given salt which governs formulation pH, since it is possible simply to adjust solution pH to a more suitable value in many cases by adding an excess of acid or base, without changing the salt form. Unfortunately, pH adjustment may be precluded by drug solubility limitations. Obviously, the pH ultimately chosen for a given solution formulation containing a salt may be a compromise between conflicting requirements.

The choice of salt form may be more critical in solid dosage forms, because then the salt form will dictate the pH of the liquid microenvironment present when the solid adsorbs trace quantities of moisture. The liquid microenvironment pH may have an important impact on the solid-state stability of the drug. Hygroscopicity is also encountered more frequently with certain salts, such as the hydrochloride and sodium salts,[2,19–21] further suggesting that alternative salt-forming agents may be favoured in some cases.

B. Predictive relationships — application to water solubility of salts

Predictive structure–solubility relationships which would enable the pharmaceutical scientist to select the appropriate counterion to achieve the desired water solubility for a given acidic or basic drug would be highly desirable. Unfortunately, only qualitative 'rules of thumb' are generally found and these may not be totally reliable. Sometimes, for example, it is observed that increasing the hydrophobicity within a series of salt-forming counterions decreases water solubility, as seen for salts of erythromycin[22] and lincomycin,[23] and, conversely, that more hydrophilic salt-forming ions such as polyhydroxy-containing acids or amines confer increased water solubility to a salt.[9]

However, structural effects on salt solubility within a series of salt-forming counterions must be considered in terms of their separate contributions to the crystal lattice energies and solvation energies. Thus, the molar free energy of solution on dissolving a salt in water, ΔG_{soln}, may be represented by

$$\Delta G_{\text{soln}} = \Delta G_{\text{cation}} + \Delta G_{\text{anion}} - \Delta G_{\text{lattice}} \tag{9}$$

where ΔG_{cation} and ΔG_{anion} are the molar free energies of hydration of the salt cationic and anionic species, respectively, and $\Delta G_{\text{lattice}}$ is the crystal lattice free energy. Both the lattice energy[24] and the hydration energies[25] increase with an increase in cation or anion charge and decrease with an increase in ionic radius. Similarly, both would be expected to increase with the polarity or hydrogen-bonding nature of the counterion. Thus, the overall effect of a given structural change on water solubility will depend on which terms, the lattice energy or the hydration energies, are most sensitive to the change in structure.

Consider, for example, the water solubilities of the alkali and alkaline-earth metal salts of the four organic carboxylic acids depicted in Fig. 34.7.[5,26] The logarithms of the solubilities of the free acids and the sodium, potassium, magnesium and calcium salts are compared graphically in Fig. 34.8. Clearly, the rank order solubilities within a given series (carboxylic acid structure fixed) fluctuate, with the potassium salt solubilities exceeding those of the sodium salts in three of four cases and the magnesium salts exhibiting higher solubility than the calcium salts in two cases, similar solubility in one, and lower solubility in another series. These observations led Chowhan to suggest that not even qualitative trends could be found between structure and water solubility of alkali metal or alkaline earth salts of organic carboxylic acids.[26] Nevertheless, an examination of Fig. 34.8 does illustrate that for these *structurally similar* carboxylic acids there are some significant qualitative trends. Note that the magnitudes of the salt solubility increases are approximately uniform, regardless of the intrinsic solubility of the free acid, for example. Mean values of log $(S_{\text{salt}}/S_{\text{free acid}})$ obtained from Fig. 34.8 are 4.1 ± 0.8 (Na^+ salt), 4.6 ± 0.3 (K^+ salt), 2.5 ± 0.3 (Mg^{2+} salt), and 2.6 ± 0.3 (Ca^{2+} salt). The scatter which is seen

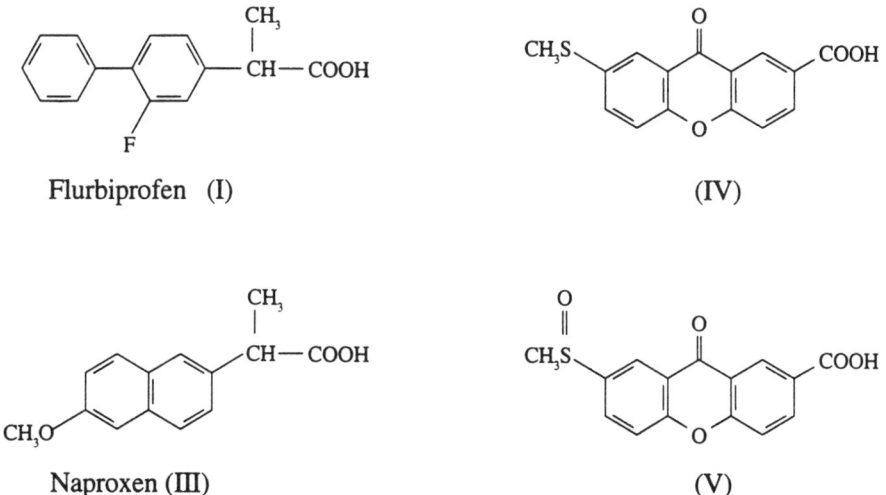

Fig. 34.7   Structures of various carboxylic acids whose solubilities are compared graphically along with their salts in Fig. 34.8.

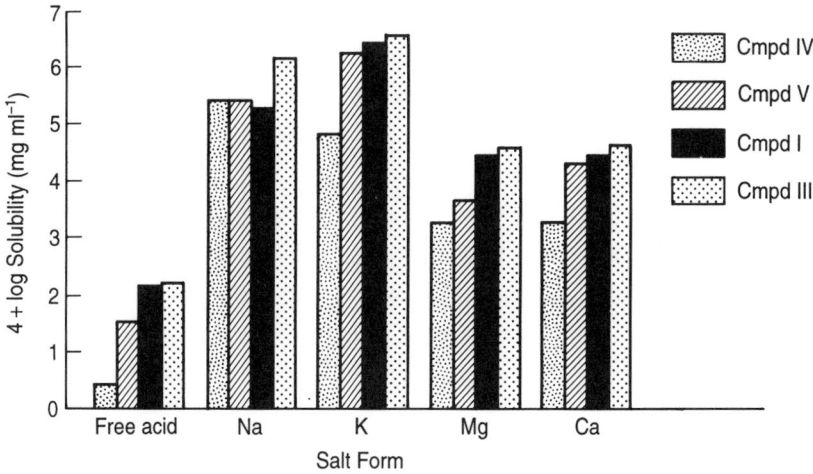

Fig. 34.8   Water solubilities of several free acids (see structures in Fig. 34.7) and their sodium, potassium, magnesium, and calcium salts.

may be due in part to the possibility that different hydrated forms may have been compared in some cases. The flurbiprofen salts were typically mono- or dihydrates, for example, whereas the hydration states for the other salts were not reported.

If the solubility changes within a given *structurally related* series of salts are due predominantly either to effects on the hydration energies or on the lattice energy term, then it may be reasonable to explore relationships between solubility and counterion attributes such as hydrophilicity (i.e. partition coefficient) or crystal properties. The relationship between the ideal mole fraction solubility of a solid, X_{ideal}, and its melting point, T_m, is given by

$$\ln X_{ideal} = -\frac{\Delta H_f}{R}\left(\frac{1}{T} - \frac{1}{T_m}\right) \tag{10}$$

where ΔH_f is the enthalpy of fusion.[27] Although many assumptions and approximations are involved, this equation implies a relationship between solubility and melting point for a series of compounds.[28] The series of ammonium salts of flurbiprofen listed in Table 34.3 allow us to search for such relationships. The counterions vary from the highly lipophilic adamantanamine to the hydrophilic tromethamine (with three OH groups). The rank order relationship between K_{sp} and melting point illustrates the importance of crystal lattice forces. Within this series, higher melting points and lower K_{sp} values were observed for the more symmetric counterions. Interestingly, the tromethamine salt ($K_{sp} = 2.9 \times 10^{-3}$ mol^2 l^{-2}) was not the most soluble among the tertiary amine salts despite being the most hydrophilic, presumably because the symmetry of this counterion led to stronger crystalline forces and a higher melting point.

Table 34.3 Solubility products (K_{sp}) and melting points (MP) of various ammonium salts of flurbiproten.

Cation	K_{sp} (mol^2 l^{-2})	MP (°C)
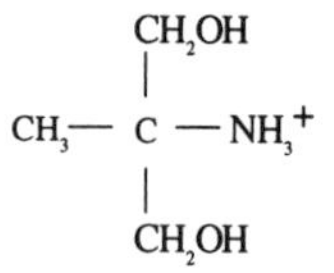 CH$_3$—C(CH$_2$OH)(CH$_2$OH)—NH$_3^+$	9.5×10^{-3}	119.0–121.0
NH$_4^+$	7.1×10^{-3}	131.0–134.6
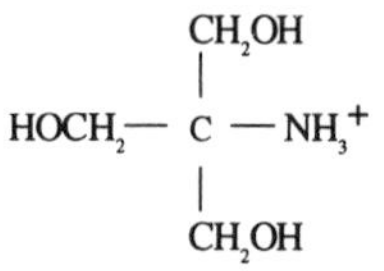 HOCH$_2$—C(CH$_2$OH)(CH$_2$OH)—NH$_3^+$	2.9×10^{-3}	148.1–150.0
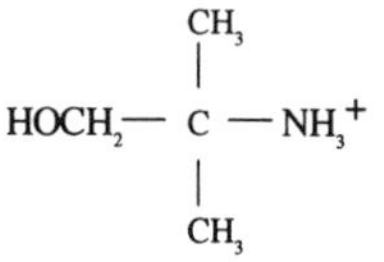 HOCH$_2$—C(CH$_3$)(CH$_3$)—NH$_3^+$	2.0×10^{-3}	151.2–153.7
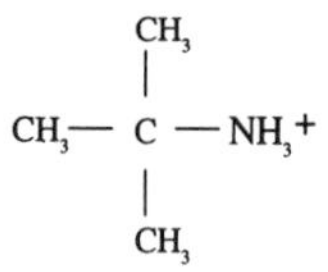 CH$_3$—C(CH$_3$)(CH$_3$)—NH$_3^+$	1.3×10^{-4}	183.0–189.8
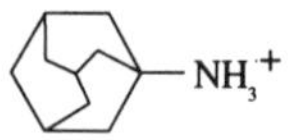 (adamantyl)—NH$_3^+$	1.8×10^{-7}	233.5–237.0

Several studies have identified relationships between salt solubilities and melting points or between salt melting points and the melting points of the conjugate acid or conjugate base salt-forming agents.[2,8] Relationships of the latter type suggest that those structural features leading to high melting (e.g. planarity, symmetry, etc.) or low-melting (chain flexibility, assymetry, etc.) salt-forming agents will be carried over in determining the crystal lattice energies of the salt.

V. OPTIMAL SALT SELECTION CRITERIA

While our focus has been primarily on identifying water-soluble salts of partially soluble drug candidates, there are a number of additional criteria by which a given water-soluble salt would have to be evaluated before a decision could be made to continue its development. These criteria, and the formulation of strategies for expeditiously selecting the optimal salt form, have been the subject of recent publications by Morris *et al.*[3] and Gould.[2] Morris and co-workers identified four primary criteria for the selection of the optimal salt form of a novel HMG-CoA reductase inhibitor including (1) low hygroscopicity, (2) integrity of the crystal form under different storage conditions, (3) aqueous solubility, and (4) chemical stability. As aqueous solubility has been amply covered in previous sections, this section will examine case histories which illustrate the importance of the remaining criteria.

A. Hygroscopicity/crystal integrity under different storage conditions

Salts having a high tendency to adsorb or desorb moisture under the ambient relative humidity conditions encountered during manufacturing (30–50% RH), or when subjected to higher temperatures during drying or tablet compression, are undesirable from a formulation standpoint. Excessive changes in the state of hydration of salts during processing may cause batch-to-batch variation in potency, handling and manufacturing difficulties,[2] tablet cracking,[19] chemical instability,[29] or variability in dissolution rates and bioavailability. Although general trends have been noted between the propensities of salts to form hydrates and various structural features such as counterion radius and charge,[30] a given salt may form several stoichiometric hydrates depending on the crystallization conditions. Therefore, the selection of the optimal salt form with respect to hydrate stability usually requires experimental evaluation.

The stability of hydrates can vary dramatically. Hirsch *et al.*[1] found, for example, that the sodium dihydrate of fenoprofen lost both moles of water at 25°C and 1% relative humidity, while the calcium dihydrate was stable under the same conditions, indicating that the water of hydration was more tightly bound in calcium salt crystals. The anhydrous, amorphous sodium salt absorbed excessive quantities of water at high relative humidities, while amorphous forms of the calcium salt absorbed only enough water to form the crystalline dihydrate. Mixtures of the sodium dihydrate with analgesic amine hydrochlorides demonstrated incompatibility within a few hours' storage, whereas the calcium dihydrate was compatible with these amine salts. Since fenoprofen calcium and fenoprofen sodium were shown to be bioequivalent in similar oral dosage forms,[31] the calcium salt was deemed to be superior from a pharmaceutical viewpoint.

Forbes *et al.*[30] saw similar trends in examining salts of *p*-aminosalicylic acid (PAS). The onset temperatures of dehydration of the magnesium and calcium salts of PAS were higher than that of the sodium salt, consistent with stronger ion–dipole interactions in the divalent salts. Crystal structures from X-ray diffraction data revealed a very open structure with an observable channel of water oxygens in the sodium salt which was not apparent in the divalent salts. This was suggested as a significant contributing factor accounting for the relative ease with which the sodium salt lost its water of hydration.

Although excessive moisture uptake appears to be a more frequent problem for sodium salts,[3,21] Morris and co-workers rejected a variety of metal salts owing to hygroscopicity or humidity-dependent changes in crystal structure, including the sodium, potassium, calcium, magnesium and zinc salts of the drug candidate under investigation. The arginine and lysine salts were resistant to changes in crystalline structure with changes in relative humidity. Ultimately, the arginine salt was selected for further development on the basis of its ease of synthesis, ease of analysis, potential impurities, and other factors. Gu and Strickley[21] reported that tris(hydroxymethyl)aminomethane (THAM) salts were also generally superior to the sodium salts of a variety of analgesic/anti-inflammatory agents in terms of hygroscopicity and suggested that more use of THAM salts might be warranted.

B.   Chemical stability of salts

While chemical stability, particularly in the solid state, may be closely linked to hygroscopicity, the selection of an optimal salt form from the standpoint of stability may also require consideration of other counterion-related factors such as melting point or crystal lattice energy (stronger crystal lattice forces generally result in superior solid-state stability[16]), pH of the liquid microenvironment (a function of counterion pK_a), and the possibility of counterion participation in the degradation of the candidate of interest.

The comparison in Table 34.4 of the solid-state stability of the prostaglandin derivative 6,9-deepoxy-6,9-(phenylimino)-$\Delta^{6,8}$-prostaglandin I$_1$ (Fig. 34.9) and several of its salts when stored protected from light at 33°C highlights the potentially marked dependence of solid-state stability on salt form.[32] None of the physical properties of these salts appeared to correlate with their solid-state reactivity. The sodium and potassium salts, for example, exhibited the highest melting points, but the sodium salt was the least stable while the potassium salt was the most stable of the compounds tested. More detailed information such as X-ray crystallographic data would presumably be useful in rationalizing such results.

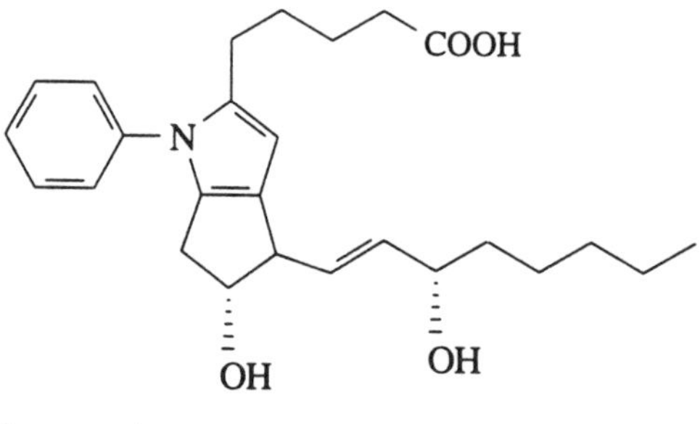

Fig. 34.9   Structure of the prostaglandin derivative 6,9-deepoxy-6,9-(phenylimino)-$\Delta^{6,8}$-prostaglandin I$_1$.

Table 34.4   Physicochemical properties and solid-state stability of 6,9-deepoxy-6,9-(phenylimino)-$\Delta^{6,8}$-prostaglandin I$_1$ and various salts.

Property	Free acid	Na$^+$ salt	K$^+$ salt	THAM salt
Water solubility	1 μg/ml^{-1}	Soluble	Soluble	Soluble
Melting point (°C)	135–140	>175 (dec.)	>175 (dec.)	95–101
Decomposition (%)[a]	>10	>>50	<2	2–3

[a]Stored protected from light for 2 months at 33°C.

A most interesting example of the importance of selecting the appropriate salt form was illustrated in a recent publication by Powell[33] comparing the stability of codeine sulfate versus codeine phosphate solutions. Codeine phosphate had been previously reported to have a room-temperature shelf-life of 1.1 years, whereas Powell found the sulfate salt to have a solution shelf-life of about 44 years under similar conditions! The difference was ascribed to catalysis of the decomposition of codeine by phosphate anion.

Morris and co-workers[3] have suggested that stability testing be conducted in the later stages of salt evaluation because it is the most time-consuming part of the process. Even so, they suggest that the entire salt-selection process, including synthesis and evaluation of solubility, hygroscopicity and crystallinity, and stability may take approximately 4–6 weeks. Therefore, consideration of salts could be included in the development programme of most candidates without adding significant delays.

REFERENCES

1. Hirsch, C. A., Messenger, R. J. and Brannon, J. L. (1978) Drug form selection and preformulation stability studies. *J. Pharm. Sci.* **67**: 231–236.
2. Gould, P. L. (1986) Salt selection for basic drugs. *Int. J. Pharm.* **33**: 201–217.
3. Morris, K. R., Fakes, M. G., Thakur, A. B., Newman, A. W., Singh, A. K., Venit, J. J., Spagnuolo, C. J. and Serajuddin, A. T. M. (1994) An integrated approach to the selection of optimal salt form for a new drug candidate. *Int. J. Pharm.* **105**: 209–217.
4. *Approved Drug Products with Therapeutic Equivalence Evaluations* (1994) US Department of Health and Human Services, Public Health Service, Food and Drug Administration, Center for Drug Evaluation and Research, Rockville, MD.
5. Anderson, B. D. and Conradi, R. A. (1985) Predictive relationships in the water solubility of salts of a nonsteroidal anti-inflammatory drug. *J. Pharm. Sci.* **74**: 815–820.
6. Kramer, S. F. and Flynn, G. L. (1972) Solubility of organic hydrochlorides. *J. Pharm. Sci.* **61**: 1896–1904.
7. Streng, W. H., Hsi, S. K., Helms, P. E. and Tan, H. G. H. (1984) General treatment of pH–solubility profiles of weak acids and bases and the effects of different acids on the solubility of a weak base. *J. Pharm. Sci.* **73**: 1679–1684.
8. Agharkar, S., Lindenbaum, S. and Higuchi, T. (1976) Enhancement of solubility of drug salts by hydrophilic counterions: Properties of organic salts of an antimalarial drug. *J. Pharm. Sci.* **65**: 747–749.
9. Senior, N. (1973) Some observations on the formulation and properties of chlorhexidine. *J. Soc. Cosmet. Chem.* **24**: 259–278.
10. Nudelman, A., McCaully, R. J. and Bell, S. C. (1974) Water-soluble derivatives of 3-oxy-substituted 1,4-benzodiazepines. *J. Pharm. Sci.* **63**: 1880–1885.
11. Hussain, M. A., Wu, L. S., Koval, C. and Hurwitz, A. R. (1992) Parenteral formulation of the kappa agonist analgesic, DuP 747, via micellar solubilization. *Pharm. Res.* **9**: 750–752.
12. Miyazaki, S., Oshiba, M. and Nadai, T. (1980) Unusual solubility and dissolution behaviour of pharmaceutical hydrochloride salts in chloride-containing media. *Int. J. Pharm.* **6**: 77–85.
13. Miyazaki, S., Oshiba, M. and Nadai, T. (1981) Precaution on use of hydrochloride salts in pharmaceutical formulation. *J. Pharm. Sci.* **70**: 594–596.
14. Bogardus, J. B. and Blackwood, J. R. K. (1979) *J. Pharm. Sci.* **61**: 188.
15. Wells, J. I. (1988) *Pharmaceutical Preformulation: The Physicochemical Properties of Drug Substances.* Ellis Horwood, Chichester.
16. Gould, P. L., Goodman, M. and Hanson, P. A. (1984) Investigation of the solubility relationships of polar, semi-polar and non-polar drugs in mixed co-solvent systems. *Int. J. Pharm.* **19**: 149–159.
17. DeLuca, P. P. and Boylan, J. C. (1984) Formulation of Small Volume Parenterals. In Avis, K. E., Lachman, L. and Lieberman, H. A. (eds) *Pharmaceutical Dosage Forms: Parenteral Medications*, vol. 1, p. 155. Marcel Dekker, New York.

18. Martindale, W. (1982) *The Extra Pharmacopoeia,* 28th edn. The Pharmaceutical Press, London.
19. Yamaoka, T., Nakamachi, H. and Miyata, K. (1982) Studies on the characteristics of carbochromen hydrochloride crystals. II. Polymorphism and cracking in the tablets. *Chem. Pharm. Bull.* **30**: 3695–3700.
20. Boatman, J. A. and Johnson, J. B. (1981) A four stage approach to drug development. *Pharm. Technol.* **5**: 46–56.
21. Gu, L. and Strickley, R. G. (1987) Preformulation salt selection. Physical property comparisons of the tris(hydroxymethyl)aminomethane (THAM) salts of four analgesic/antiinflammatory agents with the sodium salts and the free acids. *Pharm. Res.* **4**: 255–257.
22. Jones, P. H., Rowley, E. K., Weiss, A. L., Bishop, D. L. and Chun, A. H. C. (1969) Insoluble erythromycin salts. *J. Pharm. Sci.* **58**: 337–339.
23. Otsuka Pharmaceutical Co. (1971) L. Japanese Patent 7 103 600.
24. Pauling, L. (1960) The Nature of the Chemical Bond. 3rd edn, pp. 505–511. Cornell University Press, Ithaca, NY.
25. Bockris, J. O. and Reddy, A. K. (1973) *Modern Electrochemistry.* Plenum Press, New York.
26. Chowhan, Z. T. (1978) pH–solubility profiles of organic carboxylic acids and their salts. *J. Pharm. Sci.* **67**: 1257–1260.
27. Grant, D. J. W. and Higuchi, T. (1990) *Solubility Behavior of Organic Compounds,* vol. XXI. Wiley, New York.
28. Yalkowsky, S. H. (1981) Solubility and partitioning. V: Dependence of solubility on melting point. *J. Pharm. Sci.* **70**: 971–973.
29. Byrn, S. R. (1982) *Solid State Chemistry of Drugs.* Academic Press, New York.
30. Forbes, R. T., York, P., Fawcett, V. and Shields, L. (1992) Physicochemical properties of salts of p-aminosalicylic acid. I. Correlation of crystal structure and hydrate stability. *Pharm. Res.* **9**: 1428–1435.
31. Rubin, A., Rodda, B. E., Warrick, P., Ridolfo, A. and Gruber, C. M. (1971) Physiological disposition of fenoprofen in man I: pharmacokinetic comparison of calcium and sodium salts administered orally. *J. Pharm. Sci.* **60**: 1797–1801.
32. Anderson, B. D. (1985) Prodrugs for improved formulation properties. In Bundgaard, H. (ed.) *Design of Prodrugs,* pp. 243–269. Elsevier Science, Biomedical Division.
33. Powell, M. F. (1986) Enhanced stability of codeine sulfate: effect of pH, buffer, and temperature on the degradation of codeine in aqueous solution. *J. Pharm. Sci.* **75**: 901–903.

35

Preparation of Water-Soluble Compounds by Covalent Attachment of Solubilizing Moieties

CAMILLE G. WERMUTH

Ajouter à sa queue, ôter à ses oreilles
Add to her tail, remove from her ears
Jean de La Fontaine[1]

THE PRACTICE OF MEDICINAL CHEMISTRY
ISBN 0-12-744640-0

I. INTRODUCTION

The strategy described here aims to convert a water-insoluble drug into a water soluble one by attaching *covalently* an appropriate solubilizing side-chain. Surprisingly few reviews covering this subject are found in the literature .[2-5] Seen from the chemical side, the solubilizing moiety can be a neutral hydrophilic group or an ionizable organic base or acid. With the exeption of possible crystallization problems, no major difficulties are expected in the synthesis of such compounds. One problematic aspect of the solubilization approach to be taken is to decide whether the solubilizing moiety has to be fixed in a reversible manner, generating a prodrug, or in an irreversible manner, yielding a new chemical entity. In the latter case the solubilizing procedure may exact a cost in terms of the recognition mechanisms, the soluble analogue being less potent or even showing a different pharmacological profile. In some instances, changes in one part of the molecule have to be compensated by changes in another part. As Jean de La Fontaine said of the elephant, 'Add to her tail, remove from her ears'. In addition, the solubilized analogue of an already approved drug is considered by the government drug agencies as a totally new chemical entity, demanding a completely new development process. The financial investment that is then necessary can only be justified if enough sales of the solubilized form are expected. As a consequence, the attachment of solubilizing moieties has to be considered very early in the drug discovery process or else limited to drugs with sizeable markets and undertaken only when all other solubilizing stratagems fail. Despite these difficulties, many examples are found in therapy of successful drug solubilization by means of a chemical transformation of a parent drug (Table 35.1).

Table 35.1 Successful examples of drug solubilization by chemical means.

Solubilizing side-chain	Therapeutic class	Compound
Phosphoric ester	Steroids	Betamethazone
Phosphoric ester	Vitamins	Menadione
Hemisuccinate	Cardiotonics	Benfurodil
Hemisuccinate	Antibiotics	Chloramphenicol
Hemisuccinate	Steroids	Prednisolone
Hemisuccinate	Benzodiazepines	Oxazepam
Acidic	Theophylline	Etaphylline
Acidic	Antisyphilitic	Solusalvarsan
Neutral	Analgesic	Glafenine
Neutral	Bronchodilator	Dyphylline
Neutral	Antibacterial	Sulfapyridine *N*-glucoside
Basic	Antibiotics	Rolitetracycline
Basic	Flavonoids	Solurutine
Basic	Morphine	Pholcodine

Chemically solubilized active principles render possible the preparation of parenteral, and especially intravenous, forms appreciated in clinical practice. But even at the preclinical level the use of water-soluble molecules is recommended as they are effectively much easier to study by *in vitro* tests, in cell or microorganism cultures and on isolated organs. The inconveniences are that chemically modified structures may show modified pharmacological, pharmacokinetic and toxicological properties.

II.   SOLUBILIZATION STRATEGIES

Three points are decisive in terms of the solubilizing strategies: How will the solubilizing moiety be grafted? Where will it be grafted? What kind of side-chain will be utilized?

A.   How will the solubilizing moiety be grafted?

The solubilizing chain can be *reversibly* or *irreversibly* grafted to the parent molecule. In the case of reversible linkages we are dealing in fact, with prodrugs. Reversible linkages are usually provided by esters, peptides or glucosides.

Irreversible attachment of side-chains is achieved by *O*- and *N*-alkylation and creation of C—C bonds. The grafted side-chains can be basic (dimethylaminoethyl or morpholinoethyl chains), acidic (carboxylic, sulfonic, etc.) or neutral (glyceryl).

Intermediate situations are found for enol and phenol phosphates as well as for some amides. For these compounds only partial reversibility is observed *in vivo*.

B.   Where will it be grafted?

First of all a careful examination of the parent molecule must to be undertaken in order to identify the parts of the molecule that present adequate chemical reactivity and are suitable as attachment points for the solubilizing chain. Functions such as OH, SH, NH, acidic CH or CO_2H are reactive sites that furnish nucleophilic or basic entities. Conversely, aromatic double bonds are sensitive to electrophilic attack, whereas carbonyl groups and conjugated carbon–carbon double bonds are sensitive to nucleophilic attack. The second criterion that has to be considered is of a biological nature: the solubilizing chain can only be grafted to those parts of the molecule that are not involved in the drug–receptor interaction. Fixed at the wrong place, the solubilizing chain can totally inactivate the molecule.

C.   What kind of solubilizing chain will be utilized?

The size of the solubilizing chain is one selection parameter. The chains can be limited to the strict minimum and simply represent functional groups, or they can be made from larger residues containing several atoms (Table 35.2). The nature of the side chains is the second selection parameter. It has to be decided whether they will be ionizable (acidic or basic) or nonionizable.

Table 35.2   Small and large solubilizing moieties.

Small groups or simple functionalities	Larger solubilizing moieties
—CO_2H	R—OH → R—O—CH_2—CH_2—CO_2H
—SO_3H, —OSO_3H	R—NH_2 → R—NH—CH_2—CH_2—CH_2—
SO_3H	
—PO_3H_2, —OPO_3H_2	$(R)_2C{=}O$ → $(R)_2C{=}N$—O—CH_2—CO_2H
—NH_2, —NHR, —NR_2	R—OH → O-morpholinylethyl
N-oxides, *S*-oxides, sulfones	R—OH → O-glucoside
	R—OH → O—CO—CH_2—CH_2—CO_2H

Acidic ionizable moieties (e.g. carboxylic acids) yield readily crystallizable compounds and often do not alter the pharmacological profile of the parent molecule. However, owing to their amphiphilic nature, they can show haemolytic properties. In addition only a limited number of cations can be used to neutralize them. Traditional inorganic cations such as sodium, potassium or magnesium can induce mineral surcharges and are no longer recommended.

Basic ionizable moieties (e.g. substituted amines) can be neutralized by a very large number of organic and inorganic acids (see Chapter 34). The salts obtained are also readily crystallized and usually show less surface-active properties than salts from acidic chains. Their main disadvantage, which somewhat limits their utility, is their tendency to interfere with biogenic amines and neurotransmitters. In other words, attaching a basic amine functional group can seriously modify the pharmacological activity with regard to the parent drug.

Drugs with acidic side-chains cannot be mixed with drugs having basic side-chains, as it is likely that a salt formed between the two drugs might precipitate.

Nonionizable moieties (e.g. polyhydroxylated chains) do not present this disadvantage and are compatible with other drug preparations. As they can be delivered at pH values close to 7, they do not produce painful injections. The main problems encountered with nonionizable solubilizing moities is their lesser propensity to crystallize. In addition, increased cost can be expected from the necessity of added protection/deprotection steps during their synthesis.

III. ACIDIC SOLUBILIZING CHAINS

When planning solubilization by means of a carboxylic acid side-chain, one has to take into account the therapeutic properties peculiar to the carboxylic group. Thus, all arylacetic acids show more or less potent anti-inflammatory activities and many α-functionalized carboxylic acids are chelating agents. Among them we find the chelating α-amino acids[6] and antibacterial nalidixic acid-derived quinolones (for references see Hammond[7]) and probably kynurenic acid analogues acting as antagonists at the glycine site.[8]

A. Direct introduction of acidic functions

Direct introduction of a solubilizing function can be achieved by carboxylation and by sulfonation. The historical example of carboxylation is the Kolbe synthesis of salicylic acid. Sulfonation was employed to solubilize guaiacol, camphor and 7-chloro-8-hydroxyquinoline (Fig. 35.1).

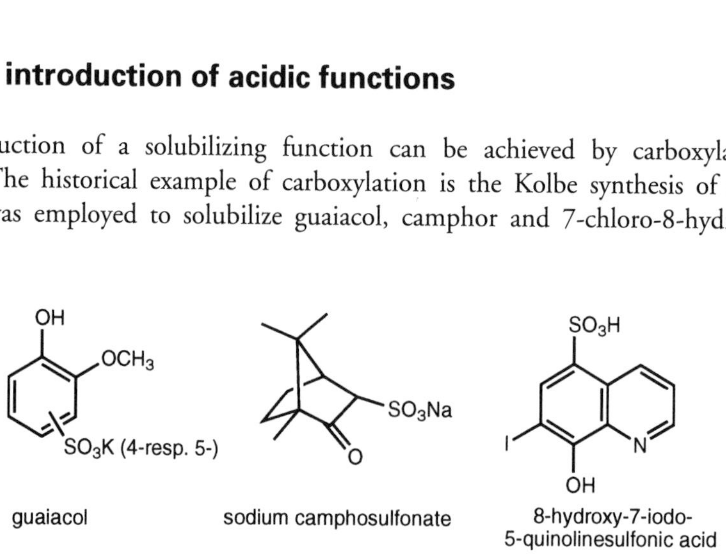

guaiacol   sodium camphosulfonate   8-hydroxy-7-iodo-
                                                  5-quinolinesulfonic acid

Fig. 35.1   Sulfonic acid solubilization.

B.   Alkylation of OH and NH functions with acidic chains

This procedure alkylates the hydroxy and the amino groups already present on the molecule with reactive intermediates bearing acidic functional residues (Table 35.3). These compounds are prepared starting from chloroacetic acid or its ethyl ester. For chains longer than acetic, cyanoethylation and hydrolysis of the nitrile obtained leads to the propionic chain; alkylation with ethyl 4-bromobutyrate and saponification leads to the butyric chain. The propanesulfonic chains are particularly accessible by means of ring-opening of propane-sulfone.

Table 35.3   Alkylation of OH and NH functions with acidic chains.

Starting derivative	Solubilized analogue	Example	Reference
Ar—OH	Ar—O—CH$_2$—CO$_2$H	Solusalvarsan	3
Ar—NH$_2$	Ar—NH—CH$_2$—CO$_2$H	Acediasulfone	9
Ar—NH$_2$	Ar—NH—CH$_2$—CO$_2$H	Iodopyracet	10
Ar—NH$_2$	Ar—NH—CH$_2$— SO$_2$H	Sulfoxone sodium	11

Dihydroartemisinin ethers. A water-soluble derivative of artemisinin, the sodium salt of artesunic acid (the succinic half-ester derivative of dihydroartemisinin; Fig. 35.2), can be administered by intravenous injection, a property that makes it especially useful in the treatment of advanced and potentially lethal infestation with *Plasmodium falciparum*. Sodium artesunate is capable of rapidly reversing parasitaemia and causing the restoration to conciousness of the comatose cerebral malaria patient. The utility of sodium artesunate, however, is impaired by its poor stability due to the facile hydrolysis of the ester linkage. To overcome the ease of hydrolysis of the ester function in sodium artesunate, Lin *et al.*[12] prepared a series of analogues in which the solubilizing moiety is joined to dihydroartemisinin by an ether rather than an ester linkage. One of the compounds prepared, artelinic acid (Fig. 35.2), is both soluble and stable in 2.5% K$_2$CO$_3$ solution and possesses superior *in vivo* activity against *Plasmodium berghei* in comparison to artermisinin or artesunic acid.[12] Other ether-linked artemisinin-solubilizing chains containing asymmetric centres did not show activities superior to that of artelinic acid.[13]

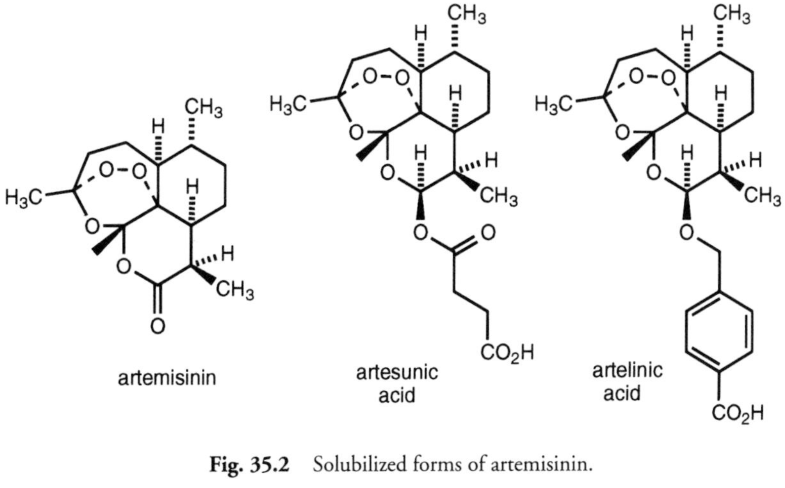

Fig. 35.2   Solubilized forms of artemisinin.

C. Acylation of OH and NH functions with acidic chains

The acylation of OH and NH functions with acidic chains is probably the most popular mode of acidic solubilization. Alcohols and phenols are converted into half-esters such as hemisuccinates, hemiglutarates, hemiphthalates[14] and *m*-benzenesulfonates[15] but also into phosphates or even sulfates (Fig. 35.3). All these derivatives can give water-soluble sodium or amine salts. Similar acylation possibilities exist for amines, but peptide-like derivatives are often preferred because the enzymatic regeneration of the parent molecule *in vivo* is easier.

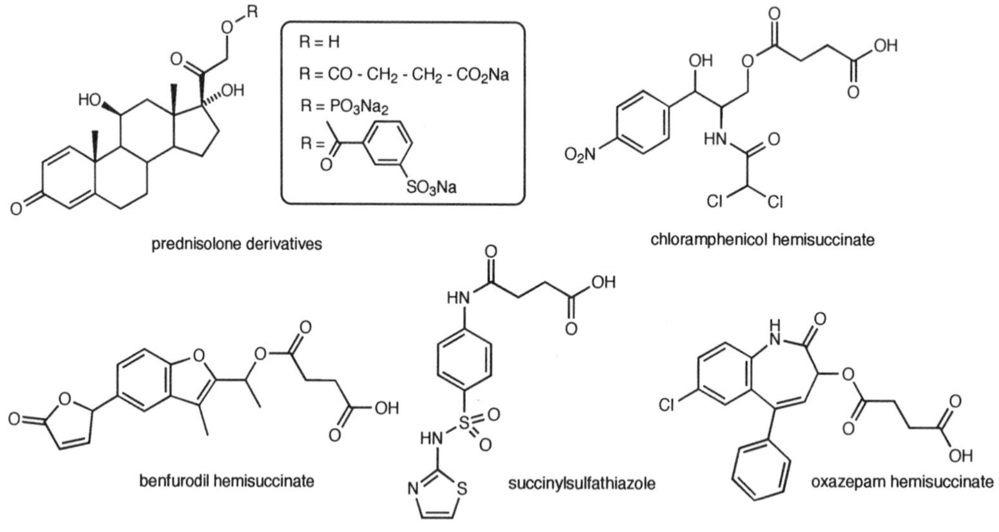

Fig. 35.3   Acylation of OH and NH functions with acidic chains.

Carboxylic half-esters (e.g., hemisuccinates) of phenols are easily hydrolysed in aqueous solution and are therefore not recommended for the solubilization of phenolic compounds. Even hemisuccinates of alcohols suffer somewhat from stability problems and must be supplied as lyophilized (freeze-dried) powders for reconstitution in water and used within 48 hours. (See, for example, the monograph Chloramphenicol Sodium Succinate or Hydrocortisone Sodium Succinate in *The Handbook of Injectable Drugs*,[16] see also Anderson et al.[17,18])

An additional difficulty occurring with hemisuccinates was discovered by Sandman et al.[19] These authors, in studying the stability of chloramphenicol succinate, found an unusual partial acyl transfer reaction of the succinyl group to give a cyclic hemiorthoester (Fig. 35.4).

In the search for an improvement in solution stability, i.e. in minimizing the ester hydrolysis and decreasing the acyl migration, Anderson and co-workers[20] synthesized a series of more stable water-soluble methylprednisolone esters. Several of the analogues were shown to have shelf-lives in solution of greater than 2 years at room temperature. Ester hydrolysis studies of these compounds in human and monkey serum indicated that derivatives having anionic solubilizing residues such as carboxylate or sulfonate are more slowly hydrolysed by serum esterases then compounds with a cationic solubilizing moiety (tertiary amine).[21]

Phosphoric esters (Fig. 35.5) are generally more stable. They have been used in the steroid[22,23] and vitamin fields (vitamin C,[24] vitamin B$_1$,[25] benfotiamin,[26,27] riboflavin,[28] dihydrovitamin K$_1$[29]).

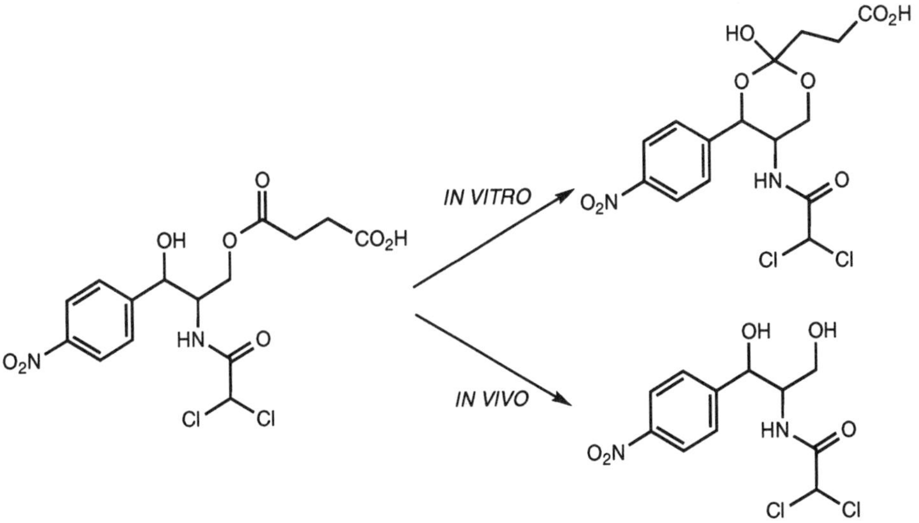
IN VITRO
IN VIVO

Fig. 35.4 Formation of cyclic hemiorthoesters from a hemisuccinate.[4,19]

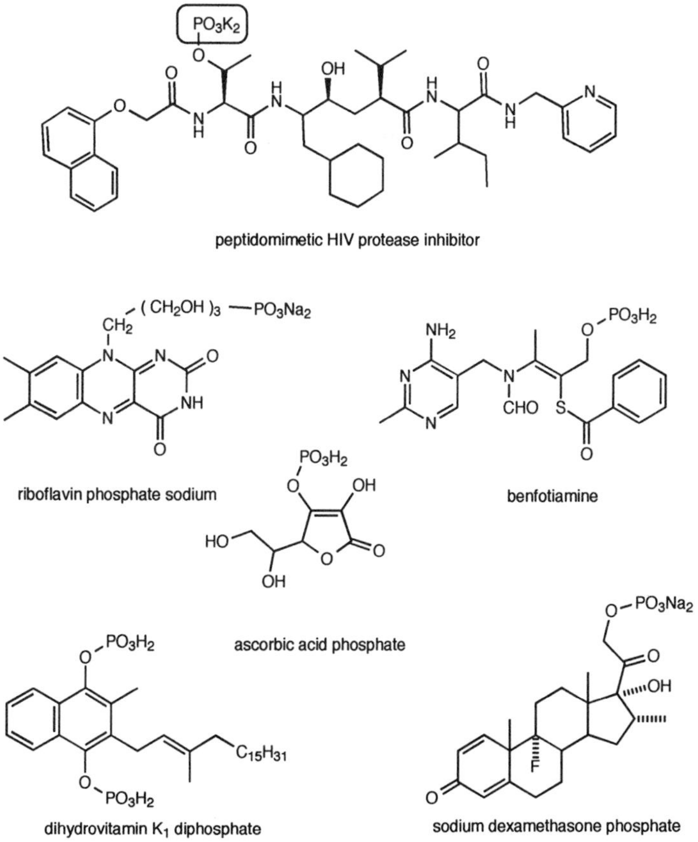
peptidomimetic HIV protease inhibitor
riboflavin phosphate sodium
benfotiamine
ascorbic acid phosphate
dihydrovitamin K1 diphosphate
sodium dexamethasone phosphate

Fig. 35.5 Phosphate esters.

Riboflavin-5′-phosphoric acid dihydrate, for example, has a solubility in water of $112\,\mathrm{g\,l^{-1}}$ at pH 6.9, compared to 0.06–$0.33\,\mathrm{g\,l^{-1}}$ for riboflavin itself. Phosphoric esters of trichloroethanol, diphenylhydantoin (open form) and clindamycin are discussed in Chapter 38.

A large number of reported peptidomimetic compounds possess very low aqueous solubility at physiological pH owing to the high lipophilicity inherent in these structures. Phosphorylation can yield improved biological activities for such compounds. This is at least the case for the HIV protease inhibitor of Fig. 35.5 described by scientists from Upjohn.[30]

Clean phosphorylation methods are now available: some of them are shown in Fig. 35.6.

Formation of sulfate esters is one of the metabolic conjugation reactions (phase II reactions,

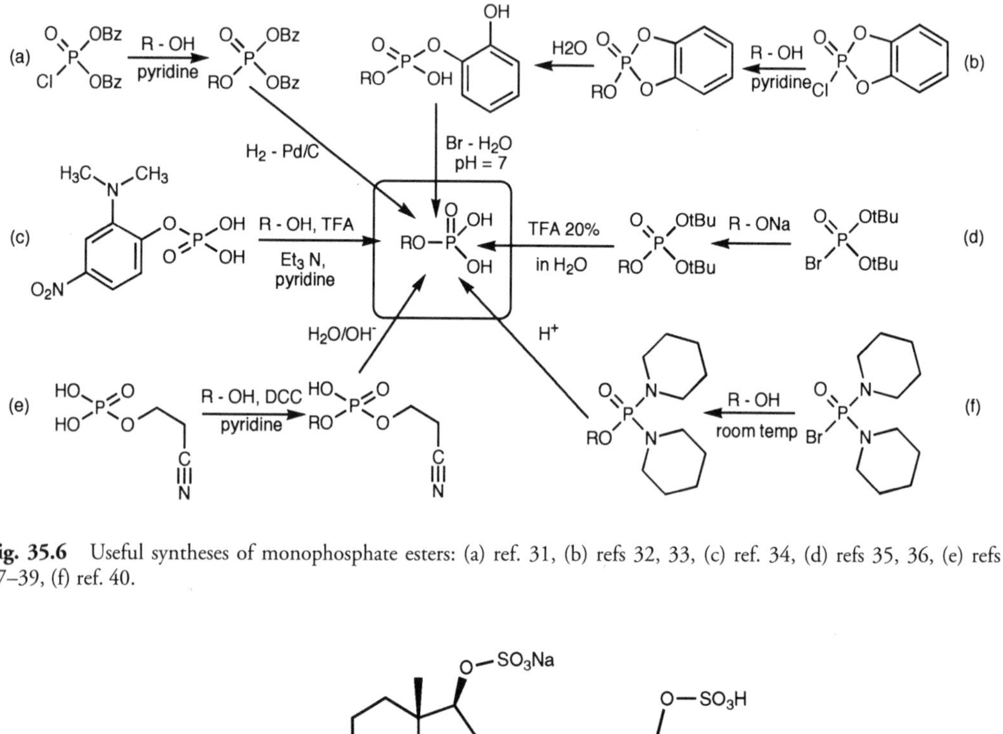

Fig. 35.6 Useful syntheses of monophosphate esters: (a) ref. 31, (b) refs 32, 33, (c) ref. 34, (d) refs 35, 36, (e) refs 37–39, (f) ref. 40.

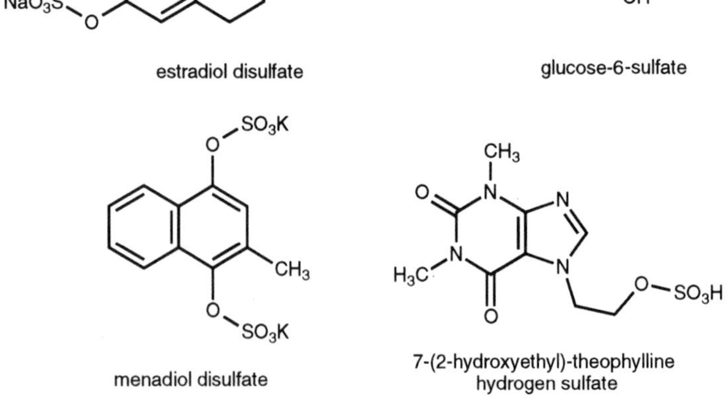

estradiol disulfate

glucose-6-sulfate

menadiol disulfate

7-(2-hydroxyethyl)-theophylline
hydrogen sulfate

Fig. 35.7 Sulfuric acid esters.

see Chapter 29). Sulfates of estradiol,[41] glucose,[42] menadiol,[43] and hydroxyethyltheophylline[44] have been prepared (Fig. 35.7). As a rule, sulfuric acid esters, compared to their phosphoric analogues, are resistant to enzymatic hydrolysis *in vivo*[45,46] and their conversion to the parent drug is questionable.

Sulfonic acids can be prepared by direct sulfonation (see above, Fig. 35.1). Compounds containing conjugated double bonds have been solubilized by addition of sodium bisulfite. Treatment of menadione (vitamin K$_3$) with sodium bisulfite leads to two addition compounds (Fig. 35.8). Mild warming of the reactants for a short time predominantly affords adduct (a), which arises from attack of bisulfite ion at carbon-2. Heating at reflux for an extended period yields adduct (b) from addition of bisulfite ion to carbon-3.[47]

In a similar way the treatment of N^4-cinnamylidenesulfanilamide (prepared from cinnamic

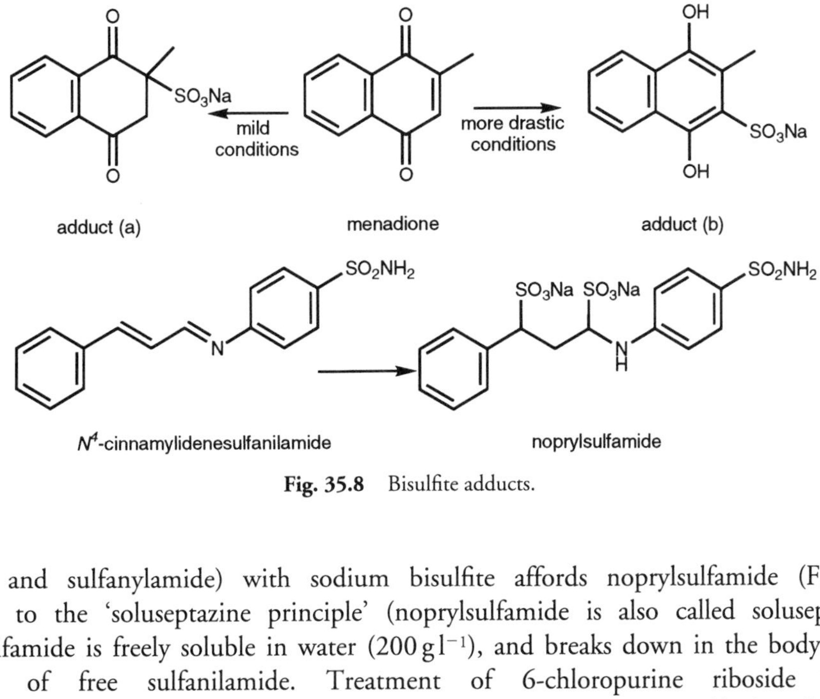

adduct (a) mild conditions menadione more drastic conditions adduct (b)

N^4-cinnamylidenesulfanilamide noprylsulfamide

Fig. 35.8 Bisulfite adducts.

aldehyde and sulfanylamide) with sodium bisulfite affords noprylsulfamide (Fig. 35.8) according to the 'soluseptazine principle' (noprylsulfamide is also called soluseptazine).[48] Noprylsulfamide is freely soluble in water (200 g l^{-1}), and breaks down in the body with the liberation of free sulfanilamide. Treatment of 6-chloropurine riboside with *p*-aminobenzenesulfonic acid leads to the highly water-soluble N^6-(*p*-sulfophenyl)adenosine (solubility >1.5 g ml^{-1}, ≈ 13 M). This compound (Fig. 35.9) is a potent A$_1$ adenosine agonist in receptor binding, in inhibitory electrophysiological effects in hippocampal slices, and in inhibition of lipolysis *in vivo*.[49]

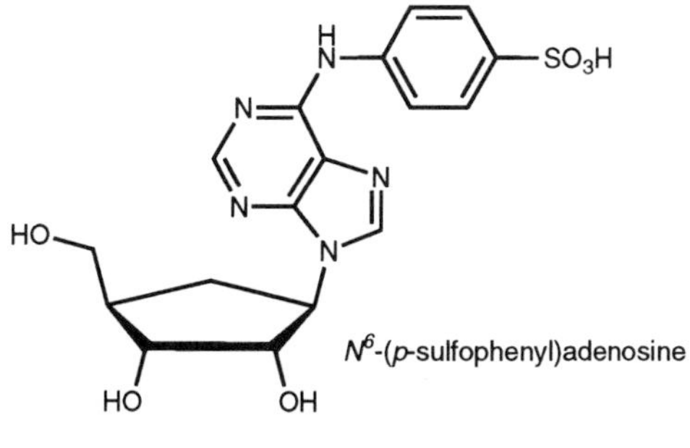

N^6-(*p*-sulfophenyl)adenosine

Fig. 35.9 N^6-(*p*-Sulfopehnyl)adenosine, a freely water-soluble adenosine A$_1$ receptor agonist.[49]

Treatment of primary and secondary amines with formaldehyde and sodium bisulfite generates stable methanesulfonates that can also act as solubilizing groups. The first example of this reaction found in the literature is the conversion of *p*-phenetidine into the corresponding methanesulfonate.[50] The compound obtained (Fig. 35.10) still possesses antipyretic properties and is much less toxic than *p*-phenetidine. Nevertheless it did not break into a new market.[3]

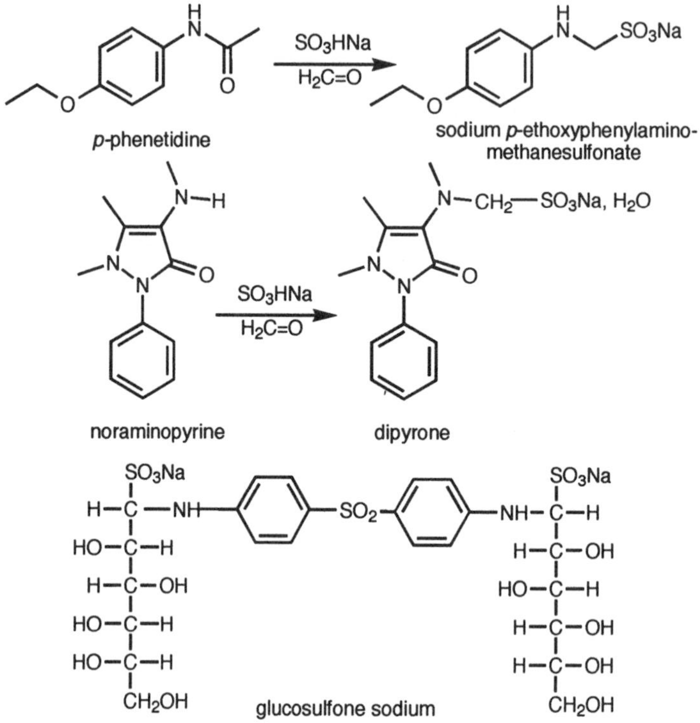

Fig. 35.10　Sulfonates.

Applied to noraminopyrine, the same solubilization strategy led to dipyrone,[51,52] a water-soluble (1 g/1.5 ml), injectable form of aminopyrine (Pyramidon®) used worldwide. Replacement of formaldehyde by acetaldehyde to yield ethanesulfonates has been claimed to lead to compounds with faster hydrolysis kinetics *in vivo*.[53] Replacement of formaldehyde by glucose afforded glucosulfone sodium, a soluble preparation of the leprostatic 4,4'-diaminodiphenylsulfone.[54,55] Replacement of formaldehyde-bisulfite by formaldehydesulfoxylate is also claimed in some references.[3,56]

Ketones can be solubilized as carboxymethoximes (Fig. 35.11). Menadoxime is freely water-soluble, can be sterilized by autoclaving and, like menadione itself, shows high antihaemorrhagic activity.[57] The carboxymethoxime of griseofulvin, on the other hand, is devoid of activity *in vitro* as well as *in vivo*.[58] This may be due either to an absence of conversion to the parent molecule or to rapid renal elimination. Unsubstituted oximes can be converted enzymatically to their corresponding ketones.[59] For carboxymethoximes, intramolecular assistance should even facilitate the hydrolysis to the initial carbonyl function. This was shown to be the case for the carboxymethoxime of naloxone.[60] Other substituted oximes seem to be rather resistant as is apparent from the metabolic stability of noxiptilin.[61]

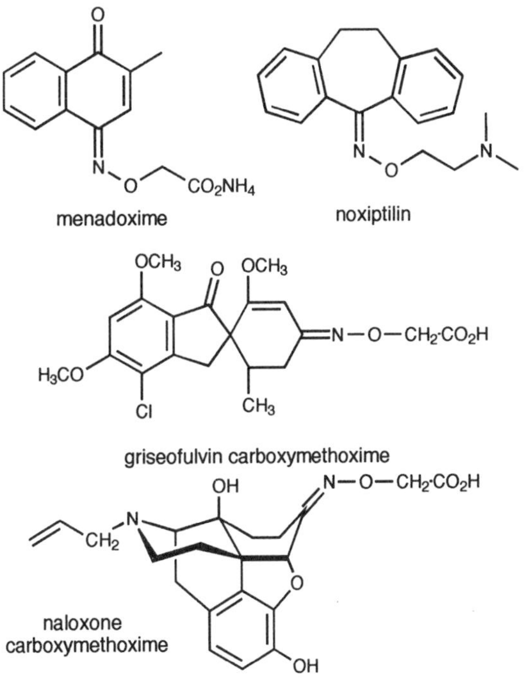

Fig. 35.11 Carboxymethoximes as (reversible?) solubilizing chains for carbonyl-containing molecules.

IV. BASIC SOLUBILIZING CHAINS

Solubilization with basic side chains involves two essential strategies: either direct binding of the amine function on a carbon atom of the parent molecule, or linking it to a function already present: alcoholic or phenolic hydroxyl, carboxylic acid, amine or amide.

A. Direct attachment of a basic residue

Simple tertiary amines can be grafted to a carbon skeleton, either by exchange reactions or by Mannich reactions. The hydrochloride salt of the camptothecin derivative (**a**) (Fig. 35.12) is soluble in water at concentrations up to $1\,mg\,ml^{-1}$; the comparable value for camptothecin itself is $0.0025\,mg\,ml^{-1}$.[62] Similar results were obtained in solubilizing the benzodiazepine (**b**)[63] and the quinazolinone (**c**).[64] The adenosine A_1 antagonist KW-3902 (**d**) was solubilized in an original manner by converting it to an amidinic and cyclized bioisostere (**e**).[65]

B. Attachment of the solubilizing moiety to an alcoholic hydroxyl

Esterification of an alcoholic hydroxyl with dialkylglycine or its analogues is a very popular mode of solubilization of alcohols. It is illustrated (Fig. 35.13) by soluble esters of forskolin,[66] of

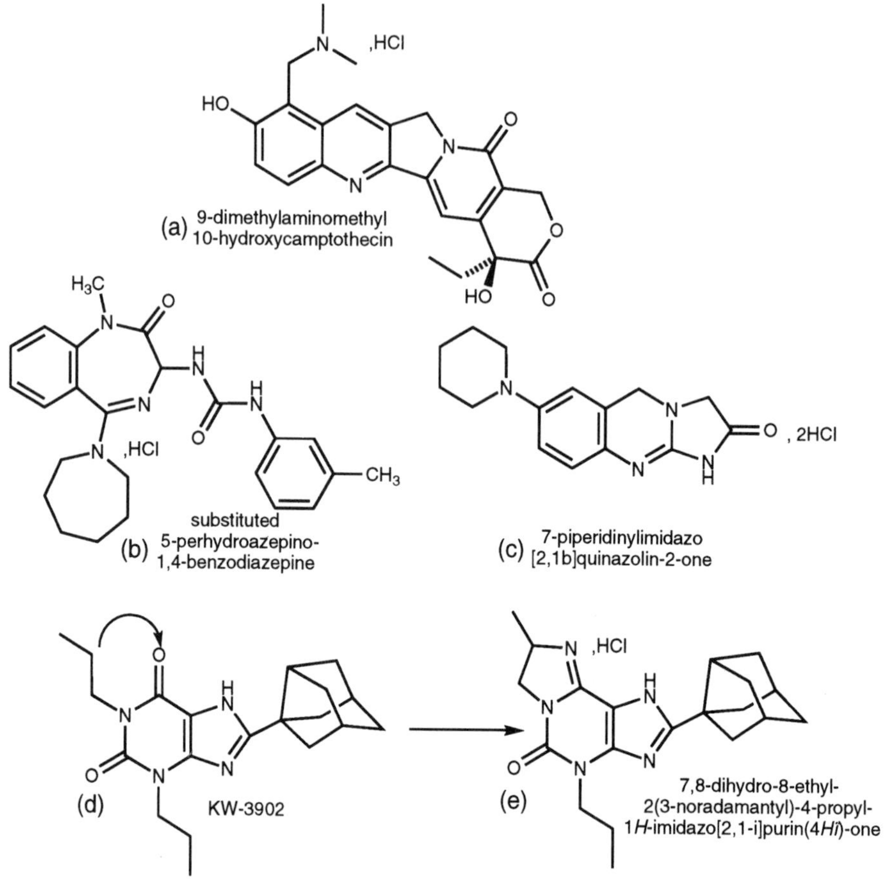

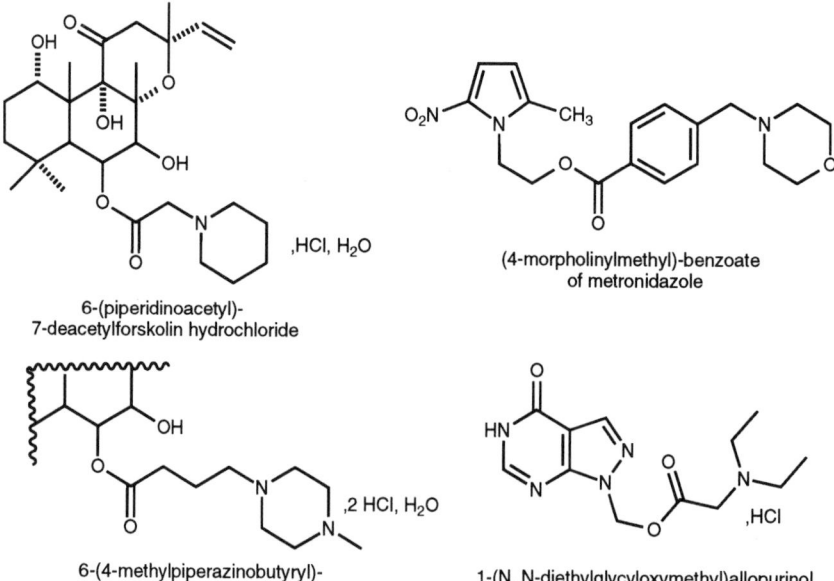

Fig. 35.12   Solubilization by means of basic side chains.

(a) 9-dimethylaminomethyl 10-hydroxycamptothecin

(b) substituted 5-perhydroazepino-1,4-benzodiazepine

(c) 7-piperidinylimidazo [2,1b]quinazolin-2-one

(d) KW-3902

(e) 7,8-dihydro-8-ethyl-2(3-noradamantyl)-4-propyl-1*H*-imidazo[2,1-i]purin(4*Hi*)-one

6-(piperidinoacetyl)-7-deacetylforskolin hydrochloride

(4-morpholinylmethyl)-benzoate of metronidazole

6-(4-methylpiperazinobutyryl)-7-deacetylforskolin dihydrochloride

1-(N, N-diethylglycyloxymethyl)allopurinol

Fig. 35.13   Dialkylglycines and related aminoesters.

allopurinol[67] and of metronidazole.[68] This mode of solubilization can also be applied to phenols such as paracetamol (see Chapter 31).

Many α-amino acid esters or related short-chained aliphatic amino esters show satisfying hydrolysis kinetics in plasma, but exhibit poor stability in aqueous solution.[68] This poor stability is predominantly due to electron withdrawal by the positively charged amino group, but may also involve intramolecular catalysis or assistance of the ester hydrolysis by the neighbouring amino group. The replacement of the glycine unit by its benzologue, as shown for the metronidazole derivative of Fig. 35.13, prevents the hydrolysis-facilitating effect of the amino group. Alternative solutions place the amino group more distant from the ester linkage in using 6-aminocaproic acid esters and sebacic acid-derived spacer groups[20] or render the ester function more resistant by replacing it by a carbonate or a carbamate function.[69]

C.   Attachment of the solubilizing moiety to an acidic NH function

The NH group in theophylline is reactive and can easily be alkylated, yielding, among others, etamiphyllin (Fig. 35.14), which is rendered water-soluble as hydrochloride or as camphosulfonate.[70] Rolitetracycline, the Mannich base derived from the carboxamide function of tetracycline, formaldehyde and pyrrolidine,[71] is surprisingly stable and is used as an injectable form of tetracycline.

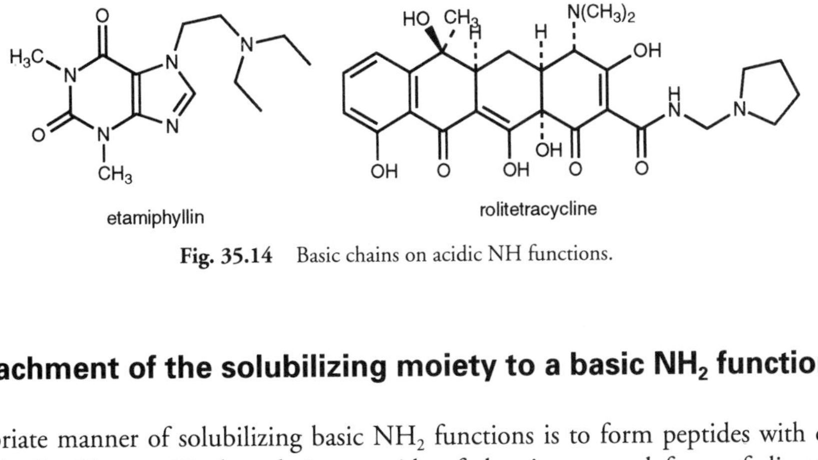

etamiphyllin   rolitetracycline

Fig. 35.14   Basic chains on acidic NH functions.

D.   Attachment of the solubilizing moiety to a basic NH₂ function

An appropriate manner of solubilizing basic NH_2 functions is to form peptides with common amino acids. In Chapter 31 the L-lysine peptide of the ring-opened form of diazepam was described. Similarly acylation of the 3-amino group of the pyrrolidine ring in a series of quinolone antibacterial agents yielded interesting compounds (Fig. 35.15).

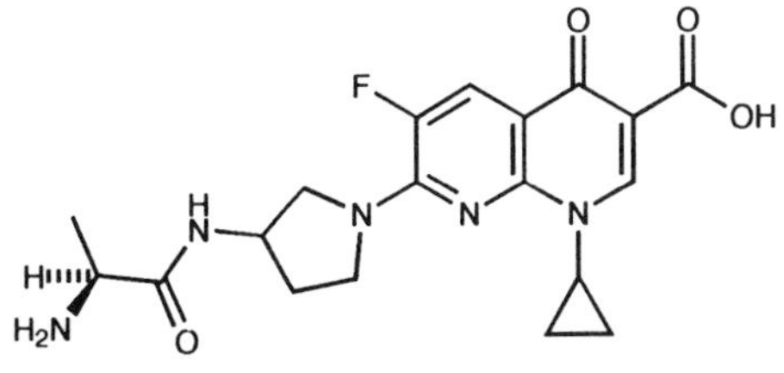

compound PD131112

Fig. 35.15   S-Alanine-derived peptide of a quinolone antibacterial agents confers high water-solubility and is sensitive to enzymatic cleavage *in vivo*.[72]

The amino acid analogues were less active *in vitro*, but had equal or increased efficacy *in vivo*. Indeed, it was shown that these compounds, which were stable to acid and base under the reaction conditions for their preparation, were rapidly cleaved in serum to give the parent quinolones. The amino acid derivatives showed a 3–70 times improved solubility when compared with the parent compounds.[70]

E. Attachment of the solubilizing moiety to carboxylic acid functionalities

As carboxylic esters of amino alcohols are usually too sensitive to hydrolysis, amides with aminoalkylamines are preferred (Fig. 35.16). The water-soluble E-lactone ring-modified 7-ethylcamptothecin analogue bearing a dimethylaminoethyl amidic chain compares favourably with the sodium salt resulting simply from the lactone ring opening.[73] Introduction of basic substituents into modified hydroxyethylene dipeptide isosteres gave inhibitors with improved solubility as well as improved potency against human plasma renin.[74]

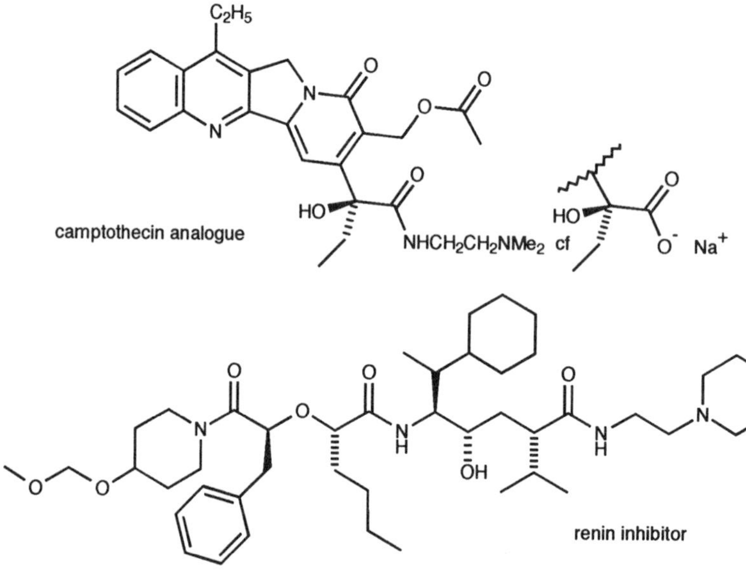

Fig. 35.16   Basic amides of carboxylic acids.

V.   NONIONIZABLE SIDE-CHAINS

The most frequently employed solubilization approaches using nonionizable moieties involve hydroxylated and polyoxymethylenic side-chains or glucosides and their analogues.

A.   Glycolyl and glyceryl side-chains

These chains are present in some classical drugs such as the muscle relaxant mephenesin[75] and the bronchodilator dyphylline (diprophylline)[76] (Fig. 35.17).

More recent applications are found in the venotropic troxerutin[77] and in the analgesic anti-inflammatory drugs glafenine,[78,79] and etofenamate.[80]

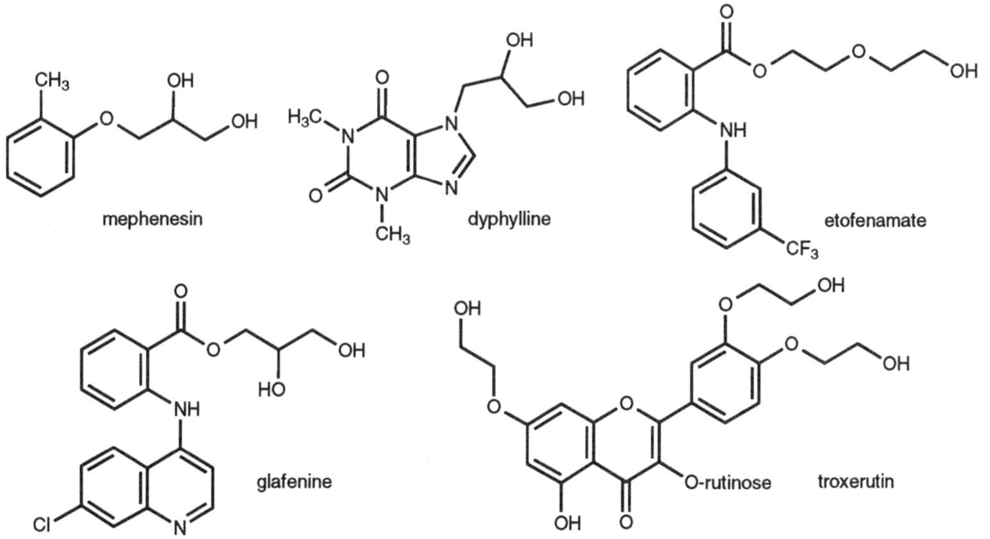

Fig. 35.17   Glycolyl and glyceryl side-chains.

B.   Poly(ethylene glycol) derivatives

Only a few examples of solubilization involving esters or ethers of poly(ethylene glycol) are found in the literature and it is not always clear whether the main purpose of the polyoxyethylenic chain grafting was to increase the aqueous solubility or to produce another improvement such as sustained release. One of the most representative examples is the antitussive benzonatate[81] (Fig. 35.18). In a similar way, Nagakawa and colleagues prepared

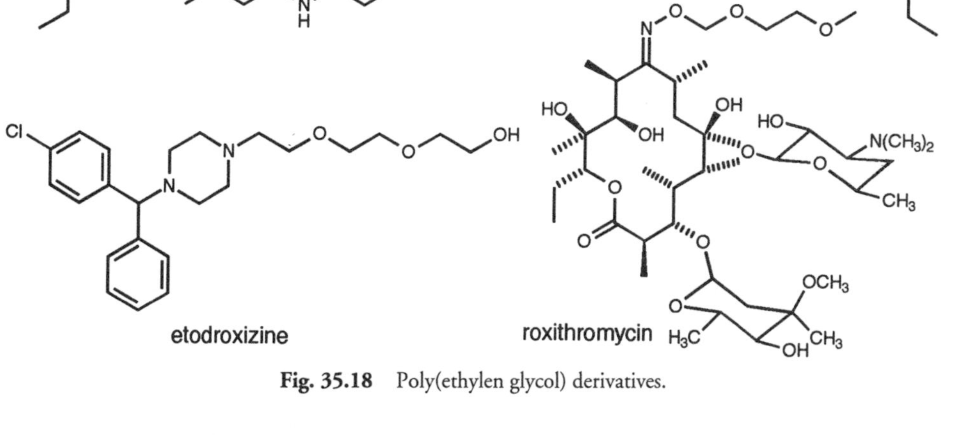

Fig. 35.18   Poly(ethylen glycol) derivatives.

soluble forms of vitamins A and E, as well as various steroids (prednisolone, testosterone, hydrocortisone, gitoxin).[82,83]

The symmetrical attachment of the local anaesthetic procaine to poly(ethylene glycol) increases the duration of action[84] and probably improves water-solubility. The hypnotic etodroxizine bears a three-ethylene-oxy-unit chain but is nevertheless used as a dimaleate.[85] In roxithromycin the oxygenated side-chain is attached to the oxygen atom of the oxime of the antibiotic erythromycin.[86]

C.   Glucosides and related compounds

Despite their ubiquitous distribution in plants, man-made glucosidic derivatives of alcohols or phenols are rarely prepared in medicinal chemistry. An old-timer is the sedative-hypnotic α-chloralose (Fig. 35.19), which is presently used only as a surgical anaesthetic for laboratory animals.

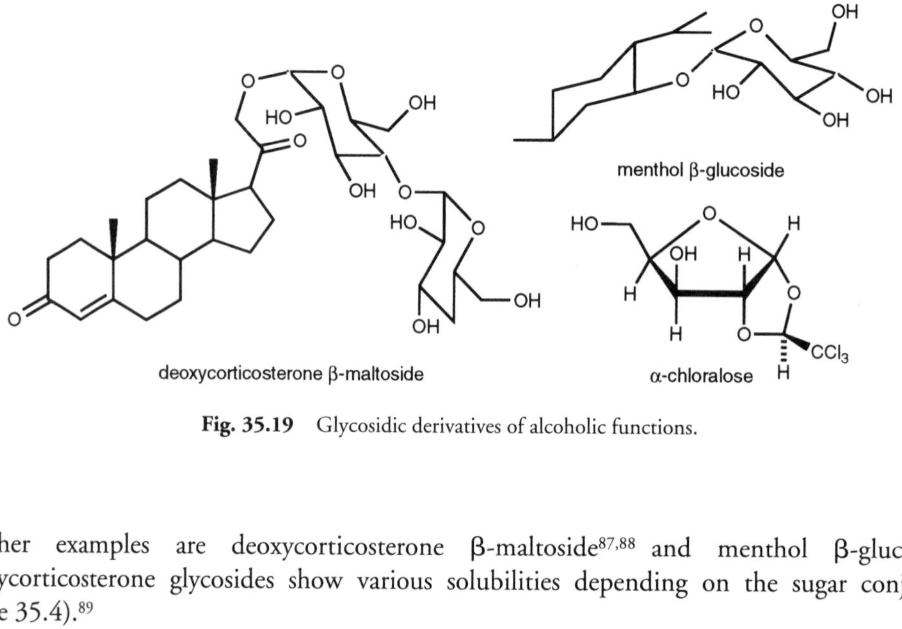

menthol β-glucoside

deoxycorticosterone β-maltoside

α-chloralose

Fig. 35.19   Glycosidic derivatives of alcoholic functions.

Other examples are deoxycorticosterone β-maltoside[87,88] and menthol β-glucoside. Deoxycorticosterone glycosides show various solubilities depending on the sugar conjugate (Table 35.4).[89]

Menthol β-glucoside is a water-soluble, nonirritating prodrug of menthol that can be used, like glucovanillin, the β-D-glucoside of vanillin, as a pharmaceutical flavour adjuvant.[90] The use of sugar moieties as drug carriers has been reviewed by Chavis and Imbach.[91]

Table 35.4   Solubilities of deoxycorticosterone glycosides[90]

Deoxycorticosterone glycoside	Solubility in water
Glucoside	1.2%
Galactoside	2.2%
Lactoside	3.4%
Lactosidoglucoside	Unlimited

Attachment of the sugar moiety to nitrogen atoms of amine, amide or hydrazine functions is much more frequently encountered (Fig. 35.20). Prontoglucal is the N^4-β-D-glucoside of sulfanylamide,[92] the tuberculostatic glyconiazide is the isonicotinoylhydrazone of D-glucuronic acid lactone,[93] and glucometacin results from the amidification of indomethacin with D-glucosamine.[94]

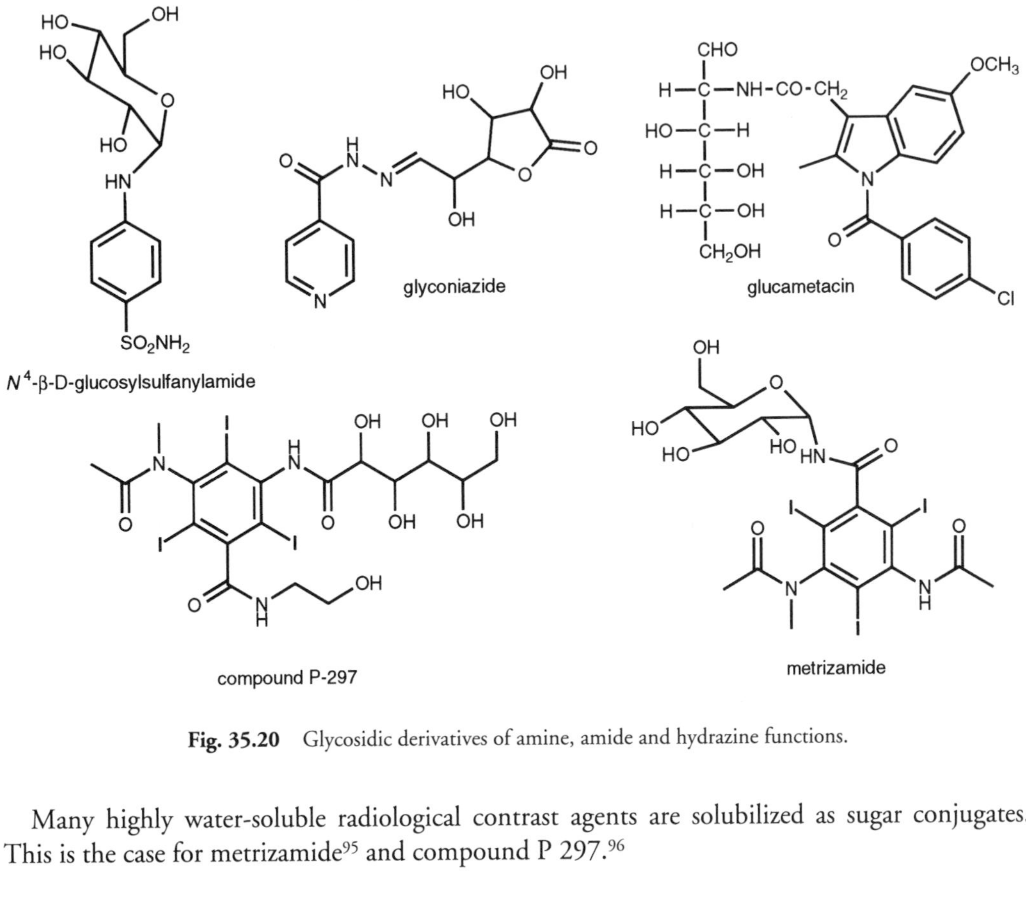

glyconiazide

glucametacin

N^4-β-D-glucosylsulfanylamide

compound P-297

metrizamide

Fig. 35.20 Glycosidic derivatives of amine, amide and hydrazine functions.

Many highly water-soluble radiological contrast agents are solubilized as sugar conjugates. This is the case for metrizamide[95] and compound P 297.[96]

VI. CONCLUDING REMARKS

The different chemical solutions to solubilization problems discussed in this chapter reveal that in many cases the chemical transformation used also improves the activity profile of the parent molecule. This can be due to purely *pharmacokinetic* factors such as a better resorption from the organism and faster transport and diffusion. These factors also explain why solubilized drugs are generally more rapidly eliminated and therefore show fewer symptoms of toxicity. But the *pharmacological* profile can also be affected. Chlorpromazine, for example (Fig. 35.21), has neuroleptic properties, whereas the parent phenothiazine possesses anthelmintic properties. In this example the attachment of the basic moiety has totally modified the pharmacological profile. However, the replacement of the basic moiety by its carboxylic counterpart yielded a compound totally inactive as a neuroleptic (C. G. Wermuth, unpublished result).

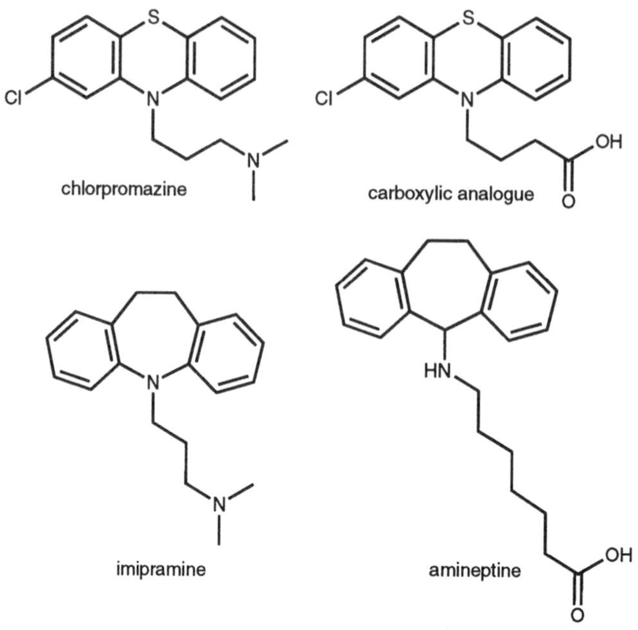

Fig. 35.21   Acidic and basic side-chains on tricyclic skeletons.

Conversely, in the tricyclic antidepressant series, the passage from the basic imipramine to the acidic amineptine conserved the antidepressant properties. In other words, there are no general rules available for the selection of the most appropriate solubilizing moiety. It is therefore recommended that for each new solubilization problem, acidic, basic and neutral solubilized versions of the parent molecule be prepared.

REFERENCES

1. La Fontaine, J. de La Besace (1993) *Fables, Livre I,* Fable VII, pp. 42–43. Florilège, Paris.
2. Marini-Bettolo, G. B. (1948) Metodos modernos de solubilizacion de medicamentos organicos. *Ann. Asoc. Quim. Pharm. Urugay* **50**: 3–17.
3. Büchi, J. (1963) *Grundlagen der Arzneimittelforschung und der Synthetischen Arzneimittel,* pp. 220–235. Birkhaüser Verlag, Basel.
4. Stella, V. (1975) Prodrugs: an overview and definition. In Higuchi, T. and Stella, V. (eds) *Prodrugs as Novel Drug Delivery Systems,* pp. 1–115. American Chemical Society, Washington D.C.
5. Silverman, R. B. (1992) *The Organic Chemistry of Drug Design and Drug Action,* pp. 358–360. Academic Press, San Diego.
6. Albert, A. (1979) *Selective Toxicity,* pp. 403–440. Chapman and Hall, London.
7. Hammond, M.L. (1993) Recent advances in anti-infective agents. In Bristol, J. A. (ed.) *Ann. Rep. Med. Chem.,* pp. 119–130. Academic Press, San Diego.
8. Leeson, P. D., Carling, R. W., Kulagowski, J. J., Mawer, I. M., Moore, K. W., Moseley, A. M., Rowley, M., Smith, J. D., Stevenson, G. I., Williams, B. J., Baker, R., Foster, A. C., Kemp, J. A. and Tricklebank, M. D. (1993) Drugs Interacting with the Glycine Binding Site. In Testa, B., Kyburz, E., Fuhrer, W. and Giger, R. (eds), *Perspectives in Medicinal Chemistry,* pp. 239–257. Verlag Helvetica Chemica Acta/VHC, Basel/Weinheim.
9. Jackson, E. L., (1948) Certain *N*-alkyl, *N*-carboxyalkyl and *N*-hydroxyalkyl derivatives of 4,4′-diaminodiphenyl sulfone. *J. Amer. Chem. Soc.* **70**: 680–684.

10. Reitmann, J. (1935) Aliphatic amine salts of halogenated pyridones containing an acid group. US Patent 1 993 039 (5 March, 1935; to Winthrop Chemical Company, Inc., New York).
11. Bauer, H. (1939) Organic compounds in chemotherapy. II. The preparation of formaldehyde sulfoxylate derivatives of sulfanilamide and of amino compounds. *J. Am. Chem. Soc.* **61**: 617–618.
12. Lin, A. J. Klayman, D. L. and Milhous, W. (1987) Antimalarial activity of new water-soluble dihydroartemisin derivatives. *J. Med. Chem.* **30**: 2147–2150.
13. Lin, A. J., Lee, M. and Klayman, D. L. (1989) Antimalarial activity of new water-soluble dihydroartemisin derivatives. 2. Stereospecificity of the ether side chain. *J. Med. Chem.* **32**: 1249–1252.
14. Coker, J. D., Elks, J., May, P. J., Nice, F. A., Phillips, G. H. and Wall, W. F. (1965) Action of some steroids on the central nervous system of the mouse. I. Synthetic methods. *J. Med. Chem.* **8**: 417–425.
15. Allais, A. A. and Girault, P. (1962) Process for the preparation of 21-meta-sulfobenzoates of $\Delta^{1,4}$-dehydrocorticosteroids. US Patent 3 032 568 (1 May 1962; Roussel-UCLAF, SA).
16. Trissel, L. A. (1986) *Handbook on Injectable Drugs*, 4th edn. American Society of Hospital Pharmacists, Bethesda.
17. Anderson, B. D. and Taphouse, V. (1981) Initial rate studies of hydrolysis and acyl migration in methylprednisolone 21-hemisuccinate and 17-hemisuccinate. *J. Pharm. Sci.*, **70**: 181–186.
18. Anderson, B. D., Conradi, R. A. and Lambert, J. W. (1984) Carboxyl group catalysis of acyl transfer reactions in corticosteroid 17- and 21-monoesters. *J. Pharm. Sci.* **73**: 604–611.
19. Sandman, B., Szulczewski, D., Winheuser, J. and Higuchi, T. (1970) Rearrangement of chloramphenicol-3-monosuccinate. *J. Pharm. Sci.* **59**: 427–429.
20. Anderson, B. D., Conradi, R. A. and Knuth, K. E. (1985) Strategies in the design of solution-stable, water-soluble prodrugs I: A physical-organic approach to pro-moiety selection for 21-esters of corticosteroids. *J. Pharm. Sci.* **74**: 365–374.
21. Anderson, B. D., Conradi, R. A., Spilman, C. H. and Forbes, A. D. (1985) Strategies in the design of solution-stable, water-soluble prodrugs III: Influence of the Pro-Moiety on the Bioconversion of 21-Esters of Corticosteroids. *J. Pharm. Sci.* **74**: 382–387.
22. Flynn, G. L. and Lamb, D. J. (1970) Factors influencing solvolysis of corticosteroid-21-phosphate esters. *J. Pharm. Sci.* **59**: 1433–1438.
23. Melby, J. C. and St Cyr, M. (1961) Comparative studies on absorption and metabolic disposal of water-soluble corticosteroid esters. *Metabolism* **10**: 75–82.
24. Cutolo, E. and Larizza, A. (1961) Synthesis of 3-phosphoric ester of L-ascorbic acid. *Gazz. Chim. Ital.* **91**: 964–972.
25. Wenz, A., Göttmann, G. and Koop, H. (1961) Verfahren zur Herstellung der freien Base und der Salze des Aneurin-orthophosphor-säureesters. German Patent 1 110 649 (13 July 1961; E. Merck, A. G. Darmstadt).
26. Ito, A., Hamanaka, W., Takagi, H., Wada, T. and Kawada, T. (1960) Verfahren zur Herstellung eines Acylierungsproduktes von Vitamin-B$_1$-orthophosphorsäureester und salzen davon. German Patent 1 130 811 (14 April 1960 to Sankyo Kabushiki Kaisha, Tokyo).
27. Wada, T., Tagaki, H., Minakami, H., Hamanaka, W., Okamoto, K., Ito, A. and Sahashi, Y. (1961) A new thiamine derivative, S-benzoylthiamine O-monophosphate. *Science* **134**: 195–196.
28. Viscontini, M., Ebnoether, C. and Karrer, P. (1952) Einfache Synthese kristallisierter Lactoflavin-5′-phosphorsäure (Coferment des Flavinenzyms). *Helv. Chim. Acta* **35**: 457–459.
29. Fieser, L. F. (1946) Antihemorrhagic esters and methods for producing the same. US Patent 2 407 823 (17 September 1946 to Research Corporation, New York).
30. Chong, K. -T., Ruwart, M. J., Hinshaw, R. R., Wilkinson, K. F., Rush, B. D., Yancey, M. F., Strohbach, J. W. and Thaisrivongs, S. (1993) Peptidomimetic HIV protease inhibitors: phosphate prodrugs with improved biological activities. *J. Med. Chem.* **36**: 2575–2577.
31. Fieser, L. F. and Fieser, M. (1967) *Reagents for Organic Synthesis*, p. 198. John Wiley, New York.
32. Khawaja, T. A. and Reese, C. B. (1966) *o*-Phenylene phosphochloridate. A convenient phosphorylating agent. *J. Amer. Chem. Soc.* **88**: 3446–3447.
33. Khawaja, T. A., Reese, C. B. and Stewart, J. C. M. (1970) A convenient general procedure for the conversion of alcohols into their monophosphate esters. *J. Chem. Soc. (C)*, 2090–2100.
34. Taguchi, Y. and Mushika, Y. (1975) 2-(*N,N*-Diethylamino)-4-nitrophenyl phosphate and its use in the selective phosphorylation of unprotected nucleosides. *Tetrahedron Lett.* **24**: 1913–1916.

35. Gajda, T. and Zwierzak, A. (1976) Phase-transfer-catalysed halogenation of di-*t*-butyl phosphite. Preparation of di-*t*-butyl phosphorohalidates. *Synthesis* 243–244.

36. Gajda, T. and Zwierzak, A. (1977) Di-*t*-butyl phosphorobromidate. A new selective phosphorylating agent containing acid-labile protecting groups. *Synthesis* 623–625.

37. Tener, G. M. (1961) 2-Cyanoethyl phosphate and its use in the synthesis of phosphate esters. *J. Amer. Chem. Soc.* **83**: 159–168.

38. Moffatt, J. G., (1963) The synthesis of orotidine-5′ phosphate. *J. Amer. Chem. Soc.* **85**: 1118–1123.

39. Brownfield, R. B. and Shultz, W. (1963) A direct method for the preparation of steroid-21-phosphates. *Steroids* **2**: 597–603.

40. Montgomery, H. A. C. and Turnbull, J. H. (1958) Phosphoramidic halides; Phosphorylating agents derived from morpholine. *J. Chem. Soc.* 1963–1967.

41. Fex, H., Lundvall, K. E. and Olsson, A. (1968) Hydrogen sulfates of natural estrogens. *Acta Chem. Scand.* **22**: 254–264.

42. Guiseley, K. B. and Ruoff, P. M. (1961) Monosaccharide sulfates. I. Glucose-6-sulfate. Preparations, characterization of the crystalline potassium salt, and kinetic studies. *J. Org. Chem.* **26**: 1248–1254.

43. Fieser, L. F. and Fry, E. M. (1940) Water-soluble antihemorrhagic esters. *J. Amer. Chem. Soc.* **62**: 228–229.

44. Stieglitz, E. and Matz, M. (1958) Verfahren zur Herstellung von Xanthinalkylschwefelsäuren oder deren Salze. German Auslegeschrift 1 090 669 (11 January 1958 to Arzneimittelfabrik Krewel-Leuffen GmbH, Eitorf/Sieg).

45. Miyabo, S., Nakamura, T., Kuwazima, S. and Kishida, S. (1981) A comparison of the bioavailability and potency of dexamethazone phosphate and sulphate in man. *Eur. J. Clin. Pharmacol.* **20**: 277–282.

46. Williams, D. B., Varia, S. A., Stella, V. J. and Pitman, I. H. (1983) Evaluation of the prodrug potential of the sulfate ester of acetaminophen and 3-hyroxymethyl-phenytoin. *Int. J. Pharm.* **14**: 113–120.

47. Greenburg, F. H., Leung, K. K. and Leung, M. The reaction of vitamin K_3 with sodium bisulfite. *J. Chem. Ed.* **48**: 632–634.

48. Despois, R. L. (1938) Procédé de préparation de composés aminés aromatiques solubles possédant une valeur thérapeutique. French Patent 831 366 (7 June 1938; Rhône-Poulenc).

49. Jacobson, K. A., Nikodijevic, O., Ji, X. -D., Berkich, D. A., Eveleth, D., Dean, R. L., Hiramatsu, K.-I, Kassel, N. F., van Galen, P. J. M., Lee, K. S., Bartus, R. T., Daly, J. D., LaNoue, K. F. and Maillard, M. (1992) Synthesis and biological activity of N^6-(*p*-Sulfophenyl)alkyl and N^6-Sulfoalkyl derivatives of adenosine: water-soluble and peripherally selective adenosine agonists. *J. Med. Chem.* **35**: 4143–4149.

50. Anonymous, Verfahren zur Darstellung von p-äthoxyphenylaminomethylschwefligsauren Salzen. German Patent 209 695 (8 May 1907; to Robert Lepetit, Garessio, Italy).

51. Anonymous, Verfahren zur Darstellung von ω-methylschwefligsauren Salzen aminosubstituierter Arylpyrazolone. German Patent 254 711 (21 July, 1911; to Fabwerke vorm. Meister Lucius & Brüning in Hoechst am Main).

52. Anonymous, Verfahren zur Darstellung von ω-methylschwefligsauren Salzen aminosubstituierter Arylpyrazolone. German Patent 259 503 (17 September 1911; to Farbwerke vorm. Meister Lucius & Brüning in Hoechst am Main).

53. Mutch, N. (1941) A new sulphonamide (Sulfonamide E.O.S.). *Brit. Med. J.* **2**: 503–507.

54. Jain, B. C., Iyer, B. H. and Guha, P. C. (1946) The preparation of promin. *Science and Culture* **11**: 568–569 (C.A. **40**, 4687[7], 1946).

55. Anonymous. Soluble diphenylsulfone. Swiss Patent 234 108 (1 December 1944; Aktien-Gesellschaft vorm. B Siegfried).

56. Bockmúhl, M., Krohs, W., Racke, F. and Windisch, K. N-Methylsulphites and N-methanesulphinic acid salts of 1-aryl-2,3-dialkyl-4-alkylaminopyrazolones. US Patent 2 193 788 (19 March 1940; Winthrop Chemical Company, Inc.).

57. Holland, D. O. Preparation of 2-alkyl-1,4-naphtaquinone-4-carboxy-alkoximes. British Patent 621 934 (22 April 1949; to Glaxo Laboratories Ltd).

58. Fischer, L. J. and Riegelman, S. (1967) Absorption and activity of some derivatives of griseofulvin. *J. Pharm. Sci.* **56**: 469–476.

59. Tatsumi, K and Ishigai, M. (1987) Oxime-metabolizing activity of liver aldehyde oxidase. *Arch. Biochem. Biophys.* **253**: 413–418.

60. Negwer, M. (1987) *Organic-Chemical Drugs and their Synonyms. Entry No 5760: Codoxime.* Vol. II. Akademie Verlag, Berlin.

61. Aichinger, G., Behner, O, Hoffmeister, F. and Schütz, S. (1969) Basische tricyclische Oximinoäther und ihre pharmakologischen Eigenschaften. *Arzneim.-Forsch.* **19**: 838–845.

62. Kingsbury, W. D., Boehm, J. C., Jakas, D. R., Holden, K. G., Hecht, S. M, Gallagher, G., Caranfa, M. J., McCabe, F. L., Faucette, L. F., Johnson, R. K. and Hertzberg, R. P. (1991) Synthesis of water-soluble (aminoalkyl)camptothecin analogues: inhibition of topoisomerase I and antitumor activity. *J. Med. Chem.* **34**: 98–107.

63. Showell, G. A., Bourrain, S., Neduvelil, J. G., Fletcher, S.R., Freedman, S.B., Kemp, J. A., Marshall, G. R., Patel, S., Smith, A.J. and Matassa, V. G. (1994) High-affinity and potent, water-soluble 5-amino-1,4-benzoidazepine CCKB/gastrin receptor antagonists containing a cationic solubilizing group. *J. Med. Chem.* **37**: 719–721.

64. Ishikawa, F., Saegusa, J., Inamura, K. and Sakuma, K., Ashida, S.-I. (1985) Cyclic guanidines. 17. Novel (N-substituted amino)imidazo[2,1-b]quinazolin-2-ones: Water-soluble platelet aggregation inhibitors. *J. Med. Chem.* **28**: 1387–1393.

65. Suzuki, F., Shimada, J., Nonaka, H., Ishii, A., Shiozaki, S., Ichikawa, S. and Ono, E. (1992) 7,8-Dihydro-8-ethyl-2-(3-noradamantyl)-4-propyl-1H-imidazo[2,1-i]purin-5(4H)-one: A potent water-soluble adenosine A1antagonist. *J. Med. Chem.* **35**: 3572–3581.

66. Khandelwal, Y., Rajeshwari, K., Rajagopalan, R., Swamy, L., Dohadwalla, A. N., de Souza, N. J. and Rupp, R. H. (1988) Cardiovascular effects of new water-soluble derivaties of forskolin. *J. Med. Chem.* **31**: 1872–1879.

67. Bundgaard, H. and Falch, E. (1985) Improved rectal and parenteral delivery of allopurinol using the prodrug approach. *Arch. Pharm. Chem. Sci. Ed.* **13**: 39–48.

68. Bundgaard, H., Falch, E. and Jensen, E. (1989) A novel solution-stable, water-soluble prodrug type for drugs containing a hyroxyl or an NH-acidic group. *J. Med. Chem.* **32**: 2503–2507.

69. Balkovec, J. M., Black, R. M., Hammond, M. L., Heck, J. V., Zambias, R. A., Abruzzo, G., Bartizal, K., Kropp, H., Trainor, C., Schwartz, R. E., McFadden, D. C., Nollstadt, K. H., Pittarelli, L. A., Powles, M. A. and Schmatz, D. M. (1992) Synthesis, stability and biological evaluation of water-soluble prodrugs for a new echinochandin lipopeptide. Discovery of a potential clinical agent for the treatment of systemic candidiasis and *Pneumocystis carinii* pneumonia (PCP). *J. Med. Chem.* **35**: 194–198.

70. Klosa, J. (1955) Beitrag zur Reaktionsfähigheit der 7-Stellung des Theophyllins. 2.Mitt. Über Synthesen in der Theophyllinreihe. *Arch. Pharm.* **288**: 301–303.

71. Gottstein, W. J. and Minor, W. F. and Cheney, L. C. (1959) Carboxamido derivatives of tetracyclines. *J. Amer. Chem. Soc.* **81**: 1198–1201.

72. Sanchez, J. P., Domagala, J. M., Heifetz, C. L., Priebe, S. R., Sesnie, J. A. and Trehan, A. K. (1992) Quinolone antibacterial agents. Synthesis and structure-activity relationships of a series of amino acid prodrugs of racemic and chiral 7-(3-amino-1-pyrrolidinyl)quinolones. Highly soluble quinolone prodrugs with *in vivo* pseudomonas activity. *J. Med. Chem.* **35**: 1764–1773.

73. Sawada, S., Yaegashi, T., Furuta, T., Yokokura, T. and Miyasaka, T. (1993) Chemical modification of an antitumor alkaloid, 20(S)-camptothecin: E-Lactone ring modified water-soluble derivatives of 7-ethylcamptothecin. *Chem. Pharm. Bull.* **41**: 310–313.

74. Boyd, S. A., Fung, A. K. L., Baker, W. R., Mantei, R. A., Armiger, Y. -L., Stein, H. H., Cohen, J., Egan, D. A., Barlow, J. L., Klinghofer, V., Verburg, K. M., Martin, D. L., Young, G. A., Polakowski, J. S., Hoffman, D. J., Garren, K. W., Perun, T. J. and Kleinert, H. D. (1992) C-Terminal modifications of nonpeptide renin inhibitors: Improved oral bioavailability via modification of physicochemical properties. *J. Med. Chem.* **35**: 1735–1746.

75. Morch, P. (1947) Glykresin. *Arch. Pharm. Chem.* **54**: 327–332.

76. Roth, H. J. (1959) Zur Darstellung von β-Oxyalkyl-dimethyl-purinen; Umsetzung von Theophyllin und Theobromin mit 1,2-Epoxyden. *Arch. Pharm.* **292**: 234–238.

77. Courbat, P. J. Qercetin and Quercetin Gycoside. US Patent 3 420 815 (7 January 1969; to Zyma SA).

78. Allais, A., Rousseau, G., Girault, P., Mathieu, J., Peterfalvi, M., Branceni, D., Azadian-Boulanger, G., Chifflot, L. and Jequier, R. (1966) Sur l'activité analgésique et antiinflammotoire des 4-(2'-alcoxycarbonyl phénylamino) quinolénes. *Eur. J. Med. Chem.* **1**: 65–70.

79. Mouzin, G., Cousse, H. and Autin, J. M. (1980) A new, convenient synthesis of glafenine and floctafenine. *Synthesis* 54–55.

80. Boltze, K. H. and Kreisfeld, H. (1977) Zur Chemie von Etofenamat, einem Anitphlogisticum aus der Klasse der N-Arylanthranyläurederivate. Arzneimit.-Forsch.-Drug Design. **27**: 1300–1312. Zur Chemie von Etofenamat, einem Antiphlogisticum aus der Klasse der N-Arylanthranylsürederivate. *Arzneimittel-Forsch. (Drug Design).* **27**: 1300–1312.

81. Matter, M. Polyethoxy Ethers of Isocyclic Organic Carboxylic Acids. US Patent 2 714 608 (2 August 1955; to Ciba Pharmaceutical Products, Inc., Summit, NJ).

82. Nagawaka, T., Muneyuki, T. and Mori, Y. (1961) Water solubilization by means of polyethylene glycol derivatives. Japanese Patent 7455; CA 55, 5879b.

83. Nagawaka, T., Muneyuki, T. and Mori, Y. (1961) Water solubilization of drugs. Japanese Patent 17006 (17 November 1960 to Shionogi & Co. Ltd); CA 55, 21494h.

84. Weiner, B.-Z. and Zilkha, A. (1973) Polyethylene glycol derivatives of procaine. *J. Med. Chem.* **16**: 573–574.

85. Morren, H. New derivatives of N-Mono-benzhydril-Piperazine and process for the preparation thereof. British Patent 817 231 (29 July 1959).

86. Gouin d'Ambrières, S., Lutz, A. and Gasc, J. C. Novel erythromycin A derivatives. US Patent 4 349 545 (14 September 1982; to Roussel-UCLAF).

87. Miescher, K., Fischer, W. H. and Meystre, C. (1942) 6. Über Steroide. (33. Mitteilung). Über Glukoside des Desoxy-corticosterons. *Helv. Chim. Acta.* **25**: 40–42.

88. Miescher, K. and Meystre, C. (1943) 26. Über Steroide. 34. Mitteilung. Über Sacharide des Desoxy-corticosterons II. *Helv. Chim. Acta.* **26**: 224–233.

89. Meystre, C. and Miescher, K. (1944) Über Steroide. (35. Mitteilung). Zur Darstellung von Saccharidderivaten der Steroide. *Helv. Chim. Acta.* **27**: 231–236.

90. Higashiyama, T. and Sakata, I. Mentholglykoside, Verfahren zur ihrer Herstellung, ihre Verwendung zur Entwicklung des Pfefferminzgeschmack sowie diese Verbindungen enthaltende Arzneimittel. German Offen. 2 242 237 (28 August 1972; to Toyo Hakka Kogyo Kabushiki Kaishy).

91. Chavis, C. and Imbach, J. -L. (1977) Sur une méthode de pharmacomodulation:l'utilisation du vecteur sucre. In Combet-Farnoux, C. (ed.) *Actualités de Chimie Thérapeutique*, pp. 3–28. Société de Chimie Thérapeutique, Châtenay-Malabry.

92. Bognar, R. and Nanasi, P. (1953) N-Substituted glycosylamines derived from sulphanilamide and *p*-aminosalicylic acid. *J. Chem. Soc.* 1703–1708.

93. Sah, P. (1953) D-Glucuronolactone isonicotinyl hydrazone. *J. Amer. Chem. Soc.* **75**: 2512–2513.

94. Demetrio, A., Ganzina, F., Magi, M., Serino, E., Paroli, E. and Samueli, F. Antiinflammatory di-(+)glucosamide of 1-(4-chlorobenzoyl)-2-methyl-5-methoxyindole-3-acetic acid. German Patent 2 223 051 (13 December 1973; to SIR Lab. Chimico Biologica SpA); CA 80, 83529e.

95. Almen, T. H. O., Haavaldsen, J. and Nordal, V. N-(2,4,6-Triiodobenzoyl)-Sugar Amines. US Patent 3 701 771 (31 October 1972; to Nyegaard & Co, A/S).

96. Hilae, S. K., Dauth, G. W., Hess, K. H. and Gilman, S. (1978) Development and evaluation of a new water-soluble iodinated myelographic contrast medium with markedly reduced convulsive effects. *Radiology.* **126**: 417–422.

36

Drug Solubilization with Organic Solvents, or Using Micellar Solutions or Other Colloidal Dispersed Systems

KURT H. BAUER

Die Schwierigkeiten wachsen, je näher man dem Ziele kommt.
The more you approach the goal, the more the difficulties increase
Johann Wolfgang von Goethe

I. INTRODUCTION

For the reasons discussed in preceding chapters, knowledge of the solubilities of drugs in biophases is very important, but the technological methods for their dispersion or dissolution in the dosage form should also be thoroughly understood. Dosage forms should be considered as disperse multicomponent systems of a particular dispersity. They are one-phase systems if they are homogeneous, and multiphase systems if different phases are recognizable. However, the degree of homogeneity may be defined differently depending on how it is observed — with the naked eye or with the microscope. Most colloidal disperse systems are homogeneous but microscopically heterogeneous.

THE PRACTICE OF MEDICINAL CHEMISTRY
ISBN 0-12-744640-0

Table 36.1 Coarse and colloidal dispersed systems, systematized according to the state of aggregation of the dispersion medium and the dispersed phase.

Dispersion medium	Coarse dispersions (dispersity >500 nm) Dispersed phase			Colloidal dispersions (dispersity 1–500 nm) Dispersed phase		
	Gaseous	*Liquid*	*Solid*	*Gaseous*	*Liquid*	*Solid*
Solid	Dry gelatin foam, pumic stones	Solid or dried emulsions	Tablets, lozenges, suppositories	Silica gel	Solid dispersions with included colloidal liquid droplets, e.g. opals	Melts, glasses solid colloidal solutions and dispersions, mesomorphic systems
Liquid	Foams	Emulsions	Suspensions	Microfoams	Emulsions, microemulsions	Suspensoids, solid colloids suspended in liquid, sols, gels
Gaseous	Molecular-disperse systems	Coarse sprayed droplets; coarse liquid aerosols	Powders	Molecular-disperse systems	Colloidal liquids aerosols, steam, varpours	Colloidal dusts, smoke, soot, colloidal solids, aerosols

Unquestionably, the therapeutic value of a drug substance is the fundamental factor in a medicament's efficiency, the way a drug substance is incorporated into a dosage form is also significant. The dispersity is very important. Does a drug dissolve as a molecular-disperse, true solution without any additional step, or is a solubilization step necessary? How the drug is released and subsequently absorbed depends on the form of incorporation. There are always several important technological, biopharmaceutical and therapeutical considerations.

In any system containing two or more chemical substances, these substances are dispersed one in another and result in dispersed systems (Table 36.1). The degree of dispersion, the dispersity, the type and method of dispersion and the hydrophilic–lipophilic characters of drug and excipient and of dispersion medium are essential to the therapeutical efficiency. Particularly important for drug release from such systems are coherent structures, hydrophilic–lipophilic properties, and intermolecular forces or interactions.

The finest dispersity is a molecular-disperse distribution, with particle sizes <1 nm. This means the molecules are truly molecularly dispersed (dissolved) in a suitable solvent. The next larger ranges after true solutions are colloidal dispersions with particle sizes of approximately 1–500 nm. This group comprises comminuted or dispersed colloids (e.g. colloidal gold or sulfur), colloidal solutions with molecular colloids (e.g. macromolecules having colloidal molecular sizes, such as gelatin or methylcellulose) and, thirdly, associated colloids built up from low-molecular-weight, mostly amphiphilic, compounds to colloidal dimensions. These associations or aggregates, particularly of amphiphilic or highly asymmetric molecules, are kept together in the form of micellar associates by considerable intermolecular forces and by the mutual compensation of these forces. They frequently build up micellar or supramolecular structures, micelles or mesophases. These formations may also influence the drug release.

Micelles are usually formed in liquids above a certain concentration, called the critical micelle concentration (CMC). There are also concentration-dependent transition systems of micellar arrangements (Fig. 36.1). Mesophases or mesomorphic structures are mainly more highly concentrated and more or less ordered transition systems (solutions or melts), between two extremes. These extremes are isotropic solutions or amorphous solids, such as glasses, on the one side, and anisotropic paracrystals or crystals on the other. Between these there is a range of nematic, smectic and some liquid-crystalline orders (Fig. 36.2). Within these systems, thermotropic and lyotropic states can be distinguished. Thermotropic are such transition states between crystalline solids and amorphous or glass-like melts, which change with temperature. If these changes depend on the concentration in solutions or blends, they are termed lyotropic.

Liquid colloidal solutions are designated as sols. They are mobile liquids because they have only one coherent phase, the dispersion medium, and an incoherent dispersed phase. Gels are semisolids, and their fundamental system is a bicoherent one, which means that they have both a coherent structure-forming network and a coherent mobile liquid phase. The solubility and the release of drugs incorporated in such systems can be influenced by the different phases, the interfaces and the interactions between them. As rheological properties depend on the inner structures, the viscosity is related to the release of drugs.

Systems coarser than colloidal dispersions, or dispersions in the colloquial sense of technical terminology, are emulsions and suspensions. Emulsions are defined as coarse dispersions of liquids that are homogeneously miscible or soluble, such as water and oil. The heterogeneous phases of this multiphase system are visible not only in the microscope but also with the naked eye. Owing to their relatively large particle or droplet sizes they are not transparent but milky. Suspensions are defined as coarse dispersions of an insoluble solid substance in a liquid. Such coarse dispersions exhibit particle sizes >500 nm. The limit of particle size sometimes varies in

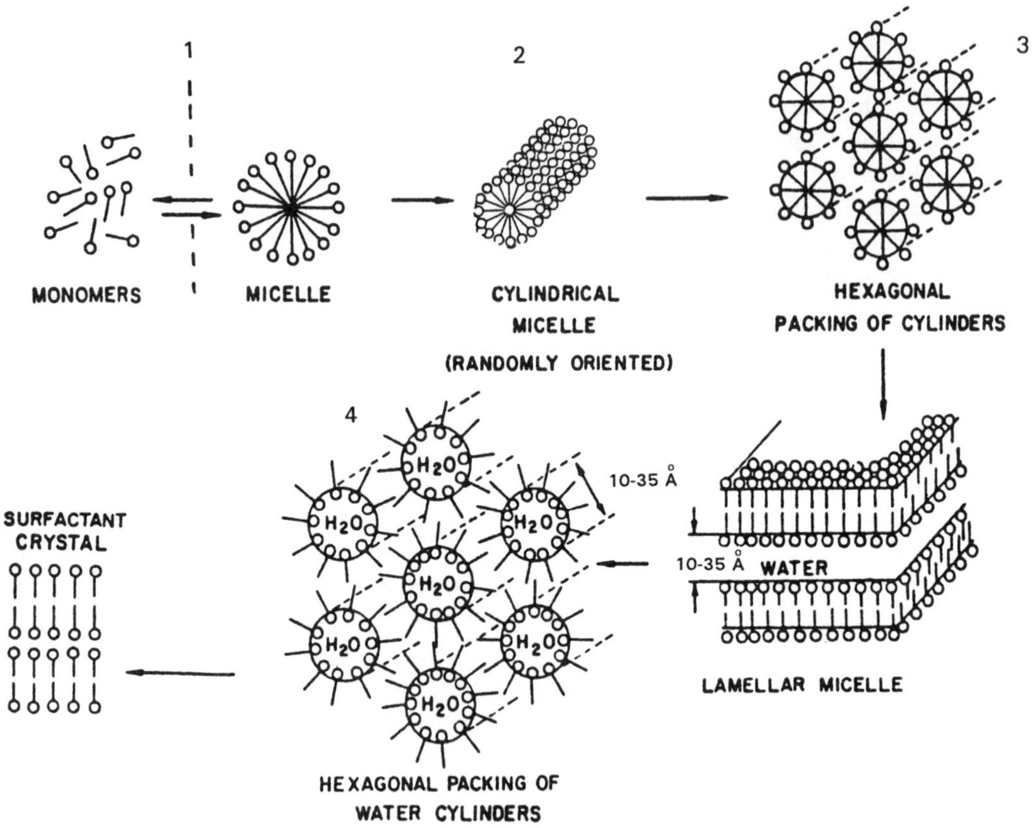

Fig. 36.1 Structure formation in surfactant solutions depends on concentration. (1) If the monomers reach a certain concentration, they initiate the formation of micelles. This is the critical micelle concentration (CMC). (2) Randomly orientated initially, the micelles can be orientated in one direction (nematic), and in one direction and in a plane (smectic). (3) Hexagonal packing of lipophilic cylinders. (4) Hexagonal packings of water cylinders (inverse micelles).

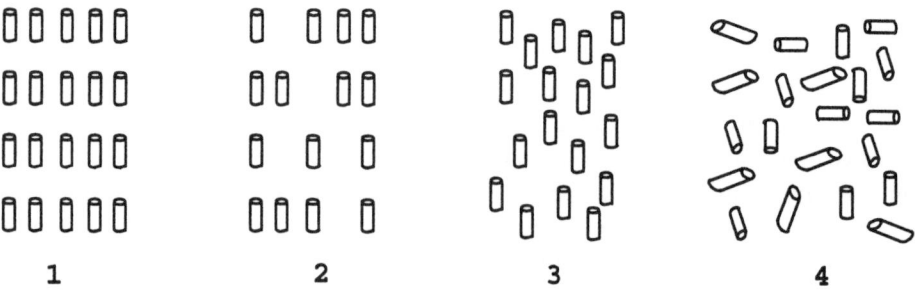

Fig. 36.2 Mesophases of rod-shaped molecules or aggregates (micelles); 1 = crystalline system; 2 = smectic mesophase; 3 = nematic mesophase; 4 = isotropic liquid.

the literature between 400 and 800 nm, since it is related with the wavelength of visible light. It is the fact that particles with diameters around the wavelength of visible light are responsible for the scattering of light; that is the reason for this characterization. This also implies that colloidal solutions are not perfectly clear: they exhibit the Tyndall effect, a slight turbidity in light scattering.

All these colloidal or coarse dispersions can be produced, or at least stabilized, by hydrotropic solvents as well as by means of amphiphilic or surface active substances — surfactants. However, for pharmaceutical formulations hydrotropic solvents are not often used. The required concentrations are mostly too high, so that the physiological benignity of such formulations cannot be guaranteed. The optimal selection of these excipients is fundamental for dissolution of the drugs or for their solubilization, and thereby for their therapeutic efficiency.

In coarser dispersions the particle sizes attain greater significance. The smaller the particles, and the larger their surfaces, the faster are their dissolution rates, so long as their surfaces are completely wetted (the Noyes–Whitney equation).

Drugs can be dissolved or solubilized by the following means.

(1) By means of hydrotropic solvents and/or cosolvents.
(2) By complexation with hydrotropic substances, for instance with polyvinylpyrrolidone (PVP) or other suitable complexing substances.
(3) With amphiphilic solubilizers by forming micellar systems, mixed micelles or microemulsions.
(4) By the preparation and stabilization of colloidal systems.

In the following, the main methods of such dissolution or solubilization are described. The release of a drug from a dosage form is an important precondition for its absorption.

II. THE USE OF HYDROTROPIC SOLVENTS AND COSOLVENTS

If a drug has a well-balanced hydrophilic–lipophilic character, and is sufficiently soluble in water or an aqueous environment, no major bioavailability difficulties are generally to be expected. But drugs insoluble or only sparingly soluble in water usually require special techniques in their pharmaceutical formulation or application.

A simple way to increase solubility is to add hydrotropic solvents or cosolvents until the drug is dissolved. In these cases, in the first instance, water can be understood as the solvent and a hydrotropic solvent as the cosolvent, but there can also be a hydrotropic main solvent, and one or more other solvents which are necessary to dissolve the drug as cosolvents.

The liquid dosage forms of the extremely insoluble compound nifedipine, a calcium-antagonist drug, provide a vivid illustration of what can be done in this respect. Nifedipine is practically insoluble in water (1:200 000); it is nonionic, and therefore cannot form soluble salts. It is also very sparingly soluble in vegetable or similar oils. Liquid poly(ethylene glycols) of the lower molecular weights were found to be a very suitable solvent for dosage forms of nifedipine. Nifedipine is soluble at concentrations of about 10% w/w in liquid poly(ethylene glycols). Such solutions of nifedipine also advantageously can be filled into soft gelatin capsules, since poly(ethylene glycol) does not attack or dissolve gelatin as do aqueous solutions or glycerol.

In the case of encapsulation, small amounts of glycerol are added to the nifedipine–poly(ethylene glycol) capsule filling solution as a cosolvent. The reason for this addition is that about 30% of glycerol needs be incorporated as a softener in the shells of soft gelatin capsules. After or during the production of soft gelatin capsules, some glycerol migrates from the capsule shell into the filling. As a result, the capsules become brittle, particularly during storage. The addition of some glycerol into the capsule filling is to establish an equilibrium between the glycerol in the filling and in the shell. In this way the development of brittleness can be prevented. This example shows that solvents may have different uses. In this case poly(ethylene glycol) is a favourable solvent, and glycerol is the cosolvent with a special function.

Cosolvents are mostly used to improve solubility if a single solvent is not satisfactory. Sometimes ethanol may also be added as a cosolvent, with the intention of lowering the viscosity of the solution. A disadvantage of this is, that in soft gelatin capsules no more than 5% addition of ethanol is possible. Higher contents will permeate across the capsule shell during the drying process and then evaporate; as a result the capsules shrink.

Actually nifedipine may also be suspended to a greater extent, though scarcely dissolved, in triglyceride oils and this suspension can also be filled into soft gelatin capsules. A general problem of such suspensions is particle or crystal growth by Ostwald ripening. The dissolution rate or the bioavailability will be decreased by crystal growth. In the case of an oily nifedipine suspension, only very small amounts of the drug are dissolved, and therefore only these small amounts are able to leave the water-insoluble capsule filling by diffusion. The main part of the nifedipine must be dissolved gradually, at about the same rate at which the dissolved fraction migrates away to be absorbed. In this respect, this dosage form exhibits no advantage over tablets. After the disintegration of tablets, the very poorly soluble nifedipine must also be wetted and then dissolved gradually in the gastrointestinal juices. If there is not complete wetting, some wetting agent must be added. Because of the slow dissolution of nifedipine, both these dosage forms are regarded as more prolonged-release or 'retard' forms. They do not have sufficiently fast onset of action compared with soft capsules of nifedipine dissolved in a poly(ethylene glycol) solution.

Commercial parenteral solutions of nifedipine contain ethanol, poly(ethylene glycol) and water. Generally, for intravenous solutions miscibility with water is strictly required, to prevent embolism due to precipitates. For intramuscular and subcutaneous applications, oils or similar non-water-miscible liquids are also permitted. Poly(ethylene glycol) is the most suitable solvent of nifedipine for parenteral solutions, but its concentration in this application should not exceed 20% w/v, as at higher concentrations injections become painful. The pain is due to the fact that the considerably hygroscopic poly(ethylene glycol) will attract and bind rather vehemently water from the tissues at the site of injection. However, if an injection solution contains enough water to compensate the hygroscopic effect, injections are relatively well tolerated. Parenteral solutions can also contain some ethanol, as a cosolvent or to produce lower viscosity. Attention must be paid to the fact that higher ethanol doses can cause problems with intoxication.

The best solvent for nifedipine is acetone (1 : 3), but for toxicological reasons it is not permitted in peroral and parenteral dosage forms; in any case, even minuscule residual amounts of acetone produce a noxious taste in dosage forms for peroral use.

These few examples illustrate from different viewpoints the important role of solubilization and the multipurpose role of the solvents' properties in pharmaceutical formulation. They additionally provide a good demonstration how to proceed with hydrotropic solvents in different dosage forms. DMSO is also a very effective all-round solvent, but health authorities do not consider it is not sufficiently inert for use as a pharmaceutical excipient. It is therefore seldom declared as a therapeutically effective substance. One disadvantage is its relatively high boiling point, particularly if it must be separated quantitatively from the final product.

Sometimes other hydrotropic, complex-forming substances can be used as solubilizers, for instance povidone (polyvinylpyrrolidone) as an electron acceptor for drugs with electron-donor properties, and caffeine with sodium benzoate or sodium salicylate. In the broadest sense, solubilizers can be characterized as lyotropic substances which are able to make drugs and other lipophilic substances soluble in water or at least to improve their solubility in hydrophilic solvents. In rare cases it may also be required to improve the solubility properties of drugs in lipophilic solvents.

Hydrotropic solvents or substances for pharmaceutical use are mainly compounds with a number of OH groups or nitrogens in the molecule, or acids or their salts. If the use of hydrotropic solvents and cosolvents is not successful, other means must be explored.

In certain cases lipophilic rather than hydrophilic solvents can or must be used. For instance, penicillins suspended in triglyceride oils produce liquid peroral suspensions which, in contrast to aqueous suspensions or solutions, are satisfactorily stable because hydrolytic reactions are practically excluded. One drawback is that there may occur laxative side-reactions caused by the influence of the antibiotic on the colonic microflora combined with the weak laxative effect of the triglyceride oil.

These examples show the value of solvents or solubilizers in pharmaceutical formulation on the basis of their physicochemical properties through to consideration of their physiological or toxicological roles. But there are only a very few hydrotropic solvents for pharmaceutical use that are accepted by health authorities.

The hydrotropic solvents most frequently used pharmaceutically are the following alcohols and ether-oxides: ethanol, isopropanol, glycerol, propylene glycol, butylene glycol, sorbitol, and poly(ethylene glycols) 400 and 600. Further pharmaceutical solvents include diethylether, acetone, glycofurol, dimethyl isosorbide, ethyl lactate, N-methylpyrrolidone, and dimethylsulfoxide (DMSO). (See Fig. 36.3.)

For topical use or as intermediates, practically all solvents are useful so long as they are toxicologically harmless and are not polluting.

III.   THE FORMATION OF MICELLAR SOLUTIONS

Besides the above-mentioned use of hydrotropic solvents as a solubilizers, insoluble drugs can in certain cases advantageously be dissolved in micellar solutions, for instance if too much solvent is necessary to produce a solution, or if the required solvent is too toxic. In the traditional sense, solubilization excipients for micellar solutions are amphiphilic surfactant substances (see Table 36.2) with high HLB (hydrophilic lipophilic balance) values.[2] They surround the insoluble or lipophilic drug particles with their lipophilic moiety orientated towards the hydrophobic surface, and their hydrophilic moiety orientated towards the aqueous medium, thus forming thermodynamically stabilized aggregates in aqueous medium, so-called micelles. These micelles, particularly in dilute aqueous solutions, mostly show colloidal dimensions; in other words, they form colloidal dispersed micellar solutions. Solubilized lipophilic substances can be incorporated into the micelles in different ways (Fig. 36.4). Examples of such micellar solubilized formulations are aqueous fragrant solutions of essential oils, solutions of hormones or oil-soluble vitamins.

From the theoretical point of view, the optimal solubilizing effect is more closely approached the more completely the hydrophobic surfaces are covered by the amphiphilic solubilizer and

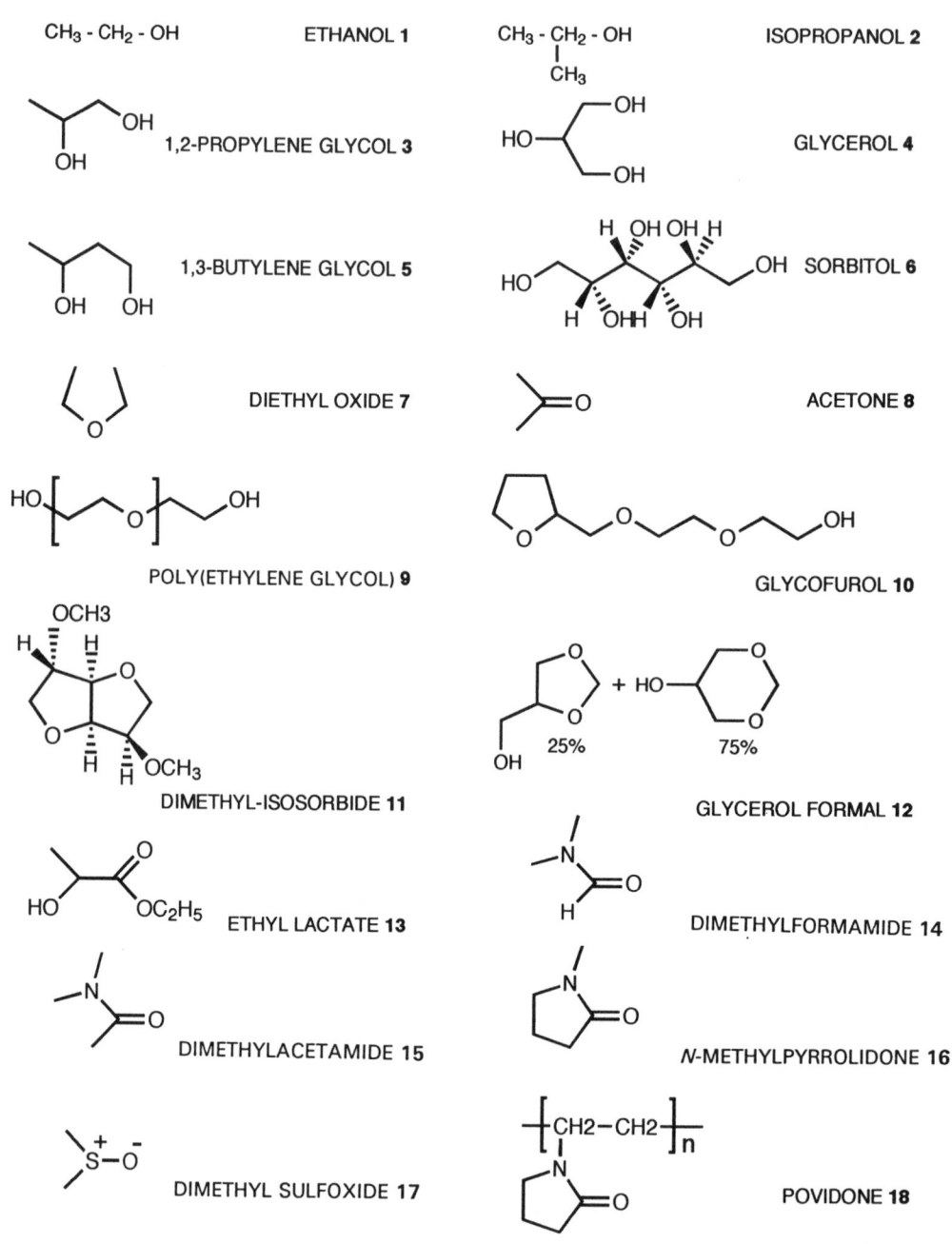

Fig. 36.3 Structures of solvents commonly used in pharmacy: 1 = ethanol, 2 = isopropanol, 3 = 1,2-propylene glycol, 4 = glycerol, 5 = 1,3-butylene glycol, 6 = sorbitol, 7 = diethylether, 8 = acetone, 9 = polyethylene glycol, 10 = glycofurol, 11 = dimethylisosorbide, 12 = glycerol formal (25% dioxalane and 75% 1,3-dioxane), 13 = diethyllactate, 14 = dimethylformamide, 15 = dimethylacetamide, 16 = N-methylpyrrolidone, 17 = dimethylsulfoxide, 18 = poly-vinylpyrrolidone.

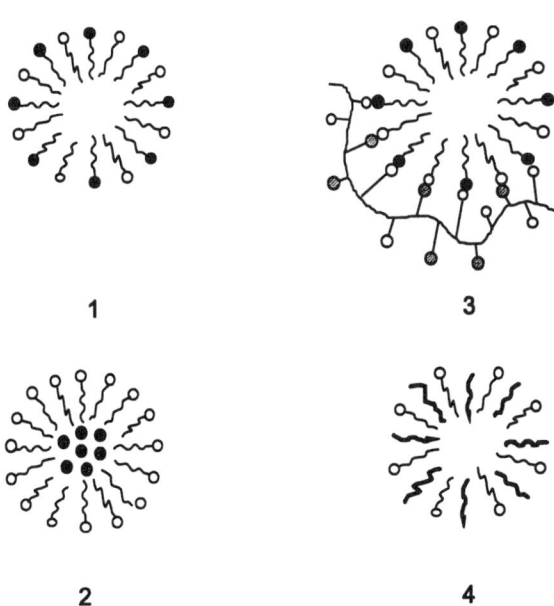

1

3

2

4

Fig. 36.4 Solubilization in micelles. 1 = micelle with anionic and nonionic surfactants; 2 = lipophilic molecules solubilized in a micelle; 3 = polymer or polymeric surfactant adsorbed on a micelle; 4 = lipophilic molecules solubilized in the lipophilic layers of the micelles.

the better the affinity between the hydrophobic surface of the drug and the lipophilic moiety of the surfactant. This means that the best micellar solubilization effect is obtained not only by a particular amount of surfactant but also by the most suitable type of surfactant. If all the surfaces completely covered, and if the concentration of the surfactant is increased further, the excess of amphiphilic molecules is forced into the surrounding aqueous phase (see Fig. 36.2).

There are manifold possibilities for forming thermodynamically stable micellar structures with relatively low energy contents, dependent on the concentration: for example, spherical or cylindric micelles and hexagonal (nematic) or lamellar (smectic) micellar aggregates. The latter more concentrated phases start to build up increasingly coherent structures, which are termed mesomeric phases. Such mesophases exist in water-in-oil emulsion-type ointments or certain other matrix dosage forms. The release of the drug is governed by the hydrophilic–lipophilic properties and the interactions in these systems, but the influence of the rheological properties must also be considered.

The mesomorphic structures of creams must also be considered from this point of view (Fig. 36.5). The release of a drug from a cream and the degree of penetration into the skin, and the correlated therapeutic effect, depend on the hydrophilic–lipophilic interplay of drug, cream vehicle and skin.

Owing to their surface-active properties, most surfactants irritate mucous membranes and they are also frequently haemolytically active.

Frequently used amphiphilic substances and surfactants which are included in the European and the US Pharmacopoeia are summarized in Table 36.2.

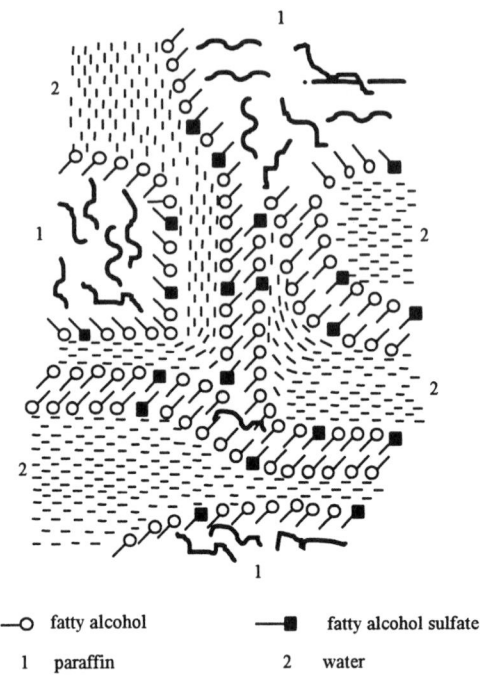

Fig. 36.5   Mesomorph structure of a hydrophilic cream. (From Bauer, K. H. Frömming, K. H. and Führer, C. (1993) *Pharmazeutische Techologie*, 4th edn. G. Thieme Verlag, Stuttgart, New York.)

The amphiphilic substances most used in pharmacy are nonionic surfactants; ionic surfactants are too reactive and anionic surfactants often show incompatibility with cationic drug substances. Cationic surfactants are insufficiently inert and are mostly used as preservatives.

HLB values,[2] a measure of the hydrophilic–lipophilic balance of surface-active substances, provide similar characterization to the partition coefficients of drugs. They should help to predict or estimate the anticipated mode of employment of surfactants. As direct determination is rather difficult, HLB values are generally calculated; they represent the relationship between the hydrophilic and lipophilic parts of the surfactant molecule. The first series of HLB values were introduced by W. D. Griffin. These series covered values up to 20 and related only to nonionic surfactants. An HLB of 10 indicates a balanced relationship between the hydrophilic and the lipophilic parts of the molecule. Values below 10 are more lipophilic, and those above 10 are more hydrophilic. As the HLB values of Griffin are not satisfactory in all cases, particularly as far as the hydrophilic properties are concerned, the method of calculation of the HLB was modified by J. F. Davies. Davies introduced a group formulation and derived positive values for the hydrophilic molecular groups and for the lipophilic groups. In this way the HLB system was extended to HLB values up to 40. So, for instance, an HLB value of 40 was attributed to sodium lauryl sulfate. A further modification was made by Rimmlinger, who tried to take into consideration different polarities, electrolyte contents and hydrophilic and lipophilic molecular masses. Despite these efforts HLB values still have certain drawbacks.

Table 36.2 The most frequently used surfactants.

Anionic surfactants	
Natrium dodecyl sulfate, Ph.Eur. =	M.p. 204–207°C, HLB ~ 40
Sodium laurylsulfate, USP/NF	
Docusate sodium, USP	M.p. 153–157°C
Cationic surfactants	
Amphoteric surfactants	
Lecithin	Soya or egg yolk lecithins
Nonionic surfactants	
Fatty alcohol or sterols	
Cetyl alcohol, USP/NF/Ph.Eur.	M.p. 46–52°C
Stearyl alcohol, USP/NF/Ph.Eur.	M.p. 55–60°C
Cetostearyl alcohol, USP/NF/Ph.Eur	M.p. 43–53°C
Cholesterol, USP/NF	M.p. 147–150°C, HLB ~ 3
Sorbitan fatty acid esters	
Sorbitan monooleate, USP/NF	Viscosity (25°C) 1200–1500 mPa s, HLB 4.3
Sorbitan monolaurate, USP/NF	Viscosity (25°C) 3500–5500 mPa s, HLB 4.3
Sorbitan monopalmitate, USP/NF	M.p. 48°C, HLB 6.7
Sorbitan monostearate, USP/NF	M.p. 51–54°C, HLB 4.7
Polyoxyethylene sorbitan fatty acid esters	
Polysorbate 20, PhEur., USP/NF	Viscosity (25°C) 250–450 mPa s, HLB 16.7
Polysorbate 60, PhEur., USP/NF	Viscosity (50°C) 75–175 mPa s, HLB 14.9
Polysorbate 80, PhEur., USP/NF	Viscosity (25°C) 375–480 mPa s, HLB 15.0
Polysorbate 40, USP/NF	Viscosity (25°C) 400–650 mPa s, HLB 15.6
Polyoxyethylene sorbitan fatty acid glycerides	
Polyoxyl 35 castor oil, USP/NF	Viscosity (25°C) 700–850 mPa s, HLB 12–14
Polyoxyl 40 hydrogenated castor oil, USP/NF	M.p. 20–30°C, HLB 14–16
Macrogol 40 hydoxystearate, Ph.Eur.	
Polyoxyethylene sorbitan fatty acid ethers	
Polyoxyl 23 laury lether, USP/NF	M.p. 36–42°C, HLB 16.9
Polyoxyl 20 cetostearyl ether, USP/NF	M.p. 38°C, HLB 15.3
Polyoxyl 10 oleylether, USP/NF	Viscosity (25°C) ~ 120 mPa s, HLB 12.4
Polymeric surfactants	
Poloxamer 188 (Poloxacol)	M.p. 50–52°C, HLB 29

IV. SPECIAL COLLOIDAL SYSTEMS: MIXED MICELLES, HYDROSOLS, LIPOSOMES, NIOSOMES, NANOPARTICLES, -SPHERES AND -CAPSULES, SOLID SOLUTIONS OR DISPERSIONS

Mixed micelles are stabilized micelles; they are employed because of the low haemolytic and irritating activities of the surfactants with the aim of reducing side-reactions. With appropriate stabilization, micelles lose their aggressivity against biological membranes. Interesting examples are the Valium MM Roche® and Konakion MM Roche® ampoules. This parenteral product contains the insoluble psychotherapeutic diazepam solubilized and stabilized by mixed micelles made with sodium cholate and lecithin. The natural surfactant sodium cholate is extremely haemolytically active, but the mixed micelles with lecithin are stable and form a colloidal system that is less aggressive towards biological membranes and exhibits almost no side-reactions. It is a general fact that haemolytic surfactants mixed with nonhaemolytic ones show no, or at least considerably reduced, haemolytic activities. There are also other parenteral dosage forms of diazepam on the market, such as Valium® ampoules containing a diazepam solution in propylene glycol and ethanol. It is recommended that this solution be cautiously injected into large veins, but despite careful and slow application irritation is possible at the site of injection. Diazepam-Lipuro® and Stesolid® Dumex are emulsions for injection that contain certain soybean oil, monoacetylglycerides, egg yolk lecithins, glycerol and sodium hydroxide. These emulsions and the mixed micelles are much better tolerated than solutions with hydrotropic solvents.

Another colloidal drug system comprises *hydrosols* with colloidal particle sizes between 1 and 1000 nm. The average particle sizes of parenteral hydrosols are below 200 nm. These systems are comparable with protective colloids, which are defined as lyophobic colloids stabilized by a coat of lyophilic colloid. Hydrosols were developed to solubilize the highly insoluble cyclosporin, and a number of other insoluble drugs.[3] There are different types of hydrosols, depending mainly on the type of the underlying colloidal drug, how the colloid is produced and how lyophobic or lipophilic its surfaces are.

The manufacturing procedures for the different hydrosols are the same in principle. The drug is dissolved in relatively high concentration in an organic solvent miscible with water. This concentrated solution is dispersed in a way that leads to colloidal particle sizes in an aqueous solution of a lyophilic colloid such as succinylated gelatin, poloxamer 188, albumins or hydroxypropylcellulose. Finally, the organic solvent is eliminated from this preparation by evaporation.

Liposomes[4] are vesicles with a wall of lecithin or some phospholipid double layer. They are spontaneously self-organizing, and the fact that the double layer is very similar to biological cell membranes prompted speculation about possible improvements of drug efficiency. Liposomal preparations are mainly found in cosmetic products on the market, mostly as hydrogels. In creams, liposomes are destroyed by the emulgators. Only few liposomal pharmaceutical formulations are known. An example worth mentioning is the liposomal antimycotic Ambisome® with the drug amphotericin B. In contrast to the conventional amphotericin B, the liposomal formulation is about twice as effective (i.e. the dose can be reduced) and this form of delivery exhibits fewer side-reactions.

In liposomes hydrophilic drugs are generally encapsulated into the aqueous inner space of the liposomes, while lipophilic drugs are incorporated in or between the double layers.

Niosomes are double-layered vesicles like liposomes but with nonionic surfactants (Table 36.2) instead of phospholipids.

Drug-loaded *nanoparticles* also belong with the colloidal solutions or colloidal drug delivery systems.[5] But while the micellar systems are predominantly intended for faster bioavailability or as better-tolerated dosage forms, nanoparticles find favour for special drug delivery or modified drug release systems. Two types of nanoparticles are distinguished: uniform material nanospheres, and nanocapsules consisting of a coat and an interior (Fig. 36.6). Nanoparticles can be loaded with the drug by adsorption, but they also can contain the drug entrapped, embedded or encapsulated. Because of the extremely fine dispersity, which lies in the colloidal size range, nanoparticles can be provided for special parenteral application. For experimental use and clinical tests, nanoparticles with hormones, enzymes, antigens, antibodies and virus preparations have been produced. Nanoparticles can be manufactured by different techniques, for instance by emulsion polymerization, coacervation or special precipitation or spraying

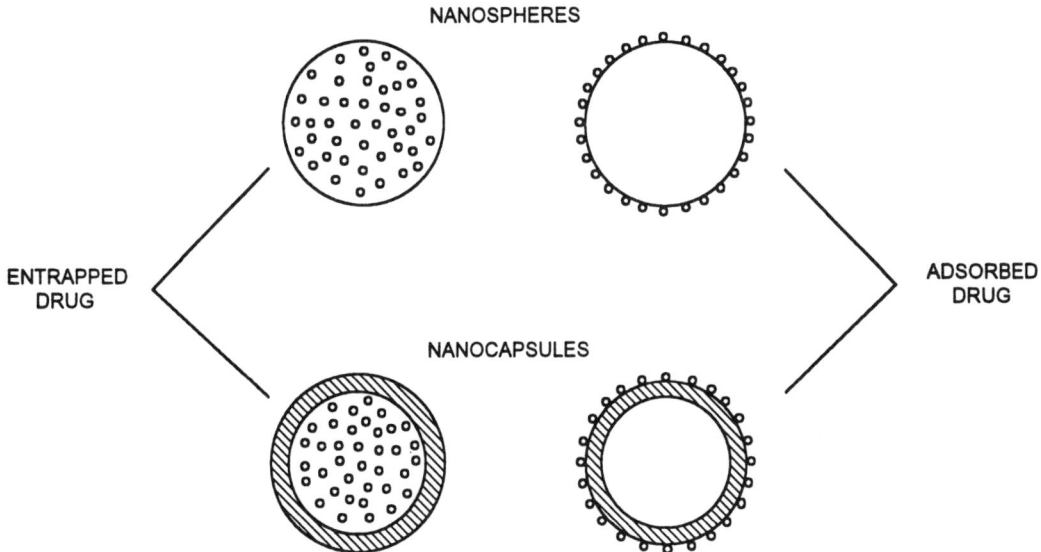

NANOSPHERES

NANOCAPSULES

ENTRAPPED
DRUG

ADSORBED
DRUG

Fig. 36.6 Nanoparticles or nanospheres, and nanocapsules, clearly divided into shell and interior, both systems with entrapped or adsorbed drug. (From Allémann, E., Gurny, R. and Doelker, E. (1993) Drug-loaded nanoparticles — preparation methods and drug targeting issues. *Eur. J. Pharm. Biopharm.* **39**: 173.)

methods. The vehicle materials can also be selected from manifold material classes, synthetic macromolecules or biopolymers, e.g. proteins, polysaccharides, cellulose derivatives, polylactides, polyglucolides, polylysin, polyacrylates, polyamides. Selection criteria are based on the intended drug delivery. The vehicle material for nanoparticles can be soluble or insoluble in physiological liquids, depending on the intended purpose. It can be a hydrophilic polymer with certain swelling properties, or it can be biodegradable. This means that there is almost infinite scope for controlling the activites — a playground for the inspiration.

Solid solutions or *dispersions*[2] are understood as solid multicomponent systems with the finest dispersed drugs in a solid carrier or vehicle. The carrier can be water-soluble or insoluble, and the corresponding drug delivery systems can exhibit fast as well as retarded onset of medicament activity. Depending on the melting point or on the solubility of the carrier, these solid dispersions or solutions can be produced by mixing, melting and congealing, particularly spray congealing, by coprecipitation or by a mixed solution and melting method. According to the operating method or conditions, eutectic blends, mixed crystals, glass-like melts or amorphous microsuspensions can be produced.

The dispersity of a given solid dispersion will result from the solubility relations in the melt or solution between the drug and the carrier or its components. They range from homogeneous one-phase systems, such as solid molecular-disperse solutions, blends or alloy-like systems, through almost transparent colloidal dispersions, up to coarse or more heterogeneously dispersed inclusions or matrices. Coarse heterogeneous systems are represented by conventional matrix tablets or suppositories. The drug can also be incorporated in much finer form, being molecularly or colloidally disperse. The homogeneity can be determined by X-ray diffraction or differential thermal analysis (DTA) methods. Using these different matrices, the drugs can be released at almost any rate (Fig. 36.7).

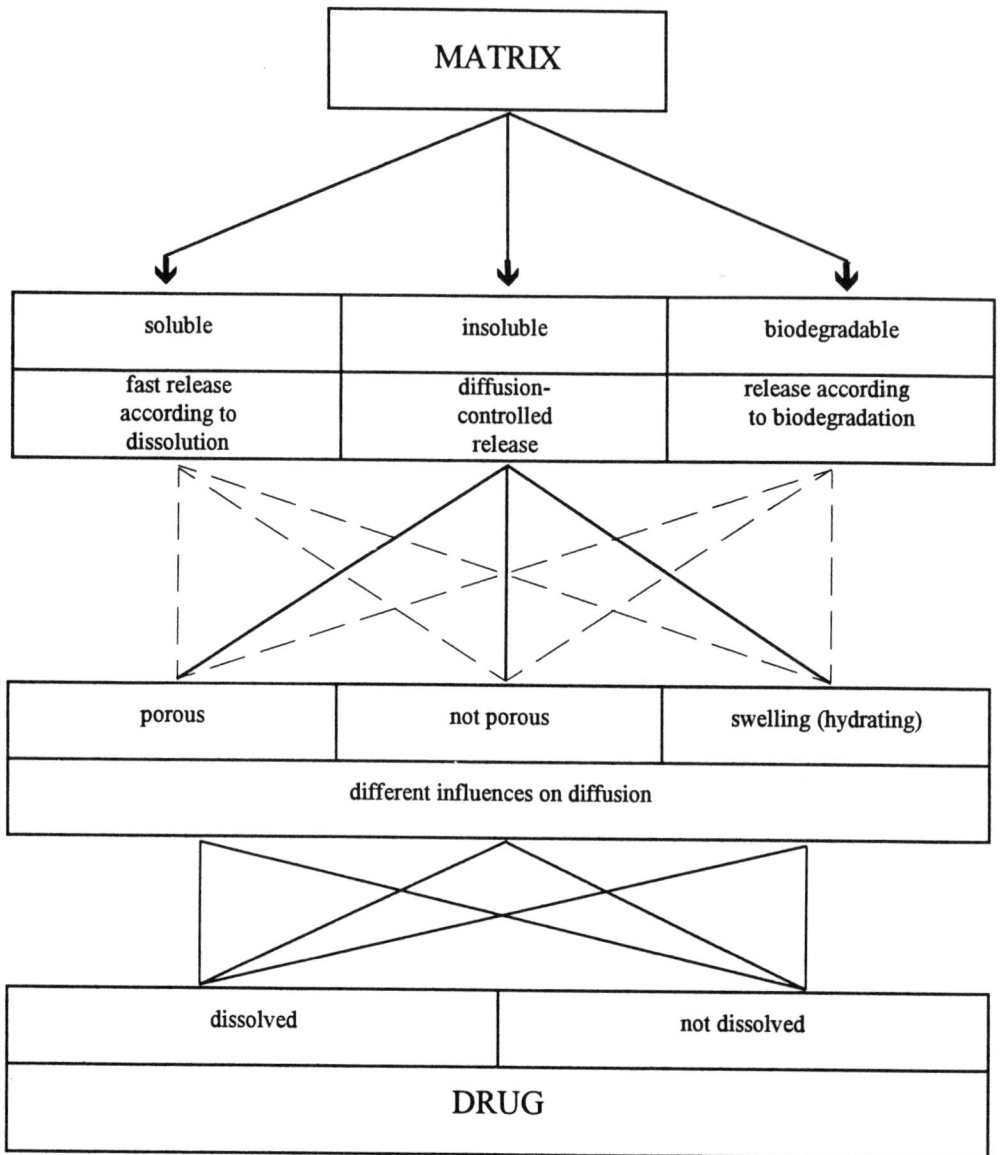

Fig. 36.7 Scheme of different types of matrices based on their building-up and function. Matrices can be built up by means of soluble, insoluble and biodegradable polymeric materials, which have different functions. The different matrices can be porous, nonporous or can exhibit different swelling properties. In all these different matrix systems the drug can be incorporated in a dissolved, undissolved or partly dissolved state. These are all points to consider when studying the drug release.

Solid dispersions or solutions can be prepared by melting or solution methods, and these methods can be combined as spray drying, spray congealing or coprecipitation. Dispersion media or vehicles used include povidone (poly(vinyl pyrrolidone)), poly(ethylene glycols), poly(vinyl alcohols), polyamides, polyacrylates, silicones, urea and adipic acid. With fast-dissolving matrices, drugs that are insoluble in water can be made bioavailable, or sometimes rapidly. The literature contains useful bioavailable solid dispersions of poorly soluble drugs like griseofulvin, sulfadiazine and cortisones.

Modified-release dosage forms can be realized by the use of insoluble matrices that swell in some way, or biodegradable matrices. In the simplest the matrix is insoluble and the drug is soluble in the vehicle; the dissolution rate then follows Fick's diffusion law. There is the question whether it is desirable, because diffusion is governed by concentration and as the concentration is reduced the dissolution rate decreases. It is more favourable if the drug is partly dissolved, so that the drug released by diffusion out of the matrix is continually replenished from the reservoir of undissolved drug. In this way a constant release is achieved, until all of the drug is dissolved and the reservoir is empty. According as the matrix is more or less porous, swellable or biodegradable, the release process can be quite complex. For several cases square-root time laws ($\sqrt{t}$) have been derived.[2] Different matrix systems allow resolution of many such modified-release problems by combination of the physical properties of drug and matrix in the most efficacious way.

V. CONCLUSION

Systems described illustrate impressively that optimal efficacy of a drug in a dosage form can be achieved by careful consideration of the chemical and physical properties of the drug in combination with an appropriate drug delivery system. This requires a fundamental understanding of the galenical formulation in terms of the vehicle, its structure and physicochemical properties, as well as the solubility and solubilization behaviour of the drug and the drug delivery system, and the path of absorption and distribution in the organism.

REFERENCES

1. (a) Hildebrand, J. H. and Scott, R. L. (1962) *Regular Solutions.* Prentice-Hall, Englewood Cliffs, NJ. (b) Hildebrand, J. H. and Scott, R. L. (1950) *The Solubility of Nonelectrolytes*, 3rd edn. Reinhold, New York. (c) Bustamente, P., Escalera, B., Martin, A. and Selles, E. (1993) A modification of the extended Hildebrand approach to predict the solubility of structurally related drugs in solvent mixtures. *J. Pharm. Pharmacol.* **45**: 253–257.
2. Stricker, H. (ed. and translator) (1987) *Physikalische Pharmazie*, pp. 37–38, 96–97, 308–310 and 516–518. Wissenschaftliche verlagsgesellschaft mbH, Stuttgart. (Translation of the original Martin, A. N., Swarbrick, J. and Cammarata, A. (1983) *Physical Pharmacy*, Lea & Febiger, Philadelphia.)
3. Gassmann, P., List, M., Schweitzer, A. and Sucker, H. (1994) Hydrosols—an alternative for parenteral application of poorly soluble drug substances. *Eur. J. Pharm. Biopharm.* **40**: 67–72.
4. Gregoriadis, G. (1993) *Liposome Technology*, 2nd edn. CRC Press, Boca Raton, FL.
5. (a) Allémann, E., Gurny, R. and Doelker, E. (1993) Drug-loaded nanoparticles – preparation methods and drug targeting issues. *Eur. J. Pharm. Biopharm.* **39**: 173–191. (b) Bornschein, M., Melegari, P., Bismarck, C. and Keipert, S. (1989) Mikro- und Nanopartikeln als Arzneistoffträgersysteme unter besonderer Berücksichtigung der Herstellungsverfahren. *Pharmazie* **44**: 585–593.

37

Improvement of Drug Properties by Cyclodextrins

KANETO UEKAMA and FUMITOSHI HIRAYAMA

THE PRACTICE OF MEDICINAL CHEMISTRY
ISBN 0-12-744640-0

I. INTRODUCTION

Cyclodextrins (CyDs) were first isolated in 1891 as degradation products of starch and were characterized as cyclic oligosaccharides (Fig. 37.1).[1] The α-, β- and γ-CyDs are the commonest natural CyDs, consisting of six, seven and eight glucose units, respectively (Table 37.1). Because of their different internal cavity diameters, each CyD shows a different degree of molecular encapsulation with different-sized guest molecules.[2,3] These CyDs have therefore been utilized for the modification of physical, chemical or biological properties of guest molecules. In the pharmaceutical field, CyDs have been recognized as potent candidates to overcome the undesirable properties of drug molecules through the formation of inclusion complexes.[4–6] Recently, a number of new dosage forms have been developed as drug delivery systems (DDS). For the design of such advanced dosage forms various kinds of CyD derivatives have been prepared to extend the physicochemical properties and inclusion capacity of natural CyDs as novel drug carriers.[7,8] This chapter deals with recent aspects of the utilization of chemically modified CyDs in pharmaceutical formulations, and will discuss some fundamental characteristics of CyDs which should be considered in the development of advanced dosage forms.

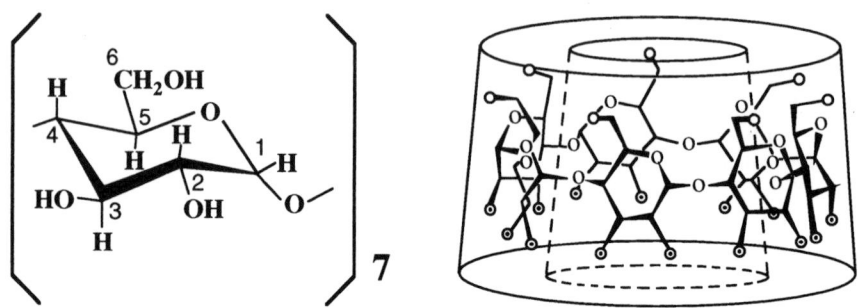

Fig. 37.1 Structure of β-cyclodextrin.

Table 37.1 Some characteristics of natural CyDs.

CyD	Number of glucose units	Molecular weight	Cavity[a] diameter (Å)	Solubility[b] (g dl^{-1})
α-CyD	6	973	5	15
β-CyD	7	1135	6	1.85
γ-CyD	8	1297	8	23

[a] Estimated by the Corey–Pauling–Koltun model.
[b] In water at 25°C.

II.   PHARMACEUTICALLY USEFUL CyDs

To obtain drug carrier properties better than those of natural CyDs, the hydroxyl groups of CyDs are available as starting points for structural modification, and various functional groups have been incorporated in the CyD molecule (Table 37.2). These chemically modified CyDs can be classified into three types: hydrophilic, hydrophobic and ionizable derivatives.[8] Hydrophilic derivatives such as methylated CyDs,[9,10] hydroxyalkylated CyDs,[11–15] and branched CyDs[16,17] deserve special attention because their solubility in water is very high, suggesting their use as solubilizers for poorly water-soluble drugs rather than the use of surface-active agents. In contrast, hydrophobic CyDs are useful as sustained-

Table 37.2   Pharmaceutically useful β-cyclodextrin derivatives

Derivative	Characteristic	Possible use (dosage form)
Hydrophilic derivatives		
Methylated β-CyD	Soluble in cold water and	Oral, dermal,
DM-β-CyD	in organic solvents,	mucosal[a]
TM-β-CyD	surface active, haemolytic	
Hydroxyalkylated β-CyD		
2-HE-β-CyD	Amorphous mixture with	Oral, dermal,
2-HP-β-CyD	different degrees of	mucosal,
3-HP-β-CyD	substitution, highly water-	parenteral
2,3-DHP-β-CyD	soluble (>50%), low toxicity	(intravenous)
Branched β-CyD		
G$_1$-β-CyD	Highly water-soluble (>50%),	Oral, mucosal,
G$_2$-β-CyD	low toxicity	parenteral (intravenous)
Hydrophobic derivatives		
Alkylated β-CyD		
DE-β-CyD	Water-insoluble, soluble in	Oral, parenteral (subcutaneous)
TE-β-CyD	organic solvents, surface-active	(slow-release)
Acylated β-CyD		
TAcyl-β-CyD	Water-insoluble, soluble in	Oral, dermal
	organic solvents	(slow-release)
Ionizable derivatives		
Anionic β-CyD		
CME-β-CyD	pK_a=3 to 4, soluble	Oral, dermal, mucosal
	at pH > 4	(delayed-release)
β-CyD·sulphate	pK_a>1, water-soluble	Oral, mucosal,
β-CyD·phosphate		parenteral (intravenous)
Al·β-CyD·sulphate	Water-insoluble	(slow-release)

Abbreviations:
DM, 2,6-di-O-methyl; TM, 2,3,6-tri-O-methyl; 2-HE, 2-hydroxyethyl; 2-HP, 2-hydroxypropyl; 3-HP, 3-hydroxypropyl; 2,3-DHP, 2,3-dihydroxypropyl; G$_1$, glycosyl; G$_2$, maltosyl; DE, 2,6-di-O-ethyl; TE, 2,3,6-tri-O-ethyl; CME; O-carboxymethyl-O-ethyl; TAcyl, 2,3,6-tri-O-acyl (C$_2$~C$_{18}$).

[a]Mucosal: nasal, sublingual, ophthalmic, pulmonary, rectal, vaginal, etc

release drug carriers of water-soluble drugs[18,19] and of peptides,[20] since they have the ability to decrease the solubility of guest molecules. On the other hand, the ionizable CyDs can modify the release rate of drug, depending on pH of the solution[21] and bind to the surface membranes of cells, which may alter the function of biological barriers.[22] Sulfates and sulfoalkyl ethers of CyDs have been evaluated as a new class of parenteral drug carriers with heparin-mimetic biological activities.[22] However, new CyD derivatives must be thoroughly characterized before practical use in pharmaceutical formulations.[23] In this section, some physicochemical and biological profiles of CyD derivatives are briefly described, comparing them with those of natural CyDs.

A.   Physicochemical profiles of CyDs

Widespread use of natural CyDs as hosts for drugs is restricted by their low aqueous solubility, particularly that of β-CyD.[24] Methylation or hydroxyalkylation of the hydroxyl groups of β-CyD has been used to obviate this problem. For example, hydroxyalkylated CyDs are amorphous mixtures of chemically related components with different degrees of substitution.[11,12] This multicomponent character prevents crystallization, and thus the hydroxyalkylated CyDs have higher solubility (>50%) in both water and ethanol. The solubility of natural β-CyD in water increases with increase in temperature. On the other hand, 2,6-dimethyl-β-CyD (DM-β-CyD) shows exothermic dissolution in water, so that the solubility decreases with increase in temperature, because of dehydration at elevated temperatures. Thus, methylated CyDs have clouding points, a behaviour similar to that of nonionic surfactants. The solubilities of maltosyl-β-CyD (G_2-β-CyD) and hydroxypropyl-β-CyD (HP-β-CyD) show a little temperature dependence.[25,26] Such information is particularly useful for the design of aqueous injectable CyD solutions which are to be heat-sterilized. The aqueous solubility of ionizable CyDs depends on the pH of the solution. O-Carboxymethyl-O-ethyl-β-CyD (CME-β-CyD), in which the hydroxyl groups of ethylated β-CyD are substituted by carboxymethyl groups, is slightly soluble in low pH regions but freely soluble in neutral and alkaline regions owing to the ionization of the carboxyl group (pK_a 3–4).[21] Thus, CME-β-CyD can serve as an enteric-type drug carrier similar to carboxylmethylethylcellulose, but may be of greater advantage than the cellulose derivatives for the stabilization of labile drugs owing to the inclusion ability.[27]

The glycosidic bonds of CyDs are fairly stable in alkaline solution, whereas they are hydrolytically cleaved by strong acids to give linear oligosaccharides.[28] The ring-opening rate of CyDs increases with increasing cavity size, and is accelerated when the ring is distorted. For example, permethylated γ-CyD (TM-γ-CyD) having a distorted ring conformation is most susceptible to acid-catalysed hydrolysis.[5] It should be noted that the ring-opening rate of β-CyD is decreased by the addition of guest molecules, the decrease being marked for guests with a close fit to the β-CyD cavity.[29] This reduction of rate can be attributed to the inhibition of access of catalytic oxonium ions to the glycosidic bond because the CyD cavity is occupied by guests. The glycosidic bonds of CyDs are cleaved by some starch-degrading enzymes with the proper substrate specificity, although the reaction rate is much slower than that of linear sugars.[17] Generally, the introduction of substituents on the hydroxyl groups slows enzymatic hydrolysis of CyDs by lowering the affinity of CyDs for enzymes or owing to the intrinsic reactivity of enzymes.

B.   Biological profiles of CyDs

α- and β-CyDs are resistant to metabolism in the body, whereas γ-CyD, having a large cavity, is hydrolysed even by human salivary α-amylase.[30] On the other hand, β-CyD is hardly hydrolysed at all in whole blood of rats, rabbits, dogs and humans, and also in rat liver homogenates.[31] In the case of G_2-β-CyD, the α-1,4 glycosidic bonds in the CyD ring and the α-1,6 bond at the junction between the CyD ring and the substituents are hydrolytically stable in human body fluids. Subacute or subchronic intravenous administration of HP-β-CyD to rats and monkeys showed no significant alteration in the morphological and clinical pathology parameters.[32] When G_2-β-CyD and HP-β-CyD were administered intravenously to rats, they disappeared rapidly from the plasma[31,33] and were recovered almost completely as a form of water-soluble G_1-β-CyD and intact HP-β-CyD, respectively. Since the nephrotoxicity of natural β-CyD at higher doses was ascribed to the crystallization of less-soluble β-CyD or its cholesterol complex in renal tissues,[34] the metabolic fates of G_2-β-CyD and HP-β-CyD are suggestive of lower renal toxicity compared with the parent β-CyD. To assess tolerance via the parenteral administration route, various blood chemistry parameters in rats and rabbits after the multiple intravenous administrations of hydrophilic β-CyDs were compared with those of the parent β-CyD.[31] Multiple injections of β-CyD or DM-β-CyD at a total dose of 900 mg kg^{-1} in rats and 1200 mg kg^{-1} in rabbits produced some kidney and liver failure, while those for HP-β-CyD, G_2-β-CyD and β-CyD sulfate at the same doses failed to induce any kidney or liver failure, suggesting that these hydrophilic β-CyDs can be safely used in parenteral formulations.

The haemolytic activities of natural CyDs are reported to be in the order β- > α- > γ-CyD.[35,36] These differences are ascribed to the differential solubilization of membrane components by each CyD. When the CyD cavity is modified by chemical derivatization, its effects on cell membranes can be changed dramatically from those of parent CyDs.[13,17] When the muscle tissue damage due to the injection of hydrophilic CyDs was compared with that of mannitol and nonionic surfactants, following a single injection (100 mg ml^{-1}) of the compounds into *M. vastus lateralis* of rabbits (Fig. 37.2), α-CyD and DM-β-CyD showed a relatively high irritation reaction, the degree of which corresponded to that of Tween 80®. On the other hand, G_2-β-CyD, HP-β-CyD and CyD sulfates showed no or only slight irritation reaction, the degree of which was comparable to those of γ-CyD, mannitol and HCO-60®.

It is generally recognized that the gastrointestinal (GI) absorption of CyDs in intact form is limited because of their bulky and hydrophilic nature. Only an insignificant amount of intact β-CyD was absorbed from the GI tract in rats.[37,38] In the case of rectal route, when oleaginous suppositories containing β-CyD derivatives were administered to the rat rectum, large amounts of intact β-CyDs were excreted into the urine up to 24 h after administration.[39] The relatively high absorption observed for β-CyDs was ascribed to a change in the permeability of the rectal mucosa and/or an interaction between the surface-active β-CyDs and glycerides, which are principle components of the suppository bases. Similarly, the hydrophilic CyDs are supposed to be hardly absorbed through the skin at all. DM-β-CyD and HP-β-CyD, however, do permeate into the skin, particularly when they are applied under occlusive-dressing conditions and/or using vehicles containing absorption-promoting agents.[40,41] Recent studies have demonstrated that HP-β-CyD, even when it is applied as an aqueous solution under nonocclusive condition, penetrates into the skin of rats and distributes homogeneously over all epidermal and dermal structures without irritation.[42]

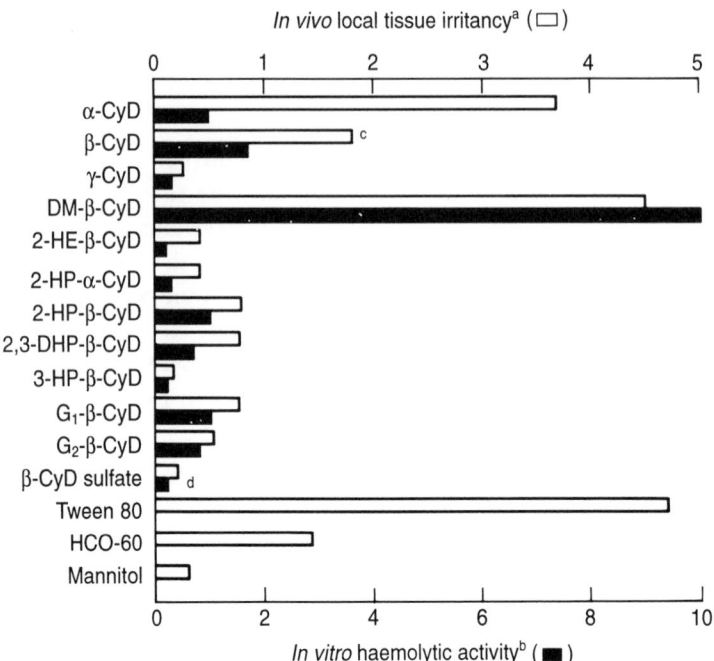

Fig. 37.2　*In vivo* local tissue irritancy and *in vitro* haemolytic activity of CyDs.
[a]Dose (100 mg ml[−1]) injected into *M. vastus lateralis* of rabbits.
[b]The reciprocal of the concentration (w/v%) of CyDs to induce 50% lysis of human erythrocytes.
[c]Used as suspension due to the limited solubility.
[d]Less than 0.2 v/w%.

III. IMPROVEMENT OF DRUG PROPERTIES

An important characteristic of CyDs is the formation of inclusion complexes in both the solution and solid states, in which each guest molecule is surrounded by the hydrophobic environment of the CyDs cavity. This can lead to the alteration of physicochemical properties of guest molecules, and can eventually have considerable pharmaceutical potential (Table 37.3). In the practical application of CyDs, attention should be directed towards the dissociation equilibrium and stoichiometry of the inclusion complex. When a CyD complex is dissolved in water or introduced into body fluids, it dissociates rapidly to free components in equilibrium with the complex. The stability constant (K_c) is a useful index for estimating the binding strength of the complex and changes in the physicochemical properties of a guest in the complex. The degree of dissociation is dependent on the magnitude of K_c, and various environmental factors such as dilution, temperature, pH and additives, will affect the K_c value. Since the formation of the inclusion complex is usually exothermic (Table 37.4), the dissociation is facilitated by raising the temperature.[40] In the case of ionizable guests, change of the pH of solutions shifts the equilibrium to such an extent and in such a direction that the un-ionized form is predominantly included in the cavity. This is due to the favouring of the inclusion of hydrophobic guests compared with hydrophilic guests. The obvious requirement

Table 37.3 Pharmaceutical products containing natural CyDs.

Drug	CyD used	Purpose	Dosage form	Efficacy
Prostaglandin E$_1$	α-CyD	Solubilization Stabilization	Injection	Chronic arteriosclerotic obstruction
Prostaglandin E$_2$	β-CyD	Solubilization Stabilization	Tablet	Labour induction
Limaprost	α-CyD	Solubilization	Tablet	Büergar, Raynaud
Benaxate hydrochloride	β-CyD	Increase of membrane-affinity Stabilization	Capsule	Antiulcer
Nitroglycerine	β-CyD	Prevention of vaporization	Sublingual tablet	Angina pectoris
Cefotiam hexetyl hydrochloride	α-CyD	Prevention of gelation	Tablet	Antibiotic
Piroxicam	β-CyD	Solubilization	Tablet Suppository	Anti-inflammatory

Table 37.4 Effect of temperature on stability constants (K_c) of inclusion complexes of ethyl 4-biphenylylacetate with various β-CyDs, and their thermodynamic parameters in water.

Complex	K_c (l mol^{-1})				ΔH	ΔS
	15°C	25°C	37°C	45°C	(kJ mol^{-1})	(J K^{-1} mol^{-1})
β-CyD	3 330	3 050	2 850	1 630	−18.2	5.7
HP-β-CyD	7 950	4 200	3 000	1 650	−37.2	−55.7
DM-β-CyD	31 500	12 500	10 000	5 700	−40.4	−57.1

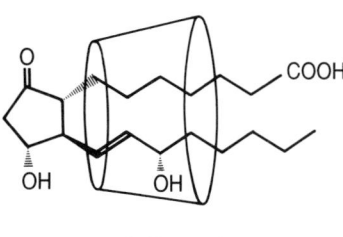

α-CyD complex

β-CyD complex

γ-CyD complex

Fig. 37.3 Cavity-size dependency of inclusion complexation of CyDs with prostaglandin E$_1$.

for inclusion complexation is that the hydrophobic moiety of a guest molecule must fit entirely or partially into the CyD cavity. In the case of prostaglandin E_1 (PGE$_1$) (Fig. 37.3), α-CyD, with a smaller cavity, preferentially includes an aliphatic chain of the PGE$_1$ molecule, while β-CyD accommodates the five-membered ring of PGE$_1$.[5] In contrast, the larger γ-CyD cavity accommodates PGE$_1$ in such a manner that the whole PGE$_1$ molecule penetrates the cavity. When a guest molecule is too large to be included in one CyD cavity or the host cavity is too small to include a whole guest, more than one CyD is available for complete inclusion. However, the inclusion complexation often shows a different stoichiometry depending on the guest/host concentration employed, which consequently affects the physicochemical properties of the guest molecules.

A.   Solubilization

The solubilizing effect of CyDs is related both to their ability to form inclusion complexes and to the intrinsic solubility of the host molecule in water. The former factor is related to the K_c values. Among β-CyD and its derivatives, DM-β-CyD shows the highest solubilizing effect for poorly water-soluble drugs, probable owing to the elongation of the cavity.[7,9,10] The steric effects of substituents also play a role in the solubilizing ability of the host molecules. For example, HP-β-CyD, similarly to DM-β-CyD, has higher complexing ability, but its solubilizing ability is lowered at very high degrees of substitution.[13] Glucose and maltose units in the branched β-CyD also hinder the inclusion of drug molecules.[17]

   HP-β-CyD can be recommended as a parenteral drug carrier because of its low toxicity, high toleration and excellent solubilizing abilities.[43] In the preparation of an HP-β-CyD-based pharmaceutical formulation, the solubility of some lipophilic drugs in water was synergistically increased with increasing temperature, suggesting that heating or heat-sterilization may be useful steps.[44] A detailed evaluation of HP-β-CyD as an excellent solubilizer and stabilizer for brain-targeting chemical delivery systems such as estradiol–dihydropyridine conjugate has been described.[45,46] The hydrophilic CyDs can solubilize some specific lipids from biological membranes through the rapid and reversible formation of inclusion complexes, leading to an increase in the membrane permeability.[35] This may allow the extended use of CyDs as adjuvants to improve the transmucosal absorption of poorly absorbable peptide and protein drugs,[47] which will be discussed in later sections.

   The solubility of guests changes according to the stoichiometry of the complexes: for example, solubilities in water of nocloprost, a derivative of PGE$_1$,[48] and sofalcon, an antiulcer agent,[49] increased on 1 : 1 complexation with β- and γ-CyDs, respectively, owing to the partial inclusion. On the other hand, the solubilities were decreased by 1 : 2 complexation at higher CyD concentrations because of the complete inclusion of the whole guest molecules within the CyD dimers, which are less hydrated.

B.   Stabilization in solution

The drug must remain sufficiently stable not only during storage but also in the GI fluids, since reactions which result in a product that is pharmacologically inactive or less active will reduce the therapeutic effectiveness. CyDs are known to accelerate or decelerate various kinds of reactions depending on the nature of the complex formed.[2,4] Generally, when a drug's active centre is included in the CyD cavity there is a deceleration effect, and the reaction rate is dependent primarily on the amount of free drug concentration resulting from the dissociation of the complex. On the other hand, if the drug does not totally fit into the cavity or is only partially included, leaving the active centre sterically fixed in close proximity to the catalysts, it experiences an acceleration effect.[28]

1. Prostanoids

Prostaglandins (PGs) are essentially long-chain unsaturated fatty acids containing a substituted cyclopentane ring system. The β-hydroxyketo moiety of E-type prostaglandins (PGEs) is extremely susceptible to dehydration under acidic or alkaline conditions to give A-type prostaglandins (PGAs), which are isomerized subsequently to form B-type prostaglandins (PGBs) under alkaline conditions. The biological activities of PGEs decrease with progress of these reactions. The chemical instability and the low aqueous solubilities of PGEs have limited dosage form design and presented a substantial challenge to pharmaceutical scientists. Natural CyDs have successfully been applied to PGEs, and stable and soluble complexes were first marketed in Japan as a PGE_2-β-CyD tablet and PGE_1-α-CyD injection (see Table 37.3). In aqueous solution, however, attempts to stabilize PGEs were rather disappointing because of the positive catalytic effect of natural CyDs (Fig. 37.4). In most cases, the stabilizing effect of TM-β-CyD is smaller than that of DM-β-CyD, preventing deep penetration of the bulky PGE_2 molecules into the narrow TM-β-CyD cavity.[50] Recently, G_2-β-CyD has been shown to improve the undesirable properties of PGE_1 in lyophilized preparations.[51] The decomposition of lyophilized PGE_1 is significantly retarded by both β-CyD and G_2-β-CyD. The rapid-dissolution property of lyophilized PGE_1 with G_2-β-CyD is maintained during storage, while it tends to decrease with β-CyD, depending on the moisture-adsorbing and wetting properties and crystallinity changes of the additives.

Prostacyclin (PGI_2) is a potent therapeutic agent in the treatment of thrombosis and relaxation of vascular smooth muscle. However, this compound undergoes an extremely facile hydrolysis of the vinyl-ether moiety to yield 6-keto-$PGF_1α$ in aqueous solution, losing its activity within a few minutes. Upon binding to CyDs, the rate of hydrolysis of PGI_2 is retarded

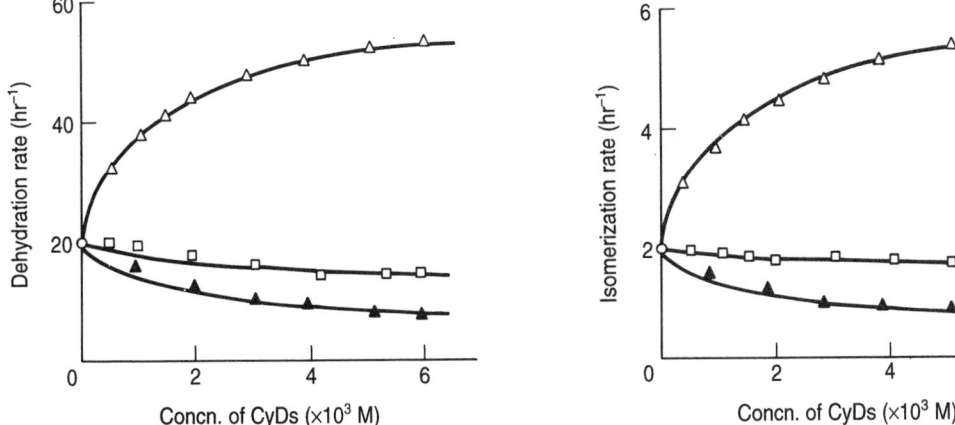

Fig. 37.4 Effects of β-CyDs on the dehydration of PGE_2 (left) and isomerization of PGA_2 (right) in phosphate buffer (pH 11.0, μ = 0.2) at 60°C. ○, PG alone; △, β-CyD; ▲, DM-β-CyD; □, TM-β-CyD.

in the order β- > α- > γ-CyD. The retardation effect of CyDs seems to be at least in part a result of the inhibition of intramolecular carboxylate ion catalysis due to the decrease in acidity of the terminal carboxyl group. Methylated β-CyDs in which the hydroxyl groups are blocked show a much greater retardation effect in the hydrolysis of PGI_2 in comparison with that of parent β-CyD.[52]

2. Cardiac glycosides

Digoxin, one of the potent cardiac glycosides, is susceptible to hydrolysis in an acidic medium, and therapeutic efficiency as well as oral bioavailability may decrease as a result. In the degradation pathways of digoxin, prevention of the appearance of digoxigenin might be clinically important because the cardioactivity of digoxigenin is about one-tenth of that of digoxin, but other digoxosides (mono- and bisdigoxosides) possess approximately the same activity. In the presence of CyDs, acid hydrolysis of digoxin is suppressed in the order β- > γ- > α-CyD, where β-CyD inhibits the conversion from digoxosides to digoxigenin almost completely. ^{1}H NMR data reveal that the A-ring of digoxin is located at the entrance to the α-CyD cavity, that it could penetrate further into the β-CyD cavity, and that it is loosely bound to γ-CyD.[53] This indicates that either a smaller (α-CyD) or a larger (γ-CyD) cavity is unfavourable for preventing the hydrolysis of digoxin. Moreover, the methylated CyDs suppressed the hydrolysis of digitoxin in the order DM-β- > β- > TM-β-CyD, where DM-β-CyD completely inhibited the conversion from digitoxosides to digitoxigenin.[54] In a dissolution study of digoxin tablets, increase in dissolution rate and decrease in acid hydrolysis were achieved by β- and γ-CyDs, where the appearance of digoxigenin was almost negligible even 60 min after the initiation of the dissolution test.[55] When tablets containing a γ-CyD complex of digoxin were administered sublingually to human volunteers, the serum levels of drug were significantly increased compared with digoxin alone, owing to the prevention of acid hydrolysis in the stomach.[56] The stoichiometric ratio is in practice responsible for the dosage form design of a drug molecule. In the case of digoxin, for example, one digoxin molecule needs four molecules of γ-CyD to form a 1 : 4 stable crystalline complex, resulting in an 8-fold increase in the molecular weight of digoxin.[53] This may facilitate the preparation of tablets containing small amounts of drug, resulting in a better uniformity of content. In the case of high-dosage drugs, the increase in molecular weight becomes a disadvantage, since the relationship between the required dose and molecular weight determines the feasibility of oral administration in CyD complexes.

C. Control of solid properties

Many solid compounds are known to exist in different crystalline modifications such as amorphous, crystalline or glassy states, affecting solubility, dissolution rate, stability and bioavailability. In order to improve the pharmaceutical potential, therefore, it is important to control the crystallization, the polymorphic transition, and whisker generation of solid drugs.[5,6]

1. Modification of crystalline states of nifedipine

The oral bioavailability of crystalline nifedipine, a potent calcium-channel antagonist, is very low because of its poor solubility and its slow dissolution rate in water. Various hydrophilic macromolecules such as poly(vinylpyrrolidone) (PVP) and poly(ethylene glycols) have been used to improve the dissolution characteristics of nifedipine.[57] However, amorphous nifedipine in these matrices gradually crystallizes during storage at high temperature and humidity, deteriorating its rapid dissolution characteristics. Recently, we have reported that crystalline nifedipine is converted to an amorphous state by spray-drying with HP-β-CyD, and the oral bioavailability is improved significantly.[52] HP-β-CD was useful in preventing the crystal growth of amorphous nifedipine, maintaining a relatively fine and uniform size of crystals even under adverse storage conditions (60°C, 75% RH). Moreover, the rapidly dissolving form of the metastable state (Form B; m.p. 163°C) transiently formed at an early stage of storage of amorphous nifedipine, and the glassy state (transition temperature at 48°C) of nifedipine could be obtained by cooling melts of stable form of nifedipine (Form A: m.p. 171°C). In the presence of HP-β-CyD, the crystallization of the glassy nifedipine and the polymorphic transition of Form B to Form A were significantly suppressed, indicating that Form B could be prepared in high yield (> 75%) by heating in the amorphous HP-β-CyD matrix. Although the initial dissolution rate of nifedipine increased in the order of glassy state > Form B > Form A, the glassy state of nifedipine was readily converted to Form A of larger crystal size at higher humidity and temperature. These facts suggest that HP-β-CyD is particularly useful for the selective preparation of the fast-dissolving Form B, and will provide a rational basis for design of formulation and storage condition in solid dosage forms of nifedipine.

2. Stabilization of carmofur

Carmofur (1-hexylcarbamoyl-5-fluorouracil, HCFU) is one of the masked forms of 5-fluorouracil (5-FU) and has been widely used to treat carcinomas of breast and GI-tract. It is expected that the highly hygroscopic character of natural CyDs may significantly influence the degradation of HCFU, because HCFU is extremely susceptible to base- and water-catalysed hydrolysis to give 5-FU. In fact, the degradation rate of HCFU in the solid CyD complex was very fast under accelerated conditions (70°C, 75% RH). This problem can be solved by adding an organic acid, such as citric or tartaric acid, as a pH-controlling agent.[59] The organic acids may provide an acidic environment around the CyD complex after moisture sorption, since HCFU is chemically stable under acidic conditions. The methylated CyDs are highly effective in preventing the decomposition of HCFU in the solid state for long periods under accelerated storage conditions (40°C, 75% RH), because they are less hygroscopic than natural CyDs. Since, the stabilizing effect of CyDs is responsible for the bioavailability of HCFU,[60,61] the acidic property of CME-β-CyD is particularly effective in improving the oral bioavailability of HCFU, preventing the degradation of HCFU into 5-FU, which irritates the GI mucosa.[27]

D. Release control

For the design of advanced oral formulations, control of drug release rate from dosage forms is of critical importance in realizing their therapeutic efficacy. Most of the slow-release preparations have been aimed at achieving zero-order release of drugs to provide a constant blood level for extended periods. For this purpose, wax-type matrices or water-soluble cellulose derivatives are generally used as slow-release carriers for water-soluble drugs. When hydroxyl groups of CyDs are substituted by ethyl, acetyl or longer alkyl groups, the solubility of these CyDs in water decreases proportionally to their degree of substitution or the length of the alkyl chains.[18,19] We have demonstrated that the ethylated β-CyDs such as DE-β-CyD and perethylated β-CyD (TE-β-CyD) are useful as slow-release carriers of isosorbide dinitrate[62] and diltiazem hydrochloride.[63] New series of peracylated β-CyDs with different alkyl chains (acetyl to octanoyl) also were prepared by acylating all hydroxyl groups of β-CyD, and their physical properties were evaluated with anticipation of more effective slow-release carriers for water-soluble drugs.[64] The concentrated solutions of peracylated β-CyDs in organic solvents were highly viscous and sticky and gelation took place upon evaporation of the solvents. Since these properties were thought to be particularly useful for a slow-release carrier, the solid complexes of peracylated β-CyDs with water-soluble drugs were prepared and their *in vitro* and *in vivo* release behaviours were examined. Drug release was markedly retarded by the complexation with peracylated β-CyDs in the decreasing order of the solubility of the host molecules. Since the peracylated derivatives with substituents longer than the hexanoyl moiety hardly released the water-soluble drugs, peracetyl- (TA-), perbutanoyl- (TB-) and perhexanoyl- (TH-)β-CyDs were used in the *in vivo* studies following oral administration of the hydrophobic complexes to dogs. As shown in Fig. 37.5, TB-β-CyD suppressed a peak plasma level of molsidomine, a peripheral vasodilator, and maintained a sufficient drug level for long periods, while other peracylated β-CyDs with shorter or longer chains were ineffective in controlling the *in vivo* release behaviour of molsidomine. It is noteworthy that the TB-β-CyD complex significantly increased the AUC and prolonged the mean residence time (MRT) of the drug. The prominent retarding effect of TB-β-CyD was ascribable to its mucoadhesive property and hydrophobicity compared with other peracylated β-CyDs.[64] These facts suggest that peracylated β-CyDs are useful as novel multifunctional carriers to modify the release rate of water-soluble drugs.

CME-β-CyD is effective in modifying the release rate of water-soluble drugs. For example, the CME-β-CyD complex of diltiazem, a potent calcium-channel antagonist, releases the drug very slowly in the stomach but rapidly in the intestine, the main absorption site. The *in vitro* release behaviour was clearly reflected in the plasma levels of diltiazem after oral administration to dogs, where the complex produced a 2-fold increase in bioavailability compared with the

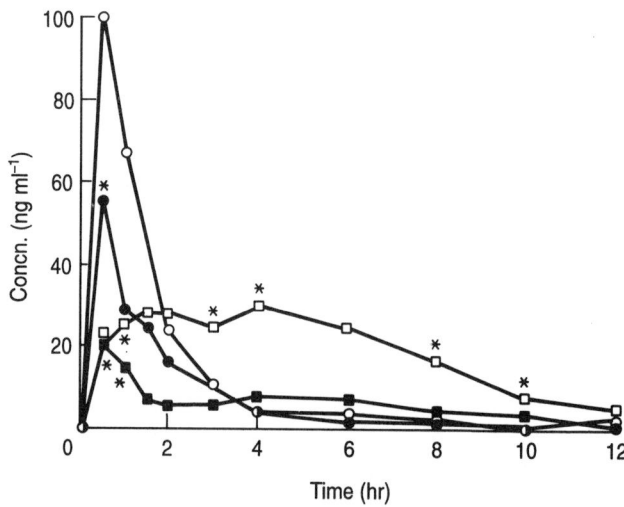

Fig. 37.5 Plasma levels of molsidomine after oral administration of capsules containing molsidomine or its peracylated β-CyD complexes (equivalent to molsidomine at 10 mg/body) in dogs.
○, Molsidomine alone (diluent: starch); ●, TA-β-CD complex; □, TB-β-CyD complex; ◆, TH-β-CyD complex. Each point represents the mean of 3–6 dogs. *$p < 0.05$ vs molsidomine alone.

drug alone.[21] Such enhancement may arise from the reduction of the first pass effect — the metabolism in the liver immediately after absorption is saturated owing to the high local concentration of the drug at the intestinal tract. To investigate the delayed-release characteristics of the CME-β-CyD complex, the *in vivo* release of diltiazem was evaluated using dogs whose gastric acidity had been controlled by pretreatment with tetragastrin or omeprazole.[65] Following oral administration of the CME-β-CyD complex tablets in dogs with high controlled gastric acidity, the absorption of diltiazem was significantly retarded, since the complex dissolved only in the intestinal fluid after passing through the stomach. In dogs with low gastric acidity, rapid absorption of diltiazem was observed owing to the dissolution of the complex in the gastric fluid. In this delayed-release formulation, a good correlation between the *in vitro* and *in vivo* release rates of diltiazem was obtained in both groups of dogs with controlled gastric acidity.[66]

A suitable combination of various CyD derivatives is effective in sustaining the release rate of drugs. For example, the release rate of theophylline, which has a narrow therapeutic range in the blood level, can be controlled by hybridizing its hydrophilic, hydrophobic and ionizable CyD complexes.[66] This formulation has many advantages in reducing the frequency of dosing, prolonging the drug efficacy and avoiding the toxicity associated with the administration of a simple plain tablet of theophylline.

The oily injection of buserelin acetate (BLA), a luteinizing hormone-releasing hormone (LHRH) agonist, with a sustained-release feature can be achieved using hydrophobic CyDs.[67] The release of BLA from the peanut-oil suspension into the aqueous phase was significantly retarded by the complexation with TA-CyDs. A single subcutaneous injection of the oily suspension of BLA containing TA-β-CyD and TA-γ-CyD in rats provided the retardation of plasma BLA levels, giving 25 and 30 times longer mean residence times, respectively, than that with BLA alone. Simultaneously, the suppression of plasma testosterone levels to induce castration, the pharmacological effect of BLA, continued for 1 to 2 weeks and significant weight reduction in genital organs was observed due to the antigonadal effect. Since TA-β-CyD and TA-γ-CyD were degraded enzymatically in rat skin homogenates, both TA-CyDs can be useful as bioabsorbable sustained-release carriers for the water-soluble peptides following subcutaneous injection of oily suspensions.[68]

E. Enhancement of drug absorption

Many factors affect drug absorption and they are largely dependent on the pharmaceutical formulation and administration route. In order to enhance drug absorption from CyD complexes, the dissociation equilibrium can be controlled by adjusting environmental factors.[69] Figure 37.6 shows the overall process of drug absorption from the complex in the presence of competing agent, where k_d is the dissolution rate constant, K_1 is the stability constant of the drug–CyD complex, K_2 is the stability constant of the competing agent–CyD complex, and k_a is the absorption rate constant of the drug. When the solid complex is administered orally, the drug is absorbed after the complex is dissolved and dissociated, since only the free form of the drug in solution is capable of penetrating the lipid barrier of the GI tract. Therefore, the absorption of the drug from the complex is mainly dependent on the magnitude of the dissolution rate (k_d) and the stability constants (K_1 and K_2) of the complexes; high dissolution rates and the relative stability of the complexes ($K_2 > K_1$) favour a free drug which is readily available for absorption. Since the displacement of drug from the cavity by exogenous and endogenous substances in the formulation and GI tract is responsible for acceleration of the drug absorption, the equilibrium can be controlled by adding an appropriate competitor and by adjusting its amount.[70] Such competition may occur not only in the body fluids containing various biological components such as lipids and sterols but also in pharmaceutical dosage forms containing various excipients.

1. Gastrointestinal absorption

The hydrophilic CyDs are useful for improving oral bioavailability of poorly water-soluble drugs, including steroids, cardiac glycosides, nonsteroidal anti-inflammatory drugs, barbiturates, antiepileptics, benzodiazepines, antidiabetics, vasodilators, etc.[1-6] These improvements are mainly due to the increase in solubility, dissolution rate and wettability of the drugs through formation of inclusion complexes. As described in Fig. 37.6, CyDs are supposed to act only as carrier materials and help to transport the drug through an aqueous medium to the lipophilic absorption site in the GI tract. Results fully confirming this view were obtained in the enhancement of the absorption of spironolactone,[71] proscillaridin,[72] prednisolone,[73] benzodiazepines,[74] cardiac glycosides,[53] acetohexamide,[75] and anti-inflammatory drugs[76] using natural CyDs. Additionally, CyDs cause some modification of the GI mucosa at high concentrations owing to the removal of membrane components such as cholesterol, phospholipids, or proteins.[77,78] Therefore, free CyDs after dissociation of the complex may alter the lipid barrier of the absorption site, which consequently facilitates drug absorption. However, despite the larger stability constant, DM-β-CyD significantly enhances both the extent and rate of absorption of drugs compared with parental β-CyD, including fat-soluble vitamins,[3,79,80] anti-inflammatory drugs,[81,82] and antitumour drugs.[83] For example, the rapidly dissolving DM-β-CyD complex of α-tocopheryl nicotinate, following oral administration to fasting dogs, resulted in the area under the plasma concentration–time curve (AUC) being about 70 times as great as that of the drug alone.[84] To explain this anomalous enhancing effect of DM-β-CyD on fatty drugs, additional factors influencing drug absorption were considered. Since highly surface-active DM-β-CyD is supposed to substitute bile in GI tract,[3] the lipophilic drugs can be finely emulsified by DM-β-CyD, which eventually provides the marked GI absorption in the fasting condition.

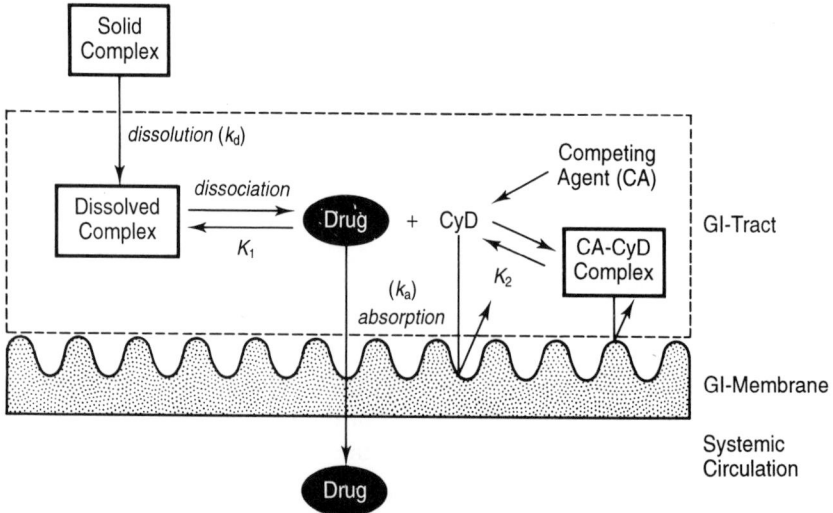

Fig. 37.6 Effect of competing agent on drug absorption from inclusion complex following dissolution and dissociation in gastrointestinal tract.

2.   Transdermal absorption

Recent studies on human volunteers demonstrated that CyDs have a significant safety margin in dermal application.[85] Optimized release of the drug from the topical preparation containing its CyD complex may be obtained by using a vehicle in which the complex is barely dissociated and maintains a high thermodynamic activity. For example, the *in vitro* release rate of corticosteroids from water-containing ointments (hydrophilic, absorptive, or polyacrylic base) was markedly increased by the hydrophilic CyDs, whereas in other ointments (a fatty alcohol propylene glycol (FAPG) or macrogol base) CyDs retarded the drug release.[86] The enhancement of drug release can be ascribed to the increase in solubility, diffusibility and concentration of the drug in the aqueous phase of the ointment through water-soluble complex formation. Moreover, the drug in the CyD complex may be displaced by some components of the ointment, depending on the stability constant of the complex.[87,88] CyDs also interact with some components of skin. For example, DM-β-CyD markedly extracts cholesterol from rabbit skin *in vitro* (Fig. 37.7), a process which may reduce the function of skin as a barrier and may eventually contribute in part to the enhancement of drug absorption.

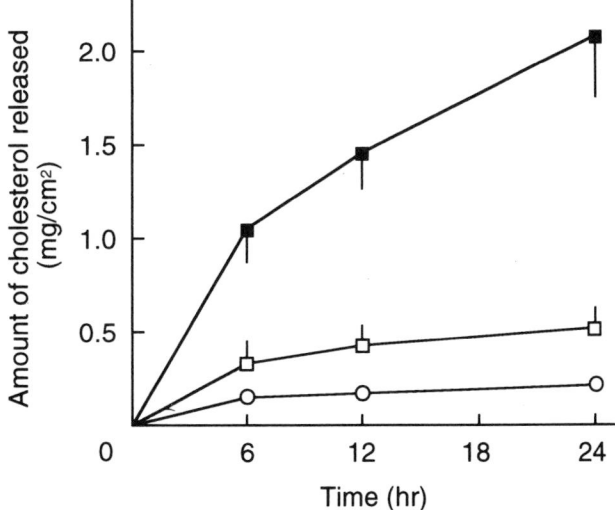

Fig. 37.7   Release profiles of cholesterol from rabbit skin treated with β-CyDs (1.2 mM) in isotonic phosphate buffer (pH 7.4) at 37°C.
○, Control; □, β-CyD; ■, DM-β-CyD. Each point represents the mean ± SE of 12 experiments.

When a hydrophilic ointment containing anti-inflammatory ethyl 4-biphenylylacetate (EBA) or its CyD complexes was applied to the skin of rats, the release of EBA from the ointment into the skin was assisted by DM-β-CyD or HP-β-CyD, while β-CyD had no appreciable effect.[41] Although the entry of CyDs into the skin made the stratum corneum more resistant to the permeation of the drug, the greater release of EBA from the vehicle compensated for the negative effect on the skin permeation of the drug and delivered the drug more effectively to the site of action. The application of EBA in the complexed form resulted in a transient rise in the total amount of EBA and its active metabolite, biphenylylacetic acid (BPAA) in the stratum corneum and in the viable skin. Interestingly, the fraction of active BPAA in the viable skin was increased when EBA was applied in the complexed form, indicating that β-CyDs assist the bioconversion of EBA to BPAA in the skin and consequently facilitate the delivery of active BPAA to subcutaneous tissues, where its action is most desired. In the model of carrageenan-induced acute oedema in rat paw, the inflammation was inhibited by pretreatment with ointments containing EBA–CyD complexes of DM-β-CyD or HP-β-CyD.[41,89]

3.   Rectal absorption

The release of drug from suppository bases is one of the important factors in the transmucosal absorption of drugs, since the rectal fluid is small in volume and is viscous compared to GI fluid. Generally, the hydrophilic CyDs enhance the release of poorly water-soluble drugs from fatty bases because of the lesser interaction of the resultant complex with vehicles,[90,91] which eventually improves the rectal absorption. For example, the methylated CyDs significantly enhance the rectal absorption of hydrophobic drugs such as flurbiprofen,[40] HCFU,[51] and BPAA.[26] The superior effect of methylated CyDs can be explained by the faster release of the drug together with the lowering of the affinity of the complexed drug for the oleaginous suppository base. HP-β-CyD is particularly useful for improving the rectal absorption of hydrophobic drugs from fatty bases. The most illuminating effect of HP-β-CyD was obtained for the enhancement of rectal absorption of EBA, a lipophilic prodrug of BPAA.[26,91] The relative potency of β-CyD analogues in enhancing the dissolution rate of EBA in water and reducing the binding affinity of drugs to the fatty base was DM-β-CyD complex > HP-β-CyD complex > β-CyD complex; this order was consistent with that of the magnitudes of the stability constants of the complexes. However, in vivo absorption of EBA was enhanced in the order HP-β-CyD complex > DM-β-CyD complex > β-CyD complex in rats after single and multiple administrations of suppositories containing the complexes. The enhancement of rectal absorption of EBA in vivo can be explained by the facts that HP-β-CyD increases the release rate of EBA from the vehicle and stabilizes it in the rectal lumen and that the drug is partly absorbed in the form of the complex. The rather small enhancing effect of DM-β-CyD was ascribable to the considerable dissociation of the complex in the vehicle together with increased viscosity of the suppository base, since DM-β-CyD is extremely surface-active and oil-soluble compared with HP-β-CyD. Consequently, HP-β-CyD had the highest potential to improve rectal absorption of EBA among the three β-CyDs tested.

4.   Nasal absorption

Highly water-soluble CyD complexes of steroid hormones are well-suited to nasal administration.[92,93] This kind of formulation may provide a rapid rise of drug levels in systemic circulation and avoid intestinal and hepatic first pass metabolism of the drugs. Inherently, the blood level of endogenous hormones rises a few times a day in episodes lasting approximately one hour. Such pulsatile release of steroids can be imitated by the nasal administration of water-soluble CyD complexes, which may provide some desirable pharmacological profiles as demonstrated in sublingual administration of a rapidly-dissolving complex of steroids with HP-β-CyD.[94] The effects of CyDs on the nasal epithelial membranes seem to be of minor importance for the absorption enhancement, because CyDs will lose their ability to interact with the membranes when their cavities are occupied by the steroids. Nasal preparations must be evaluated critically for their possible effect on the nasal mucociliary functions, which are known to defend the respiratory tract against dust, allergens and bacteria. When compared with other absorption-promoting agents and preservatives used in nasal formulations, DM-β-CyD exerted only a minor effect on the ciliary beat frequency of human nasal adenoid tissue *in vitro*.[95] This may represent an advantage of DM-β-CyD over the enhancers in promoting the nasal absorption of drugs, especially for short-term therapy. A nasal spray containing estradiol solubilized by DM-β-CyD was effective in the treatment of symptoms of estrogen deficiency in bilateral oophorectomized women, and the twice-daily administration of this formulation over a period of 6 months was well-tolerated by the patients.[96]

F. Reduction of side-effects

The molecular entrapment of a drug into the CyD cavity may prevent direct contact of the drug with biological surfaces, and both the drug's entry into the cells of nontargeted tissues and local irritation are thus decreased. Since the CyD complex eventually dissociates into its components, there is no drastic loss of the therapeutic benefits of the drug. Therefore, CyDs act as wafer-like carriers which decrease the drug-induced local tissue damage at the administration site and then deliver the drug close to the site of its action.

1. Reduction of local irritancy

CyDs alleviate muscular tissue damage following the intramuscular injection of drugs.[97,98] The protective effects of CyDs may be attributed mainly to the poor affinity of the hydrophilic complexes of drugs for the sarcolemmal membranes of muscle fibres, a situation expected from the results of *in vitro* haemolysis studies. Similarly, CyDs diminished the ulcerogenic potency of several acidic anti-inflammatory drugs when these were administered orally.[99] In addition, HP-β-CyD significantly reduced the irritation of rectal mucosa in rats caused by BPAA, both for single and multiple administrations of EBA-β-CyD complexes in oleaginous suppositories (Fig. 37.8).[91]

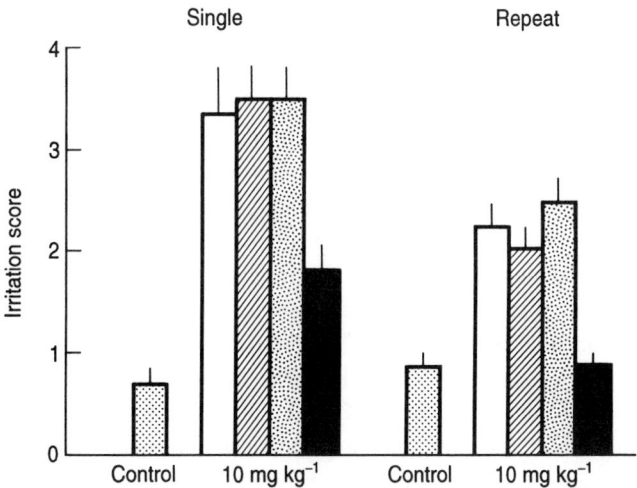

Fig. 37.8 Irritation effects of single or repeated administration (4 times, 12-h intervals) of EBA or its β-CyD complexes as suppositories (10 mg kg⁻¹ as EBA) on rectal mucosa in rats.
Open bars, EBA alone; hatched bars, β-CyD complex; tinted bars, DM-β-CyD complex; solid bars, HP-β-CyD complex. Each value represents the mean ± SE of 5 rats.

Chlorpromazine (CPZ), a typical antipsychotic agent, frequently causes cutaneous phototoxic and photoallergic responses in patients being treated with prolonged and high doses. These adverse effects may be mainly attributable to the toxic photoproducts of CPZ. We have recently reported that DM-β-CyD significantly reduced the photosensitized skin irritation caused by CPZ in guinea-pigs according to gross and histological examination.[100] The inhibitory effect of DM-β-CyD was ascribed to the alteration of the photochemical reactivity of CPZ, rather than the direct interaction of the photoproducts with DM-β-CyD. When CPZ was photoirradiated with DM-β-CyD, promazine, which is less toxic than CPZ, was produced in high yield.[101] In addition, DM-β-CyD suppresses the formation of numerous oxidation and polymerization photoproducts which are responsible for CPZ-photosensitized skin irritation. β-CyD derivatives also decreased the photoinduced free-radical production from CPZ,[102] the photodecarboxylation of benoxaprofen,[103] and the photodimerization of protriptyline,[104] resulting in the reduction of phototoxicity.

2.   Systemic detoxication

The addition of β-CyD to dialysis fluids accelerated the removal of phenobarbital by peritoneal dialysis, thereby proving effective in the treatment of drug overdose.[105] HP-β-CyD is useful not only in the administration of drugs but also in redistributing other endogenous lipophiles in the body.[145] When HP-β-CyD was infused intravenously into a patient with familial hypervitaminosis A, retinyl ester overloading in the liver was reduced.[106] Recently, the possibility of HP-β-CyD redistributing cholesterol deposited in the vascular systems of hereditary hyperlipidaemic rabbits was reported.[107] A single intravenous administration of HP-β-CyD to rabbits slightly and temporarily decreased the level of total cholesterol in the serum. Similar results were obtained using normal rats.[108] Repeated administration of HP-β-CyD to the rabbits led to a gradual increase in total cholesterol in the circulation and eventually to a slight relief of atherosclerotic lesions in the thoracic aorta. HP-β-CyD may serve as an artificial lipid carrier to catalytically augment the establishment of equilibria in lipid distribution.[109]

Gentamicin, an aminoglycoside antibiotic, is widely used in the clinical treatment of Gram-negative infections, but its use is sometimes complicated by the development of drug-induced acute renal failure. Gentamicin is thought to interact with negatively charged phospholipids of lysosomal membranes in the proximal tubular cells, the interaction of which may lead eventually to lysosomal dysfunction, resulting in necrosis of the cells. Since some polyanions such as dextran sulphates are able to interact electrostatically with gentamicin and to reduce the drug's entry into the renal cortex, the effects of CyD sulphates on development of rat renal dysfunction induced with gentamicin were studied.[110] Daily subcutaneous infection of gentamicin (100 mg kg^{-1}, 14 days) developed nephrotoxicity in the rat, as assessed by an increase in serum urea nitrogen (Fig. 37.9) and histopathological changes in the renal cortex. When CyD sulphates were given intraperitoneally at 300 mg kg^{-1} at 6-h intervals after gentamicin administration, they protected the rats against the drug-induced renal impairment, while parent CyDs were ineffective. Since the postadministration of CyD sulphates did not reduce the total amount of gentamicin accumulated in the kidney, the protection may occur through interference with intracellular events leading from the drug accumulation to nephrotoxicity. Since CyD sulphates have anti-inflammatory activity and have high affinity for growth factors and stabilize them against proteolysis, the effect of CyD sulphates on the renal regeneration processes should be considered as another possible protective mechanism. In any case, CyD sulphates may serve as potent antidotes against renal failure associated with aminoglycoside treatment.

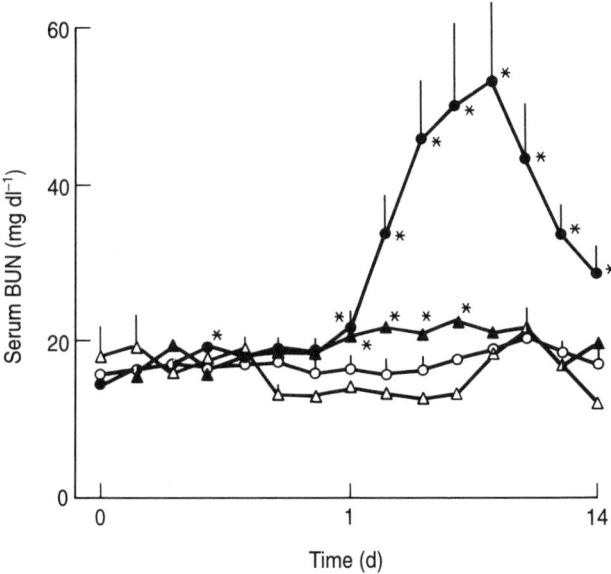

Fig. 37.9 Effect of β-CyD sulphate (300 mg kg^{-1} per day, i.p., 6 h post-administration) on serum levels of urea nitrogen in rats treated with gentamicin (100 mg kg^{-1} per day, s.c.) for 14 days. ○, Saline control; △, β-CyD sulphate alone; ●, gentamicin alone; ▲, gentamicin with β-CyD sulphate. Each value represents the mean ± SE of 3–12 rats. * $p < 0.05$ vs saline control.

G. Use in peptide and protein drugs

There are considerable hurdles in the practical use of biologically active peptides and proteins because of chemical and biological instability, poor absorption through biological membranes, rapid plasma clearance, peculiar dose–response curves, and immunogenicity. Many attempts have addressed these problems by chemical modification or by co-administration of adjuvants to promote absorption of peptides and proteins and protect them from proteolytic enzymes. The absorption-enhancing effects of CyDs mimic those of bile salts in regard to increased membrane permeability accompanied by inhibition of proteolysis, although they may differ somewhat in their manner of action on membranes. Thus, CyD complexation seems to be an attractive alternative to these approach, but the field is still in its beginnings.[69]

1. Absorption enhancement

Internasal delivery of peptide and protein drugs is severely restricted by presystemic elimination due to enzymatic degradation or mucocillary clearance and by the limited extent of mucosal membrane permeability. α-CyD has been shown to remove some fatty acids from nasal mucosa and to enhance the nasal absorption of leuprolide acetate in rats and dogs.[111] Recent studies have demonstrated the utility of chemically modified CyDs as absorption enhancers for peptide drugs in rats.[69] For example, DM-β-CyD was shown to be a potent enhancer of insulin absorption in rats,[112] and a minimal effective concentration of DM-β-CyD for absorption enhancement exerted only a mild effect on the *in vitro* ciliary movement.[113] The scope of interaction of insulin with CyDs is limited, because CyDs can only partially include the hydrophobic amino acid residues in peptides with small stability constants.[112] Under *in vivo* conditions, these complexes will readily dissociate into separate components, and hence the displacement by membrane lipids may further destabilize the complexes. The direct interaction of peptides with CyDs is therefore of minor importance in the enhancement of nasal absorption. Of the hydrophilic CyDs tested, DM-β-CyD had the most prominent inhibitory effect on the enzymatic degradation of both BLA and insulin in rat nasal tissue homogenates. Because of the limited interaction between peptides and CyDs, they may reduce the proteolytic activities of enzymes by preventing the formation of the enzyme–substrate complexes. This view was supported by the following observations. Leucine aminopeptidase in the nasal mucosa is known to cleave the B-chain of insulin from the N-terminal end. CyDs, especially DM-β-CyD and HP-β-CyD, reduce the activity of leucine aminopeptidase in a concentration-dependent manner.[114] The inhibition of proteolysis by these CyDs may participate in the absorption enhancement of peptides. Another potential barrier to the nasal absorption of peptide and protein drugs is the limitation in the size of hydrophilic pores through which they are thought to pass. The methylated CyDs significantly extracted membrane lipids, depending on the size and hydrophobicity of the CyD cavity in which lipids were included.[36] Therefore, lipid solubilization mediated by CyDs may result in transcellular processes, and these changes could be transmitted to the paracellular region, which is the most likely route for the transport of polypeptides.

The combined effect of β-CyD with absorption enhancers such as sodium glycocholate or Azone® on the nasal absorption of human fibroblast interferon-β in powder form in rabbits has been described.[115] HP-β-CyD was useful as a biocompatible solubilizer for lipophilic absorption enhancers involved in the nasal preparations of peptides.[116] When insulin was administered nasally to rats, simultaneous use of an oily penetration enhancer, HPE-101, (1-[2-(decylthio)ethyl]azacyclopentane-2-one) or oleic acid solubilized in HP-β-CyD showed a marked increase in serum immunoreactive insulin levels and a marked hypoglycaemia (Fig. 37.10). The potentiation of the enhancing effect of HPE-101 by HP-β-CyD can be explained by the

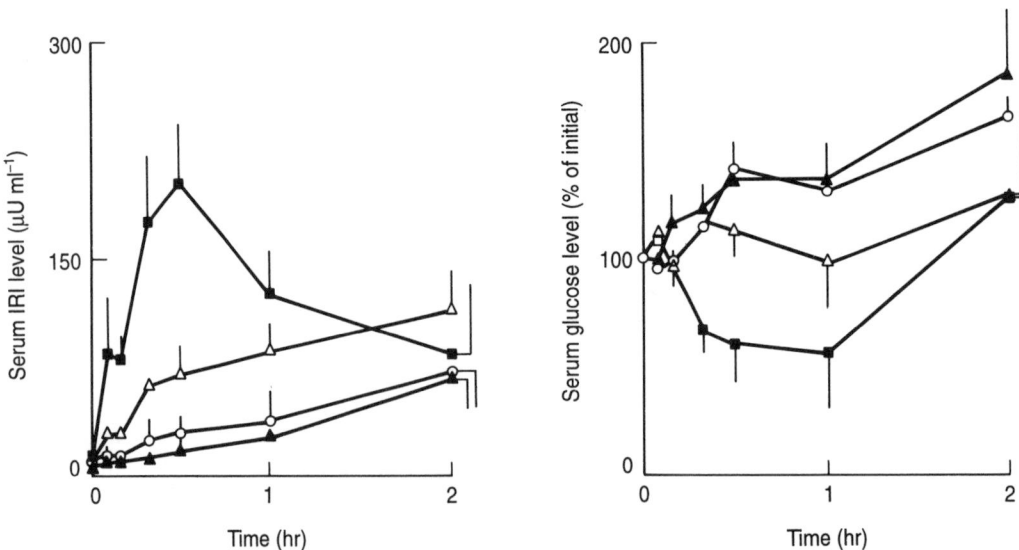

Fig. 37.10 Serum levels of immunoreactive insulin (IRI) and glucose after nasal administration of insulin (21 U/body) with HPE-101 (1% w/v) and/or HP-β-CyD (10% w/v) to rats.
○, Insulin alone; ▲, with HP-β-CyD; △, with HPE-101; ■, with HPE-101 and HP-β-CyD. Each point represents the mean ± SE of 4 rats.

facilitated transfer of HPE-101 into the nasal mucosa. Studies on the release of membrane proteins and scanning electron-microscopic observations of rat nasal mucosa indicated that the local mucosal damage due to the combination with HP-β-CyD may not be serious obstacles to their safe use.

2. Stabilization

Potential use of HP-β-CyD in peptide formulations has been reviewed.[117] For example, HP-β-CyD prevented the heat-induced charge alterations and loss of antigen-binding capacity of lyophilized monoclonal antibody (MN12) during storage.[118] Also, G_2-β-CyD has been shown to be an effective stabilizer in preventing the degradation of lyophilized tumour necrosis factor (TNF) during storage and freeze-drying processes.[119]

Basic fibroblast growth factor (bFGF) is a potent mitgen that stimulates the proliferation of a wide variety of cells and could play a crucial role in wound healing processes. The therapeutic potential of bFGF has not been fully realized, however, because of its susceptibility to proteolytic inactivation and short duration of retention at the site of action. Recent studies have demonstrated that sulphated oligosaccharides, including a sodium salt of β-CyD sulphate (Na·β-CyD·sul) have high affinity for bFGF and protect it from heat, acid and proteolytic degradation. Unfortunately, the highly hydrophilic nature of Na· β-CyD· sul is not suited to the design of bFGF formulations with controlled-release features. A water-insoluble aluminium salt of β-CyD sulfate (Al β-CyD·sul) was prepared, and its possible utility as a stabilizer and sustained-release carrier for recombinant human bFGF was evaluated. An adsorbate of bFGF with Al· β-CyD· sul was prepared by incubating the protein with a suspension of Al· CyD· sul in water.[120] The mitogenetic activity of bFGF released from the adsorbate, as indicated by the proliferation of kidney cells of baby hamster (BHK-21), was almost comparable with that of the

Table 37.5   Effects of β-CyD·suls and additives (25 mg ml^{-1}) on stability of bFGF (250 μg ml^{-1}) in the presence of pepsin (50 μg ml^{-1}, pH 1.6) for 3 h at 37°C.

CyDs	pH	Remaining bFGF (%)[a]
Without additives	1.67	ND
α-CyD	1.67	ND
β-CyD	1.60	ND
γ-CyD	1.66	ND
HP-β-CyD	1.65	ND
Na· α-CyD· Sul	1.74	1.6 ± 1.3
Na· β-CyD· Sul	1.74	3.3 ± 1.4
Na· γ-CyD· Sul	1.73	5.1 ± 1.0
Na· HP-β-CyD· Sul	1.63	4.5 ± 3.2
Al· α-CyD· Sul	3.81	96.4 ± 1.2
Al· β-CyD· Sul	3.88	99.2 ± 2.6
Al· γ-CyD· Sul	3.82	96.5 ± 3.1
Al· HP-β-CyD· Sul	3.86	93.6 ± 2.1
Dextran sulfate	1.84	20.2 ± 9.6
Sucralfate	3.78	59.5 ± 6.1

[a]Each value represents the mean ± SD of 3 determinations.
ND = not detectable.

intact bFGF. Interestingly, Al·β-CyD·sul significantly protected bFGF from proteolytic degradation by pepsin and α-chymotrypsin compared with their sodium salts and other oligosaccharides (Table 37.5). The *in vivo* release of bFGF from the adsorbate was proportional to the increase in the Al·β-CyD· sul/protein ratio in the adsorbate. Of the bFGF preparations evaluated, the adsorbate of bFGF with Al·β-CyD·sul, when given subcutaneously to rats, showed the most prominent increase in the formation of granulation tissues, owing to the stabilization and slow release of the mitogen. These results suggest that the adsorbate of bFGF with Al·β-CyD·sul has potent therapeutic efficacy for wound healing, and may be applicable to oral protein formulations for the treatment of intestinal mucosal erosions.

3. Prevention of self-association

Self-association of the insulin molecule into oligomers and macromolecular aggregates leads to complications in the development of long-term insulin therapeutic systems and limits the rate of subcutaneous absorptions, a process which is too slow to mimic the physiological plasma insulin profile at the time of meal consumption. These problems are further complicated by the tendency for insulin to adsorb on to the surfaces of containers and devices, perhaps by mechanisms similar to those inducing aggregation. Thus, many attempts have been made to prevent aggregation and surface adsorption in parenteral formulations.[119] Among the hydrophilic CyDs tested, HP-β-CyD and G_2-β-CyD significantly reduced the adsorption to containers and the self-association of insulin at neutral pH. Both hydrophilic β-CyDs facilitated the permeation of insulin through ultrafiltration membranes (Fig. 37.11). The increased permeation of insulin was much greater than that of EDTA which is known to prevent the self-association of insulin by sequestering zinc ions from insulin oligomers. By the addition of

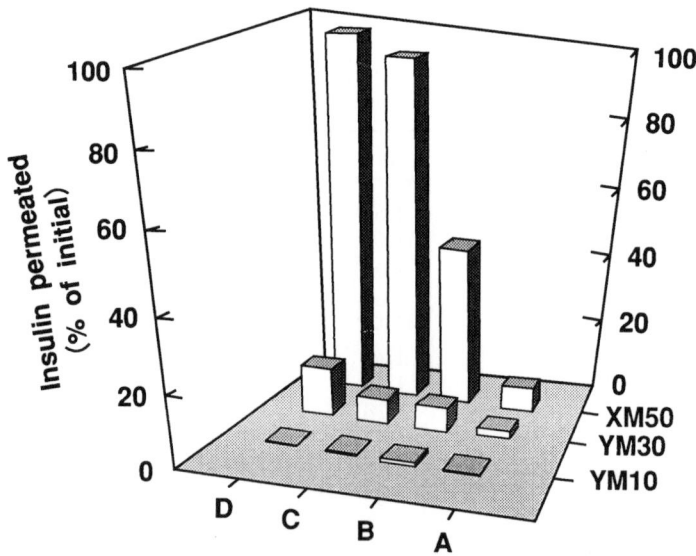

Fig. 37.11 Effects of β-CyDs (0.1 M) and EDTA (0.2 mM) on permeation of insulin (0.1 mM) through ultrafiltration membranes in phosphate buffer (pH 6.8, μ = 0.2) at 25°C.
(A) insulin alone, (B) with EDTA, (C) with HP-β-CyD, (D) with G_2-β-CyD. The membranes of YM-10, YM-30 and XM-50 were rated at pore sizes 10 000, 30 000, and 50 000 nominal molecular weight cut off, respectively.

β-CyDs, the surface tension of insulin solutions was increased, whereas decreased by EDTA. In the circular dichroism (CD) spectra of insulin, β-CyDs increased the negative CD intensity around 208 nm assigned to the α-helix structure of insulin, while decreased that around 275 nm assigned to the antiparallel β-structure of insulin oligomers. These spectral changes were in good agreement of those observed when insulin aggregates are dissociated to monomer or lower-order aggregates. In ^{1}H NMR measurements, G_2-β-CyD significantly altered the aromatic regions of insulin, particularly B24(Phe) and B26(Tyr), which are involved in the association of insulin to form an antiparallel β-sheet around the carboxyl terminal of the B-chain. The inhibition mechanism of β-CyDs seems to be different from that of EDTA: EDTA sequesters the binding zinc ions from insulin and dissociates the hexamer or higher-order aggregates to the dimer, whereas β-CyDs may interact with hydrophobic amino acid residues to prevent the direct contact of insulin molecules.

H.   Combined use of CyDs with additives

In the previous sections, the inclusion ability of CyDs has mainly been focused on modification of the pharmaceutical properties of drug molecules. However, practical formulations usually contain considerable amounts of pharmaceutical excipients and/or additives to maintain the efficacy and safety of the drug molecules. To extend their functions, attention should be given to the improvement of the properties of pharmaceutical additives by means of complexation with CyDs. Since CyDs are capable of modifying the physicochemical properties of hydrophobic guest molecules, a suitable combination of CyDs with additives will be particularly useful in the potentiation of drug efficacy.[69] In this section, therefore, a new strategy of CyDs applications will be described for the design of advanced dosage forms.

1.   Modified release of nifedipine

Conventional formulations of nifedipine must be dosed either twice or three times daily because of the short elimination half-life, due to considerable first pass metabolism, producing significant fluctuations in plasma drug concentrations. To attain a prolonged therapeutic effect and a reduced incidence of side-effects, many attempts have been made to maintain a suitable plasma level of nifedipine for long periods with much reduced frequency of administration. In the design of a modified-release formulation of nifedipine the following desirable attributes were sought: (a) the release should be at least 90% within 6–8 h, which is the average passage time of a tablet in the human GI tract after oral administration; (b) adequate release of nifedipine in the early stage is necessary to reduce the significant first pass metabolism in the intestine and liver, which may offer a more balanced bioavailability; (c) nifedipine should be released according to zero-order kinetics over an extended period, to take advantage of such therapeutic advantages as duration of pharmacological effect and reduction of side-effects. With these goals, a series of formulations of double-layer tablets containing a fast-release portion (FRP) and a slow-release portion (SRP) were designed.[121,122] The *in vitro* release rate of nifedipine from tablets containing nifedipine–HP-β-CyD (molar ratio of 1 : 1) and small amount of HCO-60®, nonionic surfactant, was much greater than those of drug or the complex alone, and this fast-release property was maintained for long periods of storage. In contrast, the release of nifedipine from hydroxypropylcellulose (HPC) solid dispersions was retarded with increasing viscosity of the HPC (L, M, H) or amount of each HPC. An optimal formulation of the double-layer tablet was

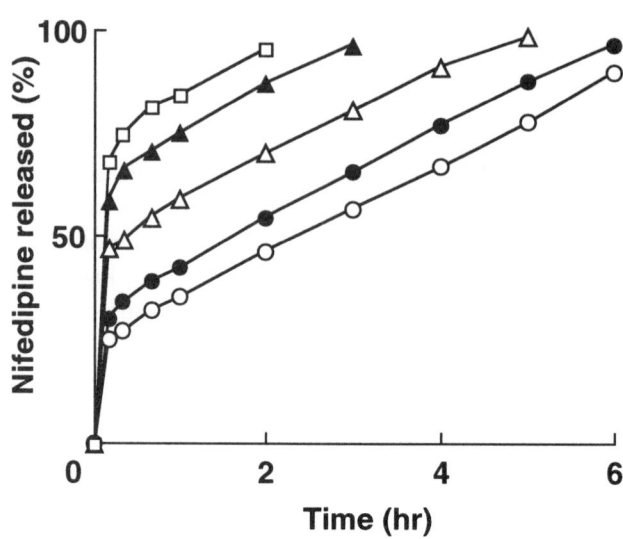

Fig. 37.12 Release profiles of nifedipine from double-layer tablets (25 mg as 5 mg nifedipine) consisting of nifedipine-HP-β-CyD with 3% HCO-60 as fast-release portion (FRP) and nifedipine-HPC-M as slow-release portion (SRP) in various weight ratios (FRP : SRP) in water at 37°C:
○, 1 : 3; ●, 1 : 2; △, 1 : 1; ▲, 2 : 1; □, 3 : 1.

tested by changing the ratios of the components (Fig. 37.12).[123] A double-layer tablet consisting of HP-β-CyD with 3% HCO-60®/(HPC-L : HPC-M) in a weight ratio of 1/(1.5 : 1.5) was found to be an appropriate modified-release formulation because it showed zero-order release from the SRP after the burst release from the FRP. This preparation exhibited prolonged plasma nifedipine levels without decrease of AUC in dogs, and the retarding behaviour was superior to that of a commercially available slow-release nifedipine product (Adalat L-20®). It is noteworthy that the release rate of nifedipine from this formulation was hardly affected by the pH of the medium and the rotation speed of the paddle in the dissolution test during accelerated storage (60°C, 75% RH). These findings suggest that a combination of HP-β-CyD, HCO-60® and HPCs can serve as a modified-release carrier of nifedipine and can be applied to other poorly water-soluble drugs with short elimination half-lives.

2. Transdermal delivery of prostaglandin E₁

Transdermal delivery of PGE₁ as an alternative to parenteral injection has engendered much recent interest in the treatment of peripheral vascular disorders. Since PGE₁ is chemically unstable and permeates poorly into the skin, a topical preparation capable of overcoming these problems needs to be devised to realize the full therapeutic potential of PGE₁. Our recent studies have shown that CME-β-CyD markedly improves the chemical stability of PGE₁ in aqueous solution and ointments.[124] Topical application of an ointment containing PGE₁–CME-β-CyD complex supplemented with HPE-101, an oily penetration enhancer, on to the skin of hairless mice resulted in a significant increase in the cutaneous blood flow owing to the vasodilating action of PGE₁.[125] The combination of CME-β-CyD and HPE-101 enhanced the percutaneous penetration of PGE₁ in a synergistic manner; CME-β-CyD assisted the release of HPE-101 from the ointment base and its entry into the skin, which may facilitate the percutaneous penetration of PGE_1.[126] Furthermore, this formulation suppressed the bioconversion of PGE_1 to give less pharmacologically active metabolites during the passage through the skin, which delivers intact PGE_1 more effectively to the site of action. Figure 37.13 shows the effects of topically applied PGE_1 or its CyD complexes in FAPG ointments supplemented with HPE-101 on the peripheral vascular occlusive sequelae induced by sodium laurate in the ears of rabbits.[127] After the intra-arterial injection of sodium laurate, vascular occlusive lesions became progressively aggravated, finally resulting in degeneration or necrosis over the entire area of the ear. PGE_1 and its CyD complexes, when supplemented with HPE-101, significantly protected against the vascular occlusive sequelae. In particular, the ointment containing PGE_1–CME-β-CyD complex supplemented with HPE-101 showed the most marked inhibitory effect on the progress of the lesions; only regional discoloration was observed on day 7 after the injection of laurate. The inhibitory effect of PGE_1 ointments was consistent with the sequence of magnitude of their vasodilating actions. Skin compatibility tests of PGE_1 ointments suggested no serious obstacles to their safe use. Accordingly, topical application of PGE_1 may be a rational choice for minimizing systemic side-effects and patient compliance for long-term therapy.

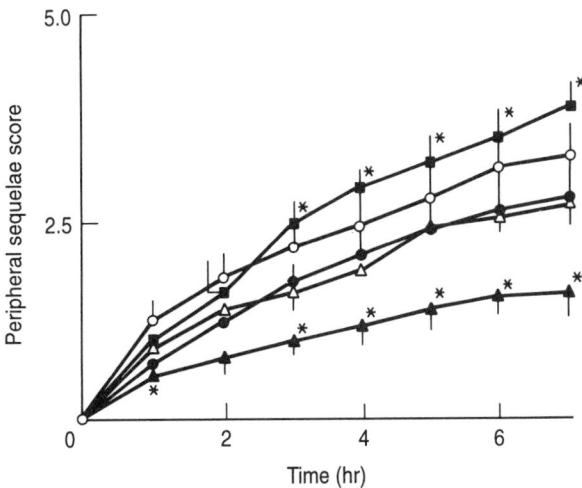

Fig. 37.13   Effects of topically applied PGE_1 or its β-CyD complexes in FAPG ointments (500 mg, 0.01% PGE_1) supplemented with HPE-101 (3 w/w%) on laurate-induced peripheral occlusive sequelae in ears of rabbits. ■, FAPG base; ○, PGE_1 alone; ●, PGE_1 with HPE-101; △, β-CyD complex with HPE-101; ▲, CME-β-CyD complex with HPE-101. Each point represents the mean ± SE of 3–6 rabbits. *$p < 0.05$ vs PGE_1 with HPE-101.

3.   *Transmucosal delivery of morphine*

The potent opioid morphine has been used for preoperative sedation and anxiolysis in paediatric patients and for the management of postoperative pain. In advanced cancer patients there is a great clinical need for the development of long-acting rectal preparations of morphine in the treatment of intractable chronic pain. However, the use of prolonged release of drugs from suppositories is limited, showing a wide interindividual variation of rectal bioavailability. We have recently demonstrated that some hydrophilic CyDs enhanced the rectal absorption of morphine in rabbits, and xanthan gum, a polysaccharide type polymer with high swelling capacity, sustained the *in vitro* release of morphine from the suppository.[128] An attempt was made to design a more effective rectal delivery system for morphine using α-CyD as an absorption enhancer and xanthan gum as a swelling hydrogel in Witepsol H-15 hollow type suppositories, and this was tested in rabbits.[129] With the combination of α-CyD and xanthan gum, the plasma morphine level was significantly sustained, with an improved bioavailability. Observation of the distribution behaviour of suppositories in rabbit rectum and colon after rectal administration showed that the xanthan gum prevented the upward spread of the drug in the rectum. This suggests that the absorption site for morphine should be limited to the lower part of the rectum so as to eliminate the first pass metabolism of morphine in the liver. In addition, gross and microscopic observations indicated that this preparation was less irritating to the rectal mucosa. From the viewpoints of safety and efficacy, therefore, this retentive opioid preparation may promise excellent therapeutic potential for the treatment of severe malignant cancer pain, offering an improvement in quality of life.

Noninvasive transmucosal routes of administration for morphine have received much current attention because these routes could bypass the gastrointestinal degradation and hepatic first pass metabolism of morphine as well as providing ease of administration. We have recently found that the nasal bioavailability of morphine in solution was greater than that of the rectal suppository in rats. Of the CyD derivatives tested, DM-β-CyD increased the rate of nasal absorption of morphine, when its plasma drug level–time profile was similar to that obtained after intravenous administration. Furthermore, DM-β-CyD increased the cerebrospinal fluid (CSF) level of morphine after nasal administration, suggesting that DM-β-CyD may facilitate the transport of morphine not only to the systemic circulation but also to CSF. Interestingly, HP-γ-CyD sustained plasma levels of morphine (Fig. 37.14), probably owing to the formation of less membrane permeable complex and/or the increase in the viscosity of the solution, since a viscosity-enhancing polymer, HPC-H, sustained plasma levels of nasally administered morphine. These findings suggest that the combination of CyDs and viscous polymers may be useful for optimizing the transmucosal delivery of morphine and potentiating its analgesic action.

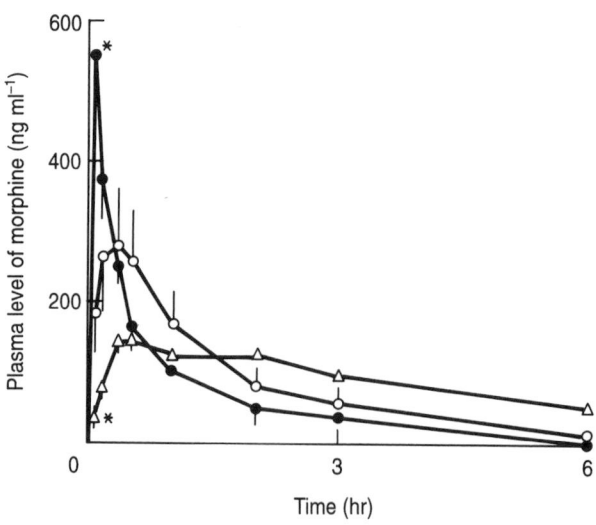

Fig. 37.14   Plasma levels of morphine after nasal administration of morphine hydrochloride (MH; 1 mg kg^{-1}) with DM-β-CyD or HP-γ-CyD in rats.
○, MH alone; ●, with DM-β-CyD (50 mM); △, with HP-γ-CyD (200 mM). Each point represents the mean ± of 2–8 rats. *$p < 0.05$ vs drug alone.

IV. CONCLUSION

The natural CyDs and their synthetic derivatives have successfully been applied to improve undesirable drug properties such as solubility, stability or bioavailability. In addition, the enhancement of drug activity and selective transfer or the reduction of side-effects has been achieved by means of inclusion complex formation. The bioadaptable CyDs can serve as potent absorption enhancers or coenhancers, and the release rate of water-soluble drugs including peptides can be appropriately modified by combination of hydrophobic, hydrophilic and ionizable CyDs. Since CyDs are also useful in extending the functions of pharmaceutical additives, the combination of molecular encapsulation with other carrier materials will be an effective and a valuable tool in the improvement of drug properties. Although the various CyDs described here have many advantages as novel drug carriers for development of advanced dosage forms, the toxicological issues together with their biological fates need to be investigated in detail.

REFERENCES

1. Szejtli, J. (1982) *Cyclodextrins and Their Inclusion Complexes.* Akadémiai Kiadó, Budapest.
2. Saenger, W. (1980) Cyclodextrin inclusion compounds in research and industry. *Angew. Chem. Int. Ed. Engl.* **19**: 344–362.
3. Szejtli, J. (1988) *Cyclodextrin Technology.* Kluwer Academic Publishers, Dordrecht, The Netherlands.
4. Uekama, K. (1981) Pharmaceutical applications of cyclodextrin complexations. *Yakugaku Zasshi* **101**: 857–873.
5. Duchêne, D. (1987) *Cyclodextrins and Their Industrial Uses.* Editions de Santé, Paris.
6. Uekama, K. and Otagiri, M. (1987) Cyclodextrins in drug carrier systems. *CRC Crit. Rev. Ther. Drug Carrier Systems* **3**: 1–40.
7. Duchêne, D. (1991) *New Trends in Cyclodextrins and Their Derivatives.* Editions de Santé, Paris.
8. Uekama, K., Hirayama, F. and Irie, T. (1991) Pharmaceutical uses of cyclodextrin derivatives. In Szycher, M. (ed.) (1991) *High Performance Biomaterials, A Comprehensive Guide to Medical and Pharmaceutical Applications,* pp. 789–806. Technomic, Lancaster, PA.
9. Szejtli, J. (1983) Dimethyl-β-cyclodextrin as parenteral drug carrier. *J. Incl. Phenom.* **1**: 135–150.
10. Uekama, K. (1985) Pharmaceutical applications of methylated cyclodextrins. *Pharm. Int.* **6**: 61–65.
11. Pitha, J. and Pitha, J. (1985) Amorphous water-soluble derivatives of cyclodextrins, non-toxic dissolution enhancing excipients. *J. Pharm. Sci.* **74**: 987–990.
12. Müller, B. W. and Brauns, U. (1985) Solubilization of drugs by modified β-cyclodextrins. *Int. J. Pharm.* **26**: 77–88.
13. Yoshida, A., Arima, H., Uekama, K. and Pitha, J. (1988) Pharmaceutical evaluation of hydroxyalkyl ethers of β-cyclodextrins. *Int. J. Pharm.* **46**: 217–222.
14. Yoshida, A., Yamamoto, M., Irie, T., Hirayama, F. and Uekama, K. (1989) Some pharmaceutical properties of 3-hydroxypropyl- and 2,3-dihydroxypropyl-β-cyclodextrins and thier solubilizing and stabilizing abilities. *Chem. Pharm. Bull.* **37**: 1059–1063.
15. Brewster, M. E., Simpkins, J. W., Hora, M. S., Stern, W. C. and Bodor, N. (1989) The potential use of cyclodextrins in parenteral formulations. *J. Parent. Sci. Technol.* **43**: 231–240.
16. Koizumi, K., Utamura, T., Sato, M. and Yagi, Y. (1986) Isolation and characterization of branched cyclodextrins. *Carbohydr. Res.* **153**: 55–67.
17. Yamamoto, M., Yoshida, A., Hirayama, F. and Uekama, K. (1989) Some physicochemical properties of branched β-cyclodextrins and their inclusion characteristics. *Int. J. Pharm.* **49**: 163–171.
18. Hirayama, F. (1993) Development and pharmaceutical evaluation of hydrophobic derivatives as modified-release drug carrier. *Yakugaku Zasshi* **113**: 425–437.

19. Hirayama, F., Kurihara, M., Horichi, Y., Utsuki, T., Uekama, K. and Yamasaki, M. (1993) Preparation of heptakis(2,6-di-O-ethyl)-β-cyclodextrin and its nuclear magnetic resonance spectroscopic characterization. *Pharm. Res.* **10**: 208–213.

20. Uekama, K., Arima, H., Irie, T., Matsubara, K. and Kuriki, T. (1989) Sustained release of buserelin acetate, a luteinizing hormome-releasing hormone agonist, from the injectable oily preparation utilizing ethylated β-cyclodextrin. *J. Pharm. Pharmacol.* **41**: 874–876.

21. Uekama, K., Horiuchi, Y., Irie, T. and Hirayama, F. (1989) O-Carboxymethyl-O-ethyl-cyclomaltoheptaose as a delayed-release type drug carrier. Improvement of the oral bioavailability of diltiazem. *Carbohydr. Res.* **192**: 323–330.

22. Folkman, J., Weisz, P. B., Joullie, M. M., Li, W. W. and Ewing, W. R. (1989) Control of angiogenesis with synthetic heparin substitutes. *Science* **243**: 1490–1493.

23. Uekama, K. (1987) Cyclodextrin inclusion compounds: effects on stability and bio-pharmaceutical properties. In Breimer, D. D. and Speiser, P. (eds) *Topics in Pharmaceutical Sciences 1987*. Elsevier, Amsterdam, pp. 181–194.

24. Coleman, A. W., Nicolis, I., Keller, N. and Dalbiez, J. P. (1992) Aggregation of cyclodextrins; an explanation of the abnormal solubility of β-cyclodextrin. *J. Incl. Phenom.* **13**: 139–143.

25. Okada, Y., Kubota, Y., Koizumi, K., Hizukuri, S., Ohfuji, T. and Ogata, K. (1988) Some properties and inclusion behaviour of branched cyclodextrins. *Chem. Pharm. Bull.* **36**: 2176–2185.

26. Arima, H., Kondo, T., Irie, T., Hirayama, F., Uekama, K., Miyaji, T. and Inoue, Y. (1992) Use of water-soluble β-cyclodextrin derivatives as carriers of anti-inflammatory drug biphenylylacetic acid in rectal delivery. *Yakugaku Zasshi,* **112**: 65–72.

27. Horiuchi, Y., Hirayama, F. and Uekama, K. (1991) Improvement of stability and bioavailability of 1-hexylcarbamoyl-5-fluorouracil (HCFU) by O-carboxymethyl-O-ethyl-β-cyclodextrin. *Yakugaku Zasshi* **111**, 592–599.

28. Bender, M. L. and Komiyama, M. (1978) *Cyclodextrin Chemistry*. Springer-Verlag, Berlin.

29. Hirayama, F., Kurihara, M., Utsuki, T. and Uekama, K. (1993) Inhibitory effect of guest molecules on acid-catalyzed ring-opening of β-cyclodextrin. *J. Chem. Soc., Chem. Commun.* 1578–1580.

30. Marshall, J. J. and Miwa, I. (1981) Kinetic difference between hydrolyses of γ-cyclodextrin by human salivary and pancreatic α-amylases. *Biochim. Biophys. Acta.* **661**: 142–147.

31. Yamamoto, M., Aritomi, H., Irie, T., Hirayama, F. and Uekama, K. (1991) Biopharmaceutical evaluation of maltosyl-β-cyclodextrin as a parenteral drug carrier. *S.T.P. Pharm. Sci* **1**: 397–402.

32. Brewster, M. E., Estes, K. S. and Bodor, N. (1990) An intravenous toxicity of study of 2-hydroxypropyl-β-cyclodextrin, a useful drug solubilizer, in rats and monkeys. *Int. J. Pharm.* **59**: 231–243.

33. Frijlink, H. W., Visser, J., Hefting, N. R., Oosting, R., Meijer, D. K. F. and Lerk, C. F. (1990) The pharmacokinetics of β-cyclodextrin and hydroxypropyl-β-cyclodextrin in the rat. *Pharm. Res.* **7**: 1248–1252.

34. Frank, D. W., Gray, J. E. and Weaver, R. N. (1976) Cyclodextrin nephrosis in the rat. *Am. J. Pathol.* **83**: 367–382.

35. Irie, T., Sunada, M., Otagiri, M., Uekama, K., Ohtani, Y., Yamada, Y. and Sugiyama, Y. (1982) Cyclodextrin-induced hemolysis and shape changes of human erythrocytes *in vitro*. *J. Pharmacobio-Dyn.* **5**: 741–744.

36. Ohtani, Y., Irie, T., Uekama, K., Fukunaga, K. and Pitha, J. (1989) Differential effects of α-, β-, and γ-cyclodextrins on human erythrocytes. *Eur. J. Biochem.* **186**: 17–22.

37. Gerloczy, A., Fonagy, A., Keresztes, P., Perlaky, L. and Szejtli, J. (1985) Absorption, distribution, excretion and metabolism of orally administered ^{14}C-β-cyclodextrin in rats. *Arzneimittel-Forsch.* **35**: 1042–1047.

38. Poelma, F. G. J., Tukker, J. J., Hilbers, H. W. and Jansen, A. C. A. (1989) Intestinal absorption of drugs II. The effects of inclusion in cyclodextrins on the absorption of dantrolene. *J. Incl. Phenom.* **7**: 423–430.

39. Arima, H., Kondo, T., Irie, T. and Uekama, K. (1992) Enhanced rectal absorption and reduced local irritation of anti-inflammatory drug ethyl 4-biphenylyl acetate in rats by complexation with water-soluble β-cyclodextrin derivatives and formulations as oleaginous suppository. *J. Pharm. Sci.* **81**: 1119–1125.

40. Uekama, K., Imai, T., Maeda, T., Irie, T., Hirayama, F. and Otagiri, M. (1985) Improvement of dissolution and suppository release characteristics of flurbiprofen by inclusion complexation with heptakis(2,6-di-O-methyl)-β-cyclodextrin. *J. Pharm. Sci.* **74**: 841–845.

41. Arima, H., Adachi, H., Irie, T., Uekama, K. and Pitha, J. (1990) Enhancement of the anti-inflammatory effect of ethyl 4-biphenylylacetate in ointment by β-cyclodextrin derivatives: increased absorption and localized activation of the prodrug in rats. *Pharm. Res.* **7**: 1152–1156.
42. Vollmer, U., Stoppie, P., Mesens, J., Wilffert, B. and Peters, Th. (1992) Hydroxypropyl-β-cyclodextrin in transdermal absorption *in vivo* in rats. In Hedges, A. R. (ed.) *Minutes of the 6th International. Symposium on Cyclodextrins*, pp. 535–538. Editions de Santé, Paris.
43. Dietzel, K., Estes, K. S., Brewster, M. E., Bodor, N. and Derendorf, H. (1990) The use of 2-hydroxypropyl-β-cyclodextrin as a vehicle for intravenous administration of dexamethasone in dogs. *Int. J. Pharm.* **59**: 225–230.
44. Hoshino, T., Uekama, K. and Pitha, J. (1993) Increase in temperature enhances solubility of drugs in aqueous solutions of hydroxypropylcyclodextrins. *Int. J. Pharm.* **98**: 239–242.
45. Brewster, M. E., Estes, K. S., Loftsson, T., Perchalski, R., Derendorf, H., Mullersman, G. and Bodor, N. (1988) Improved delivery through biological membranes XXXI: Solubilization and stabilization of an estradiol chemical delivery system by modified β-cyclodextrins. *J. Pharm. Sci.* **77**: 981–985.
46. Millard, W. J., Romano, T. M., Bodor, N. and Simpkins, J. W. (1990) Growth hormome (GH) secretory dynamics in animals administered estradiol utilizing a chemical delivery system. *Pharm. Res.* **7**: 1011–1018.
47. Merkus, F. W. H. M., Verhoef, J. C., Romeijn, S. G. and Schipper, N. G. M. (1991) Absorption enhancing effect of cyclodextrins on intranasally administered insulin in rats. *Pharm. Res.* **8**: 588–592.
48. Kurihara, M., Hirayama, F., Uekama, K. and Yamasaki, M. (1990) Improvement of some pharmaceutical properties of nocloprost by β- and γ-cyclodextrin complexations. *J. Incl. Phenom.* **8**: 363–373.
49. Utsuki, T., Imamura, K., Hirayama, F. and Uekama, K. (1993) Stoichiometry-dependent changes of solubility and photoreactivity of an antiulcer agent, 2′-carboxymethoxy-4,4′-bis(3-methyl-2-butenyloxy)chalcone, in cyclodextrin inclusion complexes. *Eur. J. Pharm. Sci.* **1**: 81–87.
50. Hirayama, F., Kurihara, M. and Uekama, K. (1984) Improving the aqueous stability of prostaglandin E_2 and prostaglandin A_2 by inclusion complexation with methylated β-cyclodextrins. *Chem. Pharm. Bull.* **32**: 4237–4240.
51. Yamamoto, M., Hirayama, F. and Uekama, K. (1992) Improvement of stability and dissolution of prostaglandin E_1 by maltosyl-β-cyclodextrin in lyophilized formulation. *Chem. Pharm. Bull.* **40**: 747–751.
52. Hirayama, F., Kurihara, M. and Uekama, K. (1987) Improvement of chemical instability of prostacyclin in aqueous solution by complexation with methylated cyclodextrins. *Int. J. Pharm.* **35**: 193–199.
53. Uekama, K., Fujinaga, T., Hirayama, F., Otagiri, M., Yamasaki, M., Seo, H., Hashimoto, T. and Tsuruoka, M. (1983) Improvement of the oral bioavailability of digitalis glycosides by cyclodextrin complexation. *J. Pharm. Sci.* **72**: 1338–1341.
54. Yoshida, A., Yamamoto, M., Hirayama, F. and Uekama, K. (1988) Improvement of chemical instability of digitoxin in aqueous solution by complexation with β-cyclodextrin derivatives. *Chem. Pharm. Bull.* **36**: 4075–4080.
55. Uekama, K., Fujinaga, T., Hirayama, F., Otagiri, M., Kurono, Y. and Ikeda, K. (1982) Effects of cyclodextrins on the acid hydrolysis of digoxin. *J. Pharm. Pharmacol.* **34**: 627–630.
56. Seo, H. and Uekama, K. (1989) Enhanced bioavailability of digoxin by γ-cyclodextrin complexation: evaluation for sublingual and oral administrations in human. *Yakugaku Zasshi* **109**: 778–782.
57. Sugimoto, I., Kuchiki, K. and Nakagawa, H. (1981) Stability of nifedipine-polyvinylpyrrolidone coprecipitate. *Chem. Pharm. Bull.* **29**: 1715–1723.
58. Uekama, K., Ikegami, K., Wang, Z., Horiuchi, Y. and Hirayama, F. (1992) Inhibitory effect of 2-hydroxypropyl-β-cyclodextrin on crystal-growth of nifedipine during storage: superior dissolution and oral bioavailability compared with polyvinylpyrrolidone K-30. *J. Pharm. Pharmacol.* **44**: 73–78.
59. Kikuchi, M., Hirayama, F. and Uekama, K. (1987) Improvement of chemical instability of carmofur in β-cyclodextrin solid complex by utilizing some organic acids. *Chem. Pharm. Bull.* **35**: 315–319.
60. Kikuchi, M., Uemura, Y., Hirayama, F., Otagiri, M. and Uekama, K. (1984) Improvement of some pharmaceutical properties of carmofur by cyclodextrin complexation. *J. Incl. Phenom.* **2**: 623–630.

61. Kikuchi, M., Hirayama, F. and Uekama, K. (1987) Improvement of oral and rectal bioavailability of carmofur by methylated β-cyclodextrin complexations. *Int. J. Pharm.* **38**: 191–198.
62. Hirayama, F., Hirashima, N., Abe, K., Uekama, K., Ijitsu, T. and Ueno, M. (1988) Utilization of diethyl-β-cyclodextrin as a sustained-release carrier for isosorbide dinitrate. *J. Pharm. Sci.* **77**: 233–236.
63. Uekama, K., Hirashima, N., Horiuchi, Y., Hirayama, F., Ijitsu, T. and Ueno, M. (1987) Ethylated β-cyclodextrins as hydrophobic drug carriers: sustained release of diltiazem in the rat. *J. Pharm. Sci.* **76**: 660–661.
64. Uekama, K., Horikawa, T., Yamanaka, M. and Hirayama, F. (1994) Peracylated β-cyclodextrin as novel sustained-release carrier for water-soluble drug, molsidomine. *J. Pharm. Pharmacol.* **46**: 714–717.
65. Uekama, K., Horikawa, T., Horiuchi, Y. and Hirayama, F. (1993) *In vitro* and *in vivo* evaluation of delayed-release behaviour of diltiazem from its O-carboxymethyl-O-ethyl-β-cyclodextrin complex. *J. Controlled Release* **25**: 99–106.
66. Horiuchi, Y., Abe, K., Hirayama, F. and Uekama, K. (1991) Control of theophylline by β-cyclodextrin derivatives: hybridizing of hydrophilic and ionizable β-cyclodextrin complexes. *J. Controlled Release* **15**: 177–182.
67. Matsubara, K., Kuriki, T., Arima, H., Wakamatsu, K., Irie, T. and Uekama, K. (1990) Possible use of diethyl-β-cyclodextrin in preparation of sustained release oily injection of buserelin acetate (LHRH agonist). *Drug Del. Syst.* **5**: 95–99.
68. Matsubara, K., Irie, T. and Uekama, K. (1994) Controlled-release of the LHRH agonist buserelin acetate from injectable suspensions containing triacetylated cyclodextrins in the oil vehicle. *J. Controlled Release* **31**: 173–180.
69. Uekama, K., Hirayama, F. and Irie, T. (1994) Application of cyclodexterin. In Boer, A. G., (ed.) *Absorption Enhancement: Concept, Possibilities and Limitations*, Vol. 3, pp. 411–456. Harwood Publishers, Amsterdam.
70. Tokumura, T., Nanba, M., Tsushima, Y., Tatsuishi, K., Kayano, M., Machida, Y. and Nagai, T. (1986) Enhancement of bioavailability of cinnarizine from its β-cyclodextrin complex on oral administration with DL-phenylalanine as a competing agent. *J. Pharm. Sci.* **75**: 391–394.
71. Seo, H., Tsuruoka, M., Hashimoto, T., Fujinaga, T., Otagiri, M. and Uekama, K. (1983) Enhancement of oral bioavailability of spironolactone by β- and γ-cyclodextrin complexations. *Chem. Pharm. Bull.* **31**: 286–291.
72. Uekama, K., Fujinaga, T., Otagiri, M., Matsuo, N. and Matsuoka, Y. (1983) Improvement of dissolution and chemical stability of proscillaridin by cyclodextrin complexations. *Acta Pharm. Suec.* **20**: 287–294.
73. Uekama, K., Otagiri, M., Uemura, Y., Fujinaga, T., Arimori, K., Matsuo, N., Tasaki, K. and Sugii, A. (1983) Improvement of oral bioavailability of prednisolone by β-cyclodextrin complexation in humans. *J. Pharmacobio-Dyn.* **6**: 124–127.
74. Uekama, K., Narisawa, S., Hirayama, F. and Otagiri, M. (1983) Improvement of dissolution and absorption characteristics of benzodiazepines by cyclodextrin complexation. *Int. J. Pharm.* **16**: 327–338.
75. Uekama, K., Matsuo, N., Hirayama, F., Ichibagase, H., Arimori, K., Tsubaki, K. and Satake, K. (1980) Enhanced bioavialability of acetohexamide by β-cyclodextrin complexation. *Yakugaku Zasshi* **100**: 903–909.
76. Miyaji, T., Inoue, Y., Acarturk, F., Imai, T., Otagiri, M. and Uekama, K. (1992) Improvement of oral bioavailability of fenbufen by cyclodextrin complexations. *Acta Pharm. Nord.* **4**: 17–22.
77. Irie, T., Tsunenari, Y., Uekama, K. and Pitha, J. (1988) Effect of bile on the intestinal absorption of α-cyclodextrin in rats. *Int. J. Pharm.* **43**: 41–44.
78. Nakanishi, K., Nadai, T., Masada, M. and Miyajima, K. (1992) Effect of cyclodextrins on biological membrane, II. Mechanism of enhancement of the intestinal absorption of non-absorbable drug by cyclodextrins. *Chem. Pharm. Bull.* **40**: 1252–1256.
79. Horiuchi, Y., Kikuchi, M., Hirayama, F., Uekama, K., Ueno, M. and Ijitsu, T. (1988) Improvement of bioavailability of menaquinone-4 by dimethyl-β-cyclodextrin complexation following oral administration. *Yakugaku Zasshi.* **108**: 1093–1100.
80. Ueno, M., Ijitsu, T., Horiuchi, Y., Hirayama, F. and Uekama, K. (1989) Improvement of dissolution and absorption characteristics of ubidecarenon by dimethyl-β-cyclodextrin complexation. *Acta Pharm. Nord.* **2**: 99–104.

81. Otagiri, M., Imai, T. and Uekama, K. (1982) Enhanced oral bioavailability of anti-inflammatory drug flurbiprofen in rabbits by tri-*O*-methyl-β-cyclodextrin complexation. *J. Pharmacobio-Dyn.*, **5**: 1027–1029.

82. Nakai, Y., Yamamoto, K., Terada, K., Horibe, H. and Ozawa, K. (1983) Interaction of tri-O-methyl-β-cyclodextrin with drugs, enhanced bioavailability of ketoprofen in rats when administered with tri-*O*-methyl-β-cyclodextrin. *Chem. Pharm. Bull.*, **31**: 3745–3747.

83. Kikuchi, M. and Uekama, K. (1988) Enhancement of antitumor activity of carmofur (HCFU) by dimethyl-β-cyclodextrin complexation in P-388 leukemia-bearing mice. *Xenobiotic Metab. Dispos.* **3**: 267–273.

84. Uekama, K., Horiuchi, Y., Kikuchi, M., Hirayama, F., Ijitsu, T. and Ueno, M. (1988) Enhanced dissolution and oral bioavailability of α-tocopheryl esters by dimethyl-β-cyclodextrin complexations. *J. Incl. Phenom.* **6**: 167–174.

85. Duchêne, D., Wouessidjewe, D. and Poelman, M. -C. (1991) Dermal uses of cyclodextrin and derivatives. In Duchêne, D. (ed.) *New Trends in Cyclodextrins and Their Derivatives*, pp. 447–481 Editions de Santé, Paris.

86. Otagiri, M., Fujinaga, T., Sakai, A. and Uekama, K. (1984) Effects of β- and γ-cyclodextrins on release of betamethasone from ointment bases. *Chem. Pharm. Bull.*, **32**: 2401–2405.

87. Orienti, I., Zecchi, V., Bertasi, V. and Fini, A. (1991) Release of ketoprofen from dermal bases in presence of cyclodextrins: effect of the affinity constant determined in semisolid vehicles. *Arch. Pharm. (Weinheim)* **324**: 943–947.

88. Uekama, K., Otagiri, M., Sakai, A., Irie, T., Matsuo, N. and Matsuoka, Y. (1985) Improvement in the percutaneous absorption of beclomethasone dipropionate by γ-cyclodextrin complexation. *J. Pharm. Pharmacol.* **37**: 532–535.

89. Arima, H., Adachi, H., Irie, T. and Uekama, K. (1990) Improved drug delivery through the skin by hydrophilic β-cyclodextrins: enhancement of anti-inflammatory effect of 4-biphenylylacetic acid in rats. *Drug. Invest.* **2**: 155–161.

90. Uekama, K., Maeda, T., Arima, H., Irie, T. and Hirayama, F. (1986) Possible utility of β-cyclodextrin complexation in the preparation of biphenylylactic acid suppository. *Yakugaku Zasshi* **106**: 1126–1130.

91. Arima, H., Irie, T. and Uekama, K. (1989) Differences in the enhancing effects of water-soluble β-cyclodextrins on the release of ethyl 4-biphenylyl acetate, an anti-inflammatory agent from an oleaginous suppository base. *Int. J. Pharm.* **57**: 107–115.

92. Hermens, W. A. J. J., Deurloo, M. J. M., Romeyn, S. G., Verhoef, J. C. and Merkus, F. W. H. M. (1990) Nasal absorption enhancement of 17β-estradiol by dimethyl-β-cyclodextrin in rabbits and rats. *Pharm. Res.* **7**: 500–503.

93. Schipper, N. G. M., Hermens, W. A. J. J., Romeyn, S. G., Verhoef, J. and Merkus, F. W. H. M. (1990) Nasal absorption of 17β-estradiol and progesterone from a dimethyl-cyclodextrin inclusion formulation in rats. *Int. J. Pharm.* **64**: 61–66.

94. Stuenkel, C. A., Dudley, R. E. and Yen, S. S. C. (1991) Sublingual administration of testosterone–hydroxypropyl-β-cyclodextrin inclusion complex simulates episodic androgen release in hypogonadal men. *J. Clin. Endocrinol. Metab.* **72**: 1054–1059.

95. Schipper, N. G. M., Verhoef, J. C. and Merkus, F. W. H. M. (1991) The nasal mucociliary clearance: relevance to nasal drug delivery. *Pharm. Res.* **8**: 807–814.

96. Hermens, W. A. J. J., Belder, C. W. J., Merkus, J. M. W. M., Hooymans, P. M., Verhoef, J. and Merkus, F. W. H. M. (1991) Intranasal estradiol administration to oophorectomized women. *Eur. J. Obstet. Gynecol. Reprod. Biol.* **40**: 35–41.

97. Yoshida, A., Yamamoto, M., Itoh, T., Irie, T., Hirayama, F. and Uekama, K. (1990) Utility of 2-hydroxypropyl-β-cyclodextrin in an intramuscular injectable preparation of nimodipine. *Chem. Pharm. Bull.* **38**: 176–179.

98. Irie, T., Otagiri, M., Uekama, K., Okano, Y. and Miyata, T. (1984) Alleviation of the chlorpromazine-induced muscular tissue damage by β-cyclodextrin complexation. *J. Incl. Phenom.* **2**: 637–644.

99. Imai, T., Maeda, T. and Otagiri, M. and Uekama, K. (1987) Improvement of absorption characteristics and reduction of irritation on stomach of flurbiprofen by complexation with various cyclodextrins. *Xenobiotic Metab. Dispos.* **2**: 657–664.

100. Ishida, K., Hoshino, T., Irie, T. and Uekama, K. (1988) Alleviation of chlorpromazine-

photosensitized contact dermatitis by β-cyclodextrin derivatives and their possible mechanisms. *Xenobiotic Metab. Dispos.* **3**: 377–386.

101. Hoshino, T., Ishida, K., Irie, T., Uekama, K. and Ono, T. (1989) An attempt to reduce the photosensitizing potential of chlorpromazine with the simultaneous use of β- and dimethyl-β-cyclodextrins in guinea pigs. *Arch. Dermatol. Res.*, **281**: 60–65.

102. Uekama, K., Irie, T. and Hirayama, F. (1978) Participation of cyclodextrin inclusion catalysis in photolysis of chlorpromazine to give promazine in aqueous solution. *Chem. Lett.* 1109–1112.

103. Hoshino, T., Ishida, K., Irie, T., Hirayama, F., Uekama, K. and Yamasaki, M. (1988) Reduction of photohemolytic activity of benoxaprofen by β-cyclodextrin complexation. *J. Incl. Phenom.* **6**: 415–423.

104. Hoshino, T., Ishida, K., Irie, T., Hirayama, F. and Uekama, K. (1987) Alleviation in protriptyline-photosensitized skin irritation by di-*O*-methyl-β-cyclodextrin complexation. *Int. J. Pharm.* **38**: 265–267.

105. Perrin, J. H., Field, F. P., Hansen, D. A., Mufson, R. A. and Torosian, G. (1978) β-Cyclodextrin as an aid to peritoneal dialysis. Renal toxicity of β-cyclodextrin in the rat. *Res. Commun. Chem. Pathol. Pharmacol.* **19**: 373–376.

106. Carpenter, T. O., Pettifor, J. M., Russell, R. M., Pitha, J., Mobarhan, S., Ossip, M. S., Wainer, S. and Anast, C. S. (1987) Severe hypervitaminosis A in siblings: evidence of variable tolerance to retinol intake. *J. Pediatr.* **111**: 507–512.

107. Irie, T., Fukunaga, K., Garwood, M. K., Carpenter, T. O., Pitha, J. and Pitha, J. (1992) Hydroxypropylcyclodextrins in parenteral use: II: Effects on transport and disposition of lipids in rabbits and humans. *J. Pharm. Sci.* **81**: 524–528.

108. Frijlink, H. W., Eissen, A. C., Hefting, N. R., Poelstra, K., Lerk, C. F. and Meijer, D. K. F. (1991) The effect of parenterally administered cyclodextrins on cholesterol levels in the rat. *Pharm. Res.* **8**: 9–16.

109. Irie, T., Fukunaga, K. and Pitha, J. (1992) Hydroxypropylcyclodextrins in parenteral use. I: Lipid dissolution and effects on lipid transfers *in vitro. J. Pharm. Sci.* **81**: 521–523.

110. Uekama, K., Shiotani, K., Irie, T., Ishimaru, Y. and Pitha, J. (1993) Protective effects of cyclodextrin sulphates against gentamicin-induced nephrotoxicity in the rat. *J. Pharm. Pharmacol.* **45**: 745–747.

111. Shimamoto, T. (1987) Pharmaceutical aspects: nasal and depot formulations of leuprolide. *J. Androl.* **8**: S14–16.

112. Irie, T., Wakamatsu, K., Arima, H., Aritomi, H. and Uekama, K. (1992) Enhancing effects of cyclodextrins on nasal absorption of insulin. *Int. J. Pharm.* **84**: 129–139.

113. Schipper, N. G. M., Verhoef, J., Romeijn, S. G. and Merkus, F. W. H. M. (1992) Absorption enhancers in nasal insulin delivery and their influence on nasal ciliary functioning. *J. Controlled Release* **21**: 173–186.

114. Irie, T., Arima, H., Abe, K., Uekama, K., Matsubara, K. and Kuriki, T. (1992) Possible mechanisms of cyclodextrin-enhanced nasal absorption of peptide and protein drugs. In Hedges, A. R. (ed.) *Minutes of the 6th International Symposium on Cyclodextrins*, pp. 503–508. Editions de Santé, Paris.

115. Maitani, Y., Igawa, T., Machida, Y. and Nagai, T. (1986) Intranasal administration of β-interferon in rabbits. *Drug Des Del.* **1**: 65–70.

116. Irie, T., Abe, K., Adachi, H., Uekama, K., Manako, T., Yano, T. and Saita, M. (1992) Potential use of 2-hydroxypropyl-β-cyclodextrin in designing nasal preparations of insulin involving lipophilic absorption enhancer HPE-101. *Drug Del. Syst.* **7**: 91–95.

117. Brewster, M. E., Hora, M. S., Simpkins, J. W. and Bodor, N. (1991) Use of 2-hydroxypropyl-β-cyclodextrin as a solubilizing and stabilizing excipient for protein drugs. *Pharm. Res.* **8**: 792–795.

118. Ressing, M. E., Jiskoot, W., Talsma, H., van Ingen, C. W., Beuvery, E. C. and Crommelin, D. J. A. (1992) The influence of sucrose, dextran, and hydroxypropyl-β-cyclodextrin as lyoprotectants for a freeze-dried mouse IgG$_{2a}$ monoclonal antibody (MN12). *Pharm. Res.*, **9**: 266–270.

119. Uekama, K., Yamamoto, M., Irie, T. and Hirayama, F. (1992) Pharmaceutical evaluation of maltosyl-β-cyclodextrin as a drug carrier in parenteral formulation. In Hedges, A. R. (ed.) *Minutes of the 6th International Symposium on Cyclodextrins*, pp. 491–496. Editions de Santé, Paris.

120. Fukunaga, K., Hijikata, S., Ishimura, K., Sonoda, R., Irie, T. and Uekama, K. (1994) Aluminium β-cyclodextrin sulphate as a stabilizer and sustained-release carrier for basic fibroblast growth factor. *J. Pharm. Pharmacol.* **46**: 168–171.

121. Wang, Z., Ikegami, K., Hirayama, F. and Uekama, K. (1993) Release characteristics of nifedipine from 2-hydroxypropyl-β-cyclodextrin complex during storage and its modification of hybridizing polyvinylpyrrolidone K-30. *Chem. Pharm. Bull.* **41**: 1822–1826.
122. Wang, Z., Hirayama, F. and Uekama, K. (1993) Design and in-vitro evaluation of a modified-release oral dosage form of nifedipine by hybridization of hydroxypropyl-β-cyclodextrin and hydroxypropylcellulose. *J. Pharm. Pharmacol.* **45**: 942–946.
123. Wang, Z., Hirayama, F. and Uekama, K. (1994) In-vivo and in-vitro evaluation of modified-release oral dosage form of nifedipine by hybridization of hydroxypropyl-β-cyclodextrin and hydroxypropylcelluloses in dog. *J. Pharm. Pharmacol.* **46**: 505–507.
124. Adachi, H., Irie, T., Hirayama, F. and Uekama, K. (1992) Stabilization of prostaglandin E$_1$ in fatty alcohol propylene glycol ointment by acidic cyclodextrin derivative, *O*-carboxymethyl-*O*-ethyl-β-cyclodextrin. *Chem. Pharm. Bull.* **40**: 1586–1591.
125. Uekama, K., Adachi, H., Irie, T., Yano, T., Saita, M. and Noda, K. (1992) Improved transdermal delivery of prostaglandin E$_1$ through hairless mouse skin: combined use of carboxymethyl-ethyl-β-cyclodextrin and penetration enhancers. *J. Pharm. Pharmacol.* **44**: 119–121.
126. Adachi, H., Irie, T., Uekama, K., Manako, T., Yano, T. and Saita, M. (1993) Combination effects of *O*-carboxymethyl-*O*-ethyl-β-cyclodextrin and penetration enhancer HPE-101 on transdermal delivery of prostaglandin E$_1$ in hairless mice. *Eur. J. Pharm. Sci.* **1**: 117–123.
127. Adachi, H., Irie, T., Uekama, K., Manako, T., Yano, T. and Saita, M. (1992) Inhibitory effect of prostaglandin E$_1$ on laurate-induced peripheral vascular occlusive sequelae in rabbits: optimized topical formulation with β-cyclodextrin derivative and penetration enhancer HPE-101. *J. Pharm. Pharmacol.* **44**: 1033–1035.
128. Tobino, Y., Torii, H., Ikeda, K., Nakamura, K., Arima, H., Irie, T. and Uekama, K. (1991) Release control of morphine hydrochloride in suppository. *Kyushu Yakugaku-Kai Kaiho* **45**: 15–20.
129. Uekama, K., Kondo, T., Nakamura, K., Irie, T., Arakawa, K., Shibuya, M. and Tanaka, J., (1995) Modification of rectal absorption of morphine from hollow-type suppositories with a combination of α-cyclodextrins and viscosity-enhancing polysaccharide. *J. Pharm. Sci.* **84**: 15–20.

38

Chemical and Physicochemical Solutions to Formulation Problems

CAMILLE G. WERMUTH

You may readily infer that such substances as agreeably titillate the sense
(of smell) are composed of smooth round atoms. Those that seem bitter
and harsh are more tightly compacted of hooked particles and accordingly
tear their way into our sense and rend our bodies by their inroads.

Lucretius, BC 47[1]

I. INTRODUCTION

Medicinal chemists aim to discover new lead compounds and to optimize them to highly potent, selective and nontoxic new drug candidates. However, the selected drug candidates can still present drawbacks of physicochemical nature (insufficient stability, inappropriate aggregation state) or which might affect the patient's compliance (causticity, irritation, painful

THE PRACTICE OF MEDICINAL CHEMISTRY
ISBN 0-12-744640-0

injections, undesirable organoleptic properties). To render the compound marketable, the pharmacists must then invent an adequate pharmaceutical formulation, stable on keeping and perfectly adapted to its clinical use. In leaving this task to the formulation pharmacists, chemists are not always aware of their own role in the formulation phase and the final presentation of a new drug. They also probably overestimate the scope for intervention of the formulation pharmacists. Of course, new pharmaceutical technologies such as microencapsulation or cyclodextrin complexation can overcome various drawbacks, but they are costly and often replaceable by simple chemical derivations. Medicinal chemists should therefore also feel concerned with these problems and tackle them early in the research stage, before the investment in a moderately satisfactory molecule has become too large for an alternative to be sought. Besides the pharmaceutical approach to formulation problems, there is place for chemical solutions.

II. INCREASING CHEMICAL STABILITY

The shelf-life of an organic chemical is the time taken for its pharmacological activity to fall by an acceptable amount. Whilst this cannot be universally defined, about 10% decomposition may be considered acceptable unless the decomposition products are toxic. Among the possible decomposition paths, the most frequent are hydrolysis, oxidation, photochemical degradations, racemization, thermal decomposition, chemical interactions and microbial degradation.[2] Usually, selected pharmaceutical prevention procedures and manufacturing practices can overcome decomposition problems. For example hydrolysis is avoided by dissolving the active principle in an anhydrous solvent; oxidation is prevented by replacing atmospheric oxygen by an inert gas or by adding antioxidants, and so on. However, it can happen that chemical derivatizations are needed to achieve satisfactory drug formulations. Some of these are illustrated by the examples described below. More detailed reviews on the basic physical and chemical principles that determine the stability of drugs are available in specialized monographs.[3, 4]

Pressing problems with prostaglandin E_2 (dinoprostone) and many other prostaglandins are chemical instability and difficulties in handling a liquid compound. Effectively, prostaglandin E_2 is a crystalline solid (m.p. 63°C), stable at room temperature for short periods, but it liquefies and decomposes rapidly after a few months. The instability of dinoprostone is due to the 9,11β-ketol system in which the activated C-11 hydroxyl undergoes facile elimination to give prostaglandin A_2. The corresponding ethylene ketal derivative (Fig. 38.1) possesses much improved solid-state stability. It might be an orally useful prodrug form, since it readily undergoes an acid-catalysed hydrolysis back to the parent prostaglandin under conditions similar to those prevailing in the stomach.[5]

The crystalline ester with *p*-hydroxyacetophenone (Fig. 38.1), or with some other phenolic compounds, represents another means of overcoming these difficulties.[6] Storage of the crystalline esters at room temperature for 22–30 months resulted in no detectable degradation as shown by silica TLC; the esters remained as white solids. The free acid, on the other hand, underwent 44–59% degradation in 12 months at room temperature.

Cycloserine forms a bioreversible condensation product with acetylacetone (Fig. 38.2). This greatly suppresses the dimerizing tendency of the parent drug, which occurs particularly rapidly in concentrated aqueous media and can even take place in the solid state.[7]

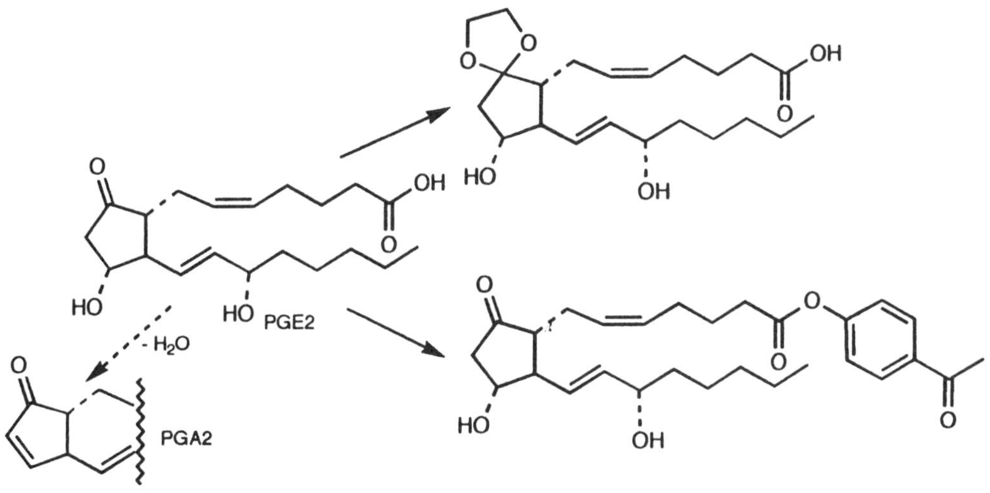

Fig. 38.1 Stabilized derivatives of prostaglandin E$_2$: ethylene ketal and crystalline ester with *p*-hydroxy-acetophenone.[5,6]

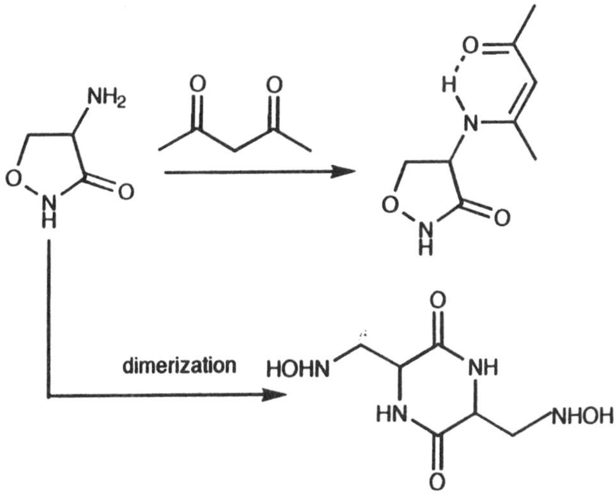

Fig. 38.2 Derivatization of the primary amino function of cycloserine. A bioreversible enamine, probably stabilized by an intramolecular hydrogen bond, is formed by reaction with acetylacetone.[7]

Pilocarpine is widely used as a topical miotic for controlling the elevated intraocular pressure associated with glaucoma. Beside its low lipophilicity, which stimulated the search for prodrugs,[8] pilocarpine has a short duration of action, its lactonic ring being rapidly opened to yield pilocarpic acid. The synthesis of its isosteric carbamate (Fig. 38.3), which is as effective as pilocarpine, has greatly improved the stability of the former lactonic ring.[9] Although the phthalimido-bearing pyridinone (1) (Fig. 38.4) is a potent reverse transcriptase inhibitor (IC$_{50}$ = 30 nM), hydrolytic instability under physiological conditions precludes the demonstration of its antiviral activity in cell culture. This instability was recognized to be due to the aminal structure of the exocyclic NH. Subsequent efforts led to the substitution of the NH with a methylene unit and the replacement of the phthalimido moiety by a benzoxazole. One of the prepared

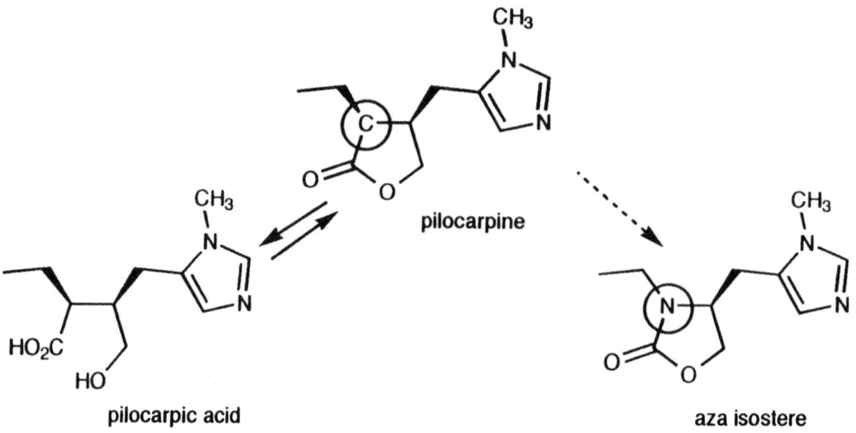

Fig. 38.3 Stabilization of the lactonic ring of pilocarpine. In preparing the carbamic analogue of pilocarpine, the sensitivity of the carbonyl group towards nucleophilic attacks is greatly decreased.[9]

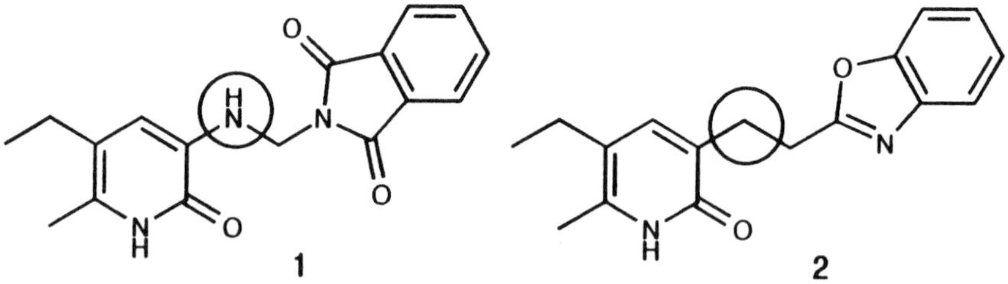

Fig. 38.4 Improved chemical stability through suppression of an aminal function.[10]

compounds, 3-[(benzoxazol-2-yl)ethyl]-5-ethyl-6-methylpyridin-2(1*H*)-one (**2**), is as potent ($IC_{50} = 23$ nM) as the phthalimido derivative but is 10 times more stable towards acid hydrolysis and shows good oral bioavailability.[10]

Cefoxitin is a broad-spectrum, semisynthetic cephalosporin antibiotic. The free acid form is a white, crystalline, practically insoluble solid and therefore the decision was made to use the sodium salt to provide a sterile solution for intravenous administration. It was soon evident that the sodium salt of cefoxitin would have limited stability in solution and would not lend itself to the formulation of a marketable solution product. Stability studies highlighted the advantages of a sterile crystalline solid over the amorphous freeze-dried product, and also the need for rubber stopper screening studies to eliminate interactions between sodium cefoxitin powder and rubber, and finally the profound effect of oxygen on the coloration rate of the product.[11]

The *N*-nitrosoureas such as lomustine, carmustine and tauromustine are important alkylating antineoplastic agents that have demonstrated activity against a wide spectrum of tumours. Although some *N*-nitrosoureas (e.g. lomustine) are sufficiently stable to be administered orally, they are generally very unstable in aqueous solutions. Addition of an equimolar amount of Tris (tris(hydroxymethy)aminomethane) forms a complex that is stable in aqueous solution and increases the shelf-life of the nitrosoureas. The rate of degradation of the drugs in the complex is 1.5–2.5 times slower than without the complex.[12]

Cyclodextrin complexation (see Chapter 37) can also represent a way of improving the stability and the solubility of sensitive drugs such as thalidomide. Thalidomide is currently in clinical use for the treatment and prevention of graft-versus-host disease in leukaemia patients after bone marrow transplantation. However, this drug is sparingly soluble in aqueous solutions $(50 \, \mu g \, ml^{-1})$ and is readily hydrolysed. Complexation with hydroxypropyl β-cyclodextrin increases the solubility to $1700 \, \mu g \, ml^{-1}$ and extends the half-life of a dilute solution from 2.1 to 4.1 h.[13] Other vulnerable and sparingly soluble drugs stabilised by means of cyclodextrin complexation are the nonsteroidal anti-inflammatory drugs diclofenac, piroxicam and indomethacin[14] and the anthracycline antibiotic daunorubicin.[15]

The presence of an alkyl substituent at N-3 in the oxazaphosphorine ring stabilizes *N*-substituted 4-(alkylthio)cyclophosphamides from 'spontaneous' decomposition. On the basis of this finding, several *N*-methyl-4-thiocyclophosphamide derivatives were synthesized and examined as prodrugs of 4-hydroxycyclophosphamide, the activated species of cyclophosphamide.[16]

All prodrugs are stable in aqueous buffer but undergo *N*-demethylation when incubated with rat hepatic microsomes, forming alkylating species. N-Methyl-4-(diethyldithio-carbamyl)cyclophosphamide particularly (Fig. 38.5) shows notable *in vitro* toxicity against mouse 3T3 cells and human tumour cells.

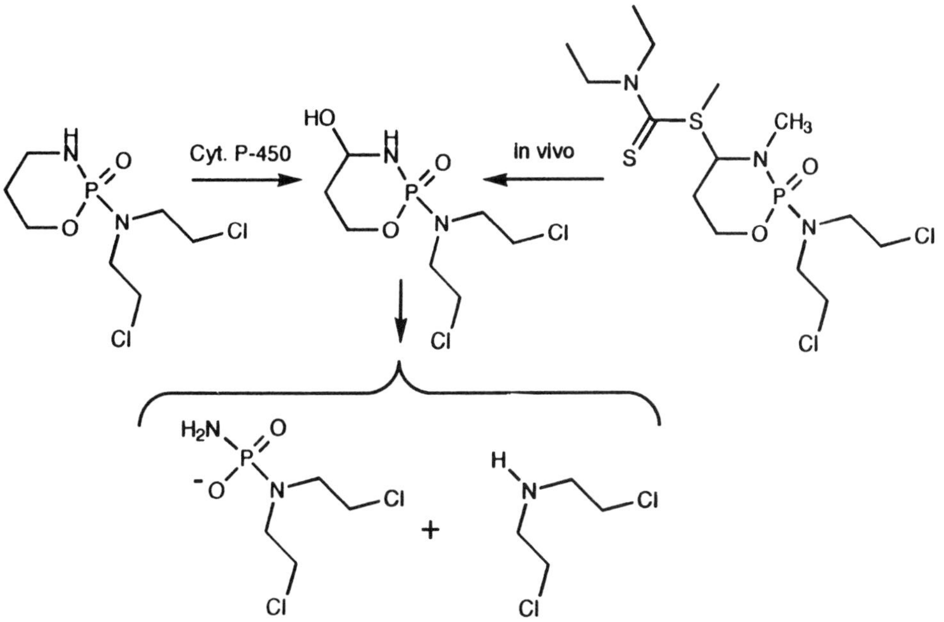

Fig. 38.5 Stable precursor of 4-hydroxycyclophosphamide.[16]

III. IMPROVED FORMULATION OF PEPTIDES AND PROTEINS

Enhancement of proteolytic stability of peptides can be achieved by well-established procedures such as synthesis of retropeptides, isosteric replacement of the peptidic bond, *N*-methylation and use of non-natural D-amino acids.[17,18] Prodrugs of peptides can also be helpful, see Chapter 31.

However, sometimes very simple derivatives can afford protection against enzymatic degradation. Thus the *N*-acetyl derivative of (Z)-glycylprolylamide (Fig. 38.6) is six times more resistant to gut prolyl endopeptidase (which normally hydrolyses the terminal primary amide) than the nonacetylated parent molecule.[19]

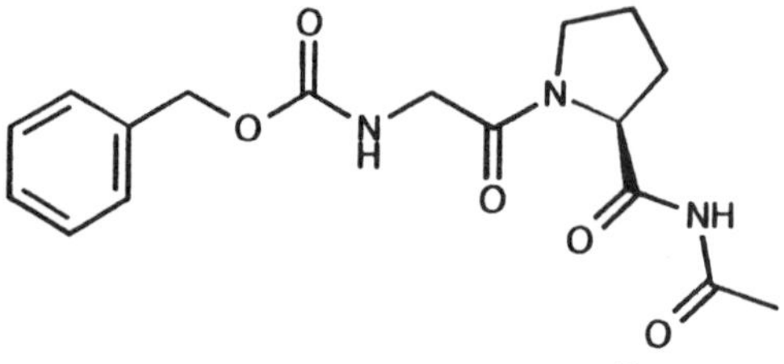

Fig. 38.6 *N*-Acetylation of (Z)-Gly-ProNH$_2$ protects against the hydrolytic activity of prolyl endopeptidase.[19]

In a analogous way, Leu-enkephalin and Met-enkephalin were rendered resistant to aminopeptidases[20] by condensation with various aldehydes and ketones to form 4-imidazoline derivatives (Fig. 38.6).

IV. DEALING WITH MESOMORPHIC CRYSTALLINE FORMS

It is well known that certain substances are able to exist in more than one crystalline state, depending on the conditions used to prepare them (nature of the solvent, crystallization temperature, presence of impurities, etc.); this property is called *polymorphism*. Some of the possible crystalline states are metastable and can be converted into more stable forms with different physicochemical properties. Two types of transformation are possible: reversible enantiotropic transformation in which the polymorphic forms can change from one into the other, and irreversible monotropic transformation, which is most often met and which involves the change from a thermodynamically unstable form to a more stable one. The different crystalline forms of a given compound can be distinguished by their melting points and solubilities, by scanning calorimetry, by thermogravimetric analysis, by infrared spectrometry, by X-ray powder diffraction, and by scanning electron microscopy.

As a rule, metastable polymorphs will tend to have increased solubility and a faster dissolution rate than a stable polymorph. Although fourfold increases in solubility are sometimes observed between the two forms,[21,22] a 50—100% increase in dissolution rate represents the most usual situation.[23] Riboflavin is an exception. It has three polymorphs with solubilities of 60 mg l^{-1}, 810 mg l^{-1} and 1200 mg l^{-1}.[24] When a metastable form is placed in contact with solvents, it can change progressively to the most stable but least soluble form. An example is provided by the acidic and amorphous form of novobiocin, which can hardly be administered as a suspension because of its tendency to turn into a much less soluble crystalline form.[25] Spray-drying of pure drugs often results in amorphous products with increased rates of dissolution, eventually an auxiliary ingredient can be added to yield solid spray-dispersions of drugs.[26]

The transformation from one crystalline form to the other can also occur during the manufacturing process. Chloroquine diphosphate crystals, for example, can be obtained anhydrous by storing the hydrate at elevated temperatures. Dehydration is favoured by grinding of the raw material. The transition of anhydrous chloroquine diphosphate into a second hydrated form is possible on storing the drug at a high relative humidity. Compression of the raw material resulted in the formation of a further crystal form.[27] In a similar way, grinding the polymorphic form A of chloramphenicol stearate in the presence of colloidal silica converts it into form B.[28] Taken together, these findings emphasize the necessity for standardization of the manufacturing processes and closer examination of the solid drug as part of the quality control.

V.   TRANSFORMING LIQUIDS INTO SOLIDS

A less frequent but none the less interesting problem arises in the chemical modification of liquid active principles into solid prodrugs suitable for tablet or capsule preparation. Indeed, solid dosage forms are still the most widely used for the administration of medicines, for reasons of patient acceptability and convenience in terms of product stability and ease of manufacture. Their preparation implies that the active principle can itself be handled as a stable solid, an objective that is usually attained by one of the following strategies: formation of a salt or a molecular complex, formation of a crystalline covalent derivative, or introduction of symmetry.

(a) Salt or complex formation.   Many basic active compound, belonging to various therapeutic classes (antihistaminics, neuroleptics, local anaesthetics, etc.) are oily liquids. Salification with an appropriate acid (hydrochloric, phosphoric, tartaric) represents a good means of converting them into the desired aggregation state (see Chapter 34). Neutral liquids can sometimes be converted into solids through formation of molecular complexes. The central and respiratory stimulant nikethamide is a slightly viscous oil or a low-melting (m.p. = 24–26°C) crystalline solid. With calcium thiocyanate it forms a solid combination made of two molecules of N,N-diethylnicotinamide and one molecule of $Ca(SCN)_2$ that can be used for tableting.[29] Chloral hydrate, another low-melting solid, yields a crystalline and odourless 2:1 complex with phenazone;[30,31] see below. Chloral formamide and chloral N-acetylglycinamide[32] are other solid complexes.

(b) Covalent derivatives.   The methodology consists in linking the liquid active principle, by means of a covalent bond, to a nontoxic moiety having a strong tendency to crystallize. Liquid or greasy fatty acids can easily be converted into phenacyl esters,[33] and, as shown above, substances related to prostaglandins give crystalline esters with p-hydroxyacetophenone (Figs. 38.1 and 38.7) or with some other phenolic compounds.[6] Chloral yields a crystalline hemiacetal (Fig. 38.14) with the phenolic hydroxyl of paracetamol.[34]

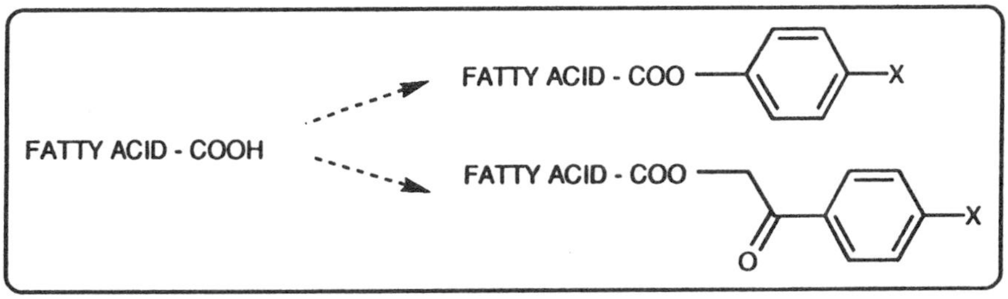

Fig. 38.7   Crystalline derivatives of fatty acids.

Trichloroethanol can be converted to its phosphate ester, which gives a crystalline monosodium salt;[35] the same possibility exists for the low-melting (m.p. = 28°C) guaiacol (guaiacol phosphate) (Fig. 38.8). Phenols can be acylated (guaiacol benzoate, phenylacetate or valerate) or alkylated (guaifenesin, guaiapate) (Fig. 38.8).

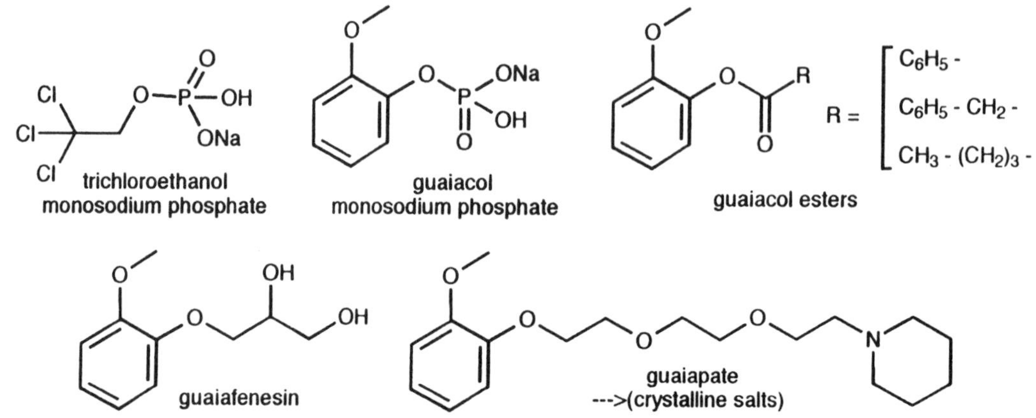

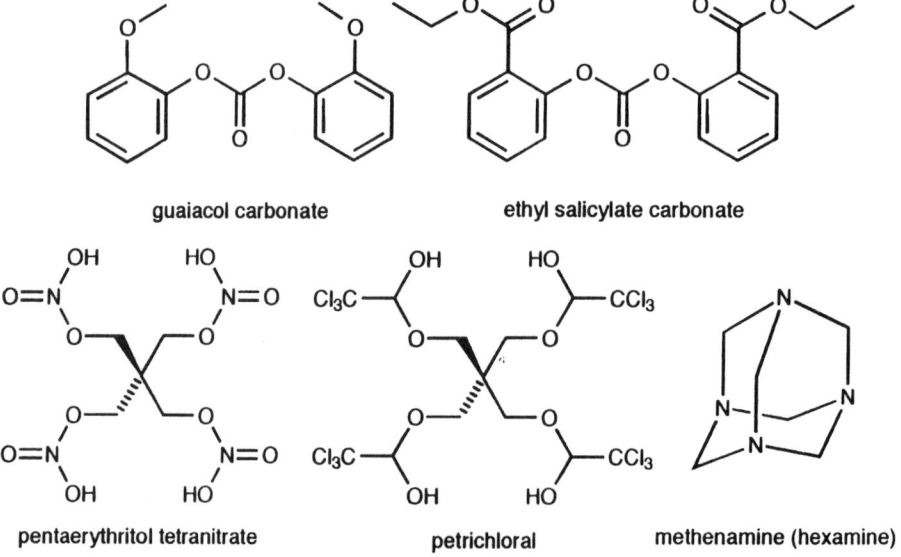

Fig. 38.8 Covalent solid derivatives of liquid active principles.

(c) Introduction of symmetry.

It is well known that symmetric molecules have higher melting points than non-symmetric ones; for example, *p*-nitrotoluene is a solid, *o*- and *m*-nitrotoluenes are liquids. For chemical formulation of pharmaceuticals, symmetry can be obtained by preparing twin drugs (see Chapter 15). Low-molecular-weight duplication reagents are formaldehyde or glyoxylic acid (methylene-bis type derivatives), phosgene or phosphorus oxychloride (carbonate or phosphate diesters), and small bifunctionalized molecules (ethylene glycol, ethylenediamine esters or amides).

guaiacol carbonate   ethyl salicylate carbonate

pentaerythritol tetranitrate   petrichloral   methenamine (hexamine)

Fig. 38.9 Compounds for which the solid state results from molecular symmetry.

Symmetric carbonates of guaiacol or ethyl salicylate are crystalline solids (Fig. 38.9), pentaerythritol tetranitrate is the solid counterpart of the liquid trinitrine, and petrichloral is again a stabilized chloral derivative. Methenamine, formulated as an enteric-coated tablet, is used as a urinary tract antibacterial. Following absorption, the compound is eliminated in the urine, where formaldehyde is generated in the acidic environment.

VI.   GASTROINTESTINAL IRRITATION AND PAINFUL INJECTIONS

A.   Gastrointestinal irritation

Gastrointestinal disturbances can occur for several reasons: (1) direct contact of the drug with the gastric mucosa, producing a localized irritating and necrotizing effect; (2) irritation of the gastric mucosa through an indirect mechanism, e.g. stimulation of gastric secretion; (3) irritation of the intestinal mucosa; (4) inhibition of mucopolysaccharide biosynthesis; (5) destruction of the intestinal flora.

Chemical formulations mainly deal with the direct irritating properties of drugs containing phenolic or acidic groups. For example, to eliminate gastric irritation produced by salicylic acid, aspirin was developed. Another possibility is given by carbonate esters (*n*-hexyl carbonate) which are rapidly hydrolysed *in vivo* and might have hydrophobic properties that allow absorption and distribution over a greater area of the GI tract, thus reducing local irritation.[36]

For nonsteroidal anti-inflammatory carboxylic acids such as mefenamic acid[37] or *N*-(7-chloro-4-quinolyl)anthranilic acid,[38] glyceryl esters are claimed as less irritating. Alternatively, the ulcerogenicity of indomethacin derivatives was reduced by formation of the ester with glycolic acid[39,40] or the peptide with serine.[41] Another indomethacin-related anti-inflammatory drug, sulindac, is an inactive sulfoxide and only becomes activated after absorption and reduction into the corresponding sulfide. Thus the initial exposure of gastric and intestinal mucosa to the active drug is circumvented (see Chapter 32).

B.   Avoidance of painful injections

When an initially painful intravenous or intramuscular injection must be administered repetitively, patient reluctance develops. Injection pains are usually accompanied by haemorrhage, oedema, inflammation, and tissue necrosis.[42] Among the factors responsible for painful injections, the most important are the drug's solubility in aqueous medium, the viscosity, the pH and the hypo- or hyperosmotic character of the injected drug solution, the amount of the injected volume, the site of injection, the pain tolerance of the patient, and the technique of administration. Other factors include precipitation of the drug at the injection site and localized cell lysis.[42]

Excessive concentrations of the active compound at the injection site (initial peak concentrations) are avoided by masking the irritating agent through complexation. The free concentrations of iron or of calcium are reduced by using calcium gluconate or laevulinate for intravenous injections and iron–sorbitol citrate for intramuscular injections.[43]

The low aqueous solubility of the antibiotic clindamycin hydrochloride is responsible for the pain experienced on intramuscular injection. Phosphorylation improves the aqueous solubility from $3\,mg\,ml^{-1}$ to $>150\,mg\,ml^{-1}$ and avoids the pain resulting from injection of the parent clindamycin[44,45] (Fig. 38.10). The phosphorylated drug possesses little or no intrinsic antibacterial activity,[46] but, owing to the enzymatic action of phosphatases, it is rapidly converted to the parent drug. The half-life for hydrolysis *in vivo* is approximately 10 min and only 1–2% of an intravenous dose is eliminated in the urine as unchanged prodrug.[47]

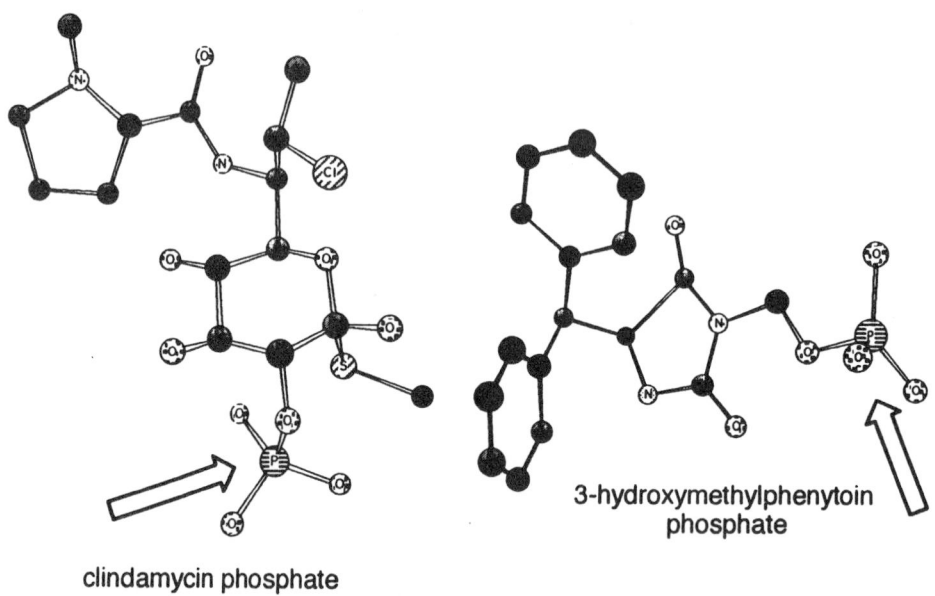

3-hydroxymethylphenytoin
phosphate

clindamycin phosphate

Fig. 38.10   Sodium salts of phosphate esters of clindamycin and of 3-hydroxymethylphenytoin are freely soluble in water and allow painless injection.

The anticonvulsant drug phenytoin (5,5-diphenylhydantoin) is sparingly soluble in water $(0.02\,mg\,ml^{-1})$ and is therefore formulated as sodium enolate for intravenous or intramuscular injections. The solvent is a mixture of 40% propylene glycol, 10% ethanol and 50% water and the pH of the solution is alkaline (pH ~12) owing to the weak acidity of the drug (pK_a = 8.3).[48] Such a formulation allows concentrations as high as $50\,mg\,ml^{-1}$, but there is a serious risk of phenytoin precipitation at the physiological pH (7.4) of the injection site. On the other hand, propylene glycol is a cardiac depressant (see Chapter 36). The disodium salt of the phosphate ester of 3-hydroxymethylphenytoin (Fig. 38.10) was found to be extremely soluble (4500 times phenytoin), pharmacologically inert and able to regenerate free phenytoin rapidly and quantitatively with no apparent irritation.[49]

VII.   SUPPRESSION OF UNDESIRABLE ORGANOLEPTIC PROPERTIES

The use of flavours and flavour modifiers represents the first attempt to improve pharmaceuticals by masking undesirable organoleptic properties such as taste, odour and 'feel' factors (for a review see ref. 50). When this approach is ineffective, chemical modifications have to be considered.

A. Odour

Despite its interesting antiseptic properties, iodoform was rejected by the medical community because of its disagreeable odour. The first historical attempt towards an odourless substitute was bismuth iodosubgallate (Airoform®), which is practically odourless (Fig. 38.11).

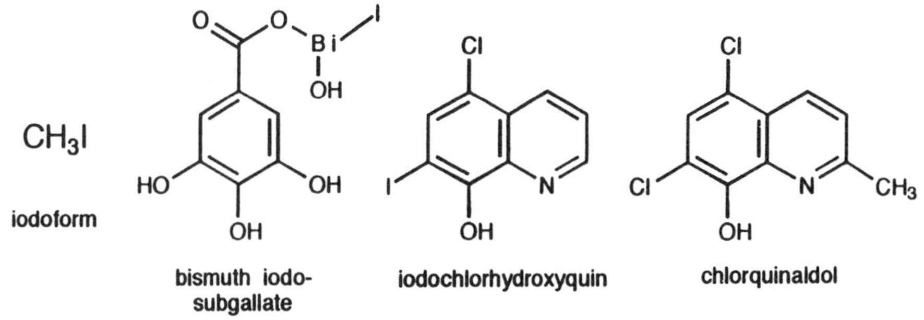

Fig. 38.11   Change from iodoform to odourless antiseptics.

Bismuth iodosubgallate was followed by the introduction of iodochlorhydroxyquin (Vioform®). Unfortunately, this latter compound has been linked with the occurrence of subacute myelo-optic neuropathy (SMON syndrome) in Japan. Decisive progress came with the iodine-free chlorquinaldol (Sterosan®).

Thiamin chloride has a slight but disagreeable and penetrating odour and often causes vomiting when incorporated in paediatric polyvitaminic preparations. The corresponding monophosphoric ester (Fig. 38.12) is totally odourless and shows increased stability.[51]

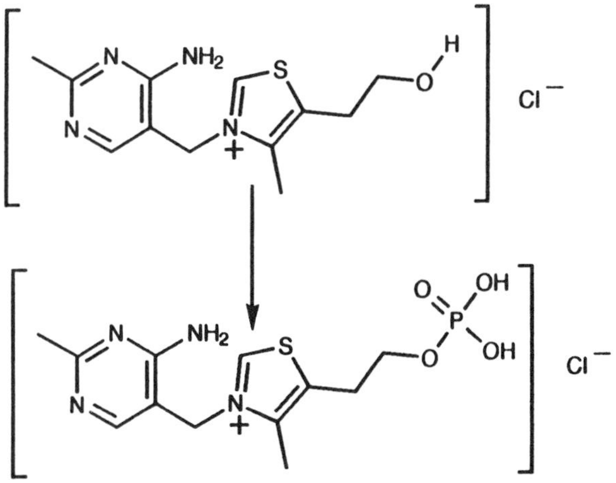

Fig. 38.12   Thiamin chloride and its odourless monophosphate ester.[51]

The development of diethyl dithioisophtalate (Etisul®) as an antituberculosis and antileprosy drug originated from the observation that ethyl mercaptan, an evil-smelling, low-boiling, inflammable liquid was active as an antitubercular agent. Among a number of derivatives prepared which would be expected to be metabolized to ethyl mercaptan *in vivo*, the most successful was diethyl dithioisophtalate (Fig. 38.13), a bland, odourless oil, which is effective in experimental tuberculosis parenterally.[52,53]

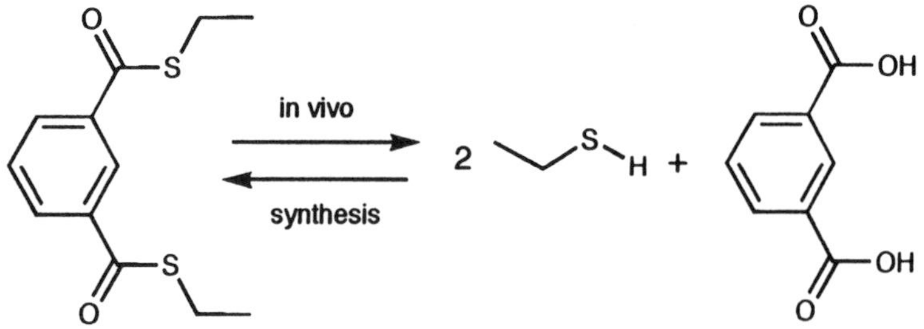

Fig. 38.13   Diethyl dithioisophtalate, an odourless administration form of ethyl mercaptan.[52,53]

Besides its bad taste and its gastric and intestinal irritating properties, chloral hydrate has an unpleasant odour. All of these disadvantages have been overcome by complexing two molecules of chloral hydrate with one molecule of phenazone to give dichloralphenazone.[30,31] Dichloralphenazone (Fig. 38.14) possesses all the hypnotic and sedative properties of chloral hydrate, and is less toxic and free from the unpleasant odour and taste of chloral. Another masked form of chloral, cloracetadol, results from a hemiacetalic bonding between chloral hydrate and paracetamol (Fig. 38.14). This combination represents three achievements: attenuation of the bad odour, obtaining of a solid state, and associative synthesis.[34] Trichloroethanol, the active metabolite of chloral, is deodorized as a symmetric ester with carbonic acid. The ester is prepared from trichloroethanol and phosgene. It is a tasteless, crystalline solid with limited solubility in water. Pharmacological comparisons show its equivalence with trichloroethanol.[54]

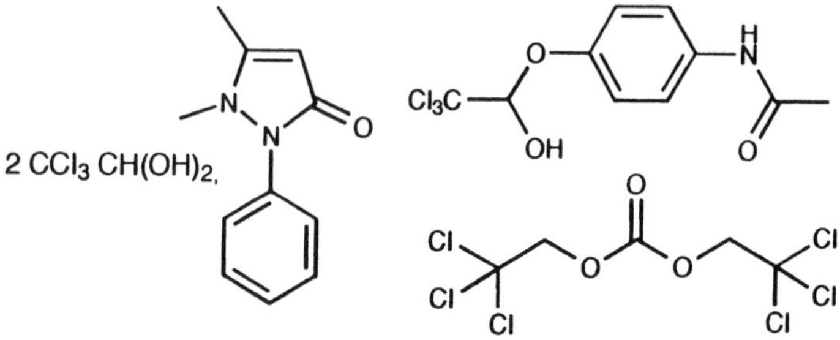

Fig. 38.14   Chloral hydrate yields an odourless 2 : 1 complex with phenazone[30,31] and a hemiacetal with paracetamol.[34] Trichloroethanol is deodorized as the carbonate ester.[54]

B.   Taste

Taste is a complex combination of sensations including gustation, olfaction, tactility, and responses to heat and cold. In humans the sensation of taste is confined primarily to the dorsal face of the tongue, the soft palate, the epiglottis, and parts of the gullet. In children, however, the taste receptors are distributed over larger areas of the mouth.[42] There are basically four so-called primary tastes: sour, bitter, salty and sweet. Others include astringent, metallic, and alkaline (soapy). For pharmaceuticals, the main problem resides in masking the bitterness of some orally administrated paediatric formulations, such as antibiotic-containing suspensions and syrups. Two strategies are possible: decreasing the drug solubility sufficiently to bring it below the threshold value for taste receptor activation, or modifing the shape and the electronic

Table 38.1   Sparingly soluble salts or esters of bitter drugs.

Parent molecule	Derivative	Reference
Dextropropoxyphene	Napsylate salt	55
Tetracycline	3,4,5-Trimethoxybenzoate salt	56
Chloramphenicol	Palmitic ester	57
Sulphafurazole (sulfisoxazole)	N'-acetyl	58
Erythromycin	Ethylsuccinate	59
Clindamycin	Dialkylcarbonate esters	60

potential of the molecule. The first strategy is well illustrated by the formation of very sparingly soluble salts or esters (Table 38.1). In the gastrointestinal tract or following absorption the derivatives are cleaved with formation of the parent drugs.

However, insolubility in water is not always a prerequisite and in some cases water-solubilizing groups achieve the suppression of bitterness. Examples are N-arylanthranilic glyceryl esters[37] or lincomycin phosphate.[61,62]

An illustration of the second strategy is provided by the p-cyano analogues of the nonnutritive sweetener suosan (Fig. 38.15). The replacement of the planar carboxylic group by the bioisosteric tetrazolyl group yields less potent but still sweet compounds.[63] However, replacement of the carboxylic group by the tetrahedral sulfonic group yields an *antagonist* of the sweet taste response which inhibits the sweetness perception of a variety of sweeteners without having any effect on the sour or salty taste response. Surprisingly the sulfonic antagonist also antagonized the bitter taste response to reference compounds such as caffeine, quinine and naringine.[64]

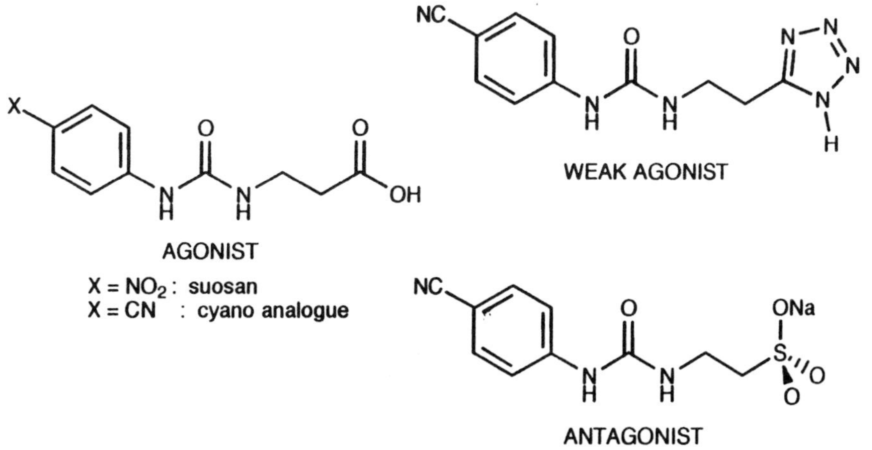

WEAK AGONIST

AGONIST

X = NO₂ : suosan

X = CN   : cyano analogue

ANTAGONIST

Fig. 38.15   Suosan analogues.[63,64]

A series of qualitative and empirical rules was collected by Sinkula.[65] These may provide some clues to the medicinal chemist for improving the taste quality of objectionable-tasting drugs (Table 38.2).

Table 38.2   Empirical and qualitative structure–taste relationships.[58]

1. Compounds containing several hydroxyl groups are usually *sweet* (glycols, sugars and other carbohydrates).
2. An increase in molecular weight, i.e. extending a homologous series, often changes from *sweet to bitter*.
    Further increases in homologation reduce drug solubility below taste threshold values.
3. Nitro groups present in a molecule are usually indicative of *bitter* taste (chloramphenicol, picric acid).
4 . Alkylation of an amine or amide usually produces a *sweet* tasting substance.
5. Alkylation of a hydroxyl soup (etherification) *destroys sweet* taste.
6. Alkylation of an imide *eliminates sweet taste*; N-alkyl saccharins are tasteless.
7. Addition of a phenyl group to a drug molecule causes or increases *bitter* taste and may be due to enhanced lipophilicity and/or preferential binding with bitter taste receptors.
8. An increase in chain branching decreases sweet taste and *increases bitter* taste.
9. Esterification *enhances sweetness*, e.g.,ethyl butyrate, aspartyl dipeptide esters.
10. Introduction of unsaturation into a molecule *increases bitterness and pungency*.
11. Primary amines *enhance sweet taste* especially if in close proximity to an electronegative group (—COOH), e.g. in certain D- and L-amino acids.
12. Secondary, tertiary amines and quaternary ammonium salts are *bitter*, especially alkaloids, antibiotics and quaternary ammonium drugs.
13. Monosubstituted ureas are usually *sweet* although some are tasteless.
    Urea itself is *bitter*. Symmetrical molecules are often *bitter*.
14. Aliphatic polyhalogenated compounds are *sweet* (chloroform, 1,2-dichloroethane, dichloromethane).
15. Aromatic halogen substitution *increases bitterness* and is a function of the atomic weight of the halogen (for example halogenated saccharins).
16. The presence of sulfur in an aliphatic molecule is usually associated with *bitterness* (—SH, —S—, —S-S—, C = S).
17. Sulfonic acids are usually *bitter or tart*.
18. Aldehydes are *sweet*. Aldehydo-semicarbazones are *not as sweet* as the parent aldehydes. Aldehydophenylhydrazones are *not sweet*.
19. Oximes are usually *sweet or tasteless*.

REFERENCES

1. Lucretius, T. C. (1951) *The nature of the Universe* (Translated by Latham). Penguin Books, London.
2. Shotton, E. and Ridgway, K. (1974) *Physical Pharmaceutics*. Clarendon Press, Oxford.
3. Connors, K. A., Amidon, G. L. and Stella, V. J. (1986) *Chemical Stability of Pharmaceutics: a Handbook for Pharmacists*, 2nd edn. Wiley, New York.
4. Essig, D., Hofer, J., Schmidt, P. C. and Stumpf, H. (1986) *Stabilisierungstechnologie – Wege zur haltbaren Arzneiform*. Wissenschaftliche Verlagsgesellschaft mbH, Stuttgart.
5. Cho, M. J., Bundy, G. L. and Biermacher, J. J. (1977) Prostaglandin Prodrugs. 5. Prostaglandin E2 ethylene ketal. *J. Med. Chem.* **20:** 1525–1527.
6. Morozowich, W., Oesterling, T. O., Miller, W. L., Lawson, C. F., Weeks, J. R., Stehle, R. G., Douglas, S. L. (1979) Prostaglandine prodrugs I: Stabilization of dinoprostone (prostaglandin E₂) in solid state through formation of crystalline C1-phenyl esters. *J. Pharm. Sci.* **68:** 833–836.
7. Jensen, N. P., Friedman, J. J., Kropp, H., Kahan, F. M. (1980) Use of acetylacetone to prepare a prodrug of cycloserine. *J Med Chem* **23:** 6–8.
8. Bundgaard, H. (1985) *Design of Prodrugs*, pp. 55–61. Elsevier, Amsterdam.
9. Saueberg, P., Chen, J., WoldeMussie, E. R. and Rapoport, H. (1989) Carbamate analogues of pilocarpine. *J. Med. Chem.* **32:** 1322–1326.

10. Hoffman, J. M., Smith, A. M. and Rooney, C. S. (1993) Synthesis and evaluation of 2-pyridone derivatives as HIV-1-specific reverse transcriptase inhibitors. 4. 3-[(Benzoxazol-2-yl)ethyl]-5-ethyl-6-methylpyridin-2(1*H*)-one and analogues. *J. Med. Chem.* **36:** 953–966.

11. Portnoff, J. B., Henley, M. W. and Restaino, F. A. (1983) The development of sodium cefoxitin as a dosage form. *J. Parenteral. Sci. Technol.* **37:** 180–185.

12. Loftsson, T. and Fridriksdottir, H. (1992) Stabilizing effect of Tris(hydroxymethyl) aminomethane on *N*-nitrosoureas in aqueous solutions. *J. Pharm. Sci.* **81:** 197–198.

13. Krenn, M., Gamcsik, M. P., Vogelsang, G. B., Colvin, O. M. and Leong, K. W. (1992) Improvements on solubility and stability of thalidomide upon complexation with hydroxypropyl-β-cyclodextrin. *J. Pharm. Sci.* **81:** 685–689.

14. Backensfeld, T., Müller, B. W. and Kolter, K. (1991) Interaction of NSA with cyclodextrins and hydroxypopyl-cyclodextrin derivatives. *Int. J. Pharm.* **74:** 65–93.

15. Suenaga, A., Bekers, O., Beijnen, J. H., Underberg, W. J. M., Tanimoto, T., Koizumi, K. and Otagiri, M. (1992) Stabilization of daunorbicin and 4-demethoxydaunorubicin on complexation with octakis(2,6-di-*O*-methyl)-γ-cyclodextrin in acidic aqueous solution. *Int. J. Pharm.* **82:** 29–37.

16. Moon, K. Y., Kwon, C. H., Shirota, F. N. and Baturay, N. Z. (1993) Design, synthesis and evaluation of *N*-methyl-4-thiocyclophosphamide derivatives as chemically stable, alternative prodrugs of 4-hydroxycyclophosphamide. In 84 Meet.

17. Fauchère, J. L. (1986) Elements for the rational design of peptide drugs. *Adv. Drug. Res.* **15:** 29–69.

18. Plattner, J. J. and Norbeck, D. W. (1990) Obstacles to drug development from peptide leads. In Clark, C. R. and Moos, W. H. (eds) *Drug Discovery Technologies*, pp. 92–126. Ellis Horwood, Chichester.

19. Møss, J. and Bundgaard, H. (1992) Prodrugs of peptides. 17. Bioreversible derivatization of the C-terminal prolineamide residue in peptides to afford protection against prolyl endopeptidase. *Int. J. Pharm.* **82:** 91–97.

20. Rasmussen, G. J. and Bundgaard, H. (1991) Prodrugs of peptides. 15. 5-Imidazolidinone prodrugs derivatives of enkephalins to prevent aminopeptidase-catalyzed metabolism in plasma and absorptive mucosae. *Int. J. Pharm.* **76:** 113–122.

21. Lin, S. L. (1972) Preformulation investigation II. Dissolution kinetics and thermodynamic parameters of polymorphs of an experimental antihypertensive. *J. Pharm. Sci.* **61:** 1423–1430.

22. Aguiar, A. J. and Zelmer, J. E. (1969) Dissolution behavior of polymorphs of chloramphenicol palmitate and mefenamic acid. *J. Pharm. Sci.* **58:** 983–987.

23. Shefter, E. (1981) Solubilization of solid-state manipulation. In Yalkowsky, S. H. (ed.) *Techniques of Solubilization of Drugs*, pp. 159–182. Marcel Dekker, Inc., New York.

24. Shotton, E. and Ridgway, K. (1974) *Physical Pharmaceutics*, p. 337. Clarendon Press, Oxford.

25. Mullins, J. D. and Macek, T. J. (1960) Some pharmaceutical properties of novobiocin. *J. Am. Pharm. Assoc., Sci. Ed.* **49:** 245–248.

26. Nürnberg, E. (1980) Darstellung und Eigenschaften pharmazeutisch relevanter Sprühtrocknungsprodukte, eine Übersicht. *Acta Pharm. Technol.* **26:** 39–67.

27. Bjerga Bjaen, A. K., Nord, K., Furuseth, S., Agren, T., Tonnesen, H. H. and Karlsen, J. (1993) Polymorphism of chloroquine diphosphate. *Int. J. Pharm.* **92:** 183–189.

28. Forni, R., Coppi, G., Iannucelli, V., Vandelli, M. A. and Cameroni, R. (1988) The grinding of the polymorphic forms of chloramphenicol stearic ester in the presence of colloidal silica. *Acta Pharm. Suec.* **25:** 173–180.

29. Büchi, J. (1963) *Grundlagen der Arzneimittelforschung und der Synthetischen Arzneimittel.* p. 206. Birkhäuser Verlag, Basel and Stuttgart.

30. Willis, G. C. and Arendt, E. C. (1954) Relative efficacy of sodium amytal, chloral hydrate and dichloralphenazone. *Can. Med. Assoc. J.* **71:** 126–128.

31. Rice, W. B. and McColl, J. W. (1956) A comparison of dichloralphenazone and chloral hydrate. *J. Am. Pharm. Assoc., Sci. Ed.* **45:** 137–141.

32. Bruce, W. F. Chloral derivatives and methods for their preparation. US Patent 2 784 237 (5 March 1957; American Home Products).

33. Vogel, A. I. (1989) In Furniss, B. S., Hannaford, A. J., Smith, P. W. G. and Tachell, A. R. (eds) *Vogel's Textbook of Practical Organic Chemistry*, pp. 1261–1265. Longman Scientific & Technical, London.

34. Anonymous (1963) Médicaments à base de paraacétylaminophénoxy-1 trichloro-2 éthanol. French Patent M 2031 (24 May 1962; Brevets Pharmaceutiques et Cosmétologiques S.A., Switzerland) *Chem. Abstr.* **60:** 9201a.

35. Hems, B.A., Atkinson, R. M., Early, M. and Tomich, E. G. (1962) Trichloroethyl phosphate. *Br. Med. J.* **1:** 1834–1835.

36. Dittert, L. W., Caldwell, H. C., Ellison, T., Irwin, G. M., Rivard, D. E. and Swintosky, J. V. (1968) Carbonate ester prodrugs of salicylic acid. *J. Pharm. Sci.* **57:** 828–831.

37. Anonymous. Glyceryl-*N*-(substituted phenyl) anthranilates in the treatment of inflammation. US Patent 3 767 811 (23 Oct. 1973; Schering Corporation).

38. Allais, A., Rousseau, G., Girault, P., Mathieu, J., Peterfalvi, M., Branceni, D., Azadian-Boulanger, G., Chifflot, L. and Jequier, R. (1966) Sur l'activité analgésique et antiinflammatoire des 4-(2'-alcoxycarbonyl phénylamino) quinoléïnes. *Eur. J. Med. Chem.*, **1:** 65–70.

39. Boltze, K. -H., Brendler, O., Dell, H. -D. and Jacobi, H. Novel substituted indole compound, process for the preparation and therapeutic compositions containing it. German Patent 3 910 952 (7 Oct. 1975; Troponwerke Dinklage & Co., Cologne).

40. Boltze, K. -H., Brendler, O., Jacobi, H., Opitz, W., Raddatz, S., Seidel, P. -R. and Vollbredht, D. (1980) Chemische Struktur und antiphlogistische Wirkung in der Reihe der substituierten Indol-3-essigsäuren. *Arzneimittal-Forsch. (Drug Res.)* **30:** 1314–1325.

41. Anonymous: Dérivés d'indolylacétylamino-acide, leur procédé de préparation et les compositions pharmaceutiques comprenant ces composés. Belgium Patent 826 711 (14 March 1975; Schering Aktiengesellschaft, Berlin und Bergkamen).

42. Sinkula, A. A. and Yalkowsky, S. H. (1975) Rationale for design of biologically reversible drug derivatives: Prodrugs. *J. Pharm. Sci.* **64:** 181–210.

43. Berger, F. M. (1952) The anticonvulsant activity of carbamate esters of certain 2,2-disubstituted-1,3-propanediols. *J. Pharmacol. Exp. Ther.* **104:** 229–233.

44. Edmondson, H.T. (1973) Parenteral and oral clindamycin therapy in surgical infections: a preliminary report. *Ann. Surg.* **168:** 637–642.

45. Gray, J.E., Weaver, R.N., Moran, J. and Feenstra, E. S. (1974) The parenteral toxicity of clindamycin 2-phosphate in laboratory animals. *Toxicol. Appl. Pharmacol.* **27:** 308–321.

46. Brodasky, T. F. and Lewis, C. (1972) An *in vivo–in vitro* comparison of the 2- and 3-phosphate esters of clindamycin. *J. Antibiot.* **25:** 230–238.

47. DeHaan, R. M., Metzler, C. M., Schellenberg, D. and Van Denbosch, W. D. (1973) Pharmacokinetic studies of clindamycin phosphate. *J. Clin. Pharmacol.* **13:** 190–209.

48. Stella, V. J., Charman, W. N. A. and Naringrekar, V. H. (1985) Prodrugs – do they have advantages in clinical practice? *Drugs* **29:** 455–473.

49. Varia, A. A. and Stella, V. J. (1984) Phenytoin prodrugs. VI: *In vivo* evaluation of a phosphate ester prodrug of phenytoin after parenteral administration to rats. *J. Pharm. Sci.* **73:** 1087–1090.

50. Adjei, A. L., Doyle, R. and Reiland, T. (1988) Flavors and flavor modifiers. In Swarbuck, J. and Boylan, J. C. (eds) *Encyclopedia of Pharmaceutical Technology,* pp. 101–139. Marcel Dekker, New York.

51. Wenz, A., Göttmann, G. and Koop, H. Verfahren zur Herstellung der freien Base und der Salze des Aneurin-orthophosphor-säureesters. German Patent 1 110 646 (13 July 1961; E. Merck A.G. Darmstadt).

52. Davies, G. E. and Driver, G. W. (1957) The antituberculous activity of ethylthiolesters with particular reference to diethyldithiol isophthalate. *Br. J. Pharmacol.* **12:** 434–437.

53. Davies, G. E. and Driver, G. W. (1958) Inhibitory action of ethyl mercaptan on intracellular tubercle bacilli. *Nature (London)* **182:** 664–665.

54. Caldwell, H. C., Adams, H. J., Rivard, D. E. and Swintosky, J. V. (1967) Trichloroethyl carbonate I. Synthesis, physical properties, and pharmacology. *J. Pharm. Sci.* **56:** 920–921.

55. Gruber, J. C. M., Stephens, V. C. and Terrill, P. M. (1971) Propoxyphene napsylate: chemistry and experimental design. *Toxicol. Appl. Pharmacol.* **19:** 423–426.

56. Rocca, G. and Rusconi, L. Procédé pour la préparation de triméthoxybenzoate de tétracycline et les médicaments qui en dérivent. French Patent 2 099 449 (17 March 1972; Officina Therapeutica Italiana, SRL).

57. Glazko, A. J., Edgerton, W. H., Dill, W. A. and Lenz, W. R. (1952) Chloromycetin palmitate: a synthetic ester of chloromycetin. *Antibiot. Chemother.* **2:** 234–242.

58. McEvoy, J. P. (ed.) (1974) *American Hospital Formulary Service*, vol. 8, p. 24. American Society of Hospital Pharmacists: Washington DC.

59. Murphy, H. W. (1954) Esters of erythromycin. *Antibiotics Annual* 500–521.

60. Sinkula, A. A., Morozowich, W. and Rowe, E. L. (1973) Chemical modifications of lincomycin: synthesis and bioactivity of selected 2,7-dialkylcarbonate esters. *J. Pharm. Sci.* **62:** 1106–1111.

61. Morozowich, W., Sinkula, A. A., Karnes, H. A., MacKellar, F. A., Lewis, C., Stern, K. F. and Rowe, E. L. (1969) Synthesis of bioactivity of lincomycin-2-phosphate. *J. Pharm. Sci.* **58:** 1485–1489.

62. Morozowich, W., Sinkula, A. A., MacKellar, F. A. and Lewis, C. J. (1973) Synthesis and bioactivity of lincomycin-2-monoesters. *J. Pharm. Sci.* **62:** 1102–1105.

63. Owens, W. H. (1990) Tetrazoles as carboxylic acid surrogates in the suosan sweetener series. *J. Pharm. Sci.* **79:** 826–828.

64. Muller, G. W., Culberson, J. C., Roy, G., Ziegler, J., Walters, D. E., Kellogg, M. S., Shiffman, S. S. and Warwick, Z. S. (1992) Carboxylic acid replacement structure–activity relationships in suosan type sweeteners. A sweet taste antagonist. 1. *J. Med. Chem.* **35:** 1747–1751.

65. Sinkula, A. A. (1977) Design of improved taste properties through structural modification. In Roche, E. B. (ed.) *Design of Biopharmaceutical Properties Through Prodrugs and Analogs,* pp. 422–445. American Pharmaceutical Association, Academy of Pharmaceutical Sciences, Washington DC.

PART VIII

Development of New Drugs:
Legal and Economic Aspects

39

From Discovery to Market Availability

JACQUES A. DANGOUMAU

> *Trouver d'abord, chercher ensuite...*
> *Discovery precedes research*
> J. Cocteau

The period between discovering a drug and launching it on the market corresponds to what is known as development. It follows research and precedes marketing. The significance of the development process is sometimes misjudged. In fact, it can be considered as the necessary and somewhat stereotyped collection of data necessary for administrative approval to be obtained. In reality, in the modern pharmaceutical industry, this is what accounts for the strength or weakness of a company.

THE PRACTICE OF MEDICINAL CHEMISTRY
ISBN 0-12-744640-0

I.   BEFORE DEVELOPMENT

A.   What is a discovery?

The starting point is the existence of a discovery. This term is rather vague as it could correspond to different realities. A discovery can be a concept or a scientific fact, for example the notion of receptor or a specific type of receptor. It could also be a hypothesis, a presumption of therapeutic interest — that of yew extracts in certain cancers, for example. By discovery we mean here the possession of a molecule (substance, compound) which can be turned into a drug. In other words, it is potentially endowed with certain curative or preventive properties with regard to human illnesses which remain to be verified; or again, it could, under certain conditions, be launched on the pharmaceutical market. Development is precisely the process which consists in transforming this molecule (the discovery) into a drug (proprietary medicinal product), that is, a chemical substance into a therapeutic agent.

B.   The initial decision

The development of a new molecule is one of the most important and difficult decisions in the life of a drug. It is no longer possible to systematically test all the molecules which appear interesting. The period of 'therapeutic dabbling' is over. Logic and regulations require the therapeutic efficacy of a drug to be demonstrated and the fulfilment of certain prerequisites before it is administered to humans. All this is costly and time consuming. In short, when a decision to develop a molecule is taken, one has sufficient reason to believe that it will become a drug. Many, of course, will fall by the wayside, but the basic assumption is that in the beginning all have reasonable chances of succeeding.

The problems to be resolved before taking a decision are as follows

- Does the molecule represent a scientific benefit? How does it contribute in treating an illness? Might it fare better than existing medication in terms of efficacy and safety? In reality, these questions are often mixed up with the following:

    Is the market share of the drug large enough for the investment to be profitable and at the end of what period? What share of the market can it possibly acquire? This would entail the assessment of several factors, such as present and future competition, solvency of patients, acceptance by social security organizations providing services, and also public health requirements.
- What is required to carry out an industrial project? What are the difficulties related to chemical synthesis, extraction, access to raw materials (for example, in the case of exotic natural products)? What are the costs involved?
- What is the extent and nature of the scientific studies to be carried out? What technical difficulties do they present? What will they cost?
- Does the company have the necessary human and financial resources and would it be able to use such resources? At what particular period could the project be undertaken?
- Since the number of projects that a company can simultaneously carry out is limited, does this molecule represent a strategic option for the company? What priority is it given?

All discoveries have potential to be developed, but not all can be selected. The company might then resort to a joint development project with another company. This, of course, would imply a sharing of expenses, risks and profits. Finally, a certain number of compounds could also be kept in reserve, to be used at a later date when needed.

The decision to develop a molecule is thus strategic, as the company would have to mobilize both human and financial means for a number of years to come. Besides, the possibility of failures should not be ruled out in pharmacology. Thus, from all points of view, this decision is of fundamental importance.

C.   Development objectives

Two objectives need to be considered at any point in the development process: obtaining the marketing authorization and determining the conditions for the compound to succeed.

In all countries, administrative authorization* is a necessary prerequisite for any proprietary medicinal product to be used. To obtain this authorization from the competent authority, an application has to be submitted, whose contents can vary depending on the country. Usually, it should contain proof that three criteria have been fulfilled: therapeutic relevance, safety when administered under usual therapeutic conditions, and pharmaceutical quality.

Success of the drug hinges on what is called its 'positioning', that is highlighting its strong points in relation to competitive drugs and playing down its weaknesses. Ideally, it should be considered an innovation; that is it should display pharmacologically unique characteristics. Moreover, efficacy, safety, quality and positioning will influence decisions during the development process. Failure to fulfil one of these criteria satisfactorily would result in the project being cast aside.

II.   DURING DEVELOPMENT

Development is a complex process entailing different kinds of operations and involving interaction between several disciplines. We shall first describe the elements involved, while emphasizing that in reality, they are largely interdependent, and then examine their organization (Fig. 39.1).

---

*This term refers to the administrative approval which is necessary before using a drug in therapeutic practice. This authorization exists in most countries and particularly in all industrialized ones. In France, it is referred to as 'autorisation de mise sur le marché (A.M.M.)' 'marketing authorization', as in the European Union directives (English version), as 'new drug application (N.D.A.)' in the United States, and so on. It is issued by a registration authority which could either be the state or a body with or without regulatory state powers (l'Agence du Médicament in France; The Food and Drug Administration in the United States; the Office Intercantonal des Médicaments in Switzerland). From 1995 onwards and for certain products only (particularly those resulting from biotechnologies), the European Medicine Agency will issue authorizations for all states of the European Union. The refusal criteria, however, are similar, owing to harmonization efforts, notably the International Conference for Harmonization (I.C.H.), grouping together the United States, Japan and the European Union.

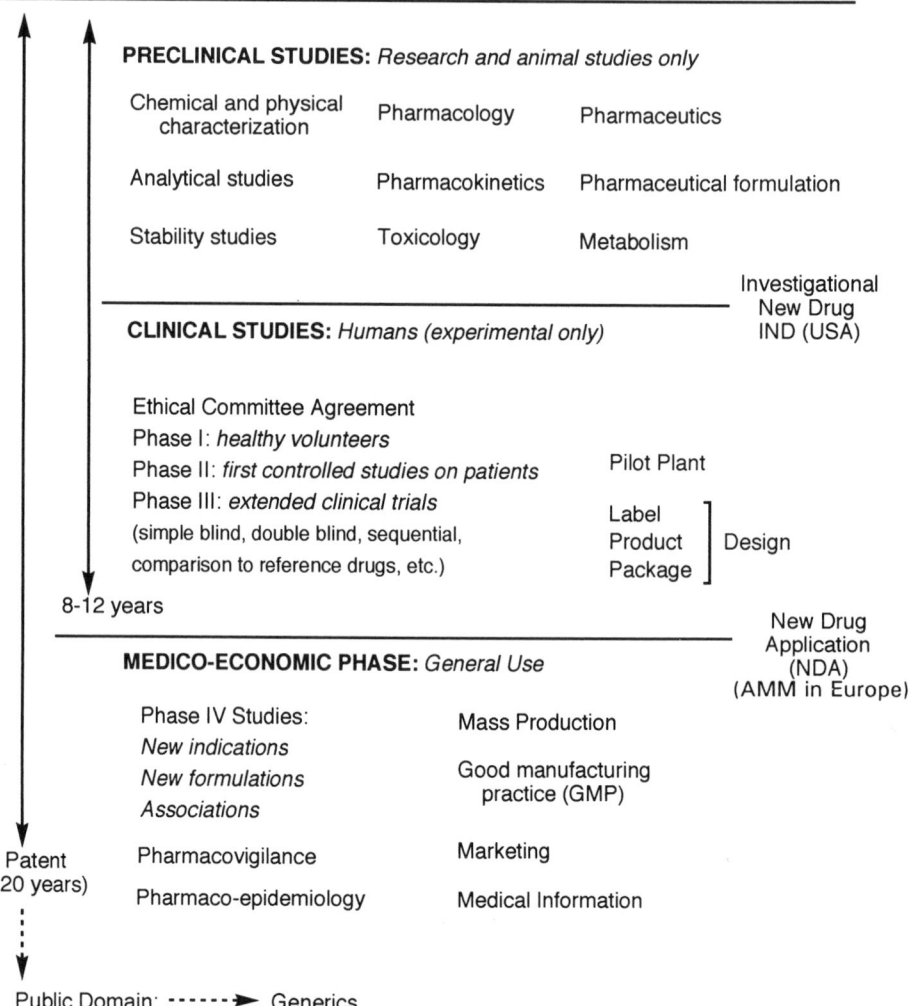

Fig. 39.1 Major steps involved in developing a new drug. A deecision to return to a previous step or to terminate development may occur at any step.

A.   Elements involved in the development process

Development consists in conducting studies.[1] *In vitro* preclinical studies can be distinguished from clinical trials on man regarding innocuousness and efficacy. Then comes the pharmaceutical and industrial development related to the drug manufacture and quality, and finally medico-economic studies pertaining to comparative costs and savings generated. These studies are carried out according to scientific methodologies established by clinical pharmacology and derived disciplines: pharmacoepidemiology, pharmacovigilance, pharmacoeconomy and pharmaceutical science. Administrative texts and registration authorities lay down a certain number of requirements concerning methods and objectives.

1.   Preclinical studies

'Preclinical studies' refer to *in vitro* studies performed before proceeding to human subjects. Their aims are to determine the nature and importance of the molecule's toxicity; reveal the pharmacodynamic effects to determine the therapeutic activity; and follow up the pharmacokinetics and the metabolic effects on animals to elucidate such effects in humans. Their role is to thus ensure the significance of biological effects determined during previous screening, as well as the possibility of and conditions for administration to humans. Regulatory texts lay down a certain number of requirements regarding the nature and number of preclinical studies.[2,3]

Preclinical studies deal with pharmacotoxicology, pharmacodynamics and pharmacokinetics. The aim of *pharmacotoxicology* is to ascertain the toxic effects associated with an overdose, and adverse effects unrelated to the dose that could occur in humans.[4] It includes toxicity, mutagenicity and cancerogenicity testing. The toxicity tests are themselves subdivided into one-dose, repeat-dose and local tolerance tests. One-dose tests study the nature and intensity of toxic phenomena and the time taken for them to appear. By means of these tests, signs of acute toxicity can be detected and the approximate lethal dose determined. They are carried out on at least two species of mammals. Repeat-dose tests help to assess therapeutic risks. Consequently, the duration of administration of the new drug in toxic studies governs the period for which the drug is administered to man; for example, two weeks for a day's treatment, four weeks for seven days', three months for thirty days', six months for anything above. They involve at least two species, one of them not being a rodent species. Three doses are administered: a strong dose provoking toxic effects; a weak dose, but strong enough to bring about a pharmacodynamic effect; and an intermediate dose (for prolonged testing, these doses are determined by means of an intermediate test of subacute toxicity). The difficulty resides in creating conditions that can be extrapolated to humans even before, at least for the initial tests, the effects of the compound on them are known.

Local toxicity tests aim to detect the physicochemical, mechanical and biological effects of the compound on the sites of contact with the organism. Studies related to effects on the reproductive function are compulsory and explore all its aspects. They deal with mating behaviour, fertility modifications, effects on embryogenesis and on the fetus (teratogenesis), interference with delivery, effects on nursing and postnatal development, and subsequent problems linked to heredity. One species of mammals is used; two for the embryo toxicity and, preferably, one whose metabolism of the compound is similar to that of humans (metabolite effects). Three doses are usually administered.

Mutagenic studies deal with possible modifications of genetic material induced by the compound. A large number of tests have been described, which can be divided into four categories: genetic mutations in bacteria, chromosomal aberrations in mammalian cells, genetic mutations in the eukaryotic system, and genetic lesions *in vivo*. Interpretation can be a tedious task if the results are inconsistent.

Most compounds considered to be carcinogenic in humans are also found to be so in animals, but the opposite is not proven. The extrapolation of an experimental cancerigenic effect to humans is tricky if there are no data available on the mechanism of the effect. Carcinogenic tests are undertaken when the drug is administered to humans over at least six months, when its chemical structure is doubtful, when it accumulates in the organism or when a mutagenic test is positive. They are conducted on two species whose metabolisms are similar to human (metabolite effects) and three doses are administered.

Pharmacodynamic tests focus on pharmacodynamic effects — measurable and reproducible modifications brought about by the compound in biological systems — and also, if possible, determine their mechanisms. These systems might be the animal as a whole, isolated organs, cell cultures, enzymatic systems, and so on. Batteries of tests are described for each type of effect. Priority is given to test(s) underlying the potential therapeutic effect, but all the major functions are reviewed to detect undesirable side-effects.

The goal of *pharmacokinetic tests* is to understand the behaviour of the compound and its metabolism in several animal species. Metabolites in particular are sought, and also the possibility of accumulation and enzymatic induction. These studies serve to determine the species, doses, modes and dosage regimens to be employed in tests on animals and assess their transposability to humans, based on the comparison of metabolisms.

Preclinical studies must be performed under Good Laboratory Practice (GLP),[5] which refers to the procedures which ensure the reliability and credibility of studies. These deal with the operative methods, computerization, filing, etc., and set forth a system of quality assurance. A European text has harmonized these procedures and made them binding in Europe.

The interpretation of preclinical tests is a complicated matter and is in no way automatic. It consists in weighing the potential benefits of the compound with the risks that patients could incur. But it must be noted that this evaluation results from a double extrapolation. Any transposition of results obtained from one animal species to another is risky. This is so, when proceeding to humans, although the retrospective examination of results of *in vitro* studies often reveals that a particular activity or toxicity could be suspected from that stage.

The difficulty is to determine when to end this series of studies and when additional studies no longer contribute anything significant. The problem consists in making the right decision regarding safety on the one hand, and time- and cost-saving factors on the other. This decision is taken within the company, but in certain countries (United States), the law requires an authorization to be issued in this respect.

It is essential to understand that this decision is relative. Everything depends on the pathology likely to be treated. If the molecule were to reveal a promising anticancerous activity, a certain degree of toxicity would be tolerated: this would not be the case for a cough mixture. Moreover, the decision maker will take into account comparisons made with reference drugs, based on the same tests. The new drug would need to have an activity and tolerance which are at least equal.

2. Clinical trials

These are trials conducted on humans[3,6] and are indispensable to ensure the efficacy and safety of the compound. At the same time, they determine the conditions of administration (route, dosage, etc.) and precautions of use.

Four phases are usually distinguished in clinical trials. This classification, however, is, subject to criticism. The distinction between phases I, II, II on the one hand and phase IV on the other, is purely administrative: phase IV includes heterogeneous studies conducted after commercialization (and so does not concern us here). The first three phases, however, which follow each other chronologically, are defined by their pharmacological nature.

Phase I concerns initial administration to humans and is done on healthy volunteers. In fact, treating an illness is not yet the main issue, but rather knowing whether the new compound can be used, in what doses, and whether the results of the animal pharmacodynamics and the pharmacokinetic parameters are also valid for the human species. For this, progressive and gradually increasing quantities are administered in succession, until signs of intolerance appear. The pharmacodynamic effects and the pharmacokinetic parameters are determined. This phase is a leap into the unknown: it cannot be known a *priori* whether humans will exhibit a particular sensitivity to the new substance. These trials are carried out in specialized centres equipped with intensive-care facilities.

Phase II concerns the first administration to patients. It needs to be known whether the compound is truly efficacious for a given indication. The optimal activity conditions, dosage regimens and duration of administration are also determined. If possible, a dose–response curve is drawn up. Detecting adverse effects is equally relevant, in order to evaluate whether the risk taken is acceptable.

Phase III provides proof of the therapeutic value of the new compound. There will be just as many studies necessary as uses claimed. Trials are conducted on patients and treatment conditions are those which will be used in actual therapy. They are comparative, that is the patients are divided into two groups, one receiving the new medication, the other serving as a reference. This reference might be either a placebo, to ascertain whether the compound influences the natural course of the illness, or a tested treatment, to determine whether the compound represents an improvement. Division into the two groups is done by randomization, so that they are identical in relation to known or unknown factors likely to influence the effectiveness of the treatment. Conducting trials under blind conditions is advised, i.e. concealing the nature of the medication actually administered either to the patient (single blind), or to both patient and doctor (double blind) in order to avoid interference of psychological factors, even if unintentional. The results are judged according to final criteria representing the anticipated benefits : mortality, morbidity, relief.

This is not always possible, especially in the case of chronic diseases where observation periods are long. Intermediate criteria are therefore used, often a biological parameter whose modification is supposed to influence or determine the course of the illness; this of course has to be validated beforehand. There are several ways, called experimental designs, of conducting these comparisons. The results are dealt with statistically according to the null hypothesis; only the differences between treatments and not their similarities are brought to light. The number of patients necessary to attain statistically significant differences is often high. Trials are therefore long, especially when the disease is rare. To reduce delays and facilitate the enrolment of patients, multicentric studies are often used. Each development is based on one or two pivotal studies, which provide the required demonstration of efficacy; other studies focus on particular points, for example the activity in a particular population of patients.

Clinical trials must also adhere to Good Clinical Practice (GCP),[7] which describes the conditions necessary for results to be reliable and credible. It also lays down a system of quality assurance. Compliance with these procedures can be controlled by official inspections.

The practice of clinical trials raises a number of ethical problems. The protection of volunteers participating in such tests, whether healthy or sick, needs to ensured. Often they are not sufficiently informed to be able to judge the utility of these studies and can be influenced. Various standards have been decreed following the Helsinki Declaration in 1964, revised by the World Health Organization in 1975 (Tokyo) and 1983 (Venice). They have, in general, been adapted by national regulatory agencies and laws. In France, the law of 28 December 1992 provides two types of guarantees, 'informed consent' and submittal of the project to an independent committee, and also the necessity of subscribing to insurance.

The organisation of a clinical trial is a complex matter involving the interaction of specialists from various disciplines: clinical pharmacologists, statisticians, computer scientists, specialists in ailments, research assistants and so on. It is a long and costly enterprise.

The conclusions drawn from clinical trials have their limits. Basically, they arise from the differences between 'experimental' trial conditions in those of the 'real' use of the drug in treatment. These conditions are controlled; there are criteria concerning inclusion and exclusion of patients, interaction with other therapies, administrative conditions, compliance and so on. Moreover, investigators are forewarned and surveillance is regular. Extrapolation to what might happen after marketing is complicated, if not impossible: the selection of patients is less strict, the marketing authorization wording is not always complied with, unforeseen drug interaction might occur, 'populations' with specific characteristics might be concerned, and not all such factors are not always foreseeable and even less controllable. Lastly, the statistical leap is considerable: from a few hundred or thousand cases at the best, to tens of thousands and even millions of cases. Some rare phenomena might then make their appearance. Thus, surveillance and the scientific collection of data do not necessarily end when the drug is launched on the market.

3.   Industrial and pharmaceutical development

The industrial and pharmaceutical aspects of development must adhere to the following objectives:

- Supply the necessary products in adequate form for tests within the proper time limits,
- Draw up the administrative application for the marketing authorization.
- Carry out the industrial project which will result in commercial production.

Preparation of the active ingredient is done according to each case, by extraction from a natural raw material, by chemical synthesis or by hemisynthesis. The preparation process is often patented. During development, the objectives aimed at are improving output, reducing and controlling impurities, but most of all adopting a process likely to produce the necessary quantities.

The pharmaceutical form is a significant development and actually constitutes part of the innovation (sustained release, for example). Usually the part which is truly pharmaceutical, i.e. preparation of the active ingredient and pharmaceutical form, must be determined before the beginning of the clinical trials. These trials should be conducted with the drug as it will be used in treatment: the criteria necessary for approval may be fulfilled for a given drug, but any modifications made are likely to cast doubt on them.

The administrative application to be submitted for obtaining the marketing authorization contains a pharmaceutical part. This is where the composition of the drug and its pharmaceutical form are described. A shelf-life is proposed on the basis of stability tests performed under regular storage conditions, or in certain cases after accelerated tests under varied storage conditions. Those which will be mentioned in the marketing authorization should be determined. The application also includes the characteristics of products used, the description of analytic methods of control and the nature and content of impurities.

From the industrial point of view, manufacturing entails a successive increase in quantitities.

The initial chemical synthesis usually involves small quantities sufficient for screening or biological assays. Thereafter, larger quantities are required for development. The manufacturing process also has to be defined. This is the role of industrial pilots. There could thus be one or several stages between the laboratory and the factory; these are indispensable as not all the processes are easily transposable.

Batches meant for clinical trials have to be manufactured under conditions similar to those for the final products. The manufacturing conditions, in particular, must adhere to Good Manufacturing Practice (GMP) in order to ensure and control the reliability of processes.[8] The inspection authorities attach great importance to this emphasis on quality.

Finally, it is during the development phase that the industrial project is implemented. When the marketing authorization is obtained, the company should be able to supply the market and the development of production capacities should correspond to the rate at which regulatory approval is granted. Usually, the factories manufacturing the active ingredient are few in number. This, of course depends on the compound and the company strategy, but one or two usually suffice for world requirements; the successive stages of synthesis might be located in different sites. However, the pharmaceutical manufacturing establishments that have to comply with GMP are usually numerous. For a long time, splitting up of markets and national overbidding resulted in the construction of almost one factory per country in the developed world. Presently, most multinational firms are reducing their overcapacities, specially in Europe with the completion of the common market. Contracting projects to outside organizations and companies, at least on a temporary basis, is another possibility. The industrial project obviously entails huge investments, which have to be carefully synchronized as the development process progresses.

4.   Medico-economic development

The notion of medico-economic development is more recent[9,10] and is a result of increasing difficulties faced by social security systems to meet health care demands financially. Industrialists have tried to demonstrate that the administration of their drugs is cost-effective for local authorities, in order to justify their prices (when freely determined) or claims. This is easy in the case of generic drugs. Rates merely have to be compared. It is much more difficult when innovations are likely to modify therapeutic habits or the prognosis of an ailment. Medico-economic studies have thus appeared as a kind of substitute for the notion of 'right price', which is extremely complex and almost impossible to define in the field of medicine.

Medico-economic studies are of several kinds:

- 'Cost–cost' studies compare treatment costs for the new drug in relation to the reference treatment(s) (drug-related or not) with equivalent therapeutic efficacy.
- 'Cost–efficacy' studies compare treatment costs on the basis of their respective efficacy in terms of mortality, morbidity, etc.
- 'Cost–utility' studies compare treatment costs according to their impact not only on objective medical criteria but also on the quality of life, including its subjective aspects.

Medico-economic studies are only valid in a given context. They are related to cost determination mechanisms and social security organizations which cover a considerable part of the expenses. Such studies also depend on cultural factors: assessment of quality of life is different in United States and in Europe. By means of such studies, a manufacturer can negotiate with a 'buyer', whether this buyer is a private or public system of social welfare, or a hospital. Such studies have to be undertaken sufficiently early for them to be available at the time of negotiation.

B.   Development strategy

Usually the development process is entrusted to a particular department of the company, the development team, sometimes associated with research. This team plays a strategic role. It takes into consideration the goal set forth (a drug is not developed for the sake of developing it) and technical and regulatory restrictions. In fact, the development process has a certain structure, which is determined by the present state of science and the administrative requirements. These have to be complied with because the registration application corresponds to them. The type of tests to be performed, especially their major aspects, is thus not freely determined.

Moreover, for a given molecule, the company defines certain objectives when it decides to develop a drug. The aim is to produce not merely a drug, but a drug which can be sold. The market is thus analysed in both health and commercial terms. Are there public health requirements which need to be fulfilled? Who are the competitors? Is there place for a new drug and under what conditions? How will the prescribers respond? The future positioning of the drug is defined in this way. Of course, it could be modified as and when test results are obtained.

On the basis of such data, a development plan will be drawn up which specifies the measures that need to be taken and when and how they should be taken. The amount and periods of necessary investments will also be evaluated.

Drawing up a development plan is a 'democratic' operation, involving the help of specialists from extremely varied disciplines. Its application, however, has to be 'dictatorial', in so far as the slightest error or delay could turn out to be catastrophic: thus, the necessity of formalizing the different stages, responsibility levels and procedures, and decision-making processes. In contrast to research, nothing should be left to chance and improvisation.

The work schedule is fundamental. A certain sequence has to be followed between studies. One could not for example start with clinical trials! Before collecting data, there are certain prerequisites to be fulfilled. In certain countries, like the United States, they even have to be submitted to the authorities in order to obtain permission to experiment on humans. However, certain studies could be conducted at the same time. When cancerogenicity testing is necessary, its cost precludes it from being performed too early so to avoid financial loss in case development is discontinued in the early phases, but it must be completed before the end of phase III so that the authorization application is not delayed. Unforeseen events must also be considered. Any delay represents an immediate and future financial loss (reduction in the real duration of patent protection), but haste of any kind could entail unnecessary expense, specially if the project is abandoned later.

Several decisions, however, need to be made,[11] depending mainly on the positioning proposed for the drug, that is, what is required of the drug and what ought to be avoided. A few examples can be mentioned. The place chosen for filing the application is important. Despite considerable efforts at harmonization in recent years, the drawing up of applications and local habits can still differ widely. The situation is changing rapidly in Europe and the setting up of the European Agency in 1995 will lead to the standardization of requirements and greater simplicity in the case of foreign studies; this is not quite the case in the United States and Japan. The choice of investigators thus still depends to a certain extent on the place chosen to file the application. Subsequent applications and studies necessary to complete the application in these new countries must also be considered. Applications prepared for European registration in particular, according to the centralized procedure, will be multinational, but will probably favour countries most likely to be interested in the drug.

These are not the only considerations determining the choice of experts. Their reputation is also exceedingly important. Tests must be performed in a centre whose competence is recognized and whose credibility is reinforced by its scientific authority. Opinion leaders in later phases could participate in launching and promoting the drug.

Choosing the criteria of comparison is not left to chance. The marketing authorization is given for the drug's own properties. Its efficacy can thus be demonstrated in relation to a placebo. If the drug is considered to represent progress in the treatment of a disease, it is not always advisable to compare it with classic treatments! It would be in the manufacturer's interest to choose as reference a drug which is expensive or poorly tolerated, rather than one which is cheap or well tolerated. In short, scientific relevance is not always the only criterion when choosing a reference drug for comparison, but this decision is often important, more for promoting the drug and establishing its price than for the marketing authorization.

The duration of the developmental phase depends, of course, on the kinds of problems raised, their complexity and novelty. In the case of a generic drug, no new process is required; in the case of a new molecule resulting from biotechnology, however, there are endless possibilities in terms of extraction, purification, control and safety. The evaluations published are not easy to compare, since it is not always evident whether the phases of applied research or administrative registration are included or excluded. They stretch from 7 to 12 years; an average of 8 to 10 years for the actual development seems likely.[12-18]

The same difficulties are encountered regarding costs.[12-15,18,19] Added to these, are problems relating to conversion of currency, the effects of inflation and the evolution of costs with time. Their regular escalation is due to regulatory and scientific changes, improved methodologies, public safety concerns and also competition and the requirements of better-informed prescribers. In the United States, estimates vary according to sources: the highest are those of the pharmaceutical industry — 230 to 500 million dollars; the lowest those of administrations — 129 to 169 million. An average estimate of the Office of Technology Assessment is 359 million dollars before taxes (1993).[19d] In France, a minimum figure of 600 million francs for a new molecule might be put forth, and this figure could reach 1.2 billion.

It must be borne in mind that drug sales not only have to bring a return on this investment but also cover investment incurred for molecules which have failed during the development process.

Development can be described as a funnel with a large opening and a narrow exit.[14,19] Here, too, the estimated figures tend to vary. It can, however, be stated that out of 10 000 synthesized molecules, only around 20 will be developed, 5 will be retained for clinical trials, and only one will become a drug. The later the elimination, the higher the costs, without taking into consideration that a rejected molecule may have taken the place of another which revealed promise. Thus, the importance of making the right choice. To develop is to choose.

Developing a molecule also involves taking risks.[19,20] Each one could lead to failure, which is all the more costly and significant if it occurs late. Such risks are not easy to evaluate and some depend on external factors that are sometimes unpredictable.

One category of risk is entirely technical: if the substance is simply incapable of fulfilling the criteria laid down by the registration authorities and presents characteristics which are inappropriate for common use in humans. To take a few examples: insufficient efficacy is a frequent cause of failure, although adequate promotion could save a drug which is no better than others. Unacceptable toxicity could make its appearance in animals: the interpretation of chronic toxicity tests that are performed late is particularly problematic, as animals tests have high predictive value but are inconsistent. The drug may also not be tolerated by humans in respect of certain effects which are difficult or impossible to detect in animals (allergies, for example). Assessment of the benefit–risk relation in the case of a limited number of subjects might be difficult to transpose to the public at large. Pharmaceutical problems that could have been solved during the development process may turn out to have no solution, for example manufacturing processes which are too costly or of low productivity, insufficient stability, or storage conditions which are too restrictive. The kinetics of the drug in humans could differ from that in animals and consequently result in administration routes or dosage regimens that are incompatible with medical practice. Moreover, an adequate pharmaceutical form may not resolve the problem. These are of course just individual cases, the drawbacks being all the more acceptable if the drug has a high therapeutic value.

A second type of risk pertains to health. Do needs exist? How important are they? It has often been noticed that this kind of consideration may lead to the abandonment of certain potentially promising compounds for rare diseases — a kind of orphan drugs. Authorities have tried to fight against this tendency by granting them special advantages (fewer administrative formalities, increased patent protection). Present and future competition must also be taken into account. Thus, the necessity of a 'scientific watch' at all times, especially since long-term planning is necessary and a number of years are required before the drug is profitable.

The third kind of risk is commercial. The aim, of course, is to have the quickest possible return on investment. This, however, requires time, the more so since development is a long and costly process. Several factors play a role: the market share to be acquired, the possibility of being directly or indirectly present in a sufficient number of markets, the possibility of patenting a drug or the manufacturing processes, the quality of this protection, and so on. A scientific success could thus very well turn out to be a commercial flop.

Financial and political implications should also to be considered. Any development project entails expenditure, and if discontinued prematurely would represent a substantial loss. The pharmaceutical industry is self-financed to a large extent and the share of public support in all countries is limited. Scientific ambitions should measure up to the company's financial capacities. Planning must be undertaken on a long-term basis. Yet an unforeseen event may suffice to disrupt plans, such as withdrawal of the product for reasons of pharmacovigilance, the arrival of a competitive drug, a change in governmental or social policy.

Finally, the crisis in the social welfare system, which is linked to the economic slump, has prompted governments to introduce cost-cutting measures and regulate expenses in the field of medical treatments. Medication is naturally affected through prescription and price controls. These kind of political decisions have repercussions on the financial capacities of companies and, consequently, on their abilities to develop their molecules.

Thus, development is a complex art, but its success determined the future progress of the drug. A development process which is too lengthy gives competitors time to establish themselves on the market; with a short process, it is easier to obtain a market niche. If the development has been successful, launching the drug will be easy and also justifiable vis-à-vis the authorities, financiers and prescribers. Development thus represents a key function in a pharmaceutical company.

The work involved is laborious, requiring a pharmaceutical and medical background and also vast experience. Its importance, which is still underestimated at times, at least in France, will continue to increase in modern companies.

III.   AFTER DEVELOPMENT

The development process ends with the marketing authorization. However, the presentation to different registration authorities is spread over time ranging from a few weeks to several years (around 30 years between France and the United States in the case of metformine, for example). Applications have to be adapted in two ways: firstly, in accordance with the different regulations and practices from one country to another. The presentation of expert evaluations by a local opinion leader is often appreciated. The application has thus to be completed according to requirements. In Europe, as a result of harmonization, it is increasingly possible to draw up a single application rather than successive ones. However, local studies are practically indispensable in the United States and Japan despite efforts to promote mutual recognition of tests, especially during international conferences of harmonization (ICH).

The marketing authorization is only a recognition of the drug's technical qualities and does not take into account any economic considerations. The situation differs depending on the country: in certain countries, prices are allowed to vary and availability on the market can immediately follow the authorization; in others, acceptance by social security organizations necessitates a specific procedure for determining prices. In France, this is done in two phases: the 'commission de transparence' (transparency commission) and the economic committee.

The transparency commission compares the advantages and drawbacks of the new drug in relation to competitive drugs. This requires the manufacturer to present scientific and medico-economic comparative studies which, as we have seen, are part of the development process. The commission evaluates the drug's medical utility and any possible improvement, and proposes coverage by the social security organs and its rate.

The economic committee for the drug asks the government to accept or refuse the manufacturer's price proposals, on the the basis of opinion of the transparency commission, following the improvement of the drug' utility or, in its absence, depending on the savings generated.

The actual marketing of the drug or its launch do not concern the development process. This is the work of the sales and/or medical team. The scientific work is reinterpreted in order to be presented to the decision-makers, prescribers, pharmacists and users, as the case may be. This launch has to be prepared in advance and thus close collaboration with the development team. Depending on these requirements, certain studies will be carried out rather than others.

Finally, during the life of the drug, the development process is often resumed and might concern new presentations, routes of administrations, pharmaceutical forms (sustained release forms for example), and dosage regimens. Sometimes, there may be new uses necessitating specific tests in phase III. Some are discovered by chance during use. Very often, a choice has already been made between potential uses. Once the product is on the market, uses kept in reserve will be developed, thanks to initial profits, thus renewing interest in the drug. These developments pertain to the final stages. From a methodological point of view, these uses have nothing in particular to offer, but still entail accurate planning.

The classical representation of a pharmaceutical company corresponds to a linear diagram:

$$\text{Research} \xrightarrow{\text{Discovery}} \text{Development} \xrightarrow{\text{Marketing authorization}} \text{Marketing}$$

From this point of view, the driving force underlying growth is innovation, a term which is considered practically identical to discovery. Innovation is the fruit of research and represents the justification of the company. This description, which can still be found in speeches and publications, can be illustrated by certain triumphs, for example the discovery of cimetidine by S.K.F.

However, there are also companies who have relentlessly striven to find the miracle molecule or renew the first market success only to be finally absorbed by more realistic competitors. There are companies which have been and remain prosperous without ever having made any 'great' discoveries, or whose innovations in certain respects have never revolutionized treatment. Certain major companies alternate the marketing of molecules resulting from their own research with drugs of outside origin which they have judiciously acquired and promoted.

It is usually said that the pharmaceutical industry is a research industry. This is, of course, true. But figures put forth are those of R&D, research and development. The respective share of each is rarely calculated. The share of development is undoubtedly far more significant than that of research. A ratio of $2:4$ could be taken for comparative costs of development and research.[16,21] The exact meaning of these terms would have to be defined. From the development point of view, what is the share of indispensable scientific studies and those necessitated by future promotion? Regarding research, what is the share of fundamental research, and that of applied research which in many respects is similar to development? Although there is general agreement within companies acknowledging the predominance of development costs, it is practically impossible to make these distinctions in financial terms.

The classical outline calls for another reflection on the utility of large research structures. There is support for the view that innovation could be inversely proportional to the means allocated and that only small teams are creative. This is a paradox in part. But is true that major research laboratories sometimes fail to discover important new drugs, whereas, in contrast, companies that are able to develop a molecule rapidly and internationally succeed, even though the drug may not be the first or the best of its class. This necessitates a review of relations between research and development.

At present, the pharmaceutical industry is undergoing major changes under the influence of regulatory requirements, the importance of necessary investment, globalization and harmonization of markets, and the crisis faced by the social security organizations (i.e. reimbursement of costs). A young industry with a pharmaceutical background experiences rapid concentration and restructuring in a typically capitalistic way. The problem is more of an economic and financial nature than related to science and health. Under these conditions one can question the adaptation of the classical model to the future of large companies.[13,22,23] Some already seem to be repositioning themselves according to a new outline for the sector:

$$\left.\begin{array}{l} \text{Research} \longrightarrow \\ \text{License} \longrightarrow \\ \text{Purchase} \longrightarrow \end{array}\right\} \text{Development} \xrightarrow{\text{Marketing authorization}} \text{Marketing}$$

The pharmaceutical company would then merely be a developing and marketing machine. The molecules and the innovation would originate not so much from their own research units, if they survive at all, but from small, more or less independent companies, universities and semipublic research bodies, who are financially and technically unable to launch their discoveries on the market. Control over distribution, promotion and the formation of scientific opinion would ensure marketing of the product. In short, as can be perceived in other fields, distribution would gain the upper hand over production. In other words, the success of large pharmaceutical companies has been due to the rapidity and quality of their development processes. Tomorrow, will this be the indispensable condition for their existence, at least in the case of international laboratories? Will we see the developer take his revenge on the researcher?

REFERENCES

1. Bouvenot, G., Eschwège E. and Schwartz D. (1993) Le médicament; naissance, vie et mort d'un produit pas comme les autres. INSERM, Nathan, Paris.
2. The rules governing medicinal products for human use in the European community (1993) In *The Rules Governing Medicinal Products in the European Community,* vol. I, Commission of the European Communities.
3. Guidelines on the quality, safety and efficacity of medicinal products for human use (1992) In *The Rules Governing Medicinal Products for Human Use in the European Community,* Vol III. Commission of the European Communities.
4. Tuchmann-Duplessis, H. (1978) Action des médicaments sur l'embryon et le foetus. In Giroud, J. P., Mathé F. and Mayniel G. (eds) *Pharmacologie Clinique; bases de la thérapeutique,* pp. 285–307. Expansion Scientifique Française.
5. *Bonnes pratiques de laboratoire* (1984) Bulletin Officiel du Ministère des Affaires Sociales, Paris.
6. Flamant. R. and Sancho, H. (1978) Méthodologie et stratégie en pharmacologie clinique. In Giroud, J. P., Mathé F. and Mayniel G. (eds) *Pharmacologie clinique; bases de la thérapeutique,* pp. 285-307. Expansion Scientifique Française.
7. *Bonnes Pratiques cliniques/Good Clinical Practices* (1987) Bulletin Officiel du Ministère des Affaires Sociales, Paris.
8. (a) *Bonnes pratiques de fabrication et de production pharmaceutiques* (1985) Bulletin Officiel du Ministère des Affaires Sociales, Paris. (b) *Good Manufacturing Practice for Medicinal Products* (1992). In *The Rules Governing Medicinal Products in the European Community,* vol. IV, Commission of the European Community. (c) Bonnes Pratiques de fabrication des médicaments (1992). In *La réglementation des médicaments dans la communauté européenn,* vol. 4, Commission des communautés européennes.
9. Dumoulin, J. (1992) L'évaluation économique du médicament par les firmes pharmaceutiques: de l'approche empirique à l'approche scientifique. *J. Eco. Med.* **10**: 191–202.
10. (a) Chicoye, A. (1992) Etudes d'évaluation économique du médicament dans l'entreprise pharmaceutique: problématique, objectifs, organisation. *J. Eco. Med.* **10**: 203–214. (b) Robinson, R. (1993) Economic evaluation and health care. *Br. Med. J.* **307**: 670–673; 726–728; 793–795; 859–862; 924–926; 994-996. (c) Souêtre, E. J., Qing, W. and Hardens M. (1994) Methodological approaches to pharmaco-economics. *Fundam. Clin. Pharmacol.* **8**: 101–107.
11. Kaniecki, D.J. and Goldberg Arnold, R. J. (1993) Integrating worldwide marketing needs and clinical research. *J. Clin. Pharmacol.* **33**: 989–992.
12. Langle, L. and Occelli, R. (1983) Le coût d'un nouveau médicament. *J. Eco. Med.* **1**: 77–106.
13. Chalchat, B. (1993) Les défis actuels pour l'industrie pharmaceutique de recherche. *Ann. Pharm. Fr.* **51**: 16–25.
14. Salinas, L. (Oct. 1991) Naissance d'un médicament, Geburt eines Medikamentes. *Optipharm.* 19–21.
15. Bridel, F. (1983) La longue et laborieuse genèse d'un médicament. Tausende vom Seiten für einige Milligramm. *Entwicklung Developpement,* (16).
16. Richard, O. (1994) Recherche et developpement: Couper ses coûts et son temps. *Pharmaceutiques* **13**: 44–49.
17. Kaitin, K. I., Di Cerbo, P. A. and Lasagna, L. (1991) The new drug approvals of 1987, 1988 and

1989: trends in drug development. *J. Clin. Pharmacol.* **31**: 116–122.

18. Kaitin, K. I., Bryant, N. R. and Lasagna, L. (1993) The role of the research-based pharmaceutical industry in medical progress in the United States. *J. Clin. Pharmacol.* **33**: 412–417.

19. (a) Lumley, C. E. and Walker, S. R. (1992) The cost and risks of pharmaceutical research. In Griffin, J. P. (ed.) *Medicines: Regulation, Research and Risk,* 2nd edn., pp. 303–318. The Queen's University of Belfast. (b) Di Masi, J. A. (1992) Rising research and development costs for new drugs in a cost containment environment. *Pharmaco Economics* **1** (supplement 1): 13–20. (c) Chirac, P. (1992) Le coût de la recherche pharmaceutique. *Prescrire* **12**: 545. (d) De Valroger, G. (Jan. 1994) Etats-Unis: polémiques autour du vrai coût d'un médicament. *Pharmaceutiques* 47.

20. Runmore, M. M. (1992) The decline in drug development. *Am. Pharm.* NS, **32**(4): 73.

21. The secret of pharma success? (1989) *SCRIP* **1411**: 18.

22. Brown, G. E. Jr. (1992) Rational science, irrational reality: a congressional perpective on basic research and society. *Science* **258**: 200–201.

23. 1993 – A year to retrench, restructure, rethink. (Jan. 1994) *SCRIPT Magazine* 2–6.

40

Drug Nomenclature

SABINE KOPP-KUBEL

Ordnung is die Verbindung des Vielen nach einer Regel
Order is the combination of amounts according to a rule
Emmanuel Kant

I. TRADE NAMES AND NONPROPRIETARY NAMES

Most products available on the market are nowadays identified by a trade name. This is also true in the pharmaceutical field. In many countries trade names, also called trade marks or brand names, are used when prescribing, dispensing, selling, promoting or buying a medicament. Trade names are usually selected by the owner of the product and registered in national trade

THE PRACTICE OF MEDICINAL CHEMISTRY
ISBN 0-12-744640-0

mark or patent offices. They are private property and can be used only with the consent of the owner of the trade mark.[1,2]

In most cases brand names are chosen for a finished pharmaceutical product, i.e. for one or various active drug substances in a defined dosage form and formulation. Consequently, pharmaceutical preparations containing the same active drug substance are frequently sold under different brand names or trade names, not only in different countries, but even within the same country (see Fig. 40.1). In practice this means that the number of trade names in one country is usually much higher than the number of active drug substances marketed and used.

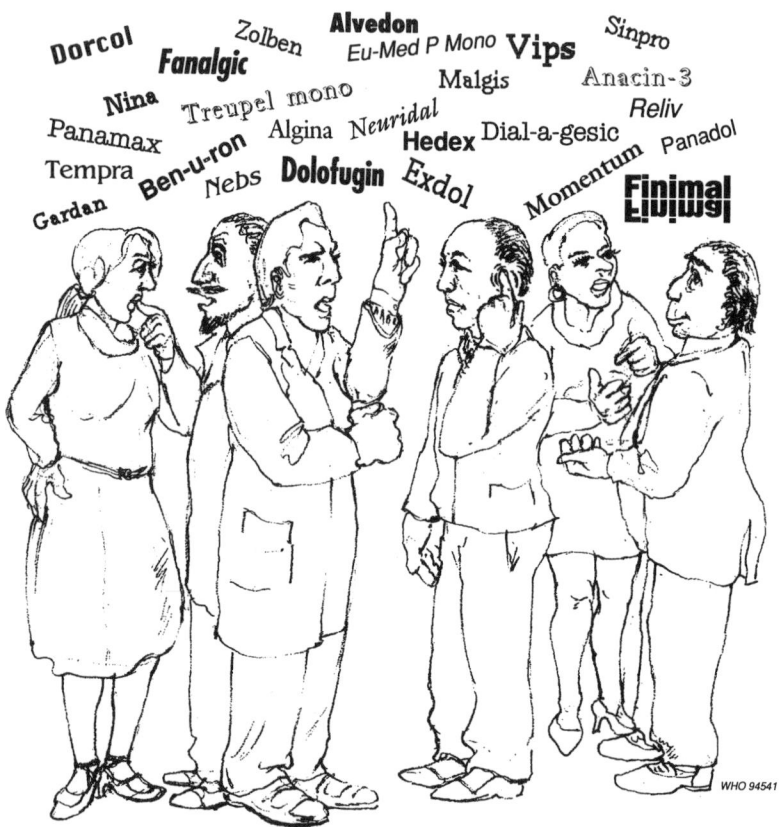

Fig. 40.1 Various trade names for one substance; example *paracetamol.*

Nonproprietary names, also called generic or common names, are intended to be used as public property without restraint, i.e. no-one should own any rights in their usage. These names are usually designated by national or international nomenclature commissions.

Both trade names and nonproprietary names are normally published first in the form of proposals. Comments may be made and objections raised for a certain period before final publication.

Although both nonproprietary names and trade names may appear similar in form to an outsider, there is, in fact, a big difference. Firstly, nonproprietary names are designations to identify the active pharmaceutical drug substance rather than the final product. Second, the selection of a nonproprietary name follows established rules, so that the name itself communicates to the medical and pharmaceutical health professional the therapeutic or pharmacological group to which the active drug substance belongs.

II.   DRUG NOMENCLATURE

A.   International nonproprietary names (INN) for pharmaceutical substances

1.   History

During the twentieth century the rapid development of pharmaceutical chemistry has brought with it the need to identify large numbers of active drug substances by unique, universally available and accepted names. The systematic chemical name, codified by international bodies, including the International Union for Pure and Applied Chemistry (IUPAC) and International

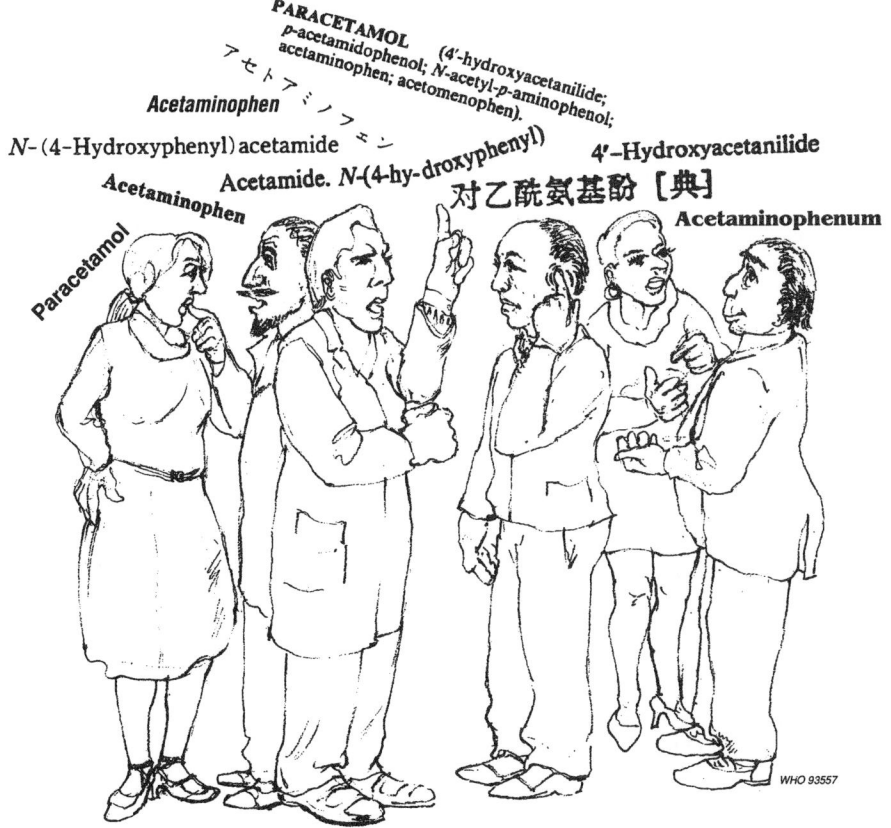

Fig. 40.2   Various common names for one substance; example *paracetamol.*

PROCEDURE FOR THE SELECTION OF RECOMMENDED INTERNATIONAL NONPROPRIETARY NAMES FOR PHARMACEUTICAL SUBSTANCES

The following procedure shall be followed by the World Health Organization in the selection of recommended international nonproprietary names for pharmaceutical substances, in accordance with the World Health Assembly resolution WHA3.11:

1. Proposals for recommended international nonproprietary names shall be submitted to the World Health Organization on the form provided therefore.

2. Such proposals shall be submitted by the Director-General of the World Health Organization to the members of the Expert Advisory Panel on the International Pharmacopoeia and Pharmaceutical Preparations designated for this purpose, for consideration in accordance with the "General principles for guidance in devising International Nonproprietary Names", appended to this procedure. The name used by the person discovering or first developing and marketing a pharmaceutical substance shall be accepted, unless there are compelling reasons to the contrary.

3. Subsequent to the examination provided for in article 2, the Director-General of the World Health Organization shall give notice that a proposed international nonproprietary name is being considered.

A. Such notice shall be given by publication in the *Chronicle of the World Health Organization*[1] and by letter to Member States and to national pharmacopoeia commissions or other bodies designated by Member States.

(i) Notice may also be sent to specific persons known to be concerned with a name under consideration.

B. Such notice shall:
(i) set forth the name under consideration;
(ii) identify the person who submitted a proposal for naming the substance, if so requested by such person;
(iii) identify the substance for which a name is being considered;
(iv) set forth the time within which comments and objections will be received and the person and place to whom they should be directed;
(v) state the authority under which the World Health Organization is acting and refer to these rules of procedure.

C. In forwarding the notice, the Director-General of the World Health Organization shall request that Member States take such steps as are necessary to prevent the acquisition of proprietary rights in the proposed name during the period it is under consideration by the World Health Organization.

4. Comments on the proposed name may be forwarded by any person to the World Health Organization within four months of the date of publication, under article 3, of the name in the *Chronicle of the World Health Organization [1959-1986 in WHO Chronicle, since 1987 in WHO Drug Information]*.

5. A formal objection to a proposed name may be filed by any interested person within four months of the date of publication, under article 3, of the name in the *Chronicle of the World Health Organization*.[1]

A. Such objection shall:

(i) identify the person objecting;
(ii) state his interest in the name;
(iii) set forth the reasons for his objection to the name proposed.

6. Where there is a formal objection under article 5, the World Health Organization may either reconsider the proposed name or use its good offices to attempt to obtain withdrawal of the objection. Without prejudice to the consideration by the World Health Organization of a substitute name or names, a name shall not be selected by the World Health Organization as a recommended international nonproprietary name while there exists a formal objection thereto filed under article 5 which has not been withdrawn.

7. Where no objection has been filed under article 5, or all objections previously filed have been withdrawn, the Director-General of the World Health Organization shall give notice in accordance with subsection A of article 3 that the name has been selected by the World Health Organization as a recommended international nonproprietary name.

8. In forwarding a recommended international nonproprietary name to Member States under article 7, the Director-General of the World Health Organization shall:

A. request that it be recognized as the nonproprietary name for the substance; and

B. request that Member States take such steps as are necessary to prevent the acquisition of proprietary rights in the name, including prohibiting registration of the name as a trade-mark or trade-name.

Fig. 40.3 Procedure for the selection of recommended international nonproprietary names (INN) for pharmaceutical substances.

Union of Biochemistry (IUB) has the advantage of unambiguously defining a specific chemical substance, but it is often very long, difficult to memorize and practically incomprehensible to the nonchemist. Moreover, it gives no indication of the therapeutic action of the substance.

In order to avoid citation of difficult chemical names, generic names came into being. However, in the beginning different names were independently assigned to the same substance in different countries. For example, not everybody would know that acetaminophen, *N*-(4-hydroxyphenyl)acetamide, 4'-hydroxyacetanilide, *p*-acetamidophenol, *N*-acetyl-*p*-aminophenol, acetomenophen and *paracetamol* are the same substance (see Fig. 40.2).

The international nomenclature programme of the World Health Organization (WHO) was established in 1953 when member countries passed a resolution at the World Health Assembly officially initiating the programme on International Nonproprietary Names for pharmaceutical substances (INN; in French, Dénominations Communes Internationales — DCI; in Spanish, Denominaciones Comunes Internacionales — DCI). Subsequently an international panel of experts developed a procedure for the selection of recommended international nonproprietary names for pharmaceutical substances (INNs) (see Fig. 40.3) and general principles for guidance in devising INNs for pharmaceutical substances (see Fig. 40.4).

When WHO's programme first started, the experts had to coordinate the activities of existing

---

GENERAL PRINCIPLES FOR GUIDANCE IN DEVISING INTERNATIONAL NONPROPRIETARY NAMES FOR PHARMACEUTICAL SUBSTANCES

1. International Nonproprietary Names (INN) should be distinctive in sound and spelling. They should not be inconveniently long and should not be liable to confusion with names in common use.

2. The INN for a substance belonging to a group of pharmacologically related substances should, where appropriate, show this relationship. Names that are likely to convey to a patient an anatomical, physiological, pathological or therapeutic suggestion should be avoided.

These primary principles are to be implemented by using the following secondary principles:

3. In devising the INN of the first substance in a new pharmacological group, consideration should be given to the possibility of devising suitable INN for related substances, belonging to the new group.

4. In devising INN for acids, one-word names are preferred; their salts should be named without modifying the acid name, e.g. "oxacillin" and "oxacillin sodium", "ibufenac" and "ibufenac sodium".

5. INN for substances which are used as salts should in general apply to the active base or the active acid. Names for different salts or esters of the same active substance should differ only in respect of the name of the inactive acid or the inactive base.

For quaternary ammonium substances, the cation and anion should be named appropriately as separate components of a quaternary substance and not in the amine-salt style.

6. The use of an isolated letter or number should be avoided; hyphenated construction is also undesirable.

7. To facilitate the translation and pronunciation of INN, "f" should be used instead of "ph", "t" instead of "th", "e" instead of "ae" or "oe", and "i" instead of "y"; the use of the letters "h" and "k" should be avoided.

8. Provided that the names suggested are in accordance with these principles, names proposed by the person discovering or first developing and marketing a pharmaceutical preparation, or names already officially in use in any country, should receive preferential consideration.

9. Group relationship in INN (see Guiding Principle 2) should if possible be shown by using a common stem. The following list contains examples of stems for groups of substances, particularly for new groups [list see text]. There are many other stems in active use. Where a stem is shown without any hyphens it may be used anywhere in the name.

Fig. 40.4   General principles for guidance in devising international nonproprietary names (INN) for pharmaceutical substances.

national nomenclature programmes, which were especially active in France, the Nordic countries, the United Kingdom and the United States. As a result of the national programmes' activities, many substances already had different well-established national names. Members of the newly established international nomenclature programme were faced with the difficulty of choosing a single name in these instances — *paracetamol* in the example given above (see Fig. 40.5). Since than, the activities of national nomenclature commissions have been coordinated in order to achieve international standardization in nomenclature under the auspices of WHO according to articles 2a and 2u of its constitution:[3]

> In order to achieve its objective, the functions of the World Health Organization shall be:
> (a) to act as the directing and coordinating authority on international health work;...
> (u) to develop, establish and promote international standards with respect to food, biological, pharmaceutical and similar products;... .

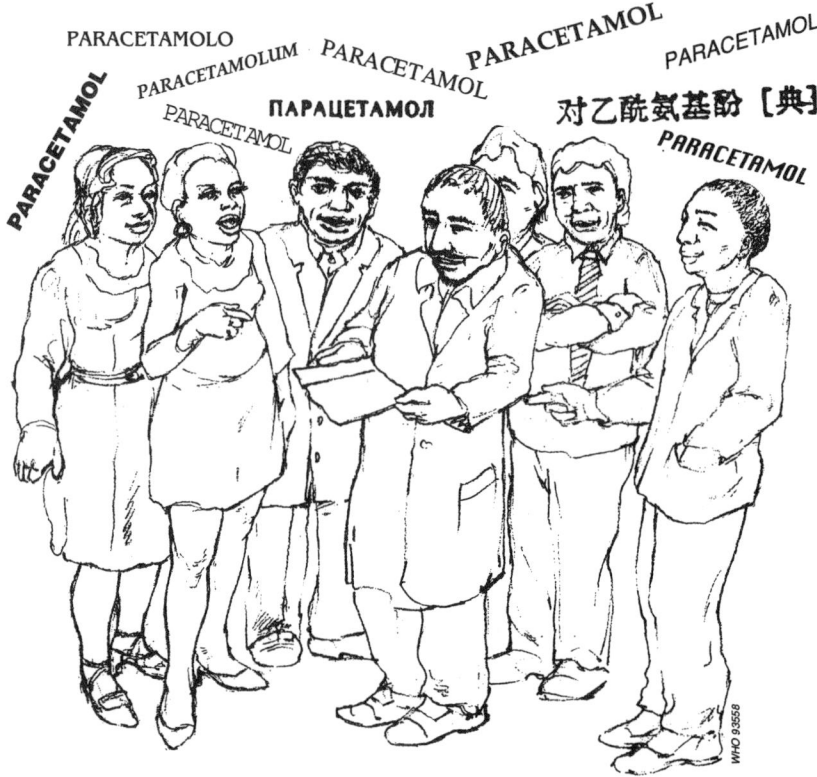

Fig. 40.5   One international name for one substance; example *paracetamol*

2.   Procedure (application, detailed steps)

Requests for recommended international nonproprietary names are submitted on a form to the World Health Organization (INN programme, World Health Organization, 20, avenue Appia, 1211 Geneva-27, Switzerland).[4] These proposals are then submitted by the WHO Secretariat on behalf of the Director General to the members of the WHO Expert Advisory Panel on the International Pharmacopoeia and Pharmaceutical Preparations designated for this purpose.

The following information has to be provided on the form:

- Name and address of manufacturer and/or originator, name of responsible person
- Suggested nonproprietary name(s) (various proposals possible)
- The chemical name (following IUPAC rules)
- The molecular formula
- The graphic formula
- Stereochemical information
- Therapeutic use and pharmacological mode of action
- Code, trade mark (known or contemplated)
- Date of commencement of phase III of clinical trials
- Agreement of the applicant to establish a new CAS registry number, if necessary.

Each name proposed by the originator of such a request is then examined to determine whether it complies with the rules and guiding principles for selection of a name. When all members of the WHO Expert Advisory Panel on the International Pharmacopoeia and Pharmaceutical Preparations designated to select nonproprietary names agree to a name, it is published first as a proposed INN. For a four-month period, any person can forward comments or a formal objection, for example on the grounds of similarity to existing trade marks. When there is no objection, the name is published a second time and the Director General of WHO gives notice to member states that the name has been selected by the World Health Organization as a recommended international nonproprietary name.

3.   Selection process and selection criteria

General rules were established at the beginning of the INN programme in order to allow health professionals to understand the rationale for a number of new names for medicaments. At first some countries used shortened chemical names as generic names, but this system was found to be very limited, since many molecules contain similar elements and groups, such as phenol, chlor, methyl or benzyl rings, in their chemical structures. In addition, in most cases a name that indicates relationship to a group of pharmacologically similarly acting substances is more meaningful to users.

The following principles should in general be applied when selecting an INN. The name should

- be distinctive in sound and spelling;
- not be too long;
- show relationship to substances with the same pharmacological action.

In addition the new name should not conflict with any existing common names or trade marks, and patients should not be confronted with nonproprietary names that are likely to have anatomical, physiological or pathological connotations; for example, a name starting *cancer-* would not be acceptable.

In principle, INNs are given only to the active base or the active acid. Names for different salts or esters of the same active substance should differ only in respect of the name of the inactive moiety of the molecule. For example, oxacillin and ibufenac are INNs and their salts are named oxacillin sodium and ibufenac sodium. The latter are also called *modified INNs* (INNM). [Note that before the existence of this rule, some INNs were published for salts; the term modified INN may, therefore, sometimes be used for a base or acid; for example, levothyroxine sodium was published as an INN and levothyroxine may thus be referred to as an INNM.]

To facilitate the translation/transliteration and pronunciation of International Nonproprietary Names for pharmaceutical substances certain letters, such as 'h' and 'k', should be avoided. Preference is given to 'f' instead of 'ph', 't' instead of 'th', 'e' instead of 'ae' or 'oe' and 'i' instead of 'y'. The INN for amphetamine is, therefore spelt *amfetamine*.

When devising an INN it is important to be aware of possible language problems. Since the name is to be used worldwide, not only should certain letters be avoided, but experts need to be aware of unsuitable connotations in the major languages spoken in the world. A name may appear excellent for an English speaker, but unacceptable in another language. For example the name 'inglicretin' could remind a French speaker of the term 'cretin Anglais' (stupid Englishman) and might therefore not be the best choice for a medicament.

As INNs should show relationship to other substances of similar pharmacological action, common stems have been created. A large number of such common stems are in use, and new stems are created whenever necessary.[5] Some examples are given in Table 40.1. Examples of INNs published for calcium channel blockers, nifedipine derivatives, include: amlodipine, barnidipine, benidipine, cilnidipine, cronidipine, darodipine, efonidipine, elgodipine, felodipine, flordipine, furnidipine, isradipine, lacidipine, levniguldipine, manidipine, mesudipine, nicardipine, nifedipine, niludipine, nilvadipine, nimodipine, nisoldipine, nitrendipine, oxodipine, palonidipine, pranidipine, riodipine, sagandipine, sornidipine, teludipine.

4. Recent developments

When requesting selection of an INN, the manufacturer has often not yet finalized the precise indications for the therapeutic use of the compound. A name is usually requested during the development phase of a new compound, which means that the request is generally submitted to WHO during the clinical trials phase. However, a name is needed as soon as an application for registration of a product is forwarded to the national authorities. This means that the naming process is close to all new scientific developments in the pharmaceutical field. External expertise is often needed for specific questions concerning new therapeutic groups and new types of products.

During the last few years the selection process has become more complex. New receptors and pharmacological actions are discovered more and more frequently. This means in many cases that new common stems have to be created. However, there is sometimes a structural relationship to existing molecules and experts have to decide whether an existing stem may be used or whether a new one must be established. Fibrinogen receptor antagonists are a recent example. These substances act as platelet aggregation inhibitors for which the stem *-grel* existed for several years. The nomenclature experts now have to decide whether the same stem should be used for the fibrinogen receptor antagonists or whether the group of new molecules is so important that a new stem needs to be established. The suffix *-fiban* has been chosen for this.

On the other hand, a new mode of action is sometimes discovered for an existing substance. If further substances are developed with a similar mode of action, the question arises whether a new stem is needed, which would mean modifying the 'old' name for the first compound in the series. For example albifylline and pentoxifylline are *N*-methylxanthine derivatives and the stem *-fylline* was therefore chosen for their names. These substances have now been found also to suppress the tumour necrosis factor-α.[6] The experts decided to retain the stem *-fylline* in this

Table 40.1   Common stems in INN formation.

Stem	Pharmacotherapeutic group
-ac	Anti-inflammatory agents of the ibufenac group
-actide	Synthetic polypeptides with a corticotropin-like action
-adol } -adol- }	Analgesics
-ast	Antiasthmatic, antiallergic substances not acting primarily as antihistaminics
-astine	Antihistaminics
-azepam	Diazepam derivatives
-bactam	β-Lactamase inhibitors
bol	Steroids, anabolic
-buzone	Anti-inflammatory analgesics, phenylbutazone derivatives
-cain-	Antifibrillant substances with local anaesthetic activity
-caine	Local anaesthetics
cef-	Antibiotics, cefalosporanic acid derivatives
-cillin	Antibiotics, derivatives of 6-aminopenicillanic acid
-conazole	Systemic antifungal agents, miconazole derivatives
cort	Corticosteroids, except prednisolone derivatives
-dipine	Calcium channel blockers, nifedipine derivatives
-fibrate	Clofibrate derivatives
gest	Steroids, progestogens
gli	Sulfonamide hypoglycaemics
io-	Iodine-containing contrast media
-ium	Quaternary ammonium compounds
-metacin	Anti-inflammatory substances, indomethacin derivatives
-mycin	Antibiotics, produced by *Streptomyces* strains
-nidazole	Antiprotozoal substances, metronidazole derivatives
-olol	β-Adrenoreceptor antagonists
-oxacin	Antibacterial agents, nalidixic acid derivatives
-pride	Sulpiride derivatives
pril(at)	Angiotensin-converting enzyme inhibitors
-profen	Anti-inflammatory substances, ibuprofen derivatives
prost	Prostaglandins
-relin	Hypophyseal hormone release-stimulating peptides
-terol	Bronchodilators, phenethylamine derivatives
-tidine	H_2-histamine receptor antagonists
-trexate	Folic acid antagonists
-verine	Spasmolytics with a papaverine-like action

case, since the 'new' action was nevertheless based on the typical xanthine-mediated inhibition of phosphodiesterase.

New approaches to naming pharmaceutical substances may be needed in the near future because of the increase of research using molecular design. 'Simple' derivatives of known compounds are becoming ever more rare. Chemistry based on receptor structure and molecular design focuses more on synthesizing compounds to fit receptor binding sites. This will mean that nomenclature will have to move in the same direction. Chemical relationship will need to be looked at from a different standpoint, and the pharmacological activity might have to be considered in almost all cases as a basic for assigning a given substance to a group.

Table 40.2   Common stems for monoclonal antibodies.

I.	General stem	*-mab*
II.	Substems for source of product	
	human	*-u-*
	rat	*-a-*
	hamster	*-e-*
	primate	*-i-*
	mouse	*-o-*
	chimeras	*-xi-*
III.	Substems for disease or target group:	
	bacterial	*-ba(c)-*
	cardiovascular	*-ci(r)-*
	immunomodulator	*-li(m)-*
	viral	*-vi(r)-*
	tumours	
	colon	*-co(l)-*
	testis	*-go(t)-*
	ovary	*-go(v)-*
	mammary	*-ma(r)-*
	melanoma	*-me(l)-*
	prostate	*-pr(o)-*
	miscellaneous	*-tu(m)-*

Whenever there is a problem in pronunciation, the final letter of the substems for disease or targets may be deleted, e.g. -co(l)-, vi(r), li(m), etc.

IV. Prefix
The prefix should be random, e.g. the only requirement is to contribute to a euphonious and distinctive name.

V. Second word
If the product is radiolabelled or conjugated to another chemical, such as a toxin, identification of this conjugate is accomplished by use of a separate, second word or acceptable chemical designation. For monoclonals conjugated to a toxin, the *tox-* stem must be included as part of the name selected for the toxin.

Substances produced by biotechnology are another challenge for the nomenclature committee.[7] New schemes and concepts need to be developed on a worldwide basis. One example is the scheme for common stems for naming monoclonal antibodies (Table 40.2). Examples of INNs include altumomab, balimomab, biciromab, dorlimomab aritox, imciromab, maslimomab, nebacumab, satumomab, sevirumab, telimomab aritox, tuvirumab.

5.   Publication

Newly selected proposed INNs are published, after the originator of the request for a name has been informed, in a list in *WHO Drug Information*, a journal published by WHO.[8] For example:

fradafibanum

fradafiban	(3*S*,5*S*)-5-[[(4′-amidino-4-biphenylyl)oxy]methyl]-2-oxo-3-pyrrolidineacetic acid
	fibrinogen receptor antagonist
fradafiban	acide 2-[3*S*,5*S*)-5-[[4′amidinobiphényl-4-yl)oxy]méthyl]-2-oxopyrrolidin-3-yl]acétique
	antagoniste du récepteur du fibrinogène
fradafiban	àcido (3*S*,5*S*)-5-[[4′-amidino-4-bifenilil)oxi]metil]-2-oxo-3-pirrolidinacético
	antagonista del receptor del fibrinógeno

$C_{20}H_{21}N_3O_4$ 148396-36-5

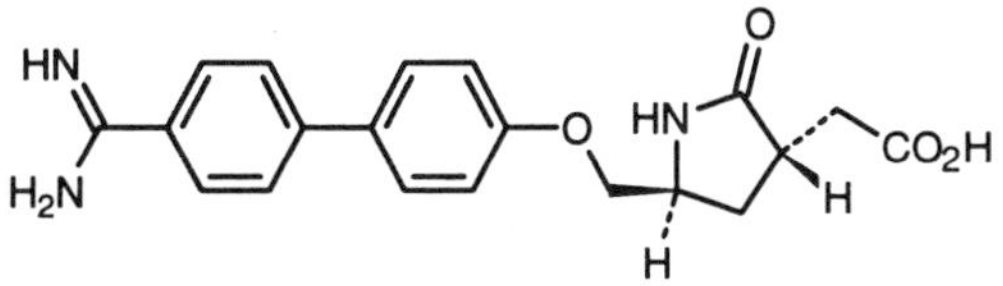

Two lists of proposed INNs are published per year. If no objection has been raised during a four-month period, the proposed name is published a second time as a recommended INN as the following example:

fradafibanum

fradafiban	(3*S*,5*S*)-5-[[(4′-amidino-4-biphenylyl)oxy]methyl]-2-oxo-3-pyrrolidineacetic acid
fradafiban	acide 2-[3*S*,5*S*)-5-[[4′amidinobiphényl-4-yl)oxy]méthyl]-2-oxopyrrolidin-3-yl]acétique
fradafiban	àcido (3*S*,5*S*)-5-[[4′-amidino-4-bifenilil)oxi]metil]-2-oxo-3-pirrolidinacético

$C_{20}H_{21}N_3O_4$

Lists of both proposed and recommended INNs are sent together with a letter signed by the Director General to WHO member states (at present 190), to national pharmacopoeia commissions and to other bodies designated by member states. In this letter the Director requests that member states should take such steps as are necessary to prevent the acquisition of proprietary rights in the name, including prohibiting registration of the name as a trade name.

Up to now more than 6600 INNs have been selected. All names that have been selected are published in a cummulative list of INNs, which is updated periodically.[9] The generic names are presented in alphabetical order by Latin name. Each entry includes

- Equivalent nonproprietary names in Latin, English, French, Russian and Spanish
- A reference to the INN list in which the name was originally proposed or recommended
- Reference to substances that have been abandoned or were never marketed
- Reference to national nonproprietary names
- Reference to pharmacopoeial monographs or similar official references
- Names issued by the International Organization for Standardization (ISO)
- The molecular formula
- The Chemical Abstracts Service (CAS) number.

Figure 40.6 illustrates the layout of the cumulative list:

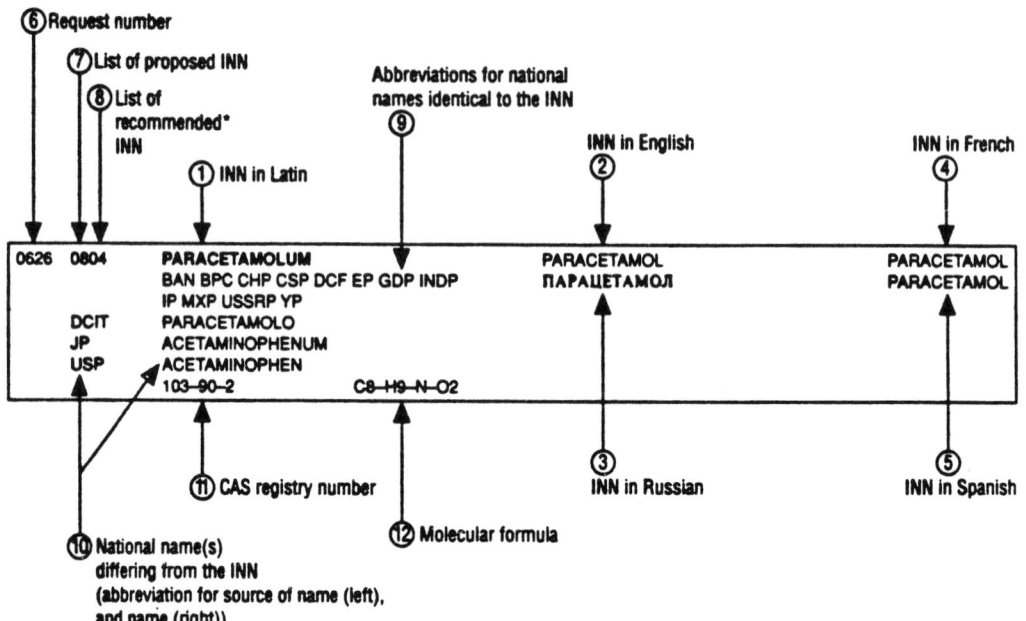

Fig. 40.6   Layout of the cumulative list of INNs.[9] An asterisk * in place of a recommended list number signifies that an objection has been raised to the proposed name.

B.   Common names selected by the International Standards Organization (ISO)

The International Organization for Standardization (ISO) has laid down principles for selecting common names for pesticides and other agrochemicals.[10] These principles are comparable to the guiding principles for selecting INNs and have a similar purpose of providing short, distinctive and easily pronounced names for substances whose full chemical names are too complex for convenient use. The names chosen should not be permitted to become privately owned trade marks. ISO names are also given for salts and complex esters, as well as mixtures of isomers. The work of the INN and ISO committees sometimes overlaps, especially in the field of veterinary medicine.

C.   National nomenclature

Since the INN programme came into existence, WHO has coordinated the activities of national nomenclature commissions. Several INN experts are Secretaries to national nomenclature commissions and in most cases the WHO Secretariat also acts as corresponding member of these commissions. Differences between national and international nomenclature have become rare.

In most countries, national nomenclature commissions are part of or are closely linked to the national pharmacopoeia. Some countries no longer have a commission and publish the INNs directly as national names in their legal publications, for example in Germany and the Nordic countries; the latter previously published Nordic Pharmacopoeia Names (NFN). In others, the national nomenclature commission adopts INNs in the language of the country as national names, e.g. the *Denominazioni Comuni Italiane* (DCIt) in Italy.

All European directives include INNs as 'usual terminology' (point 3 of Article 4(2) of Directive 65/65/EEC). The European Pharmacopoeia uses INNs in the main titles of monographs.

National nomenclature commissions select and publish the following national nonproprietary names (address of responsible authority given in brackets):

BAN — British Approved Names
(The Secretary, British Pharmacopoeia Commission, Market Towers, 1 Nine Elms Lane, London SW8 5NQ, United Kingdom).

DCF — Dénominations Communes Françaises
(Secretariat of the French Pharmacopoeia Commission at the Drug Agency, Direction des Laboratoires et des Contrôles, Unité Pharmacopée, 145–147, boulevard Anatole France, 93200 Saint-Denis, France)

JAN — Japanese Accepted Names
(Japanese Ministry of Health and Welfare, New Drugs Division, Pharmaceuticals Affairs Bureau, 1-2-2, Kasumigaseki, Chiyoda-ku, Tokyo 100, Japan)

USAN — United States Adopted Names
(United States Adopted Names Council, American Medical Association, PO Box 10970, Chicago, IL 60610, USA)

Other names:

PEN — Pharmacy Equivalent Name
A Pharmacy Equivalent Name is a short and simple name that is offered by the United States Pharmacopeia (USP) as a standardized term. The PEN name for a dosage form containing two or more therapeutic drug substances may be devised by combining portions of the official names of the component drug substances. A 'Co-' prefix indicates that the product is a combination dosage form. PEN names are not official titles in the USP pharmacopeia.

III.   USE AND PROTECTION OF NONPROPRIETARY NAMES

WHO's INN programme has been actively providing nonproprietary names since 1953. During this period more than 6600 names have been published. New pharmaceutical substances are continually being developed and some 150 to 170 new names are published every year.

In order to avoid confusion, it is strongly recommended by the World Health Organization that new drug substances are identified by codes rather than arbitrary names until nonproprietary names have been designated.

A. Use of nonproprietary names

Nonproprietary names are intended to be used in pharmacopoeias, labelling, advertising, drug regulation and scientific literature, and as product names, e.g. for generics. Some countries have defined the minimum size of characters in which the generic name must be printed under the trade mark labelling and advertising. In Canada, the United States and Uruguay, the generic name must appear prominently in type at least half as large as that used for the proprietary or brand name. Certain countries, for example Mexico, have even gone as far as abolishing trade marks for the public sector.

B. Protection of nonproprietary names

The consequence of introducing INN common stems into trade marks, which seems to be increasingly popular, hampers the selection of new nonproprietary names within the established system. Given that all new INNs should be distinctive from existing INNs, without similarity to trade marks, this practice causes confusion to the health professional, may be the source of serious errors in prescribing and dispensing, and hinders the selection of future names for compounds in the same group of substances. Based on recommendations made by the WHO Expert Committee on the Use of Essential Drugs, a resolution[11] was adopted during the forty-sixth World Health Assembly requesting Member States to

> enact rules or regulations, as necessary, to ensure that international nonproprietary names... are always displayed prominently; to encourage manufacturers to rely on their corporate name and the international nonproprietary names, rather than on trade marks, to promote and market multisource products introduced after patent expiration; to develop policy guidelines on the use and protection of international nonproprietary names, and to discourage the use of names derived from INNs, and particularly names including INN stems in trade marks.

IV SUMMARY

The existence of an international nomenclature for pharmaceutical substances, in the form of INNs, has proved since 1953 to be important for the safe prescription and dispensing of medicines to patients, and for communication and exchange of information among health professionals worldwide.

INNs identify pharmaceutical substances by unique names that are globally recognized and are public property. They are also known as generic names.

Common stems are developed for the selection of INNs to communicate to health professionals the type of pharmaceutical product in question.

National and international nomenclature commissions collaborate closely to select a single name of worldwide acceptability for each active substance that is to be marketed as a pharmaceutical.

To avoid confusion, which could jeopardize the safety of patients, nonproprietary names and their common stems should not be used in trade marks. The selection of further names within a series should not be hindered by the use of a common stem in a brand name.

The author alone is responsible for the views expressed in this article.

REFERENCES

1. Wehrli, A. (1986) Pharmaceuticals: trademarks versus generic names. *Trademark World Journal* 31–35.
2. Trademarks versus generic names for pharmaceuticals. A conflict that requires resolution. *WHO Drug Information* (1987) **1**(2): 39–40.
3. *Basic Documents*, 39th edn. World Health Organization, Geneva, 1992.
4. INN application form (WHO 5233 PHA (8/90) - 1000), World Health Organization, Geneva.
5. *The use of common stems in the selection of international nonproprietary names (INN) for pharmaceutical substances,* World Health Organization, Geneva, Switzerland, 1995 [WHOPHARM S/NOM 15 REV. 30].
6. Semmler, J., Gebert, U., Eisenhut, T. *et al.* (1993) Xanthine derivatives: comparisons between suppression of tumor necrosis factor-α production and inhibition of cAMP phosphodiesterase activity. *Immunology* **78**: 520–525.
7. Wehrli, A. (1992)Generic names for biotechnology-derived products. *Drug News & Perspectives* **5**(1): 55–58.
8. Examples of published INN lists:
   List 73 of proposed INNs: *WHO Drug Information* (1995) **9**(2).
   List 35 of recommended INNs: *WHO Drug Information* (1995) **9**(3).
   World Health Organization, Geneva, Switzerland.
9. *Cumulative List No. 8 of International Nonproprietary Names (INN) for Pharmaceutical Substances,* World Health Organization, Geneva, 1992.
10. *ISO Standard Pesticides and other agrochemicals – Principles for the selection of common names* (ISO/DIS 257, 1988), International Organization for Standardization, Geneva, 1988.
11. *Forty-sixth World Health Assembly Resolution on Nonproprietary Names for Pharmaceutical Substances* (WHA46.19), World Health Organization, Geneva, 1993.

41

Legal Aspects of Product Protection — What a Medicinal Chemist Should Know About Patent Protection

MARIA SOULEAU

I. INTRODUCTION

A patent is a grant to an inventor of the exclusive right to use and profit from his invention for a limited term. In exchange, the inventor discloses the invention in such a way that an expert could follow it without doing research. Patents play an important role in the progress of national economies and in progress in general.

THE PRACTICE OF MEDICINAL CHEMISTRY
ISBN 0-12-744640-0

During the last two centuries, the United States and some western European countries have experienced a phenomenal industrial and economic development. In this process, research and innovation played a predominant role and patents were instrumental, inasmuch as inventions were no longer kept secret but were made known to the public, thus inducing new research and innovation. The post-war development of Japan's industrial potential is an example which demonstrates the role and the importance of the patent system.

A. History of the patent system prior to 1883

Originally patents were intended to encourage the introduction of new technologies into a country so as to develop native industry, rather than to provide a just reward to the inventor. In order to encourage and reward the publication of new knowledge, privileges were granted giving the owner of the technology the exclusive right to exploit that knowledge in the relevant territory for a limited period. Until the fifteenth century, the various states were scarcely concerned with furthering the development of industry, and generally speaking manufacturing secrecy remained the rule. The statute for inventors decreed by the Council of the Venetian Republic on 19 March 1474, can be considered as the first law on patents.[1] This statute stipulated that

> whoever will make in this City [Republic of Venice] any new and ingenious artifice, not made previously in our state, will be obliged to register it at the office of our proveditors of the Commune, as soon as it will be reduced to perfection, so that it will be possible to use and apply it. It shall be forbidden to anyone else in any our land and place to make any other artifice to the image and similarity of that one without consent and licence of the author during the term of ten years.

Studies of the detailed records of early grants in other countries suggest that the idea of a patent system spread over Europe from Italy with emigrating Venetian glassworkers.

In England, from 1315, the grant of monopolies by the Crown had been widely used as a means of promoting and regulating trade and as a source of revenue. As a means of attracting new industries from overseas, letters of protection were also granted to groups of foreign workers. From the beginning, an essential condition of the validity of English patents for invention rights was that the invention should actually be worked in the country. The practice of granting patent monopolies became firmly established in England in the reign of Elisabeth I. Between 1561 and 1590 more than fifty monopolies were granted to encourage English industry and to make the country self-sufficient. Some of these patents were patents of invention for new industries, but the Queen's need for money also led her to grant other monopolies giving the right to control established industries. Such patents were clearly against the public interest and provoked vigorous protest in the House of Commons. So, in 1601, the Queen issued a proclamation revoking the objectionable patents and enforced the monopoly rights grants for invention. In 1623, under the reign of James I, the 'Statute of Monopolies' prescribed the cases for which there could be a monopoly. According to this statute, an invention had to be novel and nondetrimental to the general interest. This law also established a time limit for the 'duration of the monopoly'. After the passage of the Statute of Monopolies there was no further legislation in England on patents of invention for over 200 years.

The Statute of Monopolies was followed by similar legislation in the American colonies, where settlers began to petition the legislature or governor for monopoly patents similar to those they had been familiar with in England. In 1641 the General Court of Massachusetts adopted a 'Body of Liberties' prohibiting the granting of monopolies except for 'such new inventions as are profitable to the country and that for a short time'. After the American war of independence, the old concept of a patent granted as an act of grace and favour by the Crown began to be replaced by the idea that an inventor had a natural right to his property. In South Carolina, an act of 1784 provided for 14 years monopoly rights to inventors and most of the other new states continued and extended the colonial practice of rewarding inventors with the grant of patent rights. When the delegates of the states met to draft the Constitution of the United States of America it was recognized that it would be more effective to replace the separate state patents by a single form of protection for the whole country. In 1790 Thomas Jefferson drafted the first American law of patents. This law stipulated a monopoly to inventors of 17 years from the grant for novel inventions useful to the country.

In France, the early practice of the royal grant of patents (from 1543) for inventions was confirmed by an edict of Louis XV in 1762 which prohibited permanent privileges but provided for inventors' patents to be limited to 15 years. In 1789, with the revolution, the privileges of inventors were abolished. Nevertheless on 7 January 1791 the Constitutional Assembly passed the first law on patents. In the words of the preamble of the new French law,

> every novel idea whose realization or development can become useful to Society belongs primarily to the man who conceived it, and it would be a violation of the rights of man in the very essence if an industrial invention were not regarded as the property of its creator.

According to this French law, for a disclosure of the invention the state granted to the author a 'manufacturing monopoly' for a limited period. Under the law of 1791, French patents were granted for 5, 10 or 15 years. Patents became null and void if not worked within two years or if the patentee sought to take out a patent abroad. Examination of applications was still required, but in 1844 this was abolished. According to the 1844 law, the inventor was not obliged to delimit his monopoly by claims, but the inventor was obliged to describe his invention to the best of his ability.[2]

Thus, in the seventeenth and eighteenth centuries, with the development of commerce and the beginnings of industry, some states adopted patent laws which gave their inventors protection against the infringement of their inventions. In Europe subsequent developments in the nineteenth century were greatly influenced by competing economic interest. Industrialists who recognized the value of patents in protecting their businesses increasingly pressed for the patent system to be strengthened and expanded. A uniform patent law for the whole of Germany was adopted in 1877 with strict examination for 'novelty' and 'level of invention'.

Before enumerating the main conventions and treaties still in force, it must be noted that almost every country has now adopted a patent law.

B.   Main conventions and treaties

In the middle of the nineteenth century it was already apparent that industrial property rights should extend beyond national boundaries. In 1883, in order to facilitate the transfer of technology, a large number of states created the *Paris Convention*, an international convention. The Paris Convention established major basic rules concerning industrial property and was a remarkable piece of legislation for its time. The convention was revised in subsequent international conferences in Brussels in 1900, Washington in 1911, The Hague in 1925, London in 1934, Lisbon in 1958 and Stockholm in 1967. The main provisions which apply between the member countries are now:[3]

(1) Foreigners receive in each country the same treatment as nationals of that country.

(2) An applicant for a patent in one country receives the benefit of his original filing date for any subsequent application for that invention filed in another country within one year (this is the priority clause — *Priority Right*).

(3) Patents in different countries for the same invention are independent, so that they are not affected by refusal, revocation or expiry in any other country.

(4) Importation by the patentee of goods produced in one country is not to entail forfeiture of patent protection for those goods.

(5) Each country may take steps to prevent abuses resulting from the exclusive rights arising from patents, e.g. failure to use the invention, but the patent may be revoked only if compulsory licensing is not a sufficient remedy.

Concerning the Priority Right, no extension of the 12-month period can be allowed. After 12 months, the Priority Right is lost.

In 1978 two treaties came into force which had an impact on the world patent system unequalled since the Paris Convention of 1883. These two treaties were the Convention of the Grant of European Patents, named the European Patent Convention (signed in Munich in 1973) and set up by the Council of Europe, and the Patent Cooperation Treaty (signed in Washington in 1970) established by the World Intellectual Property Organization. Furthermore, the Council of the European Community has, for some time, been endeavouring to bring into force a Convention for the European Patent for the Common Market (the Community Patent Convention) for which the basic text was signed in Luxembourg in December 1975 by the EEC members at that time. This has been supplemented by a Community Patent Agreement, initiated by the 12 EEC countries in December 1985.

The European Patent Convention is in addition to the national patent laws which exist in each country in Europe, even though the contracting states had to modify their laws in order to harmonize it with the European Patent Convention.

The European Patent Convention and the Patent Cooperation Treaty each establishes a system for filing a single patent application to obtain, ultimately, national patents in countries designated in the application. In contrast, the Community Patent Convention, when it comes into force, will provide the granting of Community patents, as a result of filing applications under the European Patent Convention. The Community Patents will be effective in all the Community countries acceding to the Community Patent Convention by their own legal order under the Community Patent Agreement together with any further such agreement which is entered into to bring the Community Patent Convention into force.

The *European Patent Convention* (EPC) is a treaty open only to European countries and has been negotiated by 21 of them. The possibility of filing a European Patent Application is open to countries both inside and outside the EEC. According to the European Patent Convention, by means of a direct single filing at the European Patent Office (EPO) or indirect single filing through certain national patent offices, if the law of a contracting state permits, it is possible to obtain national patents in the contracting states. In 1993, the contracting states were Austria, Belgium, Denmark, France, Germany, Great Britain, Greece, Ireland, Italy, Liechtenstein, Luxembourg, Monaco, Portugal, Spain, Sweden, Switzerland, and the Netherlands.

According to the European Patent Convention, a European Patent Application is submitted to a single examination system. An applicant files a patent application in one of the official languages of the European Patent Convention, namely German, English or French. This application is examined at the EPO for formalities and then a prior art — the invention must not have been disclosed in or by prior publication or prior patents, or must not have been involved in public use or public sale, or must not have been a part of or suggested of prior knowledge — search and a search report are performed. The application and the search report are then published.

After publication of the application and the search report, the applicant has the opportunity to request substantive examination for patentability to be performed at the EPO. The examination of the application is performed by the Examining Division of the EPO. On completion of the examination, which includes an examination for inventive step as well as for novelty (novelty and inventive step are basic requirements for patentability; see Section IV), either the application is rejected or the European Patent is granted. The specification as granted is published and the grant of the European patent leads to national patents being registered in the designated countries.

Opposition can be filed at the EPO after the European Patent has been granted. The result of the opposition, i.e. amendment or revocation of the European Patent, apply equally to all the national patents resulting from the European Patent. Furthermore, each national patent can be amended or revoked under the relevant national law.

The EPO has set out to establish a practice which is a compromise between various traditions (German, British, etc.) and does not follow any existing national tradition. The officials in charge of the development procedure have attempted to avoid the worst features of the existing national systems. The EPO regards itself as having the function of granting patents rather that refusing them, and with the proviso that the claimed invention is patentable, an application will be allowed without prolonged arguments and numerous official actions.[4,5]

The *Patent Cooperation Treaty* (PCT) is open to all countries of the world which have acceded to the Convention of Paris. A great number of countries have ratified and acceded to the Patent Cooperation Treaty. The procedures of the Patent Cooperation Treaty are under the control of World Intellectual Property Organization (WIPO, Geneva). Under the provisions of the Patent Cooperation Treaty, an applicant files a single patent application called an 'international application' at the national patent office in any country which has acceded to the Patent Cooperation Treaty and in a language acceptable by that country. The national office at which the international application is filed is known as the 'receiving office'. The application must designate the countries for which national patents are required and must request a search to be performed, called an 'international search', by a competent Patent Office. It is also possible to designate a European application, so-called 'regional designation'.

The international application is examined with the required formalities. A prior art search is performed and a search report is sent to the applicant. The application and the international search report are published. This is known as the 'international phase' of the procedure.

Articles 31 to 42 PCT provide for an 'international preliminary examination' to be performed during the international phase (Chapter II of the Patent Cooperation Treaty). Countries having acceded to the Patent Cooperation Treaty can make a declaration that they will not be bound by Chapter II of the Patent Cooperation Treaty. An applicant resident in a country which is bound by Chapter II of the Patent Cooperation Treaty can make a request for an 'international preliminary examination' to be performed for selected patent offices, known as 'elected offices'.

After the issue of the search report (and the international preliminary examination, if applicable and requested) the application passes to the national patent office of each of the designated countries and this is the start of the 'national phase' of the procedure. On request of the applicant a substantive examination takes place in each of designated countries (and the EPO, if designated), under the laws of that country.

After examination in each designated country, the application can be rejected or a national patent can be granted. Opposition to the issued national patents can be filed individually and the national patents can be amended or revoked, if these courses are provided for under national laws.

Compared with direct filing at the national offices or at the EPO, the PCT route affords the advantage of postponing for at least 8 months the payment of the filing fees, and search, designation and claims fees if any, although the total cost is eventually greater.[4,6,7]

To conclude, there are currently a number of choices available for filing a patent. An applicant can file national applications. If an applicant wishes to obtain a national patent in one or more countries which are EPC contracting states or PCT contracting states, it is possible to file a PCT application designating all the selected countries which are contracting states (including a European application) or an application at the EPO designating all the selected countries which are EPC contracting states.

II. DEFINITION OF A PATENT — PATENT RIGHTS

A patent is 'piece of property' issued by a state or a state organization which grants to the owner the exclusive rights of the claimed invention.[8] In exchange for the disclosure of the invention by its owner (author), the state grants to the latter an exclusive right. In the majority of countries, a patent bestows a right of preventing any third party, from manufacturing, offering, selling, using, importing or stocking the product which is the subject of the invention without the consent of the owner of the patent.

The exclusive rights given by a patent do not extend, in general, to acts carried out in private and for noncommercial purposes, nor usually experimentation with a product when the final aim is not the marketing of the said product. In France, experimentation in order to make an improvement had not been considered as an act of infringement,[9] but experimentation with a pharmaceutical product with the aim of marketing it just after the expiry of the patent is regarded in some countries, in particular European countries, as an act of infringement. Thus, the patent can be considered as a right to 'exclude'.

On the other hand, a patent taken out in any country has several important limitations. The most significant are:

- *The territorial limitation.* The patent provides legal protection only within the frontiers of the state in which it is granted.
- *The time limitation.* A patent has a limited life which in a great number of countries is further restricted by being subjected to the payment of maintenance fees or the like, so that failure to pay such fees automatically invalidates the patent.
- *The exploitation limitation.* The invention claimed according to the patent specification may only be made, used, exercised and sold.

It must be noted that once a patent has been granted, this does not mean that the patentee is free to go ahead and make, use or sell the subject of the invention. If the invention is an improvement on an earlier product, process or piece of apparatus which is the subject of an earlier nonexpired patent having a claim which would be infringed by the improvement, it will be necessary to get a licence from the earlier patentee.

III.   KINDS OF INVENTIONS

Inventions can be divided into four main categories:

(1)   Inventions concerning products or machines
(2)   Inventions concerning processes
(3)   Inventions concerning the use of products already known for other uses (in the pharmaceutical field, primary therapeutic use and secondary therapeutic uses)
(4)   Inventions concerning compositions or combinations.

IV.   SUBJECTS OF PATENTS: BASIC AND FORMAL REQUIREMENTS FOR FILING A PATENT

Since a patent is a creation of a statute in every country, it is essential to examine the statutes for which a patent may be granted. To be able to file a patent application, a certain number of basic and formal requirements have to be met. Basic requirements are quite similar in the main industrial countries. Formal requirements vary a good deal from one country to another. Inventors, for example chemists, are mainly concerned with basic requirements and some formal requirements such as disclosure of the invention, i.e. description (see Section IV.B).

A.   Basic requirements

Depending on the country, there are two or three such requirements. Concerning the European Patent Convention, the criteria for patentability of an invention to be considered are laid down in articles 52 to 57 EPC.[4,5]

Article 52(1) EPC defines three basic criteria for an invention which must be satisfied if a patent is to be granted for the invention:

- that the invention must be susceptible of industrial application,
- that it must be new; and
- that it must involve an inventive step.

Article 52(2) EPC defines certain items which are not regarded as inventions. Discoveries, scientific theories and mathematical methods, aesthetic creations, schemes, rules and methods for performing mental acts, playing games or doing business and programs for computers and presentation of information are not considered as inventions. It must be noted that according to the wording of Article 52(2) EPC, this list is not exhaustive.

Article 52(3) is important when considering what is excluded from patentability, since it explicitly states that the exclusion relates only 'to the extent to which a European patent application ... relates to such subject matter or activities as such'. Thus, under certain circumstances other principles will apply if the subject matter or activities listed in Article 52(2) are associated with a technical use. For example, the discovery of X-rays as such is not patentable, but the use of X-rays in a process could be protected by means of a patent. A number of EPO decisions follow the general principles of the European Patent Convention in that inventions are excluded from patentability only to the extend that application relates to the excluded subject matter of Article 52(2) as such. There is no problem in patenting an invention which includes technical and nontechnical features.

Article 52(4) EPC defines certain items which shall not be regarded as inventions susceptible of industrial application. The article, which defines patentable inventions, uses the conditions of industrial application to reject a category of inventions. This article states that methods for treatment of the human or animal body by surgery or therapy and diagnostic methods practised on the human or animal body are not regarded as inventions susceptible of industrial application. A very important Decision of the Enlarged Board of Appeal of EPO is the Decision GR 01/83. With this decision the Enlarged Board of Appeal has confirmed that a claim to 'the use of a substance or composition of the treatment of the human or animal body by therapy' is not allowable, but a claim to 'the use of a substance or composition for the manufacture of a medicament for a specified new and inventive use' is allowable. Article 52(4) EPC does not exclude from being inventions susceptible of industrial applications substances or compositions for use in methods of treatment of the human or animal body by surgery or therapy. Apparatus for such treatment is also patentable.

Article 53 EPC defines certain inventions for which patents will not be granted. Two types of invention for which patents cannot be granted can be identified:

(1) Inventions the publication or exploitation of which would be the contrary to 'public order' or morality. Exploitation is not deemed to be contrary to public order or morality merely because it is prohibited by law or regulation in some or all of the EPC contracting states. This prohibition is only likely to be invoked if it is probable that the invention is regarded as so abhorrent that the grant of patent rights would be socially unacceptable.

(2) Inventions of plants or animal varieties or essentially biological processes for the production of plants or animals. However microbiological processes and the products thereof are patentable.

It must be mentioned that the patentability of animals has given rise to much discussion. The United States Patent and Trademarks Office (USPTO) following the decision in 'Ex parte Allen' 2 USPQ 2nd 1425 (1987), regards unnaturally accruing living organisms, including animals, as patentable.

The Examining Division of the EPO rejected an application for the 'Harvard mouse' *inter alia* as excluded from patentability by article 53(b) EPC. This decision was appealed and the Board of Appeal disagreed with the reasoning of the Examining Division and remitted the issue to the Examining Division for further consideration.

Article 54 EPC indicates that an invention shall be considered to be new if it does not form part of the state of the art.

Article 55 EPC defines certain disclosures of an invention which shall not be taken into consideration when determining its novelty under Article 54.

Article 56 EPC defines inventions involving an inventive step.

Article 57 EPC specifies the criteria for an invention to be considered as susceptible of industrial application.

Concerning the United States patent law (Patent – Act US Code Title 35 – Patents), Section 101 of the Patent Act states

whoever invents or discovers any new and useful process, machine, manufacture or composition of matter, or any new and useful improvement thereof, may obtain a patent therefor, subject to the conditions and requirements of this title.

Section 101 of the Patent Act expresses the novelty requirement in general terms. Section 102 attempts to spell out just what is not to be considered novel in the patent law sense. With regard to the utility, this is only considered in Section 101 and in the first paragraph of Section 112, which states

> The specification shall contain a written description of the invention, and the manner and process of making and *using,* it....

The foregoing two provisos are the only ones of the Patent Act which make mention of utility. Nevertheless, courts have almost uniformly regarded an exhibition of utility — along with novelty and unobviousness – to be the affirmative requisites of every valid patent.[10]

Section 103 of the Patent Act makes patentability depend upon, in addition to novelty and utility, the nonobvious nature of the subject matter sought to be patented.

Japanese law also defines novelty, inventive step and industrial application as the basic criteria required for an invention.

1. Novelty

Novelty is the *sine qua non* condition of every invention. The requirement for novelty is very severe since it has an absolute character and since any prior public knowledge is destructive of novelty.[11] An invention may be protected if it is new and thus enriches technology. However, within this broad definition the term may be subject to different interpretations. It appears simple enough but has developed quite differently under the various patents systems.

Articles 54(1) and (2) of the European Patent Convention stipulate:[5]

> An invention shall be considered to be new if it does not form part of the art.
> The state of the art shall be held to comprise everything made available to the public by means of a written or oral description, by use, or in any other way, before the date of filing of the European patent application.

The definition of *the state of the art* according to Article 54(2) encompasses all conceivable forms of disclosure, and expressly includes written as well as oral description as well use. In order to cover all other possible forms of disclosure, this definition also includes the making available of information.

Under European law and under the laws of most countries in the world, except the United States, disclosure of the invention by the inventor before a application is filed (first application allowing the Priority Right) will destroy novelty, i.e. patentability.

For a document 'to be made available to the public' it does not matter whether any member of the public actually reads it. The point at issue is whether, on the balance of probabilities, any member of the public had access to it. A document available to the public in a library[4,12] or in a patent office file[4,13] would represent a disclosure even if it could be proved that no member of the public had actually read the document. A document is not made available to the public upon posting but on delivery.[4]

The chemical composition of a product is state of the art when the product as such is available to the public and can be analysed and reproduced by a skilled person, irrespective of whether or not particular reasons can be identified for analysing the composition.[14]

In order to ascertain whether there is prior knowledge, three criteria are taken into account: public disclosure, sufficient disclosure, and date of disclosure. It will thus be investigated whether at the filing date of the patent application it could be known about the invention. It will be also taken into consideration whether the disclosure is sufficient for an expert to be able to perform the invention without an inventive act. Finally the date of the disclosure will be considered, which must be certain and in no doubt. In order to destroy novelty, it must of course be prior to the filing date of the patent application, or prior to the priority date, if any.

As seen, according to Article 54 EPC, the definition of the state of the art is very wide. There is no restriction as to where and when a disclosure was made available to the public, nor are there any restrictions as to the language and manner of the disclosure. There is, however, exception relating to disclosure in breach of confidence and displays at certain international exhibitions defined in article 55 EPC.[4] Since the obligation to secrecy is particularly important during licensing negotiations and demonstrations, sometimes prior to patent application filing, various principles have been adopted and are taken into consideration by the EPO (this is also the case in the law of many countries). According to the EPO's practice, the subject matter of a patent is not made available to the public if there is an express or tacit agreement to secrecy. If a person under the obligation to secrecy does make the information available to the public in abuse of this obligation, then from that moment this information forms part of the state of the art and thus destroys novelty. However, such information is not prejudicial to the invention.

A prior disclosure in a document or by use destroys the novelty of any claimed invention which is directly and unambiguously derivable therefrom.[15] The disclosure not only destroys the novelty of specifically mentioned features but also destroys the novelty of features that are implicit to one skilled in the art (an expert). A specific disclosure of a chemical compound destroys the novelty of a generic claim embracing it.[16] For example, a disclosure of the use of rubber in circumstances where its elastic properties are used would destroy novelty of the use of an elastic material in general.[17]

On the other hand, a generic disclosure does not usually destroy the novelty of a specific example falling within it or even of a subgeneric claim. Thus the disclosure of a genus does not disclose its species and the disclosure of a range does not disclose elements within that range. In this case, the claimed species or subgenus must not include, and must show an unexpected advantage over, prior disclosed species of the genus. This is similar to the situation in many countries and, concerning EPO, it was confirmed by a very first decision of the Technical Board of Appeal.[18]

Consideration must be given not only to specifically described features but also to whether by following the prior disclosure there would be an inevitable result. The Board of Appeal of EPO held that an unnamed compound which was the inevitable result of a specific starting material and a process was the closest compound in the state in the art. In this case, methyl bromide was held to be a specifically disclosed starting definition of C_{1-4} alkyl bromide.[4]

Concerning enantiomers, the EPO's Technical Board of Appeal confirmed that the disclosure of a racemate did not destroy the novelty of the enantiomers, even though they would be understood as being present in the racemate (unseparated form). According the EPO's decision, the enantiomers had not been 'individualized' in the prior art.[4,19]

To attack novelty it is not permitted to combine two or more prior disclosures.

It may in some cases be difficult to prove the date relating to oral disclosure. A written confirmation, even undated, of the oral disclosure enforces it.

The concept of absolute novelty at the filing date of the patent application is now to be found in practically all patent laws, with the exception, as mentioned before, of the law of the United States. Article 102 of the American law on patents,[20] which establishes the criteria of novelty in the United States in effect, is as follows:

A person shall be entitled to a patent unless:

(a)   the invention was known or used by others in this country, or patented or described in a printed publication in this or a foreign country, before the invention thereof by the applicant for patent, or,

(b)   the invention was patented or described in a printed publication in this or a foreign country or in public use or on sale in this country, more than one year prior to the date of the application for patent in the United States, or,

(c)   he has abandoned the invention, or

(d)   the invention was first patented or caused to be patented, or was the subject of an inventor's certificate, by the applicant or his legal representatives or assigns in a foreign country prior to the date of the application for patent in this country on an application for patent or inventor's certificate field more than twelve months before the filing of the application in the United Sates, or

(e)   the invention was described in a patent granted on an application for patent by another filed in the United States before the invention thereof by the applicant for patent, or on an international application by another who has fulfilled the requirements of paragraphs (1), (2) and (4) of section 371(c) of this title before the invention thereof by the applicant for patent, or

(f)   he did not himself invent the subject matter sought to be patented, or

(g)   before the applicant's invention thereof the invention was made in this country by another who had not abandoned, suppressed, or concealed it. In determining priority of invention there shall be considered not only the respective dates of conception and reduction to practice of the invention, but also the reasonable diligence of one who was first to conceive and last to reduce to practice, from a time prior to conception by the other.

Paragraphs (b) and (d) of this article provide a grace period of one year which enables an inventor in the United States to test an invention without such testing being regarded as destroying novelty. The invention can therefore be freely developed without the possibility of personal disclosures being counted against the inventor. During this grace period of one year, counting from the first disclosure, the inventor can then file patent application.

It must be emphasized here that all other countries in the world have opted for the criterion of absolute novelty at the filing date of the patent application and disclosures by the inventor before filing applications destroy the novelty of their own invention. Thus, an inventor in the United States taking advantage of this possibility offered by Article 102 of the American law will no longer have the chance to file in foreign countries, since there is no longer novelty at the filing date of the patent application.

Article 102 of the US law refers, moreover, to the invention and not to the filing date of the patent application. This article thus created the so-called *'first inventor system'* as contrasted with the so-called *'first depositor system'* used in almost all other countries.

Paragraph (g) of Article 102 of the US law lays down a ruling on the question of 'double patenting' different from that of other countries and the corresponding Article of EPC (Article 54(3)). According to paragraph (g) of Article 102 of the US law, in the case of 'double patenting' the patent will be granted to the inventor who not merely has the earliest date for conception and for putting the invention into practice, but who also has displayed diligence in putting the invention to use.

Under Article 54(3) EPC, the content of the art includes the content of other European patent applications filed earlier than, but published on or after, the filing date of a European application. There is no express provision in the EPC concerning co-pending application with the same priority . The EPO will allow both to proceed to the grant. But if applicants are the same, the EPO will require amendment in order to avoid double patenting.

Effect of 'priority right'.   According to the Paris Convention, a person who has filed an earlier application in any state which is party to the Paris Convention may claim for a later filed application for the same invention priority from the date of filing of the earlier application. As a result, the date of filing of the earlier application becomes the effective date of filing of the later application, if this later application is filed in a state party to the Paris Convention. This is also stipulated in Article 87(1) EPC.

Thus, a document, or oral disclosure or co-pending European patent application will be cited by the EPO as part of the state of the art if such a document or oral disclosure is believed to have been publicly available or such an application is believed to disclose matter having a priority date before the filing date of the application.[15] The test for determining whether subject matter is entitled to priority earlier than that of the date on which the application containing that matter was filled is the same as the test for novelty, i.e. the disclosure in a single earlier application from which priority is claimed must be sufficient to destroy the novelty of a claim to that subject matter in the later application, for which priority is claimed.

2.   Inventive step

A patentable invention requires the exercise of the inventive faculty or the exercise of more than the expected skill of the art. In other words, the invention must have been nonobvious to a person skilled in the art when it was made.

From the inspection of the first patent laws, the criterion of novelty was regarded as insufficient. German patent law therefore demanded that for a patent to be granted, it had to have a certain 'inventive height' (or 'inventive level') or a certain 'technical advance'. The United States patent laws speak of 'unobviousness'.

Article 52(1) EPC requires an invention to involve an inventive step if it is to be patentable, and article 56 EPC states that

> An invention will be considered as involving an inventive step if, having regard to the state of the art, it is nonobvious to a person skilled in the art. . . .

The state of the art for this purpose is defined as not including documents under Article 54(3) EPC, i.e.   patent applications which were not published at the filing date of the patent application under consideration. In fact, it is normal that it cannot really be expected that an invention 'B' should display an inventive step as compared with another invention 'A' which was totally unknown at the filing date of the application 'B' being considered. As to novelty, the contents of European patent applications still unpublished at the filling date are retained, to avoid granting two patents for the same invention (double patenting).

Since the criterion for an inventive step is expressed in a negative manner, no positive virtues are required in order to satisfy Article 56. In other words, there is no requirement for a technical advance. However a technical advance may be useful in arguing for the existence of an inventive step.[4] As noted by Dr R. Singer[21] (Chairman of the Legal Board of Appeal of the European Patent Office),

> in order to understand the term inventive step it is useful to divide technical knowledge into three levels. The first level includes all that is known, the mentioned state of the art, i.e. nothing new. The second level contains everything that is new but does not involve an inventive step, i.e. everyday developments of the state of the art. This is the so-called patent-free area. Finally, the third level includes everything that is new and which is also inventive and can be protected by patents

As with any assessment based upon a qualitative judgement, it is often a difference of opinion between the different people involved in the assessment of the inventive step (the applicant, the representative if any, the examiner, and the opponent if any).

During the examination by the EPO an inventive step may arise from devising a solution to a known problem. It may also arise from the identification of a problem to be solved and its solution, even though the solution is obvious once the problem has been identified. Each case should be carefully analysed on its own merits.

To reach a conclusion as to whether an invention includes an inventive step it is necessary to determine the difference between it and the whole of the state of the art. As cited above, the state of the art comprises everything made available to the public before the filing of the application or its priority date.

When considering whether there is inventive step, the question must always be asked: Who is the person skilled in the art? Who is presumed to know all the relevant prior art? *A person skilled in the art* is presumed to have access to the entire state of the art and, in particular, is presumed to possess common general knowledge applicable to his field of interest. Furthermore, it is part of the normal activities of the skilled person to select from the material known to him the most appropriate one. The skilled person is not regarded as having any inventive ingenuity. Thus, the teaching of a document may have narrower implications for a skilled person and broader implications for a potential inventor who first perceives the problem which the future invention is intended to solve. The skilled person is a 'practical person'. According to an EPO Decision,[22] if the problem prompts the skilled person to seek a solution in another technical field, the person of ordinary skill in that other field is the appropriate person to solve the problem. The assessment of inventive step must therefore be based on the skill of that latter person. EPO Directives[15] point out that the skilled person need not be an individual. In certain circumstances, depending of the nature of the invention, it may be more appropriate to think of a group of specialist pooling their knowledge.

The assessment of an inventive step is achieved by starting from the state of the art viewed objectively.[23] In an evaluation of the state of the art to determine an inventive step it is permissible to combine the disclosures of two or more documents, but only where to do so would have been obvious to the skilled person. Thus, documents should not be combined if it is unlikely that a skilled person would combine them to solve his problem, especially where there is an inherent incompatibility.

If an invention differs from the state of the art by the substitution of an alleged equivalent for one of its elements, it is not necessary to combine a secondary reference of the prior art in related subject matter to establish lack of inventive step, with the proviso that the type of substitution is generally known and a skilled person would expect the general effects given by the invention. But if the substitution gives an unexpectedly greater effect or a nonobvious additional effect, inventive step exists. Additionally, if the inventor was confronted with many alternative possibilities as potential solutions to his problem and he had no particular reason to select the one leading to the invention, inventive step should be recognized.

A situation encountered in chemical cases occurs when two distinct substances, each comprising two or more structural elements, have a common property and a claim is presented to a new substance combining structural elements from each of the known substances and having the same property. If the common property of the two known substances is indicated as being associated with each substance as a whole and not with the structural elements selected for the new substance, the new substance may be not obvious from the two known substances.[4,24]

In a combination of known features, an inventive step should be recognized if the combined features mutually support each other in their effect so that a new technical result is achieved.

According the EPO Guidelines[15] for examination of patent applications, there would be an inventive step 'if in a mixture of medicines consisting of a analgesic and a sedative (tranquillizer) it was found that through the addition of the sedative — which intrinsically appeared to have no analgesic effect — the analgesic effect of the analgesic was intensified in a way which could not have been predicted from the known properties of the active substances'.

An unexpected effect is one of the arguments for the existence of an inventive step. The unexpected effect must be established by evidence. Very often it is necessary to present appropriate comparative tests with materials from the closest prior art. If a particular effect or property would be expected qualitatively, applicants are often asked to supply evidence to support an inventive step by demonstrating a significant quantitative improvement. In many cases a technical advantage may be foreseeable and therefore not unexpected. In these cases there is a lack of inventive step.

The EPO Technical Board of Appeal have held that if the prior art very strongly and clearly directs the skilled person in a particular direction, there is no inventive step involved in following that direction, irrespective of the results. This is known as the 'one-way street' situation and has led to considerable discussion among commentators. 'Obvious to try' is not a standard for denying the existence of an inventive step. In accordance with recent practice in national courts in Europe and in the United States, the EPO is reluctant to maintain an 'obvious to try' objection in the face of unexpected results.

An unexpected effect in one species or subgenus selected from a known group is sufficient to render the species or subgenus patentable, because an inventive step can be acknowledged. Such inventions are called 'selection inventions'. The principle of selection invention has been upheld by the EPO in many decisions.

A chemical intermediate which has no inherent useful properties other than as a starting material for a useful end-product claimed in the same application may depend on the useful end-product for its inventive step because it is part of the same invention.[4] On the other hand, according a decision of the EPO Technical Board of Appeal, a new chemical intermediate may be inventive if it is prepared in the course of a multistage process, providing that the intermediate itself makes a contribution to the quantitative effect of the process.[25]

According the US law of patents, the criterion of inventive step is replaced by the criterion of unobviousness. Nonobvious subject matter and conditions for patentability are set forth in section 103 of the US Patent Law, which states that

> A patent may not be obtained though the invention is not identically disclosed or described as set forth in Section 102 of this title, if the differences between the subject matter sought to be patented and the prior art are such that the subject matter as a whole would have been obvious at the time the invention was made to a person having ordinary skill in the art to which said subject matter pertains. Patentability shall not be negatived by the manner in which the invention was made.

In general, in determining whether a patentable invention has been made or not, the American Patent Office (USPTO) and a court ascertain, among other points, whether the invention[1] produced new, improved or unexpected results; satisfied a long-felt want; solved an outstanding problem; was contraindicated in the prior art; succeeded over unsuccessful efforts of others; went into extensive use and enjoyed public acquiescence; and had commercial success. On the other hand, inventions are ordinarily held to be unpatentable when they involve nothing more than a change of form, size or location; a substitution of materials or equivalents; a change of proportions or ingredients of a composition without a surprising result; or superior or excellent workmanship.

3.   *The invention must be capable of industrial application*

If novelty is the *sine qua non* of invention, then industrial application or utility is its *raison d'être*. The laws of almost every country require that the invention should be capable of industrial application. Industrial application is defined by Article 57 of the EPC as follows:[5]

> An invention shall be considered as susceptible of industrial application if it can be made or used in any kind of industry including agriculture.

It would seem that the term 'industrial' will be interpreted broadly so as to include most commercial activities. For example, according to EPO Decisions,[26,27] professional use of a cosmetic process in a beauty parlour is found to fall within the meaning of 'industrial application'.

The criterion of 'utility' found in the US law is quite close to the criterion of 'industrial application' which is found in the laws of a good number of countries, and in particular in the EPC. A chemical product for which no industrial application nor any pharmacological property had been found would not be patentable under the US patent law, because it would not have any utility.

Of interest is the decision of the US Supreme Court in the 'Manson case' (383 US 519), which overruled the utility doctrine enunciated by the Court of Customs and Patent Appeals in the 'Nelson case' (47 CCPA. 1031) and which adjudicated the question of what constitutes utility in a chemical process. The invention involved a process for making certain steroids.[1] The Court held that the utility of the product must be established and that merely providing a product to be available for 'use testing' by the trade was insufficient. In the decision, it was pointed out that 'It was never intended that a patent be granted upon a product, or a process producing a product, unless such product be useful'.

The Court said that it did not mean to disparage 'the importance of contributions to the fund of scientific information short of the invention of something "useful", or that we are blind to the prospect that what now seems without "use" may tomorrow command the grateful attention of the public. But a patent is not a hunting license. It is not a reward for the search but compensation for its successful conclusion. A patent system must be related to the world of commerce rather than to the realm of philosophy'.

In view of the Supreme Court decision, it is clear that as many affirmative statements and positive results should be included in a patent specification as possible.

B.   Formal requirements

The patent application must have a single subject. This principle is known as *unity of invention*. According to EPC's Article 82:

> The European patent application shall relate to one invention only or to a group of inventions so linked as to form a single general inventive concept.

Unity of invention is required for documentary research reasons. In the United States, the requirement of unity of invention (single subject per patent application) is investigated with the greatest strictness.

If the patent application relates to more than one invention and the applicant wishes to protect two or more inventions, the 'invention or inventions' can be the subject of one or more *divisional applications.* The divisional application may be filed at any time before the grant of the 'parent application'. A divisional application cannot be filed if the parent application has been withdrawn or is deemed to have been withdrawn. Lack of unity is not a cause of invalidity of a granted patent.

The patent application must contain a *description* explaining the invention. The description shall:

(a) specify the technical field to which the invention relates;
(b) indicate the background art which, as far as is known to the applicant, can be regarded as useful for understanding the invention and preferably cite the documents reflecting such art;
(c) disclose the invention as claimed and state any advantageous effect of the invention with reference to the background art;
(d) describe in detail at least one way of carrying out the invention claimed, using examples where appropriate and referring to the drawings if any;
(e) indicate explicitly, when it is not obvious from the nature of the invention, the way in which the invention is capable of exploitation in industry; and
(f) briefly describe the figures in the drawings if any.

In fact, the patent application must explain the invention in a sufficiently clear and complete way for a person skilled in the art to be able to reproduce the invention without having to carry out research or lengthy and delicate operations.

Applications to be filed in the United States must in addition give the best method of realizing the invention.

In general it is not necessary to give detailed results of trials of use of the invention, for example biological pharmacological or clinical results for pharmaceuticals, but sometimes it can be useful to present comparative results between the products of the application and the products of the prior art, in order to demonstrate the advantage of the invention.

The patent application must contain *claims*. According to Article 84 of EPC:

> The claims shall define the matter for which protection is sought. They shall be clear and concise and be supported by the description

In fact, the claims must define the matter for which protection is sought in terms of the technical features of the invention.

The European Patent Convention enumerates four kind of claims corresponding to the four main categories of invention, but in fact there exist two basic types of claims: claims for products or machines, and claims for activities (processes, utilization).[15]

Any claim stating the essential features of an invention may be followed by one or more claims concerning particular embodiments of that invention.

It is possible to have several independent claims in a European patent application. This is in particular permitted in order to claim certain permutations of what are termed different categories.

A patent application to be filed at the EPO can have different types of claims.

The different categories permissible are:

- A product, a process adapted for the manufacture of the product and a use of the product
- A process and an apparatus or means specifically designed for the carrying out the process
- A product, a process specially adapted for making the product and an apparatus or means specially designed for carrying out the process.

In American practice, in an application for invention concerning compounds only, products and methods of use claims are generally admitted by the examiners of the Patent Office. For the process for the manufacture of the products, a divisional application is often required. In all cases, the claims cannot extend more widely than the description, completed if appropriate with the drawings.

Products claims bestow a protection that can be regarded as absolute. Until the beginnings of 1990s in most Eastern European patents systems it was not possible to claim new compounds. This was also the case, especially for pharmaceuticals, in Canada, Austria, Spain, Greece, in most Scandinavian countries except Sweden and in South American countries. Pharmaceuticals were protected only by process claims. Now the patent laws have been changed and pharmaceutical compounds can be claimed in most of countries. A product or a family of products can be defined equally well by a general chemical formula (Markush formula), as by specific chemical names.

In chemistry, *a process claim* describes a number or series of reactions leading to the production of a given chemical product. Process claims have the effect of preventing a third party from using the same process. With regard to the product, a process claim is ineffective against a third party who, in some countries, might use a different process to prepare the same product.

Sometimes, a patentable product cannot be defined by reference to its structure, composition or other reproducible property. Such products are protected (claimed) by '*product by process*' claims. A product by process claim covers a product independently of the process used to obtain it.

Concerning the *first therapeutic use*, for a compound which is shown to have a specific therapeutic use, it is possible according to the EPO's practice, to have a broad claim in a form such as 'substance or composition X for use in medicine'. Formulation of claims such as 'the use of a substance X for the therapeutic treatment of man or animals' is not permitted, because they are regarded as claims of methods of medicinal treatment.

With regard to the *second therapeutic use*, as noted above, the EPO's Enlarged Board of Appeal approved a wording such as 'the use of a substance X for the manufacture of a medicine for therapeutic application'.[15] In the United States, the patentability of 'second therapeutic uses' has long been recognized and many methods of use patents may be granted for the same product. It is now possible to protect second therapeutic uses in many countries.

Claims for second nonmedical use are also admitted by the patent laws of many countries. A claim covering a novel use of a known product will only cover the claimed use. Other uses of the compound as such are not protected.

Compositions or combinations if they yield an unexpected result of their own or a technical effect of their own are patentable, but the mere juxtaposition of two means is not by itself patentable. *Composition claims* are admitted in the patents laws of most countries. A patent covering a particular composition will cover the composition or combination effectively claimed and the obvious equivalents. Such claims are considerate as product claims.

Another formal requirement is that the patent application must *designate the true inventors*. The true inventors are the persons who have actually participated in achieving the invention. People who have only carried out routine tests (biological tests relating to screening, for example) should not be regarded as true inventors. A failure to designate any inventor in the request of a grant of a European patent creates a formal deficiency. According to the EPC there is no penalty if an incorrect designation of inventors exists, apart from procedures for correction of the designation. The resulting patent cannot be opposed or revoked merely on the grounds of wrong inventor designation. Identifying the true inventor is very important, especially in the United States. According to US patent law, any failure to designate the true inventor is a cause for invalidation of a patent. It is accordingly very important that records be properly kept, dated and identified so as not only to prove originality of invention but also to establish priority of invention by inventor.

Patent applications must be filed in the *official language* or one of the official languages of the country in which the application is filed. As mentioned above, European Patent Applications must be filed in one of the three official languages of the European Patent Office, i.e. German, English or French.

Filing a Patent Application gives also rise to *payment of fees*, i.e. filing fees, examination fees (if any) and payment of annuities. In the countries which proceed with a real examination of patentability, in addition to examination fees one should anticipate fees for answering official letters issued from the Patent Offices. Payment of annuities or periodical fees must be paid thoughout the whole life of the patent. Fees must be paid in due time. Failure to pay fees automatically invalidates the patent or the patent application.

In some cases, especially for filing in foreign countries, a *legal representative* is required for the filing of a patent application. For European patent applications, parties to proceedings may act in relation to EPO in the following alternative ways:

(a) An individual person may act for himself.
(b) An individual person may act through an authorized representative who may be a professional representative, a legal practitioner or any employee of that person.
(c) A legal person (i.e. a corporate body) may act for itself, that is to say by the actions of any responsible officer of the legal person.
(d) A legal person may act through an authorized representative who may be a professional representative, a legal practitioner or any employee of the legal person.

Individual legal persons having neither a residence nor a principal place of business in any EPC contracting state must act through a representative. This representative must be a professional representative or a legal practitioner.

Patenting is a complicated task. It is fully recommended to applicants without experience of patenting to prepare patent applications and to act through professionals (patent attorneys, patent lawyers).

V. LIFETIME OF PATENTS

At the beginning of the 1900s, the lifetime of patents varied enormously from one country to another. With the introduction of the European Patent System, the countries ratifying the EPC opted for a lifetime of 20 years from the filing date. Since then, other countries not participating in the EPC have also opted for a lifetime of 20 years. Currently, a US patent has a term of 17 years from the date of issue. Under the new law, in force from 8 December 1994, a patent issuing from an application filed on or after 8 June 1995 will have a term beginning on the date of issue of the patent and ending 20 years after the earliest effective US filing date. A patent that is in force on, or issued from a US application filed before 8 June 1995 will have a term of 17 years from the date of issue or 20 years from the applications earliest effective US filing date, whichever is longer. From January 1989, the lifetime of a Canadian patent is 20 years from filing. Some countries such as India or Egypt have special lifetimes for medicaments. Concerning Japan, the lifetime of a patent is 15 years from the publication of the application, but cannot exceed 20 years from filing. Under the new law, which will be enforced as from 1 July 1995, the lifetime of the patent will be 20 years from the date on which the patent application is filed.

Information concerning patent law and lifetime of patents for all countries throughout the world is given in the *Manual for the Handling of Applications for Patents, Designs and Trade Marks Throughout the Word* (Octroibureau Losen Stiger, Amsterdam, 1993).

In 1984, the United States adopted a law which enables the lifetime of certain American patents to be extended. According to this law, it is possible to obtain a maximum extension of five years for holders of pharmaceutical patents when the marketing of a pharmaceutical product has been delayed in its registration by the FDA. In 1988, Japan adopted a law which enables the life of patents to be extended for a period of two to five years. France and Italy, in 1990, adopted a Certificate of Complementary Protection of pharmaceutical patents. The laws concerning the French and Italian Certificate of Complementary Protection were abrogated in January 1993. Since this date the *Community Supplementary Protection Certificate* has been in force. According to the Community Certificate, it is possible to obtain a maximum extension of five years for holders of pharmaceutical patents. This certificate concerns all the EEC/EPC contracting states.

VI. OWNERSHIP OF PATENTS

A patent is a grant from the state and constitutes a property. As such, it is subject to all of the laws and regulations to property. The grant of a patent gives to the patentee a title to an intangible and incorporate right in the nature of a franchise. The title of a patent constitutes a right to the patentee until it is divested from him or by voluntary grant or by other legal means. A patent can be conveyed like any other piece of property. It can be assigned and transferred to another party.

A patent may be licensed under terms which give to the licensee the right to make, use or sell the patented invention. It is in this respect similar to a piece of property which may be leased and may be also sold. A license may be exclusive or nonexclusive. It may be restricted to a certain geographical territory, or to certain industrial fields, or may even be restricted to a certain specific factory or other place of commerce and industry.

In the United States the titular of a patent can only be the inventor, who may assign his patent application to a company, whereas in other countries the titular may be a company or an organization.

VII. INFRINGEMENT OF A PATENT

An act of infringement is an attack on the rights of the patentee in the territory where the patent is filed. A person may be guilty of 'direct infringement' when he makes, uses or sells the entire invention as defined by the claims of a patent. A person may be guilty of 'contributory infringement' if he cooperates with another in infringing a patent. For example, a chemical company which sells substances to another for the purpose of infringing a patent can be sued just like a direct counterfeiter.

An action for infringement can only be launched as from the day the patent application is published. The reason for this rule is to protect third parties who might have infringed a patent of which they are unaware. According to the laws of certain countries, it is possible to notify a suspected counterfeiter of the existence of a patent application. Concerning infringements, the Judges rule according to the claims of the patent and not according to the claims of the patent application.

Suits for the infringement of patents must be instituted in tribunals competent in matters of infringement. In each country a limited list has been established of such tribunals. Infringement actions on a European patent in the contracting states may be heard by the courts competent for infringement actions of national patents. As noted above, infringement of a European patent is dealt with under national law of the contracting states. Generally, proof of infringement must be provided by the owner of the patent. Such proof can be in the form of witnesses, documents, purchase of products, and so on.

In every case where a patent has been held to be valid and infringed, the patent owner is entitled to have an injunction issue against the counterfeiter. The injunction will restrict the counterfeiter from making, using or selling the invention. Additionally, the patent owner may obtain the payment of compensation to make up for the loss of profit or for the loss suffered. According to the law of some countries, patented articles may be withdrawn and delivered up to the proprietor of the patent. In some countries relief for the infringing action may be provided by criminal penalties, including a prison sentence.

In order to determine infringement, the subject matter protected by a patent is compared with the act alleged to constitute an infringement. Slavish reproduction of the subject matter protected by a patent constitutes an act of infringement. The reproduction of a patented invention by varying only details (variants of execution) also constitutes infringement.

VIII.   PATENTS AS A SOURCE OF INFORMATION

Patent literature is a useful source of technical, legal and commercial information. It is extremely rich in technical information. In a patent application, applicants must disclose the invention in a sufficiently clear and complete way for a person skilled in the art to be able to reproduce the invention. New and inventive concepts give rise to a considerable number of refinements, improvements and modifications. Often, the importance of an invention is related to the number of patents and patent applications which protect it.

Complete information about patentees' competitors is useful before the beginning of a new research program. Liberty of exploitation has to be evaluated before the commercialization and preferably, before the development of a new product or machine. In this case, patent applications, patents and the corresponding patent statutes of competitors must to be studied in detail.

The negotiating and conclusion of license agreements have become a specialized profession. Information obtained by patents can help companies to find new products or processes for expansion or diversification of their manufacturing activities.

IX.   PATENTING IN THE PHARMACEUTICAL INDUSTRIES

In certain trades and industries, and in particular in the pharmaceutical industries, it is generally not possible to inhibit competition effectively by keeping key formulae, products and techniques secret. Pharmaceuticals is a classic case of an industry dependent on patents. In fact, patent protection is of great importance to the pharmaceutical research and development process. Practically all new drugs which were developed after the Second World War were developed by private pharmaceutical firms in the United States, the Federal Republic of Germany, Switzerland, France, Great Britain, the Nordic European countries and Japan. These countries provide the strongest known patent protection for pharmaceuticals. Countries with similar industrial standards and possibilities, but not providing patent protection for pharmaceuticals cannot show any drug innovation of importance.

In any case, having obtained a patent, the patentee should not think he is heir to a fortune. Many worthwhile inventions have failed commercially for lack of interest or funds to promote them. Additionally, the grant of a patent is no way a guarantee that the invention is significant or that the patent is valid. It should therefore be no surprise that one of the factors considered by pharmaceutical management in deciding whether to develop a new drug, in addition to its medical and commercial potential and cost of manufacturing, is the strength and duration of patent protection.

Concerning strength, the best kind of protection, and really the only truly effective kind, is that which protects the product itself. A patent covering a product, as opposed to one covering only a process for making the product or a use for the product, can prevent others from manufacturing or selling the product for any purpose, no matter how it is made. Since chemists can often find new processes for making a compound, a patent on a process can be circumvented by use of the new processes and the owner of a patent no longer has an exclusive position with respect to the drug. The same is true concerning a patent covering only a particular use. A new use may permit a copier to sell the product free of the original use limited patent, even though the product may be prescribed and used for the original use. Patents of new use are only strong if the new use of a compound requires a special and new formulation.

Another aspect of protection, in addition to the type of protection available, is the term of the patent. In most countries the term of a patent runs from the filing date, and the maximum duration is twenty years (see Section V).

For competitive reasons, a patent application must be filed as soon as possible. In fact, a patent application for a new compound or series of compounds must be filed as soon as the new compound or series of compounds has been made and found to have significant and interesting activity. This is necessary because others may have made the same invention, and failure to file promptly may result in a total loss of patent rights (in most countries, except the United States, patents are granted to the first party to file a patent application on the subject matter — the *first depositor system,* see Section IV.A.1). There are many cases in which the same invention is made independently by more than one party within as short a period as two or three weeks.

However, in filing an application as soon as possible, many problems can be generated. The term of a patent begins starts to run even before the product is marketed. As a period of at least 7–10 years is required for the development of a new drug after a compound and its analogues have been prepared and biologically tested, the patent terms can expire before the product begins to produce any real profits. In the pharmaceutical industry many candidate products are not developed because of the short patent term that would remain after development.

Under the Paris Convention, initial filing can be followed up in other countries where protection is desired. The benefit of the initial early filing date is obtained if applications are filed within a year of this date. Thus, the choice of countries must be decided before the full importance of an invention is known. Commercial interest and the effective protection offered by the 'local' patent law must be taken into consideration in the choice of countries.

Often, at the time a patent application is filed for a new compound, research and development staff do not know which compound in a series will turn out to be the product to be developed. In addition, the chosen compound or compounds may well be chemically related to compounds patented earlier, and this might complicate the question of 'patentability.' Even before the full importance of an invention is known, a number of needs must be met at this early stage when a patent application is filed. In order to adequately protect an invention, the applicant must describe how to realize and how to use it. Normally, a chemist will invent a series of compounds all having the same type of activity to a greater or lesser degree. Inventors cannot afford to simply patent for the best compound, even if they know which compound is the best. Competitors would read the patent and make the next closest relative of the compound, thereby depriving the inventor of part of his invention. Thus examples must be described of the group of invented compounds. Moreover, a company may change its interest to another compound in the series as it learns more about the compounds. Potency, stability, side-effect profile bioavailability, availability and difficulty or cost of manufacturing may indicate that compounds prepared later in a series are preferable for development. For this reason it is necessary for a variety of compounds in the series to be described.

The other significant problem in obtaining valid and effective patent protection relates to requirements of the patent law variously referred to in different countries as the requirement for nonobviousness, or attainment of a sufficient inventive level. Normally the requirement that an invention be useful or capable of industrial application is not a problem. The novelty requirement is also not usually a problem. However, even in the usual case where compounds are novel, few compounds are of such distinctiveness that no compound of similar structure has ever previously been published. Thus, it must be established, by arguments of chemical difference or of biological properties, that the new compounds merit patent protection. Inventors' previous patents and publications often complicate the situation and it is most distressing when inventors have difficulty patenting their chosen compounds because of their earlier public disclosure of compounds long since discarded.

The opportunity for filing a patent application has to be well evaluated. Sometimes it is preferable to keep an invention secret if infringement of the intended patent related to this invention will be difficult to demonstrate. This concerns especially process patents for preparing commercially successful compounds not protected by a 'compound patent'. Infringement of such patents can generally be demonstrated by identifying impurities due to the process (if any) or by witness. If demonstration of infringement is not possible, competitors may use the process they are interested in, after the publication of the patent application, without any jeopardy or sanction.

X. CONCLUSION

Patent systems throughout the world are today based on the principle of territorial rights. As an invention will be protected in that state in which a patent has been applied for and granted, inventors and applicants are therefore forced to apply for patents for an invention in several states. This involves compliance with different laws and rules and a considerable financial outlay. Inventors and applicants are often confronted with the legalistic problems and phraseology of the world of patent protection.

Even if the phraseology can be easily understood and adopted, legalistic problems require a good knowledge of the law of the countries and the corresponding practice and jurisprudence.

There is a correlation between research and development and industrialization. Patents provide a stimulus for investment in research and development. Investment in the type of development which has brought in the world great progress in medicinal chemistry requires a healthy patent strategy.

REFERENCES

1. Greenstrat, C. H. (1972) In Liebesny, F. (ed.) *Mainly on Patents; The Use of Industrial Property and its Literature.* Butterworth, London.
2. Mathély, P. (1992) *Le droit français des brevets d'invention.* Journal des notaires et des avocats, Paris.
3. Bodeyhausey, G. H. C. (1969) *Guide d'application de la Convention de Paris pour la Protection de la Propriété Industrielle.* BIRPI, Geneva.
4. *European Patents Handbook*, Release 10 (1991) Longman, Harlow.
5. *European Patent Convention* (1993) European Patent Office.
6. *Traité de coopération en matière de brevets (PCT) et règlement d'exécution du PCT* (1993) Organisation Mondiale de Propriété Industrielle. Geneva.
7. *PCT – Guide du déposant* (1993) Publication no. 6, Organisation Mondiale de la Propriété Industrielle. Genève.
8. Chavanne, A. and Burst J. J. (1990) *Droit de la Propriété Industrielle*, 3rd edn. Dalloz, Paris.
9. *PIBD* 1982 III 235. Tribunal de Grande Instance de Paris, 8 July 1982.
10. Rosenberg, P. (1975) *Patent Law Fundamentals.* Clark Boardman, New York.
11. Decision of the Technical Board of Appeal 3.3.1 T 31/84, 4 May 1985. *Official Journal of the European Patent Office.* **11/86**: 369–372.
12. Decision of the Technical Board of Appeal 3.3.1 T 381/87, 10 Nov. 1988. *Official Journal of the European Patent Office.* **5/90**: 213–223.
13. Decision of the Technical Board of Appeal T 444/88 (1990). 12 IPD Decision IPD 13222.
14. Opinion of the Enlarged Board of Appeal G1/92, 18 Dec. 1992, *Official Journal of the European Patent Office.* **5/93**: 277.
15. *Directives relatives à l'examen pratique à l'Office Européen des brevets* (1992) Publication of the European Patent Office. Pindar Infotek, York.
16. Decision of the Technical Board of Appeal 3.3.1 T 188/83, 30 July 1984. *Official Journal of the European Patent Office.* **11/84**: 555–562.
17. Decision of the Technical Board of Appeal 3.3.1 T 181/82, 28 Feb. 1984. *Official Journal of the European Patent Office.* **9/84**: 401–414.
18. Decision of the Technical Board of Appeal 3.3.1 T.01/80, 6 April 1981. *Official Journal of the European Patent Office.* **9/81**: 349.
19. Decision of the Technical Board of Appeal 3.4.1 T, 296/87, 30 Aug. 1988. *Official Journal of the European Patent Office.* **5/90**: 195–212.
20. *Patents and Trademark Laws* (1989) The Bureau of National Affairs, Washington DC.
21. Singer, R. (1981) *The New European Patent System.* D. J. Devoys (ed.) Seminar Services International.
22. Decision of the Technical Board of Appeal 3.2.1. T 195/84, 10 Oct. 1985. *Official Journal of the European Patent Office.* **5/86**: 121–128.
23. Decision of the Technical Board of Appeal 3.3.1 T 24/81, 13 Oct. 1982. *Official Journal of the European Patent Office.* **4/83**: 133–142.
24. Decision of the Technical Board of Appeal 3.3.1 T 20/83, 17 March 1983. *Official Journal of the European Patent Office.* **9/86**: 295–301.
25. Decision of the Technical Board of Appeal 3.3.2 T 163/84, 21 Aug. 1986. *Official Journal of the European Patent Office.* **7/87**: 301–308.

26. Decision of the Technical Board of Appeal 3.3.1 T 36/83, 14 May 1985, *Official Journal of the European Patent Office.* **9/86**: 295–301.
27. Decision of the Technical Board of Appeal 3.3.1 T 144/83, 27 March 1986, *Official Journal of the European Patent Office.* **9/86**: 301–305.

42

The Consumption and Production of Pharmaceuticals

BRYAN G. REUBEN

The end of the medical art is health and that of economics is wealth
Aristotle (*Ethics*)

THE PRACTICE OF MEDICINAL CHEMISTRY
ISBN 0-12-744640-0

Medicinal chemistry is of great academic and intellectual interest. The elucidation of the arachidonic acid cascade, for example, is one of the most fascinating bits of chemistry of our generation. The study of the chemistry of the brain, so that we are able to understand how it is that we can understand, is one of the great frontiers of science. To the author, at least, it is of far greater significance than the problem of the origins of the universe, most of which is cold, inhospitable and distant, which came into being an indecently long time ago, and which will continue long after any of us are able to take an interest in it.

Unlike astrophysics, however, medicinal chemistry is an applied science. It is lavishly funded not because of its philosophical centrality but because it provides the hope that human disease can be cured or alleviated. Its paymasters intend that mankind, or at least those sections of it with access to advanced medical care, will live longer and more comfortably. Its practitioners are judged by this criterion. There are few Nobel prizes for those who discover, say, the biochemical origins of a rodent-specific dermatitis.

As the test of success is pragmatic, serendipity plays an important role in medicinal chemistry. The discoverers of sulfonamides thought that dyestuffs might prove efficacious because they bonded specifically to certain tissues, as in Ehrlich's classic experiment. In the end, Prontosil® worked not because it was a dye but because it cleaved in the gut to p-aminobenzenesulfonic acid. We still honour Domagk, just as we honour Fleming, whose chance discovery of penicillin would have been meaningless had not Florey and Chain solved the problem of its purification and Coghill and his co-workers (who did not get a Nobel prize) the problem of its large-scale production.

Medicines are thus judged by their results. A successful drug can be manufactured reasonably easily, has negligible side-effects, is widely prescribed, makes a lot of money, and is perceived as making a major contribution to health care. In this chapter, we shall discuss which drugs are important on which criteria and say something about the technical, social and economic problems of the pharmaceutical industry.

I.   THE MOST WIDELY PRESCRIBED DRUGS

From the point of view of the manufacturer, the money side is the most important. A research-oriented drug company needs adequate cash flow to maintain its organization, fund its research and keep its shareholders happy. Table 42.1 shows the 20 best-selling drugs in 1992. Most of them are still under patent or their patents have only recently expired; thus their price and profitability remain high. One of them — Omnipaque® — is not a prescription drug; it is used for X-ray imaging.

Five of the top six drugs are for heart disease, reflecting that this is the major cause of death in the developed world. Three of the drugs, including the first on the list, are for ulcers. Until the mid-1970s, ulcers could be treated only by surgery and were generally uncomfortable rather than fatal. The importance of these drugs is that they improve the quality of life rather than saving it. Four of the drugs are antibiotics, reflecting man's conquest of infectious disease. Conventional antibiotics, however, are fairly cheap and the ones listed here all have special properties to justify their prices.

Two drugs are listed for arthritis, an illness which is painful and disabling but not life-threatening. Then there are two novel compounds — acyclovir, which is the most effective herpes antiviral, and epoetin alfa, which is the human hormone erythropoietin made by

Table 42.1   The top 20 drugs by world sales, 1992.

Brand name	Chemical name	Manufacturer	Class[a]	Use	1992 sales ($US billion)
Zantac	ranitidine	Glaxo (UK)	U	H_2-antagonist for ulcers	3.44
Adalat/Procardia	nifedipine	Bayer (Germany)	H	Calcium channel blocker	1.75
Vasotec	enalapril	MSD (USA)	H	ACE inhibitor, antihypertensive	1.69
Capoten	captopril	Bristol-Myers (USA)	H	ACE inhibitor, antihypertensive	1.65
Mevacor	lovastatin	MSD (USA)	H	Hypolipaemic	1.50
Cardizem/ Herbesser	verapamil	Marion (USA)	H	Calcium channel blocker	1.25
Epogen/Procit	epoetin alfa	Amgen (USA)	M	Anaemia	1.25
Losec	omeprazole	Astra (Sweden)	U	Proton pump inhibitor for ulcers	1.22
Ventolin/ Proventil	salbutamol (albuterol)	Glaxo (UK)	As	β_2-Agonist for asthma	1.21
Ceclor	Cefaclor	Eli Lilly (USA)	A	Antibiotic	1.20
Voltaren	diclofenac	Ciba-Geigy (Switzerland)	NS	Non-steroidal anti-inflammatory	1.20
Omnipaque	iohexol	Hafslund/Nycomed (Norway)	M	X-ray contrast agent	1.14
Zovirax	Acyclovir	Wellcome (UK)	M	Antiviral	1.10
Cipro	ciprofloxacin	Bayer (Germany)	A	Antibiotic	1.10
Tagamet	cimetidine	SmithKline-Beecham (USA/UK)	U	H_2-antagonist for ulcers	1.08
Prozac	fluoxetine	Eli Lilly (USA)	CN	Antidepressant	1.07
Augmentin	amoxycillin-clavulanic acid	SmithKline-Beecham (USA/UK)	A	Antibiotic	1.03
Naprosyn	naproxen	Syntex (USA)	NS	Non-steroidal anti-inflammatory	0.95
Tenormin	atenolol	Zeneca (UK)	H	β-Blocker for angina	0.90
Rocephin	ceftriaxone	Roche (Switzerland)	A	Antibiotic	0.86

Source: Lehman Brothers.
[a]A, antibiotic; An, analgesic; As, antiasthma; CC, cold cure constituent etc.; CN, central nervous system; H, heart drug; M, miscellaneous; NS, non-steroidal anti-inflammatory; S, steroid; U, ulcer drug.

recombinant DNA technology and used mainly to counter anaemia arising from renal dialysis. Only one antidepressant is listed, reflecting the declining willingness of physicians to prescribe psychotropic drugs. Finally, there is a single drug for asthma, the only disease for which developed world mortality is rising.

The above compounds are the glamorous pharmaceuticals, the results of fairly recent research and mostly based on a clear idea of the enzyme systems they are supposed to influence. The most widely consumed pharmaceuticals, however, are aspirin, paracetamol (called acetaminophen in the United States) and vitamin C. These can all be bought over the counter. Annual world consumption is of the order of 50 000 tonnes each, an order of magnitude higher than consumption of, say, penicillin V. At the other extreme come materials such as the anticancer drug methotrexate, with annual production of about 150 kg. The prices of the large tonnage drugs are so low, however, that sales of aspirin and paracetamol together are probably less than $0.5 billion, and even that figure is achieved by producers' combining them with other drugs, dressing up the products and selling them to the consumer by extensive advertising. None the less, the number of people who take these drugs to alleviate the symptoms of colds, reduce pain and so on is astronomical. In the UK, some years ago, it appeared that consumption of aspirin-containing tablets averaged 200 per year per man, woman and child.

A. The top sixty drugs

Sometimes less profitable, but more important in terms of public health, are the drugs that are most widely prescribed. Table 42.2 shows the 60 most frequently prescribed drugs in the United States and Table 42.3 shows the same data for Germany. Table 42.4 classifies the top 60 drugs by therapeutic class and also lists the proportion of drugs in each therapeutic class in France and England.[1]

Table 42.2 Top 60 most widely prescribed drugs by chemical entity, United States, 1992.[a]

Rank	Generic name	Typical trade name[b]	Class[c]	Therapeutic class
1	amoxycillin	Amoxil	A	Antibiotic
2	conjugated estrogenic hormone	Premarin Oral	S	Hormone replacement therapy
3	ranitidine	Zantac	U	H_2-antagonist for ulcers
4	ethynylestradiol	Ortho-N 7/7/7-28	S	Steroid component of oral contraceptives
5	hydrochlorothiazide	Dyazide	H	Diuretic
6	codeine	Tylenol/codeine	An	Narcotic analgesic
7	salbutamol (albuterol)	Ventolin	As	β_2-Agonist for asthma
8	digoxin	Lanoxin	H	Cardiac glycoside for heart failure
9	penicillin V	V-cillin	A	Antibiotic
10	furosemide	Lasix Oral	H	Loop diuretic
11	L-thyroxine	Synthroid	M	Hypothyroidism
12	propoxyphene	Darvocet	An	Narcotic analgesic
13	triamterene	Dyazide	H	Diuretic
14	enalapril	Vasotec	H	ACE inhibitor
15	alprazolam	Xanax	CN	Benzodiazepine anxiolytic
16	erythromycin	E.E.S.	A	Antibiotic
17	naproxen	Naprosyn	NS	Non-steroidal anti-inflammatory
18	nifedipine	Procardia	H	Calcium channel blocker
19	diltiazem	Cardizem	H	Calcium channel blocker
20	norethindrone	Ortho-Novum	S	Steroid component of oral contraceptives
21	potassium chloride	Slow K	H	Potassium supplement used with diuretics

Continued

Table 42.2   *Continued*

Rank	Generic name	Typical trade name[b]	Class[c]	Therapeutic class
22	verapamil	Calan	H	Calcium channel blocker
23	cefaclor	Ceclor	A	Antibiotic
24	insulin	Humulin N	M	Hypoglycaemic
25	hydrocodone	Vicodin	An	Narcotic analgesic
26	glyburide	Micronase	M	Hypoglycaemic
27	prednisone	Decortisyl	S	Anti-inflammatory steroid
28	terfenadine	Seldane	AH	Non-soporific antihistamine
29	ibuprofen	Brufen	NS	Non-steroidal anti-inflammatory
30	atenolol	Tenormin	H	β-Blocker
31	norgestrel	Ovral-21	S	Steroid component of oral contraceptives
32	captopril	Capoten	H	ACE inhibitor
33	dipyridamole	Persantine	H	Coronary vasodilator
34	nitroglycerol	Nitrostat	H	Coronary vasodilator
35	cephalexin	Keflex	A	Antibiotic
36	lovastatin	Mevacor	H	HMG-CoA reductase inhibitor (hypocholesteraemic)
37	clavulanic acid	Augmentin	A	β-Lactamese inhibitor
38	lisinopril	Zestril	H	ACE inhibitor
39	cimetidine	Tagamet	U	H_2-antagonist for ulcers
40	fluoxetine	Prozac	CN	Antidepressant
41	lorazepam	Ativan	CN	Benzodiazepine anxiolytic
42	medroxyprogesterone	Provera	S	Steroid for secondary amenhorroea
43	metoprolol	Lopressor	H	β-Blocker
44	theophylline	Theo-Dur	As	Antiasthma
45	diazepam	Valium	CN	Benzodiazepine anxiolytic
46	phenytoin	Dilantin sodium	CN	Antiepileptic
47	ciprofloxacin	Cipro	A	Quinolone antibacterial
48	warfarin	Coumadin Oral	CN	Anticoagulant
49	amitriptyline	Triavil	CN	Tricyclic antidepressant
50	trimethoprim/ sulfamethoxazole	Bactrim	A	Antibacterial
51	tetracycline	Achromycin-V	A	Antibiotic
52	gemfibrizol	Lopid	H	Hypochloesteraemic
53	diclofenac	Voltaren	NS	Non-steroidal anti-inflammatory
54	glipizide	Glucotrol	M	Hypoglycaemic
55	acyclovir	Zovirax	M	Antiviral
56	nicotine polacrilex	Nicorette	M	Antismoking
57	phenylpropanolamine	Entex LA	CC	'Cold cure' constituent
58	famotidine	Pepcid	U	H_2-antagonist for ulcers
59	doxycycline	Vibramycin	A	Tetracycline antibiotic
60	propranolol	Inderal	H	β-Blocker

[a]Author's figures based on *Pharmacy Times*, April 1993.
[b]The trade name given may be a mixture of which the specified drug is only one constituent.
[c]Class abbreviations — see Table 42.1.

Table 42.3 Top 60 most widely prescribed drugs by chemical entity, Germany, 1990.[a]

Rank	Generic name	Typical brand name	Class[b]	Therapeutic class
1	mineral supplements	Calcium Sandoz Brausetabl.	M	Diet suppplement
2	paracetamol	ben-u-ron	An	Analgesic
3	diclofenac	Diclophlogont	NS	Non-steroidal anti-inflammatory
4	salicylic acid derivative ointment	Dolo-Arthrosenex	An	Non-steroidal anti-inflammatory
5	nifedipine	Adalat	H	Calcium antagonist
6	ambroxol	Mucosolvan	CC	Expectorant
7	heparin	Thrombareduct	H	Anticlotting
8	A+P+codeine	Gelonida NA	An	Analgesic
9	vitamins	D-Fluoretten	M	Diet supplement
10	xylometazolin	Olynth	CC	Nasal decongestant
11	L-thyroxine	L-Tyroxin Henning	M	Thyroid
12	hydrochlorothiazide	Esidrix	H	Diuretic
13	metoclopramide	Gastrosil	M	Antiemetic
14	isosorbide mononitrate	Ismo	H	Coronary vasodilator
15	triamterene/ hydrochlorothiazide	Dytide H	H	Diuretic
16	glibenclamide	Euglucon	M	Hypoglycaemic
17	acetylcysteine	ACC Hexal	CC	Expectorant
18	aspirin	ASS Ratiopharm	An	Analgesic
19	β-acetyldigoxin	Novodigal	H	Cardiac glycoside
20	doxycycline	Supracyclin	AA	Antibiotic
21	pencillin V	Isocillin	A	Antibiotic
22	isosorbide dinitrate	Isoket	H	Coronary vasodilator
23	plant extracts	Sinupret Drag.	CC	Combination expectorant
24	ginkgo-biloba extr.	Tebonin	H	Peripheral vasodilator
25	oxazepam	Adumbran	CN	Anxiolytic
26	estradiol	Estraderm TTS	S	Oestrogen
27	Al/Mg hydroxides	Maaloxan	M	Antacid
28	captopril	Lopirin	H	ACE inhibitor
29	allopurinol	Allopurinol-ratiopharm	M	Antigout
30	reserpine-clopamide-dihydroergicristine	Briserin	H	Antihypertensive
31	verapamil	Isoptin	H	Calcium antagonist
32	naftidrofuryl	Dusodril	H	Peripheral vasodilator
33	fenoterol	Berotec aerosol	As	Antiasthma
34	furosemide	Lasix	H	Diuretic
35	metildigoxin	Lanitop	H	Cardiac glycoside
36	pentoxifylline	Trental	H	Haemorheological agent
37	theophylline	Bronchoretard	As	Antiasthma
38	bromazepam	Lexotanil	CN	Anxiolytic
39	loperamide	Imodium	M	Antidiarrhoeal
40	dihydroergotamine	Dihydergot	H	Antihypotensive
41	human insulin	Depot H Insulin	M	Antidiabetic
42	chlormezanon	Muskel transcopal comp.	M	Muscle relaxant

Continued

Table 42.3 *Continued*

Rank	Generic name	Typical brand name	Class[b]	Therapeutic class
43	Simethicone	Lefax	M	Antiflatuent
44	dihydrocodeine	Paracodin retard	CC	Antitussive
45	cetylpyridinium chloride	Dobendan	M	Oral disinfectant
46	metroprolol	Beloc	H	β-Blocker
47	flunitrazepam	Rohypnol	CN	Hypnotic/sedative
48	conj. est. hormone	Presomen comp. drag.	S	Oestrogen
49	glyceryl trinitrate	Nitrolingual	H	Coronary vasodilator
50	hydroxyethylsalicyclate	Phlogont Salbe gel	NS	Non-steroidal anti-inflammatory
51	dihydroergotamine comb.	Ergo-Lonarid	M	Vasoconstrictor
52	cromoglycate	Allergospasmin	As	Antiasthma
53	amitriptyline	Saroten	CN	Antidepressant
54	digitoxin	Digimerck	H	Cardiac glycoside
55	doxycycline/ambroxol	Mucotectan	A	Antibiotic/expectorant
56	etofenemat ointment	Rheumon	NS	Non-steroidal anti-inflammatory
57	clenbuterol	Spasmo-Mucosolvan	As	Antiasthma
58	ranitidine	Sostril	U	H_2-antagonist
59	metamizol	Novalgin	An	Analgesic
60	diazepam	Diazepam-Ratiofarm	CN	Anxiolytic

[a]Author's data based on WIdO: Schwabe, U. and Paffrath, D. (1991) *Arzneiverordnungsreport*. Stuttgart, Gustav Fischer.
[b]Class abbreviations — see Table 42.1.

Table 42.4 Top 60 most widely prescribed drugs by therapeutic class (United States and Germany) and number of prescriptions by therapeutic class (United Kingdom and France) (subgroups shown in parentheses).

Therapeutic group	Percentage of top 60 drugs		Percentage of prescriptions	
	USA (1992)	Germany (1990)	UK (1993)	France (1992)
Heart drugs	32	32	17.2	17.5
Antibiotics and antibacterials	17	5	11.7	7.6
Gastrointestinal (ulcer drugs)	5 (5)	5 (2)	8 (2.3)	18.3
Respiratory (asthma drugs)	8 (3)	15 (7)	10.1 (5.1)	12.2
Central nervous system (analgesics)	13 (3)	15 (7)	18 (8)	19
Musculoskeletal (non-steroidal anti-inflammatories)	5 (5)	7 (5)	6 (4.6)	5.7
Sex hormones	8	3	2.2	3.7
Miscellaneous[a]	12	18	27	16

[a]USA: 3 hypoglycaemics, thyroid, antiviral, antismoking, anti-inflammatory steroid.
Germany: 2 hypoglycaemics, 2 diet supplements, antigout, antiemetic, thyroid, vasoconstrictor, oral disinfectant, muscle relaxant, antiflatuent.
Sources: USA and Germany, see Tables 42.2 and 42.3; United Kingdom: *Department of Health Statistical Bulletin* 1993/5, March 1993; France, Syndicat National de l'Industrie Pharmaceutique, *L'Industrie Pharmaceutique, ses réalités,* Paris, 1993.

On a world basis, cheap antibiotics are the most important drugs. In the developed world, heart drugs are more widely prescribed, partly because antibiotics are prescribed for a single bout of infection whereas heart drugs are generally taken for the remainder of a sufferer's life. After these two groups come drugs for the central nervous system. Nonnarcotic analgesics (aspirin and paracetamol) are usually included in this category, which remains extremely important. None the less, prescriptions for psychotropic drugs (anxiolytics, especially benzodiazepines, neuroleptics, antidepressants, and appetite suppressants) have been dropping since the mid-1980s as doctors have recognized the problems of tolerance and addiction. Drugs against asthma are increasingly prescribed, reflecting greater incidence of the disease and better diagnosis. In the respiratory drugs group, these are lumped together with drugs to ease the symptoms of coughs and colds. Prescriptions for gastrointestinal drugs have also increased in recent years, reflecting the wide range of new drugs available. Twenty years ago, only anticholinergic drugs of the atropine group were used against ulcers. Now there are H_2-

Table 42.5 Chemical groups with a range of pharmaceutical applications.

Chemical class	Example	Therapeutic use
Phenylpiperidines	meperidine (pethidine)	Opioid analgesic
	loperamide	Antidiarrhoeal
	haloperidol	Neuroleptic
	terfenadine	Antihistamine
Sulfonamides/sulphones	sulphamethoxazole	Antibacterial
	acetazolamide	Carbonic anhydrase inhibitor used in glaucoma and (infrequently) as a diuretic and in epilepsy
	glyburide	Hypoglycaemic
	dapsone	Antileprotic/antimalarial
Steroids	ethynylestradiol, norethindrone, medroxyprogesterone,	Sex hormones used in oral contraceptives and for menstrual and menopausal disorders
	prednisone	Anti-inflammatories in arthritis; immunosuppressives in transplantation operations
	beclomethasone dipropionate	Antiasthma
	estramustine phosphate	Prostate cancer
	testosterone esters	Anabolic hormones used for body-building after surgery
Prostaglandins	prostaglandin $F_{2\alpha}$ & E_2	For abortions and to induce labour. $F_{2\alpha}$ reduces intraocular pressure and may be of use in glaucoma
	misoprostol	For gastric ulcers
	prostaglandin E_1	Vasodilator used to treat vascular disease of the leg. Also for ductal-dependent congenital heart disease in newborn babies
	prostacyclin	Antithrombotic and vasodilator. Inhibits platelet aggregation. Used experimentally to inhibit clotting in operations where blood circulates outside the body

antagonists, proton pump inhibitors and cytoprotectives. Prostaglandins have not been notably successful as yet, but bismuth compounds and antibiotics are enjoying a wave of popularity.

Other widely prescribed drugs include the non-steroidal anti-inflammatories, used to counter the pain and inflammation of arthritis, hypoglycaemics for diabetes sufferers, L-thyroxine and thyroid hormone for thyroid sufferers, and antihistamines for hay fever sufferers. The chemical class of steroids plays an unusual role in the list, being the active component of oral contraceptives, some antiasthma drugs and some anti-inflammatories. Few chemical classes are therapeutically active in a number of areas and the most important of these are shown in Table 42.5.

B.   National differences in prescribing

National differences in prescribing can be identified and are related to national culture and attitudes towards the role of drugs in medical treatment. A belief in the prophylactic benefits of taking medicines is widespread in Belgium, France, Greece, Italy and Spain but less prevalent in Britain, Ireland, the Netherlands and the Scandinavian countries. Germany, Austria and the United States have a culture with elements in common with both groups.[2] Prescriptions per head per year in different countries vary dramatically, as shown in Table 42.6. The expenditure per head is also shown. Changes in rank order between the two lists reflects differences in drug prices: drugs are cheap in France and expensive in Japan.

Table 42.6   Prescriptions per person, 1990–91, and expenditure per person in 1989 US dollars.

	Prescriptions	Expenditure		Prescriptions	Expenditure
France	38.3	163	UK	8.5	91
Italy	19.6	141	Belgium	9.5	123
USA	15.5	179	Denmark	6.2	90
Spain	15.0	73	Netherlands	4.8	73
Germany	12.0	154	Japan	NA	245
Ireland	10	60			

Source: OECD (Different definitions of prescriptions may be used in different countries but the overall rank order is likely to be correct.)
NA=not available.

Precisely what constitutes the cultural differences is unclear. It has been suggested that it is related to the proportion of Roman Catholics in the population, but that scarcely explains the gap between Italy and Ireland. There is a loose correlation with climate, people from more temperate climates requiring fewer prescriptions, but that does not explain the difference between Belgium and the Netherlands. The perception of the doctor and the patient of their roles, however, is at the root of the discrepancies. A patient visiting an Italian doctor will emerge with a prescription in 95% of cases. In the United Kingdom, this drops to about 70%. The giving of a prescription is seen to a greater or lesser extent in high- and low-prescribing countries as a way of signalling the conclusion of a consultation. To hand out a prescription reinforces the doctor's image of him or herself as a doctor (that is what doctors are 'supposed' to do) and the patient's image of him or herself as a patient (patients are given medicine; by giving me a prescription, the doctor is confirming that I am ill, have not troubled him or her unnecessarily and am justified in taking the day off work to visit the doctor).

The differences between countries are less clear-cut, none the less, than the above figures imply. The drugs discussed so far are those that must be prescribed by a physician. Some drugs are classified as 'generally regarded as safe', however, which means that they can be sold direct to the public, that is over the counter (OTC) rather than on prescription. Diet supplements are apparently much more popular in Germany than in the United States but, in fact, the Americans buy them over the counter instead of having them prescribed. This reflects both culture and systems of health insurance reimbursement.

Apart from differences in quantity, there are disparities between countries in the types of drugs prescribed. In the United States and the United Kingdom, almost all the leading drugs are therapeutically active; in Germany, France and Italy, many prescriptions are for 'comfort' drugs that are generally agreed to have little therapeutic value. Estimates are given in Table 42.7. The Germans show enthusiasm for ointments based on non-steroidal anti-inflammatories and salicylic acid derivatives. They also take peripheral vasodilators and antihypotensives, drugs that are rarely used by the British and Americans. They are concerned, as are the French, with problems of the digestive system and take drugs that supposedly reinvigorate the gallbladder. The French also take peripheral vasodilators and numerous drugs for the *crise de foie*.

Table 42.7   The 'useless drugs' league.

	Top 25 products			Top 50 products			'Useless' drugs (percentage of sales)
	A	B	C	A	B	C	
Italy	11	7	7	25	15	10	21.2
France	16	4	5	26	14	10	20.5
Germany	19	5	1	35	9	6	11.9
UK	24	1	0	46	4	0	NA

Source: Health Economics Centre, Cesav, Italy, reported in *SCRIP* (1993) **1860**: 4.
NA=not applicable.
Class A: Products agreed internationally to be therapeutically effective.
Class B: Second-line therapy, open to misuse, more expensive than similar products, or combination products with no advantage over monosubstances.
Class C: Drugs with no evidence of efficacy.

In comparison, the British and Americans take large numbers of antibiotics. These are indeed therapeutically active, but the number of prescriptions compared with Germany suggests that in many cases they too are prescribed as 'comfort' drugs for conditions that are either self-limiting or viral infections insensitive to antibiotics, or both.

As noted, the above tables exclude OTC drugs. In most developed countries, the therapeutically active constituents of OTC drugs are largely confined to nonnarcotic analgesics, antihistamines, antacids and anti-inflammatory steroid ointments. In some countries, antibiotics are available without prescription and the narcotic analgesic codeine is sometimes permitted mixed with aspirin or paracetamol. As governments try to increase the proportion of drug costs paid by patients, the range of OTC drugs will probably increase. The antiviral acyclovir can now be obtained OTC in the United Kingdom, and permission was granted early in 1994 for the H_2-antagonist cimetidine.

The other major group of drugs omitted from the prescriptions list is those given in hospitals. Recent figures are not readily available, but US data from 1987 list numerous antibiotics (mainly cephalosporins) used to counter potentially resistant bacteria found in hospitals together with blood products (e.g. albumin), intravenous products (e.g. total parenteral nutrition, dextrose) and the anticoagulant heparin.[3] In the United Kingdom, anti-infectives (antibiotics and antibacterials) account for 25% by value of hospital drugs.

The proportions of pharmaceutical production at manufacturers' prices dispensed on prescription, in hospitals and OTC, are shown in Table 42.8.

Table 42.8   Sources of drugs (at manufacturers' prices, 1989).

	Percentage via:		Percentage as OTC
	Doctors	Hospitals	
Belgium	71	12	17
France	79	14	7
Germany	68	16	16
Italy	81	13	6
Netherlands	72	15	12
Spain	76	12	12
UK	70	14	16
USA	65	15	20
Japan	17	68	15

Source: Ref. 25.

II.   SOURCES OF DRUGS

Drugs are obtained from five sources: animal and vegetable extracts, biological sources, fermentation, and chemical synthesis. Our ancestors, lacking synthetic skill, drew primarily on animal and vegetable sources. Macbeth's witches brewed up 'eye of newt, toe of frog and liver of blaspheming Jew', which must have had a largely psychological effect, not to mention encouraging antisemitism, but they remembered to add pharmacological activity with 'root of hemlock picked in the dark'.

A.   Vegetable sources

Plants continue to this day to provide a range of medicinal alkaloids (e.g. papaverine, atropine, codeine, quinidine), glycosides (e.g. digoxin) steroids (e.g. diosgenin, stigmasterol, sitosterol, the raw materials for medicinal steroids), and vitamins (e.g. vitamin E from the tocopherol from the distillate from the steam deodorization of soya bean oil). This is discussed in Chapter 7. A current problem is the anticancer drug paclitaxel (Taxol® (**1**)), a diterpenoid ester produced in 0.02% yield from the stem bark of the Pacific yew tree *Taxis brevifolia*. This can never be an adequate source and a practicable synthetic route is sought.

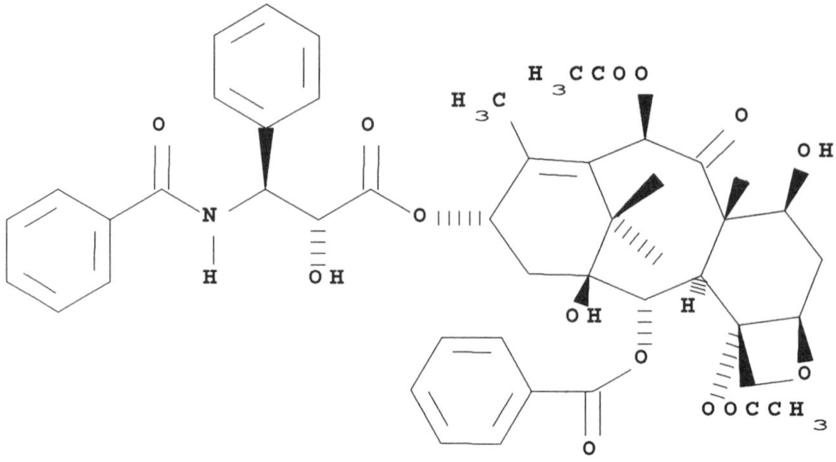

(1)

B.   Animal sources

Animal sources are less convenient than vegetable sources for production of commercial quantities of drugs, but some pharmaceuticals are obtained from slaughterhouse wastes. Heparin, cow and pig insulin, thyroid hormone and bile acids are examples. Conjugated oestrogenic hormone is obtained from the urine of pregnant mares, with the bonus that the animal does not have to be slaughtered.

Human blood, given by blood donors, is a source not only of cellular material (red cells, white cells, platelets) but of blood plasma, which is subjected to protein fractionation to give albumin, antihaemophilia factors and immunoglobulins. The possibility of transmission of AIDS if sterilization procedures fail, combined with the feasibility of manufacturing proteins by recombinant DNA techniques, means that there is uncertainty about the long-term future of the blood products industry.

C.   Biological sources

Biological sources are primarily used for vaccines. Vaccines are suspensions of living or killed microorganisms, or components or products thereof. They are produced in living systems. Eggs are the most widely used medium at present, but there is increasing use of animal cell cultures. Bacterial vaccines, for example the diphtheria vaccine, can be cultured. There is an overlap here with fermentation processes (Section II.D).

Recombinant DNA processes can be used to make subunit vaccines. These can be classified either as biological or as fermentation processes. Hepatitis B vaccines are made by genetic manipulation of yeast or animal cells. The cells then express the hepatitis B virus outer coat protein, which is harmless to the host because there is no DNA present.

There are two types of immunization, active and passive. In active immunization, the vaccine is administered to the patient, whose immune system responds by producing antibodies and cells sensitized to the vaccine and hence conferring immunity to the disease. In passive immunization, a donor who has had a specific disease donates blood and an immunoglobulin is isolated from the blood plasma. This is then injected into the patient.

Some immunoglobulins cannot be obtained from normal, healthy blood donors and are obtained instead by inoculation of volunteers so that they develop the required antibody. Such procedures are used for immunoglobulins against vaccinia, tetanus, measles, hepatitis A, Rhesus incompatibility and rabies.[4] The biological 'factory' for the immune globulin, in such cases, is the body of the volunteer.

In the future, monoclonal antibodies will have a major role in the development of new diagnostic and therapeutic products.

D.   Fermentation

Fermentation in its simplest forms, such as the production of bread or wine, is very old technology. In its application with recombinant DNA to produce pharmacologically active proteins (erythropoetin, human growth hormone, human insulin), it is central to the modern biotechnological revolution. In between, it is the method for production of antibiotics and vitamin B_{12} and provides a step in the production of vitamin C and the synthesis of cortisone from diosgenin.

Plant cell culture might be classified as fermentation or production from a biological or vegetable source. It is not yet widely applied. There were reports that a digoxin producer modified the useless glycosides from *Digitalis lanata* by plant cell culture and thus converted them to digoxin and increased yield per plant. The Japanese are certainly using plant cell culture to produce shikonin (**2**) a red pigment with anti-inflammatory properties.

(**2**)

E.   Chemical synthesis

In spite of the importance of the above methods, chemical synthesis is the most important method of drug manufacture. It is responsible for almost all heart drugs, drugs for the central nervous system, antiulcer drugs, analgesics and antihistamines. Many pharmaceuticals are made simply from readily available bulk chemicals. For example, the non-steroidal anti-inflammatory agent ibuprofen is made from toluene and propylene, two of the seven basic building blocks of the petrochemical industry.[5] Chemical synthesis is also used to modify materials made from other sources, and chemical methods of extraction are used in the downstream processing of products from other sources.

The combination of methods illustrates the eclecticism of the pharmaceutical industry. The use of fermentation in the production of vitamin C and cortisone was mentioned above. In the production of the semisynthetic penicillins, penicillin G or V is first made by fermentation. It is then cleaved to 6-aminopenicillanic acid by an immobilized enzyme, and a new side-chain is added by chemical means. With the thrombolytic drug Eminase®, a plasminogen-streptokinase activator is made by a cell-cloning biotechnological technique. This is then chemically modified by addition of a *p*-anisoyl group to give a longer-lived product that can be administered by injection rather than through a drip.

III.   MANUFACTURE OF DRUGS

The largest-tonnage organic chemical is ethylene, made in the United States on a scale of about 18 million tonnes/year. It sells for about $0.40/kg. The largest medicinal chemicals are aspirin, paracetamol (acetaminophen) and vitamin C, made worldwide on a scale of 30 000–50 000 tonnes/year. A total of about 149 000 tonnes of medicinal chemicals was manufactured in the United States in 1992, 92 000 tonnes of which were sold for $2.4 billion at an average price of $25.90/kg.[6] These medicinal chemicals were formulated into products, however, which sold for about $35 billion, amounting to almost $200/kg of raw material.

The manufacture of pharmaceutical chemicals in some ways resembles a scaled-up version of the organic chemical syntheses carried out in the laboratory and in others a scaled-down version of the processes used in the heavy chemicals industry. The heavy chemicals industry manufactures commodity chemicals that are largely undifferentiated and have to be sold at the ruling market price. The individual company, having little control over prices, is therefore preoccupied with reducing costs. A major source of cost reduction is economies of scale and those in turn are related to the use of continuous rather than batch processes, and the former are well-nigh universal in the heavy chemicals sector

The pharmaceutical industry, in contrast, manufactures a large number of chemicals in small quantities to a high level of purity. Economies of scale are relatively inaccessible. The product, especially if it is under patent, is highly differentiated and can be sold, like other speciality chemicals, at a price that reflects its value-in-use rather than its manufacturing cost. The industry is preoccupied with quality control, and this is more easily achieved in batch equipment. Purity is of greater importance than high yield. The process must always be operated in such a way that the quality of the final product is maintained, and this leads to certain design features not normally found in chemical works. An analytical department intervenes at every stage to monitor the progress of a drug through the system. There is a code of Good Manufacturing Practice (GMP) for the pharmaceutical industry, which lays down guidelines within the European Community,[7] and this is matched by similar regulations of the Food and Drug Administration (FDA) in the United States. It dominates the organization of pharmaceutical manufacturing sites.

A.   Good Manufacturing Practice

Medicinal products must be fit for their intended use, comply with the requirements of market authorization and not place patients at risk because of inadequate safety, quality or efficacy. These objectives are easy to state, but to achieve them requires a comprehensively designed and correctly implemented system of quality assurance. It is important that this is documented and its effectiveness monitored. Records must be kept that are open to inspection by validating bodies, and there must also be procedures for self-inspection and quality audit that allow appraisal of the quality assurance system. Management must be adequately trained and their responsibilities minutely defined. Two key posts are the heads of Production and of Quality Control. These posts are required by the guidelines to be independent of one another.

Quality control is part of GMP. It is concerned with sampling, specification and testing, and with the organization, documentation and release procedures that ensure that tests have indeed been carried out. No materials must be released for use or sale until their quality has been judged satisfactory. For example, the purity of most drugs is greater than 99.9% and the content of the remaining 0.1% is usually specified in the Pharmacopoeia and in the quality control specifications. Absorbent cotton fibres may present a problem and ointments are specified to contain less than 1 fibre cm^{-3}, the fibre being less than 1 mm long. Contamination by the ubiquitous *Penicillium* microorganisms is a particular problem (see below).

B. Plant design

A large pharmaceuticals manufacturer will operate several different plants. The plant for the manufacture of active ingredients by chemical synthesis will be separate from the plant that formulates the active ingredients into finished medicines. Fermentation plant will usually be on a totally different site geographically from a chemical synthesis plant. The reason for this is to minimize contamination by the *Penicillium* microorganism, among others. Penicillin concentrations in finished products must be kept below 1 ppm w/w to avoid allergic reaction in penicillin-sensitive patients. Bacteria insensitive to an antibiotic may grow in a medium containing it, and most countries demand the absence of harmful varieties (e.g. salmonella) and specify a limit for total bacterial count. Thus the US Pharmacopoeia quotes 5000 cm^{-3} for a gelatin base. The cautious manufacturer will prefer to build his chemical plant far away from the microorganism-rich environment of a fermentation plant. There is also likely to be a separation from plant making biological medicinal products and these have separate regulations.

As far as equipment is concerned, the pharmaceutical industry rarely follows the chemical industry pattern of purpose-built plant, carefully optimized and with the larger sections fabricated on site. In general, equipment is bought 'off the shelf' and assembled like a child's erector set.

Optimization is sacrificed to availability of plant items. A secondary benefit to emerge from this is that lead times (i.e. the time taken to build plant) are lower than in the chemical industry. Because kilogram quantities of a drug are required for testing before it is known whether a drug will be a success, the initial manufacturing process usually involves a batch preparation on general-purpose equipment. There may subsequently be a need for changes to the initial method on economic or safety grounds (e.g. one of the reagents may be pyrophoric), but the need to register a validated process means that there will be a conservative attitude to process change.

The equipment supplier will therefore aim to offer versatile, multipurpose equipment that can be used in a range of processes. Most of it will be stainless-steel or glass-lined to avoid problems with contamination or corrosion. In spite of its versatility, however, the plant, once built, will rarely be changed. Any new process or important modification of an existing process must be validated, and critical phases of an existing manufacturing process must be regularly revalidated. If the manufacturer wants to add a recycle stream, for example, clearance must first be obtained.

Wherever possible, a single reaction vessel is dedicated to one particular process, and usually each preparation is performed in a self-contained area. This situation has eased somewhat in recent years, and more multiuse equipment is being installed. There is still not the flexibility in equipment use that one might expect in comparison, say, with the dyestuffs industry, but there is a trend in that direction.

An exception to the rule of small, general-purpose equipment arises with fermentation processes. A reactor producing penicillin G will certainly be dedicated and may have a capacity of 250 tonnes and a 2000 kW stirrer. Because yields are so low, the weight of penicillin produced per run will be two orders of magnitude smaller. One of the problems of downstream processing is to reduce the volume of the penicillin-containing stream to more manageable proportions and to dispose of the effluent fermentation liquid without imposing an unacceptable biochemical oxygen demand on the aquatic environment.

The availability of on-line microcomputers and microprocessor-controlled equipment is extending many of the benefits of continuous processing to the batch processor. The pharmaceutical industry has been a leader in the employment of these new techniques.[8]

C. Formulation and packaging — sterile products

Plant for the production of active ingredients resembles plant for the production of other small-tonnage chemicals. Formulation and packaging plant, in which the active ingredient is converted into a saleable form, is much less familiar to the industrial chemist. The reason is the need for a controlled environment. Some straightforward chemical products to be taken by mouth do not need to be tableted in a sterile environment. For others, such as injectable antibiotics, it is essential. Although the regulations do not demand sterility for all products, most companies will carry out all their formulating in a controlled environment, the severity of which will depend on the nature of the product. Walls and floors are rounded off to allow efficient cleaning. Sinks and drains are avoided as far as possible. Packaging is carried out in individual cubicles to avoid cross-contamination if there is spillage. Production of sterile medicines is carried out in clean areas whose entry is through airlocks both for people and goods. The areas are supplied with suitably filtered air and are classified A, B, C or D according to the required characteristic of the air. These are shown in Table 42.9. The actual regulations are more detailed and the table merely summarizes a few of the points. In particular, it illustrates the need for personnel to wear suitable clothing that will prevent contamination by viruses, bacteria or particulate matter.

Manufacturing operations for sterile products are divided into two groups, one where the product is sterilized terminally, that is at the end of processing after it has been sealed in its container, and the other where some of the processing must be conducted aseptically. For terminally sterilized products, a grade C environment is usually adequate. Aseptic preparation can be performed in a grade C environment provided the product is sterile-filtered later in the process. If not, a grade A zone with a grade B background is required.

The provision of sterile areas in a packaging and formulation plant means that such a plant may cost as much as a conventional manufacturing plant for the active ingredient. The tableting

Table 42.9 Air classification system for the manufacture of sterile products.

	Maximum permitted numbers of particles per m³		Maximum permitted number of viable micro-organisms per m³	Approximate equivalent US Federal Standard 209C	Clothing for each grade
	$\geq 0.5\ \mu m$	$\geq 5\ \mu m$			
A[a]	3 500	0	<1[b]	100	
B	3 500	0	5[b]	100	Clean, sterilized protective garments provided at least once a day. Gloves disinfected during operations. Masks and gloves changed every working session. Disposable clothing a possibility
C	350 000	2 000	100	10 000	Hair covered. Two-piece non-fibre-shedding trouser suit gathered at wrists and with high neck required
D	3 500 000	20 000	500	100 000	Hair covered. Protective clothing and shoes required

Source: ref. 7.
The number of air changes should generally be higher than 20 per hour in a room with good air flow pattern and appropriate HEPA filters.
[a]Laminar-air-flow workstation. Systems should provide homogeneous air speed of 0.3 m s⁻¹ vertical and 0.45 m s⁻¹ horizontal flow.
[b]Only reliable when a large number of air samples is taken.

and packaging equipment are relatively inexpensive, and most of the money is spent on equipment to produce a controlled environment.

D. Choice of reagents

The special characteristics of the pharmaceutical industry also affect choice of reagents. In general, processing costs are higher than in the chemical industry as a whole, and capital costs are lower. Because of the high unit value of pharmaceuticals, expensive chemicals are practicable. For example, lithium aluminium hydride might be used as a reducing agent while, in the petrochemical industry, hydrogen is the only economic reagent.

Pharmaceutical companies are involved in long, multistep synthetic processes. A modest way in which they try to keep costs within bounds is by the use of standard intermediates that can be used for a number of products. For example, all the different chemically modified penicillins are based on 6-aminopenicillanic acid, which can consequently be manufactured on a much larger scale than any of the individual penicillins. Such intermediates are known as synthons.

In general, companies prefer to reduce the number of synthetic steps they have to carry out themselves by purchase of synthons — high quality raw materials, reagents and key intermediates — from fine chemical manufacturers. These manufacturers are often prepared to develop reagents and intermediates specifically for one customer in the expectation that they will have further uses in the future. Reagents that increase reaction selectivities are often identified in academic laboratories but cannot be used on a tonnage scale because of lack of availability or cost. Fine chemical companies can find niche markets by developing methods of making these reagents cheaply available. Recent examples are Hünig's base, N,N-diisopropyl-N-ethylamine[9] (i-C$_3$H$_7$)$_2$NCH$_2$CH$_3$, and oxalyl chloride[10] (COCl)$_2$. An improvement in selectivity is economically attractive not only because it gives higher yields but also because it produces less waste; the reduction of waste is currently a key environmental issue.

Companies may contract out some intermediate stages in a drug synthesis or conduct them in an isolated part of the plant if they offer particular hazards. Nitrations would probably be carried out in a special nitrating plant with equipment designed to prevent runaway reactions; phosgene would be handled only under carefully controlled conditions because of its toxicity. Experience is similarly needed with organofluorine compounds, reactions at cryogenic temperatures and fermentation routines for steroids and antibiotics. A firm that has been engaged in such operations for many years accumulates know-how, and this gives them a great advantage over new entrants to the industry.

An area of ferment at present is the question of chirality. In May 1992 the FDA published a policy statement questioning the 'commonly made assumption' that racemic mixtures of drugs will continue to be acceptable to the regulatory body. Meanwhile, the marketing of single enantiomers is not yet mandatory. Since Monsanto's pioneering asymmetric synthesis in the early 1980s of L-dopa, a drug for Parkinson's disease, chiral syntheses and separations have been of intense interest. This was accentuated by the realization that it was the D-isomer of thalidomide that was responsible for birth defects while the L-isomer was the hypnotic. More recent research has suggested that thalidomide has applications in leprosy and tuberculosis.[11] It has orphan drug status (see Section IV.C) in the former application.

Sometimes both enantiomers of a drug are pharmacologically active and in such cases there is no reason to favour one over the other. In other cases, a chiral drug, when administered, racemizes in the body anyway. None the less, there are numerous examples of drugs where the administration of a racemic mixture means that patients are needlessly exposed to pharmacologically inactive chemicals. Even if the racemic mixture is synthesized but separated in the production stage, half of the production may be wasted. It might in the end be cheaper to make the correct enantiomer to start with. Hence there is great interest in chiral intermediates and chiral catalysts. Many specialist firms are springing up to try to find niche markets in this area.

E. Downstream processing

The reagents used by the pharmaceutical industry are more complex and sophisticated than those employed by the heavy organic chemical industry. The same is true of the purification and isolation of the products. The small, simple molecules of the petrochemical industry can usually be separated from impurities by distillation. In the pharmaceutical industry, this remains true for solvents, less true for intermediates, and rarely true for end-products. In the case of medicinal products from biological sources or made by fermentation, it is never true.

Much downstream processing is performed by the well-documented but less widely used unit processes of chemical engineering — solvent extraction, filtration, leaching, adsorption and crystallization. Freeze drying, centrifugation, ion exchange and preparative chromatography are valuable options. Cross-flow filtration has become important, especially since the development of anisotropic membranes. These permit adequate flow rates but are still sufficiently robust to withstand high pressures and the wear and tear of industrial-scale operations. Cross-flow techniques may be used for microfiltration, reverse osmosis and microfiltration.

Sterilization is a unit process not found in the heavy chemical industry. The aim of sterilization is to kill and/or remove bacteria and pyrogens. Pyrogens are fragments of bacterial cell walls, which may produce fever as a reaction to foreign proteins if they enter the bloodstream of a sensitive person.

For heat-stable materials, sterilization by steam for 15 min at 121°C kills all bacteria and viruses. Pasteurization for a longer period at a lower temperature is also effective. Dry heat at a temperature above 250°C destroys pyrogens.

Heat-sensitive materials may be sterilized by radiation, providing the product and its container are not radiation-sensitive. It is particularly used with plastics and more widely used with containers than with products. An alternative is ethylene oxide gas. This presents problems in that the gas must be brought into contact with the cell walls of contaminating bacteria. Ethylene oxide is highly reactive and it can only be used when it can be proved not to react with the product.

Filtration through a 0.22 μm filter removes bacteria and moulds but not all viruses or mycoplasma. It is not considered sufficient when terminal sterilization is practicable.

IV.   SOCIAL AND ECONOMIC FACTORS

The economics of the research-based pharmaceutical industry is as remote from classical economics as its technology is from that of the heavy chemical industry. Neither the manufacturers nor the consumers conform to the concept of a free market.

Producers of pharmaceuticals are monopolists to the extent that they have patents on their products. Instead of conventional competition on price and quality, there is competition in innovation between rival producers, so that a number of manufacturers may offer, for example, different H_2-antagonists for the treatment of gastric ulcers. In so far as patients require a particular product, however, they are faced by a monopoly producer.

At the consumer's end, the situation is even more confused. Drugs are taken by the patient, prescribed by the physician and paid for (to a varying extent in different countries) by the patient, the state or by insurance companies. Thus, the usual market constraints are lacking. On the other hand, the state, insurance companies and hospitals sometimes have much of the power of monopoly purchasers — so-called monopsonists. In many countries, the state licenses individual pharmaceuticals and sets their prices. In the negotiations with drug companies, the usual price determinants of supply and demand are replaced by political considerations.

The above factors mean that the market for pharmaceuticals is subject to severe distortions. Certain aspects will be discussed in this section, notably the pattern and cost of innovation, the role of patents, orphan drugs, the rise of generic drugs, and the attempts by governments at cost containment.

A.   Pattern and cost of innovation

The modern pharmaceutical industry dates back to the discovery of the sulfonamide drugs in 1935. The industry has grown since 1950 typically at 7–15% per year, and over 95% of drugs available originated after that date. An astonishing series of innovations has increased life expectancy and improved the quality of life in developed and to a lesser extent in developing countries. The industry has moved from a 'molecular roulette' system by which new drugs were developed on the basis of trial and error to a sophisticated system hinging on an understanding of the enzyme systems the drugs are intended to influence.

The industry was surprisingly unregulated in its early days but, since the thalidomide disaster in 1960, regulation has become increasingly strict and the cost of developing new drugs has escalated. Figure 42.1 shows the number of new products launched worldwide each year since 1960, together with total spending on research and development at 1990 prices.

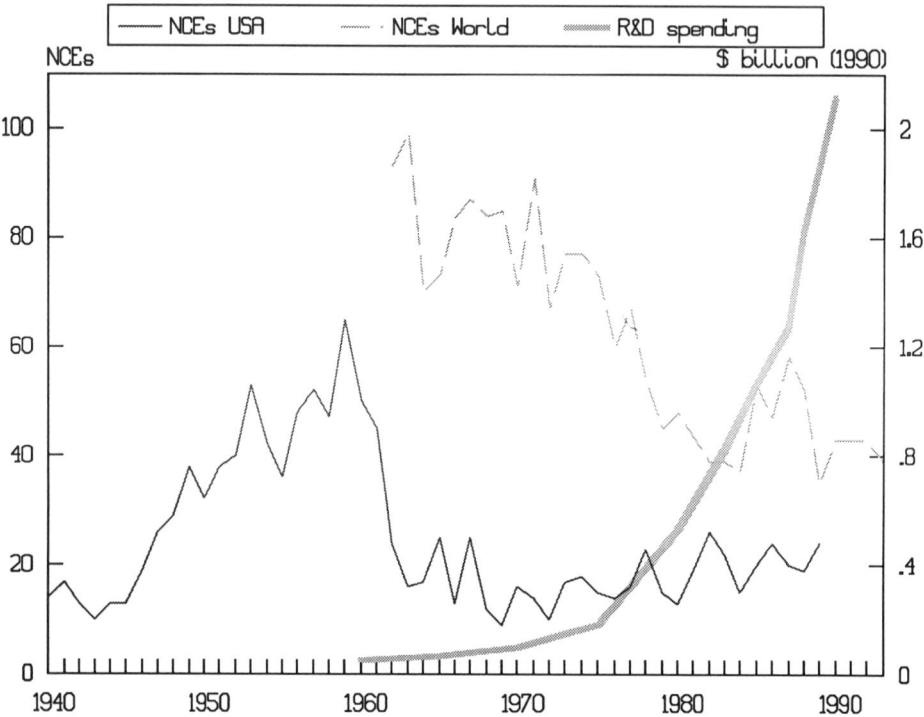

Fig. 42.1 Numbers of new chemical entities (NCEs) launched worldwide and in the United States each year and worldwide R&D expenditure at 1990 prices.

The cost of introducing a new chemical entity to the drug market in the mid-1980s has been estimated at $114 million, measured in 1987 dollars.[12] This figure includes the cost of failures, that is drugs that were eliminated during testing. This high cost is accentuated by the increased time required for drug discovery and testing. The average new chemical entity in the above survey took 11.8 years to reach launch. This had two consequences. First, the patent life remaining to the drug, during which its development costs could be recovered, was much shortened. Second, the return on the R&D outlay was delayed. To get a true cost for the development of a new drug, one must discount the expenditure to the moment of launch. If a discount rate of 9% is assumed, then a figure of $231 million is obtained.

This huge figure explains why only large multinationals with generous cash flow from other projects can be serious players in the game of pharmaceutical innovation. Smaller companies may come up with bright ideas that they sell to the multinationals, but only the giants can undertake the testing and registration procedures. Indeed, not only is pharmaceutical innovation confined to large companies, it is also confined to countries that can provide the resources and manpower for such high-technology operations.

The countries where drug discovery takes place are shown in Table 42.10. The leading countries would appear to be those at the top of the list with the greatest number of discoveries, notably the United States, France and Japan. This is misleading. Genuine advances in drug therapy are marketed worldwide, or at least in major markets outside their country of discovery. By this criterion, the big players are the United States, the United Kingdom, Germany, Japan, Switzerland and Belgium. France drops from third to eighth place and the United Kingdom rises from seventh to second. In terms of foreign sales of pharmaceutical products,[13] Switzerland, Germany, the United Kingdom, the United Stastes, France and Sweden are the only countries showing a positive balance of trade, although Japan in the 1990s has shown a positive balance on intellectual property for the first time.

Table 42.10   Country of discovery of new chemical entities (NCEs), 1975–89.

	All NCEs	International[a]	Worldwide[a]
USA	207	115	47
Japan	160	22	5
France	94	18	3
Germany	86	38	9
Italy	72	10	2
Switzerland	45	23	5
UK	35	22	14
Belgium	30	20	5
Sweden	21	13	4
Others	18	7	1
Netherlands	7	5	2

Source: Quoted in Syndicat National de l'Industrie Pharmaceutique, *L'Industrie Pharmaceutique, ses réalités*, Paris, 1993, p. 16.
[a]'worldwide' entities are those marketed in the seven major markets, USA, Japan, Germany, France, Italy, UK and Sweden. 'International' entities are marketed in at least four of the seven. Products are attributed to the country in which they were discovered even if it was by a foreign firm having a research centre in the country.

The governments of the leading drug-producing countries are in a curious position. On the one hand, they are anxious to limit the social security costs of drugs at home. On the other hand, they are anxious to promote foreign trade in pharmaceuticals and to ensure that their industry remains prosperous. The countries with less drug-producing capability may have ambitions to build up their own industry but otherwise are more determined to limit drug expenditure. Until recently, the drug companies have been successful in fighting off cost containment measures, but there is evidence now that governments are collaborating on global measures which, they hope, will save money for governments without wrecking the industry.[14,28] Whether this will be successful remains to be seen.

B.   Patents

'I knew that a country without a patent office . . . was just a crab', said Mark Twain, 'and couldn't travel any way but sideways or   backwards'. Patent protection is recognized as a cornerstone of the success of the industrialized market economies of Western Europe and North America in the nineteenth and twentieth centuries. Without it, individuals would have been discouraged from investing in innovation, fearing that, even if their research was a success, they would never recover development costs because of cut-price competition from imitators.

As described in Chapter 41, a patent provides the discoverer of a 'non-obvious' invention with a monopoly to exploit it for a specified period after its registration in return for disclosure of details of the invention. The period in the United States is 17 years from the granting of the patent, while the European Community has adopted a European Patent Convention that grants 20 years from the filing of the patent application. This applies also in some countries outside the Community, for example Sweden and Switzerland. In Japan, a patent lasts for 20 years from filing or 15 years from publication, whichever is shorter. As there is an interval between the filing and granting of a patent, all these patent lives are similar. Some countries, especially in the third world, do not have patent laws and their citizens are not bound by foreign patents. Such countries have difficulty gaining access to first-world technology and are unable to export to countries that subscribe to patent conventions. Trade sanctions may be imposed on offenders, for example the United States took action against Brazil in 1988. Mexico has promised to introduce product patents in 1997.   Countries trying to industrialize find it worthwhile to introduce patent laws at some stage, but even Italy did not legislate until 1978.

The pharmaceutical industry invariably seeks patent protection for new drugs. The problem is that the time taken to develop and test a new drug has lengthened. In 1962, the process of invention and testing took on average only 2 years. By the late 1980s, this had lengthened to 11.8 years. The effective patent life of a drug varies from country to country and drug to drug. The detailed picture is provided by Lis and Walker[15,16] and their broad conclusion is that it has shortened to between 6 and 8 years. Thus, the time for a company to recoup its investment has been more than halved while the cost of development has risen exponentially.

The industry campaigned with some success for patent term restoration. The US Federal Food, Drug and Cosmetic Act was amended in 1984. It extended the patent term of pharmaceuticals and biologicals by half the time from which the first investigational new drug application (IND) became effective until the date of filing of the new drug application (NDA) plus all the time the FDA takes to review the new drug application, up to a maximum of 5 years. A limitation is that a company cannot have more than a 14-year patent life by this method, and time can also be subtracted if the FDA feels the company is not pursuing the project with sufficient diligence.

A new Japanese patent law came into effect in 1988 which allows patent term restoration up to a maximum of 5 years. Restoration is applicable only to products that have taken more than 2 years to obtain marketing authorization after patent grant. The effect of this is similar to that of the US legislation.

The European Community has lagged behind in legislation, partly because of the legal difficulties in amending the European Patent Convention. Agreement was reached on a maximum of 15 years protection from the date of first marketing. After patent expiry, companies can apply for a supplementary protection certificate for up to 5 years. A series of court rulings on data protection make it likely that some innovators will gain an extra 3–4 years' marketing exclusivity on top of this, but the total protection must not exceed 15 years.

C.   Orphan drugs

The spiralling cost of drug development has also created problems with drugs for rare diseases. About 4000 rare diseases are described in the literature. Many are known by the names of those who first described them — Huntington's chorea, Paget's disease, Tourette's syndrome and so on. Many might or do respond to chemotherapy. It is in the public interest that such diseases should be treated, but the problem is who should pay.

The cost of developing a new drug has been estimated at $231 million. If a 15-year patent life is assumed (patent term restoration!) and a 9% discount rate assumed, then, to cover the development costs alone, a worldwide income of about $30 million/year is required, about a quarter of this in the European Community. There are about 20 000 sufferers from Huntingdon's chorea in the Community, which means $1500 per person. Add in the other costs of drug production and the patient is being asked to pay about $5000 annually.

Such a sum is lower than the cost of the antihaemophilia Factor VIII in the massive doses that need to be administered to patients who have developed antibodies to Factor VIII. It is of the same order of cost as a week in hospital. One might argue that social security funds should be willing to pay large sums for the relief of a tiny minority of the population. The fact remains that a debate on reimbursement of Factor VIII expenditure is raging in Germany at the time of writing. Whatever the outcome, research on rare diseases — and there are many that are rarer than Huntingdon's chorea — must appear uneconomic to pharmaceutical companies planning their research expenditure. A project focusing on migraine or arthritis is bound to appear more attractive.

There is little question that the high cost of development inhibits speculative research. Drug companies may well refuse to carry out research on a particular disease because, even if they find a drug to cure it, the disease is so rare that they cannot hope to recoup their expenditure. Alternatively, a drug may be available but no one may want to produce it, either because the drug is not patentable or because the cost of testing is too high. For a truly rare disease, there are problems in assembling enough patients for statistical analysis of test results. Add to these factors that the companies fear litigation, damages and loss of their good name if things go wrong.

Compounds that no one wants to develop are known as orphan drugs.[17] Because of the difficulties surrounding their development, there was a vigorous campaign in the United States to alter the law. One of the principal spokesmen was David Abelow, who suffered from neurofibromatosis, which became widely known as a result of the film *The Elephant Man*. John Merrick, the subject of the film, had it in a severe form.

As a result of the campaign, the 'Orphan Drugs Act' was passed in 1983, which allows for grants, provides tax credits, eases regulatory pressures and permits 7 years' exclusive marketing rights for nonpatentable drugs to companies making them. It is possible for the US Secretary of State to hold the product licence and for the supplier not to be responsible for the safety of the product. In the United Kingdom, drugs can be given a clinical trials certificate, which allows patients under close supervision to be given a drug that has not been fully tested. An orphan drug is defined in the United States as one used for the treatment of a disease or condition affecting fewer than 200,000 people there. If more than 200 000 people are affected, it could alternatively be shown that the cost of developing the drug and making it available would not be covered by sales in the United States.

By January 1991, 50 orphan products had been approved for the treatment of 58 rare conditions.[18] Companies had received $12 million in tax credits for orphan research. The 'classic' orphan drug cases had been sorted out. For example, trientine hydrochloride,

$H_2N(CH_2)_2NH(CH_2)_2NH(CH_2)_2NH_2 \cdot 2HCl$, a chelating agent used to remove excess copper in Wilson's disease for patients who did not respond to penicillamine, and which had been a major concern of J.M. Walshe[19] in Cambridge, was licensed in 1985.

The US Congress became concerned in 1990 about what they saw as abuse by some companies of the Orphan Drugs Act, or at any rate that the act was not always working as intended. In some cases, compounds were registered as orphan drugs when a disease was rare, but then the disease became epidemic and the number of sufferers rose well above the 200 000 mark. For example, the AIDS virus was identified in 1981. By 1986 there were only 23 000 cases in the United States and the drug azidothymidine (AZT) was genuinely orphan. Since then, many millions of cases have been diagnosed worldwide. Sales of AZT in 1992 amounted to a little under $200 million. A similar rise in demand applied to drugs for the commoner side-effects of AIDS. Epoetin alfa, one of the best-selling drugs listed in Table 42.1, obtained orphan drug status for treatment of anaemia associated with AZT therapy, prematurity and end-stage renal disease in both dialysed and nondialysed patients.

Legislation to amend the Orphan Drugs Act has been slow. Early in 1994 a compromise proposal was introduced which would reduce the period of marketing exclusivity from 7 to 4 years, allow more than one version of an orphan drug if they were developed simultaneously, and allow withdrawal of exclusivity for orphan products when the patient population exceeds 200 000. Orphan drugs 'of limited commercial potential' could be granted an additional 3 years exclusivity if sales information and related data justified it.[20]

An interesting scientific question raised by the new regulations was the point at which two drugs should be regarded as 'identical'. The definition affects not only whether a novel drug could be patented as a new chemical entity but also whether an out-of-patent generic drug (see Section IV.D) could be approved on the basis of an abbreviated new drug application.

With small molecules, there was no problem. If structures were different, apart from salts and esters, then the drug was a new chemical entity. With macromolecules, however, small and insignificant differences might occur which, it was felt, did not constitute genuine innovation. For example, two protein drugs would be considered the same if the only difference between them was due to post-transitional events, infidelity of transcription or translation, or minor differences in amino acid sequence. Different glycosylation patters or tertiary structures would only be considered significant if the drug were shown to be clinically superior.

Even allowing for government grants and tax concessions, the cost of developing orphan drugs is high and the price is bound to be substantial. The original price set for azidothymidine drew widespread protests and was, in fact, reduced on the grounds that sales were likely to be much higher than had been anticipated.

There are other diseases whose incidence is likely to remain static. Cystic fibrosis is the commonest genetic disorder in Caucasian populations. It afflicts between 1 person in 1600 and 1 in 8000. In the United Kingdom, about 400 infants a year are born with the disorder and fewer than 25% would be expected to live until their thirties. The population of sufferers depends on survival rates but, with a United States incidence of 1 in 3800,[21] a figure of the order of 10 000 is probable, well within the orphan drugs limit. Recombinant DNase, Pulmozyme® (dornase alpha) is an orphan drug that is claimed to break down the thick mucous secretions associated with the disease. It is expected to gain regulatory approval in 1994, but estimates are that it will cost each patient $10 000 per year.[22]

The orphan drug that has caused the greatest furore is alglucerase (Ceredase®), a treatment for Gaucher's disease. Gaucher's disease is characterized by the presence of enlarged lipid-containing histiocytes (Gaucher cells) in the bone marrow. The cells cause bone pain and necrosis of some bones and make the patient liable to bone fractures. The disease (to which Ashkenazi Jews are genetically disposed) is due to a deficiency of the enzyme glucocerebrosidase. There are about 2000–3000 sufferers in Europe and a similar number in the United States who can benefit from enzyme replacement therapy. Ceredase® is a modified preparation of glucocerebrosidase derived from placentas. It was approved in the United States in April 1991, in Israel in 1992 and in the European Union in 1994.[23] Supplies are limited and it was estimated in 1992 that a year's supply might cost $350 000. It was described as 'the orphan drug that broke the camel's back'.[24]

Thus the Orphan Drugs Act has been a success in that companies have been encouraged to develop drugs for rare diseases. On the other hand, the US government is currently paying the bill and in certain cases feels that it is being asked to pay excessively for drugs that could legitimately be asked to stand on their own Whether it proves possible to 'fine-tune' the legislation to make it more cost-effective remains to be seen.

D.   Generic pharmaceuticals

Innovative drugs, particularly orphan drugs, present economic problems for health administrators. The same is true at the other end of the spectrum, for drugs that have been on the market for many years and are out of patent. The original manufacturer is then open to imitation and competition. Out-of-patent pharmaceuticals fall into four categories:[25]

(1) Those manufactured by their inventors under their brand names. For example, Hoechst still sells Lasix® even though furosemide is out of patent.

(2) Those marketed by nonoriginating companies under their own brand names. For example, ampicillin is sold as Amcill®, Omnipen®, Polycillin® and Principen®, as well as under the originator's name, Penbritin®. These are known as branded generics.

(3) Out-of-patent pharmaceuticals marketed by nonoriginating companies under a generic name plus a company name or prefix or suffix. Furosemide is sold under its own name by Geneva, Lederle and Rugby, and the company name features on the label. The companies undertake limited promotional activity. In some statistics these are included in branded generics.

(4) Out-of-patent pharmaceuticals marketed by nonoriginating companies under a generic name with minimum mention of the company's name. The bottle may be labelled furosemide BP or furosemide USP and the producer appears only in small letters.

Categories 1 to 4 are known as multisource drugs; 2 to 4 are the true generics. Group 4 (minimum-name generics) are illegal in most European countries since the doctor must specify the source, and hence the generics category is limited to groups 2 and 3.

Although some generics companies try to develop new dosage forms, calendar packs and so on, generic drugs in general sell entirely on price. This is resented by the research-based companies who see their profit margins being eroded after what they regard as an inadequate period of patent protection. They present the public with a picture of hole-in-the-wall generics companies flooding the market with inferior, inadequately tested drugs made on the cheap. In 1988, three multinationals sent key legislators in the United States a 'memorandum in opposition' that featured photographs of modern pharmaceutical manufacturing plant compared with the garbage-strewn vacant lot of a 'New York generics manufacturer'.[26]

Grotesque as the attack was, it is only fair to note that shortly afterwards the generics industry was rocked by a series of revelations that indeed showed serious failure among some firms to comply with testing standards. Among other infringements, various producers had apparently submitted samples for testing of drugs not made by them but by the originators.

In fact, most generics are made by the same companies that manufacture ethical pharmaceuticals. About 80% of multisource drugs in the United States are made by the approximately 60 member companies of the Pharmaceutical Manufacturers' Association. If one excludes category 4, then the proportion drops to 70%. The figure is anyway rising as research-based companies take over generics companies as an insurance against government measures to contain pharmaceutical prices.

Furthermore, it is the originating companies who can manufacture out-of-patent products on the cheap. They have already amortized their plant, they have personnel already available, they have optimized the process and the product can share analytical and distribution facilities with in-patent products. The reason the research based companies *appear* to have higher costs is an accounting convention that loads the costs of research and development of *new* products on to products already being sold. This is legitimate in that the cash flow for research and development must come out of current income, but it is an illusion to see it as a higher cost. Rather it is a question of cross-subsidy.

Until the past decade, the issue of generics was not significant. Doctors in general prescribed drugs by the names they knew and loved, which were usually the brand names given by the originators. In the United States, the situation was revolutionized by the Waxman–Hatch Act of 1984. Generics companies were granted the right to market out-of-patent drugs under their generic names without having to repeat all the tests performed by the originator. Instead, they were able to submit an abbreviated new drug application (ANDA) in which they had to prove that the chemical composition and bioavailability of the drug matched the standards previously agreed by the FDA and the originator. Products regarded as equivalent are listed in the 'Orange Book'.[27] The proportion of *new* prescriptions written generically in the United States (probably minimum-name generics are meant here) has remained static at 14% for over ten years but well over 50% (30% by value) are being filled generically. The reason is that laws in all 50 states permit the pharmacist to substitute a less-expensive generic even when the doctor prescribes a brand name. In some states, doctors must write 'prescribe as written' if they want the patient to receive the branded product and in other states they must sign on one of two lines. Always they must specify that the branded product be supplied if that is what they wish.

In UK medical schools, doctors are trained to write generic names rather than brand names. By 1991, the proportion of prescriptions written generically had risen to 41% and the number dispensed generically to 35%, the difference being where the prescription was written with a generic name but the product was still under patent. Because it is the older, cheaper products that are available as generics, only 27% of prescriptions *by value* were written generically and 14% dispensed generically.

In France, the generics market has been largely confined to hospitals. Perhaps 2–3% of prescriptions are filled generically. Even in-patent drugs in France are cheap, and French doctors have hitherto been hostile to generics, although this is changing.

Generics established themselves from the early 1980s in Germany, and by 1989 they accounted for 21.9% of all prescription. Multisource products accounted for 50.4%. The extensive and complicated health service reforms since then have probably given a further boost to the generics sector.[28]

From a simplistic viewpoint, the distinction between originators' drugs and generics looks like the difference between, say, Kellogg's corn flakes and a supermarket's own brand. Two factors modify this picture. First, the consumer is able to tell whether one brand of corn flakes tastes as good as another and how much the difference is worth financially. Second, if the consumer does not pay directly for the product, then there is no reason to choose a cheaper one with an unpromoted brand name. As in all economics problems, it is the organization that pays that complains, and governments are anxious to promote cheaper drugs whether generic or otherwise.

E.   Cost–benefit analysis

The organisations that actually pay for medicines — governments, insurers and so on — have only recently started to use the power conveyed by their expenditure. A consequence is that a drug company has not only to show that its new product is safe and works but also that it is cost-effective. In Australia, this has been spelled out in legislation. Since 1993, any drug submitted for approval there must be accompanied not only by the results of clinical trials but also by an economic impact analysis.

The analysis must be based on comparisons with existing treatments. It must cover not only the spending on the drug but possible savings on other medical services, for example the cost of a period in hospital or of providing social services for an elderly patient at home.

The exercise is relatively simple if a drug is only a marginal improvement on its competitors. Small improvements in hospital bed occupancy and so on can readily be computed. On the other hand, drugs that offer only marginal improvements will rarely be able to command a high enough price to justify development costs. Thus the exercise is mainly of importance to companies trying to justify very high prices for 'breakthrough' products.

Economic impacts can be measured in a variety of ways.[29] Cost-effectiveness studies measure the cost in relation to outcome. The classic cost-effectiveness study was carried out on the pioneering antiulcer drug cimetidine. The figures are shown in Table 42.11. The major saving in cimetidine-treated patients was in hospital costs. It was also shown that among nonhospitalized patients who were on older drugs, two days of work per week were missed on average, while among the cimetidine-treated group only one day was missed. A similar study showed the benefits of the anticancer drug carboplatin in spite of its costing ten times as much as the older drug cisplatin. The point is that the latter has to be given to inpatients while the

Table 42.11   Costs and benefits of cimetidine. Annual average Michigan Medicaid expenditures per patient with duodenal ulcer.

	Control group (US$)	Cimetidine treated group (US$)
Physician	109	57
Hospital	602	97
Drugs	10[a]	66
Total	721	220

Source: Patterson, M. L. (1983) *Management and Decision Economics.* **4**: 50.
[a]Does not include antacids that are excluded from Michigan Medicaid.

former can be used as outpatient therapy. When hospital costs are taken into account, the more expensive drug offers higher cost-effectiveness.[30]

A third example compared the cost in Sweden of treating patients who had had myocardial infarction with the β-blocker metoprolol. The direct health service costs for treatment were reduced from 17 120 to 12 310 Swedish Kröner, a saving of 28%.[31] A fourth example was used to justify hepatitis B vaccination in Japan. A net saving of 16 billion yen was estimated as a result of vaccination costing 1.3 billion yen.[32]

The problem for hospital administrators is that the largest savings come from a reduction in time spent in hospital. In countries with long hospital waiting lists, such as the United Kingdom, however, beds do not remain empty. They are reoccupied at once. During a patient's stay in hospital, the first few days are the most expensive, and subsequently only minimal care and nursing are required. Consequently, by hastening the turnover of patients, a hospital will have more patients in the early, expensive stage of their stay. Although the average cost per patient treated will decrease, the overall hospital costs will increase and so will the cost per patient per day. Governments might complain and the efficient hospitals will be the ones that are criticized. With 'inefficient' care, one patient is treated at a cost of $x. With efficient care, three patients are treated at a cost of $2x. More patients benefit but at higher total cost. (In a country with too many hospital beds, such as France, the unoccupied bed might remain empty in which case, although the direct costs of hospitalization are saved, the overheads and depreciation will be spread among fewer patients and the cost per patient per day will again appear to rise.)

The Health Service reforms in the United Kingdom in 1991 avoided this trap and used instead the cost-utility concept. Cost-effectiveness takes into account only the cost of a single standardized outcome; cost-utility looks at the costs of a range of different outcomes, such as extra years of survival and improved quality of life. A Dutch study of two cholesterol-lowering drugs, for example, showed that cholestyramine cost 131 000 Dutch Guilders per year of life saved compared with simivastatin, which cost 31 500 Dutch Guilders.[33]

The above example is attractive in that it compares two forms of therapy. What it does not do is place a value on an extra year of life gained or indeed on the quality of life. Economists have worked hard at producing measures to quantify these two concepts. A number of indexes have been produced, the meaning of which is uncertain and discussion of which is beyond the scope of this chapter. They include the Nottingham Health Profile, the American 'Sickness Impact Profile' and the Rosser Health Index.[34] The Rosser Index has been used to produce a 'Quality Adjusted Life Year' or QALY. Each year of life is discounted by a factor reflecting the disability and distress suffered during the year. The factor is obtained by asking people to estimate what number of years of perfect health would be equivalent to ten years of life in a particular state of disability.

The technique is clearly subjective and there is room for much development and validation. None the less, it makes possible some worthwhile comparisons. Table 42.12 shows the treatment costs per QALY produced by different types of health intervention. Simple preventive measures such as changing diet or giving up smoking produce the cheapest benefits. Reduction of blood pressure to avert strokes and selective testing for cholesterol are also cost-effective. Hospital haemodialysis for renal failure is much less cost-effective than kidney transplantation. That, together with erythropoeitin treatment for dialysis patients and brain surgery for malignant tumours, comes at the most expensive end of the list.

The final type of analysis is the full cost–benefit study. The term is often used to cover all methods described above, but strictly it applies only to studies where every cost and every benefit is taken into account. This includes such things as the contribution to the national economy of people whose lives are saved or prolonged. Such a study would be immensely

Table 42.12   Treatment costs at 1990 prices and technology of various interventions.

Treatment	Cost/QALY (£)	Treatment	Cost/QALY (£)
Cholesterol testing and diet only (all adults aged 40–69)	200	Kidney transplantation	4710
Neurosurgical intervention for head injury	240	Breast cancer screening	5780
GP advice to stop smoking	270	Heart transplant	7840
Neurosurgical intervention for subarachnoid haemorrhage	490	Cholesterol testing and treatment (incrementally, all adults aged 25–39)	14 150
Antihypertensive therapy to prevent stroke (ages 40–69)	940	Home haemodialysis	17 260
Pacemaker implantation	1100	Coronary artery bypass graft (one-vessel disease, moderate angina)	18 830
Hip replacement[a]	1180	Hopital haemodialysis	21 970
Valve replacement for aortic stenosis	1410	Erythropoetin treatment for anaemia in dialysis patients (assuming 10% mortality reduction)[b]	54 380
Coronary artery bypass graft (left main disease, severe angina)	2090	Neurosurgical intervention for malignant intercranial tumours	107 780

Source: Maynard, A. (1990) The Upjohn Lecture, quoted in *SCRIP* **1568**: 8.
[a]Does not alter survival but improves QALY.
[b]Before epoetin alfa became available.

complicated, but a partial study of hypertension and stroke in Britain has been performed.[35] Between the mid-1950s and the mid-1980s, new cases of stroke dropped from 2.4 to 1.75 per 1000 population. The cost of stroke to the Health Service in 1984 was £550 million. Had the incidence been at the 1950s level, it would have cost 550 × 2.4/1.75 = £754 million. In addition there was a contribution to the national economy of £322 million through a reduction in premature mortality. A total gain of £526 million can be set against the cost of antihypertensive drugs (at manufacturers' prices) of £185 million. The social benefit of control of hypertension is evident.

Economics is not an exact science and the question of the cash value of a year of life or a quality adjusted year of life (whose? where? under what conditions?) is one that no one would find it easy to answer, if there is an answer, and many would find it offensive even to ask the question. The problem is that with limited resources a community has to channel cash to where it will do the most good. The analyses above show some of the directions that are being taken.

V.   THE FUTURE OF THE PHARMACEUTICAL INDUSTRY

The years since 1935 have seen the rise of the pharmaceutical industry to its present eminence. Despite the thalidomide disaster and a handful of other tragic episodes, the industry has flourished. A formulary of life-saving and life-improving drugs has been discovered. Two questions are now paramount. First, can society go on spending ever more of its national product on health care and, second, can the momentum be maintained? Have all the easy illnesses been dealt with so that only the difficult ones are left?

A.   Cost containment measures

Governments are increasingly worried about the rise in health care expenditure. The pharmaceutical industry would say that drugs provide the best possible value within that system and permit treatment at home of patients who would otherwise be costing much more in hospital. Drugs in the United States and Europe average about 7% and 10% of health care spending respectively, so that savings on drugs have to be huge to make much impact on overall health care costs. Much smaller cuts in hospital costs in percentage terms would have a larger effect. On the other hand, medical and paramedical personnel enjoy high status and public support. The pharmaceutical industry does not: its reputation is equivocal and its very success in commercial terms makes it more vulnerable to attack. Official controls on pharmaceutical expenditure are found everywhere in Europe and North America.[36]

Most European countries control the permitted prices of individual prescription drugs. A price is agreed at the time a new product is introduced and it may not be increased even to compensate for inflation without official permission. The exceptions to this system are Denmark, which permits free pricing and Ireland, which permits free pricing of new drugs but restricts the price of those on the market. Germany and Netherlands permit free pricing but have reference prices (see below). The United Kingdom regulates prices indirectly via limits on profitability. The United States has free pricing but stimulates generic competition. In all countries, OTC drugs and prescription drugs that are not reimbursed by the national health care system are free from controls.

The UK Department of Health negotiates with companies a maximum rate of return on capital employed in their sales to the National Health Service. An overall rate is fixed for the industry as a whole and within this figure an individual firm is awarded a particular rate 'having regard to the scale and nature of the company's relevant investments and activities and the associated long-term risks'. The system may perhaps have to be changed because of EC legislation.

The German and Dutch reference pricing systems set reference prices for three groups of pharmaceutical products:

(1)   those containing the same active ingredients (i.e. multisource products);
(2)   those containing active ingredients that are comparable therapeutically and pharmacologically (e.g. benzodiazepine anxiolytics);
(3)   those having comparable effects, especially if combination products (e.g. anti-hypertensive–diuretic combinations).

The reference price is related to the average price of the various products on the market. A physician may prescribe as he or she pleases, but if the product costs more than the reference price, the patient has to pay the difference. The result of reference pricing was that virtually all producers dropped their price to the reference price and, where they were in a position to do so, raised the price of their in-patent (therefore not reference-priced) products. This did not necessarily work to the advantage of the generics producers, because the cut in the price of the branded product undermined their own major selling point.

An alternative to price controls is stimulation of competition from generics producers and this is the path that has been followed in the United States and Canada. This was discussed in Section IV.D. In Europe, Germany, Denmark and the Netherlands permit generic substitution.

Pharmaceutical spending may also be controlled by regulation of the drugs that may be prescribed. Denmark, France, Germany and Japan have positive lists. The United Kingdom, the Netherlands and Germany have negative lists. Both reduce the proportion of prescriptions that are reimbursed. In principle a positive list should indicate a more considered approach to prescribing than a negative list, but in practice other factors seem much more important. It is difficult to deny reimbursement to popular drugs of doubtful efficacy.

A way for governments to save money is for part of the burden to be shifted to the patient through patient co-payments. These are more or less universal. Two systems operate: a flat-rate co-payment unconnected with the price of the drug, as in Ireland, the Netherlands and the United Kingdom, or a proportion of the price of the drug, as in Spain, Denmark, Belgium and France. Exemptions are common. For example, in the United Kingdom 80% of prescriptions were exempt in 1991. Encouragement of OTC drugs is another way in which patients can be encouraged to contribute. Self-diagnosis and prescription worries doctors, but there has been an increase in the scope of drugs licensed for OTC sale and this may be expected to increase.

The final method for discouraging lavish prescribing is drug budgets for general practitioners. These have been introduced in Germany and the United Kingdom. In Germany the effects were immediate and considerable. In the first quarter of 1993, drug volume fell by 17% and spending by 24% compared with 1992. There was a substantial drop in sales volume by the large research-based companies and massive increases by the bottom of the market generics producers.[37] There was also a serious effect on the pharmacists, whose turnover in 1993 was reported to be down by 13%. In the United Kingdom, not all general practitioners are budget holders. Furthermore, the level of generic prescribing in the United Kingdom has always been relatively high and there is smaller opportunity for switching. Hence any pattern has been swamped by other factors.

Directorate-General III of the European Commission[38] concluded in 1993 that price controls had failed to control health spending and, by stifling competition, had succeeded in rigidifying the market. It felt that there was a need for convergence in the area of pricing but stressed the importance of the industry to the EC economy. The three major policy recommendations were:

(1) To contain growth in pharmaceutical expenditure by measures specific to reimbursement rather than direct price controls
(2) To enhance competition by making the market more transparent and allowing generics to stimulate price competition
(3) To step up involvement of health professionals and raise the cost-awareness of patients by better informing them of the cost/benefit ratios of therapeutic alternatives

These recommendations are in line with the Commission's long-term policy, which has been to increase the transparency of pharmaceutical transactions rather than trying to legislate across the Community

The research-based pharmaceutical industry has fought vigorously against cost-containment measures. To some extent, the patent term restoration legislation was intended as a sweetener to diminish industry anxiety about the other initiatives. Financial pressures have persuaded a number of research-based companies to take over generics companies to provide them with some sort of insurance against a swing in that direction. The irony of this is that the added respectability given to generics by such policies has increased their rate of penetration of the market.[39] In addition to takeovers, there have been a number of mergers that will enable companies to spread the research risk. In the end, however, the industry will continue to flourish only if it continues to produce a stream of innovative drugs. What are the possibilities?

B.   Trends in pharmaceuticals

Technological forecasting of pharmaceutical progress is as risky as, if less expensive than, drug research itself. There have been bitter disappointments in the past 15 years in areas where success was confidently expected. For example, success in understanding the role of endorphins and enkephalins in the perception of pain by the brain gave the hope that effective but nonaddictive substitutes for morphine would be available by the mid-1980s. In the event, no drugs based on such structures have been developed. Instead, slow-delivery forms of morphine have become available so that pain can be 'titrated'. The success of the technique has meant the United Kingdom alone now consumes as much morphine as did the world 20 years ago.

Prostaglandins have been another disappointment. They have orphan drug status in a number of applications but developments have been slow. Our understanding of the arachidonic acid cascade, the biosynthetic route to prostaglandins, has led to advances in the development of prostaglandin inhibitors (e.g. the non-steroidal anti-inflammatories). Prostaglandin analogues, on the other hand, have at present only a handful of indications (Table 42.5). Leukotriene inhibitors were seen as the next generation of antiasthma drugs, but none has yet been registered, although four launches are planned between 1995 and 1997. Asthma therapy is certainly an area where intensive research is in progress and advances can be hoped for.

Statistics on the compounds in research at present are shown in Table 42.13 by therapeutic category. These give a picture of how the major players see the future. A fuller list appears in ref. 40.

Drugs against cancer head Table 42.13 under therapeutic category and recur in fourth position. Cancer is second only to heart disease as a cause of death in the developed world. Cancer drugs are registered more readily than other drugs because they are the only hope for many sufferers. Progress has been made to the extent that the five-year survival rate increases steadily. New cancer drugs will continue to reach the market but it is unlikely that one drug will be the answer to more than a handful of cancers. None the less, the introduction of Taxol® (paclitaxel) against ovarian cancer in 1993 will prove a breakthrough if it can be produced in adequate quantities. The second-ranking category is anti-inflammatories, with other antiarthritis drugs in position 18. Antiasthma drugs appear in third place. The reasons were mentioned in Section I.

Antiviral drugs come fifth and ninth. They are an important research area, but again progress has been slow. Acyclovir (herpes) and azidothymidine (AIDS) have been the main drugs on the market for a surprising length of time. Other antiviral drugs are in development, and famciclovir and stavudine were launched in 1994. Unfortunately, viruses have the ability to modify themselves in unpredictable ways. An antiviral that would cure influenza or the common cold would be a best seller, but the problem seems too difficult. Most research focuses on AIDS and herpes.

An area where progress seems certain is the development of new protein-based drugs made by

Table 42.13   Drugs in research by therapeutic category and mode of action, 1993.[a]

Rank	Therapeutic category	Number of compounds	Mode of action[b]	Number of compounds
1	Anticancer, other (K6Z)	338	Protein synthesis antagonist	83
2	Anti-inflammatory (M1A1)	277	Platelet aggregation antagonist	72
3	Antiasthma (R8A)	255	Calcium channel antagonist	70
4	Anticancer, immunological (K3)	253	Cell wall synthesis inhibitor	67
5	Antiviral, anti-HIV (J5A)	231	DNA antagonist	59
6	Recombinants, other (T2Z)	210	RNA-directed DNA polymerase inhibitor	54
7	Vaccine (J7A)	202	DNA topoisomerase ATP hydrolysing inhibitor	52
8	Cardiovascular (C9Z)	201	Cyclooxygenese inhibitor	46
9	Antiviral, other (J5Z)	189	Prostaglandin synthetase inhibitor	46
10	Nonrecombinant antibody (TIB)	188	Bone formation stimulant	39
11	Memory enhancer (N6D)	188	Angiotensin II antagonist	38
12	Neuroprotective (N7C)	181	5-Lipoxygenase inhibitor	36
13	Antithrombotic (B1B9)	176	DNA synthesis inhibitor	35
14	Immunosuppressant (I5)	172	Sodium channel antagonist	31
15	Antihypertensive, other	155	RNA synthesis inhibitor	31
16	Monoclonal antibody (I4A1)	153	PAF antagonist	30
17	Hypolipaemic/ antiatherosclerotic (B4A)	147	Plasminogen activator stimulant	27
18	Antiarthritic, other (M2Z)	133	Phosphodiesterase inhibitor	27
19	Alimentary/metabolic (A16)	131	Thrombin inhibitor	26
20	Antianginal (C1D3)	127	HIV protease inhibitor	24

Source: Pharmaprojects database, December 1993, quoted in *SCRIP Magazine* (Jan. 1994): 47.
[a]The number of compounds listed by mode of action is smaller than those listed by therapeutic category because four coding categories have been omitted: unidentified pharmcological activity 488; immunostimulant 217; immunosuppressant 141; 'not applicable' 193.

recombinant DNA technology (categories 6 and 10). Interferon-β was introduced in 1993 to counter multiple sclerosis. Two recombinant Factor VIII (antihaemophilia) products were launched in the succeeding two years and in the long term could replace the material extracted from blood plasma. Indeed, genes have been cloned for most of the proteins obtained from plasma, but the products are very expensive. The plasma-derived material is likely to be used for some time, depending on the number of future scandals about infected blood products. Extracellular haemoglobin, which in 1992 looked to be a couple of years away, has now receded to the end of the century as it appears that the nitric oxide pathway is not adequately understood.

Alzheimer's disease and senile dementia leading to memory loss (position 11) are escalating problems in the developed world. Cognex® (tacrine), a cerebral vasodilator, has recently been licensed and has sold well, but more effective drugs are required. Velnacrine® is expected to be launched in 1995. Osteoporosis and prostate enlargement are two other penalties of ageing. A large market exists. Proscar® (finasteride), a testosterone antagonist, is the only prostate drug on the market at present, but others are nearing launch.

Antibiotics are registered relatively quickly because they are taken for short times, and long-term toxicity tests are not as important. New quinolones and cephalosporins will be developed and will find niche markets. The ability of quinolones to counter 'tourist's tummy' could result in substantial sales in the developed world and an improvement in the quality of life in the third world.

Ranking of compounds in research by mode of action is also shown in Table 42.13 Discussion of these mechanisms appears elsewhere in this book.

C. Conclusion

There is still a large number of interesting and important problems to be solved by the pharmaceutical industry. Many of them can be solved, but at a cost. All drugs are expensive to develop and drugs for rare diseases are prohibitively expensive on a *per capita* basis unless there is a government subsidy. In recent years, for the first time as an overt policy issue, society has questioned the amount of money spent on health care. There is general agreement that some sort of rationing is inevitable but none on who is to do the rationing or how. Will a balance will be struck on the basis of ability to pay or on some sort of cost–benefit analysis? Consider the following situation. It appears that the consumption of health care increases exponentially with age and is 5–10 times higher at age 80–84 than at 60–64.[28,41] The number of old people is increasing rapidly throughout the developed world. Demand for additional health care comes and will come increasingly in the future from the elderly. On a cost–utility analysis, however, treatment of the elderly is not an attractive option. The elderly are less likely to recover from their illnesses. If they do, the fact that they are elderly to start with means that the years of life gained will be smaller. The elderly will have already retired so that their contribution to national income is zero or (because of their pensions) negative.

If health care is to be rationed by cost, then doctors will have the task of turning away patients who cannot pay (and if the doctors are soft-hearted, then the hospitals will turn them away instead). If care is to be allocated on a cost–utility basis, then the doctor will have to find out the patient's age before deciding whether to offer a coronary bypass, a packet of antiangina pills or a loaded revolver.

There is thus an ethical challenge to governments, to economists and, worst of all because they are the ones to see the patients, the medical profession. Doctors do not want to be the people to do the rationing, particularly if it is to be done overtly against a series of guidelines, so that they can be criticized afterwards. They have taken the Hippocratic oath[42] and are committed to 'carry out regimens for the benefit of the sick and keep them from harm and wrong'. But if a doctor does not take the decision, will it be taken by an economist or a politician? Will a patient abandoned by a doctor be permitted to seek a second opinion, and at whose expense? Will there be a health care sector for people whose treatment under the social security system would not be cost-effective but who are able and prepared to pay?

At the beginning of this chapter, I quoted Aristotle's distinction between health and wealth. My late father, Jacob Victor Reuben, to whom this chapter is dedicated, qualified as a doctor in 1922. For his first 13 years in practice, there was scarcely a drug he could prescribe that would cure disease. The most he could do in many cases was to advise patients to stay in bed, take some aspirin and plenty of fluids, and allow nature to run its course. If the patients died, he could say in all honesty that he had done everything in his power to save them. Is his successor 85 years later going to have to say to patients, at any rate the elderly ones, that there are many things he or she *could* do to save them, but they are all too expensive, and why not stay in bed, take some aspirin and plenty of fluids, and allow nature to run its course?

REFERENCES

1. The methods by which these figures have been derived are outlined in Reuben B. G. and Wittcoff, H. A. (1990) *Pharmaceutical Chemicals in Perspective,* Appendix 1. Wiley, New York.
2. (a) O'Brien, B. (1984) *Patterns of European Diagnosis and Prescribing.* Office of Health Economics, London. (b) Payer, L. (1991) *Medicine and Culture.* Gollancz, London. (c) Teeling-Smith, G. (1991) *Patterns of Prescribing.* Office of Health Economics, London.
3. *SCRIP* **1310**: 18.
4. Myllylä, G. (1991) Whole blood and plasma procurement and the impact of plasmapheresis. In Harris, J. R. (ed.) *Blood Separation and Plasma Fractionation.* p. 38. Wiley-Liss, New York.
5. Wittcoff, H. A. and Reuben, B. G. (1980) *Industrial Organic Chemicals in Perspective,* p. 39. Wiley, New York, also ref. 1, Section 12.1.1.
6. *Synthetic Organic Chemicals, US Production and Sales 1992.* US International Trade Commission, Washington DC, 1994.
7. Commission of the European Communities (1992) *Rules Governing Medicinal Products in the European Community,* vol. IV, *Good Manufacturing Practice for Medicinal Products.* Office for Official Publications of the European Community, Luxembourg.
8. Last, P. E. (1987) *Chem. Br.* **23**: 1073.
9. Brathwaite, M. J. and Ketterman, C. L. (1993) *Chem. Ind.* 1042–1044.
10. Jackson, A. and Angoh, G. (1993) *Chem. Ind.* 1046–1048.
11. Fox, J. (1993) *Chem. Ind.* 270.
12. DiMasi, J. A., Hansen, R. W., Grabowski, H. G. and Lasagna, L. (1991) *J. Health Econ.* **10**: 107.
13. *International Trade Statistics Year Book,* United Nations, New York, published annually. See also Reuben, B. G. (1991) Pharmaceuticals. In Meyers, R. A. (ed.) *Encyclopedia of Physical Science and Technology, 1991 Yearbook.* Academic Press, New York.
14. Reuben, B. G. and Burstall, M. L. (1995) Pricing and reimbursement regulation in Europe: the industry perspective. *DIA Journal* **29**: 273–283.
15. Lis, Y. and Walker, S. R. (1989) *Pharmaceutical Patents.* Centre for Medicines Research, Carshalton, Surrey.
16. Lis, Y. and Walker, S. R. (1989) In Griffith, J. P. (ed.) *Medicines: Regulation, Research and Risk.* Queen's University, Belfast.
17. For general background, see (a) Asbury, C. H. (1985) *Orphan Drugs: Medical versus Market Value.* Lexington Books, Lexington, MA; (b) Asbury, C. H. (1991) The Orphan Drug Act: the first seven years. *J. Am. Med. Assoc.* **265**: 893.
18. A full list of orphan drugs up to 1991 appears in *Drug Evaluations Annual 1992.* American Medical Association, Chicago, IL, 1992.
19. Scheinberg, I. H. and Walshe, J. M. (eds) (1985) *Orphan Diseases and Orphan Drugs.* Manchester University Press, London.
20. *SCRIP* (1 Apr. 1994) **1910**: 15.
21. *Cystic Fibrosis.* Office of Health Economics, London, 1986.
22. *SCRIP Magazine* (Jan. 1994): 48.
23. *SCRIP* (29 March 1994) **1909**: 21.
24. Tobias, G. and Faigen, N. (1992) *SCRIP Review.* 12
25. Reuben, B. G. and Burstall, M. L. (1989) *Generic Pharmaceuticals – The Threat.* Economists Advisory Group, London.
26. *Consumers Reports* (1987) **8**: 80. (Magazine published in USA.)
27. *Approved Drug Products with Therapeutic Equivalence Evaluations.* US Department of Health and Human Services, Rockville. MD, published annually and updated by monthly supplements.
28. Burstall, M. L. and Reuben, B.G. (1992) *Cost Containment in the European Pharmaceutical Market.* MarketLetter, London.
29. Teeling Smith, G. (ed.) (1990) *Measuring the Benefits of Medicines: The Future Agenda.* Office of Health Economics, London.
30. Tighe, M. and Goodman, S. (1988) Carboplatin versus cisplatin. *The Lancet.* **2**: 1372.
31. Olsson, G., Levin, L.A. and Rehnquist, N. (1987) Economic consequences of post-infarction prophylaxis with β-blockers. *Br. Med. J.* **294**: 339.

32. *Technological Assessment of Drug Therapy – Analysis of Cost-benefit Studies on Pharmaceuticals.* Institute of Statistical Studies, Tokyo, 1988.

33. Martens, L. L. and Finn, P. (1991) In Teeling Smith, G. (ed.) *Patterns of Prescribing.* Office of Health Economics, London.

34. Rosser, R. M. (1984) A history of the development of health indicators. In Teeling Smith, G. (ed.) *Measuring the Social Benefits of Medicine.* Office of Health Economics, London.

35. Teeling Smith, G. (1989) The economics of hypertension and stroke. *Am. Heart J.* **119**(3) pt 2: 725.

36. Burstall, M. L. and Reuben, B. G. (1990) *Critics of the Pharmceutical Industry,* especially pp. 19–69. REMIT Consultants, London.

37. Munnich F. (1993) IIR Pharma Pricing Meeting '93. *SCRIP* **1861**: 6.

38. *SCRIP* (1993)**1860**: 3, **1857**: 2. The communication is the work of the services of Directorate-General II and has still to be adopted by the Commission. Objections could be raised by other Directorates.

39. *SCRIP* (1994) **1916**: 15.

40. Pharmaceuticals research and development. *Financial Times,* 23 March 1994.

41. (a) Olsson, G. J. (1988) *R.. Soc. Med.* **81**: 242. (b) Goldman, L., Sia, B., Cook, F., Rutherford, J. D. and Weinstein, M. C. (1988) *N. Engl. J. Med.* **319**: 152.

42. *British Medical Journal* (1994) **309**: 952–953.

Index